W0080747

CARE

of the

NEWBORN

NINTH EDITION

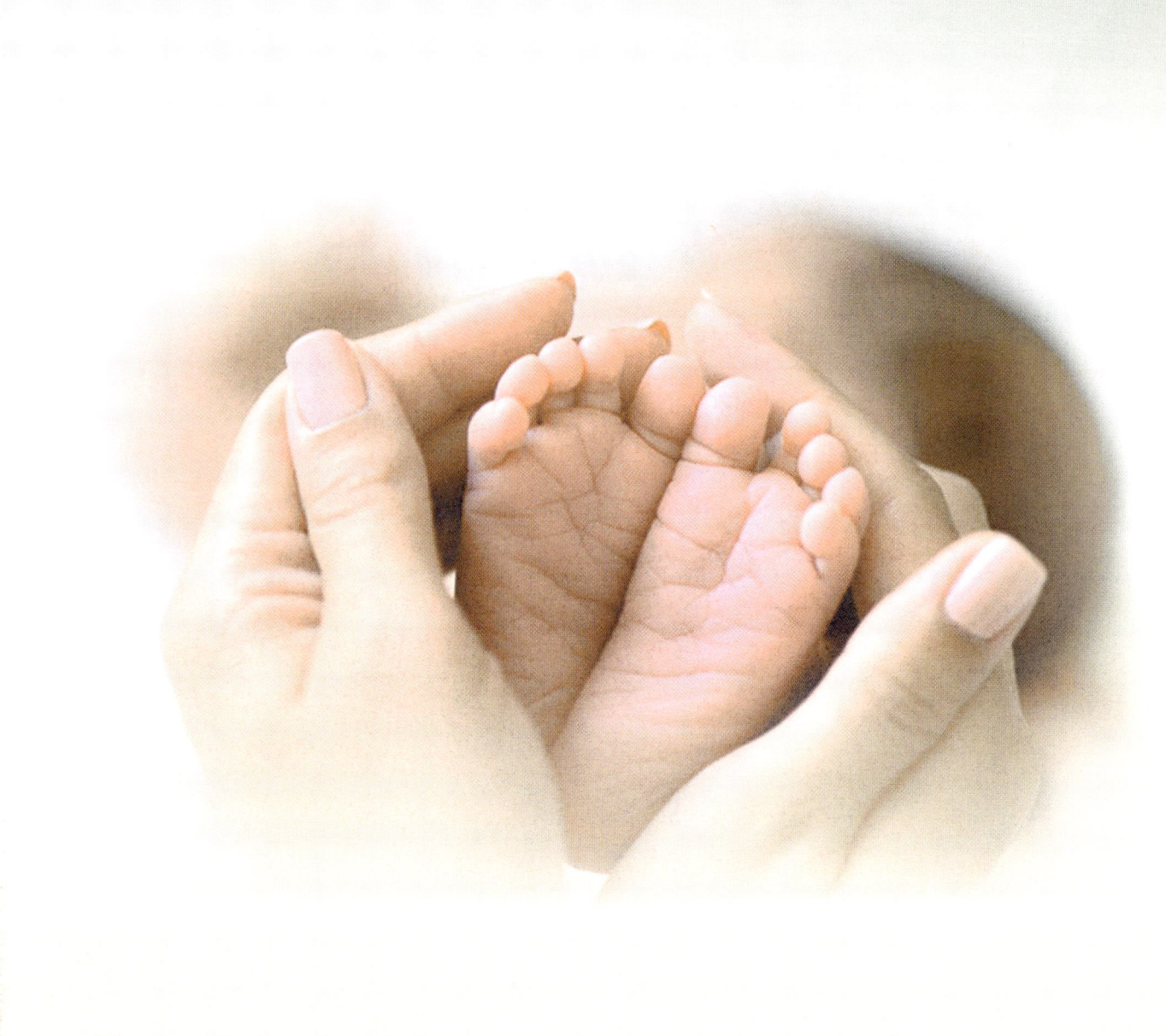

CARE
of the
NEWBORN

NINTH EDITION

Meharban Singh

MD, FAMS, FIAP, FIMSA, FNNF, Hony. FAAP

Former Professor and Head
Department of Pediatrics and Neonatal Division
WHO Collaborating Center for Training and
Research in Newborn Care
All India Institute of Medical Sciences
New Delhi

CBSPD

CBS Publishers & Distributors Pvt Ltd

New Delhi • Bengaluru • Chennai • Kochi • Kolkata • Lucknow • Mumbai
Hyderabad • Jharkhand • Nagpur • Patna • Pune • Uttarakhand

Disclaimer

Science and technology are constantly evolving and dynamic. The author has taken care to ensure that the doses of drugs and schedules of treatment are accurate and in accordance with standard recommendations at the time of publication. There is, however, a constant research and progress to identify more effective therapeutic agents or revise existent recommendations for dosages to improve therapeutic efficacy. It is, therefore, desirable to consult the package insert especially in case of a new therapeutic agent or infrequently used drug to make certain that there has been no changes in the recommended dose of the drug or in the indications and contraindications for its administration.

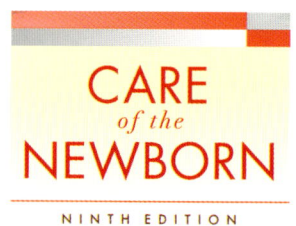

CARE
of the
NEWBORN

NINTH EDITION

ISBN: 978-93-90709-25-0

Copyright © Meharban Singh

Ninth Edition: 2021
   Reprint: 2024
First Edition: October 1976
Second Edition: January 1979
Third Edition: February 1985
Fourth Edition: April 1991
Fifth Edition: August 1999
Sixth Edition: August 2004
Seventh Edition: April 2010
Eighth Edition: January 2015
   Revised Eighth Edition: 2017

All rights reserved. No part of this book may be reproduced or transmitted in any form or by any means, electronic or mechanical, including photocopying, recording, or any information storage and retrieval system without permission, in writing, from the author and the publisher.

Published by Satish Kumar Jain and produced by Varun Jain for

CBS Publishers & Distributors Pvt Ltd

4819/XI Prahlad Street, 24 Ansari Road, Daryaganj, New Delhi 110 002, India.
Ph: 011-23289259, 23266861

Website: www.cbspd.com
e-mail: delhi@cbspd.com

Corporate Office: 204 FIE, Industrial Area, Patparganj, Delhi 110 092
Ph: 011-49344934   Fax: 011-49344935   e-mail: publishing@cbspd.com; publicity@cbspd.com

Branches

- **Bengaluru:** Seema House 2975, 17th Cross, K.R. Road, Banasankari 2nd Stage, Bengaluru 560 070, Karnataka, India
  Ph: +91-80-26771678/79   Fax: +91-80-26771680   e-mail: bangalore@cbspd.com
- **Chennai:** 7, Subbaraya Street, Shenoy Nagar, Chennai 600 030, Tamil Nadu, India
  Ph: +91-44-26680620, 26681266   Fax: +91-44-42032115   e-mail: chennai@cbspd.com
- **Kochi:** 42/1325, 1326, Power House Road, Opp KSEB, Ernakulum, Kochi 682 018, Kerala, India
  Ph: +91-484-4059061-65,67   Fax: +91-484-4059065   e-mail: kochi@cbspd.com
- **Kolkata:** 147, Hind Ceramics Compound, 1st Floor, Nilgunj Road, Belghoria, Kolkata-700056, West Bengal, India
  Ph: 033-25633055/56   e-mail: kolkata@cbspd.com
- **Lucknow:** Basement, Khushnuma Complex, 7 Meerabai Marg (Behind Jawahar Bhawan), Lucknow-226001, UP, India
  Ph: +91-522-4000032   e-mail: tiwari.lucknow@cbspd.com
- **Mumbai:** PWD Shed, Gala no 25/26, Ramchandra Bhatt Marg, Next to JJ Hospital Gate no. 2, Opp. Union Bank of India, Noorbaug, Mumbai-400009, Maharashtra, India
  Ph: +91-22-66661880/89   e-mail: mumbai@cbspd.com

Representatives

- **Hyderabad**   0-9885175004
- **Jharkhand**   0-9811541605
- **Nagpur**   0-9421945513
- **Patna**   0-9334159340
- **Pune**   0-9923910676
- **Uttarakhand**   0-9716462459

Printed at Magic International Pvt. Ltd., Greater Noida, UP, India

Affectionately dedicated
to my parents
and
my wife Kaushal
for her courage,
compassion and confidence
and
our children Sonia and Manik
and
our grandchildren
Ishita, Ishrat, Karan and Kabir
who taught me the subtle nuances
of neonatology

Newborn indeed is a "seed", endowed with an immense potentiality. You can't do anything to alter its genome but you can provide optimal nurturing, nutrition, safe environment and global health care to unfold myriads of human capabilities to help him evolve as a robust citizen of the society.
Meharban Singh

It is a great pleasure to write a foreword for this first textbook of pediatrics from South-East Asia devoted entirely to the care of the newborn infants. In the last two decades, university departments of pediatrics have rapidly advanced in the countries of South-East Asia so that practice, teaching and research for the care of sick children by pediatricians is now well established almost everywhere. Much more recently the problem of overpopulation has been recognized as a serious threat to family health and national progress, so that in many of these countries, programs for population control are being urgently and energetically implemented. Inevitably when every baby is a wanted baby, which is the aim of these efforts, tremendous demands are made on pediatricians to reduce the very high neonatal mortality rate which prevails throughout this region. Not only the chances of survival of neonates should be improved but the survivors must have a good quality of life by ensuring prevention, early diagnosis and effective treatment of those hazards of the fetus and newborn infant which produce long-term handicaps in children.

The pediatricians of South-East Asia have responded with enthusiasm to this new challenge so that the discipline of neonatology with its great emphasis on prevention has been successfully launched and the time is ripe for launch of this book. The author is well known and has been involved in pediatric teaching and research in India for many years and has developed a special interest in neonatology with the recognition of the great scope it provides for new knowledge. Nevertheless, he has wisely recognized that the emphasis in this book must be on prevention and early recognition of disorders and the acquisition of good clinical skills associated with meticulous attention to detail which is the basis of all successful neonatal care. He must be congratulated on the production of a book which is so compact in size and concisely written but significantly comprehensive to be an invaluable working guide for all those involved in regular care of the newborn, including the nursing profession.

Although this book has been written with extensive knowledge of the background of newborn care in South-East Asia and their special requirements, care of the newborn infants is a universal problem and the same principles apply everywhere so that this book should be an equally valuable working guide for use by the health care professionals in other regions.

Bristol
12th September, 1976

Beryl D Corner
MD, FRCP (London)

"Neonates constitute the foundation of a nation and mothers are its pillars. And no sensible government can afford to neglect their needs and rights."
UNICEF

Preface to the Ninth Edition

The rapid strides and advances in the art and science of medicine demand that textbooks must be revised and updated to incorporate latest information in order to optimally serve the needs of physicians. This indeed is a stupendous and challenging task especially for the writer of a single author book. The overwhelming interest, enthusiasm and response accorded by a large number of postgraduate students and consultants in pediatrics and obstetrics, to the previous editions, provided me the necessary impetus and inspiration to take up the onerous task of bringing out yet another edition. There has been an upsurge of interest in neonatology in India coinciding with the publication of the first edition of this book which was released in 1976. Like the speciality of neonatology, the book has grown from a manual to a comprehensive textbook of neonatology over the years. It is indeed a matter of great satisfaction to me that over the years this book has served as a useful catalyst to initiate and enthuse young pediatricians to take interest in the care and welfare of newborn babies. Most pediatricians have rightly realized that perinatology is indeed the core or true pediatrics. Neonatology is unique and distinctive from the rest of pediatrics due to special problems and disorders because of extrauterine adaptations, anatomical, physiological and biochemical immaturity, subtle and gross developmental disorders and enhanced vulnerability to infective and chemotherapeutic agents leading to an alarmingly high morbidity and mortality among newborn babies.

This edition of the book has been extensively revised and updated to include recent advances in the art and understanding of perinatal disorders. Most chapters have been rewritten to incorporate additional evidence-based information to make it an up-to-date and a comprehensive textbook. The physiological basis for common neonatal diseases has been provided and current concepts regarding pathogenesis of common disorders, such as meconium aspiration syndrome, persistent pulmonary hypertension, periventricular–intraventricular hemorrhage, necrotizing enterocolitis, oxygen toxicity, bronchopulmonary dysplasia, apneic attacks and patent ductus arteriosus, have been highlighted. Apart from extensive revision, a large number of additional topics have been included in the appropriate chapters, for example, antenatal diagnosis, universal precautions, neurological sequelae of hypoxic-ischemic encephalopathy, transfusion of blood and blood products, ethical, social and legal issues in perinatal medicine, analgesia and sedation, peritoneal dialysis and follow-up program for high-risk babies. The book provides an up-to-date information regarding neonatal advanced life support and assisted ventilation with special focus on continuous positive airway pressure which is being increasingly harnessed in the care of newborn babies with respiratory distress syndrome. The newer modes and modalities of mechanical ventilation and details of ventilator settings in different clinical situations have been comprehensively discussed. A large number of new clinical photographs, illustrations, algorithms and flowcharts have been included. The references have been updated by inclusion of recently published original and review articles. Above all, the basic attributes of the earlier editions, i.e. brevity, clarity and problem-oriented approach, have been maintained. Without any offense to the feminists and girl child activists, I have uniformly referred to the newborn baby as 'he' for sake of convenience and to avoid the confusion by using 'he', 'she', 'it' at different places.

I am thankful for the enthusiasm and support of Mr SK Jain (CMD) and Mr Varun Jain (Director), CBS Publishers & Distributors Pvt Ltd to publish the revised book in an improved style and format. I am obliged for continuous support from Mr YN Arjuna (Senior Vice-President—Publishing, Editorial and Publicity) and his entire team, especially Ms Ritu Chawla (GM—Production), Mr Neeraj Prasad (graphic artist), Mr Vikrant Sharma (DTP operator) and Mr Surendra Jha (copyeditor). I appreciate the entire team of CBS Publishers & Distributors for composing and improving the format of the book.

I am greatly indebted to my erstwhile colleagues Dr Vinod K Paul and Dr Ashok K Deorari for their suggestions, guidance and active support during the preparation of the revised edition. The cover design has been created by our grand-daughter Ms Ishita Singh. I would like to thank my understanding and enterprising soulmate Ms Kaushal for her encouragement and inspiration to shed my procrastination to revise the book.

I am confident that *Care of the Newborn* would continue to meet the high expectations and felt needs of the pediatricians and obstetricians working in India and South-East Asia region to improve the survival and neuromotor outcome of newborn babies.

26th January, 2021

Meharban Singh MD

Child Care Center
625, Arun Vihar, Sector 37
Noida 201 301
Tel: 0120-4346451, Mob: 9818888772
e-mail: drmbsk@gmail.com

Preface to the First Edition

Perinatal mortality is alarmingly high in most developing countries. Many avoidable handicaps during childhood such as cerebral palsy, mental subnormality, learning disabilities and recurrent seizures, have their origin in the perinatal period. It is possible to increase the perinatal survival and improve the quality of human life through prompt and effective management of newborn babies. The immaturity, fragility, vulnerability and dependence of the perinates demand high degree of skills and collaborative efforts on the part of the obstetricians and pediatricians.

The life begins much before the actual birth. The concept of prevention, therefore, must be extended up to and even before conception. It is hoped that the chapter on preventive neonatology would meet these needs and requirements of the obstetricians. The epidemic proportion of neonatal bacterial infections and their contribution to the preventable neonatal mortality in the developing countries, has been accorded due emphasis and a detailed coverage of the guidelines to prevent neonatal infections have been discussed. The book was conceived to serve as a guide to the resident staff so that the approach is basically problem, rather than system-oriented. A significant proportion of the physician's time is spent on physical examination and evaluation of apparently healthy babies, detection of minor developmental peculiarities, supervision of feeding, reassurance and guidance to the mother, which have been given adequate coverage in the text. In view of our priorities and financial constraints, a greater emphasis has been accorded to the needs of the Special Care Nursery rather than a detailed discussion on Intensive Care Neonatal Unit with sophisticated monitoring equipment and ventilatory assistance.

Perinatology is an actively expanding field and new knowledge is accumulating fast. This book is not intended to be a comprehensive textbook but aims at providing a useful practical manual for those who care for the healthy and sick newborns.

14th October 1976
New Delhi

Meharban Singh MD

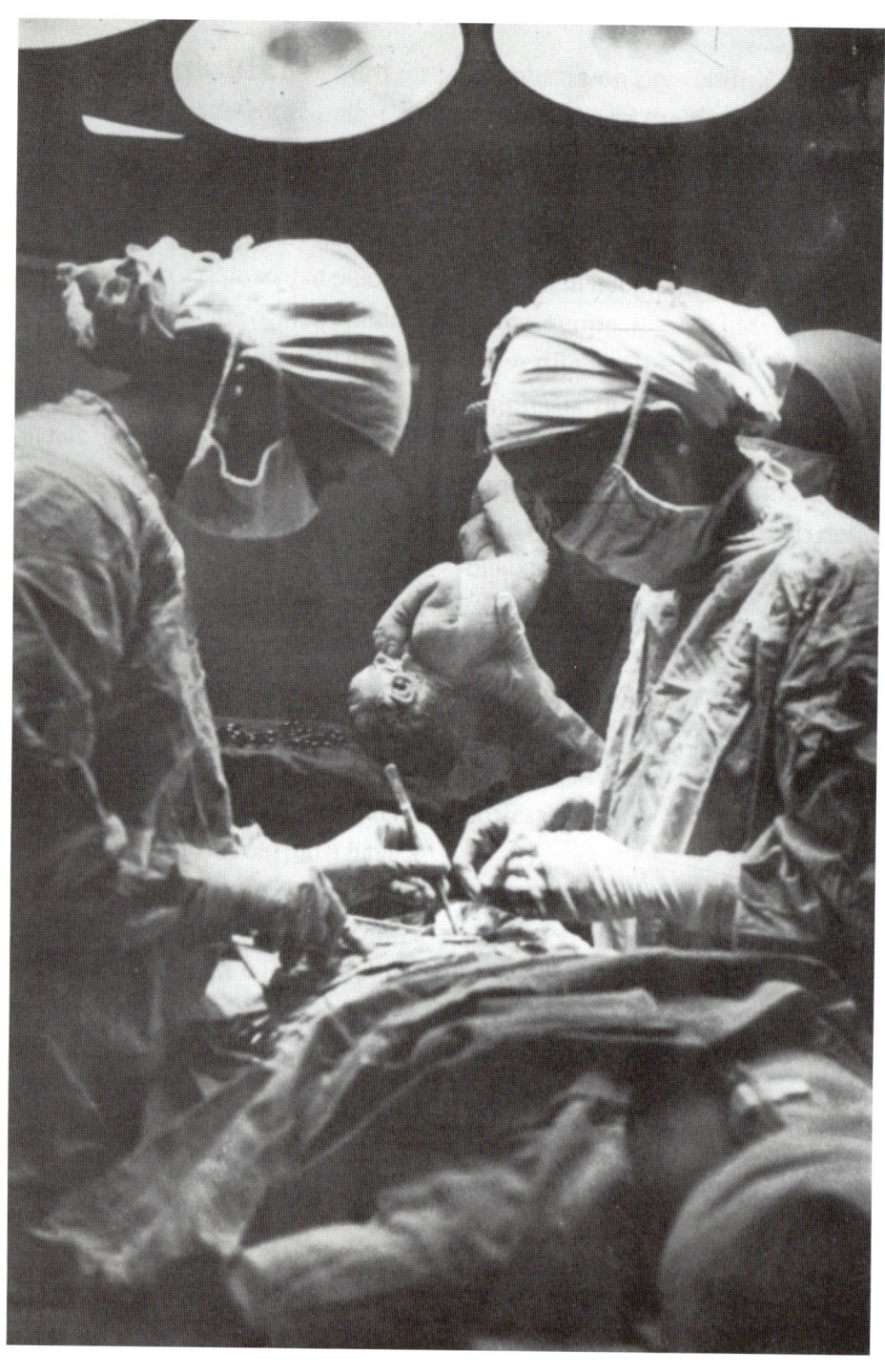

"In every child who is born under no matter what circumstances, and of no matter what parents, the potentiality of the human race is born again, and in him too, once more our terrific responsibility towards human life."

James Agee and Walker Evans

Contents

Contents

Contents

Other Popular Titles by Prof Meharban Singh

- **A Manual of Essential Pediatrics**
  (2nd Edition, 2013)

- **Medical Emergencies in Children**
  (6th Edition, 2021)

- **Pediatric Clinical Methods**
  (6th Edition, 2019)

- **Essential Pediatrics for Nurses**
  (4th Edition, 2017)

- **Medical Quotations
  by Eminent Physicians and Philosophers**
  (4th Edition, 2016)

- **Drug Dosages in Children**
  (10th Edition, 2019)

- **Neonatal Emergencies**
  (2nd Edition, 2021)

- **Celestial Principles: The Mystical Laws of Living**
  (1st Edition, 2016)

- **The Art and Science of Baby and Child Care**
  (4th Edition, 2014)

- **Textbook of Pediatric Nursing**
  (1st Edition, 2019)

- **A to Z Child Care**
  (1st Edition, 2015)

- ***Bachon Ka Swasthya Aur Unkee Dekhbhal*** **(Hindi)**
  (1st Edition, 2015)

Introduction to Care of Newborn Babies

Infants between birth and first 28 days of life are called newborns or neonates. They truly constitute the foundation of human life. *Just as children are not mini-adults, neonates are not mini-children.* They have unique health issues and problems due to structural and functional immaturity of various body organs depending upon their gestational age and birth weight. Newborn period is the most vulnerable phase of life and deaths during first 28 days of life account for around 70% of all infant deaths and 56% of all deaths of under-5 children.

Most healthy term neonates can be managed at home under the guidance and supervision of mother or health care professional. On the other hand, low birth weight and premature babies are fragile and vulnerable, and they demand high degree of skills and technology in a special care nursery or neonatal intensive care unit (NICU) for their intact survival. Apart from high neonatal mortality rate of 22.7 per 1000 live births, many avoidable handicaps during childhood, such as cerebral palsy, mental subnormality, learning disabilities and recurrent seizures, have their origin in the perinatal period. Based on "thrifty gene" or "developmental origins of adult diseases" hypothesis by Barker, there is evidence to suggest that infants with intrauterine growth restriction are at an increased risk to develop certain adult-onset diseases like hypertension, coronary artery disease, obesity, type 2 diabetes mellitus and hyperlipidemia. *The aim and goal of newborn care is not only to reduce neonatal mortality but more importantly to ensure their intact survival.* The enhancement of neonatal and infant survival is truly the key to the success of family welfare program and stabilization of population dynamics. And to achieve that goal, the task must be pursued like a mission.

EVOLUTION OF NEONATOLOGY

The concept and practice of neonatology evolved about 50 years ago and since then we have made outstanding advances in the care of newborn babies. It is amazing that a newborn baby with a birth weight of 1.0 kg had a mortality risk of 95% in 1960 and now has a 95% probability of survival! Neonatology has evolved from a state of passive or "hands-off years" (1920–1950) through aggressive or "heroic years" (1950–1970) and has reached a phase of "experienced years" (1970–2000) by promoting evidence-based neonatology. Due to integration of science and art of newborn care, the practice of neonatology has now reached the "years of wisdom" (middle path concept) and focus has shifted from mere survival to "intact" survival. Major advances in neonatology include effective resuscitation at birth, prevention of hypothermia and infections, rational use of antibiotics and promotion of optimal nutrition with human milk and parenteral nutrition. Availability of microsampling of blood has ensured frequent monitoring and correction of abnormalities in blood gases, acid–base parameters, electrolytes, glucose, bilirubin and other biochemical parameters. It is possible to monitor vital signs and arterial oxygen saturation with the help of noninvasive technology. The outcome and survival of preterm babies has improved by use of antenatal corticosteroids, administration of exogenous surfactant, and respiratory support (CPAP, assisted ventilation, iNO, ECMO). Pharmacological manipulation of ductus arteriosus, support of blood pressure, portable or point-of-care echocardiography, use of inhaled nitric oxide (iNO), interventional cardiology, newer modalities of assisted ventilation (PTV, SIMV and high frequency ventilation) and extracorporeal membrane oxygenation (ECMO) have revolutionized the cardiopulmonary management of critically sick neonates. Phototherapy has reduced the need for exchange blood transfusions and risk of bilirubin encephalopathy. A number of therapeutic misadventures or disasters of our good intents, like retinopathy of prematurity (ROP), pulmonary air leaks, bronchopulmonary dysplasia (BPD), kernicterus (sulfisoxazole prophylaxis, synthetic vitamin K, novobiocin), "gray-baby" syndrome (chloramphenicol over dose), pyloric stenosis (prokinetics like erythromycin), intraventricular hemorrhage (aggressive handling, bolus administration of sodium bicarbonate), cerebral palsy (corticosteroids) and pumonary air leaks, due to aggressive assisted ventilation are prevented or recognized early and managed effectively. It is important that we must exercise restraint and caution while introducing newer therapeutic interventions while keeping in mind their safety and cost effectiveness.

THE ART OF NEONATOLOGY

"The art of newborn care should not be sacrificed at the altar of technology. Art and science should provide an hormonious blend to ensure holistic care".

Meharban Singh

The technology has revolutionized the practice of neonatology and we have moved from an exceedingly "passive" or gentle hands-off approach to an over enthusiastic technology-oriented "aggressive" or "robotic" approach. It is a sad reality that nobody knows the ultimate or absolute truth. Science only provides a tentative or partial truth or truth for the time being. Neonatology is dynamic and we are likely to find new facts and data in due course of time. Therefore, we should not be dogmatic and we must work with humility, common sense and compassion. Evidence-based neonatology or Cochrane data base is probably closest to the truth but it must be integrated with personal experience or expertise, and common sense to transform these recommendations into best neonatal practices in order to harness best dividends. It is better to adopt and follow a balanced "middle path" approach in the care of newborn babies instead of having an extremely passive or balatantly aggressive approach. We should exercise restraint with a checks and balances on the pace of change to ensure that the knowledge is transformed into wisdom and it should be effectively harnessed keeping in mind the existent social constraints and realities. Technology should not be allowed to further dehumanize neonatology and we must treat babies not only with our heads but also with our hearts. Babies should be provided comfort, cuddling and gentle care by promoting best newborn care practices which are safe and cost-effective. We should not merely try to satisfy our ego in trying to save "previable premies" but our aim should be to ensure their "intact survival" so that the baby grows to become an asset to the nation rather than a liability to the society. Every newborn unit must have an integrated follow-up program to assess the quality of life of their NICU graduates and provide them with early stimulation.

In the best pediatric tradition, the approach in perinatal medicine should be oriented towards prevention, early identification and prompt management of common perinatal disorders. The art and science of newborn care should be integrated to provide holistic care to preterm babies. Babies should not be handled as "objects" and instead they should be provided with humanized developmentally supportive care. The nurses should provide individualized supportive care to preterm babies by adopting a "flexible" approach. They should feel connected and tuned with babies under their care. All the health care professionals in the neonatal intensive care unit (NICU) should be gentle, considerate and compassionate in providing care to preterm babies. The nature is supreme the way it looks after all the needs of the baby in the womb. The physiological needs of comfort, protection (against hypothermia and infection), oxygenation, nutrition and excretion are admirably met by the uteroplacental unit. *Womb is our gold standard for care of preterm babies and we should try to create a baby-friendly womb-like ambience and ecology in the NICU.* Despite several attempts, scientists have failed to fabricate an incubator with all the qualities and characteristics of the womb.

MATERNAL HEALTH AND NEWBORN SURVIVAL

Mothers are the creators and sustainers of progeny. The health and wellbeing of children is intimately linked with the health, nutrition, education and status of their mothers. Healthy and well-informed mothers are likely to produce healthy and normal weight babies while undernourished and high-risk mothers are likely to produce high-risk and low birth weight babies. Healthy mothers are in a much better position to look after the health and wellbeing of their children. Nutrition during fetal life and early infancy (exclusive breastfeeding) is entirely transmaternal and

"The health and wellbeing of the fetus is dependent upon the health and nutrition of the mother (not the father!) because she is both the seed as well as the soil wherein the baby is nurtured for 9 months".

Meharban Singh

its adequacy depends upon the nutritional status of the mother. *Mother is the best primary health worker because of her strong motivation, concern and commitment.* She must be provided with information, knowledge and skills of mothercraft to handle her baby with ease and confidence. She can provide skin-to-skin contact or kangaroo mother care which is credited to reduce the risk of nosocomial infections and hypothermia with improved survival of LBW babies. Over one-third of women in India are undernourished with a body weight of less than 40 kg or height of less than 145 cm. They are prone to develop a variety of infections, genital colonization, bacterial vaginosis with high prevalence of pelvic inflammatory disease and unsatisfactory reproductive health. Around one-half of women in our country are illiterate, they lack personal and financial independence and empowerment. The situation is further complicated by early marriages, teenage and frequent pregnancies. Despite Child Marriage Act 1978, almost 30% girls in India are married off before the age of 18 years without their consent. No wonder every fourth baby is a low birth weight in our country. In India, antenatal care of questionable quality is available to 85% of pregnant women and less than 50% of deliveries are conducted by skilled birth attendants.

GLOBAL NEONATAL HEALTH

Globally 130 million babies are born every year and of these 4 millions die during the newborn period, i.e. first 4 weeks of life. A similar number of babies are stillborn accounting for 8 million perinatal deaths per year, i.e. 15 lives are lost every minute. Most neonatal deaths occur in first week of life (75%) and almost 25% during first 24 hours. The risk of mortality during neonatal period is 30-fold higher than during the post-neonatal period. Almost 99% of neonatal deaths occur in low-middle income countries (LMICs). India accounts for the highest number of annual births (26 million) and neonatal deaths (0.75 million or 30% of global burden). Neonatal deaths account for two-thirds of all infant deaths and 56% of under-5 child deaths. The millennium development goal 4 (reducing under-5 mortality by two-thirds) cannot be achieved without substantial reduction in neonatal mortality. The situation is further worsening due to global epidemic of HIV and COVID-19. According to analysis of 3.6 million neonatal deaths from 192 countries in 2010, the main direct causes of neonatal deaths include preterm births (29%), severe infections (29%), birth asphyxia (23%) and congenital malformations (8%). The direct causes of global neonatal deaths are listed in Figure 1.1. The common correlates of adverse neonatal outcome include poor health status of women, illiteracy, lack

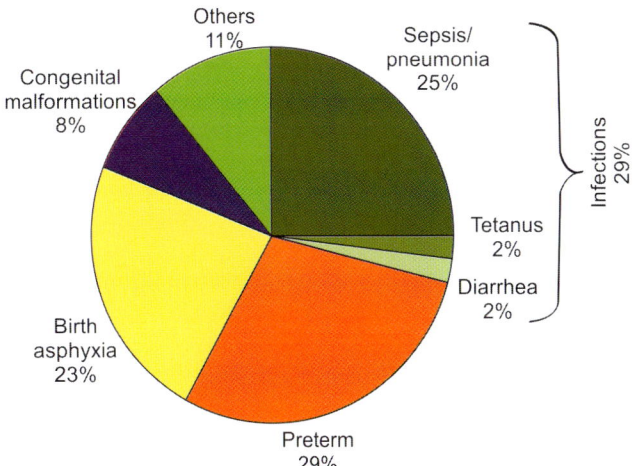

Figure 1.1 Estimated distribution of direct causes of global neonatal deaths (Adapted from Lawn JE, Cousens S, Zupan J. 4 million neonatal deaths: When? Where? Why? *The Lancet* 2005, 365:891–900.

of empowerment, early marriages and frequent pregnancies. In developing countries, lack of resources, poor infrastructure, lack of antenatal care, deliveries by unskilled attendants or relatives and poor accessibility and credibility of the facility-based health care services are the leading causes of dismal situation of newborn health.

MYTHS AND MISCONCEPTIONS REGARDING NEWBORN CARE

There are a number of myths and misconceptions regarding newborn care which can discourage health care professionals in initiating effective interventions to improve newborn survival.

1. *Newborn mortality can be reduced only by developed countries with high gross domestic product (GDP):* Several countries with low GDP, like Sri Lanka, Indonesia, Vietnam, Cuba, Honduras, and Nicaragua, have reduced neonatal mortality rates (NMR).

2. *High-tech interventions are needed to improve newborn survival:* Many countries have reduced NMR to about 15 per 1000 live births with community-based interventions without use of complex technology. There are minimum technology needs for care of newborn babies in the community (Box 1.1).

3. *Newborn care is expensive and not cost-effective:* Several low-cost interventions are effective to reduce neonatal mortality, like administration of tetanus toxoid to pregnant women, exclusive breast-feeding, kangaroo mother care for LBW babies, prevention and early use of antibiotic therapy for prompt treatment of infections.

Introduction to Care of Newborn Babies

1

Box 1.1 The technology needs for care of newborn babies in the community

- Birth attendant "disposable delivery kit"*.
- Mask for providing mouth-to-mask resuscitation.
- Five cleans (surface, hands, blade, cord tie, cord care).
- Promotion of early and exclusive breastfeeding.
- Home-based strategies for prevention of hypothermia (postpone bath, provide effective clothing, closeness with mother, warm room, external heat source).
- Kangaroo mother care.
- Ensuring hygienic practices (hand washing skills, clean blade, cord care, clean environment, clean sun-dried clothes).
- Gavage and spoon or *paladay* feeding of LBW babies.
- Availability of oral and injectable antibiotics.
- Distribution of information, education and communication (IEC) material on care of normal and LBW babies and identification of sick babies (danger signs).

---

*According to NFHS-4, disposable *dai kit* was used in 50% of home deliveries.

4. *Newborn health is not a priority in a developing country because high neonatal mortality is a blessing in disguise to control population dynamics*: Newborn survival is indeed the greatest assurance and incentive to parents to adopt family planning measures and achieve desired population goals.

5. *Neonatal-specific interventions are not needed because current safe motherhood and child survival strategies are sufficient to reduce deaths of newborn babies.*

Till recently, Child Survival and Safe Motherhood (CSSM) and Reproductive and Child Health (RCH) programs focused on reduction of post-neonatal deaths by promotion of breastfeeding, immunizations, ORS for treatment of diarrhea and antibiotics for acute respiratory infections. The need for specific neonatal interventions is being addressed in India by launch of Integrated Management of Neonatal and Childhood Illnesses (IMNCI) program and India Newborn Action Plan (INAP) so that newborn diseases are tackled through simple algorithms. There is a need to create a network of good quality level II newborn care units throughout the country which are more cost-effective and less technology or labor-intensive and can bring down the neonatal mortality rate to less than 20 per 1,000 live births.

ESSENTIAL NEWBORN CARE

Every year about 26 million babies (20% of global births) are born in India and almost 0.75 million die during newborn period accounting for 30% of global deaths. *India has the dubious distinction of having the highest number of annual neonatal births and deaths among all countries in the world.* In order to reduce neonatal mortality, essential or basic newborn care services should be available at all the health care levels because they are highly cost-effective. The components of essential newborn care services include good quality antenatal care (at least 4 ANC contacts), safe delivery and optimal care at birth, promotion of exclusive breastfeeding, prevention and early treatment of hypothermia and bacterial infections. The moderately low birth weight babies (birth weight >1800 g) and/or late preterms with a gestation >34 weeks account for 90% of LBW babies and they should be provided essential care at home or primary health care facility. There is a need for greater focus on the preventive rather than curative strategies because a large number of neonatal deaths occur due to potentially preventable disorders, like birth asphyxia, hypothermia and septicemia. The provision of essential newborn care is the most urgent key health care priority in our country and saving newborn babies in India is a national priority in order to achieve further reduction in infant mortality rate.

NEONATAL MORBIDITY

The health problems of newborn babies are unique and distinctive compared to diseases of infants and older children. Neonates are prone to develop health problems due to transition from dependent fetal to independent neonatal physiology, disorders due to structural and functional immaturity of various body organs and a variety of iatrogenic disorders because of aggressive use of technology in the NICU. The salient health problems of newborn babies are listed below.

"The seeds of neonatal morbidity are sown in the labor room".
Meharban Singh

1. **Disorders due to unsatisfactory adaptation from fetal to neonatal physiology** Fetus is totally dependent and at the mercy of placental integrity and maternal wellbeing. After birth, baby must breathe, clear all the fluid from the lungs and promptly make a change over from fetal to neonatal cardiorespiratory physiology for survival. Birth asphyxia, wet lungs (transient tachypnea of the newborn), patent ductus arteriosus and persistent pulmonary circulation are some of the manifestations of unsatisfactory transition from fetal to neonatal physiology.

2. **Disorders of body temperature** Most babies rapidly lose body temperature because they are

born naked and wet and they come from a warm womb to a cold room. If a baby is not promptly dried or effectively covered or kept under a radiant warmer, he is likely to develop hypothermia and its consequences. Fever is the commonest signal of infection in a child, while a neonate, especially a preterm baby, may succumb to sepsis without exhibiting any fight and instead becomes sluggish, cold and apneic.

3. **Vulnerability to infections** Newborn babies are extremely vulnerable to develop bacterial infections because from a relatively aseptic uterine abode they make entry into a room which is teeming with microbes. They are endowed with suboptimal immunologic responses with a relatively poor localization of infection leading to sepsis and adverse outcome. Some babies may be born with intrauterine infections (TORCH infections) or develop infection during their passage through the infected birth canal leading to development of early-onset sepsis. Most neonatal infections are nosocomial and are acquired from the hospital or from the community.

4. **Respiratory difficulties** Idiopathic respiratory distress syndrome or hyaline membrane disease due to deficiency of surfactant is limited to preterm babies. Availability of surfactant and assisted ventilation facilities have improved the survival of premature babies. Apneic attacks due to immaturity of respiratory center is also limited to preterm or sick babies. Meconium aspiration syndrome is an important cause of RDS in post-term or growth-retarded term babies with placental dysfunction. Premature babies are prone to develop aspiration of feeds in the absence of skilled nursing.

5. **Gastrointestinal disorders** Incoordination between sucking and swallowing, and laxity of gastroesopha-geal sphincter may lead to intolerance of oral feeds, frequent episodes of regurgitation and aspiration into the lungs. Necrotizing enterocolitis due to GI stasis and poor motility of gut is known to occur in preterm babies.

6. **Cardiac disorders** Congenital cardiac malformations may present as congestive heart failure or shock as a life-threatening emergency in newborn period. Many cardiac malformations are duct-dependent and palliative relief can be provided by administra-tion of prostaglandins. Functional patency of ductus arteriosus, which can be managed with medical therapy, is peculiar to preterm babies having RDS.

7. **Neonatal jaundice** The causes and spectrum of jaundice in newborn babies are unique compared to older children. Almost two-thirds of neonates manifest physiologic jaundice which does not need any investigations or treatment. Hyperbilirubinemia due to blood group incompatibility between the mother and her baby (Rh or ABO system) is unique to newborn babies. Hyperbilirubinemia due to elevated levels of unconjugated bilirubin may seep through the blood–brain barrier and cause damage to basal ganglia (acute bilirubin encephalopathy or kernicterus). It is managed by unique therapeutic modalities, like phototherapy and exchange blood transfusion which are not applicable to older children. Jaundice (with some elevation of direct bilirubin) may occur as a manifes-tation of urinary tract infection, sepsis and cholesta-sis in neonates. Some breast-fed babies may develop prolonged jaundice (breast milk jaundice) which is harmless and does not need any therapy. Viral hepatitis is the commonest cause of jaundice in an older child while it is rare in a newborn baby.

8. **Hematological problems** Because of relative hypoxia during fetal life, average hemoglobin in newborn babies is around 16–18 g/dL with a high risk of symptomatic polycythemia and hyper-viscosity. Hemorrhagic disease of the newborn due to vitamin K deficiency is limited to newborn babies. Disseminated intravascular coagulation (DIC) is a common complication in critically sick, hypoxic and hypotensive preterm babies.

9. **CNS disorders** There is high incidence of seizures in newborn babies due to hypoxia, hypoglycemia, birth trauma, sepsis and congenital malformations. Unlike older children, most seizures are sympto-matic rather than idiopathic. Intraventricular hemorrhage due to immaturity of capillaries is limited to preterm babies. Administration of cortico-steroids in newborn babies may lead to neuronal damage with increased risk of cerebral palsy. The seeds of cerebral palsy and neuromotor disorders during childhood are sown in the perinatal period.

10. **Congenital malformations** Congenital malfor-mations, developmental defects, chromosomal disorders and inborn errors of metabolism due to genetic defects are limited to newborn babies and infants.

11. **Iatrogenic disorders** Because of liberal use of technology and greater vulnerability of neonates,

1

the incidence of disasters due to acts of omissions and commissions by doctors and nurses is much higher during neonatal period. Iatrogenic disorders may occur due to administration of drugs (kernicterus due to administration of vitamin K and sulfisoxazole, gray baby syndrome due to chloramphenicol, deafness due to aminoglycosides, intraventricular or pulmonary hemorrhage due to bolus administration of intravenous sodium bicarbonate), oxygen therapy (ROP and bronchopulmonary dysplasia) and procedures (premature delivery, skin burns, necrotizing enterocolitis, pneumothorax, bronchopulmonary dysplasia, electric shock, etc.).

THE LEVELS OF NEWBORN CARE

Based upon birth weight and gestational age, a three-tier system of neonatal care is proposed for developing countries.

Level I Care

Over 80 percent of newborn babies require minimal care which can be provided by their mothers under the supervision of basic health care professionals. Neonates weighing above 1800 g or having gestational maturity of 34 weeks or more (late preterms) belong to this category. The care can be provided at home, subcenter and primary health center level. Basic care at birth, provision of warmth, maintenance of asepsis and promotion of exclusive breastfeeding form the mainstay of level I care. Traditional birth attendants and community health workers must be trained in the art of esssential perinatal care.

Level II Care

Infants weighing between 1200 and 1800 g or having gestational maturity of 30–34 weeks need specialized neonatal care supervised by trained nurses and pediatricians. First referral units, district hospitals, teaching institutions and nursing homes should be equipped to provide intermediate neonatal care. Equipment for resuscitation, maintenance of thermo-neutral environment, intravenous infusion and gavage feeding, phototherapy and exchange blood transfusion should be available. There should be no compromise on the basic needs of adequate space, nursing staff and maintenance of asepsis including round the clock handwashing and hand sanitization facilities, provision for disposable gamma-irradiated suction catheters, feeding tubes, endotracheal tubes, and small-vein infusion sets. Intermediate neonatal care is needed for about 10 to 15% of newborn population and should be available at all hospitals catering to 1000 to 1500 deliveries per year.

Level III Care

Intensive neonatal care is required for babies weighing less than 1200 g or those born before 30 weeks of gestation. Apex institutions or regional perinatal centers equipped with centralized oxygen and suction facilities, servo-controlled open care systems and incubators, vital sign and transcutaneous monitors, ventilators and infusion pumps are best suited to provide intensive neonatal care. Skilled nurses and neonatologists especially trained in the art of neonatal intensive care are required to organize this service. About 3 to 5% of newborn population qualify for intensive care. Establishment of neonatal intensive care unit (NICU) demands a sound infrastructure and should be envisaged only when optimal intermediate neonatal care facilities have already been in existence for some time. The capital and recurring expenditure for level III care is exorbitant and it is not cost-effective unless service is regionalized.

IMPROVING THE QUALITY OF MATERNAL AND NEWBORN CARE

World Health Organization has launched a global initiative to improve quality of maternal and neonatal health care, especially in the low and middle income countries (LMICs). The improvements in the quality of health care are essential to meet the health-related targets of the Sustainable Development Goals (SDGs). The quality assurance (QA) and quality improvement (QI) efforts are crucial for improving the maternal, fetal, neonatal and child survival at all levels of health care. The QI initiative aims to increase the probability to provide safe, timely, effective, equitable and patient-centered health services to mothers and their offsprings. The "Every Newborn Action Plan" (ENAP) and Ending Preventable Maternal Mortality (EPMM) initiatives have been launched to end all preventable maternal and neonatal deaths and stillbirths by 2035. Monitoring the performance of the health care system and implementation of quality improvement activities need reliable systems for data collection, analysis and interpretation.

India and other LMICs have launched QI initiatives for providing safe, effective, patient-centered and equitable maternal and neonatal health care services at various levels of health care facilities. World Health Organization has provided an eight-point directive to provide quality assured services in the field of maternal and perinatal health. These domains include (i) evidence-based practices for essential care of mothers and their children, (ii) early recognition of complications and their management, (iii) actionable information system, (iv) robust referral system, (v) effective communication, (vi) respect and dignity, (vii) emotional support with the help of (viii) motivated human resources and functional health care infrastructure. A conceptual framework is useful to develop QI parameters in the field of health care. The framework proposed utilizes two approaches for delivery of good quality health care. The Donabedian model divides the health care into structure, processes and outcomes, while the Institute of Medicine's (IOM) initiatives focus on the needs to provide *safe, timely, effective, efficient, equitable* and *people-centered* health care services.

The QI Initiatives

The QI approaches try to narrow the gap between current knowledge and actual practices in various health care facilities. They share four core principles. First, to identify the gap between expected outcomes of various clinical situations versus the actual outcomes achieved by the first-line health workers providing the clinical care. Second, understanding the local health care systems to identify various barriers preventing delivery of quality health care. Third, to implement the classic problem-solving small steps of change under the format of Plan-Do-Study-Act (PDSA). To initiate the cycle of change under PDSA, the intervention is Planned, it is carried out (Do), its outcome is evaluated (Study) and whether any modifications are required for the intervention (Act). The PDSA intervention should be feasible, effective and adaptable in the local context before it is launched for universal implementation. Fourth, the salient health problems should be identified on the basis of available data and to assess whether interventions are achieving their objectives. Various health care issues can be studied under PDSA to promote the concept of QI. Various outcomes of quality measures like vision, hearing, neuromotor disability, seizures, etc. can be studied to achieve best dividends.

The Health Care System

The health care system includes essential physical infrastructure and availability of adequate number of competent health care providers. Shortage of skilled manpower is an important correlate of poor quality of care in the LMICs. The quality of care can be improved by providing adequate physical and human resources. The facility-based resources should be specifically tailored to prevent and manage prematurity, infections and perinatal asphyxia, which are three leading causes of neonatal morbidity and mortality in LMICs. The framework of quality improvement of perinatal services is summarized in Box 1.2. The performance of health care system, the success and failure of QI efforts is largely dependent on availability of health care workers, their motivation level, burnout, teamwork and leadership skills.

Health Care Processes

The vision of World Health Organization for improvement of quality of care of mothers and there children is summarized in Figure 1.2. The QI depends on availability of sound health infrastructure, and evidence-based processes to ensure improved outcomes. The components of health care processes in neonatal resuscitation include identification of neonates who need resuscitation, the need for positive pressure ventilation, criteria for adequacy of bag and mask ventilation and administration of drugs. Data about health care processes are best measured by direct observations. However, this is prone to Hawthorne effect wherein alteration of behavior is likely to occur when it is known that you are being observed. The Hawthorne effect should be reduced by installing CCTV cameras and monitoring by regular staff members. Data about processes can be retrieved from digital records and personal interviews.

Box 1.2 The framework for quality improvement of perinatal services

- Establish core set of essential perinatal services at all levels of health care facilities.
- The WHO has outlined a set of quality of care indicators and standards for improving quality of maternal and newborn health care facilities. These standards and indicators can be adapted on the basis of national needs.
- There is a need to establish the processes for measurement of core set of quality of care indicators for neonatal-perinatal care.
- There should be a robust system of data collection for perinatal morbidities and outcomes by establishing state level and national level neonatal-perinatal quality monitoring and improvement of resource facilities.
- The existing health information management systems and digital electronic patient record systems should be modified to include quality of care indicators.
- There is a need to develop quality improvement activities by incorporating QI training in pre- and in-service curriculum for assessment of quality of care on a day-to-day basis, quarterly and yearly appraisal.

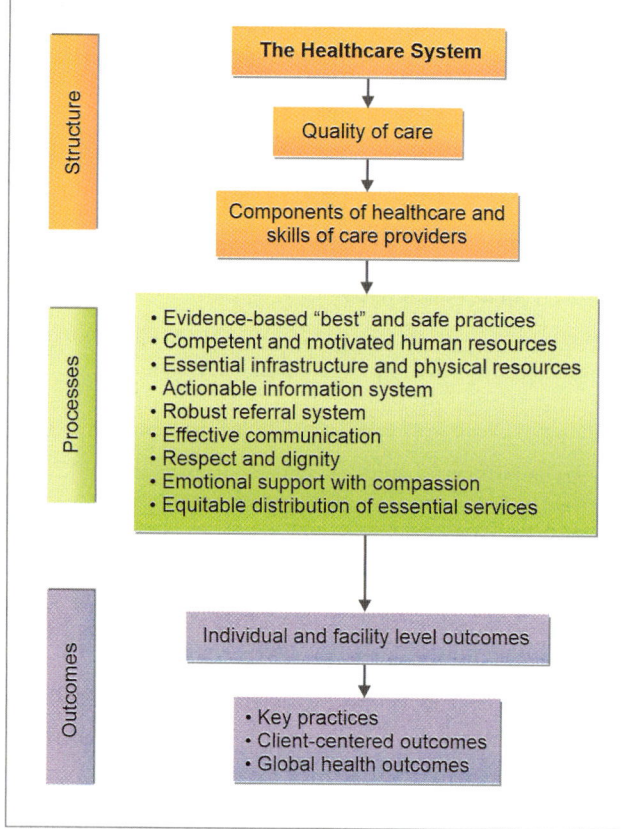

Figure 1.2 WHO vision for quality of care of mothers and their neonates

Health Outcomes

The morbidity and outcome of a disease process is the best parameter of quality of care. Apart from adequacy of preventive and curative health care services, genetic predisposition, developmental abnormalities, environmental exposures and care-seeking behavior influence the outcomes. Examples of health care outcomes in neonatal care include incidence of morbidities like hypoxia, RDS, infections, hypothermia and hypoglycemia. The parameters of quality improvement of perinatal services are summarized in Box 1.2. The health care facilities and monitoring agencies should invest in collection and analysis of reliable data to assess the dividends of quality assurance and quality improvement activities.

Future Developments and Perspectives

A large number of newer interventions are in the pipeline to further revolutionize the practice of neo-natology. A number of multicentric randomized controlled trials (RCTs) have been launched to identify evidence-based, reliable, and safe newborn care practices. Skin surface electrodes are being developed for non-invasive monitoring of blood gases, glucose, bilirubin, electrolytes and pH. There is a need to develop ultramicrotechniques for assessment of complete biochemical parameters with the help of a drop of blood. Newer diagnostic techniques with the help of polymerase chain reaction (PCR) are being developed for the diagnosis of a variety of infective and genetic disorders. Neonatal screening for inborn errors of metabolism is likely to become universal. Efforts are being made to develp specific monoclonal antibodies for prevention and treatment of life-threatening infective disorders. There is availability of a variety of sophisticated lasers for treatment of birth marks. Vaccines are being developed for prevention of Group B streptococci (GBS), cytomegalovirus (CMV), human immunodeficiency virus (HIV) and novel coronavirus infections. Tailor-made drugs are being formulated with the help of pharmacogenetics and attempts are being made to deliver the drugs to the site of disease with the help of liposomes.

There is increasing use of homologous blood obtained from placenta and possibility of storing cord blood has become a reality for future use as "totipotent" stem cells for repair of any organ and treatment of malignant or genetic disorders in the donor, siblings or parents. Genetic engineering is being exploited to replace a "bad" gene with a "good" gene by tagging it to the carrier viruses. Assisted reproductive technologies (ARTs) are being harnessed to produce genetically normal babies, flawless designer babies, surrogacy and gender selection raising several moral and ethical issues. There is a need to develop strategies to prevent premature birth of babies who are structurally normal. Prolongation of gestation and improvement of fetal nutrition are important interventions to improve birth weight which is the single most important correlate of improved survival and outcome of a neonate. However, the ultimate dream of a neonatologist, which has defied all attempts till date, is to prevent premature births to improve the birth weight and to develop a prototype of a uteroplacental unit to provide all the virtues of the womb to nurture babies who are born prematurely.

NOMENCLATURE AND DEFINITIONS

It is essential to have uniformly accepted definitions to express perinatal–neonatal morbidity and mortality. The data pertaining to perinatal audit should conform to a universal format for ease of comparison with other national and international studies. The adoption of standard nomenclature is essential for generating meaningful data and for surveillance of impact of interventional strategies. Accuracy of record keeping is mandatory for generation of meaningful data for perinatal audit. The data is collected from antenatal records, specialized neonatal proformas and admission/discharge registers. It is essential to maintain separate registers for NICU (one each for intramural and extramural babies) and rooming-in babies. A software should be created to store the data in the computer. The data should be checked and reviewed weekly, monthly and yearly in the joint meetings between the staff members looking after the mothers and babies. The analysis and retrieval of data can be greatly augmented by computer facilities. The majority of definitions and terminologies described below are based on the standard sources, such as tenth revision of International Statistical Classification of Diseases (ISCD) by WHO and they are duly approved and adapted by the Taskforce of National Neonatology Forum of India.

Fetus

Fetus is a product of conception, irrespective of the duration of pregnancy, which is not completely expelled or extracted from its mother. Up to 9 weeks of gestation, it is designated as embryo.

Live Birth

Live birth is defined as complete expulsion or extraction from the mother of a product of conception (irrespective of the duration of pregnancy) and which after such separation, breathes or shows any other evidence of life, such as beating of the heart, pulsation of umbilical cord or definite movements of the voluntary muscles irrespective of the attachment of placenta and/or cord. In a community setting, cry and breathing efforts alone may be used as a criterion of live born. In 1970, WHO recommended that babies weighing less than 500 g at birth should show signs of life for at least one hour before they are designated as live born.

Fetal Death

Death prior to the complete expulsion or extraction from its mother of a product of conception irrespective of the duration of pregnancy, the death being indicated by absence of any signs of life.

Early fetal death Death at a gestational age of less than 22 weeks or of a fetus weighing less than 500 g or crown-heel length of less than 25 cm.

Intermediate fetal death Death at a gestational age of 22–27 weeks or of a fetus weighing 500–999 g or crown-heel length between 25 cm and less than 35 cm.

Late fetal death Death at a gestational age of 28 weeks or more or of a fetus weighing 1000 g or more or crown-heel length of at least 35 cm. The body may be fresh or macerated.

Early fetal deaths are called abortions while intermediate and late fetal deaths are designated as stillbirths.

Birth Weight

Birth weight is the first weight of a live or stillborn baby which should preferably be taken within the first hour of life and certainly during the first day of life before any significant postnatal weight loss has occurred. If weight is recorded after 24 hours, the age at which the weight is taken should be specified. The average birth weight of newborn babies in India is around 3.0 kg.

Birth Weight Groups

Low birth weight (LBW) babies Babies with a birth weight of less than 2500 g (up to and including 2499 g) irrespective of the period of gestation are designated as LBW babies. These include preterm (one-third) and small-for-dates term (two-thirds) babies. In India, for purposes of according specialized care, babies with a birth weight of less than 1800 g are considered as high risk and are admitted to the special care neonatal unit (SCNU). The current incidence of LBW babies in India is around 28% (lowest incidence of 7.6% in Mizoram) accounting for 8 million LBW babies (40% of global burden) every year. However, over 80% of LBW babies are good-sized and weigh between 2000 and 2499 g, and 15% infants weigh between 1500 and 1999 g.

Very low birth weight (VLBW) babies Babies with a birth weight of less than 1500 g (up to and including 1499 g) are designated as VLBW babies. In India, around 3% babies are VLBW babies.

Extremely low birth weight (ELBW) babies Babies with a birth weight of less than 1000 g (up to and including 999 g) are classified as ELBW babies. They account for <1.0% of all live births.

Micropremies Infants with a birth weight of less than 750 g.

Gestational Age

Gestational age is calculated from the first day of the last normal menstrual period till the date of birth and is expressed in weeks and days. For example, 30 2/7 weeks of pregnancy means 30 completed weeks plus 2 days. It is also called menstrual age. On the other hand, the conceptional age is the true fetal age and it refers to the length of pregnancy from the time of conception and is generally 2 weeks less than the menstrual age.

The American College of Obstetricians and Gynecologists (ACOG) and the Society for Maternal and Fetal Medicine have revised the classification based on the gestational age.

Preterm (premature) Neonates between 20 weeks and 36 6/7 weeks (<37 completed weeks) are classified as preterm. Around 10–15% babies are born preterm in India.

Late preterm 34 0/7 weeks through 36 6/7 weeks of gestation.

Extremely preterm Babies born before 28 completed weeks of gestation.

Full term (or "Term") Babies between gestational age 39 0/7 weeks through 40 6/7 weeks. According to new definition, a pregnancy is "full term", only in the narrow two-week window between 39 and 41 weeks. The outcome of babies is best during this narrow window. It is recommended that elective cesarean section should not be done before 39 weeks of gestation.

Early term Babies between 37 0/7 weeks through 38 6/7 weeks of gestation.

Late term Babies between 41 0/7 weeks through 41 6/7 weeks of gestation.

Post term Babies with a gestation of 42 0/7 weeks and beyond are classified as post term and postmature.

Classification by Birth Weight and Gestational Age Groups

Small-for-dates (SFD) babies (Small-for-gestational age, light-for-dates). Babies with a birth weight of less than 10th percentile for their gestational age population-based weight data are designated as SFD babies. For purposes of specialized care and monitoring of blood glucose levels, babies with a birth weight of less than 3rd percentile for the period of their gestation are admitted in the NICU.

Ideally, regional intrauterine growth charts should be constructed from a population belonging to high socioeconomic level with optimal maternal nutrition, and after excluding known maternal and fetal conditions, which cause intrauterine growth retardation. It also appears justified to employ one universally accepted international reference standard for purposes of comparison of the data. The terms intrauterine growth restriction (IUGR) and small-for-gestational age (SGA) are often used interchangeably but they are actually distinct. The fetus is diagnosed to have growth restriction, if the intrauterine growth is less compared to the predetermined growth potential of healthy fetuses. An infant with IUGR may be SGA or his birth weight may be appropriate-for-gestational age.

Appropriate-for-dates (AFD) babies (Appropriate-for-gestational age). Babies with a birth weight between 10th and 90th percentile for the period of their gestation are called appropriate-for-dates babies.

Large-for-dates (LFD) babies (Large-for-gestational age, heavy-for-dates). Babies with a birth weight of more than 90th percentile for the period of their gestational age. The babies with a birth weight of more than 97th percentile for their gestation are considered high risk and monitored for hypoglycemia.

By combining classification of the babies on the basis of gestational age alone and gestational age with birth weight, the newborn population can be divided into the following 9 subgroups (Figure 1.3).

1. Preterm	SFD, AFD, LFD
2. Term	SFD, AFD, LFD
3. Post-term	SFD, AFD, LFD

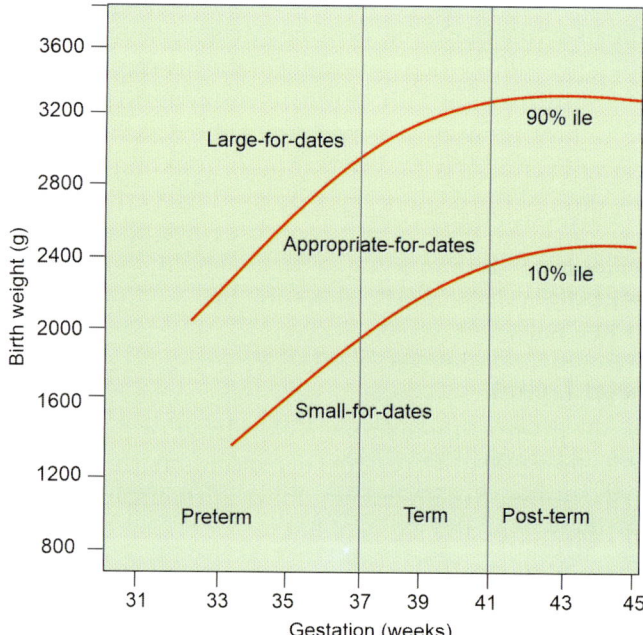

Figure 1.3 Classification of neonates on the basis of birth weight and gestational age. (Adapted from Singh M, Giri SK and Ramachandran K. *Indian Pediatr* 1974,11:475)

The neonatal mortality is high among preterm babies due to anatomical and functional immaturity of various body organs. The least neonatal mortality is seen in term appropriate-for-dates babies. In each gestational group (whether preterm, term or post-term), mortality is higher among LFD and SFD babies as compared to AFD babies.

Perinatal Period

Perinatal period extends from the 28th week of gestation (or more than 1000 g) to the 7th day of life (early neonatal period). In view of the increasing survival of the babies weighing less than 1000 g in many centers as a result of improvements in the perinatal care, the concept of *extended perinatal period* has been introduced. This period extends from 22nd week of gestation (or more than 500 g) to 7th day of life.

Perinatal Mortality Rate (PMR)

It is defined as late fetal plus early neonatal (first week) deaths of babies weighing more than 1000 g at birth (or 28th weeks of gestation or more) per 1000 total births weighing over 1000 g. It is suggested that for international comparisons, the numerator as well as the denominator in perinatal-neonatal statistics should be restricted to fetuses and infants weighing 1000 g or more.

$$PMR = \frac{\text{Total perinatal deaths}}{\text{Total number of births}} \times 100$$

$$\text{Extended PMR} = \frac{\begin{array}{l}\text{Intermediate stillbirths}\\ + \text{Late stillbirths}\\ + \text{Early neonatal deaths}\end{array}}{\text{Total number of births}} \times 100$$

The perinatal mortality rate within various birth weight groups and due to specific causes should be expressed. Population attributable risk of various adverse perinatal factors and idealized PMR by exclusion of non-salvageable causes of perinatal deaths should be calculated.

On the basis of NFHS-4 community-based studies, it is estimated that stillbirth rate in India is 9.7 per 1000 births. This rate is much lower than the modelled estimate of 22 per 1000 births by INAP.

Neonatal Period

Neonatal period extends up to 28 days of life. Infants up to 28 days of life are called newborns or neonates. Early neonatal period refers to first 7 days or under 168 hours of life while late neonatal period extends from 7 days to under 28 completed days of life.

Neonatal Deaths

First day deaths are defined as deaths occurring within 24 hours of age (exclude if baby had completed 24 hours of age). Early neonatal deaths include deaths within first week or <168 hours of age (exclude if baby has completed 168 hours of age). Neonatal deaths include all deaths within 28 days of age (exclude if baby has completed 28 days).

In case of premature babies, it would appear more logical to count 28 days of neonatal period from post-menstrual maturity of 40 weeks instead of date of birth. In any case, all neonatal deaths that occur before discharge from the NICU should be included in the statistics.

Neonatal Mortality Rate (NMR)

Early NMR Neonatal deaths of babies weighing over 1000 g during first 7 days per 1000 live births.

Late NMR or unspecified NMR Neonatal deaths of babies weighing over 1000 g during 28 days of life per 1000 live births.

The extended neonatal mortality rate can be calculated by including babies weighing up to 500 g. It is suggested that hospital-based neonatal–perinatal statistics may be presented separately for booked and unbooked cases.

The current NMR in India is around 22.7 per 1000 live births and it accounts for 70% of infant deaths (IMR 32) and 56% of under-5 child mortality (U5MR 42). NMR in rural areas is over one and a half times of the urban areas.

Birth Weight Classification for Perinatal–Neonatal Data

The morbidity and mortality can be expressed by weight intervals of 500 g, i.e. 1000–1499 g, 1500–1999 g, 2000–2499 g and so on.

Gestational Age Classification for Perinatal–Neonatal Data

Less than 28 weeks (less than 196 days)
28–31 weeks (196–223 days)
32–36 weeks (224–258 days)
37–41 weeks (259–293 days)
42 weeks and more (294 days and more)

Calculation of Incidence

The incidence of neonatal conditions (e.g. LBW babies, preterm, and birth asphyxia, etc.) should be calculated per 100 live births, while that of pregnancy and labor

Care of the Newborn

1

related conditions (e.g. toxemia, maternal anemia, cesarean deliveries, etc.) should be calculated per 100 total births.

Maternal Mortality

The maternal death is defined as a death of a woman known to be pregnant within 42 days of termination of pregnancy, irrespective of the duration or site of the pregnancy. The death may be due to any cause related to or aggravated by the pregnancy or its management but not from accidental or incidental causes. The maternal mortality rate is expressed as maternal deaths per 100,000 live births. The current adjusted MMR in India is 122 per 100,000 live births accounting for 25% of global maternal deaths. The common correlates of high maternal mortality include poor socioeconomic status, unsatisfactory health and nutrition of women, illiteracy, early or delayed pregnancy, obesity, lack of antenatal care and delivery by untrained birth attendants.

Direct obstetric deaths Deaths resulting from complications of pregnancy, child birth or puerperium including interventions, omissions, incorrect treatment or from a chain of events resulting from any of the above causes. The common direct causes of maternal deaths include induced abortions, sepsis, hemorrhage, anemia, thrombosis and thromboembolism, amniotic fluid embolism, pre-eclampsia and eclampsia, ectopic pregnancy and obstructed labor.

Indirect obstetric deaths Deaths resulting from previous existing disease or a disease that developed during pregnancy, child birth or the puerperium which was not due to direct obstetric causes but which was aggravated by physiologic effects of pregnancy. The most common causes of indirect deaths include cardiac illnesses and psychiatric disorders.

CLINICOPATHOLOGICAL CLASSIFICATION OF PERINATAL DEATHS

There is a lack of unanimity and considerable confusion exists regarding the most acceptable method for classification of deaths during perinatal period. It is essential that all perinatal centers should adopt an identical or uniform protocol for clinicopathological classification of perinatal deaths so that mortality data is comparable in order to identify any regional differences. During perinatal period, many deaths cannot be classified merely on the basis of clinical findings unless it is complemented by autopsy data. Efforts should always be made to obtain an autopsy

in each and every case of perinatal death. It is generally easier to obtain permission for autopsy in a case of perinatal death because of relatively less emotional bondage of parents and their concern for having a normal healthy baby during next pregnancy. A routine autopsy performed by an adult-oriented pathologist may not be informative and may be unable to identify the cause of death.

NEONATAL AUTOPSY

Identification of cause(s) of death, elucidation of pathogenetic mechanisms and assessment of quality of clinical management are the key objectives of autopsy examination at any age. Neonatal autopsy, in addition, is expected to guide the clinician to provide genetic counseling to the parents. Information derived from the stereotyped, adult-oriented, routine necropsies is very limited, and such a procedure is not cost-effective. Hence, a specially designed protocol should be developed for newborn autopsies at each center by the combined efforts of pediatricians and pathologists. Neonatal autopsy should be performed by a trained perinatal pathologist well-versed with its methodology. It is mandatory to accord due importance to anthropometry, assessment of gestation and recording of accurate weights of various body organs. Appropriate radiological, cytogenetic and metabolic studies should be undertaken, if dysmorphic features or congenital malformations are present.

Prerequisites for an Autopsy

Both maternal and neonatal case notes should be reviewed before commencing the postmortem examination. It is always helpful, whenever possible and in all complicated deaths, to discuss the case personally with the treating physician. This shall allow the pathologist to pay special attention to certain organs and plan appropriate additional investigations, like karyotyping, metabolic and microbiological studies.

The perinatal autopsy should commence after the pathologist has established from the available notes the maturity of the baby, birth weight, postnatal age (if live born) and probable cause and mode of death.

Anthropometry and Visceral Weights

The size of the baby and its organs varies with maturity and birth weight of the infant and these must be measured accurately and compared with known standards. It is often misleading to state that an organ is enlarged without taking into consideration these facts. The organ weights may be affected in certain characteristic ways by malformation syndromes, placental insufficiency and diabetes mellitus.

Organ weights of each of the following internal organs should be independently and accurately taken; brain, heart, lungs, liver, spleen, thymus, kidneys and adrenals. The norms of standard weights of these organs at different gestations and birth weights should be available for ready reference (Tables 1.1 and 1.2). It is desirable to record weights of large organs to the nearest gram and that of smaller ones to the nearest 0.1 g by using an accurate weighing scale. Accuracy of weights of organs in neonatal autopsies is of great importance since some of the specific diagnoses, like hypoplasia of an organ, can be made only on the basis of weight.

In case of small-for-dates infants and babies born to diabetic mothers, it is important to compare the organ weights with that of normal appropriately grown infants of the same maturity. In small-for-dates babies, the brain appears to be relatively large while liver and thymus are atrophied. The weight of the heart and lungs is unaffected. The brain to liver ratio is usually more than 5 in growth retarded babies. In large-for-dates babies, all viscera weigh more than normal except the brain.

External Examination

The pathologist should do a thorough external examination, keeping in mind that there are a large number of syndromes with a typical phenotype. The general features, such as cyanosis, pallor, edema,

TABLE 1.1 Organ weights in grams by groups of body weights (mean ±SD)								
Body weight (g)	Brain	Heart	Lungs (combined)	Liver	Spleen	Adrenal glands (combined)	Kidneys (combined)	Thymus
1000	143 ±34	7.7 ±2.0	24 ±8	47 ±12	2.6 ±1.5	3.5 ±1.6	10.4 ±3.4	3.7 ±2.0
1250	174 ±38	9.6 ±3.3	30 ±9	56 ±21	3.4 ±1.8	4.0 ±1.7	12.19 ±3.9	4.9 ±2.1
1500	219 ±52	11.5 ±3.3	34 ±11	65 ±18	4.3 ±2.0	4.5 ±1.8	14.9 ±4.2	6.1 ±2.7
1750	247 ±51	12.8 ±3.2	40 ±13	74 ±20	5.0 ±2.5	5.3 ±2.0	17.4 ±4.7	6.8 ±3.0
2000	281 ±56	14.9 ±4.2	33 ±13	82 ±23	6.0 ±2.7	5.3 ±2.0	18.8 ±5.0	7.9 ±3.4
2250	308 ±49	16.0 ±4.3	48 ±14	88 ±23	7.0 ±3.3	6.0 ±2.3	20.2 ±4.9	8.2 ±3.4
2500	339 ±50	17.7 ±4.2	48 ±15	105 ±21	8.5 ±3.5	7.1 ±2.8	22.6 ±5.5	8.3 ±4.4
2750	362 ±48	19.1 ±3.8	51 ±15	117 ±26	9.1 ±3.6	7.5 ±2.7	24.0 ±5.4	9.6 ±3.8
3000	380 ±55	20.7 ±5.3	53 ±13	127 ±30	10.1 ±3.3	8.3 ±2.9	24.7 ±5.3	10.2 ±4.3
3250	395 ±53	21.5 ±4.3	59 ±18	145 ±33	11.0 ±4.0	9.2 ±2.4	27.3 ±6.6	11.6 ±4.4
3500	411 ±55	22.8 ±5.9	6.3 ±17	153 ±33	11.3 ±3.6	9.8 ±3.5	28.0 ±6.5	12.8 ±5.1
3750	413 ±55	23.8 ±5.1	65 ±15	159 ±40	12.5 ±4.1	10.2 ±3.3	29.5 ±6.8	13.0 ±4.8
4000	420 ±62	25.8 ±5.1	67 ±20	180 ±39	14.1 ±4.0	10.8 ±3.4	30.2 ±6.2	11.4 ±3.2

Adapted from Gruenwald P, Minh HN. *Am J Clin Pathol* 1960, 34:247–253.

TABLE 1.2 Organ weights in grams by groups of gestational age (mean ±SD)								
Gestation (weeks)	Brain	Heart	Lungs (combined)	Liver	Spleen	Adrenal glands (combined)	Kidneys (combined)	Thymus
28	139 ±48	7.6 ±2.3	23 ±7	46 ±16	2.6 ±1.4	3.7 ±1.7	10.4 ±3.6	3.8 ±2.1
30	166 ±55	9.3 ±3.3	28 ±11	53 ±19	3.4 ±2.0	4.2 ±2.2	12.3 ±3.9	4.6 ±2.3
32	209 ±44	11.0 ±3.7	34 ±11	65 ±22	4.1 ±2.1	4.3 ±2.3	14.5 ±4.8	5.5 ±2.3
34	246 ±58	13.4 ±3.9	40 ±13	74 ±27	5.2 ±2.1	5.5 ±2.3	17.7 ±5.3	7.5 ±3.8
36	288 ±62	15.1 ±4.8	46 ±16	87 ±33	6.7 ±3.0	6.4 ±3.0	21.6 ±6.7	8.1 ±4.2
38	349 ±56	18.5 ±5.5	53 ±15	111 ±40	8.8 ±4.2	8.4 ±3.5	23.8 ±7.0	9.7 ±4.8
40	362 ±55	20.4 ±5.3	56 ±15	130 ±45	10.0 ±3.9	8.6 ±3.4	25.6 ±6.5	9.5 ±4.4
42	405 ±54	21.9 ±6.2	56 ±18	139 ±45	10.2 ±4.3	9.1 ±4.0	25.8 ±7.5	10.4 ±4.4

Adapted from Gruenwald P, Minh HN. *Am J Clin Pathol* 1960, 34: 247–253.

Introduction to Care of Newborn Babies

1

jaundice and autolysis, should be looked for. Evidence of trauma in the form of bruises, punctures, forceps marks and incisions should be diligently searched for. All drainage tubes and catheters should be left *in situ* till the exact location of their tips is checked internally.

In a few centers, routine radiographs (whole body) are taken before each neonatal autopsy. They are of great help in the diagnosis of chondrodysplasias, osteogenesis imperfecta, intrauterine infections, meconium ileus, etc. In addition, they provide useful guidelines to assess the gestational age.

Thorax The thorax must be opened under water in a sink or a tub in all cases in order to detect pneumothorax especially in babies dying following resuscitation attempts and artificial ventilation. The presence of air can also be checked by aspirating the serosal cavities through a water-filled syringe before opening the chest and abdomen. It is useful to incise the heart under water, so that presence of air in the cardiac blood is revealed. Intracardiac air may be caused by air embolism following an exchange blood transfusion or by interstitial emphysema rupturing into the pulmonary vessel. Thoracic viscera are removed en bloc along with upper abdominal organs. Delineation of cogenital cardiac defects needs a systematic examination. If lungs appear solid, a piece of lung tissue should be dropped in a jar of water to see whether it floats or sinks. If it sinks, it is atelectatic (possible hyaline membrane disease), but if it floats in water, it is indicative of aerated lungs. Each lung should be weighed separately. If the weight is greater than +1SD, it is suggestive of pneumonia or massive pulmonary hemorrhage.

Umbilical vein, liver, stomach, pancreas and spleen should be removed in one block. The umbilical vein should be opened up to the liver and examined. The stomach and duodenum are dissected, and patency of bile passages confirmed by squeezing the gallbladder and observing for free flow of bile. If there is no flow of bile, biliary tracts should be dissected with precision.

The aorta is opened and umbilical arteries are examined for their number and distribution. If an umbilical artery catheter is *in situ*, position of its tip should be checked and thrombus looked for. Patency of renal arteries is checked. The adrenals are large in the newborn and may weigh up to half of the kidney. They regress in size during the first few days after birth. The congestion of the fetal zone may sometimes be mistaken for hemorrhage.

Head Newborn baby's head is very soft, and it deserves special treatment from the pathologist. Skull is opened by Beneke's technique avoiding damage to meninges and blood vessels. Before opening the vault of the skull, the contents of the posterior fossa should be examined by cutting down between the occipital bone and the atlas. Increased pressure of CSF can be recognized, if there is bulging of the meninges exposed through this gap, and blood or pus can be readily seen when the meninges are incised.

Each cerebral hemisphere may be removed separately cutting through the cerebral peduncles. Alternatively, the whole cerebrum can be removed by cutting through the midbrain, after freeing the anterior attachment of the falx, and then lifting the body till feet are over the head. The pons, medulla, and cerebellum may be removed after cutting through the tentorial leaflets and severing the cranial nerves and spinal cord.

After the brain has been weighed, it should be fixed in formalin for two or three weeks and then sectioned with a large knife. By placing the brain on its vertex, make cuts just in front of the temporal poles, in front of the midbrain, behind the midbrain, and in the occipital region. Hemorrhage should be identified and differentiated from choroid congestion. The pons, medulla and cerebellum are also incised. The definitive diagnosis of periventricular–intraventricular hemorrhage is made by cutting the brain after fixation.

Vertebrae and spinal cord Fracture or evidences of injury should be looked for. The state of vertebral vessels may be ascertained by histological section. In case of hydrocephalus associated with spina bifida, posterior cranial fossa and cervical spine should be examined for Arnold-Chiari malformation.

The Placenta

No fetal necropsy is complete until the placenta has been examined macroscopically and microscopically. Diseases of decidual vessels and extensive infarction may be an important cause of fetal death *in utero*. Inflammation of the placenta is always present in fetal pneumonia following prolonged rupture of membranes. The umbilical cord should be inspected for knots, ruptured vessels, number of umbilical arteries and their insertion. Placenta may be large in syphilis, hemolytic disease of the newborn while it is small in cases of placental insufficiency. Maternal surface of placenta should be looked for blood clots, infarcts, or malformations. Placenta should also be fixed for 2 to 3 weeks before sectioning. Four to five blocks of tissue should be taken from the central slices and membranes for microscopic examination.

Histopathology

Histopathology of lung (one block from each lobe) is important because macroscopic diagnosis of pulmonary lesions is difficult. Hyaline membranes, which are pathognomonic of HMD, have been described as early as 3 hours of age. The diagnosis can be made in the presence of atelectasis with characteristic clinical course even in the absence of hyaline membranes. In the absence of recognizable macroscopic abnormality, sections of other organs seldom yield diagnostic information. Any tissue which appears abnormal should be examined microscopically. It should be remembered that postmortem preservation of fetal and neonatal tissues is far better compared to the adult tissues because of lower enzyme activities, more rapid cooling of body on refrigeration and less chances of bacterial proliferation.

Microbiological Studies

Blood culture should be obtained by collecting a sample from the heart under aseptic precautions. Blood may be obtained from the sagittal sinus through the anterior fontanel. The cultures must be routinely taken from the lungs.

Chromosomal Studies

Chromosomal analysis is indicated in the presence of facial dysmorphism, multiple malformations and dysmaturity. Sterile, anticoagulated blood prior to or at the time of death should be collected. Lymphocytes can be cultured up to 48 hours in such samples kept at room temperature. Tissues (skin, thymus, gonad) can be sent for karyotyping under special circumstances.

Biochemical Studies

Analysis of body fluids or frozen tissue or both for abnormal metabolites or enzymes is diagnostic in certain cases of otherwise unexplained neonatal deaths. Inborn error of metabolism should be suspected whenever unexplained neurologic, electrolyte or acid–base abnormalities are seen in an otherwise normal baby or if an earlier sib had died at an early age. Urine and serum samples should be lyophilized and sent for analysis to a well-equipped advanced biochemistry laboratory.

Final Diagnosis

The postmortem examination itself may not always give the information regarding the immediate cause of death. It is essential to correlate the gross autopsy, histological and microbiological findings with the clinical details of the mother and her infant to arrive at the primary cause and terminal event leading to death. Free and frank scientific interaction and discussion among pathologist, obstetrician and pediatrician in the form of a clinicopathological conference is an exceedingly useful exercise. The parents should be informed about the findings of autopsy by the consultant pediatrician and given an appropriate advise and guidance for future pregnancies.

For the purposes of classification of perinatal deaths, perinatal period is defined to include newborn babies dying within 7 days after birth and stillborn infants weighing 500 g or more, regardless of their gestational period. The following clinicopathological classification of perinatal deaths appears to be most comprehensive and should be followed. The cause of all perinatal deaths can be classified into the following four subgroups.

Primary Causes of Neonatal Deaths

They include major conditions which have directly or indirectly lead to the neonatal death. If there is more than one primary cause of death, they should be identified and the one which appeared to be the most significant in terms of lethality should be given priority. At times it may indeed be difficult to choose the cause of death among several primary causes of deaths in a given case. For example, if an infant with perinatal hypoxia develops aspiration syndrome at birth and subsequently dies from pneumonia, it may be difficult to identify the incriminating event which was actually responsible for death.

Extrinsic perinatal hypoxia It refers to perinatal hypoxia as evidenced by presence of features of fetal hypoxia and birth asphyxia (5-minute apgar score of ≤3) and occurs mostly due to complications of pregnancy or delivery. It excludes those conditions which cause intrinsic anoxia due to disorders in the infant, such as hyaline membrane disease, pneumonia PPHN, and cyanotic congenital heart disease. Pathologically, it is characterized by anoxic encephalopathy, congestion with or without focal petechial hemorrhages in the medulla of kidneys, adrenals, liver, and mucosa of gut. There may be evidences of massive amniotic fluid or meconium aspiration in the lungs.

Infections Sepsis is diagnosed on the basis of clinical, laboratory and pathological findings. Appropriate culture studies from blood and infected organs must be obtained at the time of autopsy to identify causative microorganisms. Infected infants should be further subclassified into transplacental, intrapartum and postnatal depending upon timing of infection. Postnatal or nosocomial infection is diagnosed when infant is asymptomatic for at least 48 hours after birth and there is no evidence of intrapartum infection in the form of prolonged rupture of membranes, foul smelling liquor amnii, and polymorphs in the gastric aspirate of the neonate.

Hyaline membrane disease The diagnosis is based on characteristic predisposing factors, typical clinical and radiological picture and atelectasis with presence of diffuse hyaline membranes in the lungs. When it is associated with patent ductus arteriosus, intraventricular hemorrhage, subarachnoid hemorrhage, pneumonia or pneumothorax, bronchopulmonary dysplasia, the death is attributed to HMD.

Congenital malformations Those malformations which are severe enough and directly responsible for neonatal death are considered in this category.

Immaturity Immaturity as a cause of death is assigned to infants having birth weight of less than 750 g where no other primary cause of death is found on autopsy. These infants are grossly immature and are unable to maintain ventilation due to hyaline membrane disease, and die because of recurrent apneic attacks, intraventricular hemorrhage, and histologically their lungs are immature.

Miscellaneous causes Numerically less significant primary causes of neonatal deaths include erythroblastosis fetalis, necrotizing enterocolitis, massive primary pulmonary hemorrhage (in a relatively healthy infant), birth trauma (birth injury with fracture, massive subdural hematoma, visceral rupture), primary hemorrhagic disease of the newborn, and non-immunologic hydrops fetalis.

Cause unidentified Depending upon the experience of the neonatologist and pediatric pathologist and availability of investigative facilities, it may be difficult to assign a primary cause of death in about 10 to 20% of perinatal deaths. At times, stillborn baby may be so macerated that no meaningful information is obtained on autopsy.

Secondary Complications of Primary Disease

After identifying the primary cause of death, efforts should be made to identify the complications or terminal events which actually proved lethal. This is based on information regarding the mode of death and supportive pathological findings. The common complications during neonatal period which must be screened and specially looked for, both clinically and pathologically, include disseminated intravascular coagulation (secondary hemorrhagic disease of the newborn), intraventricular hemorrhage, patent ductus arteriosus, kernicterus, intestinal perforation, shock, sclerema, anemia, and metabolic complications.

Associated Fetal and Neonatal Conditions

The underlying fetal or neonatal conditions which may have accounted for development of primary disease and death should be identified. A large number of serious neonatal disorders are limited to immature infants, such as hyaline membrane disease, intraventricular–periventricular hemorrhage, nosocomial infections, and necrotizing enterocolitis. Infants with severe intrauterine growth retardation are predisposed to suffer from perinatal hypoxia, meconium aspiration syndrome, hypoglycemia, and pulmonary hemorrhage. Some non-lethal congenital malformations may be associated with life-threatening infections.

Associated Maternal Conditions or Complications of Pregnancy

They may account for primary cause of stillbirths in several cases. Infants of high-risk mothers are predisposed to develop several complications leading to increased morbidity and mortality. Those maternal conditions which are indirectly or directly responsible for unfavorable neonatal outcome must be identified so that strategies for reduction of perinatal mortality can be formulated in a proper perspective. The important maternal conditions or complications of pregnancy which must be specifically looked for in the antenatal case records including pregnancy-induced hypertension, essential hypertension, antepartum hemorrhage (placenta previa or abruptio placentae), chronic systemic disease, endocrinal disorders especially diabetes mellitus, nutritional status, drugs and infections during pregnancy, polyhdramnios or oligohydramnios.

BIBLIOGRAPHY

Editorial. Every newborn, every mother, every adolescent girl. *Lancet* 2014, 383:755.

International classification of the diseases. 11th revision, WHO, *Geneva* 2018.

Lawn JE, Cousens S, Zupan J. Four million neonatal deaths. When? Where? Why? *Lancet* 2005, 365: 891–901.

Lawn JE, Blencowe H, Pattinson R, *et al.* Stillbirths. Where? When? Why? How to make data count? *Lancet* 2011, 37:1448–1463.

Lawn JE, Kerber K, Enweronu-Laryea C, Cousens S. 3.6 million neonatal deaths: what is progressing and what is not? *Semin Perinatol 2010, 34, 371–386.*

Manchester DK, Shikes RH. The perinatal autopsy: special considerations. *Clin Obstet Gynecol 1980, 23: 1125.*

National Family Health Survey 2015-16 (NFHS-4), Ministry of Health and Family Welfare, Government of India.

Philip AGS. The evolution of neonatology. *Pediatr Res 2005,* 58: 799–815.

Robertson AF. Reflections on errors in neonatology:1. The "Hands-off" years 1920 to 1950. *J Perinatol 2003, 23: 48–55.*

Robertson AF. Reflections on errors in neonatology II. The "Heroic" years, 1950 to 1970. *J Perinatol 2003, 23:154–56.*

Robertson AF. Reflections on errors in neonatology III. The "experienced" years 1970–2000. *J Perinatol 2003, 23: 240–9.*

Singh M, Paul VK, Bhakoo ON. Neonatal nomenclature and data collection. National Neonatology Forum, Delhi 1989.

Singh M. Perinatal services in India: current status and future perspectives. *Natl Med J India 2003, 16 (Suppl 2): S1–S4.*

Singh M. The art, science and philosophy of newborn care. *Indian J Pediatr 2014, 81(6):552–559.*

Singh M. Health and welfare of women and child survival: a key to nation building. *Indian J Pediatr 2018,85(7):523–527.*

Spong CY, Mercer BM, D'Alton M, Kilpatrick S, Blackwell S, Saade G. Timing of indicated late preterm and early-preterm birth. *Obstet Gynecol 2011, 118:323–333.*

State of India's Newborns. Public Health Foundation of India, All India Institute of Medical Sciences and Save the Children, New Delhi, India 2014.

United National Children's Fund. The State of the World's Children 2018, *UNICEF, New York.*

Organization of a Neonatal Intensive Care Unit

The organization of a good quality special care neonatal unit (SCNU) is essential for reducing the neonatal mortality and improving the quality of life among the survivors. During the past four decades, improvements in the diagnostic and therapeutic approaches in the care of high-risk infants have influenced their prognosis favorably. Unfortunately, many neonatal centers in the developing countries are unplanned and merely improvised. The pediatrician and nurse incharge of neonatal services should be taken into confidence during the planning stage so that the neonatal intensive care unit (NICU) is based on their opinions for meeting the special needs of critically sick infants. It is a welcome move that government of India has launched an initiative to establish special care newborn units (SCNUs) at district hospitals. The SCNU at the district hospital is envisaged to provide; (i) care at birth including resuscitation of asphyxiated newborns, (ii) identification of a sick neonate, (iii) management of sick newborns, (iv) referral and transport services for babies needing mechanical ventilation and major surgical intervention, (v) postnatal care and immunization services and (vi) follow-up of high-risk newborns.

Adequate space, availability of running water round-the-clock, centralized oxygen and suction facilities, maintenance of thermoneutral environment and ready availability of plenty of linen and disposables are mandatory requirements to provide optimal level II newborn care. Facilities for prevention and management of common neonatal problems, viz. perinatal hypoxia, hypothermia, LBW babies, respiratory distress syndrome, septicemia, hyperbilirubinemia and life-threatening congenital malformations, should be established. The emphasis should be laid on developing a sound infrastructure to ensure safe delivery, promote asepsis, provide warmth and adequate

nutrition with human milk. The lop-sided enthusiasm to acquire sophisticated electronic gadgets including ventilators, in the absence of basic infrastructural facilities, must be discouraged. At the present state of our development, level III or neonatal intensive care unit (NICU) should be established in a phased manner in regional centers selected on the basis of available infrastructure and professional expertise. Effective and optimal management of newborn babies at birth, prevention of hypothermia and bacterial infections and feeding of all babies with human milk should be ensured before establishing neonatal intensive care facilities. Intensive care of the newborn is highly cost-intensive and demands considerable inputs of staff, equipment and time. The philosophy of specialized conservative management of high-risk newborn babies should be fully exploited to bring down the neonatal mortality rate to less than 20 per 1000 live births before intensive care facilities are launched (Figure 2.1).

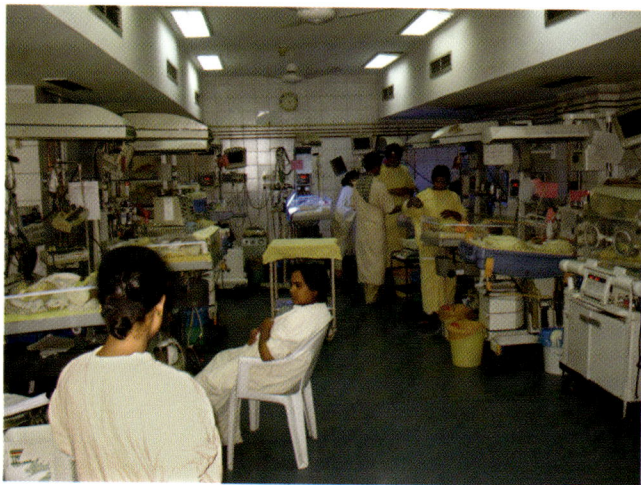

Figure 2.1 NICU of All India Institute of Medical Sciences, New Delhi.

PHYSICAL FACILITIES

Space

The size of the unit is related to the expected population intended to be served. In India, about 15 to 20% of newborn babies need special care, depending upon the criteria for antenatal booking for confinement. In addition, if the center is to serve as a referral unit for the infants born outside the hospital (extramural babies), allowance should be made for additional physical facilities and space. In a maternity unit having 2,000 deliveries per year, facilities for special care of 6–8 high-risk infants should be available. Each infant should be provided with a minimum area of 100 sq. ft. or 10 m². However, additional space would be needed to provide for special facilities as outlined below in the floor plan. There should be no compromise on space and its adequacy is crucial for reduction of nosocomial infections. Space should be allocated within the nursery complex for promotion of breastfeeding, expression of breast milk and its storage.

Location

The neonatal unit should be located as close as possible to the labor rooms and obstetric operation theater, to facilitate prompt transfer of sick and high-risk infants. The presence of an elevator in close proximity is desirable for transport of outborn infants. In tropical countries, the nursery should not be located on the top floor of the hospital but there should be feasibility for the sunlight to peep into the nursery to enhance brightness and provide ultraviolet rays to augment asepsis.

Nursery Design

The unit design may be in a square space or a single corridor-based rectangular unit. A split unit, i.e. on either side of the hospital corridor, should be avoided for ease of mobility and for prevention of infections. A unit design occupying one side of the corridor with a nurses control room in the center, from where all the babies can be viewed, is preferred (Figure 2.2). Apart from constant surveillance of all babies, the design should ensure minimal walking distance for the staff.

Baby Care Area

The unit should be provided with areas and rooms for inborn or intramural babies, stepdown nursery, outborn or extramural babies, examination area, mother's area for breastfeeding and expression of breast milk, nurses station and charting area. The floor and walls should be made of washable glazed or vitrified tiles and windows should have two layers of glass panes to ensure some measure of heat and sound insulation. The obviously infected infants with open sepsis (especially those with diarrhea and abscesses) should be isolated in a septic nursery, which should be located away from the NICU and manned by different nursing and resident staff. A large number of ancillary services are needed and should be identified and designed during the planning stage.

Handwashing and gowning room Handwashing and gowning facility should be located at the enterance. It should be provided with abundant space with self-closing doors. A positive air pressure should be maintained in the NICU so that corridor air does not enter the NICU. Street shoes are changed with nursery slippers, followed by handwashing and gowning. The use of mask is controversial and is best avoided. Hand-free elbow-operated handwashing sink with liquid soap dispenser is recommended. Sink should be made of porcelain or stainless steel. Pictorial handwashing instructions should be provided on the wall next to the sink. WHO recommend 2-minute thorough hand washing before entry to the NICU. The recommended steps include (i) remove wrist watch, rings and bracelets, (ii) wet the hands with water and apply enough liquid soap to produce a good lather, (iii) rub hands palms to palms and then palms to dorsums, (iv) rub with fingers interlocked, (v) rub finger tips to opposing palms, (vi) do rotational rubbing of thumbs of both hands and (vii) rinse the hand and forearm thoroughly with water (Figure 2.3). Hands should be dried with single use or disposable napkins. Walls adjacent to the sink should be made of non-porous or non-absorbent material to prevent growth of molds. Sinks should not be provided with slabs or countertops which are a potent source of infection. The unit should be provided with 24-hour uninterrupted water supply by having dedicated over head tank with a capacity of 1000–2000 liters.

Examination area A small comfortable room with examination table, comfortable seating, sufficient light, and warmth is needed for assessment of baby before admission to the nursery. The baby is cleaned and provided with nursery garments in this room.

Mother area The room should be provided with comfortable seating and privacy to the mother to breastfeed and express the breast milk with the help of a lactation nurse.

Care of the Newborn

2

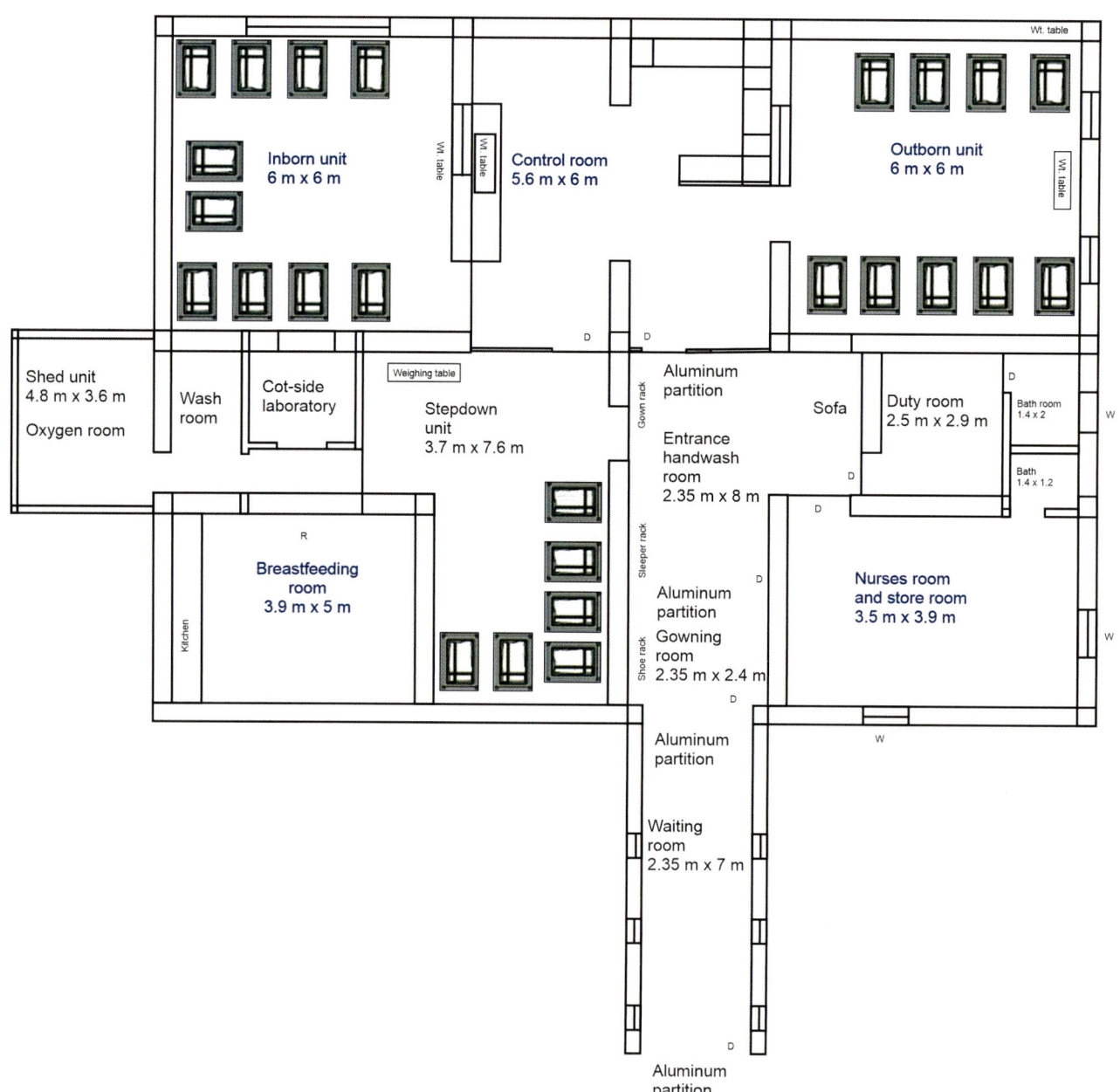

Figure 2.2 The conceptual layout for a neonatal intensive care unit for 25 babies. Adapted from tool kit for setting up special care neonatal unit, UNICEF.

Handwashing stations Handwashing sinks should be provided within 20 feet (6 meters) of every newborn bed. The sink should be large and deep (24″ wide × 16″ front-back and 10″ deep) and made of porcelain or stainless steel and without any counter or shelf. Single use cotton or disposable paper napkins should be available for drying the hands. Alternatively, antiseptic sanitizing solution (sterillium) can be used for disinfection of hands in-between the babies.

Preparation of intravenous fluids A separate area should be earmarked and provided with a laminar flow system for preparation of intravenous fluids, parenteral nutritional formulations, enteral feeds and medications. Boiling and autoclaving facilities should be available next to this area.

Nurses station Nursing station and charting area for nurses and residents should be located in a central area from where all the babies can be observed. Newborn charts, hospital forms, computer terminals, telephone lines should be located in this area. It is preferable to use electronic or digital medical recording of clinical notes and retrieval of laboratory reports.

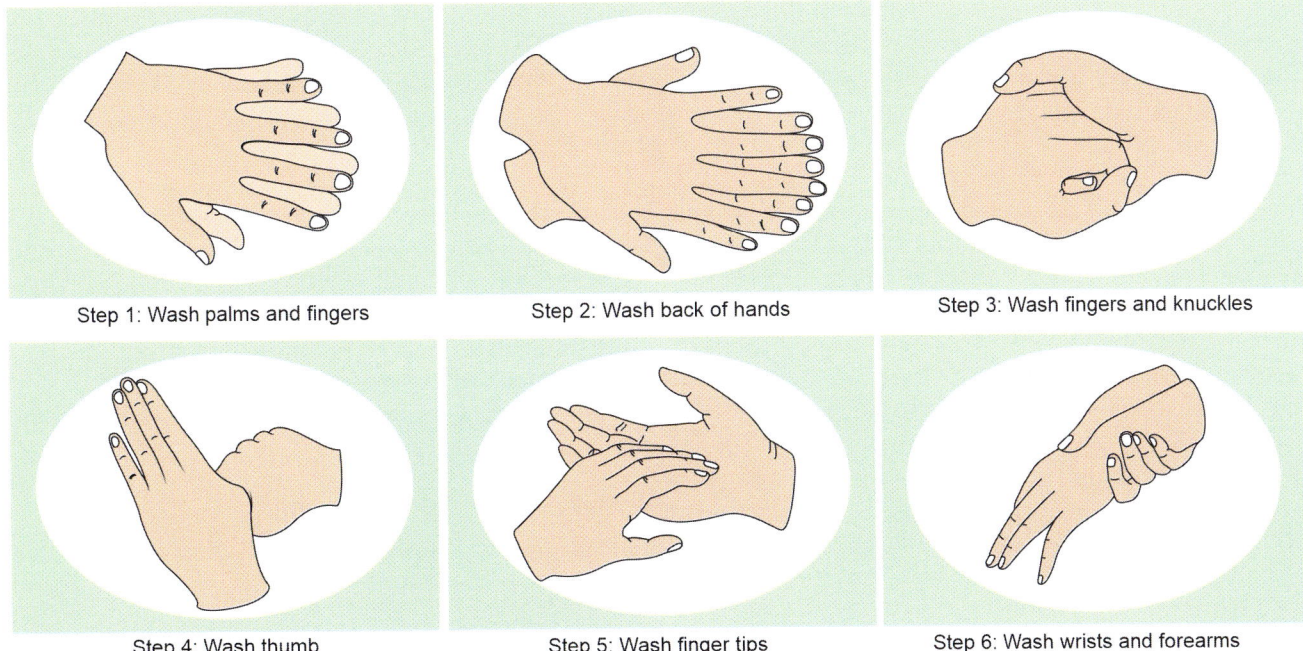

Step 1: Wash palms and fingers Step 2: Wash back of hands Step 3: Wash fingers and knuckles

Step 4: Wash thumb Step 5: Wash finger tips Step 6: Wash wrists and forearms

Figure 2.3 WHO protocol for handwashing

Clean utility and soiled utility holding rooms There should be enough space for stocking clean utility items and sterile disposables, and for disposal of dirty linen and contaminated disposables. Built-in wall wooden cabinets with foldable covers are useful for stacking purposes. The ventilation system in the soiled utility or holding room should be engineered to have negative air pressure with all air being exhausted to the outside. The soiled utility room should be so located that it enables removal of soiled material without passing through the baby care area.

Staff rooms Space should be provided within the unit to meet the professional, personal and administrative needs of resident staff on duty. A comfortable room with intercom, telephone and computer terminal and WC facilities is mandatory. Nurse's change room is required for changing from formal street clothes to a smart shirt and trouser dress stipulated by the NICU.

Growing nursery A separate bay in the lying-in ward should be earmarked for transitional care of high-risk babies by their mothers before they are discharged from the hospital. The entry of visitors to this area should be restricted and it should be kept adequately warm. Facilities for monitoring asepsis and weighing the babies should be available in the transitional care room (TCR) or growing nursery (GN). The growing nursery is used with advantage for educating the mothers in child craft activities and promoting the practice of exclusive breastfeeding.

Ventilation

Effective air ventilation of nursery is essential to reduce nosocomial infections. The most satisfactory ventilation is achieved with laminar air flow system which is rather expensive. When centralized air-conditioning is used, minimum of 12 changes of room air per hour are recommended. There should be no draughts of air on and near the newborn beds. The air-conditioning ducts must be provided with millipore filters (0.5 μ) to restrict the passage of microbes. A simple method to achieve satisfactory ventilation consists of provision of exhaust fan in a reverse direction near the ceiling for input of fresh uncontaminated air and fixation of another exhaust fan in the conventional manner near the floor for air exit. A constant positive air pressure should be maintained in the nursery so that contaminated air from the corridors does not gain access into the nursery. The use of chemical air disinfection and ultraviolet lamps are no more recommended.

Lighting

The nursery must be well illuminated and painted white or slightly off white to permit prompt and early detection of jaundice and cyanosis. It is best achieved by cool white fluorescent tubes or LED (light-emitting diodes) to provide at least 100 foot-candle, shadow-free illumination at the infant's level. The number and exact location of fixtures can be worked out taking into account size of the nursery, height of the ceiling, and availability or otherwise of sunlight. Spot illumination for various procedures can be provided by a portable angle-poise lamp having two 15 watt fluorescent bulbs which when held at a distance of about one foot from the infant, produce about 100 foot-candle intensity of light. Most open care systems are equipped with in-built source of overhead spot lights. In places where electrical failure is frequent and prolonged, the electrical system of the nursery complex must be attached to a generator. Exposure of preterm babies to strong light has been incriminated as a risk factor for the development of retinopathy of prematurity. The nursery light should be dimmed at night to simulate day-night pattern to promote hormonal surge and growth of babies. Bedside lights with dimmer switches should be provided to create specialized microenvironment for each baby.

Environmental Temperature and Humidity

The temperature of the nursery complex must be maintained between 26 and 28°C (78.8–82.4°F) in order to minimize effects of thermal stress on the babies (see Chapter 15). This is best achieved by centralized air-conditioning having temperature control knobs in the nursery. The air movement should be so designed that draught is minimized. In places where air-conditioning is not feasible, room temperature can be reasonably well maintained in winter by use of radiant heaters and hot air blowers. The external windows of nursery should be glazed to minimize heat gain and heat loss and baby beds should be located at least 2 feet (0.6 meter) away from the wall or window. In most parts of India, relative humidity averages above 50%, which is quite satisfactory for routine needs of newborn babies. Humidity level can be raised for preterm babies nursed in an incubator. High and effective humidity level is useful to reduce insensible water loss but is associated with increased risk of nosocomial infection.

Acoustic Characteristics

The ventilation system, incubators, air compressors, suction pumps and many other devices used in the nursery produce noise. Sound intensity in the nursery should not exceed 75 dB to protect hearing of nursery personnel and infants. Excessive noise may lead to hearing loss, physiological and behavioral disturbances, such as sleep disturbances, startles and crying episodes, hypoxia, tachycardia and increased intracranial pressure. The fabrication and redesigning of

nursery equipment should take into account the desirability of minimizing noise by dampening the sounds by acoustic or other means. It is desirable to have effective soundproofing of ceilings, walls, doors and floor when a new nursery is designed. Telephone rings and equipment alarms should be replaced by blinking lights. Instead of air compressors, centralized sources of compressed air, oxygen and suction should be provided. Decibel meters should be installed to monitor sound levels in the nursery. The beneficial and soothing effects of meaningful sounds, such as gentle music or recordings of parent voice, should be harnessed to provide physiologic stability to the babies.

Handling and Social Contacts

Excessive and rough handling of delicate newborn babies is associated with several adverse physiological consequences, such as excessive crying, sleep disturbances, tachycardia or bradycardia, hypoxia and rise in blood pressure and intracranial pressure. Handling should be gentle and kept to the barest minimum without compromising care. Soothing words, gentle stroking and rocking should be practised after a painful procedure. Gentle caressing, cuddling and touching by the mother are desirable to provide comfort and confidence to the baby and aid the process of healing. Infants should be exposed to gentle and soothing tactile, kinesthetic, vestibular, motor, auditory and visual experiences to provide opportunities for early learning and improvement in behavior. Parents should be allowed unrestricted entry to the nursery to provide these useful sensorimotor stimuli. It enhances the process of bonding between the baby and the family.

Communication System

The nursery complex should be provided with an intercom system so that additional person can be called for help in case of an emergency without leaving the sick infant. A direct line external telephone is mandatory so that parents have an easy access to inquire about welfare of their infants and in turn they can be readily contacted whenever needed. Mobile phones should not be used near the vicinity of the nursery because the electromagnetic waves are likely to interfere with the functioning of the electronic equipment. The family should be kept constantly informed about the condition of their baby including therapeutic interventions being given. They should be given emotional support and pragmatic view of the likely outcome.

Electrical Outlets

There should be adequate number (8–12 electrical points at the height of 4–5 feet) of 5 amperes and 15 amperes electrical points attached to a common ground. Each infant must be provided with at least eight electrical outlets, 4 should be 5 amperes and another 4 of 15 amperes. The use of adapters and extension boards should be discouraged. The electrical equipment used in the nursery must be checked at least once a month for leakage of current and adequacy of grounding. If possible, special fittings with safety devices should be installed. The unit should have round-the-clock uninterrupted servo-stabilized power supply. There should be round-the-clock power back-up including provision of UPS system for the sensitive equipment.

PERSONNEL

It is important, that while allocating nursing, medical and paramedical staff to the hospital, the needs of the neonatal unit are not ignored. It is unfortunate that newborn babies are not counted as patients requiring nursing and medical care while expressing the bed strength of a hospital. The census of the hospital bed is administratively based on dieted beds. In fact, the situation is paradoxical because the neonates need rather specialized and sophisticated nursing and medical care. Therefore, the highest priority in the organization of the NICU is the availability of sufficient number of adequately trained personnel especially the nurses. The survival of newborn babies depends upon the availability of specially trained nurses. The Nursing Council of India has not outlined any special guidelines for this purpose. It has been recommended by the American Academy of Pediatrics that one nurse is needed to offer special or intermediate nursing care to 3 babies or intensive care to one infant. In countries where monitoring devices are not routinely available, relatively larger number of nurses are necessary for undertaking manual monitoring. It is generally not appreciated by the hospital administrators that a considerable time of the nurse is spent in rigorous housekeeping rituals to maintain asepsis in the nursery. The frequent toilet care, expression of breast milk, formula preparation and feeding are time consuming and unassisted by any attendant. Whenever adequate number of nurses are not available, these rituals are compromised resulting in outbreak of epidemic of infection in the nursery. The nursery complex must, therefore, be considered as an independent nursing unit under the charge of a fully qualified nursing superintendent. The 6Cs qualities of neonatal nurses viz. Care, Compassion, Competence, Communication, Confidence and Commitment must be harnessed to provide the state-of-the art nursing care.

The National Neonatology Forum of India has recommended that at least one trained nurse should be allocated to provide coverage to four babies in the special care neonatal unit. The allowance should be kept for additional 25% staff to provide for the exigencies of day off and leave. Therefore, for a 8-bedded SCNU, eight nurses should be sanctioned to ensure availability of two nurses in each shift along with one additional sister incharge in the morning shift. In NICUs providing tertiary care, one nurse should be allocated for a baby on assisted ventilation. The continuity of service can be maintained, if at least 50% of the nurses are rather permanent and not transferred frequently as is the usual practice in general hospitals. There must be equal distribution of nurses in the three duty shifts during 24 hours. The nurses must be imparted continuing in-service training in the art of neonatal nursing and preventive maintenance of a variety of electronic equipment used in the NICU. They should not be rotated to other area of the hospital. Each nurse should be allocated "specific babies" to provide developmentally supportive care. The NICU should be managed by an independent nursing unit under the supervision of a "tough" nursing superintendent. They should participate in the monthly perinatal morbidity and mortality meetings. It is desirable to have services of public health nurses and social workers for follow-up and home care of low birth weight babies after their discharge from the hospital.

A pediatrician specially interested in the care of newborn babies should devote his full time to improve the existing standards of neonatal special care services in the country. The unit must also have an independent senior resident and one junior resident round-the-clock for every 8 babies requiring special care. The resident doctors must work in these units for at least 3 months to maintain continuity of medical care. All deliveries in the hospital should preferably be attended by a pediatrician trained in the care of newborn. A laboratory technician should be available to operate bilirubinometer, glucometer, microcentrifuge, CRP kits and blood gas analyzer. A biomedical technician or a link person is essential to maintain a liaison with suppliers of equipment to ensure their smooth functioning, prevent breakdowns and reduce the downtime. The resident staff and nurses working in the NICU must be trained to properly handle and use the equipment. When ventilatory facilities are established, respiratory therapist is a useful member of the neonatal team to monitor ventilatory settings, provide tracheal suctioning and chest physiotherapy. A pediatric pathologist, who is specially trained for conducting and interpreting neonatal autopsies, is desirable to complement the functioning of the neonatal team.

EQUIPMENT

During the last 3–4 decades, a large number of monitoring devices for diagnostic and therapeutic use for the high-risk newborn infants have been developed. These have considerably improved their intact survival. Several basic prerequisites must be fulfilled before any center invests in purchase of expensive equipment involving foreign exchange. The fundamental needs of the unit are availability of adequate space, freedom from congestion and presence of a sufficient number of adequately trained nurses. A reasonable level of asepsis must be achieved and facilities for maintaining thermoneutral environment should be established. The feeding of babies should be associated with minimal risk of aspiration.

Acquisition of new equipment does not necessarily ensure better services and outcome. *Machines cannot replace men. The best monitors with us are dedicated nurses and resident doctors involved in the care of newborn babies with their observational skills sharpened by experience.* Therefore, they need continued in-service training, teaching and encouragement for achieving the best results. In view of the exorbitant cost of imported equipment and problems faced in their maintenance, there is a constant need to promote indigenous fabrication of equipment required for neonatal care.

The maintenance of the existing equipment in proper working condition is more important than acquiring newer and sophisticated gadgets. Before placing an order, check with existent consumer/s regarding reliability of the equipment and quality of after sales service provided by the local dealer. The supplier must install the equipment and provide training to the staff for proper use and maintenance of the equipment. Date of installation and expiry of warranty period should be recorded. After expiry of mandatory warranty period, you should enter into a yearly maintenance contract with the local dealer for preventive maintenance and emergency repairs in the event of breakdowns. In case of sophisticated and expensive equipment, a counter-guarantee of service should also be taken from the foreign principals. Inventory of spares should be maintained and essential spares should be purchased and kept in stock while ordering new equipment. Photocopies of working and service manuals should be available in the NICU while original documents should be kept in a safe custody. Maintain a log book containing postal and e-mail addresses, telephone and fax numbers of local dealers and suppliers of equipment. When telephonic complaints are not heeded by the local supplier, you should send a written complaint and endorse a copy to the foreign principals. The use of cell phones should not be permitted near the vicinity of NICU because electromagnetic waves can lead to malfunctioning of various electronic gadgets.

Preventive Maintenance and Emergency Repairs

After-sales technical services including annual maintenance contract (AMC) should be a mandatory requirement at the time of purchase of the equipment. At the time of installation, the supplier should provide technical training, hands-on training for clinical use of the equipment and its proper maintenance to the nurses and resident doctors. A qualified in-house biomedical technician should be available to maintain an inventory of equipment and spares, ensure optimal preventive maintenance and take prompt action to call the service engineer to ensure maximum uptime of the life saving medical equipment. The in-house technician should have up-to-date information regarding the proper use of the equipment, should be able to undertake first-line corrective intervention that does not require any spare parts and when required he should be able to report correctly the nature of technical malfunctioning of the equipment to the on-call service engineer of the company.

The objectives of preventive maintenance include that the equipment should be functional most of the time and should operate with accuracy, efficiency and safety. The maintenance engineer should undertake at least two technical visits per year to check the wear and tear, and performance of the device as per manufacturer's technical check list. The equipment should be cleaned and defective components replaced by spare parts. He should interact with in-house technician and end-users to provide necessary guidance for correct use of the equipment to ensure effective preventive maintenance and upkeep.

Despite careful use of the equipment, the average lifetime of most electronic equipment is about 5–7 years. In the event of breakdown, when contacted the service engineer should report to the NICU without delay to ensure that the downtime of the equipment is minimum. In case the device cannot be repaired on-site and the machine is taken to the workshop, a replacement model should be provided by the company for the period of the repair.

The equipment listed below are by and large arranged in the order of their usefulness and priority. *The maintenance of existing equipment in proper working condition is more important than acquiring additional gadgets.*

Resuscitation Equipment

The equipment needed for resuscitation of asphyxiated baby at birth are discussed in detail in Chapter 6. Emergency tray should be available in each infant care room of NICU containing Ambu bag and mask, infant laryngoscope, tracheal tubes of different sizes, sterile suction catheters, oral mucus suction traps, and emergency drugs.

Bag and Mask Resuscitator

Self-inflating bag of 250–500 mL capacity is ideal for resuscitation of a newborn baby. There are four components of self-inflating bag, i.e. air inlet, oxygen inlet, patient outlet and valve assembly (Figure 2.4). It should be provided with a pop-off valve or with a facility to attach a pressure gauge. An oxygen reservoir in the form of a corrugated tube or rubber bladder, helps to increase the oxygen concentration to 90 to 100%. When self-inflating bag is used without an oxygen reservoir, it delivers 40–60% oxygen because room air enters the bag with each inflation. A one-way valve allows delivery of oxygen at the outlet when bag is squeezed but closes as soon as the bag is released so that the exaled air cannot re-enter the bag. A peep valve can be attached to the valve assembly to deliver required PEEP. The self-inflating bag cannot be used for providing free-flow oxygen to the baby unless it is equipped with closed bladder reservoir. The silicone rubber bags of Laerdal make are more sturdy and can withstand autoclaving and cleaning with antiseptic solutions. Indigenously manufactured bags and masks are highly unsatisfactory due to poor quality of rubber, lack of oxygen inlet, absence of any safety features and loss of re-expansion capabilities of the bag.

A resuscitation trolley equipped with radiant warmer, timer, electrical suction, observation light and manual facilities is an essential equipment for the labor

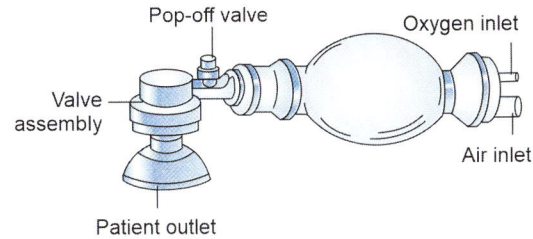

Figure 2.4 The components of a self-inflating bag.

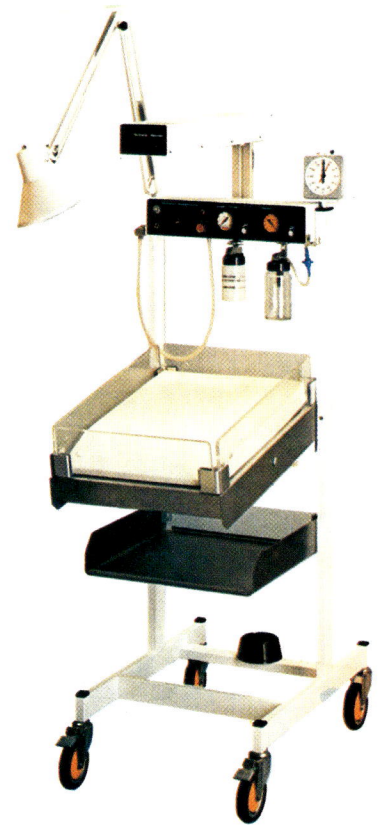

Figure 2.5 Resuscitator for receiving babies at birth. Note the stop clock which is useful to time the events during resuscitation.

room (Figure 2.5). In-built pulse oximeter is extremely useful to monitor heart rate and oxygen saturation. Face masks (size 0, 1 and 2) should be rigid with a cushioned rim to form a tight air-seal fit on the face enclosing the mouth and nostrils. Anatomical shaped masks are avoided due to the potential risk of causing local trauma due to pressure.

Oxygen and Suction Facilities

A centralized source of oxygen, compressed air and suction outlet consoles (50 psi) affixed on the walls is ideal. By mixing variable quantities of compressed air and oxygen, one can obtain oxygen concentrations ranging between 25 and 100%.

DeLee trap for a single use oral suction with 12 Fr catheter should be avoided because of potential risk of transmission of HIV infection. A soft plastic catheter or nozzle with a suction bulb is a good alternative but difficult to clean. Suction machines using recoil springs are bulky and complex to operate and difficult to clean. A foot-operated suction machine is useful in rural health care facilities because of non-availability or erratic power supply (Figure 2.6). In hospitals, centralized suction, venturi suction and electrical suction

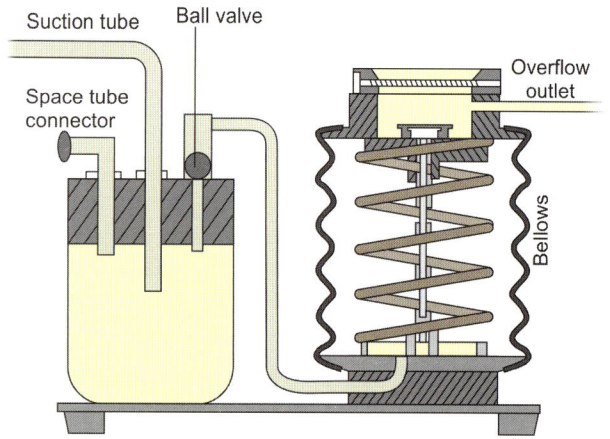

Figure 2.6 Diagrammatic view of a foot-operated suction machine.

machines are used. The suction pressure is regulated with a pressure dial. Facility should be available for intermittent suction because continuous suction may cause bradycardia and mucosal damage. The suction pressure should be limited to 60–80 cm H_2O (1.0 mm Hg = 1.3 cm H_2O). Slow suction devices are used for continuous suction of chest cavity and upper pouch of infants with esophageal atresia.

Catheters, Syringes and Needles

Nasogastric polyethylene feeding tubes (Fr 5, 6 and 8), suction catheters (Fr 10 and 12), umbilical vein catheters, small-vein infusion sets (G 23), medicaths (neoflon), and exchange transfusion sets are now freely available in India at a reasonable cost. They are prepacked sterile by a process of gamma-irradiation. These should not be reused after boiling. As relatively small volume of parenteral medications are needed for low birth weight babies, it is desirable to use tuberculin or insulin syringes for injections to ensure ease and accuracy of administration. Only single-use syringes and needles should be used. *The availability of liberal supplies of disposables is crucial for reduction of nosocomial infections.*

Feeding Equipment

Glass or stainless steel bowls of adequate size (120 mL capacity) should be available in the nursery for collection of expressed breast milk, mixing and preparing the formula. A hot air autoclaving oven or a pressure sterilizer should be provided for auto-claving feeding equipment. Storage facility, like a refrigerator, should be available in the nursery. The formula room should be equipped with working shelves having laminated plastic surfaces or preferably these should be made of stainless steel so that they can be easily washed and cleaned.

Laminar Flow System

The laminar flow system is useful for safe and aseptic formulation and mixing of drugs, parenteral fluids and nutrients. It is equipped with high efficiency particulate aggregate (HEPA) filter to filter out bacteria, a blower and plenum. HEPA filters are effective in trapping 99.97% of all the particles of >0.3 μ size including dust and bacterial pathogens. Two types of systems are available. In a vertical type system, the air flows from above downwards and it is recommended for use in the NICU. The horizontal flow type system is used for tissue culture and microbiologic techniques. Ultraviolet light source in the chamber is kept on for 30 minutes before use to make the area of operation free of bacteria. The vertical flow of bacteria-free filtered air maintains a positive pressure of 15 mm Hg to prevent entry of contaminated air into the chamber. Strict asepsis should be ensured by wearing a mask, sterile gown and disposable gloves while operating the laminar flow system. The critical work area and accessible surfaces should be disinfected with bacillocid or 70% isopropyle alcohol.

Weighing Machine

Accurate weight record of babies is a sensitive index of their wellbeing and availability of a sturdy and reliable weighing machine fulfills a fundamental need. A sensitive beam-type weighing scale with a precision of ±10 g is a useful equipment in the SCNU. It must be calibrated frequently against standard one kilogram weight. The chances of cross-infection should be minimized by using a sterile paper or a towel over the pan before weighing each infant. Electronic weighing machine (resolution either ±5 g or ±1 g) with a digital read-out though expensive is desirable for use in the NICU (Figure 2.7). Availability of a reliable

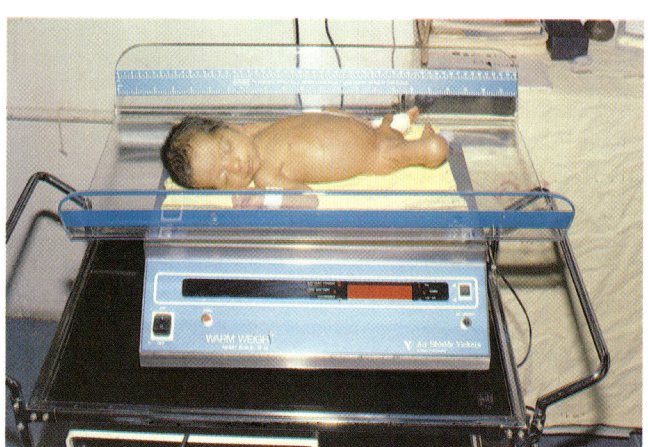

Figure 2.7 Electronic weighing scale with an accuracy of ±1.0 g.

and sensitive electronic weighing scale is more useful and desirable than acquiring a ventilator which is kept as a showpiece in the nursery because of lack of experienced medical and nursing staff to operate it.

Bassinets

A variety of bassinets are available for routine use in the nursery. It is desirable to use bassinets, which can be easily cleaned and are equipped with a locker and head tilting mechanism (Figure 2.8). The locker can be used to hold the supplies of an individual baby, such as diapers, frocks, sterile gauze, cotton, thermometer, feeding equipment, drugs, etc. Plastic plexiglass or fiberglass bassinets with relatively low walls and placed at a convenient height are desirable for ease of observation and examination of the infant. They can be easily cleaned and disinfected by antiseptic solutions. Alcohol or organic solvents should not be used to clean the plastic or plexiglass material due to risk of opacification.

Incubators

The incubators are essential to provide an ideal microenvironment for high-risk babies. About one-third of nursery beds should comprise of incubators. The main functions of an incubator are isolation, maintenance of thermoneutral ambient temperature, desired humidity and administration of oxygen. It is desirable to nurse extremely low birth weight (<1000 g) stable babies in the incubator. The sensory stimuli, like light, sound, touch and pain, should be kept to the barest minimum without compromising the quality of care. It is essential that an incubator should not interfere with observation of an infant, should offer easy access to the baby and be readily cleanable. Even when sterile water is used in the humidity tank, incubators are a potential source of infection. The water in the humidity tank should be changed daily and 1–2 mL of glacial acetic acid or vinegar should be added to prevent bacterial colonization. Most centers are now using incubators without adding any water in the humidity chamber, while in some countries incubators are used to provide 100% humidity akin to *in utero* environment.

The incubator may be of portable type for transport of sick babies or stationed in the nursery. The open box type (Armstrong) incubators are incapable of maintaining thermoneutrality due to alterations in the temperature when lid is opened. They are equipped with an inefficient thermostat and do not provide for entry of filtered air in the incubator. The intensive care or closed type (isolette) incubators are equipped with portholes for access to the infant (Figure 2.9). The front panel can also be opened and bassinet can be pulled out for unhindered access to the infant for examination and various procedures. These incubators are equipped with an air pump for circulation of filtered air for uniform distribution of heat throughout the incubator. They are also provided with partitioned circuit which allows for gradual changes in heat current as opposed to conventional on-off thermostat. A double wall incubator is preferred because radiant heat loss is reduced by 50%. A servo-control system is ideal for automatic adjustments in the ambient temperature to keep the infant homeothermic. Skin sensor or thermocouple is affixed to the abdominal

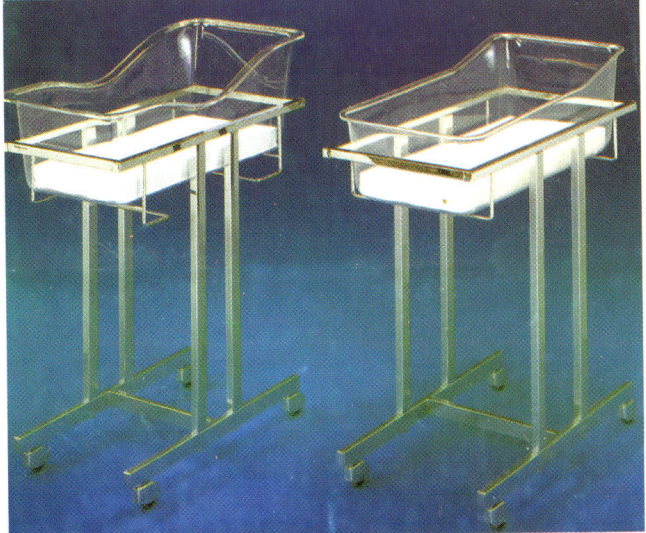

Figure 2.8 Plexiglass bassinets for keeping stable babies. They are aesthetic and easy to clean.

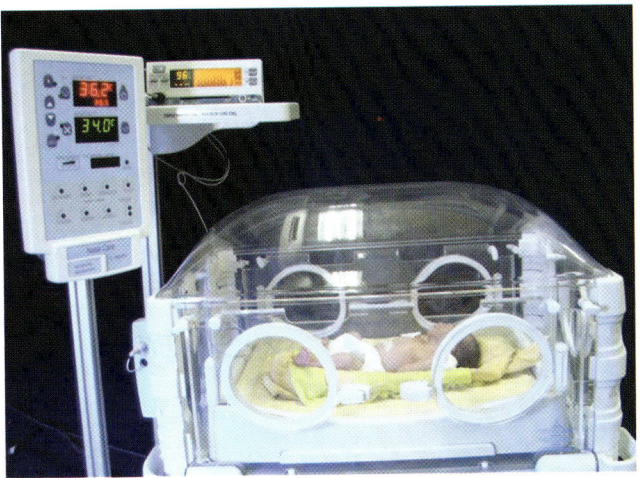

Figure 2.9 Intensive care double-walled incubator. It is provided with portholes and circulation of filtered air.

skin midway between umbilicus and xiphisternum and incubator is set for maintenance of skin temperature at 36.5°C. The skin sensor feeds the information regarding temperature of the baby to the thermostat which automatically regulates the output of heat to maintain the desired skin temperature. Infants nursed under servo mode should be watched to ensure that skin probe is in place. If skin probe inadvertently gets dislodged, infant may get overheated because ambient temperature delivered to the baby would approach 36.5°C. They should be provided with in-built audio and visual alarms for set temperature, high body temperature, air flow, probe or sensor failure, etc. When fever develops in a baby nursed on skin servo mode, there will be repeated activations of the alarm unless the baby is shifted to the manual mode. The built-in heater output monitor provides information regarding the amount of heat generated by the incubator warmer to keep the infant homeothermic. When heater output reading is minimal or nil, it suggests that infant is capable of generating enough metabolic heat to keep himself warm and the baby can be taken out of the incubator and nursed in an open cot.

Radiant Warmer/Open Care System

During various procedures, the infant loses body temperature, unless he is kept warm by use of radiant heat warmer. The infrared heat is preferable because it directly warms the subject without affecting the temperature of intervening environment. When an overhead radiant warmer is intended to be used for a prolonged period, it should be combined with a skin sensor and a servo-control system.

Open care systems which are equipped with an overhead radiant warmer and skin thermister or thermocouple with servo-control are now the most useful and popular equipment. They are equipped with a narrow band proportional heat controllers which can rapidly cycle up and down the temperature. They are provided with audio and visual alarms for high and low temperature and heater output. Recently, talking warmers have been introduced which provide verbal warning to the nurses regarding low temperature, high temperature and out of reach temperature. The steps followed in using an open care system are summarized in Box 2.1. Unless baby is extremely small or gravely sick, open care system is preferable over an intensive care incubator because of easy access to the infant and less chances of nosocomial infection. Skin probe is applied over the

> **Box 2.1: Steps for using open care system**
> - Switch on the unit.
> - Select manual mode with heater output of 100% for 10–15 minutes for rapid warming of the bassinet covered with linen.
> - Select servo mode to maintain skin temperature of the baby at 36.5°C.
> - The skin probe site (right hypochondrium in a supine baby and flank when baby is nursed prone) is prepared by using surgical spirit.
> - Fix the probe with an adhesive tape and cover it with a reflective pad.
> - Ensure that the skin sensor is kept affixed to baby's skin at all times.
> - When a hypothermic baby needs to be rapidly warmed, select the manual mode and the desired heater output.
> - Record baby's axillary temperature after 30 minutes and then 2 hourly.
> - Respond to the alarm immediately, identify the fault and rectify it.

liver area in the epigastrium and shielded with a foil-covered foam adhesive pad. When a baby is nursed prone, skin probe is applied over the flank. The probe should not be allowed to come in contact with the bed. These units also have a provision for overhead light source and phototherapy unit and are most suitable for undertaking any prolonged procedure, like assisted ventilation, exchange blood transfusion or surgery (Figures 2.10 and 2.11). Babies nursed in the open care system have excessive evaporative fluid losses and have significantly higher metabolic rate compared to babies kept in the incubator. After stabilization of the baby kept in the open care system, it is preferable to cover the baby with clothes or thin polythene sheet to reduce evaporative fluid losses. Application of sterile liquid paraffin or non-irritating oil on the skin is associated with reduced evaporative losses from skin.

Therapeutic Cooling Devices

High technology whole baby cooling devices (Blanketrol, Tecotherm Neo, Meditherm) are equipped both for cooling and rewarming the baby by virtue of a heater, a compressor, water circulating pump and a microprocessor board. The baby is placed on a blanket which is designed to circulate cold or warm distilled water which is pumped from the unit. The equipment functions in three modes, manual mode, automatic or servo mode and monitor only mode. The water hoses of the blanket are connected to the cooling unit.

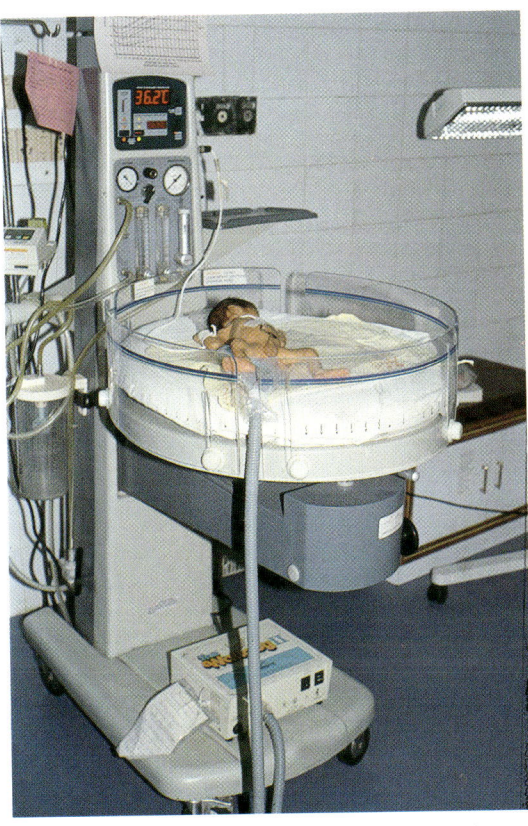

Figure 2.10 Open care system. It is equipped with overhead heat and light source along with servo-control facility.

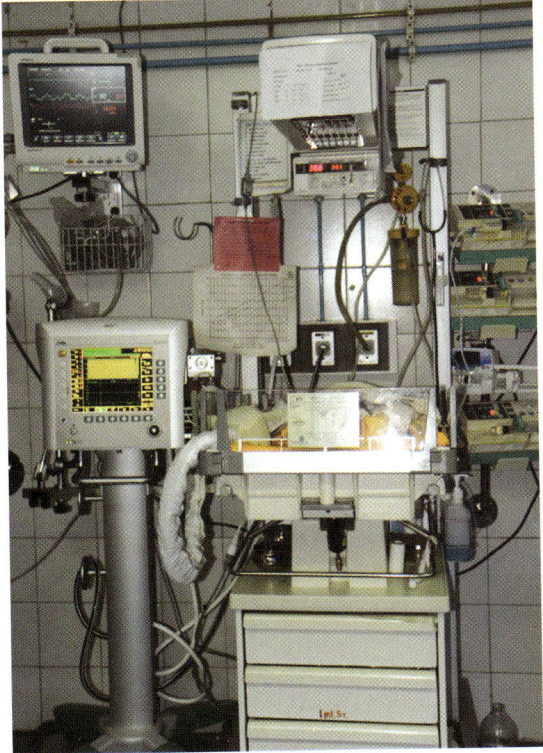

Figure 2.11 Premature infant in an open care system on ventilator and multichannel vital sign monitor.

The manual control mode is used to pre-cool the blanket by circulating sterile or distilled water cooled to the set temperature of 5°C. The baby (<6 hours of age) fulfilling the inclusion criteria for whole body cooling, is placed in a supine position on the blanket to ensure that complete body including occiput is touching the blanket (Figure 2.12). The radiant warmer or any other source of exogenous heat should be put off.

A disposable temperature Steri-Probe is placed in the esophagus or rectum to automatically maintain core temperature of the baby to 33.5°C. Esophageal probe is inserted through the nose and placed in the lower third of esophagus and securely taped. During automatic or servo mode, the unit maintains the set temperature of the baby either by cooling or warming the water circulating in the blanket. After the blanket is completely filled with water, check and maintain the level of sterile water in the reservoir at the desired level. Selective head cooling devices (Olympic cool cap) are available which are associated with reduced immediate adverse effects because core body temperature is maintained at a safe level by use of a radiant warmer. However, selective head cooling is less effective in improving survival and reducing the risk of neuromotor disability in neonates with severe hypoxic-ischemic encephalopathy (HIE).

The infant is provided with state-of-the-art NICU care by monitoring vital signs, biochemical parameters, maintenance of fluids and electrolytes, blood gases and acid–base parameters with the help of assisted ventilation, high-frequency oscillations (HFO) and inhaled nitric oxide (iNO). Antibiotics should be given as per the protocol of the NICU. The neurologic status

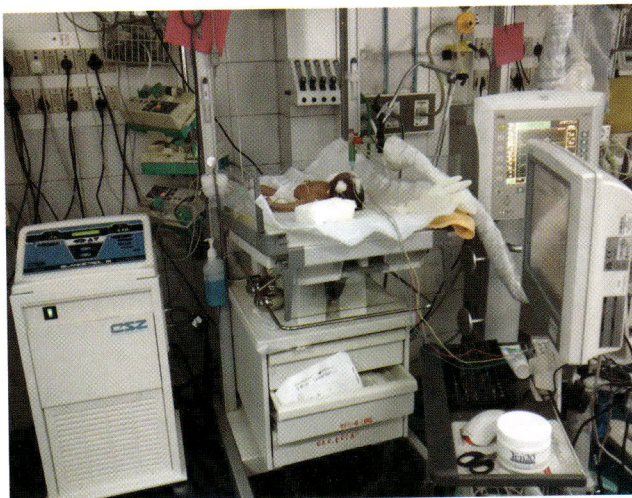

Figure 2.12 Infant with grade 3 HIE being nursed on a cooling blanket and attached with various monitoring devices.

Organization of a Neonatal Intensive Care Unit

2

is checked clinically, with the help of an aEEG and neurosonography. The infant is nursed on the cooling blanket for 72 hours and then gradually warmed by raising the set temperature by 0.5°C every hour to achieve skin temperature of 36.5°C in a period of about 6 hours.

In low and middle income countries (LMICs), simple cost-effective low-tech cooling devices like ice packs, frozen gel packs, cold water bottles, etc. have been used with variable results. Recently mattresses fabricated with phase changing materials (PCM) have been used effectively. The PCM consist of salt hybrid, fatty acids, and esters or paraffin that melt at a set temperature. During this process, they can store or release large amounts of energy to produce cooling. The PCM cooling mattress (Climator™) has been used with favorable results in studies conducted in Kerala.

Thermometers

Low reading (30–40°C) rectal thermometer is essential to assess the severity of hypothermia. The severity of hypothermia in small babies may be over-looked, if only conventional thermometers are used. Electronic or tele thermometers with skin censors or rectal probes with an accuracy of ±0.1°C are ideal for continuous atraumatic monitoring of body temperature. These temperature monitors are also equipped with acoustic and visual alarms set at a desired low and high temperatures. Simultaneous monitoring of core and toe temperature can provide useful information regarding state of peripheral perfusion. When a baby gets overheated in the incubator, both core and peripheral skin temperature rises while in an infant with circulatory failure, peripheral skin temperature may be more than 1°C lower than core temperature. This offers quantitation and objectivity to the time honored clinical observation of finding warm trunk and cold extremities in infants with septic shock. Cold extremities, in the absence of shock, suggest that the baby is under cold stress and expending extra oxygen and calories for metabolic thermogenesis and thus compromising the weight gain and mental growth of the baby.

Oxygen Concentrator

Portable oxygen cylinders are expensive and not readily available in a district hospital or community health center. Oxygen concentrators are being indigenously manufactured and they work both on a battery and mains. The atmospheric air is passed through a chemical zeolite (aluminum silicate) which absorbs all gases except oxygen. It can increase the concentration of oxygen in the air from 21% to about 90%. The oxygen

sensor device (OSD) shows a green signal when oxygen concentration in the outlet exceeds 90%. It is possible to treat simultaneously up to four infants (flow rate 0.5–1.0 liter/min) at a time by using an oxygen flow-splitting device. The equipment is provided with four filters to eliminate dust, humidity and bacteria. Depending upon the flow rate, various concentrations of oxygen can be delivered to the patient. Oxygen-air blender with an oxygen analyzer can be interposed to deliver a precise concentration of FiO_2 but it considerably enhances the price of the device. Oxygen must be warmed (36.0–36.5°C) and humidified before administration to the baby. Oxygen concentrators are cost-effective and promoted by WHO in developing countries. The unit cost is high (around INR 50,000–00) but recurrent costs are low. They are useful in domiciliary practice for administration of oxygen to preterm neonates with chronic lung disease (CLD) and children with chronic interstitial lung disease.

Oxygen Head Box (Oxihood)

A square-shaped box made of transparent plastic or perspex which can enclose the head of the infant is useful for administration of higher concentration of oxygen. The box should be made of unbreakable material molded as a single piece without any joints. It can be used whether the baby is nursed in an open cot or incubator. It should be provided with an adjustable neck port or flexible occluding collar to create an effective seal to prevent free entry of environmental air. The oxygen concentrations which are likely to be achieved with different flow rates should be printed on the box.

Oxygen Analyzer

This is useful for monitoring ambient oxygen concentration in order to protect the infant against oxygen toxicity. It helps in regulating the flow rate of oxygen so that desired concentration of oxygen is delivered to the infant depending upon his clinical condition and oxygen requirements. The Beckman's paramagnetic oxygen analyzer of earlier days has been replaced by newer oxygen sensors which operate on galvanic cell principle. The electric current generated between two electrodes is proportional to the partial pressure of oxygen. Cathode is gold plated while anode is made of lead and filled with potassium hydroxide. The newer oxygen analyzers provide continuous digital display of oxygen concentration and trigger off audiovisual warning signal when environmental concentration of oxygen falls or rises beyond the safety levels (Figure 2.13). The instrument

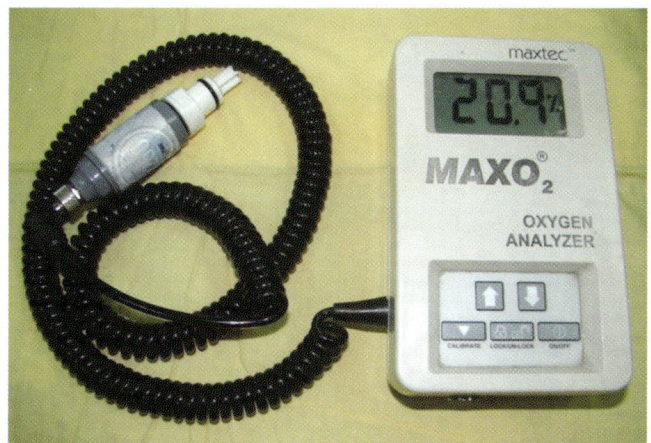

Figure 2.13 Oxygen monitor. It provides continuous digital display of ambient oxygen concentration.

is calibrated by checking the oxygen concentration of room air which is usually constant at 21%. The sensor life is about 9 months only and would need replacement once a year.

Perspex Heat Shield

Heat shield made of perspex or transparent plexiglass measuring 18″ × 10″ × 8″ in a dome shape is a very simple and useful device to reduce the heat loss by radiation and evaporation. When a sick infant with respiratory distress is nursed naked in the incubator, he must be enclosed in the perspex heat shield to limit fluctuations in his body temperature. It reduces insensible water loss by about 25%. Based on this analogy, the currently available intensive care incubators are double-walled, which are credited to reduce radiant heat loss by 50%.

Transilluminator

It is a useful, cheap, non-invasive device for point-of-care use in a number of situations in NICU. Fiberoptic light source is used to provide up to 12,000 candles with a halogen quartz lamp, LED light source or xenon arc. The shorter wavelengths (up to 470 nm) of visible light which produce heat are filtered out to provide "cold light" at the tip of the cable. The efficacy of transillumination is enhanced by competence of the operator, intensity of light and by maintaining the room as dark as possible. Thermal injury to the skin can be minimized by reducing the duration of contact of light to the skin between 15 and 30 seconds. The halo of light around the probe is visualized, measured and compared on two sides.

It is a useful device for point-of-care prompt diagnosis of air-leaks (pneumothorax, pneumomediastinum and pneumopericardium), hydrothorax and chylothorax. Cranial transillumination is useful for the diagnosis of subdural hematoma or effusion, hydrocephalus, hydranencephaly, cystic hygroma and craniocervical meningocele. Transillumination of abdomen and pelvis can be used for diagnosis of hypertrophic pyloric stenosis, necrotizing enterocolitis, hydronephrosis, inguinal hernia and hydrocele. It can be used for delineation of bladder for suprapubic aspiration of urine. Transillumination is a useful aid for venous and arterial cannulation in neonates.

Phototherapy Unit

Phototherapy is now generally accepted as a safe and effective method for treatment of neonatal hyperbilirubinemia. A light source designed to give an irradiance or flux of 10–30 $\mu W/cm^2/nm$ between 400 and 520 nm wavelength range at the level of mattress is ideal. Blue light is more effective than the white light but former interferes with the observation of the infant. Special blue lamps with a peak output at 425 to 475 nm are most efficient for phototherapy and these do not emit harmful ultraviolet rays. To enhance irradiance or flux, four blue compact fluorescent tubes (F 20 T12/BB and Philips TL 20 W/52) and two white fluorescent tubes can be used because excessive blue color makes evaluation of the baby difficult and is uncomfortable to the eyes (Figure 2.14). It is preferable to use 40 W 2 feet long tubes which are economical with reduced recurring expenses. These units provide irradiance of 20–30 $\mu W/cm^2/nm$ in the 400–520 nm range. Cooling fan is required to reduce radiant heat exposure to the baby. The nude infant may be exposed under a portable or fixed light source kept at a distance of about 18 inches (45 cm) from the skin. Double-light system, where total baby is exposed from below and

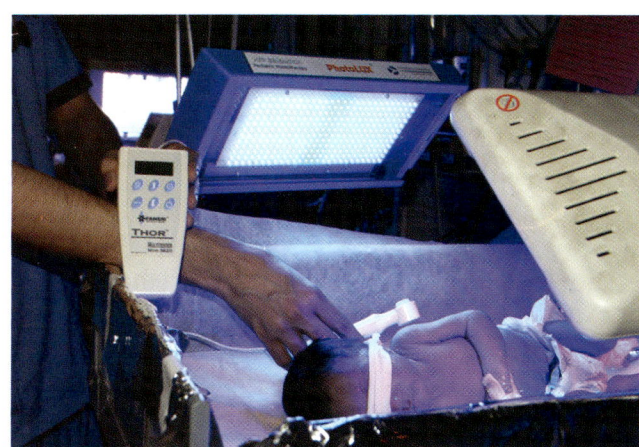

Figure 2.14 A compact fluorescent light phototherapy unit.

above, has been used for more effective light exposure. The conventional double surface phototherapy is uncomfortable and unfriendly to the baby who is made to lie on a cold and hard perspex sheet. Instead, intensive single surface phototherapy can be given by using tubes providing greater irradiance (40 W, 2 ft, TL-52) and by reducing the distance between the tubes and the baby to 15–20 cm. The tube light should be covered with plexiglass or plastic sheet to screen out ultraviolet rays. The flux density reduces with time and average rated life of tubes vary between 1000 and 2000 hours. The tubes should be replaced when their ends become black or spectral radiant energy ('flux') at the level of skin is less than 8 $\mu W/cm^2/nm$.

Spotlight phototherapy units are available which are equipped with a 150 watt 21 volt halogen bulb with a specially coated reflector which absorbs harmful infrared waves. The latest phototherapy units are based on the principle of fiberoptics in which an illuminated blanket is wrapped around the baby. It ensures exposure of greater surface area and is ideal for providing double-surface light exposure. The baby is placed on the fiberoptic biliblanket or light-emitting diode (LED) mattress and additional phototherapy is provided with blue compact fluorescent tubes from the top. The effect of phototherapy unit can be enhanced by using slings or curtains made of white cloth or aluminum to reflect light on the baby. Newer phototherapy units are equipped with a dosimeter to calculate cumulative exposure of phototherapy. Recently, gallium nitride light-emitting diode units have been launched to provide intense phototherapy benefits. They produce minimal heat and provide narrow luminous spectra in the blue-green range of visible spectrum of light with massive delivery of irradiance up to 200 $\mu W/cm^2/nm$.

The efficacy of phototherapy unit is not dependent upon the intensity of light but on the irradiance or flux (Figure 2.15). Most phototherapy units in the country are suboptimal because their flux is not monitored. In a large NICU, in-house fluxmeter should be available or the supplier should be asked to periodically check the flux and replace the tubes when irradiance drops below 8 $\mu W/cm^2/nm$. The phototherapy unit is put on for at least 10 minutes. The irradiance is measured by placing the sensor probe of the fluxmeter at a distance of 50 cm. The total irradiance read-out given by the fluxmeter is averaged to $\mu W/cm^2/nm$ by dividing it by the bandwidth, i.e. for the instrument providing waveband range 425–475 nm, it is divided by 50.

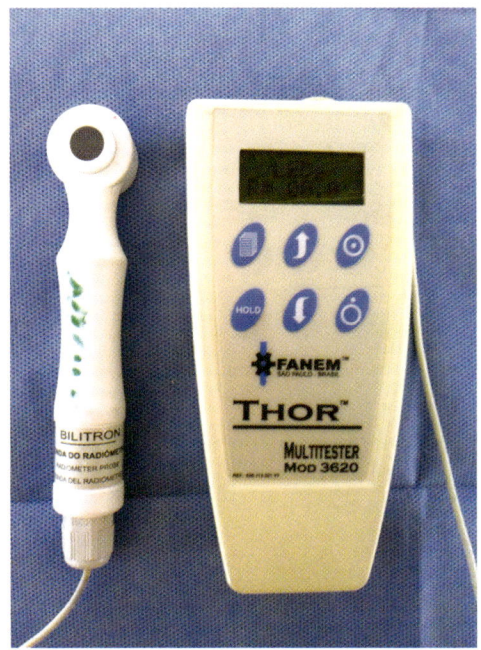

Figure 2.15 Irradiance meter.

Heart Rate Monitor

Among various electronic gadgets for monitoring vital signs, cardiac monitor showing digital display of heart rate (along with audible beep) or an electrocardiographic configuration on an oscilloscope or both, is most useful. Generally an apneic attack is followed by bradycardia within 20 seconds so that heart rate monitor (with an alarm set at heart rate of less than 80 per minute) can be used with advantage over an apnea monitor. They are ideal to monitor high-risk infants and are especially useful during prolonged procedures, such as exchange blood transfusion and surgery (Figure 2.16).

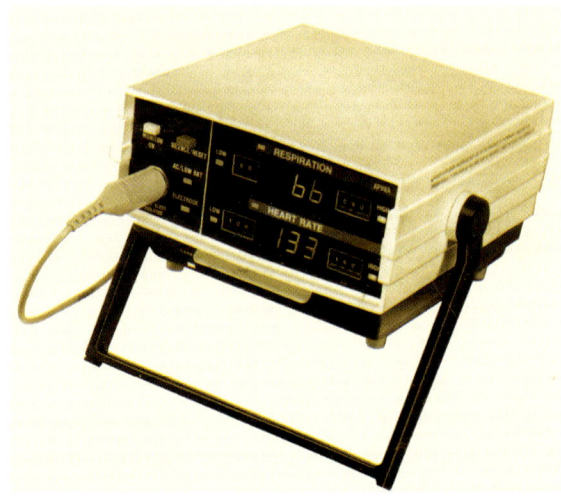

Figure 2.16 Heart rate and respiration monitor.

Respiratory Rate and Apnea Monitor

The respiratory monitor based on impedance technique measures changes in the electrical resistance during breathing. The electrode is fixed on the chest wall to pick up signals which are digitally displayed as respiratory rate. The respiratory excursions can also be displayed on the oscilloscope. The conventional apnea monitors are based on air mattress having plethysmographic sensor. The mattress is placed underneath the chest of the infant and mechanical alterations produced by the respiratory movements of the infant are recorded and displayed. When infant stops breathing, after a variable interval of 10 to 20 seconds depending upon the preset lag, the instrument emits a beep and displays red light warning signal.

Blood Pressure Monitor

Recording of blood pressure by flush or conventional method is inaccurate and time consuming in newborn babies. Direct arterial pressure can be recorded by introducing a transducer into umbilical artery but this method is invasive and fraught with complications and should be reserved for critically sick VLBW babies on assisted ventilation. Doppler system based on the principle of ultrasound waves provides an accurate and non-invasive means for recording blood pressure in newborn babies. The ultrasonic waves are picked up by the transducer located in the cuff. The usual cuff size to cover two-thirds of the upper arm of newborn baby varies between 2.5 and 4.0 cm depending upon the birth weight. The blood pressure reading may be unreliable, if baby is crying or moving. The blood pressure instruments based on oscillometric technique are more accurate and should preferably be used. They are more reliable and are not affected by the movements of the baby. The instrument provides continuous digital display of heart rate, systolic, diastolic and mean blood pressure. There is a provision for alarm or warning signal when blood pressure falls or rises beyond certain preset limits (Figure 2.17). In future, finger plethysmography with the help of a small cuff and a light source may provide a constant display of mean blood pressure, heart rate and arterial oxygen saturation.

Multi-channel Vital Sign Monitor

The multiple channel complex monitors are available to display and record all the vital signs on an oscilloscope. They are very useful but extremely expensive. They are equipped to record temperature at different

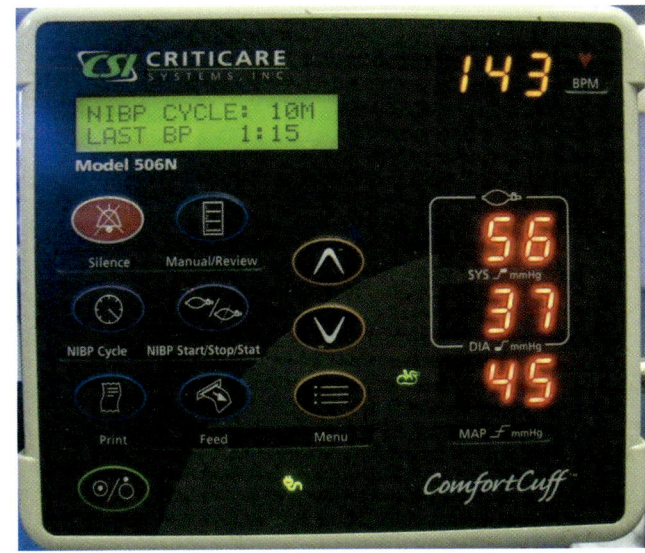

Figure 2.17 Non-invasive blood pressure monitor.

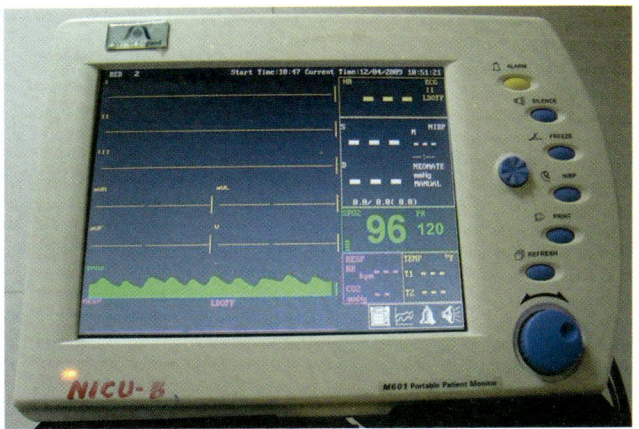

Figure 2.18 Multi-channel vital sign monitor.

sites, heart rate, respiratory rate with apnea alarm, invasive and non-invasive blood pressure and pulse oximetry. ECG, pulse waves and respiratogram are displayed on the oscilloscope. There is a need to have a computer based monitor to analyze all the information provided by complex vital sign monitors (Figure 2.18).

Infusion Pump

In view of the fact that relatively small quantities of fluids need to be infused and minor errors in rate of administration may prove lethal to low birth weight babies, constant infusion pumps with an accurate control are essential to meet these requirements. In centers where parenteral nutrition is used for the care of sick babies, the use of infusion pumps has become obligatory. The infusion pump is a sophisticated electronic micropump which displaces fluid and a microprocessor or pressure transducer controls the

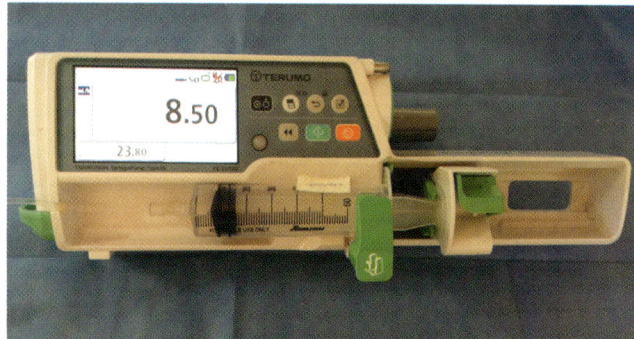

Figure 2.19 Syringe-based infusion pump. The flow rate of drip can be regulated between 1.0 and 99.9 mL/hour with this device.

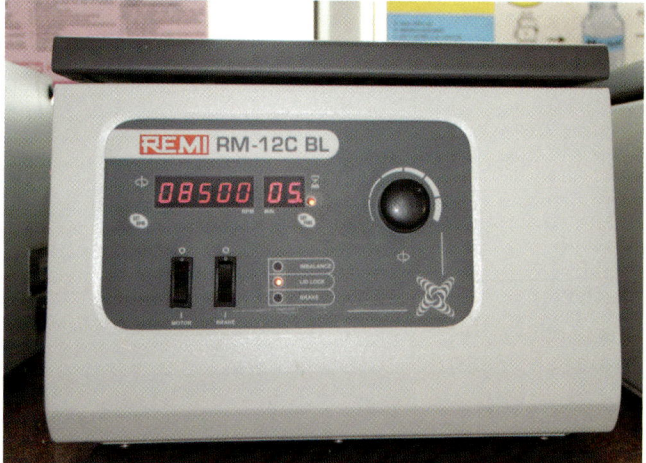

Figure 2.20 Laboratory microcentrifuge.

rate of fluid delivery. Various devices used for accurate administration of fluids in neonates include gravity-dependent drip rate regulators, volumetric infusion pump and syrings pumps accepting a wide range of syringes. The rate of infusion is either depicted as drops/minute (1–99 drops/minute) or in terms of volume (1.0–99.9 mL/hour) through a disposable cassette or plastic syringe. The syringe-based infusion pumps are ideal for administration of drugs or intralipid. It is desirable to buy an infusion pump which accepts syringes of different sizes (20, 50, 100 mL) and all makes and should work both on mains and Ni-Cd batteries. The syringe and tubing must be changed every 24 hours to reduce the risk of nosocomial infection. The latest infusion pumps have inbuilt alarms to signal occlusion of flow, air in the system, system failure and low battery charge (Figure 2.19). The infusion site must be watched diligently for any extravasation because infusion will not stop due to the effect of pumping force. The new generation "smart" infusion pumps are available which are equipped with computerized prescriber order entry (CPOE) and automatic or programmed medication system to reduce the risk of adverse drug events.

Microcentrifuge

Centrifugation is done to separate solid particles or cells suspended in a liquid medium, like blood, urine and various body secretions (CSF, gastric aspirate) and serosal transudates and exudates. Laboratory microcentrifuge is used for measuring hematocrit or packed cell volume (PCV) and for separation of plasma from cellular elements of blood for estimation of bilirubin in a microcapillary sample (50–70 μL). The main components of the centrifuge include a rotor with slots for placing capillaries, a lid with a lock, a timer and a knob for adjusting the speed. The microcapillaries made

of borosilicate glass and certified for centrifugation at a high speed of 10,000–15,000 rpm are recommended for use. Heparinized microcapillaries with internal diameter of 1.0 mm and length of 7.0 cm are used. After taking the blood sample in the tube, one end is sealed with plasticine. The placement of tube/s in the slots should be balanced on two sides by placing blood or water-filled capillary tubes on the identical or corresponding slots on the opposite side of the rotor. The instrument should be kept at least 30 cm away from the wall for proper dissipation of heat. The motor is provided with a blower to ensue that the temperature of the machine is not allowed to cross 40°C. After placing the capillary tubes in slots (including balancing capillaries), the centrifuge is turned on and set to rotate at 10,000 rpm for 5 minutes (Figure 2.20). The instrument should be kept clean and any blood spills should be wiped off with a wet gauze piece or 10% bleach solution. The instrument should be kept lubricated and its motor brush should be checked every 3 months.

Bilirubin Analyzer

The spectrometric bilirubinometer works on the principle of two-wavelength direct spectrometry with the help of a light source that emits a narrow beam of light at 465 nm and 540 nm. The light beam passes through a slit in the microcapillary tube holder or a couvette and the unabsorbed light is detected by a photodedector. The microcapillary tube containing 50–70 μL of baby's blood is blocked at one end with plasticene and centrifuged at 12,000 rpm for 5 minutes to separate out the plasma or serum. The serum or plasma column should cover the entire length of the slit through which the light waves pass. The capillary

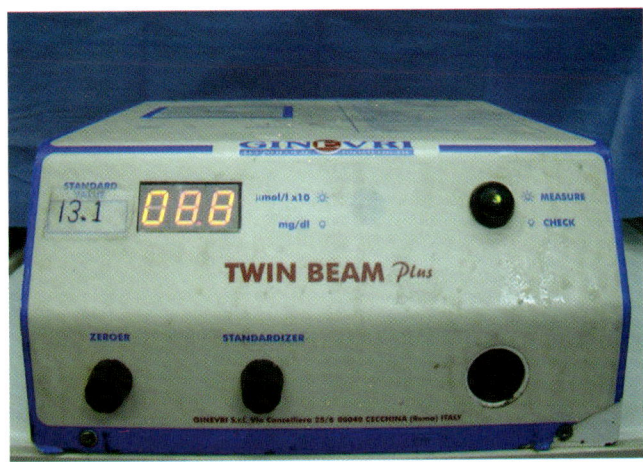
Figure 2.21 Twin beam bilirubin analyzer.

slit must be kept clean of any dust or particles of plasticene to ensure accuracy of results. The instrument provides direct read-out of total serum bilirubin which is reliable for taking therapeutic decisions for the management of neonatal hyperbilirubinemia. The hematocrit can be read off from the same sample and serum can be subsequently used for determination of C-reactive protein or other biochemical tests; thus minimising the need for blood sampling (Figure 2.21).

Apart from bilirubin, there are several other components in the plasma, like oxyhemoglobin, transferrin, methemalbumin and lipids which can interfere with absorption of light. The instrument is so calibrated by using complex mathematical equations and correction factors, that the bilirubinometer gives a reliable estimate of total bilirubin. Nevertheless, beta-carotene levels of blood can interfere with test results but fortunately carotenoids are not present in the serum of newborn babies. However, after an exchange blood transfusion with adult blood, transfused carotene may provide falsely high values of bilirubin. Hemolysis does not interfere with the reliability of spectrometry method of bilirubin estimation unlike conventional Diazo method.

Transcutaneous Bilirubinometer

The yellow discoloration of skin and subcutaneous tissues can be quantitated and equated to total bilirubin value with the help of a photoprobe. The probe is pressed against forehead or sternum. The light passes through inbuilt fiberoptics and reflectometer and is analyzed by computerized spectro-photometer to provide immediate digital display of total bilirubin. It is useful bedside screening method for the young resident doctor to assess the degree of jaundice. There is a good correlation between transcutaneous

and biochemically assessed bilirubin values. It gives an estimate of only total bilirubin which, however, is quite satisfactory because there is hardly any elevation of direct-reacting bilirubin during first week of life. Skin pigmentation of black babies may interfere with transcutaneous bilirubin evaluation. In such cases, photoprobe placed against a drop of blood taken on a filter paper, has given reliable estimate of serum bilirubin. The latest multi-wavelength reflectance meter (BiliChek by Norcross) or dual wavelength reflectance meter (JM-103 by Minolta/Air Shields) provides reliable estimate of total serum bilirubin without any interference by skin pigmentation or gestational age of the baby. According to the guidelines of American Academy of Pediatrics, transcutaneous bilirubinometry (TcB) can be used as a surrogate of serum total bilirubin (STB) for screening of jaundice in term and near-term neonates. However, bilirubin level must be confirmed by a spectrometric bilirubin analyzer or Diazo method before starting any therapeutic intervention. During phototherapy, a small area of skin should be kept covered to serve as a reference point to reliably monitor transcutaneous bilirubin levels. Icterometer is a plastic strip depicting different shades of yellow color and can also be used to match the yellowness of the skin of the baby to roughly assess the degree of jaundice.

Transcutaneous Blood Gas Monitor

Sick preterm infants with respiratory difficulties require frequent arterial blood sampling for blood gases and acid–base analyses. Arterial electrode placed in umbilical artery has been successfully used for continuous monitoring of PaO$_2$ but it is complicated by inherent hazards of umbilical vessel catheterization with indwelling catheter. The availability of non-invasive transcutaneous monitor is indeed a useful technological advance in the field of bioengineering during the last decade. This has simplified constant monitoring of oxygen tension *in vivo* with the hope that sequelae of hypoxia and hyperoxia in the newborn can be reduced. It utilizes a miniature Clarks' electrode which can be heated to 44°C. The sensor is slipped over the membrane assembly and is affixed over the chest or upper abdomen. The heated skin electrode produces local hyperthermia causing vasodilation, thus arterializing the capillary bed under the electrode. Molecular oxygen diffuses from the dilated capillaries towards the cathode (platinum) of the electrode where it is reduced. The resultant current generated by the flow of electrode is proportional to the partial pressure of oxygen which is continuously displayed on the digital read out. The transcutaneous PO_2 values are quite reliable and comparable to simultaneous PaO_2 which should be cross-checked every 4 to 6 hours. Due to risk of skin burns, the site of sensor should be changed every 2 hourly. When the electrode becomes loose, room air may leak under the sensor to produce spuriously high $TcPO_2$ values (usually above 150 torr). Transcutaneous oxygen monitoring is essential for optimal management of infants with respiratory distress syndrome and frequent apneic attacks. It provides diagnostic information in several clinical situations. In infants with cyanotic congenital heart disease, $TcPO_2$ cannot be raised above 100 torr by administration of 100% oxygen. The right-to-left shunting at the ductal level can be suspected by using two skin sensors, one placed over the right upper chest (pre-ductal) and the other placed over left lower abdomen (post-ductal). A discrepancy of greater than 20% in $TcPO_2$ value obtained by two skin sensors is indicative of significant right-to-left shunt. Lastly, if $TcPO_2$ value is considerably lower than simultaneous PaO_2 level, it is suggestive of peripheral vasoconstriction or impending shock. Transcutaneous oxygen monitors have lost the initial enthusiasm because they are time consuming and cumbersome to use.

Transcutaneous carbon dioxide monitors are also available though they are very expensive. The $TcPCO_2$ sensor is larger in size and work on the principle of Stowe and Severinghaus. Like the oxygen sensor, CO_2 sensor also needs to be kept heated at 44°C and its site is changed every 3 to 4 hours. Technology is also available for continuous monitoring of tissue PCO_2 with a mass spectrometer and infrared method. The continuous monitoring of tissue pH is also feasible but it is rather invasive and requires insertion of an indwelling electrode either over the surface of a muscle or in the subcutaneous tissue.

Pulse Oximeter

Pulse oximeter provides a simple, convenient and non-invasive method for continuous monitoring of hemoglobin saturated with oxygen. It has virtually replaced the transcutaneous monitors. The arterial blood oxygen saturation (SpO_2 or SaO_2) can be determined transcutaneously by measuring the absorption of two selected wavelengths of light. The light generated in the sensor (probe) passes through the blood and tissues and is converted into electronic signals by a photodetector located in the sensor. The oxyhemoglobin and reduced hemoglobin allow different amounts of light at selected wavelengths to reach the photodetector. The monitor gives the digital display

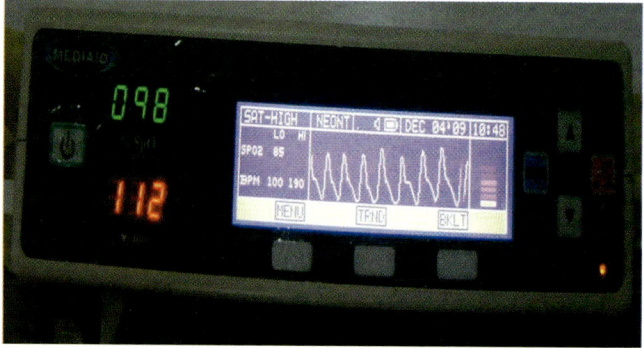

Figure 2.22 Pulse oximeter for monitoring arterial oxygen saturation and heart rate.

of arterial oxygen saturation, pulse rate and audible pulse tone (Figure 2.22). There are two pulse oximeter technologies, signal extraction technology (SET) and resistor calibration technology (RCAL). The SET pulse oximeter picks up oxygen saturation values faster than the oximeters based on RCAL technology. Most instruments have a facility to set alarm limits for SaO_2 (low and high) and for pulse rate which can provide a dual function of an apnea alarm. A hand-held pulse oximeter which runs on batteries can be used during transport of sick babies. The flex probe (sensor) can be affixed on the dorsum of the foot of the baby. The sensor containing the photocell is extremely sensitive to light and must be shielded from strong external light sources, like observation light and phototherapy. Do not apply cuff of blood pressure monitor on the same limb where sensor is affixed. The probe site should be periodically changed to prevent damage to the skin. Pulse oximetry provides a simple, convenient and non-invasive method for continuous monitoring and display of SaO_2. It is ideal for early detection of hypoxia in critically sick newborn babies but it has its own limitations to identify hyperoxia because oxygen dissociation curve is displaced to the left in newborn babies. To safeguard against the risk of hyperoxia and retinopathy of prematurity, it is recommended that the upper limit of alarm for oxygen saturation should be set at 95%. Arterial oxygen saturation should be maintained between 90 and 95% for acute conditions and 85 and 90% for chronic situations. Shock and peripheral vasoconstriction is associated with unreliable display of SaO_2.

Capnography or End Tidal CO_2 ($EtCO_2$) Monitor

This is a simple, non-invasive and quick method to assess alveolar CO_2. Apart from water vapor, CO_2 is the only component of alveolar gases which absorbs infrared rays. When water vapor is eliminated, infrared analyzer provides a good measure of CO_2 concentration. Carbon dioxide, an end product of cellular metabolism, is transported from the cells via circulation, diffuses into the alveoli and exhaled through the airways. Thus $EtCO_2$ values reflect metabolism, pulmonary perfusion, alveolar diffusion and ventilatory efficacy. In normal subjects, $EtCO_2$ is an accurate approximation of "average" mixed alveolar gas composition. In spontaneously breathing infant, nasal cannula is used for air sampling while in a baby on assisted ventilation, an adaptor is placed between endotracheal tube and the ventilator circuit. It is preferable to buy the mainstream analyzer (instead of sidestream analyzer) because couvette can be mounted directly in line with the endotracheal tube without any risk of blockage.

The $EtCO_2$ range varies between 0 and 99 mm Hg with an accuracy of ±2 mm Hg for values between 0 and 40 mm Hg and ±5 mm Hg for values between 41 and 99 mm Hg. It is a useful modality to assess whether endotracheal tube has gone into the esophagus or it is kinked/blocked giving $EtCO_2$ value of near zero. The gradient between arterial carbon dioxide and $EtCO_2$ ($PaCO_2 - EtCO_2$) should be calculated. In infants with normal lungs, the gradient is usually up to 5 mm Hg. In neonates with V/Q abnormalities, the gradient may be 10–20 mm Hg. Even when there is a wide gradient, $EtCO_2$ is a reliable predictor of $PaCO_2$ because gradient is usually constant over a long period of time. A sudden increase in the gradient is indicative of an increase in the dead space with a decrease in pulmonary perfusion. When the gradient between $PaCO_2$ and $EtCO_2$ drops to less than 10 mm Hg, it is indicative of improved lung function and feasibility of weaning. However, due to various limitations and availability of more reliable monitoring modalities, capnography is rarely used in newborn babies.

CPAP Delivery System

Continuous positive airway pressure (CPAP) is a useful and affordable technology to manage neonates with RDS and respiratory insufficiency. In contrast to assisted ventilation, it conserves surfactant, improves functional residual capacity (FRC) and reduces the risk of bronchopulmonary dysplasia. Infant on CPAP can be fed with an orogastric tube. The feeding tube is kept plugged for 20 to 30 minutes after the feed to prevent efflux of milk. However, most of the time, OG tube is kept open to prevent distension of abdomen or CPAP belly.

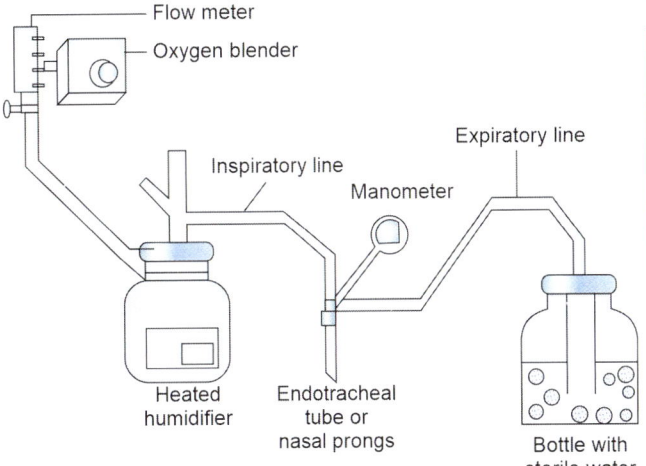

Figure 2.23 The components of bubble CPAP.

CPAP can be delivered through nasopharyngeal tube or face mask but is best provided through nasal prongs. The minimum requirements of CPAP include pulse oximeter (to maintain SpO_2 between 90 and 95%), FiO_2 monitor for mixing air and oxygen; and effective warm humidification. CPAP can be provided through a ventilator but in resource constrained situations, stand alone CPAP machine and bubble or water seal CPAP can be used. The salient components of bubble CPAP are shown in Figure 2.23. The distal end of expiratory tube is immersed in sterile water and its depth in water can be varied to provide CPAP between 5 and 10 cm H_2O. CPAP pressure is adjusted to control chest retractions and grunting, and maintain SpO_2 between 90 and 95%. In general, CPAP pressure and FiO_2 go hand in hand, e.g. 5 cm CPAP and 50% FiO_2, 7 cm CPAP and 70% FiO_2, 10 cm CPAP and 100% FiO_2 and so on so forth. Bubble CPAP with combined effects of CPAP and pressure oscillations from the bubbles provide a lung protective, safe and effective method of providing respiratory support to spontaneously breathing sick neonates. The common complications of CPAP include abdominal distension, retention of carbon dioxide and pneumothorax.

Neonatal Ventilators

Assisted ventilation is required in several babies with respiratory failure. It is irrational to procure a ventilator unless adequate basic facilities, such as skilled nurses and residents, blood gas analyzer, monitoring devices, microchemistry and portable X-rays are available. Till such time, the financial resources may be more usefully expended in augmenting more urgent needs of the NICU. Centralized supply of oxygen and purified air (alternatively air compressor of 50 PSI) is

Organization of a Neonatal Intensive Care Unit

2

mandatory for assisted ventilation. Continuous positive airway pressure (CPAP) apparatus can be readily fabricated to improve the medical care of infants with hyaline membrane disease and recurrent apneic attacks (*see* Chapters 19 and 27).

Ventilators are sophisticated electronic mini-air pumps. The type of ventilator being used is not as important as the level of training and experience of personnel using it. Practical experience and thorough understanding regarding the use of a particular type of a ventilator is more important than having the theoretical knowledge of various ventilators. Basically there are two types of intermittent positive pressure ventilators, they are either pressure generator or flow generator modules. The pressure generator ventilators regulate the pressure gradient at the airway and flow changes are determined by the compliance and resistance of lungs. The flow generator ventilator may have a constant or variable flow rate during two phases of respiration. In flow generator ventilator, the flow of gases in the airways is predetermined while pressure changes depend upon the physical characteristics of lungs. On the basis of their built-in control principles for termination of inspiratory phase, the ventilator may be pressure-cycled, volume-cycled or time-cycled. There are mixed forms of ventilators where more than one type of cycling is utilized, viz. time-controlled, pressure-limited ventilator. All modes of ventilation should be available including intermittent positive pressure ventilation (IPPV), continuous positive airway pressure and synchronized intermittent mandatory ventilation (SIMV).

There are inherent advantages and disadvantages of various types of ventilators. A small leak in the circuit can be adequately compensated in a pressure-cycled ventilator while in a volume-cycled ventilator tidal volume can be maintained adequately even when there is severe reduction in lung compliance. A suitable infant ventilator should be able to deliver adequate gas volume and compensate for any loss of gas volume due to compression, leaks and dead space (Figures 2.24 and 2.25). It should have a sensitive patient triggering mechanism and high cycling frequency. The ventilator should be equipped to supply a wide range of air-oxygen mixtures and provided with a mechanism to vary inspiratory–expiratory ratios. The essential accessories, like humidifier, probe for recording temperature of air-oxygen mixture, air compressor, and infusion pump, must be ordered along with the ventilator. In order to reduce the risk of nosocomial infection, disposable patient circuits compatible with the ventilator should be used.

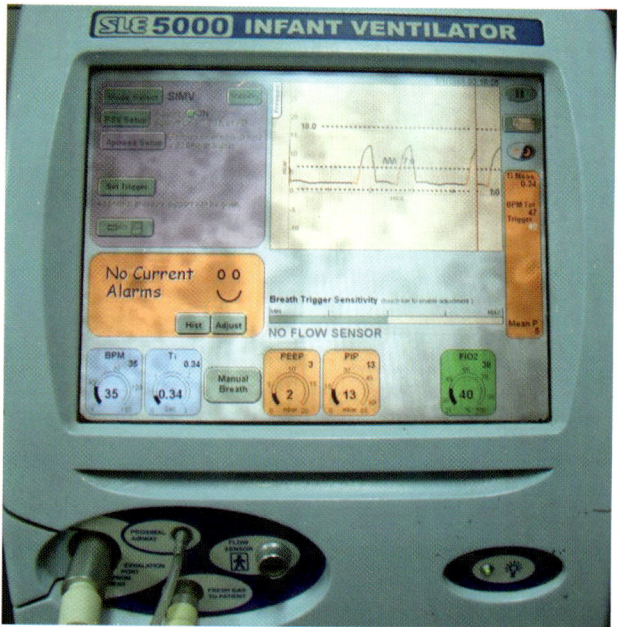

Figure 2.24 SLE 5000 infant ventilator.

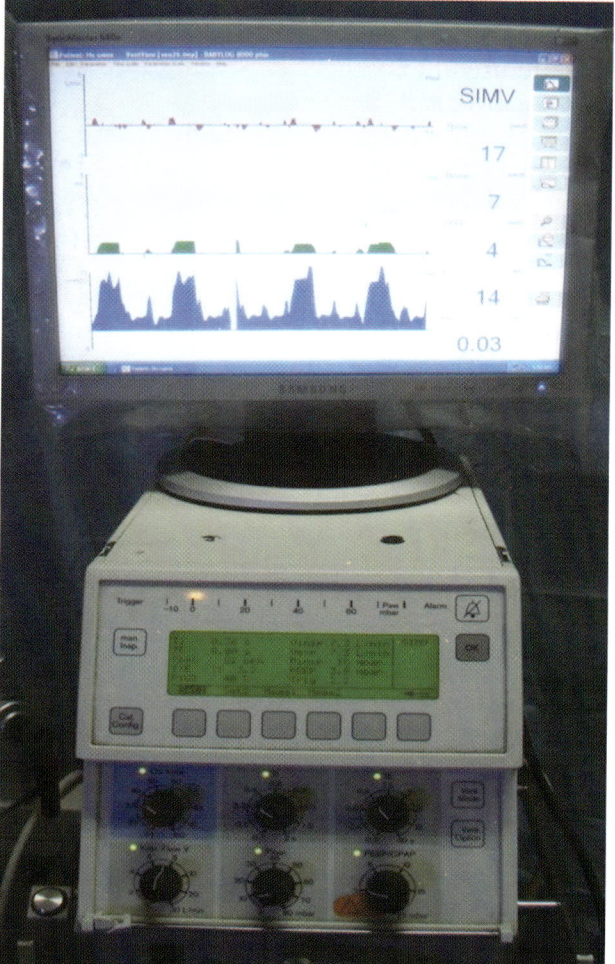

Figure 2.25 Babylog 8000 ventilator with pulmonary graphics.

When conventional ventilation fails or baby has persistent pulmonary hypertension (PPHN) and pulmonary air leaks, high frequency ventilators (HFV) are used. These ventilators use extremely low tidal volume and operate between 150 and 2,400 breaths/min. They are exorbitantly expensive and should be acquired by the state-of-the-art NICUs when their staff has achieved excellence in handling conventional ventilators.

Intermittent negative pressure ventilators are less popular due to hazards of abdominal distension. They are cumbersome and difficult to operate in very low birth weight babies and access for nursing procedures and blood sampling is difficult. The respirator is divided into two compartments to enclose the head and body with the help of sealing around neck. Intermittent negative pressure operates at chest wall resulting in the intermittent gas flow down the airway. Oxygen-air mixture is allowed to flow in the chamber enclosing the head. Endotracheal intubation may be needed in some infants.

Neonatal Pulmonary Function Tests

They are useful to assess infants with cardiopulmonary disease but are mostly used for research purposes at present. The equipment includes a pneumotach to measure air flows and volumes and an esophageal balloon catheter and transducer to measure transpulmonary pressure. These are integrated with a computer and printer. The pulmonary function profile enables the neonatologist to obtain data on tidal volume, compliance, airway resistance and work of breathing. Baseline and daily pulmonary function studies on an infant evaluates changes in lung function, adjustments in mechanical ventilation and ability to wean. It is a useful modality to monitor the therapeutic response to pharmacologic agents, such as bronchodilators, corticosteroids and diuretics in infants with bronchopulmonary dysplasia and chronic lung disease.

Cranial Ultrasonography (CUS)

Ultrasonography with real-time portable ultrasound is the method of choice for evaluation of size of ventricles and possible intraventricular hemorrhage in very LBW babies. The linear-array ultrasonic scanner is used by directing ultrasound waves through anterior fontanel which serves as an acoustic window to obtain best images or echoes. A multi-frequency sector probe providing 5–8 MHz resolution is ideal. It is difficult to transport high-risk LBW babies on assisted ventilation or other life supportive

measures to the specialized radiodiagnosis laboratory for CT scan or MRI studies. Instead cot-side or point-of-care testing (POCT) ultrasound in the nursery can provide equally reliable information (Figure 2.26). The second generation ultrasound machines with color Doppler facility are available which are useful to study blood flow and perfusion. It can be repeated frequently (because it is non-ionizing) as and when indicated depending upon the condition of the infant. At present, ultrasonography appears to be the safest, cheapest and most convenient technique for imaging the intracranial contents in the newborn. A single ultrasound scan performed on day 7 of life will detect almost all the infants who may have developed intraventricular hemorrhage.

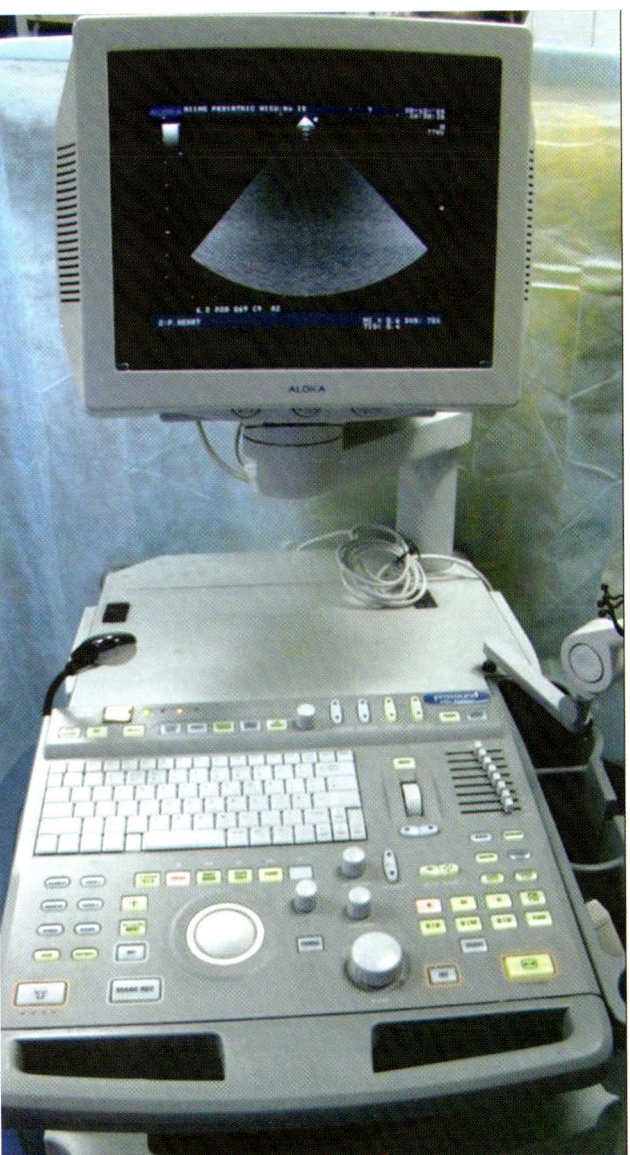

Figure 2.26 Portable ultrasound machine with color Doppler.

2

Routine screening cranial ultrasound (CUS) should be performed on all infants with birth weight <1250 g or gestation of <30 weeks at 7–14 days of age followed by a repeat ultrasound at 36–40 weeks of post-menstrual or postconceptional age. Other indications for doing CUS include (i) hypoxic–ischemic encephalopathy, (ii) neonatal seizures, (iii) suspicion of intracranial hemorrhage and (iv) enlarging head size. The neonatologist should have adequate training and skills to do cot-side cranial ultrasound evaluation. It is a useful, reliable and safe modality for diagnosis and follow-up of infants with intraventricular hemorrhage, cystic periventricular leukomalacia (PVL), ventriculomegaly and certain congenital malformations, like hydrocephalus, agenesis of corpus callosum, and AV malformation. In infants below 1000 g or <28 weeks, cranial ultrasound may be done on day 1 to rule out severe intraventricular hemorrhage or antenatal brain injury to make a decision whether aggressive management should be given or denied.

Intracranial Pressure Monitor

Measurement of intracranial pressure in infants with birth asphyxia, intracranial hemorrhage, meningitis and hydrocephalus can provide useful information to guide therapy and predict prognosis. Several non-invasive techniques have been developed to measure intracranial pressure in the newborn. Oscillographic technique or air tonometer placed over anterior fontanel has been used with variable success. A technique based on fiberoptic system and air bellows gives reliable results with good correlation with direct intraventricular measurements. Caution is advised while placing the sensor on the anterior fontanel because excessive force can lead to spuriously high values. Most of the instruments are still experimental and are used for research purposes.

Neonatal Brain Monitor (aEEG)

The neonatal brain or cerebral function monitor (CFM) is a point-of-care equipment for monitoring back-ground activity of the brain by recording an amplitude-integrated EEG (aEEG) with the help of three electrodes, one placed over the vertex and two biparietal or bifrontal electrodes. It selectively picks up <2 and up to 15 Hz frequencies of cerebral discharges by filtering out artefacts. It is preferable to use low impedance needle electrodes which are placed subdermally and secured with a tape. To ensure close contact between the electrode and brain, the impedance should be kept below 20 Z (ohms). The CFM record is evaluated for amplitude, background activity, burst suppression (flat tracing between 5 and 10 µ volts) and seizure activity.

The CFM is useful to continuously monitor CNS activity in neonates with (i) perinatal asphyxia to grade the severity of HIE, assess the need for whole body cooling and therapeutic response to anticonvulsants, (ii) encephalopathy or non-convulsive seizures due to any cause, (iii) monitoring the effects of anticonvulsants, and (iv) assessment of prognosis. It does not replace the conventional 19-lead EEG which is essential for diagnosis and management of seizures in newborns. Fetal EEG can be recorded by attaching electrodes directly on the scalp of fetus after surgical removal of fetus, attaching electrodes on the abdomen or cervix of the mother or by attaching electrodes to the scalp of infant during labor.

BERA Phone

It is a cot-side device to screen hearing of babies in the NICU by recording automated brainstem evoked response audiometry (BERA). It consists of a hand-held headphone unit having a set of three fixed touch electrodes and a preamplifier (Figure 2.27). The NICU should be noise-free and the baby should be asleep or calm and at least 34 weeks of gestation. The BERA phone is placed gently over one of the ear and electrodes are affixed with the help of gel. The mastoid electrode is placed below the ear lobe, the ground electrode is kept just above the ear lobe and vertex electrode is positioned higher up over the vertex. The correct position of BERA phone is checked by recording impedance which should be between 250 and 10,000 Ohm for each electrode pair, i.e. mastoid-ground and vertex-ground. A USB cable connects

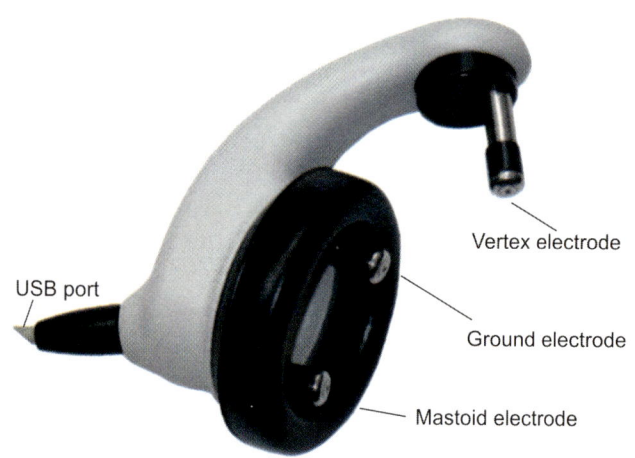

USB port

Vertex electrode

Ground electrode

Mastoid electrode

Figure 2.27 BERA phone with integrated electrodes.

BERA phone with a USB port of a notebook PC or desktop computer. The instrument delivers 35 dB sound stimuli or clicks to see whether wave V of automated auditory brainstem response (AABR) is present or absent. The result of screening is either PASS or REFER which is displayed on the computer. Both the ears are tested separately one after the other. When test result indicates REFER, the infant should be evaluated by an audiologist.

Extracorporeal Membrane Oxygenator (ECMO)

In seriously sick infants with persistent fetal circulation and diaphragmatic hernia, when conventional mechanical ventilation has failed, ECMO has been used with variable results. The technology requires appropriate instrumentation for cardiac bypass and a membrane of an appropriate size for the infant. The blood is drawn from a catheter in the right internal jugular vein or right atrium, it is oxygenated as it crosses the membrane, and then returned to the patient via the right common carotid artery or the femoral vein. The infant is kept heparinized and ventilated at low pressures, rates and oxygen concentrations. It is highly cost intensive modality demanding close cooperation and coordination of neonatologists with pediatric surgeons, nurses, trained technicians (perfusionists) and respiratory therapists. The ECMO may be venoarterial (VA) or venovenous (VV).

Venoarterial (VA) ECMO

The blood is drained from a vein (internal jugular vein, femoral vein) and returned into the arterial system (internal carotid artery). This extracorporeal right-to-left shunt unloads the failing heart by preload reduction. In order to ensure circulatory support, VA cannulation is performed. It is indicated for primary cardiac failure or respiratory failure combined with secondary cardiac failure. The patient's total cardiac output (CO) is the sum of the native CO and the pump flow generated by the circuit.

Venovenous (VV) ECMO

During VV ECMO, deoxygenated blood is drained from a large vein, it is oxygenated and decarboxylated in the extracorporeal device and returned to the right atrium. The blood is drained and returned to the jugular vein through a double-lumen cannula. The internal jugular vein has to be large enough for a 14-Fr double-lumen cannula. VV ECMO supports only the respiratory system and is indicated for isolated respiratory failure. It can be considered for respiratory failure combined with hypotension and cardiovascular instability, if hypoxemia is the sole cause of the hemodynamic instability. VV ECMO is changed to VA modality, if infant develops hypotension, cardiac failure or metabolic acidosis or when there are technical difficulties because of large recirculation in the venous cannula.

Placenta Prototype

The ultimate objective of bioengineers is to fabricate a sophisticated "uteroplacental unit" so that extrauterine survival of a fetus, which is born early is assured with least hazards and greater certainty. It appears to be an extremely difficult task because placenta is not merely a membrane oxygenator and renal dialyzer but has multiple additional biological roles. Apart from passive transport of oxygen and urea, placenta actively transports a variety of substances including amino acids, calcium, glucose and maternal antibodies. The placenta also functions as an important endocrine organ, secreting hormones that affect both mother and the fetus.

COT-SIDE LABORATORY FACILITIES

Satisfactory facilities for routine radiological examination should be available in the nursery round-the-clock. A good portable 3-phase generator X-ray machine of at least 200 milliamperes with extremely short exposure time (1/120 seconds) should preferably be housed in a small room adjacent to the NICU. In-house EKG, ultrasound, aEEG and echocardiography facilities should be available.

A side laboratory for routine analysis of blood, urine, amniotic fluid, gastric aspirate for shake test and cytology, Kleihauer-Betke count, glucose, bilirubin, hematocrit and arterial blood gases and acid–base parameters should be available. Centralized facilities for microbiochemical techniques especially for estimation of total and direct serum bilirubin, blood glucose, arterial PO_2, PCO_2, pH and base deficit are desirable. Facilities for analysis of serum sodium, potassium, calcium, magnesium and total serum proteins, and albumin should be available round-the-clock. The collection of venous blood is often difficult and hazardous in sick preterm babies. These babies often require frequent biochemical estimations. It is generally not appreciated that removal of 10 mL of blood from a 1,500 g infant amounts to about 8% of his total blood volume. This is equivalent to removal of about 400 mL of blood in an adult. Thus a microchemical laboratory which can carry out investigations on very small samples of blood obtained in heparinized capillary tubes or microcentrifuge tubes from heel puncture, should be considered as an essential facility for NICU.

TRANSPORT OF SICK NEONATES

Satisfactory transportation facilities are needed, whether a baby is being transported from one hospital to a regional or referral intensive care unit or simply within the hospital from NICU to the operation theater, imaging department or diagnostic laboratory. The short distance transport within the hospital can be accomplished in a transport incubator. The use of a plastic basket with perforated sides coupled with careful placing of hot water bottles or warm gel matresses is recommended for use in the rural setting. The baby can be wrapped in tin foil or covered with several layers of cotton and carried next to skin. Thermocole (polystyrene) box is an effective insulator and can be used in the community for transport of babies. Skin-to-skin contact with mother or a caretaker is a useful modality for transport in rural setting and resource poor situations. It is a sad reality that most transports in India are accomplished either by parents in their own vehicle or by utilizing private ambulances without any dedicated equipment or trained staff. It is no wonder that most babies are cold, blue or hypoglycemic when they reach the referral NICU. Regionalization of perinatal services cannot be achieved unless a network of efficient neonatal transport services are established.

Indications for Neonatal Transport

When a high-risk mother is identified, it is best to transfer her to a center having NICU facilities because uterus is an ideal transport incubator. It is desirable that delivery should take place in a tertiary care center so that a sick or high-risk baby is not exposed to the risks of neonatal transport. The neonate is transferred to the nearby NICU, if the parent hospital is not equipped to look after the health care needs of the infant. Depending upon the facilities available at the birthing hospital, the following neonates are transferred to a NICU providing tertiary care facilities.

- Preterm infants with a birth weight <1500 g or gestation <32 weeks.
- Respiratory distress requiring CPAP or assisted ventilation.
- Severe hypoxic–ischemic encephalopathy.
- Life-threatening sepsis.
- Intractable seizures.

- Severe jaundice with a need for exchange blood transfusion.
- Bleeding neonate.
- Cardiac failure or arrhythmia
- Major congenital anomalies or surgical neonate.
- Infants suspected to have inborn errors of metabolism.
- Procedures or diagnostic facilities unavailable at the parent hospital.

Pretransport Stabilization

Metabolic derangements like hypoglycemia, hypothermia, poor perfusion and oxygenation are reliable predictors of mortality in transported neonates. Pretransport stabilization basically includes maintenance of vitals and correction of metabolic derangements before start of journey. There are acronyms like STABLE (Sugar, Temperature, Artificial breathing, Blood pressure, Laboratory work-up, Emotional support) and TOPS [Temperature, Oxygenation (airway and breathing), Perfusion, Sugar] which are useful to remember important steps of pretransport stabilization. The STABLE program is a widely accepted pretransport neonatal stabilization educational and clinical tool. TOPS, a simplified assessment of neonatal acute physiology also gives a good prediction of mortality in sick neonates.

Airway

This includes maintaining a neonate's head in a slightly extended position or intubating the baby depending upon the respiratory and neurological status of the neonate. The infant can be transported without intubation, if the gestation is greater than 30 weeks, vital signs have been consistently stable in an FiO_2 of <0.5 and $PaCO_2$ is normal. If the infant is extremely preterm (<30 weeks), clinically unstable, has high oxygen requirement (FiO_2 of 0.5 or more), and rising $PaCO_2$, with recurrent apneic attacks, endotracheal intubation and respiratory support must be provided during the transport. If an infant is already intubated, it is better to transport the baby with a tube *in situ* and endotracheal tube position confirmed radiologically or by $EtCO_2$ monitoring. It is better to sedate an intubated baby during transport to prevent accidental tube dislodgement.

Breathing

Breathing is assessed by chest movements and good bilateral air entry. A portable ventilator in a good working condition is required to provide assisted breathing to an intubated infant. The blood gas parameters like PaO_2, $PaCO_2$, pH and SaO_2 should be satisfactory before commencement of journey. If an infant with pneumothorax is being transported, it is important to make sure that the chest drain is functioning.

Circulation

Sick infant should have secure and dependable venous access. A well positioned umbilical venous catheter is a safe and reliable route for the delivery of fluids and drugs, especially inotropes and prostaglandins. Baby's perfusion (color, capillary refill time, blood pressure) should be assessed prior to transport. Bolus of normal saline and inotropes should be initiated as per need. Severe anemia should be corrected by administration of packed RBCs. Arterial access is required for infants who are ventilated or who have an unstable circulation for invasive blood pressure and ABG monitoring. The umbilical artery, radial and posterior tibial arteries are the preferred sites. All lines and connections must be visible and marked with the site of insertion and details of the infusates and drugs being administered.

Temperature

Small and sick preterm infants rapidly lose heat. Hypothermia increases oxygen consumption and caloric requirements with increased risk of hypoxia, hypoglycemia, acidosis and intraventricular hemorrhage. It is important to warm the transport incubator to the correct temperature before the start of journey. After placing the infant in the incubator, affix the temperature sensing probe over right hypochondrium. On arrival at the referral hospital, connect the transport incubator to the mains supply, set the desired temperature and keep the access ports closed. Bubble sheet or polythene wraps can be used to cover smaller infants but without obscuring the sites of probes and cannulae.

Metabolic

Before transporting the baby, it is important to stabilize the sugar, electrolytes, blood gases and acid–base status. In the presence of metabolic acidosis, baby's perfusion should be assessed and shock should be managed. Antibiotics should be started when sepsis is suspected on clinical grounds or screening tests.

Transport Team and Equipment

The neonates needing special or intensive care should preferably be transported by a skilled transport team.

The receiving tertiary care NICU should have a dedicated team and a protocol for providing transport services. At least one senior resident and a specially trained neonatal nurse should report to the referring hospital to pick up the baby. The transport vehicle should be checked for availability of all equipment which should be in working order and should be equipped with essential supplies, disposables and life-saving drugs (Table 2.1). Customized transport ambulance should be equipped like a "mini-NICU" and should have a multi-channel vital sign monitor, portable incubator and a ventilator. The ambulance should be air conditioned, smooth in motion without any shaking and draughts of air. In India, most neonatal transports are executed in a road vehicle; while in some tertiary care centers in the West, helicopter or aircraft services are used for a long distance transport. The neonate needing transport should be transported with the quickest available transport through the shortest possible route.

The condition of the baby should be assessed before transfer. The goal of every transport is to bring a sick neonate to a specialized neonatal center in a stable condition. To avoid complications during transport, the infant should be as stable as possible before leaving the referring hospital. Hypothermia, hypovolemia,

---

TABLE 2.1 Equipment and supplies required during neonatal transport

- Transport incubator with multi-channel vital sign monitor for recording temperature, heart rate, blood pressure and oxygen saturation.
- CPAP facility with nasal prongs and portable ventilator (integral part of incubator or stand alone system).
- Airway equipment: Suction device, oral airway, T-piece device, nasal prongs, self or flow inflating bag and mask, laryngoscopes (size 00,0 and 1 blades) and endotracheal tubes (2.5, 3.0, 3.5, 4.0 mm), etc.
- Infusion facilities: Infusates, infusion pumps, glucometer.
- Oxygen and compressed air cylinder, oxygen hood, heat and light source, electrical power points and adaptors and a power backup with a dedicated generator or an inverter.
- Disposables: Catheters (5, 6, 8, 10, 12 Fr), syringes, needles, feeding tubes (8, 10 Fr), surgical alcohol, betadine swabs, micropore tape and gloves, etc.
- Instrument tray for endotracheal intubation, vascular access, insertion of chest tube and nasogastric tube, etc.
- Life-saving drugs.

1. All the equipment should have a battery backup and should be kept fully charged all the time.
2. Enough oxygen supply should be carried which should last during the duration of journey.

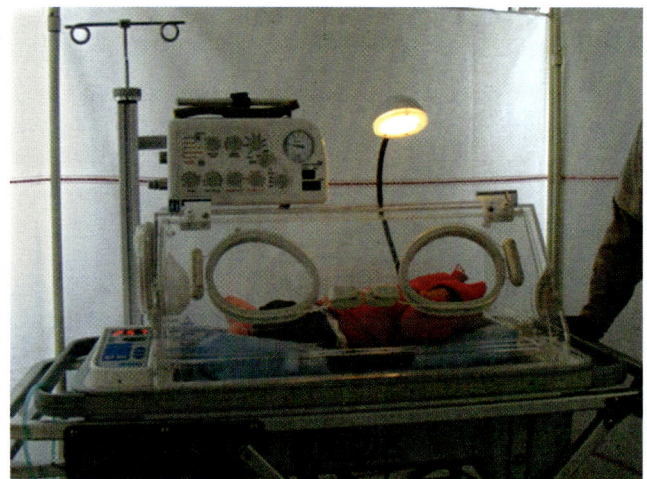

Figure 2.28 Battery-operated transport incubator with built-in oxygen supply and portable ventilator.

hypoglycemia, acidosis and seizures should be treated before baby is shifted to the transport vehicle. Oral feeding should be stopped and an IV line established at a peripheral site or through umbilical vein for administration of 10% dextrose. Add 1 unit of heparin per mL of fluid, if infusion is given through an umbilical catheter. The infant with history of frequent apneic spells or severe respiratory distress syndrome should be decompressed and intubated before the start of journey. The baby should be placed in a prewarmed transport incubator and administered oxygen. The portable incubator provides an ideal microenvironment during transport. It is battery operated and has built-in system for oxygen supply (Figure 2.28). The transport incubator should be light in weight but sturdy and should allow sufficient access to manage a critically ill baby. The transport team should estimate the amount of oxygen and air required during transport by assessing the distance, time required for journey and needs of the infant. The ambulance should be warm and well illuminated for observation of the baby. Temperature and color of the baby should receive due attention. Early transfer of a mildly ill baby is preferable to the transfer of a baby, whose condition has deteriorated to a state, when there is little hope for survival.

Air Transport

Air transport assures expedient and high quality care, and safe delivery of a critically sick infant to a tertiary care center. The first civilian hospital-based air medical helicopter service was established at St Anthony's Hospital in Denver, Colorado, in 1972. The two primary modes of air transport are helicopters (or rotor-wing aircraft, RWA) and airplanes (fixed-wing aircraft, FWA) with their own merits and demerits. Specialized air ambulances are not available in India and a modified nine-seater FWA is used for air transport because of safety, availability of pressurization, less noise and vibrations and feasibility for its use during long distance transport of 800–1500 km.

Air medical physiology Air transport is associated with changes in body physiology by virtue of altitude, noise and vibrations. As altitude increases, barometric pressure decreases requiring adjustments in FiO_2. Air expands at a higher altitude. It is mandatory that pneumothoraces are drained and a chest drain is *in situ* during air transport. Abdomen should be decompressed before transporting the infant in an aircraft. Because of changes in heart rate and peripheral vasoconstriction due to noise, it is desirable to insert ear muffs before the start of journey. Special precautions should be taken to harness the incubator firmly during take off and landing.

Equipment issues during air transport Hospital-based equipment may cause electromagnetic interference with aircraft navigation or communication system. Ventilators must have the operational tables, indicating changes in performance and corrective actions required at various altitudes. The oxygen analyser must have an altitude conversion table, indicating equivalent oxygen percentage concentrations at different altitudes. Non-invasive blood pressure readings may be inaccurate in a helicopter transport posing therapeutic issues. Pressure changes in intravenous solution containers can affect flow rates of fluids, intravenous lines should be operated on volume-regulated infusion pumps. All monitoring equipment and displays must be clearly visible from a variety of heights and angles by the transport personnel.

Protocol to be followed by the Referring Hospital

The neonate should be stabilized under the guidance of transport team of the referral NICU. The following management steps should be implemented and recorded.

- Maintain airway, oxygenation, thermal stability and tissue perfusion. In infants with RDS requiring long-distance transport, it is desirable to start CPAP through nasal prongs or nasopharyngeal catheter. It is recommended to intubate the baby before transport, if (i) infant with RDS needs ambient oxygen concentration of more than 40% (FiO_2 >0.4), (ii) recurrent apneic attacks, (iii) persistent seizures, (iv) shock, (v) infant receiving prostaglandin E_1 infusion for congenital heart lesions and (vi) congenital diaphragmatic hernia.

- Ensure umbilical or peripheral venous access and insert a nasogastric tube and decompress the stomach.
- Circulatory volume deficits of fluids and electrolytes should be replenished.
- Maintain adequate blood glucose level.
- Obtain culture samples and administer first dose of an appropriate antibiotic.
- Obtain a recent chest skiagram as a baseline and to check the position of catheters and tubes.
- Take the family member or parents along with the baby whenever feasible.
- When required, the transport team should undertake life-saving procedures (like endotracheal intubation, drainage of pneumothorax) and administer life-saving drugs, like surfactant and prostaglandin E_1.
- The referring hospital should prepare a detailed transport note including copies of obstetric and neonatal charts for the transport team (Box 2.2).

Care and Concerns during Transport

It is desirable to have a dedicated transport vehicles which should be adequately equipped to function like a mini or a portable NICU. The transport incubator

---

Box 2.2: Salient data to be recorded in the referral note prepared by the referring hospital

- Name, address and contact details of the referring and referral hospitals.
- Detailed perinatal history, labor, delivery and neonatal resuscitation.
- Name of the baby (mother's name), date and time of birth, mode of delivery, gestational age, birth weight and weight at transfer.
- Neonatal problems, complete diagnosis, and treatment given before transfer.
- Condition of the baby at the time of transfer: Vital signs, arterial blood gases (ABG), complete blood counts (CBC), blood sugar, bilirubin, blood urea nitrogen (BUN), imaging studies, supportive care and medications being given before transfer.
- Mode of transport.
- The possible needs for emergency procedures during the transport.
- Reason/s for transport.
- Duly signed consent form by parents.
- The name/s and contact number/s of key personnel at the referral NICU.

---

and portable ventilator or stand alone CPAP facility should be securely fixed to the vehicle rails to avoid unnecessary jolts and jumps. The oxygen cylinder/s, air tanks and monitoring equipment should be securely fastened. Depending upon the condition of the baby and duration of the journey, there should be sufficient supply of oxygen and air. There should be uninterrupted power source (dedicated generator, inverter, batteries) to operate the incubator, ventilator and monitoring equipment. Necessary adapters should be available to access the ambulance power source. The ambient conditions in the vehicle should ensure temperature stability, avoidance of excessive noise and vibrations and prevention of infection. The transport journey should be rapid and smooth without compromising the safety.

The ambulance temperature should be maintained above 26°C. In order to ensure optimal thermal control, availability of a transport incubator is ideal. When transport incubator is not available, thermal stability can be ensured through various improvisations like skin-to-skin contact, polythene covering, thermocole box or basket and use of phase-change warm gel mattress. Enteral feeds should be avoided in critically sick infants and they should preferably be given intravenous fluids. Infant should be positioned with slight extension of neck to maintain patency of the airway. Depending upon the respiratory studies and arterial oxygen saturation, infant may be provided with nasal CPAP through a T-piece resuscitator or attached to a ventilator. If tissue perfusion is poor (cold extremities, capillary refil time ≥2 sec or low blood pressure), infant should receive intravenous fluids with inotropes. The transport team should carefully observe the infant and various monitoring parameters so that corrective intervention/s are undertaken without any delay. The transport team should remain in constant touch with the nodal staff of the referral NICU to inform them about the latest condition of the baby and seek their expert guidance and advice during the course of transport.

Complications during Transport

Complications during transportation of sick neonates on life support measures may arise either due to failure of equipment, excessive movement and worsening of the clinical condition of the baby. The common complications encountered during transport are listed below.

- Hyperventilation during manual ventilation may cause respiratory alkalosis, cardiac arrhythmias and hypotension.
- The loss of PEEP may result in hypoxemia.

- Inadvertent disconnection of intravenous drugs like inotropes or prostaglandins may lead to hypotension or hypoxemia.
- Movements due to rough ride may result in accidental extubation, disconnection from ventilator support, dislodgement of vascular access and bleeding.
- Equipment failure, and exhaustion of oxygen cylinder may occur.

Special Clinical Circumstances

The basics of organization of transport and monitoring remain the same with some specific components of care during special clinical situations as mentioned below.

Respiratory distress syndrome Infant should be provided with CPAP through nasal prongs or intubated and provided assisted ventilation during transport. FiO_2 should be adjusted to maintain SpO_2 between 85 and 90%. Resuscitation facilities and adequate supply of oxygen should be available for the duration of transport. The referral unit should be fully prepared to administer surfactant as soon as the neonate is received.

Congenital diaphragmatic hernia Baby should preferably be intubated and ventilated during transport with large bore nasogastric tube *in situ* for continuous decompression of stomach. These infants should never be ventilated with a bag and mask. If baby is having features of persistent pulmonary hypertension and shock, inotropes and vasodilators should be started.

Spina bifida with myelomeningocele Position the infant either prone (preferable) or on the side and dress the lesion with a sterile non-adhesive dressing and cover it with a sterile gauze.

Necrotizing enterocolitis Fluid resuscitation, antibiotics, securing the airway and ventilation are important interventions when transferring babies with NEC. Bowel should be decompressed and continuous nasogastric drainage is mandatory. A tension pneumoperitoneum should be aspirated prior to transfer to allow adequate ventilation.

Esophageal atresia and tracheo-esophageal fistula During transfer, the proximal pouch is decompressed using a sump drain (10 Replogle tube) with continuous suction.

Gastroschisis or exomphalos Nasogastric decompression should be done. The exposed herniated bowel is a source of heat and fluid loss. The baby should be covered with a cling film and bowel wrapped with sterile gauze. To prevent stretching or twisting of the mesentery and possible vascular compromise, the infant should be nursed in lateral decubitus.

Congenital heart disease During first few weeks of life, the duct-dependent cardiac malformations present as worsening cyanosis, hypoxemia, metabolic acidosis and shock. In these infants, it is critical to maintain patency of duct by prostaglandin infusion. It is preferable to intubate and ventilate these infants because of the risk of apnea during prostaglandin infusion.

Cooling during Transport

Therapeutic hypothermia is the standard treatment to decrease adverse consequences of hypoxic-ischemic encephalopathy and improve the survival of infants with moderate to severe birth asphyxia. Because hypothermia must be initiated within first six hours of life, cooling during transport is an important issue in developing countries when infant is born in a peripheral center and needs to be transported to a tertiary care center for further management. As per 2015 NRP recommendations, therapeutic hypothermia in resource-limited settings may be considered and offered but only under clearly defined protocols and in facilities having capabilities for multidisciplinary care and long-term follow-up. Servo-controlled active cooling improves thermal control, avoids temperature fluctuations and reduces stabilization time compared to passive cooling. If active cooling facilities are not available, passive cooling with continuous rectal temperature monitoring is advocated during transport.

Medicolegal Issues Associated with Transport

Excellent communication between transporting team and the parents is important to avoid any medicolegal issues. In case of cardiorespiratory arrest during transport, ambulance should be stopped and baby should be resuscitated according to the NRP guidelines. In case of the death of the baby, team should approach a nearby health facility and a death certificate should be issued by the transporting team after emergency admission. Parents should be constantly kept informed.

Quality Assurance

Quality management program should be an integral part of development of transport system. It assesses all the aspects of transport including patient care, communication, training of manpower, maintenance of required certifications, ambulance maintenance, safety issues and establishment of patient care guidelines. The institution providing transport services should have predefined quality indicators and should follow local standards of operation and regional standards of care.

Arrival at the Receiving NICU

The transport team should remain in constant touch with the referral NICU during the course of journey. The referral center should have a dedicated communication facility with mobile helplines operating 24 hours a day for ease of constant communication. The team should brief the NICU caregivers regarding the status of the baby and immediate clinical concerns. The clinical documents including referral note, copies of charts, consent form, radiographs and investigation reports, etc. should be handed over to the receiving unit. The referring hospital and parents of the baby (if not accompanying during transport) should be informed about the safe arrival and latest condition of the baby. The inventory of transport equipment should be checked, medications and essential supplies should be restocked for the next transport service. When infant has recovered from the underlying emergency and is stable for several days and he does not require intensive care, he is discharged or transported back (reverse transport) to the referring hospital.

PROCEDURE MANUAL FOR THE NICU

In view of the fact that many personnel working in the NICU are relatively floating, it is essential to have a procedure manual to establish continuity and uniformity of service. It should offer ready guidance to the new nurses and resident physicians so that the routines and policies for neonatal care are maintained at an optimal level.

The manual should outline detailed instructions regarding care of the baby in the labor room. Indications for admission to the NICU should be stated. The routines to be followed in the lying-in ward regarding bath, feeding, prophylaxis, etc. should be outlined. A detailed description of various house keeping rituals for prevention of infection in the NICU is most rewarding. Detailed instructions should be provided regarding temperature control of the nursery, incubator care, keeping babies warm, nurses observations, weight record and working knowledge of various equipment. The nurses should be conversant with various danger signs in the babies. The policy regarding mother–baby contact, discharge, aftercare and what to do when a baby dies, should be clearly defined. It is essential to have various charts, such as intrauterine growth charts, postnatal growth charts, feeding routines, thermoneutral ambient temperature ranges for low birth weight babies, drugs and dosages, etc. for ready reference. The resident doctors should be given guidelines for the management of common neonatal emergencies, such as birth asphyxia, hypothermia, respiratory distress syndrome, jaundice, sepsis and bleeding. A complete protocol and guidelines should be available for the transport team.

A computer with an internet facility should be available in the NICU. It can be used to download reports of laboratory investigations. The details of various equipment, their spares and accessories, addresses and telephone numbers of suppliers can be stored in the computer. It can be used for printing discharge summaries and analyzing the data regarding the morbidity, mortality and follow-up of NICU babies.

COOPERATION BETWEEN OBSTETRICIANS AND NEONATOLOGISTS

For effective delivery of perinatal services and to improve the management and outcome of newborn babies, the neonatologist should establish a close interaction and collaboration with a large number of specialists especially obstetrician, pediatric surgeon, anesthetist, pediatric pathologist, pediatric radiologist, biochemist and biomedical engineer. Each one of these sub-specialists provides important and crucial links but cooperation and interaction with obstetricians is most vital to upgrade and improve the perinatal services in the teaching institutions and corporate hospitals. The neonatologists should not merely provide care to the newborn baby after their birth but must actively involve themselves with issues pertaining to fetal diagnosis, fetal therapy and over all fetal wellbeing.

The purpose of pregnancy is to produce a baby which should be healthy, good-sized, and free from any malformations. The obstetrician should ensure that this physiological function is achieved with minimal hazards to the mother. The pediatrician expends his efforts to make certain that the baby survives the hazards of delivery, cardiorespiratory adaptation, biological inadequacies and environmental insults after birth. It is often forgotten that discredit for the death of a baby or credit for his ultimate survival, usually goes to the obstetrician because mother has reposed her confidence and full faith in her obstetrician who had provided all the care to her before conception, throughout pregnancy and during delivery. It is but natural that the obstetrician cannot suddenly sever her/his links with the family after delivering the baby. Indeed, the pediatricians must appreciate the magnanimity and faith that the obstetricians repose in them by handing over the baby, whom they had nurtured and tendered for nine long months. It is, therefore, desirable that pediatricians and obstetricians must join hands with each other not only to enhance neonatal survival but also to improve the quality of life among the survivors. The cooperation is particularly desired in the following areas of perinatal care.

Antenatal Care and Fetal Diagnosis

Pediatricians should be actively involved so that they can give their advice and expert guidance in the field of fetal diagnosis and fetal therapy by attending fetal medicine or high-risk mothers antenatal clinic. The responsibility for assessment of severity of rhesus isoimmunization, use of antenatal anti-D immunoglobulins, timing of delivery in various high-risk situations, assessment of the risk of continuing in utero existence versus extrauterine care (on the basis of available facilities in NICU) should be jointly shared and decision taken by weighing all the pros and cons.

Perinatal Hypoxia

Adequate infrastructural facilities must be made available to the pediatrician in the delivery room and maternity OT in order to provide resuscitation facilities to all babies in every birthing room. The potentially harmful drugs, like pethidine, morphine, diazepam, etc. should be avoided during labor. The neonatologist should maintain constant liaison with expectant mothers by visiting the pre-delivery suites. Infants with fetal hypoxia must be promptly delivered and pediatrician must be informed well in time so that he/she is available at the time of delivery. The obstetricians must also be trained in the skills and art of neonatal resuscitation to handle the exigencies of unexpected or precipitate deliveries. It is important that level III perinatal facilities must evolve in paripassu with level III neonatal care services by creating facilities for improved monitoring of fetus before birth and during labor. The widening gap between the quality of obstetrical and neonatal services must be narrowed. The delivery complex of the hospital should be designated as perinatal intensive care unit and administrators should be approached for adequate inputs of space, staff, and equipment.

Promotion of Feeding with Human Milk

The mother must be physically and emotionally prepared for breastfeeding during antenatal visits. The problems of retracted or cracked nipples must be managed before the baby is born. Additional room, attached to the nursery, should be available to promote the feeding of all preterm and high-risk babies with expressed breast milk (EBM). The mothers are encouraged to visit this facility round-the-clock for promotion of breastfeeding and expression of breast milk with the help and guidance of a lactation nurse. The mother should be allowed to stay in the lying-in ward as long as her baby is being managed in the NICU so that the baby is provided with all the therapeutic advantages of mother-infant bonding, EBM and skin-to-skin contact. The medications which are known to produce hazards to the suckling infant should be avoided during lactation. Above all, there should not be any contradiction between the advice of the obstetrician and pediatrician regarding feeding of babies to avoid any confusion in the minds of mothers. The feeding advice should be uniform and unambiguous. The policies and practices to be followed in the rooming-in ward should be finalized after mutual discussion. The instruction manual should be available for the benefit of residents and nursing staff.

Supervised Care of LBW Babies

The policy of early discharge from NICU is desirable to decongest the nursery in order to reduce the risk of nosocomial infections. The extended nursery concept should be utilized by providing an area with adequate physical facilities, warmth, asepsis and weighing scale, etc. in the rooming-in ward. After initial management of life-threatening disorders, once the baby is stabilized, he/she can be managed in the "growing nursery" by the mother under the supervision and guidance of a nurse. The mother can be taught basic principles of Kangaroo mother care and home care of a LBW baby before she is discharged from the hospital. During follow-up, the mothers are likely to be more receptive and responsive to the pediatrician, who must share responsibility and concern to give advice and guidance to the mother regarding birth spacing and family welfare.

BIBLIOGRAPHY

Alberman E, Collingwood J, Pharoah POD, Vaizey J, Oppe TE. Arrangements for special care and intensive care of the newborn. Brit Med J 1977, 2: 1045.

American Academy of Pediatrics. Guidelines for Perinatal Care. 4th Ed. Illinois/Washington: *American Academy of Pediatrics and American College of Obstetricians and Gynecologists,* 2002.

American Academy of Pediatrics. Guidelines for Air and Ground Transport of Neonatal and Pediatric Patients. Chicago: *American Academy of Pediatrics*, 2003.

American Academy of Pediatrics. Committee on Fetus and Newborn. Levels of neonatal care. *Pediatrics* 2012, 130(3): 587–597.

Bergman I. Questions concerning safety and use of cranial ultrasonography in the neonate. *J Pediatr* 1983, 103: 855.

Blix E, Kumle M, Kaergaard H, Oian P, Lindgren HE. Transfer to hospital in planned home births: A systematic review. *BMC Pregnancy and Child Birth* 2014, 14: 179.

Chandrasekaran M, Swamy R, Ramji S, Sankaran S, Thayyil S. Therapeutic hypothermia for neonatal encephalopathy in Indian neonatal units: A survey of national services. *Indian Pediatr* 2017, 54:969–70.

Cornette L. Contemporary neonatal transport: Problems and solutions. *Arch Dis Child Fetal Neonatal Ed* 2004, 89: F 212.

Cornette L. Transporting the sick neonate. *Current Pediatr* 2004, 14: 20–25.

Deorari AK, Paul VK. Neonatal Equipment: Everything that you would like to know. *Sagar Publications, New Delhi* 4th edition, 2010.

Dingle RE, Grady MD, Lee JA, Paul S. Continuous transcutaneous oxygen monitoring in the neonate. *Amer J Nurs* 1980, 80: 890.

Gluck L (Ed.). Organization of perinatal care. *Clin Perinatology* 1976, 3: 267.

Gluck L. Design of perinatal center. *Pediatr Clin N Amer* 1979, 17: 777.

Hegyi T. Transcutaneous bilirubinometery: A new light on old subject. *Pediatrics* 1982, 69: 124.

Jeyapal S, Kommu PPK, Manikandan M, Krishnan L. Performance of two different pulse oximeters in neonatal transition. *Indian J Pediatr* 2017, 84(1): 7–12.

Lagler U, Duc G. Systolic blood pressure in normal infants during the first 6 hours of life: Transcutaneous Doppler ultrasound technique. *Biol Neonate 1980,* 37: 243.

Long GJ, Lucey JF, Philip AGS. Noise and hypoxemia in the intensive care nursery. *Pediatrics* 1980, 65: 143–145.

Malhotra AK, Deorari AK, Paul VK, Bagga A, Singh M. A new transport incubator for primary care of low birth weight babies. *Indian Pediatr* 1992, 29: 587–593.

Murdoch DR, Darlow BA. Handling during neonatal intensive care. *Arch Dis Child* 1984, 59: 957–961.

Orr RA, Felmet KA, Han Y, *et al.* Pediatric specialized transport teams are associated with improved outcomes. *Pediatrics* 2009, 124(1): 381–383.

Philip AGS. Bio-invasive diagnostic techniques in newborn infants. *Pediatr Clin N Amer* 1982, 29: 1275.

Raghu Raman TS. NICU environment—A need for change. *Indian Pediatr* 1997, 34: 414–419.

Segal S, Pirie GE. Equipment and personnel for neonatal special care. *Pediatr Clin N Amer* 1970, 17: 793.

Shellhaas RA, Chang T, Tsuchida T, *et al.* The American Clinical Society Guidelines on continuous electroencephalography monitoring in neonates. *J Clin Neurophysiol* 2011, 28(6): 611–7.

Singh M, Paul VK, Deorari AK. Biomedical equipments: Status and perspective. *National Neonatology Forum,* New Delhi 1990.

Singh M. Neonatal care perspectives in India (Editorial). *Indian J Pediatr* 1998, 65: 243–247.

Steggerda S, Leijser L, Walther FJ, Van Wezel-Mei Jhu G. Neonatal cranial ultrasonography: How to optimize its performance. *Early Human Development* 2009, 85: 93–99.

Thayyil S. Cooling therapy for neonatal encephalopathy in low- and middle-income countries. *Indian Pediatr* 2018, 55:197–8.

Thayyil S, Oliveira V, Lally PJ, Swamy R, Bassett P, Chandrasekaran M, *et al.* Hypothermia for encephalopathy in low and middle-income countries (HELIX): Study protocol for a randomized controlled trial. *Trials* 2017, 18:432.

Tyne MD. Concepts for improved nursery design. *Hospitals* 1974, 48: 66.

Vidyasagar D, Raju TNK. Non-invasive technique of measuring intracranial pressure in the newborn. *Pediatrics* 1977, 59 (suppl.): 957.

Woodward A, Insoft R, Kleinman N (Eds). Guidelines for Air and Ground Transport of Neonatal and Pediatric patients. 3rd edition, *American Academy of Pediatrics* 2007.

Preventive Neonatology

In the best pediatric tradition, the approach in perinatal medicine should be oriented towards prevention. Throughout the lifespan of an individual, perinatal period is of greatest danger as regards survival and occurrence of handicaps. As opposed to geriatrics, deaths during this period truly represent a nipping of life in the bud and sequelae of various neonatal hazards manifest as a lifelong disability. The aim of preventive neonatology is to reduce perinatal and neonatal mortality and to ensure complete freedom from physical and mental handicaps among those who survive.

PRENATAL CARE

The health of the baby must be guarded from the day of conception. Maternal health before conception, the genetic endowments of sperms and ova, maternal milieu and maternal infections, like rubella, have profound influence on the outcome of pregnancy.

Premarital Health Check-up

A girl should undergo a complete medical check-up before getting married so that she is fully equipped to meet the needs of her baby when she gets pregnant. The ideal age of 18–35 years for bearing children needs to be emphasized to discourage too early and late marriages. Despite Child Marriage Act 1978, about 30% girls in India are married off before the age of 18 years and without their consent. The government of India has launched a scheme *Apni beti apna dhan* in order to give an incentive of ₹ 25,000-00 to the family who has a daughter who is unmarried on her 18th birthday. There is increasing trend for late marriages or delayed pregnancy due to career concerns by the working couples. Advanced maternal age is associated with declining fertility, increased risk of miscarriage and stillbirth, chromosomal abnormalities, hypertensive complications and prematurity. A detailed systemic examination should be conducted to identify and treat any underlying systemic disorder, like hypertension, heart disease, bronchial asthma, diabetes mellitus, hypothyroidism, urinary tract infection, pelvic inflammatory disease and sexually transmitted disease. Prospective mother should be informed about the harmful effects of smoking or chewing tobacco, excessive intake of alcohol, and substance abuse on the growing fetus.

Healthy women produce healthy babies while undernourished and sick women are likely to produce LBW and high-risk babies. According to National Nutrition Monitoring Bureau of India, 75% of adolescent girls are anemic with high incidence of deficiency of iron, folic acid and other micronutrients. The average weight and height of rural women in India are 42 kg and 152 cm, respectively. One-third of 18-yr-old women in India have a body weight of <40 kg and height of <145 cm and they are vulnerable to produce LBW babies. Special emphasis should be placed on the health care and nutrition of girl children during infancy and adolescence. Nutritional deficiencies, if any, should be recognized and corrected before pregnancy is contemplated. Adequacy of iron stores should be ensured before pregnancy rather than trying to correct the deficiency state during pregnancy. Adolescent girls should be provided with supplements of iron to maintain hemoglobin and serum ferritin levels above 12 g/dL and >35 ng/L, respectively. Premarital genetic counseling and recognition of metabolic carrier states in the would-be couples help to reduce the incidence of genetic disorders. All girls should preferably be immunized against rubella and tetanus before marriage. There is a genuine need to produce an effective vaccine against cytomegalovirus infections.

Physiological and Metabolic Changes during Pregnancy

During pregnancy, there is a gradual expansion of plasma volume and increase in cardiac output. The peak expansion of plasma volume of 50% is achieved at 28 weeks of gestation. There is reduction in hemoglobin, albumin and water-soluble vitamins. The iron requirements during pregnancy are enhanced by 100% (30 mg of elemental iron/d) due to borderline iron status of Indian women and to meet the iron requirements of fetus and placenta and replenish the anticipated loss of 600–1000 mL of blood at delivery. There is enhanced calcium and iron absorption and increased nitrogen retention during pregnancy. There is increased risk of gestational diabetes mellitus due to increased release of stress hormones. There are increased levels of placental hormones (estrogen and progesterone) with elevation of triglycerides, cholesterol, vitamin E, carotene and blood clotting factors, like fibrinogen. Apart from increased sex and stress hormones, there is greater elaboration of T_3, T_4 and insulin during pregnancy.

CARE OF THE MOTHER DURING PREGNANCY

Pregnancy is a physiological process but it can impose considerable risks both to the mother and her unborn child. Adequate antenatal care and maintenance of optimal nutrition by proper dietary advice are crucial for favorable outcome of pregnancy. She should avoid taking any drugs, as far as possible, during first trimester of pregnancy which is a period of organogenesis. During pregnancy, the mother must eat for two, for herself and for her growing infant. She should consume additional 350–500 kcalories and 20 g proteins by taking fresh green vegetables, pulses and legumes, milk and milk products and seasonal fruits. Pregnant women should take at least 2.6 g of omega-3 fatty acids and 300 mg of docosahexaenoic acid (DHA) to ensure adequate growth of fetal brain. Intake of folic acid 400 μg/day during periconceptional period is recommended to reduce the risk of neural tube defects. Women with previous history of neural tube defects are advised to take 5 mg folic acid daily when planning for pregnancy and during first 3 months of gestation. The total energy cost of pregnancy is around 80,000 kcal. The deficiency of micronutrients during pregnancy is associated with increased risk of abortions, neural tube defects and stunting of fetal growth. There is some evidence to suggest that adequate intake of calcium, riboflavin, vitamin C, vitamin E and omega-3 fatty acids is associated with reduced incidence of pre-eclampsia. Vitamin D deficiency is common in pregnant women and nursing mothers throughout the world. The endogenous production of vitamin D in the skin by effect of sunlight is compromised due to several factors. They include lifestyle changes, urbanization, lack of outdoor activities, overcrowding, over clothing, skin pigmentation, etc. The dietary sources of vitamin D like fatty fish, fortified dairy product and egg yolk are expensive and poorly consumed. When a nursing mother is given 5000–6000 i.u. of vitamin D everyday, her breast milk content of vitamin D is adequate to meet the RDA of her exclusively breastfed infant without any supplements. During second half of pregnancy, she should receive regular supplements of iron and folic acid daily to maintain hemoglobin above 11 g/dL. When adequate intake of protein and micronutrients cannot be ensured by consumption of balanced nutritious food, commercially available nutritional supplements should be given during pregnancy. It is important to remember that up to 25% of energy should come from protein sources because excessive intake of protein has no additional benefits and has been shown to adversely affect the fetal growth. The recommended dietary allowances of key nutrients during pregnancy and lactation are shown in Table 3.1.

In order to conserve the energy expenditure, mother should be advised adequate physical rest and relaxation during last trimester of pregnancy so that energy is spared for the growth of the fetus. Every pregnant woman must receive two doses of tetanus toxoid four

TABLE 3.1 Recommended dietary allowances during pregnancy and lactation*

Nutrient	Pre-pregnancy	Pregnancy	Lactation
▪ Calories (kcal)**	2200	2500	2700
▪ Proteins (g)	45–50	60	75
▪ Vitamin A (mg)	800	800	1300
▪ Vitamin C (mg)	60	75	90
▪ Vitamin D (iu)	800	1000	5000–6000
▪ Folate (μg)	180	400	280
▪ Calcium (mg)	800	1200	1200
▪ Phosphorus (mg)	800	1200	1200
▪ Iron (mg)	15	30	15
▪ Iodine (μg)	60	75	90
▪ Zinc (mg)	12	15	19

*Food and Nutrition Board, National Research Council, RDA's 10th Ed; Washington DC 1989.

**The caloric cost of pregnancy is 80,000 kcal while caloric cost of 6 months of exclusive breastfeeding is around 100,000 kcal.

Preventive Neonatology

3

weeks apart as a safeguard against development of tetanus neonatorum. Tetanus toxoid may be given any time during the pregnancy but the second dose must be received at least 4 weeks before the anticipated time of delivery. She must be emotionally and physically prepared and motivated for breastfeeding by paying proper attention to her breasts and nipples during pregnancy. The underlying systemic problems and pregnancy-induced disorders must be identified early and managed appropriately. Mothers with high-risk factors should be recognized early and given special care in the antenatal clinic. The pediatrician must be involved with the care of the unborn baby during the antenatal period to ensure enhanced survival of newborn babies.

Stimulation of the Fetus

Fetus is fully aware and perceptive in the womb. Fetus can hear sounds as early as 20 weeks and ears are structurally well formed by 24 weeks of gestation. Apart from physical connection, there is an ethereal or spiritual bond between the mother and her baby in the womb. Every emotion experienced by the mother is transmitted as vibrations and vibes to her baby. Her thoughts and perceptions have a profound effect on her unborn baby. The "mother in making" should be meditative and have positive and vibrant thoughts of love, peace and hope to touch the soul of her baby. It is well known that babies respond to their mother's heart beats and voice while still in the womb. There is research evidence to suggest that thoughts and actions of a pregnant woman have a profound effect in molding the character of the child in the womb. The fetus is most alert and perceptive during the night. It seems when the tired mother lies down for rest, her baby wakes up and kicks around. This *in utero* behavior of the baby may continue even after birth, that is why babies are usually more active, awake and playful at night for several weeks after birth. In order to take advantage of this *in utero* behavior, the mother can stimulate her baby. Every night she can touch and communicate with her baby, for example by saying Hi this is your mummy calling. I love you Kabir (any assumed pet name), you are going to be a smart and happy baby. You are going to be a kind, generous and compassionate human being. Mother can hum a soothing song, recite a nursery rhyme or sing a lullaby. Audio cassettes of classical or instrumental music, stories of bravery or compassionate acts are available which can be played through mummy's tummy. Researchers in Spain have invented a device called Babypod™, an intravaginal device, emitting 54 decibel sound which is equivalent to the sound of a conversation. The mother can insert a small pink speaker in her vagina and control it by using a phone app to play music and messages at her convenience especially when her fetus is most perceptive.

HIGH-RISK PREGNANCIES

The high-risk factors may be preconceptional and these may be present at the time of the first visit to the antenatal clinic or they may appear subsequently during the course of pregnancy.

Primary Selection of High-Risk Pregnancy

1. Poor socioeconomic status and maternal illiteracy.
2. Maternal undernutrition, short stature (<145 cm), under weight (<40 kg) or obese (BMI >30) and anemic (hemoglobin of less than 8 g/dL) mother.
3. Interpregnancy interval of <24 months
4. Primigravida or grand multipara (>4)
5. Maternal age of less than 18 years or more than 35 years.
6. Presence of chronic systemic illness including kidney disease, hypertension, heart disease, bronchial asthma, autoimmune disease and endocrinal disorders, such as diabetes mellitus, hypothyroidism and thyrotoxicosis.
7. Past obstetrical history of difficult or operative deliveries, abortions, stillbirths, genetic disorders, neonatal deaths, low birth weight babies and developmental defects.
8. Rhesus negative blood group
9. Sexually transmitted disease (STD)
10. Substance abuse

Secondary Selection of High-Risk Pregnancy

The appearance of any of the following disorders during the course of pregnancy should receive immediate attention of the obstetrician. The key time for reassessment of these secondary high-risk factors is around 28th week of gestation.

1. Pregnancy-induced hypertension or pre-eclampsia
2. Gestational diabetes mellitus
3. Rhesus isoimmunization
4. Maternal infections
5. Slow growth of the fetus
6. Antepartum hemorrhage
7. Anemia (hemoglobin <8 g/dL)
8. Abnormal presentation, like unstable lie, breech presentation, vertex malposition, face presentation, etc.

9. Multiple pregnancy
10. Poly- and oligohydramnios
11. Cephalopelvic disproportion
12. Fetal distress
13. Prelabor rupture of membranes (PROM) or preterm premature rupture of membranes (PPROM) when ROM occurs before 37 weeks of gestation.
14. Early onset of labor

FETAL MONITORING

During the last two decades or so, greater concern has been shown to monitor and ensure the welfare of unborn child. Several technological advances, like ultrasound and continuous fetal heart rate monitoring, have improved the outcome of high-risk pregnancies.

Fetal Maturity

Date of last menstrual period (LMP) provides the most accurate means of computing the gestational age of the fetus. Human gestation averages 280 days and expected date of delivery is calculated by adding 9 calendar months +7 days to the first day of the last menstrual period. The actual duration of pregnancy is two weeks shorter than this period because conception occurs around midpoint of menstrual cycle. The gestational age is reliable, if mother had regular periods, kept record of LMP and was not using oral contraceptives prior to conception. Due to ignorance and illiteracy, many Indian women do not keep record of their menstrual history thus denying this vital landmark of pregnancy to the obstetrician.

Physical Examination

Pelvic examination around 8 to 10 weeks of gestation can accurately date the pregnancy by assessing uterine size, if there are no uterine fibroids or retroversion and excessive obesity. Accurate measurement of height of uterine fundus from symphysis pubis can provide estimate of gestational age within ±4 weeks. The uterine height averages 20 cm at 20 weeks of gestation and 28 cm at 28 weeks of gestation in the absence of obesity, polyhydramnios, fibroids, and twins. Uterine fundal height as an index for assessing duration of pregnancy becomes unreliable after 28 weeks due to high incidence of disorders of fetal growth during third trimester of pregnancy.

Quickenings or fetal movements are perceived around 18 to 20 weeks of gestation but may be unreliable in an inexperienced primigravida mother. Fetal heart sounds are first heard between 16 and 20 weeks of gestation with a conventional fetoscope. They provide a useful landmark, if mother is examined at weekly intervals after 12 to 14 weeks of gestation.

Radiologic Examination

Distal femoral epiphysis is usually present by 36 weeks and proximal tibial epiphysis by 40 weeks of gestation. Therefore, the absence of distal femoral epiphyses indicates prematurity and the presence of proximal tibial epiphyses connotes maturity. However, because of variability in the time of appearance of epiphyses, delay in their appearance in infants with intrauterine malnutrition and hazards of ionizing radiation to the developing fetus, radiological examination for assessment of fetal maturity is not recommended.

Ultrasound

During early pregnancy, measurement of the crown-rump and crown-heel length with real-time or B-mode ultrasound can date the pregnancy within one day. Measurement of fetal biparietal diameter (BPD) is accurate within ±3 days up to 28 weeks of gestation. Subsequently, assessment of fetal maturity on the basis of BPD is unreliable and it increases at a rate of about 1.8 mm/week during the last 10 weeks of pregnancy. BPD around 38 weeks of gestation averages 9 cm in Indian babies. Femoral length is a more reliable ultrasonographic parameter of fetal age during later gestation with an accuracy of ±8 days. Fetal length/ head circumference is a more robust parameter to characterize fetal proportions compared to fetal length/biparietal ratio.

Amniotic Fluid Analysis

Please refer to **Chapter 29** for procedure of amniocentesis.

Surfactant The word surfactant is an abbreviation for surface active agent. The appearance of surfactant in the fetal lung is related to gestational maturity and it provides protection to the infant against occurrence of hyaline membrane disease (HMD) after birth. The principal pulmonary surfactant is a specialized phospholipid, dipalmitoyl lecithin or phosphatidyl choline, synthesized by type II alveolar cells of lungs. Surfactants are usually organic compound that are amphiphilic, meaning they contain both hydrophobic groups (their tails) and hydrophilic groups (their heads). Therefore, a surfactant contains both a water-insoluble (or oil-soluble) component and a water-soluble component. The surface active material is available in adequate quantities around 35 weeks of

Preventive Neonatology

3

gestation and can effectively lower the surface tension so that alveoli do not completely collapse during expiration. Fetal lung fluid containing surfactant travels up to hypopharynx with the help of respiratory mucosal cilia. It is partly swallowed by the baby and partly washed away by the amniotic fluid. Therefore, before birth, the amniotic fluid surfactant levels reflect the concentration of surfactant elaborated in the fetal lung. Lecithin and sphingomyelin are present in identical concentrations until the middle of third trimester. At this point, the level of lecithin begins to increase whereas that of sphingomyelin remains relatively constant. Around 35 weeks of gestation, average L/S ratio approximates 2 which is indicative of satisfactory fetal lung maturity. The results of L/S ratio may be unreliable, if specimen of amniotic fluid is contaminated with meconium or blood, diluted due to polyhydramnios, advanced maternal age, diabetes mellitus, Rh-isoimmunization, multiple gestation, sample stored too long or centrifuged at high speed.

Amniotic fluid *bubble stability or shake test* is a reliable bedside screening test to assess fetal lung maturity. Undiluted amniotic fluid and its various saline dilutions are taken in test tubes and shaken for 15 seconds with an equivalent volume of 95% ethanol. The tubes are allowed to stand for 15 minutes and test is read as positive, if a complete ring of bubbles persist at the meniscus. Positive shake test in dilutions of 1:2 or greater correlates well with mature L/S ratios and reduced risk of HMD. Another simple test to assess the maturity of fetus is to determine amniotic fluid optical density at 650 nm. An optical density of 0.15 or greater correlates well with mature L/S ratio. The negative shake test or optical density test should be rechecked by performing L/S ratio or other definitive test because of high incidence of false-negatives. Recently, it has been shown that estimation of phosphatidyl glycerol in amniotic fluid especially in mothers with diabetes mellitus is the most reliable test to assess fetal lung maturity and its presence would assure that infant would not develop HMD. While monitoring high-risk pregnancy, as far as possible, induction or operative intervention should be delayed till amniotic fluid examination has confirmed fetal lung maturity.

Creatinine Amniotic fluid creatinine is mostly derived from fetal urine and its increasing levels as gestation advances probably reflects maturing renal function rather than growth of fetal muscle mass. Creatinine concentration of 2 mg/dL or more is indicative of gestational maturity of at least 37 weeks. A 'mature' creatinine level does not ensure the absence of HMD. Maternal diabetes mellitus and severe Rh-isoimmunization may be associated with failure of progressive increase or even decline in amniotic fluid creatinine values.

Cytology Lipid-containing epithelial cells from sebaceous glands of fetal skin are shed into the amniotic fluid. As gestation advances, more lipid-containing orange-staining epithelial cells are seen when amniotic fluid deposit is stained with 0.1% Nile blue sulfate or hematoxylin-eosin. When proportion of orange-staining cells is more than 20% it is indicative of full maturity.

Fetal Growth

Assessment of fetal growth is essential for early diagnosis and management of a pregnancy complicated by intrauterine growth retardation. Intrauterine growth restriction (IUGR) does not become clinically evident before 20 weeks and seldom before 28 weeks. Accurate information regarding duration of pregnancy is mandatory before data regarding uterine or fetal size can be interpreted. A fetus is diagnosed to have growth restriction, if the intrauterine rate of growth is less than the predetermined ideal growth potential. The IUGR baby may be small-for-gestational age or appropriate-for-gestational age on the basis of his birth weight and gestational age.

Maternal Weight Gain

Steady and progressive weight gain during pregnancy is a reliable indicator of satisfactory fetal growth. Static or falling maternal weight is ominous and suggests unsatisfactory fetal growth. The average weight gain during pregnancy among healthy pregnant women varies between 6 and 10 kg of which about half is contributed by weight of the fetus and uteroplacental unit and the other half by laying down of extra fat by the mother to provide nutritional support during lactation. The weight gain during pregnancy depends upon pre-pregnancy health, nutrition and body mass index of the mother (Table 3.2.). The lean or malnourished mother is likely to gain more weight compared to over nourished or obese mother.

Uterine Size

In a single pregnancy uncomplicated by polyhydramnios, uterine malformations and fibroids, increase in uterine size provides reliable estimate of fetal growth. During each prenatal visit, fundal height above symphysis pubis should be measured accurately with a tape. Like intrauterine growth charts, uterine growth charts are available which provide useful reference

TABLE 3.2 Weight gain during pregnancy in relation to pre-pregnancy body mass index*	
*Body mass index***	*Weight gain*
■ <19.8 (under weight)	12–18 kg
■ 19.8–25 (normal weight)	11–16 kg
■ 26–29 (over weight)	7–11 kg
■ >29 (obese)	up to 6 kg

*National Academy of Sciences, 2001
**Body mass index = Weight in kg/(height in meters)^2

curves to plot uterine measurements in order to make early diagnosis of fetal growth retardation in a community setting (Figure 3.1).

Abdominal Girth

Changes in abdominal girth measurement relate closely to increasing uterine size and they are easier to obtain and much less influenced by the skill of different examiners. After 20 weeks of gestation, abdominal girth increases by about 1 cm every week. Obesity, abnormalities in the volume of amniotic fluid and fibroids may interfere with the reliability of this parameter.

Ultrasonography

Rapid advances in the field of imaging technology have vastly simplified visualization of fetus and other gestational products. Ultrasonography is a non-invasive,

non-ionizing method and has completely replaced radiographic techniques for antenatal diagnosis and assessment and fetal maturity, physical growth and malformations. The energy levels employed in diagnostic B-scanning (brightness mode) are of low intensity sound waves at frequencies above human hearing (above 18,000 cycles/second). The presence of a full bladder is a desirable prerequisite for satisfactory gestational sonography as it lifts up the gravid uterus above symphysis pubis and provides useful uterovesical landmark for localization of placenta.

Pregnancy can be diagnosed and timed accurately before the appearance of a positive conventional pregnancy test. Gestational sac can be identified and direct Doppler beaming of a sac can detect fetal heart beats as early as 6 weeks of gestation. Linear array real-time ultrasound can easily localize cardiac pulsations to confirm that fetus is alive. Fetal sex can be identified as early as 8–10 weeks of gestation. Fetal cephalometry by measurement of fetal biparietal diameter (BPD) provides useful information regarding fetal maturity or size but it is desirable that each institution should establish its own BPD growth curves on a pattern identical to intrauterine growth or anthropometric curves (Figure 3.2). A BPD diameter of 8.5 to 9.0 cm later in the course of pregnancy is indicative of a term-AGA infant. Serial BPD measurements every

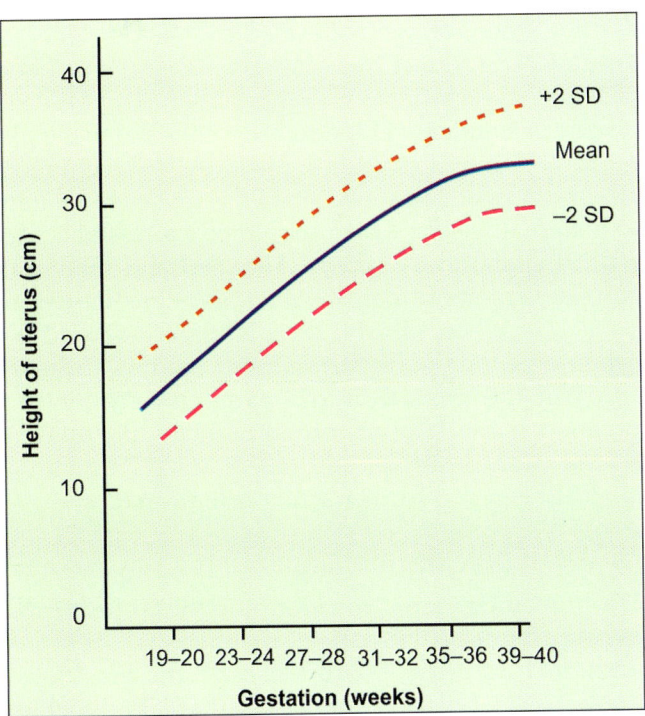

Figure 3.1 Uterine growth chart for early clinical detection of intrauterine growth retardation.

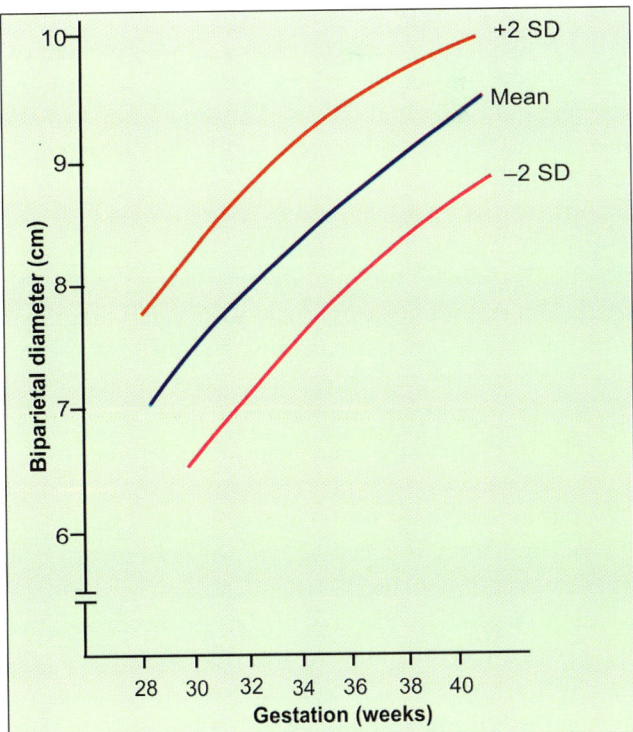

Figure 3.2 Ultrasonographic fetal biparietal diameter curves based on AIIMS data.

Preventive Neonatology

3

3–4 weeks can provide useful information regarding fetal growth but is handicapped by the fact the fetal brain growth is usually not effected by intrauterine malnutrition. Instead fetal head/abdomen or head/femur ratios are increased and they are more reliable for early diagnosis of intrauterine growth retardation because of disproportionately greater adverse effects of fetal malnutrition on linear growth and abdominal visceral growth. Ultrasonography can accurately diagnose fetal position and their number. The procedure also provides accurate means for localization of placenta and identification of serious placental abnormalities. Reliability and safety of amniocentesis during early pregnancy can be ensured once fetal parts and placenta are accurately localized by prior ultrasonography. Accurate diagnosis of incompetent cervical os can be made during first trimester of pregnancy by ultrasonography.

IDENTIFICATION OF GENETIC AND DEVELOPMENTAL ANOMALIES

About 3–6% neonates may be born with congenital anomalies despite liberal use of medical termination of pregnancies for lethal or severe developmental anomalies and inborn errors of metabolism. A routine antenatal ultrasound (3D high resoluble fetal ultrasound) performed at 18–20 weeks of gestation can pick most of the common anomalies.

Early diagnosis of fetal chromosomal and biochemical disorders has raised the unique possibility of reducing the birth of abnormal babies. There is a hope in the near future that following early identification of genetic abnormality in the fetus, one may be able to a channelize and achieve normal growth with the aid of genetic engineering. In the meantime, fetus with life-threatening developmental defects is managed with medical termination of pregnancy. Prenatal diagnosis with the help of various procedures should be made and medical termination of pregnancy is recommended, if the following prerequisites are satisfied:

1. The treatment of the disorder is not available or is unsatisfactory or very expensive.
2. In the event of the fetus being affected, termination of pregnancy is acceptable to the couple.
3. The risk of genetic disorder is sufficiently high or is greater than the risk of diagnostic procedure (Trisomy syndromes, neural tube defects).
4. Accurate prenatal diagnostic test is available.

A large number of inborn errors of metabolism (genetic disorders), chromosomal disorders and congenital malformations can be diagnosed prenatally.

Intrauterine infections can also be reliably diagnosed by examination of fetal blood obtained through cordocentesis or percutaneous umbilical blood sampling (PUBS).

Biochemical Screening

Alpha-Fetoprotein (AFP)

AFP is a glycoprotein which is produced by the yolk sac and fetal liver during beginning of second month of gestation. The hepatic contribution of AFP increases as pregnancy advances. It has a molecular weight of 68,000 daltons and can cross the placenta. Peak fetal serum AFP levels are achieved around 14 weeks of gestation and its production gradually wanes off as pregnancy advances. After birth, synthesis of AFP ceases within a few days except when infant develops hepatocellular injury due to any cause. The exact role of AFP in fetal life is unknown but it acts as a carrier protein and has immunologic capabilities. The main source of amniotic fluid AFP is the fetal urine while fetal skin also allows seepage of small amounts of AFP.

Maternal Serum Alpha-Fetoprotein (MSAFP)

Radioimmunoassay of maternal serum for AFP provides a useful non-invasive screening test to monitor high-risk pregnancies. Fetal AFP is transferred to the maternal circulation through placenta and amniotic membranes. The median MSAFP level is around 25 ng/mL at 16 weeks and increases by about 15% every week till 30 weeks gestation. The MSAFP levels are maintained for next 5–6 weeks and then falls rapidly. The optimum time for MSAFP screening is 16–20 weeks of gestation. MSAFP is inversely related to maternal weight which should be expressed along with the laboratory report. The fetal and maternal correlates of abnormal MSAFP values are shown in Table 3.3. When MSAFP level is high, it should be repeated along with ultrasound examination to confirm the gestation and to exclude multiple pregnancy and fetal abnormality. If the ultrasound examination is normal and repeat MSAFP is within normal range, no further action is indicated.

Human Chorionic Gonadotropin

The human chorionic gonadotropin (hCG) produced during pregnancy helps in the maintenance of corpus luteum. It is initially produced by the blastocyst trophoblastic cells and later by the placental syncitiotrophoblast. hCG assays are useful for the diagnosis and monitoring of pregnancy. During normal pregnancy,

TABLE 3.3 MSAFP levels and fetal abnormalities

Elevated MSAFP levels

(a) Fetal causes
- Open neural tube defects*: Anencephaly, open meningomyelocele
- Multiple pregnancy
- Missed or threatened abortion or fetal death
- Exstrophy of bladder
- Omphalocele and gastroschisis
- Meckel's syndrome
- Congenital nephrosis
- Fetal infections
- Turner syndrome
- Sacrococcygeal teratoma
- Cystic hygroma
- Fetal cutaneous disorders
- Hemangioma of cord/placenta
- Underestimated gestation

(b) Maternal causes
- Below average maternal weight
- Maternal diseases, like hepatocellular carcinoma, viral hepatitis and systemic lupus erythematosus

Low MSAFP levels
- Fetal autosomal aneuploidy (Down syndrome, trisomy-18)
- Nonviable gestation
- Over estimated gestation
- Molar pregnancy
- Diabetes mellitus
- Above average maternal weight

*Check amniotic fluid total and acetylcholinesterase (AChE) which is elevated in open neural tube defect.

there is exponential increase in serum hCG levels until the eighth week after the last menstrual period followed by a gradual decline. Subnormal hCG levels in early pregnancy may herald abortion. In molar pregnancy, hCG levels continue to rise beyond eighth week of pregnancy. The diagnosis of hydatidiform mole can be established by determination of hCG level and ultrasonography. Serum hCG levels are also elevated in mothers carrying a baby with Down syndrome.

Unconjugated Estriol

The unconjugated estriol (uE3) produced by the fetal adrenal gland is handled by the placenta and conjugated by the fetal liver. uE3 levels in the maternal serum are lower by 25% in pregnancies with Down syndrome as early as 9–11 weeks of gestation. The proteins which are elevated in the maternal serum with Down syndrome include hCG, pregnancy-associated placental protein A and neutrophil alkaline phosphatase.

Triple and Quadruple Test

In a high-risk pregnancy, especially elderly (>35 years) pregnant woman, evaluation of three maternal serum factors namely alpha-fetoprotein (AFP), human chorionic gonadotropin (hCG) and unconjugated estriol (uE3) is useful for prenatal diagnosis of Down syndrome. In quadruple test, dimeric inhibin A (DIA) is also tested. The test is performed around 15–20 weeks of gestation. When fetus is afflicted with Down syndrome, maternal serum levels of AFP and uE3 are decreased while levels of hCG and inhibin A are increased. The test should not be performed in all pregnancies because it may cause considerable mental stress to the mother due to high chances of false positive reports. Other proteins that may be elevated in the maternal serum of a mother carrying Down syndrome fetus include pregnancy-associated plasma protein A (PAPP-A) and neutrophil alkaline phosphatase. Quad screen has a sensitivity of 81% for detection of Down syndrome. When Quad test at 16 weeks of gestation is complemented with first trimester maternal pregnancy-associated plasma protein A (PAPP-A) and nuchal translucency measurements of fetus, the detection rate of trisomy 21 approaches 90–95%. The diagnosis can be confirmed by amniocentesis and chorionic villus sampling (CVS).

Naked Eye Single Tube Red Cell Osmotic Fragility Test (NESTROF Test)

This is a simple and cheap screening test to detect carriers of beta thalassemia. In populations with high incidence of beta thalassemia, all antenatal women should be screened with naked eye single tube red cell osmotic fragility (NESTROF) test. Two mL each of freshly prepared 0.36% buffered saline and distilled water (control) are taken in two test tubes. 20 μL of maternal blood is added to each tube, the solution is mixed well and kept for 5 minutes. Hemolysis in the two tubes is compared visually by holding them against black line drawn on a white background. In a normal subject, the blood would hemolyze in both the tubes and the black line would be easily visible. In women with thalassemia trait, the red blood cells resist hemolysis. The blood mixed in 0.36% buffered saline remains turbid with RBCs' settling at the bottom of the tube. The black line will not be visible and the test would be considered as positive for thalassemia trait. In case the NESTROF test is positive, red cell indices are determined and HbA_2 estimation is done. When mother is found to have thalassemia trait, her husband's blood sample should be taken and tested. If husband is not carrying thalassemia trait, then nothing further need to be done. When both the parents are having thalassemia trait, the molecular studies should be undertaken to characterize DNA mutations in the globin gene and prenatal diagnostic tests should be offered to carry out fetal diagnosis of beta thalassemia major.

Fetal Blood Sampling

Fetal blood sample can be obtained through cordocentesis or percutaneous umbilical blood sampling (PUBS) which is a skill based invasive procedure. A needle is introduced through the pregnant woman's abdoman into the umbilical cord under the guidance of real-time ultrasonography. The common indications for undertaking the procedure are listed below:

- Karyotyping and fluorescence *in situ* hybridization (FISH).
- DNA microarray studies for genetic disorders
- Assessment of severity of Rh-isoimmunization
- Evaluation of fetal infection
- Evaluation of a fetus suspected to have non-immune hydrops
- Assessment of fetal thrombocytopenia in alloimmune thrombocytopenia
- Administration of fetal medications and blood transfusion.

Prenatal Cytogenetics

Abnormalities of number of chromosomes (aneuploidies) and many structural chromosomal abnormalities (deletion, translocation) can be diagnosed prenatally. Indications for prenatal cytogenetic studies include advanced maternal age, previous child with aneuploidy, parental chromosomal abnormalities and fetal abnormalities detected on ultrasound. The cells used for prenatal cytogenetic analysis include chorionic villus samples (CVS), amniocytes obtained by amniocentesis and fetal blood collected by cordocentesis. The result of fetal karyotype is available within 72 hours with CVS or cord blood and in 2 to 3 weeks with amniotic fluid.

The combination of molecular genetics and cytogenetic techniques has evolved into a useful technology of fluorescent *in situ* hybridization (FISH). A fluorescently labeled DNA probe is hybridized to a standard chromosome preparation on a microscope slide. This method is useful for detecting chromosomal abnormalities involving both numerical and micro-deletion syndromes which may not be picked up by G-band analysis. The technique is currently used for detecting chromosomal aneuploidy involving X, Y, 13, 18 and 21 chromosomes. FISH technique has also been used for diagnosis of contiguous gene syndrome and for detection of carrier status for Duchenne or Becker muscular dystrophy in females whose affected male relatives have a known specific gene deletion. In Down syndrome, apart from karyotype, a large number of biochemical correlates and evidences of dysmorphism on ultrasound examination provide useful supportive evidence for the diagnosis. The various sampling procedures used for antenatal diagnosis of molecular, cytogenetic and biochemical disorders are listed in Table 3.4.

Prenatal Molecular (DNA), Biochemical and Genetic Studies

A large number of inborn errors of metabolism can be diagnosed by identification of biochemical or enzymic abnormalities and, more specifically with the help of DNA probes. The principle of DNA probes is based on the fact that DNA complement is identical in every cell of the body and, therefore, a genetic defect detectable at the DNA level should be found in all the nucleated cells of the affected individual. The DNA studies can be done on CVS obtained at 9–12 weeks, amniotic fluid cells obtained at 16–18 weeks or fetal

TABLE 3.4 Commonly used sampling procedures for antenatal diagnosis			
Procedure	*Timing*	*Risks*	*Indications*
CVS	i. 9–12 weeks (transcervical)	Fetal loss 3–5%, fetomaternal hemorrhage and limb defects	Molecular, cytogenetic, and biochemical studies
	ii. 12 weeks (transabdominal)		
Amniocentesis (conventional)	16–18 weeks	Fetal loss 0.5–1%, fetomaternal hemorrhage and respiratory problems	Cytogenetic, molecular and biochemical studies
Cordocentesis	>18 weeks	Fetal loss 1–5%	Hematological indices, intrauterine infections and cytogenetic studies

*CVS: Chorionic villus sampling.

TABLE 3.5 Single gene diseases amenable to prenatal diagnosis by DNA analysis

Autosomal dominant
- Neurofibromatosis
- Polycystic kidney disease
- Huntington's disease
- Myotonic dystrophy

Autosomal recessive
- Beta thalassemia
- Sickle cell anemia
- Hemoglobin E
- Phenylketonuria
- Cystic fibrosis
- Alpha-1-antitrypsin deficiency
- Wilson disease
- Albinism
- Congenital adrenal hyperplasia
- Spinal muscular atrophy

X-linked recessive*
- Hemophilia A and B
- Duchenne muscular dystrophy

*These disorders can be inferred indirectly by fetal sexing, if advanced diagnostic facilities are not available.

blood obtained at 18 weeks (Table 3.5). Transabdominal CVS is safer, less traumatic and has a lower risk to the fetus compared with vaginal or transcervical CVS. The nucleated fetal red blood cells circulating in the maternal blood can also be utilized for DNA extraction and prenatal tests. These tests can be done in the first trimester of pregnancy for population screening and they carry no risk of maternal infection or miscarriage. The fetal nucleated red blood cells, leukocytes and trophoblasts circulating in the maternal blood are isolated by flow cytometry, monoclonal antibodies and PCR. In view of limited number of fetal cells in the maternal circulation, efforts are being made to extract and process free fetal DNA from maternal blood which is likely to be present in significant amount.

Direct Mutation Analysis Techniques

The following techniques are used to directly identify mutant genes.

Restriction Enzyme Studies

Restriction endonucleases are bacterial enzymes that recognize and cleave short specific base sequences in the double-stranded DNA. They are used to identify mutant genes, deletions within a gene and for characterization of DNA polymorphism.

Polymerase Chain Reaction (PCR)

This technique is used when molecular basis of a disease is known. The specific region of DNA is amplified by PCR technology to synthesize microgram quantities of DNA copies from template segment present in a single molecule. A number of inherited diseases including phenylketonuria, Duchenne muscular dystrophy, alpha-1-antitrypsin deficiency, fragile X syndrome, etc. can be diagnosed by PCR.

Allele-specific Oligonucleotide Probes

This technique employs two synthetic oligonucleotides, one specific for a normal gene and the other specific for the unknown genetic mutation. In autosomal recessive disorders, in the affected individual, there will be two copies of mutated genes while the carriers would have one mutated gene and one normal gene.

Expanding Trinucleotide Repeats

This form of mutation is seen in fragile X syndrome, myotonic dystrophy and Huntington's disease. In these disorders, the polymorphic trinucleotide repeat sequences found at the disease locus expand beyond the normal size range in the affected individual.

Indirect Mutation Analysis Techniques

Linkage

In most genetic disorders, the mutation is unknown. By using certain markers, that are close to the mutant gene, one can indirectly infer about the existence of a mutant gene.

Restriction Fragment Length Polymorphism (RFLP)

In this technique, specific enzymes are used to cut the DNA molecule. The measurement of the fragment length to which a DNA probe will hybridize can be used to track the transmission of DNA variations (polymorphism) in the affected family. About 80–85% of thalassemic mutations can be detected by this method. The other types of polymorphisms which are being increasingly used for diagnostic linkage analysis are microsatellites or simple sequence repeats.

The list of genetic disorders which are amenable to reliable prenatal diagnosis is rapidly increasing. Table 3.5 provides list of selected single gene diseases which are amenable to prenatal diagnosis by DNA analysis. Many of these diseases can be diagnosed antenatally by the specialized genetic centers which have been established in the country in the metroplitan cities.

Preimplantation Genetic Diagnosis (PGD)

It is a highly specialized and cost-intensive technique available only in a few centers in the world. The embryonal cells are sampled after *in vitro* fertilization. Following several embryonic cell divisions, one or more cells are removed from the embryo, DNA is amplified and analyzed for a single gene disorder. The defective embryo is discarded while the healthy embryo is implanted in the uterus. In women who are at risk for X-linked recessive disorders, determination of XX-containing embryos by fluorescent *in situ* hybridization (FISH) can enable transfer of only female embryos through assisted reproduction.

Visualization of Fetus

Ultrasonography is an important tool to detect major malformations in the fetus (Figure 3.3). Pregnancies complicated by slow fetal growth, polyhydramnios or oligohydramnios and previous history of serious congenital malformation should be subjected to ultrasonographic evaluation by an experienced and reliable sonologist. The optimal timing for prenatal diagnosis of various congenital anomalies is given in Table 3.6.

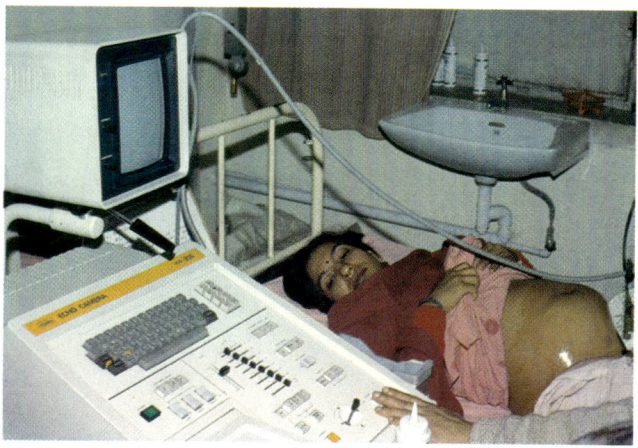

Figure 3.3 Ultrasound scan during pregnancy for diagnosis of fetal anomalies

TABLE 3.6 Optimal timing for fetal ultrasound examination

Anomaly	Timing
Anencephaly	10–12 weeks
Hydrocephaly/microcephaly	16 weeks onwards
Limb abnormalities	16 weeks onwards
Spina bifida	16–18 weeks
Renal anomalies	16 weeks onwards
Anterior abdominal wall defects	16–18 weeks
Cardiac abnormalities	18–22 weeks
Face and mouth anomalies	18–22 weeks

TABLE 3.7 Prenatal diagnosis of neural tube defects

Investigation	Findings
■ Maternal serum	Raised AFP
■ Amniotic fluid	Raised AFP and acetyl-cholinesterase
■ Ultrasonography – Transvaginal (1st trimester) – Transabdominal (2nd trimester)	The skull vault is absent in anencephaly. Spina bifida is diagnosed by splaying of spine, evidences of hydrocephalus, lemon sign*, banana sign** and lower limb defects.
■ Chromosomal studies	When NTD is associated with a chromosomal disorder.

*Lemon sign: Forward scalloping or indentation of the frontal bone. It is classically seen in Arnold Chiari II malformation and fetuses with spina bifida.
**Banana sign: Banana-shaped abnormal cerebellum.

The characteristic ultrasonographic findings along with other diagnostic markers for prenatal diagnosis of neural tube defects are given in Table 3.7.

The indications for fetal echocardiography include family history of congenital heart disease, diabetic mother, intrauterine infection, exposure to teratogen, non-immune hydrops fetalis and unexplained polyhydramnios. Transvaginal and transabdominal ultrasonography done at 11–14 weeks and 18–20 weeks respectively can detect developmental heart defects. Esophageal or small gut atresias, pulmonary hypoplasia, diaphragmatic hernia and ventral wall defects can be diagnosed during second trimester of pregnancy.

An experienced sonologist can diagnose chromosomal disorders on ultrasonography by looking for evidences of facial dysmorphism and other associated abnormalities. Characteristic ultrasonographic features and antenatal diagnostic correlates of Down syndrome are depicted in Table 3.8. Trisomy 18 syndrome can be suspected on the basis of strawberry-shaped head, choroid plexus cyst, facial cleft, micrognathia, exomphalos and complex abnormalities of hands and feet.

The direct visualization of the fetus is also possible with the help of a fetoscope. A fine caliber endoscope is inserted into the uterus for inspection of fetus and collection of fetal blood and tissue samples. This technique is rarely used because of high risk of abortion due to the invasive nature of the procedure.

ASSESSMENT OF FETAL WELLBEING

Fetal Activity Record (Count-to-ten)

This is a simple innovative method by which the mother herself plays an important part in checking the health

TABLE 3.8 Prenatal diagnosis of Down syndrome

Investigations	Findings
Maternal serum markers*	
■ AFP (14–16 weeks)	Decreased
■ uE3 (14 weeks)	Decreased
■ hCG (14 weeks)	Increased
■ DIA (14 weeks)	Increased
■ PAPP-A (1st trimester)	Increased
■ Neutrophil alkaline phosphatase	Increased
Amniocentesis	
■ Early	Karyotype on cultured amniocytes
■ Conventional (16–18 weeks)	FISH on uncultured cells
Chorionic villus sampling (8–11 weeks)	Short-term culture or direct preparation for karyotype
Cordocentesis (18 weeks)	Culture of fetal lymphocytes for karyotype and FISH on non-dividing cells
Ultrasound (11–20 weeks)	Nuchal fold >4 mm thick, double-bubble in abdomen, short femur, clinodactyly, macroglossia, renal pyelectasis
Fetal echocardiography	Atrioventricular canal defects
Fetal cells in maternal circulation	FISH

*When three maternal serum markers are abnormal, the validity for detction of Down syndrome goes above 60%. Figures in parentheses indicate the appropriate time for the test. AFP: alpha-fetoprotein, UE3: unconjugated estriol, hCG: human chorionic gonadotropin, DIA: dimeric inhibin A, PAPP-A: pregnancy-associated placental protein A, FISH: fluorescent *in situ* hybridization.

of her own baby. It involves counting the number of movements or 'quickenings' made by the baby during third trimester of pregnancy. She is advised to count the number of fetal movements every day starting at 9 AM in the morning until the total movements equals ten. It is recorded in the chart as shown in Figure 3.4. The recording indicates that by 2 PM she had felt ten fetal movements. No more counting is done until the following day when she starts counting again. If she feels less than ten movements per day for two consecutive days, she must report to the doctor on the following day (Figure 3.4B). In case she does not appreciate any fetal movements in a day, she must contact the doctor immediately (Figure 3.4C). Alternatively, the mother is asked to watch for fetal movements during morning, noon and evening for a period of one hour each. The total fetal count is multiplied by 4 to get a fetal movement count for 12 hours. The fetus must produce at least one movement per hour. The method is quite reliable in an experienced mother as long as she is honest and maintains an accurate record. In view of its simplicity and reliability, it needs to be popularized in resource-poor countries.

Uteroplacental Unit

A number of biochemical agents and hormones, such as diamine oxidase, alkaline phosphatase, urinary pregnenediol, human placental lactogen and estriol elaborated by uteroplacental unit, have been employed to assess its status. Because of wide range of variability in their levels during pregnancy, their utility is limited.

Human Placental Lactogen (HPL)

HPL concentrations in maternal serum increase as pregnancy advances and a level of less than 4 µg/mL after 30 weeks of gestation is associated with fetal jeopardy.

Estriol

Estriol production during pregnancy progressively increases as pregnancy advances. Its normal level is indicative of integrity of both fetus and placenta, because fetal adrenal androgen precursor (dehydro-epiandrosterone) is converted to estriol by the placenta. Estriol can be measured in the maternal plasma or urine, but both measurements have their limitations. The mean unconjugated plasma estriol increases from 6 ng/mL at 28 weeks to 18 ng/mL at term. Isolated estriol levels are of no significance and this must be estimated at least twice weekly. A decline of more than 30% in serial plasma estriol level or in 24-hour urine assay, is indicative of fetal distress. Urinary estriol may be falsely lowered by maternal intake of ampicillin, mendelamine, and phenolphathalein. Persistently low levels of plasma estriol may

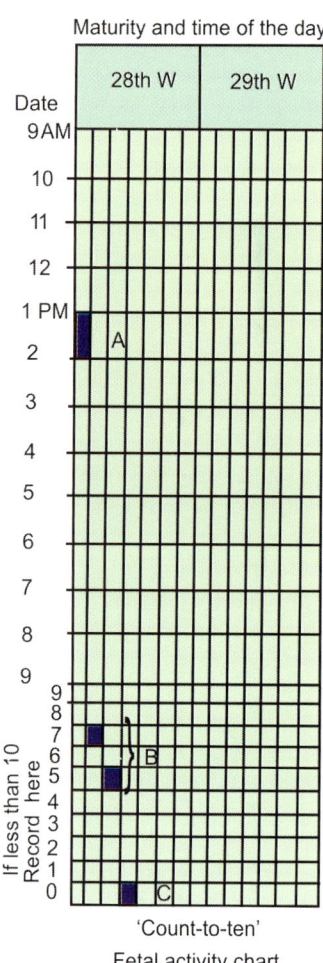

Figure 3.4 Fetal activity chart. Refer to text for details.

be seen in a mother carrying anencephalic infant or if she has received high doses of corticosteroids during pregnancy.

Nonstress Monitoring

Simultaneous and continuous records of fetal heart rate, uterine contractions and fetal movements provide useful information (Figure 3.5). Fetus is considered as 'reactive' and without any distress, if he can demonstrate acceleration of his heart beats by 15 or more for 15 seconds in association with fetal movements at least twice in a 20-minute record period. In case he does not show fetal movements or cardiac acceleration, fetus should be stimulated and watched for another 20-minute spell. To reduce observation time, fetal movements can be produced by acoustic stimulation. If fetus remains non-reactive even after stimulation, he should be subjected to oxytocin challenge test. A persistently slow fetal heart rate without any variability in response to fetal movements or uterine contractions, is indicative of fetal hypoxia.

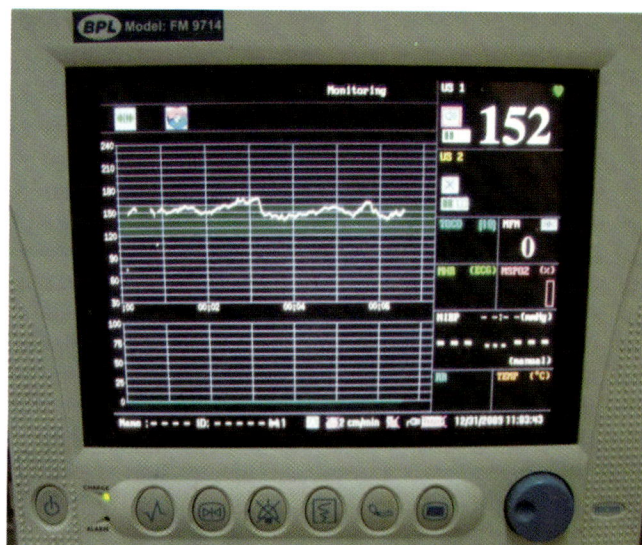

Figure 3.5 Cardiotocometer for monitoring of fetal heart rate and uterine contractions.

Oxytocin Challenge Test (OCT)

It is a useful test to biologically assess integrity of ulteroplacental unit. Uterine contractions are induced with oxytocin and their effects on fetal heart rate is monitored which is akin to exercise tolerance studies in patients with suspected coronary artery disease. When uteroplacental unit is optimal, uterine contractions as assessed with tocodynamometer are unlikely to critically affect the circulation or oxygenation of the fetus and they would not lead to fetal bradycardia. When there is fetal hypoxia, FHR begins to decelerate 15–30 seconds after the onset of uterine contraction, reaches its nadir well after the peak of the contraction and does not return to the baseline even after cessation of uterine contraction. This heart rate pattern is called *late deceleration* or type 2 deceleration or deceleration of uteroplacental insufficiency (Figure 3.6). Early deceleration is benign and may occur due to compression of the fetal head while variable fetal heart deceleration is indicative of cord compression and carries adverse prognosis.

The patient is positioned in the semi-fowler position and oxytocin is delivered intravenously by an infusion pump at an initial dose of 0.5 mU/minute. The dose is doubled after every 20-minute to obtain at least three uterine contractions in a 10-minute period. Cardiotocometer is affixed to simultaneously and continuously record fetal heart rate, uterine contractions and fetal movements. A negative-OCT is extremely reliable indicator of adequacy of uteroplacental unit and test can be safely repeated every week. If OCT shows persistent late deceleration, the baby should be

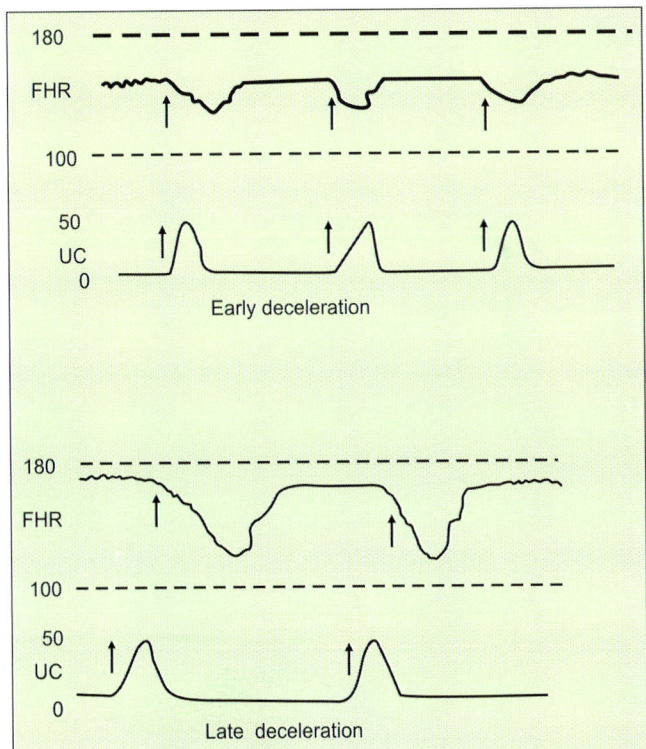

Figure 3.6 Diagrammatic representation of changes in fetal heart rate pattern in relation to uterine contractions following oxytocin challenge test. Each deceleration of fetal heart rate at the beginning of uterine contraction is benign and may occur due to compression of fetal head. Late deceleration following uterine contraction is ominous and indicative of uteroplacental insufficiency.

delivered, if amniotic fluid L/S ratio is indicative of fetal maturity. When L/S ratio is less than 2.0, the pregnancy should not be terminated unless both OCT and estriol levels are indicative of compromised uteroplacental unit.

Oxytocin challenge test is fairly safe and without any undue risk of premature labor. It is contraindicated in patients with placenta previa and in situations associated with high risk of premature labor, viz. twins, ruptured membranes and incompetent cervical os. In view of its potential risk to the fetus and several contraindications, it is preferable to monitor fetal biophysical variables with the help of real-time ultrasound which is non-invasive and more informative.

Fetal Biophysical Profile

Fetal biophysical profile is the most accurate and non-invasive parameter of fetal wellbeing and is assessed by real-time ultrasound. A combination of five ultrasonically monitored fetal biophysical variables, i.e. fetal posture, fetal breathing movements, gross body movements, reactive fetal heart rate, and volume of amniotic fluid are used to assess and assign fetal

risk. Each variable is scored by coding it normal and abnormal (Table 3.9). The fetus is observed ultrasonically for at least 30-minute or earlier, if normal criteria are visualized. On the basis of biophysical score, the following management protocol is followed:

Score 10 Normal fetus but test should be repeated at weekly intervals. The test may be repeated twice weekly in high-risk situations especially in case of diabetic and post-term pregnancy.

Score 8 Normal fetus with low risk of chronic asphyxia. Repeat the test weekly or twice weekly in diabetic and post-dated. If oligohydramnios is present, it is an indication for delivery, if baby is mature.

Score 6 It is indicative of chronic asphyxia. Repeat the test after 4–6 hours. If oligohydramnios is present, immediate delivery is indicated.

Score 4 Compromised fetus and baby should be delivered immediately, if amniotic fluid L/S ratio is >2. Otherwise repeat the test after 24 hours. If score is still 4 or less, delivery is mandatory.

Score 0–2 It is suggestive of severe degree of chronic asphyxia and baby should be watched over an extended period of 120 minutes. If score remains <4, the baby should be delivered without further delay irrespective of gestational age and pulmonary maturity.

Doppler Velocimetry Studies

Doppler velocimetry studies of umbilical and uterine artery are reliable to assess the adequacy of uteroplacental circulation to the fetus. There is a good correlation between Doppler-measured resistance to the flow of blood in the uterine and umbilical arteries and fetal hypoxia or acidemia. The normal flow of blood is from the mother to the fetus to provide oxygenation and nutrition to the baby. Absence of umbilical artery end-diastolic flow (AEDF) and reversal of umbilical artery end-diastolic flow (REDF) are ominous. It has been documented that singleton fetuses with REDF are likely to die *in utero* within 7 days, if no intervention is done.

Partograph

Partograph or partogram is a graphic information about the progress of labor in which the salient information about the fetal wellbeing, maternal

Preventive Neonatology

3

TABLE 3.9 Fetal biophysical profile score (Manning score or planning score)

Biophysical variable	Normal (score 2)	Abnormal (score 0)
1. Posture	Flexed	Extended
2. Fetal breathing movements	At least one episode of FBM of at least 30 sec duration in 30 min	Absent FBM or their duration <30 sec
3. Gross body movements	At least 3 discrete body/limb movements in 30 min	2 or fewer body/limb movements in 30 min
4. Reactive FHR	At least 2 episodes of FHR acceleration of 15 bpm of at least 15 sec duration in a period of 30 min	Less than 2 episodes of acceleration of FHR >15 bpm in 30 min
5. Amniotic fluid volume	At least one pocket of AF measuring 1 cm or more in two perpendicular directions	No AF pocket or <1.0 cm in two perpendicular directions

FBM; fetal breathing movements, FHR; fetal heart rate, AF; amniotic fluid.

wellbeing and the progress of labor are recorded against time on a single sheet of paper. It is considered as the "gold standard" labor monitoring tool being used universally. It is a useful tool to monitor the progress of labor and for taking timely decision to deliver the baby safely without any undue risk either to the baby or mother. A partogram or partograph should be recorded in all women who are in labor, whether they are low or high risk. The three components of partogram, from top to bottom, include evidences of fetal wellbeing, progress of labor (rupture of membranes, effacement and dilatation of cervix, uterine contractions, descent of fetus) and wellbeing of the mother.

Fetal wellbeing Timing of rupture of membranes, amniotic fluid whether clear or meconium stained, fetal heart rate especially after uterine contraction, degree of molding or over lapping of skull bones.

Progress of labor Timing of onset of labor, timing of each vaginal examination, effacement and dilation of cervix, uterine contractions, descent of fetal head and adequacy of pelvic outlet. When progress of labor is satisfactory, the plotting parameters will remain on or to the left of the *alert line* on the partogram. The labor pattern is recorded as normal labor, prolonged latent phase (cervical dilation 2 cm or less), primary dysfunctional labor and secondary arrest of labor. WHO has modified the partogram and color-coded it into green representing the normal progress, red indicating dangerously slow progress and amber color indicating the need for greater vigilance.

Maternal wellbeing Record name, age, parity, brief antenatal history, gestational period, vital signs, features of exhaustion, medications being given

(oxytocin, pethidine, pudendal block), episiotomy, urine examination for output, albumin, sugar and ketones.

All events should be written legibly, dated and timed. The mode of delivery, any evidence of fetal hypoxia and birth asphyxia (including Apgar score at 1-minute and every 5-minute till >7) should be recorded.

Fetal Scalp Blood Sampling

Prolonged fetal hypoxia leads to anerobic metabolism resulting in metabolic acidosis and fall in pH. Fetal scalp sample can be obtained transvaginally with the help of an amniosocope in a vertex presenting fetus when membranes are ruptured and cervix is well dilated. The procedure is rather invasive, and interfered by caput or scalp edema. Blood sample is collected under direct vision in a heparinized polyethylene capillary tube. Maternal acidemia should be ruled out by simultaneous sampling of maternal blood as it can get reflected in the fetal blood. There is a good correlation between fetal scalp pH of less than 7.15, positive OCT and severe asphyxia at birth. The abnormal fetal heart rate pattern assumes more ominous significance, if there is associated fetal acidosis. If the scalp pH is less than 7.10, the baby should be delivered immediately either by forceps or cesarean section depending upon the stage of cervical dilatation. Local infection and intractable bleeding after birth from sampling site may complicate the procedure. The procedure is contraindicated, if mother is HbsAg or HIV-positive because of increased risk of materno-fetal transmission of these viral infections. Many obstetric units have replaced fetal scalp blood sampling with non-invasive techniques to assess the fetal status.

FETAL DIAGNOSIS AND THERAPY

Neonatologists are increasingly concerned with the welfare of fetus from the day of conception. They are seeking collaboration and active partnership with their obstetric colleagues in the specialized antenatal clinics for the care of high-risk pregnancies. Infact a team of specialists comprising of obstetricians, neonatologists, geneticists, endocrinologists and surgeons is now working together for early diagnosis and management of fetal disorders. Sophisticated intrauterine diagnostic techniques have been introduced to diagnose inborn errors of metabolism, developmental and chromosomal defects, fetal infections and other life-threatening fetal disorders. When a fetus is affected with a lethal non-correctable congenital malformation or genetic disorder, medical termination of pregnancy with the consent of couple is an acceptable option. At times, fetal therapy is instituted to sustain life and enhance gestational maturity of the fetus before delivery. Fetal surgery has been undertaken for a number of non-lethal but progressive congenital malformations. The initial enthusiasm has not been sustained due to unsatisfactory outcome of most of the procedures. Fetal therapy is unwarranted, if fetus has already achieved a maturity of 32 weeks and when mother is carrying a twin pregnancy due to potential risk of harm by therapy/procedure to the unaffected fetus.

Preventive Fetal Therapy

Acceleration of Fetal Maturation

Administration of betamethasone 12 mg IM two doses 24 hr apart or dexamethasone 6 mg IM every 12 hr for 4 doses to a pregnant woman between 24 and 34 weeks of gestation at least 24 hr to 7 days before delivery enhances lung maturity and reduces the incidence and severity of hyaline membrane disease, intraventricular hemorrhage, necrotizing enterocolitis and retinopathy of prematurity. Betamethasone is preferred by virtue of its greater efficacy and lesser side effects. Antenatal administration of thyrotropic-releasing hormone (TRH) for enhancing lung maturity is still in experimental stage and not recommended for clinical use. Administration of phenobarbitone sodium 60 mg oral single dose at night to an Rh-isoimmunized mother daily for two weeks before the anticipated time of delivery enhances fetal hepatic maturity and is associated with reduced severity of neonatal hyperbilirubinemia.

Prevention of Intracranial Hemorrhage

A number of antenatal obstetric strategies, like administration of vitamin K, phenobarbitone sodium and indomethacin, are not associated with any consistent benefit and are thus not recommended. Antenatal administration of steroids to enhance fetal lung maturity is also credited to reduce the risk of intraventricular hemorrhage.

Prevention of Fetal Hemorrhage

The mother receiving anticonvulsants during pregnancy should be administered vitamin K during last two weeks of pregnancy to reduce the incidence of early-onset hemorrhagic disease of the newborn.

Prevention of Fetal Infections

Early-onset group B streptococcal (GBS) infection is fortunately rare in India as compared to the West where 10–30% pregnant women are colonized with GBS in the genital tract. In high-risk populations with invasive GBS infection, administer crystalline penicillin G 5 million units IV followed by 2.5 million units IV every 4 hourly till delivery. Alternatively, ampicillin 2.0 g IV loading dose followed by 1.0 g IV every 4 hr till delivery is equally effective. For prevention of vertical transmission of HIV infection to the fetus, refer to Chapter 16 for details. Administration of large doses of vitamin A to the mother and vaginal douches with povidone-iodine are of doubtfull utility to reduce transmission of HIV infection. The baby should be delivered by elective cesarean section. Infant should be given zidovudine 2 mg/kg orally every 6 hr for 6 weeks. These strategies have reduced perinatal transmission of HIV from 25% to 8%. For prevention of other TORCH infections, refer to Chapter 16.

Prevention of Neural Tube Defects

There is convincing evidence to suggest that periconceptional intake of folic acid is associated with reduced risk of neural tube defects. The protective and preventive utility of folic acid is best during earliest phase of conception when pregnancy is still undiagnosed (even before missing the period). Therefore, when a married couple is planning for a pregnancy or having unprotected sex, the woman should start taking folic acid and continue for 4 months after conception. The optimum dose of folic acid is unknown but it would appear that 0.4 mg (400 µg) folic acid per day is sufficient to afford effective protection. In a woman with previous birth of a child with NTD, the daily prophylactic dose of folic acid is 4.0 mg.

Fetal Therapy

Fetal therapy must be safe for the mother (her safety must be a greater concern than the survival of the

Preventive Neonatology

3

baby) with an acceptable risk-benefit odds. The therapy should be instituted, if it is well known that in the absence of *in utero* intervention, the condition of fetus would progressively deteriorate to such an extent that either he would die *in utero* or he would die soon after birth despite intensive management. Before undertaking fetal therapy, it is mandatory to evaluate the fetus for any structural malformations, abnormal karyotype, gestational and functional maturity and evidences of intrauterine infection by ultrasonography, amniocentesis, cordocentesis and chorionic villus biopsy. The fetal disorders may be treated either by administration of drugs (transuterine or direct delivery of drugs to the fetus) or by a surgical procedure.

Medical Therapy

Congenital Adrenal Hyperplasia (CAH)

Following birth of a child afflicted with CAH, subsequent pregnancies should be monitored by chorionic villus sampling (CVS) at 8 to 9 weeks for CAH due to 21-hydroxylase deficiency which can be diagnosed by PCR-DNA technology. Elevated levels of pregnanediol or 17-hydroxyprogesterone in the amniotic fluid is also diagnostic of CAH. If fetus is affected, mother should receive oral dexamethasone 1.0 mg daily throughout pregnancy to prevent masculinization of female fetus. In centers where facilities for CVS are not available, when there is high risk for birth of CAH affected child (due to birth of previously affected sibling), maternal dexamethasone therapy should be started at 10 weeks of gestation. The therapy is continued throughout pregnancy, if fetus is found to be female by amniotic fluid examination around 15–16 weeks of gestation.

Cardiac Arrhythmias

Fetal tachyarrhythmia with impending congestive heart failure can be treated by oral administration of digoxin to the mother in a dose of 0.75 to 1.0 mg/d. Other drugs, like verapamil, propranolol, procainamide and quinidine, have been used but are potentially hazardous. Fetal cardiac decompensation by complete heart block has been successfully managed by administration of sympathomimetic drugs and *in utero* fetal pacemaker.

Congenital Hypothyroidism

Congenital hypothyroidism due to iodine deficiency is totally preventable by consumption of iodized salt or injection of depot preparation of iodine deep IM to the pregnant women residing in iodine deficient endemic areas.

Inborn Errors of Metabolism

It is hoped that fetal therapy of certain inborn errors of metabolism may reduce mental damage and ensure intact survival. Methylmalonic acidemia is responsive to vitamin B_{12} therapy and multiple carboxylase deficiency responds to large doses of biotin. These diseases are amenable to antenatal diagnosis. The women carrying affected fetus can be administered large doses of these vitamins (vitamin B_{12} 5000 μg IV daily) during last trimester of pregnancy. It is also recommended that if a mother is carrying a baby afflicted with galactosemia, she should be given galactose-free diet during pregnancy to reduce CNS damage during fetal life. These therapeutic modalities need to be subjected to multicentric trials to evolve uniform recommedations.

Thrombocytopenia

Mothers with active ITP should receive corticosteroid therapy during last 2 weeks of pregnancy. In iso-immune type of fetal thrombocytopenia (as evidenced by platelet antigen PLA_1 and history of previous affected sibling), transfusion of maternal platelets and immunoglobulins through the umbilical vessels by cordocentesis have been shown to prevent the risk of fetal hemorrhage. High doses of weekly intravenous immunoglobulins (IVIG 1.0 g/kg) to the mother can prevent fetal thrombocytopenia, if cordocentesis is not technically feasible.

Thyrotoxicosis

Euthyroid pregnant mothers, who had undergone subtotal thyroidectomy for thyrotoxicosis, should be investigated for the presence of human thyroid-stimulating immunoglobulins (HTSI). Carbimazole or propylthiouracil therapy is advocated, if there is fetal tachycardia and elevated maternal levels of HTSI. In order to prevent hypothyroidism in the mother, supplemental thyroxine therapy is given.

Surgical Interventions

Fetal *ex utero* intrapartum treatment (EXIT) procedures are conducted for a number of life-threatening disorders with variable results. The indications for fetal interventions are rapidly evolving and changing.

Intrauterine Blood Transfusion

Intrauterine blood transfusion is life saving to treat severe anemia due to Rh-isoimmunization so that fetal gestation is enhanced till *ex utero* viability is assured.

Fetal intraperitoneal transfusions have been replaced by fetal intravascular transfusion by cordocentesis. Intrauterine transfusion is indicated when fetal hematocrit drops to 20–25%. The volume of blood transfused depends upon the hematocrit and the estimated blood volume of the fetus. The aim of intra-uterine transfusion is to raise fetal hematocrit to 45–50%. Hematocrit usually falls at a rate of approxi-mately 1.0% per day, thus repeat transfusions are required after every 15 to 20 days till gestational matu-rity of 32 weeks is achieved. Even partial exchange blood transfusion has been done through the cord to reduce central venous pressure and cardiac over-load. Infants who have undergone multiple intra-uterine transfusions will be born with adult O-Rh negative RBCs because all their fetal red blood cells have been destroyed.

Nonimmune Hydrops Fetalis

After excluding major life-threatening cardiac and other malformations, fetal abdominal paracentesis and thoracocentesis have been done successfully. Albumin transfusion can be given through the umbilical vessels or peritoneum to improve the vascular oncotic pressure.

Obstructive Uropathy

In severely affected fetus with bladder neck obstruc-tion, marsupialization of the urinary bladder with vesicoamniotic shunt (VAS) has been performed with variable results. In advanced cases with oligohydram-nios, the outcome is poor because of development of hypoplastic lungs. In these cases, administration of physiological saline into the amniotic cavity is associa-ted with reduced severity of lung hypoplasia and improved outcome. Cystoscopic ablation of posterior urethral valve has been successful done by an *ex utero* intrapartum treatment (EXIT) procedure.

Congenital Hydrocephalus

Fetal ventriculoamniotic shunt has been done in some rapidly progressive cases of hydrocephalus around 20 weeks of gestation. *In utero* management of this condition is controversial and initial enthusiasm has not been sustained due to unsatisfactory outcome with severe neurological impairment. Many centers have abandoned the procedure.

Congenital Diaphragmatic Hernia (CDH)

Despite aggressive postnatal management of infants with CDH, outcome is unsatisfactory with high mortality due to hypoplasia of lung. Attempts have been made to retract the hernial contents into abdominal cavity around 26–28 weeks of gestation. The success of the procedure is limited. The concept of lung expansion by tracheal occlusion gave birth to the fetal endoscopic tracheal occlusion technique (FETENDO). Fetal trachea is occluded endoscopically using a clip or balloon which is removed at the time of delivery. The results of fetal intervention are poor and there is high risk of premature delivery.

Pleural Effusion

Pleuroamniotic shunt has been created *in utero* to relieve pleural effusion and prevent development of hypoplasia of lung.

Cardiovascular Disorders

A number of fetal cardiac interventions have been done successfully. They include aortic valve dilatation for critical aortic stenosis, atrial septostomy or stent placement for intact atrial septum with hypoplastic left heart syndrome and vascular photocoagulation of twin-to-twin transfusion syndrome or twin reversed arterial perfusion (TRAP) syndrome.

Future Hope

The myth that fetus is inviolable has been shattered. But the currently available modalities pertaining to fetal therapy require considerable inputs of skills and technology to make them useful, acceptable, safe and cost-effective. The role of hyperalimentation through umbilical vein cannulation, to improve the nutrition and growth of fetus compromised by severe placental dysfunction, needs to be evaluated. There is a possibility of undertaking fetal bone marrow and stem cell transplantation in certain crippling and life-threatening hematological diseases and immuno-deficiency states. There is encouraging experimental evidence that closure of spina bifida and resection of encephalocele in fetal monkeys is associated with vastly improved outcome. There is a hope, that by the dawn of 21st century, the "fetal surgeons" are likely to tamper with the embryo under the dissecting micro-scope to replace a bad gene or RNA with a healthy one, with the help of rapidly evolving technology of genetic engineering.

COMMON CAUSES OF PERINATAL DEATHS

Perinatal deaths include late fetal and early neonatal (first week) deaths. The exact estimate of perinatal mortality in India is not known due to gross under reporting of late fetal deaths but is estimated around 26 per 1000 births. There is almost equal contribution by stillbirths and early neonatal deaths. A large majority of stillbirths are attributable to placental insufficiency due to pregnancy-induced hypertension and maternal malnutrition, fetal and intranatal hypoxia, antepartum hemorrhage and congenital malformations.

Nearly one-half of early neonatal deaths occur during first 24 hours of life. Neonatal mortality is directly related to birth weight and gestational maturity of the infant. In India, it varies between 0.5% among healthy term infants and about 30% in preterms or infants with a birth weight of less than 2000 g. It is estimated that about 16.4% infants born in India are LBW (<2500 g at birth) and about 85% of all neonatal deaths occur among them. The neonatal mortality among LBW babies is about twenty times of mortality in term-AGA (appropriate-for-gestational age) infants. Generally several factors operate in most perinatal deaths. Data from various hospital-based studies in India suggest that the three leading causes of neonatal deaths in India include prematurity, infections and perinatal hypoxia. Major congenital malformations, and rhesus isoimmunization account for 10%, and 5% of neonatal deaths, respectively.

In the best pediatric tradition, preventive neonatology is the key for newborn survival. Prevention, early diagnosis and prompt management is the mantra to enhance newborn survival and reduce the risk of neuromotor disability. The neonatal conditions which are amenable to preventive strategies include prematurity, perinatal hypoxia, hypothermia, hypoglycemia, bacterial infections, respiratory distress syndrome and hyperbilirubinemia. A number of congenital malformations and iatrogenic disorders like anemia, retinopathy of prematurity, necrotizing enterocolitis, airleaks and bronchopulmonary dysplasia are by and large preventable.

REDUCTION OF PERINATAL MORTALITY

Almost two-thirds of perinatal deaths due to obstetrical factors, perinatal hypoxia and infections are preventable. Adequate nutrition and antenatal medical care with early recognition of at-risk pregnancy are crucial for reduction of perinatal mortality. High-risk mother must be referred to a center equipped with higher level of perinatal care for confinement. Transport of a woman in labor or high-risk infant after birth is associated with poor outcome. Traditional birth attendants and accredited social health activists (ASHAs) must be adequately trained in the art of essential perinatal care and provided with disposable delivery kits to ensure asepsis at birth. Efforts must be made to establish intermediate neonatal care facilities at all district and community hospitals.

REDUCTION OF LBW BABIES

Most LBW babies in the West are preterm. In India, about two-thirds of LBW babies are born at term but are small-for-dates. The mortality in preterm babies is higher compared to the neonatal mortality among term small-for-dates babies. The greatest impact on further reduction of perinatal mortality can be made by recognizing various factors that initiate normal labor and application of this knowledge for arrest of labor which starts before term. The prolongation of gestation in the absence of any recognizable adverse fetal factors improves the chances of survival of the baby after birth.

There is a need to provide basic or essential perinatal care to all pregnant women through existing health infrastructure. In view of limited resources, it is desirable to adopt at-risk approach in order to provide adequate perinatal care to high-risk mothers. Traditional birth attendants, ASHAs and auxiliary nurse midwives should be provided with simple guidelines to identify high-risk pregnancy before 20 weeks of gestation. Adequate nutrition and provision of supplements of iron and folic acid during second half of pregnancy are associated with improvement in birth weight. In order to conserve the meagre resources of energy, the mother should be advised to take complete physical rest during the last 4–6 weeks of pregnancy. Maternal infections during pregnancy should be identified early and treated adequately. Appropriate antimicrobial intervention to combat genital mycoplasma, chlamydiae and other pathogens may offer a simple technology to reduce incidence of preterm and small-for-dates babies.

Nutritional supplements during pregnancy alone cannot reverse the adverse biological effects of malnutrition which have operated over several generations. The existing cycle of low birth weightness in India should be viewed in the context of birth of a LBW female infant, who "grows" under the constraints of prevailing female neglect and discrimination, is provided with left over food, suffers from a variety of infective illnesses, lacks optimal adolescent growth spurt and evolves into a small woman. She gives birth to a small baby thus perpetuating the cycle of low birth weight babies with its attendant health consequences to the nation. There is an urgent social, cultural, religious and political need to upgrade the status of women in our society. *The present sense of despair at the* birth of a female child should be replaced by the awareness and reality that she is the creator and sustainer of life. If we wish to improve the health of human progeny, we must ensure optimal nutrition of girls during childhood, adolescence, pregnancy and lactation. Social awareness also needs to be created to ensure that no girl enters motherhood before 18 years of age. There is a need to launch a national drive to enhance female literacy both in the formal and non-formal settings. These measures would yield far more dividends as compared to ad hoc nutritional supplementation programs during pregnancy. Table 3.10 summarizes various strategies to reduce the incidence of LBW babies in low-middle income countries (LMICs).

Reduction of Perinatal Hypoxia and Birth Trauma

Early recognition of pregnancy, adequate antenatal care, prompt recognition and management of pregnancy-induced disorders are crucial for reducing morbidity and mortality due to perinatal hypoxia. Most deliveries in developing countries are conducted by untrained traditional birth attendants. It is essential that they should be trained to conduct a delivery safely with reduced hazards to the mother and the baby. The knowledge and skills pertaining to basic care and

TABLE 3.10 Strategies to reduce incidence of LBW babies
■ Women should be considered as the creators of progeny and accorded due health care, education, status and empowerment in society.
■ Provide optimal nutrition and health care to girl children throughout their life cycle viz. childhood, adolescence, pregnancy and lactation.
■ Impart family life and mother-craft education to teenage boys and girls.
■ Avoid early marriage and teenage pregnancy.
■ Provide pre-pregnancy health check-up, general and nutritional guidance, and essential vaccines.
■ Ensure inter-pregnancy interval of at least 3 years.
■ Provide optimal and good quality antenatal care to all pregnant women.
■ Enhance caloric intake, ensure balanced protein intake and provide supplements of iron, folic acid and micronutrients during pregnancy.
■ Avoid smoking, tobacco chewing, intake of alcohol, and substance abuse especially during pregnancy.
■ Early recognition and management of incompetent os, PIH, placental dysfunction, malaria, tuberculosis, urinary tract infection, diarrhea, dysentery, genital colonization and bacterial vaginosis, etc.
■ Avoid physical labor, emotional stress and sex during third trimester.

resuscitation of newborn baby at birth should be taught with flip charts, simple colored illustrations and practical demonstrations. As a long-term policy, it should be ensured that all deliveries are conducted in a health care facility. A national crusade should be launched to spread the message of "give a breath, save a life" to the grass root level health workers. Early recognition of signs of fetal hypoxia (clinically and by judicious use of monitoring equipment) and prompt measures to deliver the child with speed and safety are of fundamental importance. In borderline cases of cephalopelvic disproportion and malpresentation, the decision for instrumentation or manipulation and cesarean section should not be unduly delayed but executed with a sense of urgency and purpose. All deliveries in the hospital must be attended by a pediatrician who should be adept in resuscitation of asphyxiated babies at birth. The high-risk deliveries must be attended by a pediatrician.

PREVENTION OF NEONATAL INFECTIONS

Neonatal bacterial infections are one of the leading causes of neonatal mortality in developing countries. Measures for reducing neonatal infections deserve high priority and should be enforced at all levels where deliveries are conducted and newborn babies are being looked after. Most neonatal infections are preventable, if strict asepsis is maintained in the nursery. The vigilance and strict aseptic routines that are enforced in the operating theaters must be followed in the neonatal intensive care unit.

Prophylaxis

The prophylactic use of antibiotics to newborn babies is not recommended because of risk of emergence of resistant strains of bacteria. Prompt antibiotic therapy should be instituted at the first sign or suspicion of infection. If a mother is known to have untreated N. gonorrhoeae infection, the infant should receive a single dose of ceftriaxone 25–50 mg/kg (up to a maximum of 125 mg) IM or IV at birth. To protect against gonococcal ophthalmia, 1% silver nitrate or 2.5% povidone-iodine solution, or 1% tetracycline or 0.5% erythromycin eye ointment or single injection of benzyl penicillin is recommended amongst population with high incidence of gonorrhea. Irrigation of the eyes with normal saline following instillation of silver nitrate does not reduce the risk of chemical conjunctivitis but may compromise its antibacterial effectiveness. Erythromycin ophthalmic ointment provides the added advantage of preventing infection with C. trachomatis.

Preventive Neonatology

3

If more than one infant develops acute gastro-enteritis in the nursery, prophylactic neomycin or colistin should be administered to all babies and the unit should be closed to all further admissions until the situation is brought under control. When epidemic of thrush occurs in the nursery, all babies should receive oral application of gentian violet or nystatin for one week. The routine administration of immunogolobulins to low birth weight babies is of doubtful protective utility and may interfere with the development of infant's own immune response. Artificial bacterial colonization with deliberate introduction of non-virulent strains of a coagulase-negative staphylococci has not sustained the initial enthusiasm. These supposedly non-virulent bacteria have, at times, caused serious infections in some babies. Efforts to modify gut microbial ecology in preterm babies by oral administration of probiotics has been found to be useful for prevention of NEC. Hepatitis immune globulins (HBIG) and hepatitis B vaccine (HBV) should be administered within 48 hours of birth to babies born to HbsAg positive (especially e-antigen positive) mother. In countries with high incidence of tuberculosis and poliomyelitis and hepatitis due to HBV, BCG, first dose of OPV and HBV are given during first week of life.

Barrier Techniques in the Nursery

Policy Guidelines

The provision of plenty of space, adequate number of air exchanges or ventilation in the air-conditioning ducts, and availability of adequate number of well-trained nurses is essential for prevention of noso-comial infections. *The nursery complex must be accorded with similar facilities and high standard of asepsis as in the case of operation theater.* All the personnel working in the NICU should make conscious and determined efforts to enforce aseptic techniques at all times. Individuals with an acute infective illness (diarrhea, skin infection, ARI) or recent exposure to chickenpox should not enter the nursery. The nurse-incharge of the NICU should have the authority and mandate to ensure that every member of the team (including chief neonatologist!) honors the stipulated code of conduct during the discharge of his/her responsibilities.

Each unit should establish its own dress code for its personnel depending upon local needs and requirements. Nursery slippers should be worn before entering the nursery. It is preferable for the resident doctors and nurses, who spend most of their time in the nursery, to wear short sleeved gowns or pant suits which are laundered daily by the hospital. If a gown is used in the care of a neonate, it should be changed after every eight hours. Short-sleeved airy gowns should be used to cover the street clothes by visitors or personnel entering for brief periods. The routine use of mask is not recommended because improper use, such as frequent fingering, touching and displacing the mask, is fraught with hazards of infection. Hands should be restrained against unnecessarily touching one's own body parts especially nose or any object in the nursery. When hands get contaminated, they should be washed or sanitized immediately.

Handwashing

Effective and thorough handwashing before entering the nursery and after touching each baby is the **single most important** strategy for prevention of nosocomial or health care-associated infections (HCAIs). Obsessive handwashing is far more important for prevention of hospital-acquired infections compared to the ritual of using a mask and gown.

The WHO guidelines should be followed for effective handwashing (refer to Chapter 2). Rings, wrist watch, bracelet, bangles, etc. should be removed before entering the nursery. Nails should be kept trimmed and no nail polish should be used. Wash hands and arms up to elbows by using liquid soap and running water. Soap cakes may get colonized and are more likely to be stolen. Soapy antiseptic preparations containing povidone-iodine or chlorhexidine are available in dispensers (betadine scrub, gramophen) and are ideal for handwashing. Lather thoroughly by covering all areas including nails, webs and sides of fingers which are known to harbor pathogens. A thorough two-minute handwashing is mandatory before entering the nursery, before performing an invasive procedure and after providing care to an infected baby (Figure 3.7). A half-minute handwash is recommended for in-between touching the babies. The use of alcohol-based antiseptic solutions, like sterillium (ethyl-hexadecyl-dimethyl ammonium-ethyl sulfate in propanol), is useful before touching any baby during the round. The hands should be dried with single-use autoclaved napkins, disposable sterile paper napkins or allowed to dry spontaneously. The use of a common towel for drying the hands is a dangerous practice and is condemned.

Housekeeping Routines

The environment of NICU may be more heavily contaminated with bacteria compared to other hospital wards unless rigorous housekeeping routines are enforced. Dirt and organic matter may inactivate

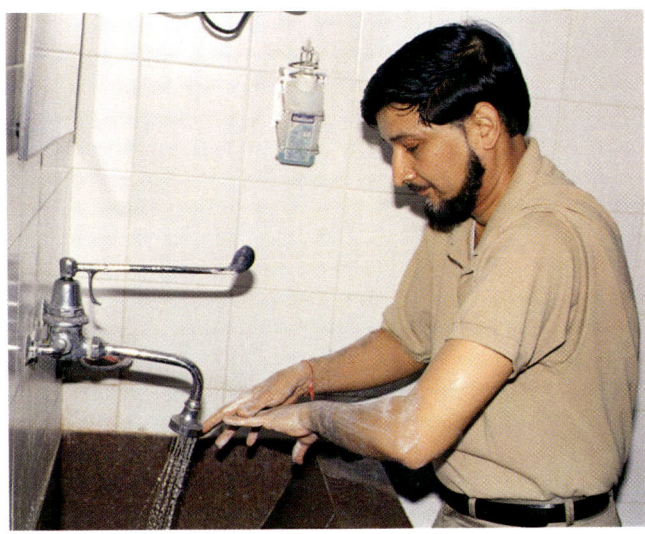

Figure 3.7 The correct technique of handwashing.

many chemical disinfectants, and therefore thorough cleaning and scrubbing with soap or detergent and water is necessary. Dry dusting and sweeping should be avoided due to risk of dissemination of bacteria. It is preferable to use vacuum cleaners to suck the dust from the floor, walls and equipment. Wet mopping of floors with soap and water containing 3% phenol should be carried out at least thrice daily (once during each duty shift). The waxing of surfaces and use of oil in water for mopping may limit dissemination of microorganisms. The sinks should be washed with 3% phenol (carbolic acid) or 5% lysol at least once a day. The utility of ultraviolet light for sterilization of nursery is of limited value and expensive. The policy guidelines for housekeeping and disinfection routines should be available in the form of a manual in the NICU (Table 3.11).

Disposal of Waste and Soiled Linen

There must be adequate provision of foot-operated bins adjacent to each baby unit for disposal of used material and soiled linen. Plastic bags should be kept as hampers in the dustbins. They should be sealed before their removal. The dustbins should be mopped with 3% phenol everyday.

Disinfection of Equipment

Disinfection is defined as the process of destruction of all pathogenic microorganisms and their toxins. Sterilization is the process of destruction of all microorganisms including vegetative forms, like spores. The commonly used disinfectants and germicides in the NICU are listed below:

1. **Bacillocid** It contains formaldehyde, glutaraldehyde, alkylurea derivative and benzalkonium chloride. Use 2% solution by dissolving 200 mL of the concentrate in 10 liters of water. It is used for disinfecting surfaces and for spraying rooms. The fans and air conditioners should be put off for 30 minutes and surfaces should be kept wet with bacillocid for 30 minutes for optimal efficacy.

2. **Korsolex** It contains formaldehyde and glutaraldehyde. One part of the concentrate is mixed with 9 parts of water to prepare 10% solution. For disinfection, the solution should remain in contact for 20 minutes and for sterilization for 4 hours.

3. **Cidex** It is a 2% solution of glutaraldehyde with an activator. The solution should remain in contact for 20 minutes for disinfection and 4 hours for sterilization.

4. **Savlon** It is a mixture of cetrimide, chlorhexidine gluconate and isopropyl alcohol. Use 1:100 solution for equipment and furniture and 1:30 solution for treating dirty wounds and disinfecting catheters or thermometers.

5. **Sterillium** It contains 2-propanolol, 1-propanolol, and ethyl-hexadecyl-dimethyl ammonium-ethyl sulfate. Rub 2–3 mL of sterillium on the palms and backs of hands for 30 seconds and allow it to dry for disinfection of hands. It can be used in-between nursing care or after handling the babies.

6. **Sodium hypochlorite (NaOCl or NaClO)** It is sodium salt of hypochlorous acid. It is available as TetraClean camphor disinfectant™ or Milton 5% solution for spray of fomites and cleaning of floors.

7. **Betadine** It is 7.5% solution of povidone-iodine and used for preparation of skin and disinfection of wounds. It should be applied in circular movements by moving from center towards periphery and allowed to dry for 60 seconds before wiping with 70% isopropyle alcohol.

8. **Formalin** (40% formaldehyde aqueous solution) is used for fumigation.

9. **Hydrogen peroxide** (100 mL H_2O_2 10% V/V solution diluted with 900 mL distilled water) is used for sanitization of equipment and fomites against COV-2 viruses which are highly contagious.

Resuscitation equipment Resuscitation bags and masks should be disinfected in cidex after every use. Silicon bags and masks can withstand autoclaving. Laryngoscope should be wiped cleaned with 70% isopropyl alcohol after each use. Oxygen hood should be cleaned daily or after each use with a detergent or soap and water. Alcohol should not be used for cleaning as it will cause opacification.

Preventive Neonatology

3

Care of the Newborn

3

TABLE 3.11 Housekeeping and disinfection routines

Area/item	Disinfection method and frequency	Other measures and remarks
Floors	Use chlorophore cleanser (3% phenol or 5% lysol) during every shift. Pesticide spray and anti-cockroach measures should be used once a week.	Do not sweep or do dry dusting. Avoid use of cidex. The holes and crevices in the floors, walls and ceilings should be sealed.
Walls	Wipe with 2% bacillocid once in two weeks	Fumigation is done when infection rate goes up.
Fans	Wet mop with soap and water once a month.	
Air conditioner	Vacuum cleaning is done once in two weeks. Window AC should be sprayed with 2% bacillocid once a week.	Thorough cleaning and change of filters by AC maintenance staff twice a year.
Sinks	Clean once a day with detergent powder and chlorophore cleanser	Tiles under the sink should be cleaned daily. Avoid sink top or shelf adjacent to the sink.
Entrance wash area	Daily mopping with chlorophore cleanser and 2% bacillocid spray twice a week	Switch off fans and AC and close the area for one hour after spray
Refrigerator	Defrost and clean with soap solution once every 2 weeks	
Buckets and dustbins	Wash daily with soap and water	The buckets and bins should be lined with polythene bags which should be changed after each disposal
Baby linen, cotton, gauze, etc.	Wash and autoclave	
Baby blankets and blanket covers	Wash or dryclean and autoclave between babies	
Feeding utencils	Boil for 15 min or autoclave before each use	
Swab containers, injection and medicine trays	Clean daily with soap or cleanser	Use a separate tray for each baby
Steel drums	Autoclave after every 48 hours	They should be kept closed properly and replaced, if broken
Cheatle forceps	Autoclave daily and keep in a sterile bottle containing 5% savlon or dry sterile cotton	
Stethoscope, measuring tape, thermometer, cuff of sphygmoma-nometer, and electronic probes, etc.	Clean daily with 70% isopropyl alcohol or sterillium	Keep a separate stethoscope for each baby. Keep thermometer in a bottle containing sterile cotton
Laryngoscope blade	Clean with 70% isopropyl alcohol or sterillium after each use	Never use cidex because it may be harmful to the baby
Oxygen hood	Wash daily with soap and water. Dry with an autoclaved linen	
Face mask	After each use, clean with a detergent and immerse in cidex for 20 min. Rinse in sterile water and dry it with autoclaved linen	

(contd.)

TABLE 3.11 Housekeeping and disinfection routines (*contd.*)

Area/item	Disinfection method and frequency	Other measures and remarks
Ambu bag and its reservoir, ventilator tubing, oxygen tubings, water taps, humidifier bottles, bottle and tubings of suction machine	Dismantle and clean with a detergent. Keep immersed in korsolex or cidex for 4 hours, rinse in sterile water, dry it and reassemble. Ambu bag and its reservoir should be cleaned once a week while other items should be cleaned daily.	Change ventilator circuit and oxygen tubing daily. Use distilled water in the humidifier and change it daily. Discard suction catheter after single use. Put 100 mL savlon in suction bottle up to the blue line. Keep the suction connector covered with a sterile gauze piece.
Weighing machine and radiant warmer	Mop daily with 2% bacillocid	Place an autoclaved sheet on the scale before weighing the baby.
Incubator	Clean daily with a detergent and water followed by 2% bacillocid. Do not use alcohol to clean the canopy because it will make the perspex foggy. After discharge or death of a baby, fumigation is done by adding 50 mL of formalin in 50 mL of water in the humidity tank of the incubator and plugging it on for 4 hours.	Do not keep the baby in the same incubator for more than one week.
Nursery equipment	Wet mop with sterile water once a day.	Keep them covered with a clean polythene sheet when not in use.

Note: Always discard disposables after a single use and do not compromise. Terminal disinfection should be done after discharge or death of a baby.
Bacillocid: Mixture of formaldehyde, glutaraldehyde and benzalkonium chloride by Raman and Weil.
Cidex: Glutaraldehyde 2% W/V by Johnson and Johnson.
Korsolex: Combination of glutaraldehyde and chemically bound formaldehyde by Raman and Weil.
Lysol: Mixture of ethanol, isopropyl alcohol, p-chloro-o-benzylphenol, potassium hydroxide, alkyl-dimethylbenzyl-ammonium chloride by Reckitt Benckiser.
Savlon: Mixture of 3.0 g cetrimide and 0.3 g chlorhexidine gluconate per 100 mL by Johnson and Johnson.
Sterillium: Alcoholic antiseptic and sanitizer containing 2-propanol, 1-propanol and mecetronium ethyl sulfate by Bode Chemie Hamburg.

Open care systems and cots They should be cleaned everyday with 3% phenol or 5% lysol. Mattresses should have intact plastic covers which should be cleaned daily with an antiseptic solution. The blankets used for cot-cared babies must be enclosed in autoclaved cotton covers which should be changed in-between babies.

Incubators The baby should not stay in an incubator for more than 7 days after which it should be dismantled and thoroughly disinfected. The surface of the incubator should be washed with soap and water and wiped with Milton hypochlorite solution or 2% bacillocid. The surface of the canopy and mattress should be cleaned everyday with liquid soap and water. Alcohol should not be used to clean the canopy as it will opacify. Humidification unit should be emptied daily and disinfected with cidex for 10 minutes. It should be filled with sterile water.

Add 6 mL of vinegar or acetic acid to every 2 liters of sterile water in the humidity reservoir, to prevent bacterial colonization. After discharge or death of a baby, fumigation is done by adding 50 mL of formaline in 50 mL of water in the humidity tank of the incubator and plugging it on for 4 hours.

Ventilators There is a lack of agreement on the best way of sterilizing more complex machines. The fumigation with hydrogen peroxide or ethylene oxide by means of an ultrasonic nebulizer is probably the most effective. It is desirable to have central sterilization facilities for routine intensive cleaning and sterilization of incubators and ventilators.

Rubber and plastic tubing The tubes connected with incubators, oxygen equipment and suction apparatus should be changed daily. The humidity bottles in the oxygen circuit and suction bottles should be boiled or autoclaved daily. Infant face masks should be cleaned

Preventive Neonatology

3

with 70% isopropyl alcohol after use. The polyethylene suction catheters, feeding tubes and scalp vein infusion sets should never be reused after boiling. It is desirable that ventilator circuit should not be reused and should be discarded after single use.

Feeding utencils The bottles and teats should be washed with soap and water immediately after feeds. They should be either boiled for at least 15 minutes or preferably autoclaved. The use of hypochlorite solution for chemical sterilization of bottles is not uniformly effective and not recommended for hospital practice. The formula should preferably be prepared by the nurse who does not handle the babies. She should observe strict asepsis by wearing sterile gown, mask and gloves. Terminal sterilization of in-bottle feeds at 10 to 15 lbs/inch pressure for 15 minutes is desirable. It is recommended that feeding bottles should be replaced by cup and spoon/*paladay* feeding in the NICU. The cups and spoons/*paladays* should be boiled for at least 15 minutes before use.

Infusion set Gamma-irradiated disposable infusion set, cannulae, needles, etc. should be used. The infusion set should be changed everyday while the intravenous cannula should be changed after every 48–72 hours. The tip of the cannula should not be covered with leucoplast so that it can be observed for signs of inflammation every 2 to 4 hours. The medications should not be administered through the rubber tubing of the IV set. Instead they should be given through a three-way stopcock attached to the cannula or through a side port meant for administration of drugs. The neck of the ampoule should be wiped with alcohol before breaking. Top of the vial should be wiped with alcohol before inserting the needle. Needles should not be left vented to atmosphere in the stoppers of infusion bottles due to risk of contamination. A new disposable needle should be used each time the fluid is withdrawn. The mixing of IV fluids and TPN solutions should be undertaken inside the laminar flow system. Avoid using stock solution of heparinized saline for flush purposes. It is recommended to use single-use normal saline ampoules for flushing the IV cannula.

Procedures

Strict asepsis should be ensured while performing any procedure in the nursery. Apart from thorough handwashing *vide supra*, sterile gloves should be worn for obtaining blood culture samples, endotracheal suction and emergency drainage of pneumothorax. Mask and sterile gloves should be worn for performing lumbar puncture and suprapubic aspiration of bladder. During more invasive procedures, like umbilical vessel catheterization, exchange blood transfusion, insertion of intercostal tube, establishing TPN lines, etc. mask, sterile gloves and gown should be worn.

Disinfectant Solutions

Many disinfectant solutions in current use get contaminated with Gram-negative bacteria particularly *Pseudomonas aeruginosa*. The use of benzalkonium chloride, cetrimide (cetavalon) and chloroxylenol (dettol) should be avoided because of their limited efficacy against Gram-negative organisms. *The cold sterilization solution must be freshly prepared daily.* Cheatle forceps and thermometers should be kept in 5% savlon or 2% cidex. Gamma-irradiated disposable catheters, feeding tubes, endotracheal tubes and small-vein infusion sets should be used only once and discarded. Venipuncture or medicath skin puncture site is an important portal for entry of micro-organisms. It should be thoroughly cleaned with savlon, tincture iodine (povidone-iodine) and ethly alcohol. The bottles containing disinfectant should never be closed with bark bungs or screw caps with cork liners because these contain substances which may inactivate the antiseptic.

Surveillance of Bacterial Flora

The routine suveillance of bacterial flora of nursery, personnel, equipment and infants is of limited value and involves too much of laboratory work. Whenever there is an outbreak of infection, the efforts should be made to identify the organisms and its possible source. The cold sterilization solutions and water in the humidifier should be cultured from time to time to identify any contaminants. Hands, nasal and throat swabs of personnel are cultured as and when needed.

Screening of Admissions

The infants referred from elsewhere should not be admitted to the neonatal intensive care unit when they are suffering from acute gastroenteritis or discharging abscess. The provision of a septic nursery is essential for admission of such infants and isolation of all infected babies. If mother is suffering from acute gastroenteritis, her baby should not be transferred to the nursery.

Fumigation

In centers where excellent housekeeping and aseptic routines are maintained, fumigation does not provide any additional benefit. However, most special care neonatal units in India undertake periodic fumigation whenever feasible during low occupancy phase and following an epidemic of infection. Doors, windows, walls and floors are scrubbed thoroughly with soap and water. The oxygen and central suction lines are shut off. The fans and air conditioners are put off. The ventilator outlets, air conditioner vents and gaps in doors and windows should be sealed airtight. For effective fumigation, 500 mL of formalin (40% formaldehyde) is needed for a room of 30 cubic metres capacity. Formalin can be sprayed with the help of a vaporizer (Oticare) for 6 hours. After fumigation, the doors and windows are kept open till all the formalin fumes are allowed to escape. The left over formalin should be removed and 4–6 ounces of ammonium hydroxide is poured in the vaporizer which is plugged on for faster elimination of formalin fumes. When vaporizer is not available, formalin can be boiled or treated with 250 g potassium permanganate and allowed to evaporate for 12 hours. Formalin should not be poured over potassium permanganate as this may lead to an explosion.

Isolation Policies

Availability of adequate number of trained nurses is crucial for prevention of nosocomial infections. The neonates with septicemia, meningitis and pneumonia do not need any isolation. Infants with acute gastroenteritis or draining abscesses must be isolated and managed by different nurses. Whenever, there is an epidemic of diarrhea or thrush in the NICU, further admissions should be stopped and all babies treated with an appropriate antibiotic or topical antifungal agent. The infected mother (if not gravely sick) should be advised to continue breastfeeding her baby. She should be taught general principles of hygiene and importance of handwashing for prevention of spread of infection. The use of a surgical mask while feeding will reduce the chances of droplet infection.

Congenital Infections

Babies with cytomegalovirus (CMV) infection, rubella, syphilis and chickenpox are highly infectious. Depending upon the nature of infection, they may continue to discharge the infecting agent in the nasopharynx, mucous membranes, urine and skin, sometimes for several weeks and months. Female health care personnel working in the NICU are at great risk. These neonates should be isolated and looked after in a separate room. The use of sterile gloves and thorough handwashing is essential while nursing these babies.

Neonate of Hepatitis B Positive Mother

There is a risk of vertical transmission of hepatitis B virus, if mother is HBsAg positive (especially if e-antigen positive). Babies born to mothers who are HBsAg positive or having acute hepatitis (or born to HIV positive mother) should be bathed as soon as possible to wash off the maternal blood and secretions contaminating their skin during birth. Health personnel who handle these infants should protect themselves by wearing gloves. Mothers can breastfeed and handle their babies safely. Hepatitis B immunoglobulin (HBIG) 0.5 mL should be given IM as early as possible but within 48 hours of age. Hepatitis B vaccine (HBV) should be given as per the standard protocol. The first dose of vaccine is given at the same time when HBIG is given but injected at a different site.

Infant of a Mother with Hepatitis A Infection

The baby born to a mother with acute HAV infection within 2 weeks of delivery should be given 0.5 mL immune globulin IM within 72 hours of birth. Breastfeeding is allowed but mother should follow strict handwashing routines to prevent fecal-oral contamination and risk of infection.

Infant of a Mother having Chickenpox

If mother gets chickenpox five days before or within five days of delivery, the baby should be isolated during 21 days of incubation period. If a mother develops chickenpox on the day of delivery, the baby should be isolated from the mother for at least one week and given formula feeds. Varicella zoster globulin (VZIG) 125 units/kg IM should be given to the baby as soon as possible after delivery. If baby develops chickenpox, isolation is continued till the scabs are formed.

UNIVERSAL PRECAUTIONS FOR HIV

Due to burgeoning epidemic of acquired immunodeficiency syndrome (AIDS), every health care professional is at risk of acquiring infection due to human immunodeficiency virus (HIV). It is desirable that all health care personnel must follow *universal precautions* in handling all patients on the premise that every patient is potentially infected with HIV (and HBV). Table 3.12 summarizes the protocol for universal precautions.

Ensure Protective Barrier

Intact skin forms an excellent barrier against HIV and HBV infections. If there is any cut or wound on the skin, apply occlusive water-tight dressing (band-aid) over it. Wear gloves, gown and plastic apron when

TABLE 3.12 Universal precautions

- Treat every specimen of blood or body fluid as potentially infectious.
- Wear gloves for handling all bodily fluids and while performing phlebotomy.
- For all procedures where splashing of body fluids or droplets may occur, wear waterproof gown, mask and goggles.
- Avoid re-capping, bending or breaking of needles, but when recapping is unavoidable it should be done with a single hand to avoid accidental needle stick injury to the finger.
- Wear gloves for patient care, if exudative or weeping dermatitis is present.
- Handwashing is a must in-between examination of patients, after any procedure and on removal of gloves.
- Promptly clean any blood spills or bodily fluids by pouring 1% bleach solution or 5% sodium hypochlorite over the spill and leave it soaked for at least 10 minutes.
- Disinfect or sterilize re-usable devices as recommended.
- Dispose the needles and other sharps safely into puncture resistant containers. The puncture resistant disposable container should be discarded for decontamination or incineration when three-quarters full.
- Wear heavy-duty rubber gloves for cleaning instruments, handling soiled linen or dealing with spills of blood and body fluids.

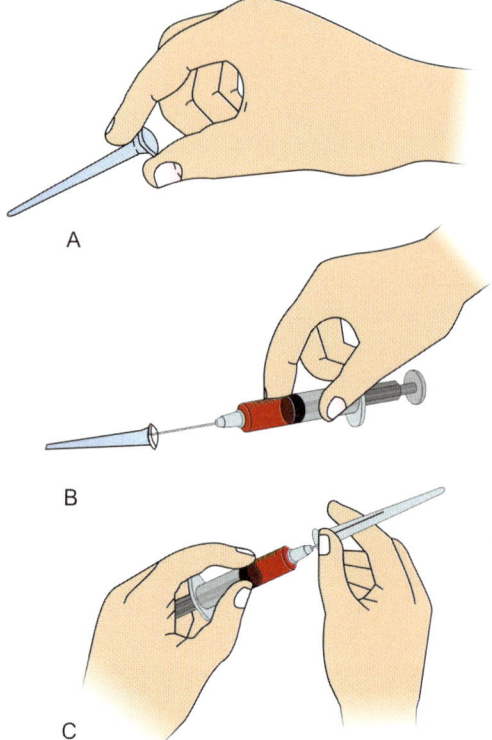

Figures 3.8 A to C The steps for recapping the needle with one hand to avoid needle stick injury to the fingers. (A) Place needle cap on a flat surface. (B) With one hand, hold syringe and use needle to scoop up the cap. (C) When the cap covers the tip of the needle, use the other hand to secure the cap firmly on the needle hub.

handling a newborn baby until blood and amniotic fluid have been wiped off. Wash hands thoroughly with soap and water when contaminated with blood, amniotic fluid, vaginal secretions and other body fluids. Wash hands after removing the gloves as a matter of routine. A mask or protective eyewear must be worn while performing any procedure where there is a likelihood of splashing of blood or other body fluids.

Prevention of Injuries

After using the disposable needles, never recap them due to potential risk of injury. They should be disposed off uncapped. When recapping is unavoidable, the proper procedure should be followed (Figures 3.8A to C). Injection file and cotton swab should be used for breaking ampoules. Scissors and blades should be handled with extreme care. The infusion bottles should be opened carefully with a bottle opener or tin cutter. Heavy duty gloves should be worn while handling and washing sharp instruments and glass ware. The needles, scalpel blades and other sharp objects should be disposed off in puncture resistant containers immediately after use. Needles should never be left on the bed, table, chair, nurses station, etc. In case of an accidental injury due to needle or

scalpel, allow local bleeding to occur to discharge any infective material. Wash the wound thoroughly with soap and water and apply betadine. Postexposure prophylaxis with antiretroviral drugs should be followed without delay as per standard protocol.

Handling the Laboratory Specimens

It is a good policy to consider every specimen as potentially infectious. The specimen should be collected in screw-capped plastic disposable containers without soiling laboratory forms. You should never pipette blood or other body fluid with your mouth.

Handling of Blood Spill

The spill should be covered with cotton, newspaper or other absorbent material. Pour 5% bleach solution or sodium hypochlorite over the spill. Wipe the spill-soaked area after 20 minutes. Discard the soiled material in a polythene-lined waste bag. The soiled floor should be cleaned with detergent. The gloves should be discarded into a polythene-lined waste bin and hands washed with soap and water.

Handling the Garbage and Soiled Linen

The soiled garbage, like soaked dressings and blood-stained sanitary napkins, should be collected in polythene bags, tied up carefully, labeled as "infection risk" or "biohazard" and sent for burning in an incinerator. The soiled linen should be sorted with gloved hands, placed in polythene bag and washed in the laundry with soap and bleaching powder for 25 minutes at 70°C. The surgical instruments should be sterilized by autoclaving. The liquid waste, like suction fluids, excretions and secretions, should be carefully poured down a drain without splashing.

PREVENTION OF CONGENITAL MALFORMATIONS

Majority of congenital malformations are not associated with any predisposing etiologic factors and are not preventable with the current state of our knowledge. During the first trimester of pregnancy, all medications and irradiation should be avoided as far as possible. Girls should be given rubella vaccine before they get married. The incidence of chromosomal disorders in infants of elderly mothers is high. These can be reduced by discouraging active reproduction beyond the age of 35 years. The incidence of genetic disorders can be brought down by avoiding consanguineous marriages. There is evidence to suggest that administration of high doses of folic acid during periconceptional period may lower the incidence of neural tube defects and cleft lip/palate. Prenatal diagnosis of genetic and chromosomal disorders and induction of therapeutic abortion of abnormal fetuses is being increasingly practised.

PREVENTION OF RHESUS ALLOIMMUNIZATION

The prophylactic utility of anti-D immunoglobulins for the prevention of rhesus alloimmunization or isoimmunization has been widely used during the past four decades. The administration of anti-D immunoglobulins to Rh-negative non-immunized mother soon after the delivery of an Rh-positive baby would immediately destroy the Rh-positive fetal red blood cells, which might have seeped into the maternal circulation, and thus prevent the development of sensitization. If Rh status of the fetus or stillborn baby is unknown or cannot be determined, anti-D immuno-globulins should be administered to the mother, if her indirect Coombs' test is negative. The protective efficacy of the procedure is up to 98% but occasional failures may occur due to one of the following reasons:

1. The prior sensitization of the mother may have been undetected by the insensitive anti-globulin technique employed for detection of anti-D antibodies. The enzyme treated red blood cells are preferred for detecting low levels of antibodies.
2. The occurrence of fetomaternal leak early in the course of pregnancy or an unusually large fetomaternal hemorrhage may be followed by sensitization, if only routine dose of anti-D immuno-globulin is administered.
3. Rarely, presence of antibodies against anti-D immunoglobulin may neutralize the latter.

The injection of anti-D immunoglobulins (300 µg) should be given intramuscularly into the deltoid or anterolateral region of thigh (avoid in the gluteal region due to delayed and slow absorption) to the mother within 72 hours of delivery. This dose is generally enough to provide protection against 15 mL of transplacental hemorrhage of fetal red blood cells. In exceptional circumstances of excessive fetomaternal hemorrhage, proportionately larger dose of anti-D immunoglobulin would be required (10 µg for each additional 0.5 mL of fetomaternal hemorrhage). When an Rh-negative woman is carrying more than one fetus, she should be given double the dose of anti-D immunoglobulin. All unsensitized Rh-negative women should receive prophylactic injection of anti-D immunoglobulins in following situations:

1. After birth of each Rh-positive baby.
2. After abortion or miscarriage of Rh-positive conceptions.
3. The situations and procedures which are associated with increased risk of fetomaternal hemorrhage (amniocentesis, chorionic villus biopsy, cordocentesis, intrauterine transfusion or surgical procedure, antepartum hemorrhage, ectopic pregnancy, abdominal trauma, podalic version, etc.) should be managed by administration of anti-D immuno-globulins.

To further enhance its efficacy, it has been recommended to administer 300 µg of anti-D immunoglobulins to all unsensitized Rh-negative women around 28–32 weeks of gestation. If delivery occurs more than 4 weeks later, and the infant is Rh-positive, the mother should receive additional 300 µg anti-D immuno-globulins intramuscularly, within 72 hours of delivery. The dose of anti-D immunoglobulins is 150 µg when given before 12 weeks of gestation.

The extent of fetomaternal hemorrhage (FMH) should be assessed by doing Kleihauer-Betke count on the maternal blood in infants with unexplained anemia at birth, intrauterine death, manual removal of placenta and amniocentesis. Flow cytometry is more reliable to quantify the severity of FMH but is not readily available in our country. The rosetting technique is a relatively simple serological method which can also be used to quantify the extent of FMH following an intervention or procedure. The appropriate dose of anti-D immunoglobulin (20 µg for each mL of fetal red blood cells) should be administered depending upon the estimated amount of fetal red blood cells in the maternal circulation.

A number of monoclonal anti-D (Rho) immunoglobulin preparations are available (125 µg and 300 µg/mL), such as Rhoclone (Bharat Serums), Rhogam (Johnson and Johnson) and Imogan (Ranbaxy). The prophylactic utility of anti-D immunoglobulins for prevention of rhesus isoimmunization is exceedingly high and reliable but it is grossly under utilized in developing countries due to cost constraints and logistic difficulties.

BIBLIOGRAPHY

American Academy of Pediatrics. Committee on Genetics. Prenatal Genetic Diagnosis for Pediatricians. *Pediatrics* 1994, 93:1010–1015

American Academy of Pediatrics. Committee of Fetus and Newborn: Decontamination of fomites in neonatal units. *Pediatrics* 1966, 38: 142.

American College of Obstetricians and Gynecologists (ACOG). ACOG Practice Bulletin No. 62. Intrapartum fetal heart rate monitoring. *American College of Obstetricians and Gynecologists,* Washington DC, 2005.

Ayliff GAJ, Collins BJ, Lowbury EJL. Cleaning and disinfection of hospital floors. *Brit Med* J 1966, 2: 442.

Beatrice K. Control of Gram-negative bacilli in a hospital nursery. *Amer J Dis Child* 1974, 107: 363.

Bowman JM. Prevention of hemolytic disease of the newborn. *Brit J Hemat* 1970, 19: 653.

Campbell S, Pearce JM. Ultrasound visualization of congenital malformations. *Brit Med Bull* 1983, 39:322–331

Concensus conference on anti-D prophylaxis. Royal college of Physicians of Edinburgh and Royal College of Obstetricians and Gynecologists. *Transfusion* 1998, 38: 97–99.

Dalal AR, Purandare AC. The partograph in child birth. An absolute essentiality or a mere exercise. *J Obstet and Gynecol of India* 2018, 68(1):3–14.

Gilbert F, Marinduque B. DNA prenatal diagnosis. *Curr Opinion Obstet Gynecol* 1990, 2: 226–235.

Haddow JE, Polomaki GE, Knight GJ, *et al.* Prenatal screening for Down syndrome with use of maternal serum markers. *N Engl J Med* 1992, 327: 588–593

Kulkarni ML, Vengalath S. Prenatal diagnosis of genetic disorders. *Indian Pediatr* 1995, 32:1229–1238

Singh M, Paul VK. Strategies to reduce perinatal and neonatal mortality. *Indian Pediatr* 1988, 25(6):499–509.

Singh M, Deorari AK, Khajuria RC, Paul VK. Perinatal and neonatal mortality in a hospital. *Indian J Med Res* 1991, 94:1–5.

Singh M. Housekeeping rituals and routines in the NICU. In: Essential Pediatrics for Nurses. *CBS Publishers & Distributors Pvt. Ltd, New Delhi, Fourth edition, 2017, p 44–49.*

Wang L, Shi Y, *et at.* Chinese Working Committee on Perinatal and Neonatal Management for the Prevention and Control of the 2019 Novel Coronavirus infection. *Ann Transl Med.* 2020,8(3):47.

Maternal Disorders and Fetal Outcome

The maternal wellbeing, optimal nutritional status and freedom from systemic disorders are essential to provide an optimal *in utero* environment for proper growth and development of the fetus. In general, fetus is well protected and insulated against adverse physical, chemical and biological insults. Uterus is a unique portable incubator with thermostatically controlled system for temperature regulation, provision for ready supply of oxygen and nutrients and prompt disposal of waste products through the vital link of placenta. The following maternal conditions, some of which are peculiar to a pregnant woman, may jeopardize fetal safety and provide useful clues for the diagnosis of certain neonatal disorders. Drugs given to the mother for the management of her illness may also adversely affect the fetus.

DISORDERS PECULIAR TO PREGNANCY

Pregnancy-induced Hypertension (Toxemia of pregnancy, pre-eclampsia and eclampsia)

Hypertension during pregnancy or gestational hypertension is a major cause of prematurity, intrauterine growth retardation and perinatal deaths and is responsible for 20–30% of all maternal deaths. Pre-eclampsia is characterized by hypertension (blood pressure 140/90 mm Hg or more) after 20th week of gestation, proteinuria (>0.3 g/24 hr) or spot urinary protein to creatinine ratio (PCR) ≥0.3 or a urine dipstick reading of 1+ or greater and/or edema. The usual time of onset is 32 weeks of gestation, but it may present earlier in women with pre-existing kidney disease, hypertension or hydatidiform mole. The blood pressure must be elevated on at least two occasions 6 hours apart and should return back to normal within 6 weeks of delivery. Isolated edema is of no significance while proteinuria of more than 1.0 g/L in a random sample is suggestive of severe toxemia and adversely affects the prognosis.

'Roll-over-test' has been proposed for early diagnosis of pregnancy-induced hypertension and prediction of small-for-gestational age infant. During antenatal visits, between 28 and 34 weeks of gestation, blood pressure is first recorded in a supine position. The woman is then asked to lie in left lateral recumbent posture for one to two minutes and blood pressure is rechecked in the same arm. 'Roll-over-test' is considered as positive, if in supine position diastolic pressure is 20 mm Hg or more higher than in the left lateral position. It has a good correlation with subsequent development of pre-eclampsia and birth of SGA infant. HELLP syndrome (hemolysis, elevated liver enzymes and low platelets) is suggestive of advanced and ominous pre-eclampsia with disseminated intravascular coagulation. Eclampsia is diagnosed when pre-eclamptic clinical picture is complicated by seizures. Almost one-third cases of eclampsia develop during pregnancy, one-third during labor and one-third within 48 hours of delivery.

The incidence of toxemia of pregnancy varies between 5 and 8%. Its incidence is higher among primigravida, and very young or elderly overweight women. Family history of toxemia in her mother or sisters is associated with increased risk of the disease. Diabetes mellitus, chronic hypertension, polyhydramnios, multifetal gestation and hydatidiform mole are additional associates of pregnancy-induced hypertension. Its exact etiopathogenesis is uncertain. Adrenomedullin, a potent vasodilator, is produced in diminished quantities by the placenta in pre-eclampsia. Various workers have postulated increased ratio of thromboxane to prostacyclin, elevated circulating lipid peroxide, nitric oxide, endothelins and endothelial cell injury or vasculitis due to circulating immune complexes.

There is recent evidence to suggest that elevated levels of soluble receptors for vascular endothelial growth factor (VEGF) and transforming growth factor-beta (TGF-β) namely soluble fms-like tyrosine kinase-1 (SFlt-1) and soluble endoglin respectively in the maternal blood. This leads to reduced bioavailability of VEGF and TGF-β in maternal circulation leading to increased arterial tone (hypertension) and enhanced leakage in the capillaries (edema, proteinuria and pulmonary congestion). A woman with early and severe pre-eclampsia may have an underlying metabolic disorder, such as factor V Leiden mutation, antiphospholipid antibody syndrome, hyperhomocys-teinemia or protein S deficiency. Antiphospholipid syndrome (Hughes syndrome) is associated with hypercoagulation state, thrombotic complications, eclampsia, preterm delivery and stillbirth. There is elevation of immune antibodies, like lupus anticoagu-lant, anticardiolipin and anti-β_2-glycoprotein-1. There is some evidence to suggest that intake of DHA, calcium and riboflavin supplements and low dose aspirin may reduce the incidence and severity of pre-eclampsia. There is some controversial evidence to suggest that supplementation with calcium, ribofla-vin, vitamin C, vitamin D, vitamin E and omega-3 fatty acids is associated with reduced risk of pre-eclampsia.

Hypertension during pregnancy is the commonest cause of chronic placental insufficiency leading to chronic fetal hypoxia, oligohydramnios and intra-uterine growth restriction and its consequences in the newborn. At times, IUGR and reduced urinary estriol may precede development of eclampsia. There are higher levels of markers of oxidative stress in maternal and cord blood in pregnancies complicated by pre-eclampsia. Incomplete reduction of oxygen produces a series of molecules called reactive oxygen species (ROS). Free radical damage to tissues plays an important role in the pathogenesis of a number of neonatal disorders including periventricular leukomalacia, bronchopulmonary dysplasia and necrotizing enterocolitis. Fetal outcome is related to the duration and severity of hypertension and degree of proteinuria. Perinatal mortality and stillbirth rate is extremely high in severe pre-eclampsia and eclampsia. Accidental hemorrhage due to abruptio placentae leads to acute fetal hypoxia, birth asphyxia and respiratory distress due to meconium aspiration.

Management

Hypertension appears to be a compensatory pheno-menon to maintain placental circulation and patient may not be given any specific treatment unless diastolic blood pressure rises above 100 mm Hg. Hydralazine, labetalol and nifedipine are safe while other antihypertensives should be avoided during pregnancy due to their adverse effects on the fetus. There is a risk of development of sudden hypotension, if calcium channel blocker is used in conjunction with magnesium sulfate infusion. Diuretics are contra-indicated due to reduced intravascular volume. Pregnancies complicated by hypertension demand considerable skill and experience on the part of obstetrician to monitor fetal growth and utero-placental status in order to accurately time the delivery both in the interest of the mother as well as the fetus.

Fetal wellbeing should be closely monitored by non-stress test, biophysical profile and Doppler ultrasonography. It would appear that prostaglandin E_2 may be preferable for induction of labor in pre-eclamptic hypertensive high-risk patient because it has lowering effect on blood pressure and lacks the antidiuretic effect of oxytocin. Antiphospholipid syndrome with a risk of widespread thrombosis is treated with low molecular weight heparin. Warfarin or coumadin is not recommended during pregnancy because of its potential risk of teratogenicity and fetal hemorrhage (Figure 4.1). Nasal hypoplasia and stippled bone epiphyses may associated with upper airway obstruction which is relieved with an oral airway. Antenatal corticosteroids should be given, if delivery can be delayed by 48 hours. When there are evidences of fetal distress or impending eclampsia, baby should be delivered without delay. In women with impending or established eclampsia, magnesium sulfate infusion is started (6 g IV loading dose followed

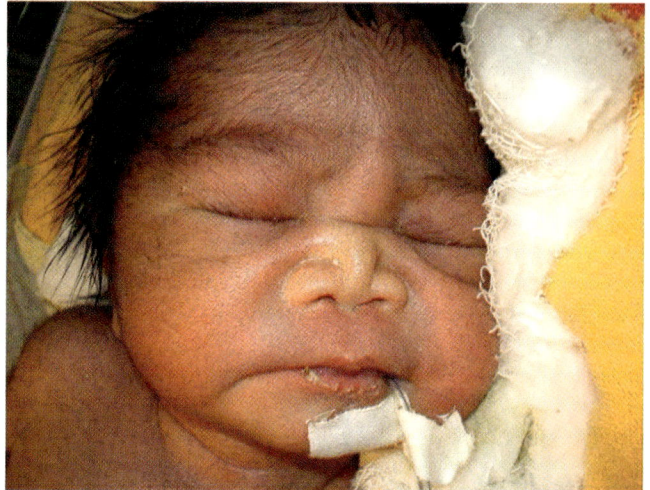

Figure 4.1 Infant with typical nasal deformity due to warfarin embryopathy.

by 2 g/hr constant infusion) and continued at least 24 hours postpartum. There is reduced risk of neuro-motor disability in babies born following magnesium sulfate therapy to the mother.

A close watch should be kept on respiratory status, deep tendon reflexes and urine out put to monitor maternal magnesium toxicity. If there are any side effects, magnesium sulfate infusion should be discontinued and calcium gluconate administered. Infants born to pre-eclamptic mothers are at risk to suffer from consequences of placental dysfunction. They are likely to have intrauterine growth retardation, perinatal asphyxia, polycythemia and hypoglycemia. They are at risk to develop RDS due to meconium aspiration syndrome. Sedatives given to the mother may cause respiratory depression and hypotonia. Antihypertensives especially beta-blockers may aggravate development of intrauterine growth retardation and hypoglycemia. About one-third of infants born to mothers with pre-eclampsia may have transient thrombocytopenia and neutropenia with increased risk of neonatal infections.

Abnormal Quantity of Liquor

The dynamics of amniotic fluid are not well understood. During first trimester (<14 weeks), there is bidirectional diffusion of amniotic fluid between fetal skin and transudation of extracellular fluid from amnion, placenta and umbilical cord. When fetal skin gets keratinized (around 20 weeks), amniotic fluid is mostly contributed by fetal urine and efflux of lung secretions. Fetus swallows liquor, absorbs and retains some and voids the excess through the urine. There is a small contribution from oral, nasal and tracheal secretions. The volume of amniotic fluid is related to the gestational age and is maintained within a narrow range. The exact factors regulating the volume of amniotic fluid are ill understood. The vascular endothelial growth factor (VEGF) is believed to regulate the endothelial growth of network of blood vessels located on the fetal surface of placenta which result in transudation of extracellular fluid into the amniotic cavity. Alterations in the quantity of amniotic fluid are related to the presence of certain fetal disorders which may either interfere with swallowing and absorption of amniotic fluid or with the production of urine, besides certain maternal conditions.

The amniotic fluid provides nutrients and growth factors that facilitate fetal growth. It contains significant amounts of epidermal growth factor (EGF), transforming growth factor beta-1 (TGF-β_1), insulin-like growth factor-1 (IGF-1), granulocyte colony-stimulating factor (G-CSF) and erythropoietin. It provides mechanical cushioning and antimicrobial factors that protect the fetus. It has an important role in the development of gastrointestinal, pulmonary and musculoskeletal systems and is a useful source of stem cells and diagnostic studies.

Polyhydramnios There is excessive amount of amniotic fluid (>2 liters) and it occurs in 1 in 1000 pregnancies. The diagnosis is based on the discrepancy between size of the fetus and the volume or size of the uterus, increased amniotic fluid index (≥20 cm) and a large gap between the fetus and the anterior and posterior uterine walls on ultrasonography. To calculate the amniotic fluid index (AFI), the anteroposterior diameters of the largest empty fluid pocket (no umbilical cord or fetal parts) in each quadrant are added together. The AFI is normally 7–25 cm. In addition, each individual pocket of fluid should be 2 to 8 cm. Polyhydramnios may occur due to some maternal disorders, such as diabetes mellitus, syphilis and chronic renal or cardiac disease. Pre-eclamptic toxemia is commonly associated with polyhydramnios. The presence of excessive amniotic fluid should alert the pediatrician to the possibilities of anencephaly, high intestinal obstruction, omphalocele, gastroschisis and ectopia vesicae. Twins and hydrops fetalis may be associated with polyhdramnios.

Oligohydramnios Oligohydramnios (amniotic fluid index ≤5 cm) is often associated with placental insufficiency and postmaturity. The fetal disorders which interfere with passage of urine, such as bilateral renal agenesis, renal dysplasia, polycystic kidney disease and obstructive uropathy, may have associated oligohydramnios. To compensate for oligohydramnios, the fluid from fetal lungs egress from trachea into the amniotic sac. This leads to hypoplasia of the lungs because aspiration of amniotic fluid is essential for growth of lungs. Due to loss of buffering effect of amniotic fluid, the baby may get compressed or squashed *in utero* and develop typical flat facies or Potter facies, limb deformities and hypoplastic lungs.

Antepartum Hemorrhage

Antepartum hemorrhage whether due to placenta previa or abruptio placentae may lead to fetal hypoxia and intrauterine death, premature delivery, severe birth asphyxia and anemia. Bleeding from rupture of marginal sinus, circumvallate placenta and vasa previa as a result of velamentous cord insertion is also associated with identical hazards. The vaginal blood can be examined to find out whether it is of fetal or maternal in origin by estimation of fetal hemoglobin.

Maternal Disorders and Fetal Outcome

4

Rhesus and ABO Incompatibility

The severity of rhesus alloimmunization may be assessed by the history of previous pregnancies and their outcome, zygosity of the father, titer of anti-D antibodies during pregnancy and optical density of the amniotic fluid when severely affected baby is anticipated. Following the routine use of anti-D immune globulins for prophylaxis, rhesus isoimmunization has become uncommon.

Mothers with O group may develop ABO hemolytic disease in the fetus, though its occurrence or severity cannot be predicted before birth. When Rh-negative woman has ABO incompatibility, the severity of rhesus isoimmunization is reduced because fetal RBCs are rapidly hemolyzed. Isoimmunization of the mother against fetal leukocytes and thrombocytes is also documented.

Premature Rupture of Membranes

Amniotic membranes constitute an effective barrier against ascending infection from the birth canal. The membranes usually rupture after the onset of labor but in around 10% of pregnancies they may rupture before the onset of labor. The marked delay (>24 hours) between the rupture of membranes and the birth of the baby may predispose the fetus to develop bacterial infection by swallowing or aspirating infected amniotic fluid especially when the mother is exposed to unclean vaginal examinations. The mother may develop clinical evidences of amnionitis in the form of fever, tachycardia (both maternal and fetal), leukocytosis, uterine tenderness and foul smelling amniotic fluid.

Preterm prolonged rupture of membranes (PPROM) is a major risk factor for occurrence of preterm delivery and perinatal infections. It is preferable and safer to deliver the baby, if there are evidences of chorioamnionitis or when gestational maturity is 34 weeks or more. If expectant management is chosen in a woman with preterm PROM, strict bedrest is advised. High vaginal swab should be taken for culture and antibiotics (ampicillin and aminoglycoside) are started, if there are evidences of chorioamnionitis. There is no role of tocolytic agents to delay labor and corticosteroids to accelerate fetal pulmonary maturity. Pregnancy should be closely monitored for evidences of fetal hypoxia because of umbilical cord compression and chorioamnionitis.

NUTRITIONAL STATUS OF THE MOTHER

Relatively high incidence of low birth weight babies in developing countries is related to early marriages, socioeconomic deprivation, maternal ill-health and malnutrition. Chronic starvation of the mother operating over several generations adversely affects the fetal growth and birth weight. It is well known that a short or light mother tends to produce a small baby. Maternal height of less than 145 cm and a weight of less than 40 kg is considered as an important maternal high-risk factor adversely affecting fetal growth. Fetus is a parasite and during short period of acute gestational starvation in healthy mothers, maternal tissues are catabolized or sacrificed to meet the nutritional needs of the fetus. However, when food deprivation is more severe or prolonged and mother is having marginal nutritional status, it would have deleterious effects on the growth of the fetus. It has been documented that during calamities, like famine and war when intake of food is limited or denied during last weeks of gestation, the birth weight is reduced by about 200 g of the expected weight when compared with mean birth weight of infants born before and after the disaster. Intervention studies have also shown that when mothers in a community are provided additional 200 kcal and 25 g proteins/day during last 6–8 weeks of pregnancy, the birth weight of their offsprings was on an average 110 g more compared to non-supplemented controls.

The incidence of LBW babies can be halved by food supplementation during pregnancy. It is likely that the salutary effects of food supplements during pregnancy are greater in populations with lower nutritional status and higher incidence of LBW babies. Anemia is a frequent complication of pregnancy and significant correlation exists between degree of anemia and birth weight. Supplementation of iron and folic acid during last trimester of pregnancy is associated with increased mean birth weight. Maternal iron deficiency during pregnancy does not exercise any adverse effect on the hemoglobin of the baby at birth but these infants are liable to develop serious iron deficiency anemia by the age of 5 to 6 months due to poor stores of iron.

Zinc deficiency usually co-exist with iron deficiency and it is also known to adversely affect the fetal growth. There is evidence to suggest that adequate intake of essential fatty acids especially docosahexaenoic acid (DHA) which is metabolic end product of omega-3 fatty acid (alpha-linolenic acid) is mandatory to optimize brain growth during fetal life. It is recommended that supplements of omega-3 fatty acids (2.6 g/day) and DHA (100–300 mg/day) should be taken by pregnant women to ensure optimal physical growth and mental development of their offsprings.

Recently, startling observations have been made to suggest that deficient iodine intake during pregnancy in endemic areas may be associated with increased prevalence of hypothyroidism at birth. Vitamin overdosage, especially of the fat-soluble vitamins, has been implicated to produce fetal abnormalities. Vitamin A overdose has been associated with kidney malformations, neural tube defects and hydrocephalus and vitamin D overdose with cardiac, neurologic and renal defects.

CHRONIC SYSTEMIC DISORDERS

Bronchial Asthma

Chronic intractable asthma during pregnancy may be associated with fetal growth retardation. Iodide containing expectorant mixtures during pregnancy may lead to the development of fetal goiter and hypothyroidism.

Chronic Cardiac Disease

There is an increased risk of maternal cardiovascular complications in the form of thromboembolism and sudden death during pregnancy. Rheumatic heart disease with congestive heart failure or cyanotic congenital heart disease in a pregnant woman is often associated with increased risk of abortion, prematurity, intrauterine growth retardation and perinatal asphyxia. The drugs used for the management of cardiovascular disorders may produce serious side effects to the fetus. Administration of warfarin is associated with risk of embryopathy (15–25%) and fetal hemorrhage. Uterine contractions may be initiated by maternal ingestion of quinidine, disopyramide and propranolol. Other neonatal consequences of maternal propranolol therapy during pregnancy include intrauterine growth retardation, birth asphyxia, sedation, bradycardia, hypoglycemia, polycythemia and hyperbilirubinemia. The use of thiazide diuretics during pregnancy is known to cause neonatal liver damage and thrombocytopenia.

Hypertension

Chronic hypertension is diagnosed when it precedes pregnancy or occurs within 20 weeks of gestation and it does not resolve by the 6-week postpartum checkup. Essential hypertension of a long-standing duration may adversely affect the fetal growth because of placental vasculopathy. Chronic or pre-pregnancy hypertension is becoming a common problem due to delayed childbearing. In almost 50% cases, preeclampsia may be superimposed on chronic hypertension. Methyldopa is the antihypertensive of first choice during pregnancy because it has no adverse effects on uteroplacental blood flow. Labetalol and calcium channel blockers are useful alternatives. Atenolol should be avoided while ACE-inhibitors are contraindicated due to risk of cardiovascular and CNS congenital anomalies. Diuretics should be used with caution, if there is associated pre-eclampsia. Chronic hypertension is associated with high maternal and perinatal morbidity and mortality. There is high risk of prematurity, intrauterine growth restriction, fetal hypoxia, placental abruption and stillbirths.

Chronic Renal Disease

Chronic nephritis and nephrotic syndrome may lead to premature delivery and fetal growth retardation probably by virtue of associated hypertension. Urinary tract infection or bacteriuria during pregnancy may be associated with prematurity and low birth weight. Pregnancy following renal transplantation is associated with high risk of preterm delivery and overall 30% risk of neonatal complications including RDS, congenital anomalies, adrencortical insufficiency, hyperviscosity, seizures and septicemia.

Viral Hepatitis

Jaundice is not common during pregnancy except during epidemics. Most cases are either due to viral hepatitis or because of recurrent intrahepatic cholestasis of pregnancy. Hepatitis during pregnancy carries higher maternal morbidity and mortality. The fetal consequences of maternal jaundice are related to its etiology, gestational timing and severity. There is increased risk of abortions, stillbirths, prematurity and higher perinatal mortality rate among pregnant women having hepatitis. If mother had severe unconjugated jaundice before delivery, neonate is likely to be jaundiced at birth due to fetomaternal transfer of bilirubin. There is an increased risk of transplacental transfer of infection to the fetus but more often transfer is perinatal, mostly during delivery and soon after birth through handling. At birth, the baby should be cleaned off any blood and secretions. Infants born to mothers who suffered from hepatitis A during pregnancy should be given 0.5 mL/kg of pooled human gammaglobulins intramuscularly at birth. Effective measures should be taken to minimize the risk of fecal-oral spread of virus from the infected mother to her baby. The vertical transmission of hepatitis B is variable but if mother is HBe antigen positive, there is 90% risk of fetal and neonatal infection. It is preferable to deliver such women by cesarean section. It is recommended that infants born to mothers positive for Au antigen should receive 0.5 mL of hepatitis B immunoglobulin (HBIG) intramuscularly within 12 hours of birth along with three doses of hepatitis B vaccine at 0, 1 and 6 months of age. The first dose of hepatitis B vaccine and HBIG can be given simultaneously but at two independent sites. There are no contraindications to breastfeeding.

Systemic Lupus Erythematosus

Pregnancy complicated by maternal systemic lupus erythematosus (SLE) may lead to fetal death, prematurity, intrauterine growth retardation and transient neonatal lupus erythematosus. Approximately, one-third of patients with SLE have antiphospholipid (anticardiolipin) and anti-RO (anti-SSA autoantibodies) antibodies which serve useful markers for passively acquired fetal and neonatal disease. The common manifestations of neonatal lupus include photosensitive maculopapular rash on the face, trunk and proximal extremities which is aggravated by phototherapy or exposure to sunlight. Mild thrombocytopenia, anemia, hepatosplenomegaly and carditis may occur. Congenital complete heart block may be diagnosed *in utero* and may serve as the first clue to maternal disease. Complete heart block does not require any therapeutic intervention except when it leads to congestive heart failure, syncope or seizures because of intermittent asystole. The clinical condition resolves in 10 to 12 weeks without any corticosteroid therapy.

MATERNAL INFECTIONS

In developing countries, due to unsatisfactory sanitary conditions and poor sense of personal hygiene, significantly higher perinatal morbidity and mortality is related to infectious diseases. A variety of viral, bacterial, protozoal and spirochetal maternal infections during pregnancy pose a serious threat to the wellbeing and survival of the fetus, though their overall incidence is low. A mild or even unrecognized maternal illness may produce crippling or fatal consequences in the developing embryo. Broadly speaking, fetal infections are manifested by intrauterine growth retardation, meningoencephalitis, hepatitis, congenital malformations and abortions or stillbirths. Most live viral vaccines are contraindicated during pregnancy because they may cause fetal infection and death *in utero*.

During second half of pregnancy, asymptomatic bacteriuria is common and occurs in about 4–7% women. The relationship between asymptomatic bacteriuria of pregnancy to perinatal morbidity is controversial. About one-third of women with asymptomatic bacteriuria develop symptomatic pyelonephritis which is associated with higher incidence of low birth weight babies. There is some controversial evidence to suggest that vaginal colonization with mycoplasma and chlamydiae is also associated with higher incidence of LBW babies due to prematurity and fetal growth retardation. Malaria during pregnancy is an important cause of intrauterine growth retardation in endemic areas. Placental malaria without any symptoms or laboratory evidence of infection in the mother, is an important cause of fetal wasting. Among first born, it has been found that birth weight of infants may be 150–200 g lower in those with malarial parasites in the placenta as compared with birth weight of infants without placental infection. During delivery, a number of infections may be contracted by the baby during its transport through an infected birth canal, viz. gonococci, *Listeria monocytogenese, Group B streptococci, Escherichia coli, Candida albicans and herpes virus hominis, hepatitis B virus and human immunodeficiency virus* (HIV).

Human immunodeficiency virus (HIV) can be passed from the mother to her baby during pregnancy, delivery and through breastfeeding. Although HIV infection has been detected in an aborted fetus of 8 weeks gestation but almost 90% of transmission occurs during last 2 months of pregnancy and around 65% occur perinatally. There is some evidence that infants who acquire the infection in early gestation *in utero* are likely to have more severe disease compared to those who acquire the infection perinatally. When positive-HIV status of the mother is known during early pregnancy, she can be given the option of medical termination of pregnancy.

The median rate of transmission of HIV from an infected mother to her newborn baby is 25% with a range of 15–35%. The risk of vertical transmission of HIV from mother to her baby is increased when there is acute viremia during pregnancy and maternal viral load is high or maternal CD4 count is below 400/mm^3. Additional factors which are recognized to increase the risk of materno-fetal transmission of virus include chorionic villus sampling, cordocentesis, fetal scalp blood sampling, chorioamnionitis, presence of another sexually transmitted disease and vaginal delivery. Vaginal delivery, especially when episiotomy is done, is associated with greater risk of transmission compared to delivery by cesarean section. The risk of transmission of HIV through breast milk is around 5–15%. The risk of transmammary transmission of HIV increases, if there are cracks or bleeding from nipples.

Antiretroviral therapy to the infected mother during pregnancy and her baby during newborn period has been shown to reduce the risk of perinatal transmission of HIV by 70%. Zidovudine is given after 28 weeks of pregnancy in a dose of 100 mg 5 times/day orally. At the onset of labor, a combination of single dose (Sd) NVP, AZT and 3TC followed by postpartum ART, with AZT and 3TC are given to the mother for 7 days. Newborn baby is started on oral zidovudine in a dose of 2 mg/kg every 6 hourly, Sd-NVP 2 mg/kg single daily dose and therapy is continued for a period of 4 weeks. The baby should preferably be delivered by elective cesarean section. In view of 15% risk of transmission of HIV through breastfeeding, the mother should be given all the facts so that she can make an informed decision whether to breastfeed or give formula feeds to her baby. When decision for breastfeeding is made, exclusive breatfeeding without any formula feed poses less risk of transmammary transmission of HIV.

ENDOCRINAL DISORDERS

Thyroid Disorders

Independent pituitary–thyroid relationship is maintained by the fetus and the mother. Iodine and thyrotropin-releasing hormone (TRH) readily cross the placenta. Thyroid-stimulating hormone (TSH) does not cross the placental barrier, while long-acting thyroid stimulator (LATS) and human thyroid-stimulating immunoglobulins (HTSI) elaborated in the lymphoid tissue of thyrotoxic mother, can cross through the placenta. Thyroxine does cross the placental barrier but its concentration depends upon the level of thyroid-binding globulin. It may provide some protection to the fetus with congenital hypothyroidism. The relatively higher level of thyroid-binding globulins in the maternal blood favors the distribution of thyroid hormones toward the maternal side.

There is a surge of TSH at birth resulting in the release of T_4 due to stress of labor and exposure to cold. TSH may be elevated up to 40 mU/L during first 48 hours of life and declines to less than 20 mU/L by the age of 3 days. For definitive diagnosis of congenital hypothyroidism, blood sample for TSH and T_4 should be collected after 3 days of age.

Maternal Hypothyroidism

Maternal myxedema is associated with relative sterility and early fetal deaths. In adequately treated cases, physiological situation prevails and no untoward effects are noted. In women with thyroiditis,

placental transfer of thyroid-blocking immunoglobulins (TBIs) may cause fetal hypothyroidism which can be prevented by increasing the dose of thyroxine to the mother. There is an increased iodine turnover and elevation of thyroxine-binding globulins (TBGs) during pregnancy. During pregnancy, the dose of thyroxine should be increased to maintain TSH within normal range. Treatment with triiodothyronine (T_3) can be theoretically hazardous because it does not saturate all the binding sites of thyroxine-binding protein which may lead to "leaching" of thyroid hormones from fetus to mother thus causing hypothyroidism with or without goiter in the fetus. Apart from tests of thyroid function, thyroid-blocking immunoglobulins (TBIs) and thyroid-stimulating immunoglobulins (TSIs) should be checked during third trimester of pregnancy.

Neonatal hypothyroidism does not produce any characteristic facial appearances or skin changes at birth and needs high index of suspicion for diagnosis. The infant may be large in size and may show diffuse goiter. Baby is often sluggish, placid and may not cry for feeds. The cry may be hoarse. Skin mottling due to intolerance to cold and constipation are common. Physiological jaundice is often exaggerated and prolonged beyond 2 weeks of age. Cranial sutures may be wide and anterior fontanel is large. Skeletal survey shows epiphyseal dysgenesis, retarded bone age and deformity with beaking of 12th dorsal and first and second lumbar vertebrae. Elevated serum TSH (>20 mU/L) levels and decreased T_4 (<6 µg/dL) after 3 days of age are diagnostic. Therapy with sodium l-thyroxine (10–15 µg/kg single dose per day) must be initiated during neonatal period to ensure intact survival and improved quality of life.

Thyroxine doses should be adjusted every 2-month during first year and every 6-month subsequently to maintain T_4 in the 10–16 µg/dL range and TSH below 5 mU/L. Therapy may be stopped for a brief period after the age of 2 years to assess whether it is transient hypothyroidism or needs lifelong treatment. Radionuclide scintigraphy can be performed within 2 to 5 days of starting therapy or when therapy is temporarily stopped around 2 years of age. When radionuclide scan shows absent uptake, ultrasound examination should be done to differentiate between thyroid agenesis (no thyroid tissue) and defective thyrogenesis (goiter). Physical growth, mental development and skeletal maturation should be closely monitored during therapy.

Maternal Thyrotoxicosis

High doses of antithyroid drugs during later pregnancy may cause fetal goiter and hypothyroidism because they readily cross the placental barrier. Propylthiouracil (PTU) is the preferred antithyroid drug due to its reduced passage across the placenta and limited excretion in the breast milk. Iodides are also potent goitrogens. Therefore, after initial stabilization with antithyroid drugs, sub-total thyroidectomy is recommended as the treatment of choice for thyrotoxicosis during early pregnancy.

In some infants of thyrotoxic mother, transplacental passage of LATS may result in transient neonatal thyrotoxicosis. It has been recently recognized that long-acting thyroid stimulator (LATS) is detectable in about two-thirds of cases while human thyroid-stimulating immunoglobulins (HTSI) are invariably present in all mothers having thyrotoxicosis. Elevated maternal thyroid-stimulating antibodies (>300%) are usually associated with development of neonatal thyrotoxicosis. The symptoms may be delayed for a few days due to controlling effect of maternal antithyroid drugs before they are excreted by the infant. The clinical picture of fetal thyrotoxicosis is characterized by intrauterine growth retardation, microcephaly (due to craniosynostosis), hypertension, tachycardia, intractable congestive cardiac failure, diffuse enlargement of thyroid, exophthalmos (if also present in the mother), jitteriness, excessive crying, diarrhea, and poor weight gain inspite of ravenous appetite. Advanced skeletal maturation, T_3 uptake of red blood cells and demonstration of HTSI either in the mother or baby's blood support the diagnosis.

Treatment consists of management of congestive heart failure, propranolol 2 mg/kg per day in three divided doses, Lugol's iodine one drop every 8-hourly orally and propylthiouracil 2.5 mg 8 hourly for a few weeks. Sodium ipodate (oragrafin) in a dose of 600 mg/m²/day is preferred to iodine solution. Iodine is given for about 2 weeks and propranolol is stopped once tachycardia is controlled. Therapy is usually required for 4–12 weeks. Breastfeeding should be allowed, if nursing mother is receiving propylthiouracil which is sparingly excreted in the milk.

Diabetes Mellitus

Diabetes mellitus is the commonest endocrinal disorder during pregnancy. In fact, many prediabetics and potential diabetics may show chemical evidences of diabetes mellitus during the course of metabolic stress of pregnancy. Gestational diabetes, wherein glucose homeostasis returns back to normal after delivery, is also fraught with risk to the fetus and newborn. Risk factors for gestational diabetes mellitus (GDM) include advanced maternal age, obesity, multifetal gestation and strong family history of diabetes. Women diagnosed with GDM have a 50% lifetime risk of developing overt type 2 diabetes mellitus. The duration and severity of maternal diabetes, and quality of its control during pregnancy determine the outcome of the offspring. During pregnancy, diabetes should be effectively controlled with insulin by frequent monitoring of blood glucose levels. Oral hypoglycemic agents are contraindicated during pregnancy due to risk of teratogenesis and intractable hypoglycemia in the newborn baby. Strict maintenance of normoglycemia (fasting glucose <120 mg/dL) can significantly reduce the incidence of neonatal morbidity and mortality.

Insulin does not cross the placenta but high maternal blood levels of glucose are reflected in the fetal circulation and lead to islet-cell hyperplasia of fetal pancreas. In the presence of fetal hyperglycemia, insulin acts as a primary anabolic hormone for fetal growth. Macrosomia in the fetus is reflected by increased body fat, muscle mass and organomegaly but there is no increase in the size of brain and kidneys. After birth, infant no longer receives placental glucose, and hypoglycemia often supervenes because of excessive release of insulin from beta-cells of pancreas. Level of glycosylated hemoglobin in the maternal blood truly reflects the plasma glucose concentrations over the previous 12 weeks. The level of glycosylated hemoglobin (HbA1c) expressed as percentage of total hemoglobin is dependent upon the average glucose concentrations to which red blood cells have been exposed and thus provides a useful parameter to assess adequacy of diabetic control. Fetal macrosomia is directly related to the levels of glycosylated hemoglobin in the maternal blood during third trimester while incidence of congenital malformations is related to periconceptional or early first trimester levels of glycosylated hemoglobin.

Infants of Diabetic Mothers

Infants of diabetic mother (IDM) and gestational diabetes mellitus (IGDM) are characteristically large, plethoric and moon-faced. Between 15 and 45% of newborns of mothers with gestational diabetes mellitus are macrosomic with a birth weight of ≥4.0 kg. They have hypertrichosis and hairy-pinna is pathognomonic and should be looked for in all large babies (Figures 4.2 and 4.3). Their head circumference corresponds to the gestational age rather than birth weight. Due to large size, they may be delivered preterm and are susceptible to shoulder dystocia, birth trauma, bruises and birth asphyxia. Various birth injuries include cephalhematoma, subdural hemorrhage, facial

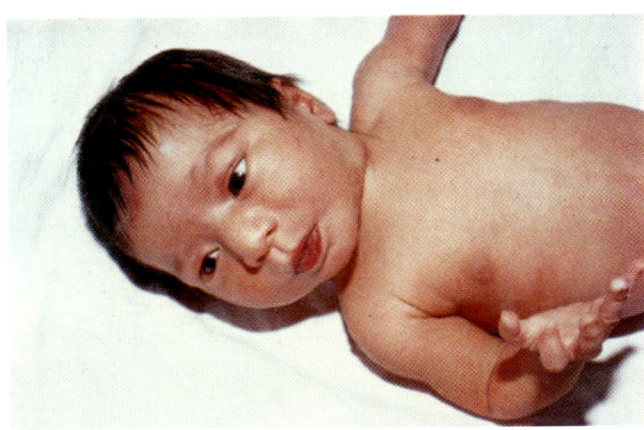

Figure 4.2 Typical appearances of an infant of a diabetic mother (gestation 38 weeks, birth weight 4100 g). All large-for-dates babies must be screened for hypoglycemia.

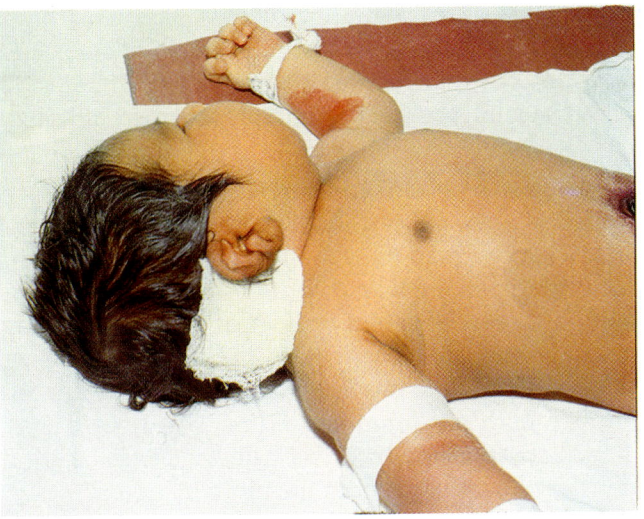

Figure 4.3 Hairy-pinna in an infant of a diabetic mother.

palsy, clavicular fracture and brachial plexus injuries. About 75% of IDMs and 25% of IGDMs suffer from first-day asymptomatic hypoglycemia. Hypocalcemia and hypomagnesemia are frequent but their pathogenesis is unclear. Hypocalcemia probably occurs due to delay in the appropriate parathyroid hormone response after birth and hypomagnesemia because of maternal magnesium losses in the urine. Approximately 50% of infants born to insulin-dependent diabetic women develop hypocalcemia (total serum calcium <7 mg/dL) during first three days life. The contributory factors appear to be prematurity, birth asphyxia and inappropriate response of parathormone to hypocalcemia. These biochemical abnormalities may contribute to excessive tremulousness, excitability, apneic attacks and hypotonia.

These infants are at a greater risk to develop respiratory distress due to hyaline membrane disease because of immaturity and hypoxia. It is postulated that increased fetal levels of insulin interfere with incorporation of choline into lecithin producing deficiency in saturated phosphatidyl choline (SPC) in the lungs and amniotic fluid. The amniotic fluid L/S ratio is unreliable predictor of hyaline membrane disease in IDMs because a ratio of more than 2.0 may be associated with development of hyaline membrane disease. Therefore, estimation of amniotic fluid SPC is mandatory for assessing fetal lung maturity, before deciding induction of labor in diabetic women. When premature delivery is planned, antenatal cortico-steroids should be given for induction of fetal lung maturity. Corticosteroid-induced hyperglycemia is managed by continuous intravenous infusion of insulin until the effect of the steroids wear off. Other causes of RDS in IDMs include cardiomyopathy, transient tachypnea of the newborn and polycythemia. Hyperbilirubinemia may occur due to immaturity, polycythemia, hypoglycemia and excessive bruising. Venous hematocrit of 65% or more has been observed in 20–40% of IDMs which may be associated with symptoms of hyperviscosity in the form of jitteriness, seizures, tachypnea, cyanosis and priapism. These infants are susceptible to develop renal vein thrombosis and its consequences due to polycythemia, hyperviscosity and osmotic diuresis. Coagulability of blood is enhanced by increased platelet aggregation because of increased synthesis of prostaglandin endoperoxides. Poor feeding without any obvious cause is seen in one-third of IDMs and often leads to prolonged hospital stay.

The incidence of congenital malformations is three- to four-fold in the offsprings of diabetic women which is a major contributor to increased perinatal mortality. Exact etiology of developmental defects is controversial but appears to be related to hyperglycemia during embryonic phase and placental vasculopathy in women with long-standing diabetes mellitus. The infants with congenital malformations may be small-for-dates. The common malformations include congenital heart abnormalities, neural tube defects, musculoskeletal deformities, caudal regression syndrome and renal agenesis. Almost one-half of all cases of caudal regression syndrome (sacral agenesis) are seen in IDMs. It is characterized by spinal abnormalities and syringomyelia with various degrees of developmental failure involving legs, lumbar, sacral, coccygeal vertebrae and corresponding segments of spinal cord with urinary incontinence and dribbling. Small left colon syndrome presents as generalized abdominal distension because of inability to pass meconium. Small colon syndrome occurs during the second half of gestation, after organogenesis is complete. Its exact cause is uncertain but is related to large changes in the maternal and fetal serum glucose concentrations. The diagnosis can be confirmed by gastrografin enema which should be performed after ensuring good hydration of the baby. There is almost fivefold increased incidence of congenital heart defects. About 30% of infants of diabetic mothers have cardiomegaly in the absence of structural malformations of heart and about 10% show evidences of cardiac dysfunction. Hypertrophic cardiomyopathy with asymmetric septal hypertrophy causing outflow obstruction to the left ventricle has been extensively documented. Echocardiography in these infants show that septal to left ventricle free wall ratio is greater than 1.3. The septal hypertrophy reverts back to normal by six months of age.

Management

Apart from expert medical management of diabetic pregnant women, the delivery should be timed depending upon fetal wellbeing (estriol, non-stress and oxytocin challenge test) and pulmonary maturity based on amniotic fluid SPC levels. Amniotic fluid L/S ratio of >3.5 and the SPC level of >1000 µg/dL are suggestive of mature indices. Large baby should preferably be delivered by cesarean section. Early feeding and prophylactic use of phenobarbitone is recommended for prevention of hypoglycemia and hyperbilirubinemia. Enteral feeding needs skill and patience in these infants. Almost one-third of IDMs demonstrate poor feeding behavior without any underlying cause. Biochemical monitoring is essential for early recognition of hypoglycemia, hypocalcemia and hypomagnesemia. Symptomatic hypoglycemia is managed by administration of 2–4 mL/kg of 25% dextrose solution IV at a rate of 1.0 mL/kg/min. This is followed by continuous infusion of glucose at a rate of 6–8 mg/kg/min. Special attention should be paid to early recognition and management of respiratory distress syndrome.

These infants should receive special care in keeping with their gestational maturity, even though they may have a deceptively healthy appearance. Exchange transfusion with plasma or physiological saline is indicated for correction of severe polycythemia and hyperviscosity. Congenital malformations should be screened by a thorough clinical examination and relevant imaging studies. Cardiac dysfunction due to asymmetric hypertrophy of septum with subaortic obstruction is best treated with furosemide and propranolol because

digoxin may be deleterious in these infants. Cardiac symptoms usually disappear by 2 weeks of age and septal hypertrophy resolves by 4 months. Sluggish bowel activity due to small left colon syndrome is managed by enemas with meglumine diatrizoate (gastrografin) or half-normal saline (5 mL/kg) and glycerine suppositories.

Disorders of Adrenal Cortex

Independent pituitary-adrenal axes are maintained in the fetus and the mother. Adrenocorticotropic hormone (ACTH) does not cross the placenta while cortisol transfer is dependent upon the relative amounts of transcortin, a specific cortisol binding globulin.

Maternal hyperadrenocorticism Corticosteroid therapy during pregnancy or maternal Cushing's disease may cause fetal death, premature labor and fetal growth retardation. The symptoms of steriod withdrawal in the baby should be watched although they are rarely manifest.

Maternal hypoadrenocorticism Mother with Addison's disease is unlikely to carry pregnancy to term without replacement therapy. Because of increased concentration of transcortin during pregnancy, administration of potent analogues of cortisone, may not fully saturate the carrier globulin thus producing leakage of cortisol from fetus to mother. The infant of a mother with autoimmune Addison's disease may manifest Addisonian crisis due to transplacental transfer of antibodies from the mother.

Parathyroid Disorders

Maternal hypercalcemia due to hyperparathyroidism is reflected in the fetal circulation with suppression of fetal parathyroid glands. After birth, baby may manifest hypocalcemic fits or tetany.

MISCELLANEOUS DISORDERS

Uterine Disorders

Cervical incompetence, fibroids and bicornuate uterus may lead to premature delivery.

Epilepsy

Epilepsy during pregnancy is seen in about 3 per 1000 women. Epileptic mothers on anticonvulsant therapy have two to three times greater risk of congenital heart disease and a five to ten times increased risk of giving birth to babies with cleft lip and cleft palate than the general population. It is uncertain whether this teratogenic predisposition is related to anticonvulsant drugs, epilepsy or genetic factors. If a woman has been seizure-free for several years, medications should be gradually withdrawn before she plans for a pregnancy. In case anticonvulsants are inescapable, phenobarbitone, carbamazepine and newer antileptics are relatively safe as far as risk of congenital malformations is concerned. Those women who seek advice later than three months of pregnancy, should be advised to continue their prescribed anti-seizure medications. They should be reassured that the risk of anticonvulsants to the fetus is rather small. Untreated seizures during pregnancy can lead to fetal death, brain damage because of hypoxia, and neuro-logical sequelae in later life. Epileptic women have an increased risk of seizures during pregnancy. The anti-convulsants are cleared more rapidly from the plasma during pregnancy. The dose of anticonvulsants may have to be increased during pregnancy to maintain adequate plasma levels. Vitamin K should be routinely administered at birth to newborn babies who have been exposed to anticonvulsants during pregnancy.

Malignant Disorders

Duration, timing and mode of therapy determine fetal outcome. Metastatic spread to the fetus is rare but may occur in cases of malignant melanoma and chorio-epithelioma arising from placenta. Virilizing ovarian tumor in the mother may result in female pseudo-hermaphroditism in the offspring.

Thrombocytopenic Purpura

Idiopathic or drug-induced autoimmune thrombo-cytopenic purpura in the mother may be associated with transient thrombocytopenia in the baby. Mother should be given prednisolone 10 to 20 mg 4 times in a day 10 to 14 days before delivery. High-dose intravenous IgG therapy, corticosteroids and platelet transfusion are indicated in infants with severe thrombocytopenia.

Myasthenia Gravis

Transient neonatal myasthenia gravis may occur in about 12% of infants born to mothers with myasthenia gravis. After 1 to 3 days of birth, baby develops marked flaccidity, excessive accumulation of oral secretions due to poor swallowing, and mask-like facies with open eyes and mouth. The baby remains alert but is unable to suck and swallow and may get choked during feeds. The condition is treated by administration of neostigmine methyl sulfate 0.1–0.5 mg/dose IM 10 minutes before each feed for 1 to 2 days followed by oral neostigmine bromide 1.0 – 4.0 mg half an hour before each feed. The disorder is transient and therapy may be tapered off in 3 to 4 weeks.

Pemphigus Vulgaris

Transient neonatal pemphigus due to passively trans-ferred humoral factors has been documented in infants of mothers suffering from pemphigus during preg-nancy. The condition resolves spontaneously.

BIBLIOGRAPHY

ACOG Committee on Practice Bulletins. ACOG Practice Bulletin. Chronic hypertension in pregnancy. *Obstet Gynecol* 2001, 98 (Suppl): 177–185.

American Diabetes Association. Gestational diabetes mellitus. *Diabetes Care Supplement* 25 (Suppl 1), 2002: S94–S96.

American College of Obstetricians and Gynecologists. Practice Bulletin 33: Diagnosis and Management of Preeclampsia and eclampsia. January 2002.

Cleveland, WW. Maternal-fetal hormone relationship. *Pediatr Clin N Amer* 1970, 17: 273.

Cowet RM, Schwartz R. The infant of the diabetic mother. *Pediatr Clin North Amer* 1982, 29: 1213.

Davies AM. Epidemiology of the hypertensive disorders of pregnancy. *Bull WHO* 1979, 57: 373.

Deorari AK, Saxena A, Singh M, Shrivastava S. Echocardiographic assessment of infants born to diabetic mothers. *Arch Dis Child* 1989, 64: 721.

Drimikis SM, Munro DS. Placental transmission of thyroid-stimulating immunoglobulins. *Brit Med J* 1975, 2: 665.

Hofmeyr GJ, Lawrie TA, Atallah AN, *et al*. Calcium supple-mentation during pregnancy for preventing hypertensive disorders and related problems. The *Cochrane Database of Systematic Reviews* 2014, 6: CD001059.

Kamana KC. Shakya S, Zhang H. Gestational diabetes mellitus and macrosomia: A literature review. *Ann Nutr Metab* 2015, 66 (Suppl 2): 14–20.

Kochupillai N, Godbole MM, Pandav CS, Karmarkar MG, Ahuja MMS. Neonatal thyroid status in iodine deficient environments of the sub-Himalayan region. *Indian J Med Res* 1984, 80: 293.

Lockshin MD, Qamar T, Drazin ML. Hazards of lupus pregnancy. *J Rheumatol* 1987, 14 (suppl. 13).

Mandel SJ, Cooper DS. The use of antithyroid drugs in pregnancy and lactation. *J Clin Endicrinol Metab* 2001, 86: 2354–2359.

Mersha AG, Abegaz TM, Seid MA. Maternal and perinatal outcomes of hypertensive disorders of pregnancy in Ethiopia: A systematic review and meta-analysis. *BMC Pregnancy Childbirth* 2019, 19:458.

Maternal Disorders and Fetal Outcome

4

North AF, Mazumdar S, Logrillo VM. Birth weight, gestational age and perinatal deaths in 5,471 infants of diabetic mothers. *J Pediatr* 1977, 90: 444.

Obeid N, O'Kelly R, Saadeh FA, Crowly V, Daly Sean. A comparison of spot urine protein-creatinine ratio with 24 hours urine protein excretion for prediction of proteinuria in preeclampsia. *Res Rep Gynaecol Obstet* 2018, 2(1):11–15.

Owens A, Yang J, Lizhou N, *et al.* Neonatal and maternal outcomes in pregnant women with cardiac disease. *J Am Heart Assoc* 2018, 7(21): e009395.doi:10.1161/JAHA.118.009395.

Pasricha JS, Seetharam KA, Singh M. Passively transferred pemphigus in a newborn. *Indian J Dermat Venerol Leprol* 1989, 55: 116.

Paul VK, Gupta U, Singh M, *et al.* Association of genital mycoplasma with low birth weight. *Internat J Gynec Obstet* 1998, 63: 109–114.

Reece EA, Homko CJ. Infant of the diabetic mother. *Semin Perinatol* 1994, 18: 459.

Ruiz-Ivastorza G, Crowther M, Branch W, Khamashta MA. Antiphospholipid syndrome. *Lancet* 2010, 376: 1498–1509.

Singh M. Neonatal myasthenia gravis. *Indian Pediatr* 1974, 11: 831.

Singh M, Kumar A, Paul VK. Hairy pinna: A pathognomonic sign in infants of diabetic mothers. *Indian Pediatr* 1987, 24: 87.

Stump D. Anticonvulsant use during pregnancy. *Clin Ther* 1985, 7: 258.

Toft AD. Thyroxine therapy (Review). *N Engl J Med* 1994, 331: 174.

van Wassenaer AG, Westera J, Houtzager BA, *et al.* Ten year of follow-up of children born at < 30 weeks gestational age supplemented with thyroxine in the neonatal period in a randomized controlled trial. *Pediatrics* 2005, 116 (5): e613–e618.

Verma VL, Tejani NA, Chaterjee S, Weiss RR. Screening for SGA by the "Roll-over-test". *Obstet and Gynecol* 1980, 56: 275.

Perinatal Pharmacology

Physiological, biochemical and metabolic handicaps predispose the fetus and the newborn baby to the toxic effects of drugs, which may be relatively safe in older children and adults. Fetus and the newborn baby are exposed to the hazards of drugs administered to the mother during pregnancy and lactation.

MATERNAL MEDICATIONS AND FETAL OR NEONATAL HAZARDS

The developing fetus is immature both structurally and functionally. When a pregnant woman is administered a chemotherapeutic agent, there is unwanted and unavoidable exposure of her unborn child to the same agent. *A drug which is apparently safe and well tolerated by the mother, may be harmful and damaging to the fetus.* No drug is entirely safe for the fetus especially during embryonic period. Therefore, the pediatrician should always be alert to recognize and manage the baby who shows effects of *in utero* medication.

The drugs reach the developing fetus through the placenta and to a lesser extent via the amniotic fluid and rarely by direct accidental administration during paracervical block. The exact mechanism of placental transport is uncertain. Experimental evidence suggests the following modes of materno-fetal transport.

Simple Physical Diffusion

Lipid solubility, degree of ionization, uterine blood flow, concentration gradient at placenta and the molecular size of the drug determine its penetration through the cell membrane by physical diffusion. The smaller molecules diffuse more readily than the larger ones. In general, substances with a molecular size of less than 1,000 readily cross the placenta by diffusion.

Active Transport

Substances, like iodides, isoniazid, thiouracil and digoxin, are actively transported against the chemical placental gradient. Thus a greater concentration may be achieved in the fetal blood as compared to the maternal levels. Active transport is regulated by the uterine blood flow and placental drug metabolizing enzymes.

Pinocytosis

Certain immune globulins can be englufed by the cells lining the chorionic villi and are then released into the fetal circulation. The permeability of the placenta increases as the pregnancy advances but the vulnerability of the fetus decreases as the maturity proceeds. The first trimester of pregnancy is the most vulnerable period as it is characterized by organo-genesis and any alterations in the fetal environment during this phase may lead to developmental defects. Some mothers may be unable to carry a pregnancy successfully to term without the use of drugs and in fact active treatment of a serious infective maternal disease by antibiotics protects and safeguards fetal wellbeing. The enzyme inducers, such as pheno-barbitone and corticosteroids when given during the last weeks of pregnancy, have been shown to lessen the incidence and severity of neonatal jaundice and hyaline membrane disease, respectively. It also needs to be borne in mind that at times the maternal disease for which the drugs are administered may harm the unborn child.

However, the fetal hazards and disadvantages far outweigh the possible benefits of maternal medications. Some of the important toxic effects of the maternal drugs to the fetus and newborn are listed below but some of the effects recorded have been reported very rarely or even as single case reports. The drugs have been arranged alphabetically after giving a brief outline of chemotherapeutic agents causing fetal deaths and congenital malformations.

Drugs which may Cause Fetal Death

As many as one-third of pregnancies are known to end in abortion and in vast majority the precise cause remains unknown. Quinine, lead, aloes and certain other substances may produce abortion by their oxytocic action and these agents are at times used to produce criminal abortion. They have to be administered in a dose high enough which may be toxic to the mother before the abortifacient effect is produced. Large doses of antifolic acid agents and dicumarol may result in fetal death. Corticosteroids in high doses have been shown to cause abortion in experimental animals.

Teratogenic Agents

The "periconceptional period" is most vulnerable and challenging time because most women do not realize that they are pregnant until they miss the period. *Therefore, married women of reproductive age should avoid unnecessary medications during two weeks preceding menstruation.* The period of organogenesis is most vulnerable to teratogenic effects of drugs. Different organ systems differentiate at a precise or specific time during embryogenesis. Organogenesis or differentiation of various organs is essentially complete around 8 to 10 weeks postconception except in case of brain and genital system which continue to differentiate throughout pregnancy.

The cause of majority of congenital malformations remains unknown but in about 10% of cases it is induced by the alterations in the fetal environment during the period of embryogenesis. A large and ever increasing number of chemotherapeutic agents have been shown to be teratogenic in different species of experimental animals. This includes high doses of cortisone, insulin, oral hypoglycemic agents, salicylates, caffein, thyroxine, trypan blue, nicotinic acid, vitamin A, vitamin D, penicillin, streptomycin, tetracycline, antihistamines, and meprobamate, etc. It is true that the results of animal experiments cannot be extrapolated to human beings and alarmist attitude is unwarranted but on the analogy of Koch's postulate, Smithells has suggested similar criteria in the human beings for labeling a particular malformation as drug induced.

1. The drug should be associated with a specific malformation more frequently than is expected by chance.

2. The history of the drug having been taken during the first trimester of pregnancy should be available in a significantly higher proportion of mothers of malformed babies than the controls.

3. The drug should be able to induce the characteristic malformation in the susceptible strain of the laboratory animal.

The assessment of teratogenic effects of drugs in experimental animals is both labor and cost-intensive. In view of the fact that a limited number of pregnant women are likely to use the drug, most pharmaceutical companies are reluctant to launch large-scale studies. The drug manufacturers, therefore, protect themselves legally by saying that "safety during pregnancy is not established". The following chemotherapeutic agents have been definitely shown or strongly suspected to induce congenital malformations in the human fetus.

Antifolate agents and cytotoxic drugs In large doses, they cause fetal death but if small doses are used there is a high probability of inducing malformation. Chemotherapy for malignancy during pregnancy is associated with risk of abortion and congenital malformations. Aminopterin and methotrexate are associated with cranial dysostoses, micrognathia, ear anomalies and growth retardation. Chromosomal abnormalities and bone marrow suppression may occur, there is a prolonged exposure of fetus to cytotoxic drugs. Administration of azathioprine and cyclosporin following renal transplant during pregnancy is safe to the fetus without any risk of congenital malformations.

Thalidomide The current interest in human teratology dates back to thalidomide disaster. Till 1962, more than 3500 "thalidomide babies" had been born with a wide-spectrum of congenital malformations including phocomelia, hemangioma over the forehead, absent external ear, duodenal and anal atresia, congenital cardiac defects and mental retardation (Figure 5.1).

Miscellaneous drugs There is some evidence to suggest that meclizine, tetracyclines (producing cataract) and tolbutamide may be teratogenic in the human beings and caution should be exercised in their use in early pregnancy. An association between maternal intake of diazepam, diphenyl hydantoin, imipramine and occurrence of cleft palate in their offsprings has been suggested. These infants may have, in addition, a variety of other unrelated anomalies in various systems. There have been several reports of neural tube defects (anencephaly and spina bifida) amongst children born to mothers who received chlomiphene for induction of ovulation immediately prior to or unwittingly at the time of conception (Figure 5.2).

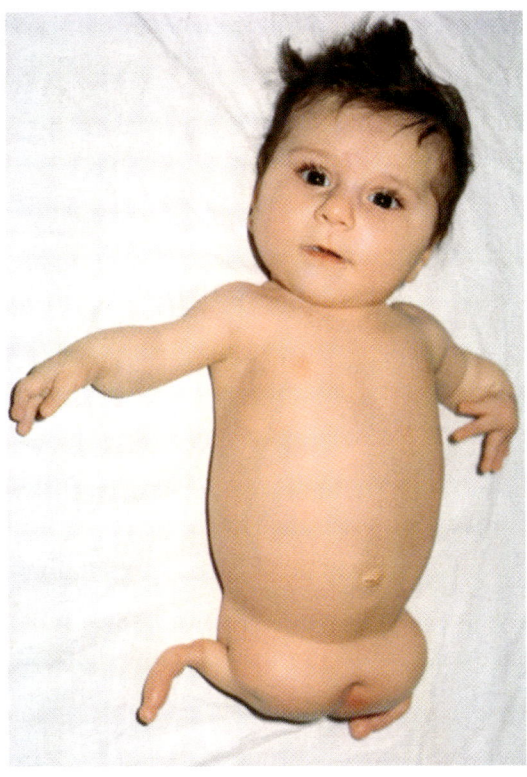

Figure 5.1 Classical thalidomide baby.

Severe birth defects in the form of absence of fore-arm bones, fingers and toes amongst offsprings born to mothers who received haloperidol during early first trimester of pregnancy have been reported (Figure 5.3). Lithium during pregnancy is associated with increased risk of fetal cardiovascular malformations (Ebstein's anomaly), bradycardia, hypotonia and cretinism with goiter. There is some evidence to suggest that maternal intake of dicumarol and/or warfarin may be associated with skeletal hypoplasia. Isotretinoin for acne should be avoided during pregnancy due to risk of causing dysmorphism and mental retardation. There is controversial evidence to suggest an higher incidence of maternal intake of salicylates amongst mothers who give birth to babies with a variety of malformations as compared to the controls. The incidence of congenital malformations is also higher among offsprings of mothers addicted to alcohol, LSD, diazepam, meclizine and dexamphetamines.

Irradiation In addition to above chemotherapeutic agents, irradiation during pregnancy is fraught with dangers to the offspring. Though the follow-up studies of pregnancies during Hiroshima and Nagasaki atomic bomb explosion have failed to show any increased

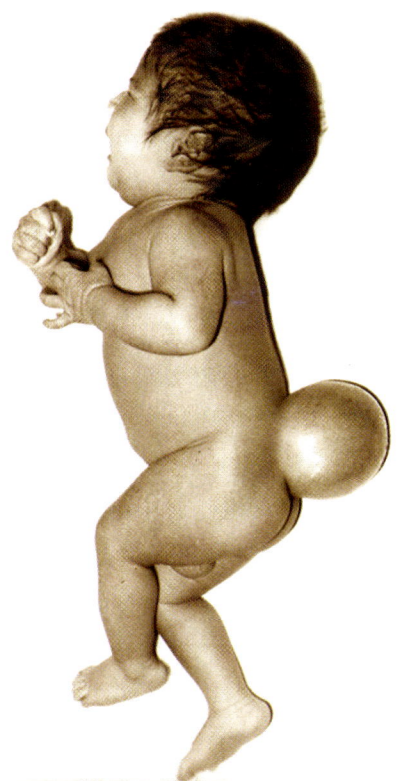

Figure 5.2 Spina bifida with covered meningocele in an infant of a mother who received clomiphene before and during early gestation.

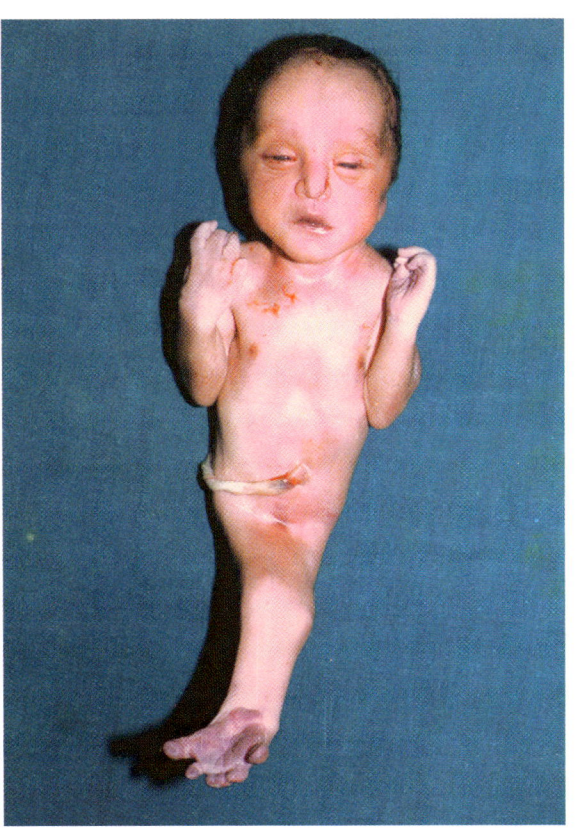

Figure 5.3 Mermaid like features due to intake of haloperidol during pregnancy.

Perinatal Pharmacology

5

incidence of congenital malformations but there is an increasing experimental evidence to suggest that human chromosomes grown in tissue cultures are damaged by exposure to irradiation. Higher incidence of leukemia and cancer amongst children born to mothers exposed to diagnostic irradiation during pregnancy has been documented. Every married woman in the reproductive age group is potentially capable of becoming pregnant and may expose her offspring unwittingly to an environmental hazard before she becomes aware of the fact that she has conceived. *It is, therefore, recommended that in married women, the diagnostic radiological studies should be restricted to the 2 weeks of post-menstruation period and no pelvic X-rays should be taken during first trimester of pregnancy.*

Addicted Mother

Drug abuse among youth has assumed epidemic proportions in the west and many youngsters in low-middle income countries (LMICs) are aping the habit. During intrauterine life, fetus is totally at the mercy of mother and is at risk to suffer from deleterious effects of various addictions. Drug abuse during pregnancy is associated with increased fetal wastage and perinatal mortality. There is higher incidence of congenital malformations, twining, intrauterine growth retardation with slow postnatal physical and mental growth. Higher incidence of LBW babies may be due to direct effect of drug on the fetus or poor nutrition of addicted mothers. Infants of drug addict mothers are more liable to suffer from intrauterine infections especially syphilis, Au antigen associated hepatitis, AIDS and sepsis.

Fetal alcohol syndrome is seen in about 50% infants of chronic alcoholics. It is characterized by intrauterine growth retardation, microcephaly with slow postnatal physical and mental growth. Facial dysmorphism includes maxillary hypoplasia, short palpebral fissures, epicanthic folds, short upturned nose, indistinct or smooth philtrum, thin upper lip, shortened lower jaw, strabismus and ptosis. Cardiac malformations, ear anomalies, small nails, restricted joint movements, large hemangiomata and altered palmar dermatoglyphics may be associated. High levels of fatty acid ethyl esters (FAEE) in the first stool of the newborn, because of maternal intake of alcohol during pregnancy, is a reliable marker of development of cognitive dysfunction in the child.

Smoking is associated with IUGR and increased perinatal mortality which needs to be highlighted in all campaigns against cigarettes. The adverse effects have been shown experimentally to be due to nicotine rather than smoke. Smoking is not associated with fetal malformations but delayed neuromotor development, hyperkinetic syndrome and sudden infant death syndrome (SIDS) have been linked to smoking during pregnancy. Chewing of tobacco which is prevalent in certain rural communities in India, is also associated with retarded fetal growth. Opium, morphine and its derivatives including pethidine and methadone, heroin and cocaine have been shown to be associated with higher incidence of congenital malformations and behavior changes in experimental animals due to alterations in fetal neuronal processes. Incidentally, some of these agents, especially heroin, are associated with enhanced or accelerated maturation of lungs and liver resulting in reduced incidence of hyaline membrane disease and jaundice in the infants of addicted mothers. Intake of marijuana during pregnancy may be associated with thymic hypoplasia resulting in higher incidence of recurrent respiratory infections, diarrhea and moniliasis during infancy. Lysergic acid diethylamide (LSD) has been shown to cause chromosomal damage leading to stunted fetal growth. Cocaine may lead to abruptio placenta, fetal tachycardia, hypertension, CNS irritability and cerebral infarcts. The effects of marijuana (cannabis, *hashish*, *charas*, *bhang*) use during pregnancy are variable. Some studies have demonstrated long-term cognitive deficits and neurobehavioral abnormalities.

Infants of substance abuse mothers may also show manifestations of narcotic withdrawal syndrome during early neonatal period. After birth, the infant no longer receives the drug to which he got "addicted" *in utero*. These children are characteristically over-alert, irritable, overactive, excessively fretful, crying and jittery. Due to constant rubbing and fretting, they may develop skin abrasions at elbows and ankles. Hyperthermia due to muscular overactivity, sweating, yawning and sneezing are common. Severe diarrhea may produce life-threatening dehydration and electrolyte disturbances. Their weight gain is poor in spite of excessive appetite and satisfactory caloric intake.

Anesthetic Agents

General anesthetics In accordance with other central nervous system depressants, general anesthetics may cause respiratory depression and difficulty in initiating the breathing at birth. Halogenated hydrocarbons, such as halothane and trichlorethylene, reach the fetus more easily than nitrous oxide because of high lipid solubility.

Local anesthetics Accidental injection of local anesthetics into the fetal scalp during the paracervical block can result in development of apnea, hypotonia, brady-cardia, fixed and dilated pupils, loss of oculocephalic reflexes (doll's eyes) and intractable convulsions in the baby soon after birth. In seriously sick babies, forced diuresis and repeated stomach wash with continuous gastric aspiration may be life-saving. The therapeutic utility of exchange blood transfusion is doubtful. Citanest for local analgesia is unsafe as it can cause fetal methemoglobinemia.

Spinal anesthetics Sudden maternal hypotension due to spinal anesthetics may result in fetal hypoxia. Bupivacaine has been documented to be associated with increased risk of jaundice in the newborn baby.

Analgesics

Acetaminophen Paracetamol is the analgesic of choice during all stages of pregnancy. There is recent data to suggest that when paracetamol is taken for more than 28 days during pregnancy, the offspring may develop poor gross motor and communication skills, and increased risk of behavior problems including ADHD. The behavioral effects may be mediated by increased production of cannabinoid in the CNS during intake of paracetamol.

Salicylates Aspirin in low doses (75 mg/d) used for prevention of pre-eclampsia and intrauterine growth retardation has been shown to be safe. In therapeutic doses, salicylates may cause neonatal bleeding due to deficiency of vitamin K-dependent coagulation factors. By virtue of their ability to bind with albumin, they can reduce the bilirubin binding capacity of albumin and predispose the infant to bilirubin toxicity at lower levels of serum bilirubin. Salicylates are also known to cause methemoglobinemia and platelet dysfunction in the fetus.

Nonsteroidal anti-inflammatory drugs (NSAIDs) They should preferably be avoided during pregnancy due to risk of causing miscarriage, fetal renal dysfunction and oligohydramnios. It is safe to use indomethacin for 3 days as a tocolytic agent when labor starts before 34 weeks of gestation. Prolonged use of indomethacin during pregnancy is associated with risk of oligohydramnios, premature closure of ductus arteriosus, renal insufficiency, pulmonary hypertension, necrotizing enterocolitis and ileal perforation. NSAIDs may cause closure of ductus arteriosus leading to pulmonary hypertension in the newborn.

Morphine and pethidine These analgesics when given to the mother during labor may cause severe respiratory depression of the newborn. Nalorphine is a potent antagonist of these depressants and should be administered to the mother in a dose of 5 to 10 mg intravenously about 5 minutes before the expected time of delivery. This can also be administered to the neonate in a dose of 0.1–0.2 mg per kilogram through the umbilical vein, if a baby is depressed at birth. "Morphine addiction syndrome" is reported in newborns of morphine addict mothers. It is characterized by withdrawal symptoms of progressive restlessness, irritability, incessant shrill cry, diarrhea and convulsions. The treatment consists of giving small amounts of either morphine derivatives, phenobarbitone or chlorpromazine.

Antibacterial Agents

In general, antibiotics are safely tolerated by the fetus and would safeguard fetal wellbeing in a seriously infected mother. Sulfonamides and nitrofurantoin may cause hemolytic anemia in G-6-PD deficient babies. The long-acting sulfonamides, in addition, may consume bilirubin binding capacity, thus predisposing the baby to bilirubin brain damage at lower serum bilirubin levels. Tetracycline molecule chelates with calcium and gets deposited in the bone and teeth resulting in intrauterine growth retardation and brownish staining of future primary teeth. Cotrimoxazole should preferably be avoided during early pregnancy due to its theoretical teratogenic potentiality in view of its ingredient trimethoprim which is a potent folic acid antagonist. Aminoglycosides may cause damage to the acoustic nerve. Metronidazole has no known teratogenic effects in humans.

Anticoagulants

Thrombosis in the deep veins during pregnancy raises the issue of safety of different anticoagulant agents. Dicumarol and its derivatives may result in intra-uterine fetal death or severe bleeding manifestations in the neonate due to deficiency of vitamin K-dependent coagulation factors. The offsprings of mothers receiving warfarin during early pregnancy have been shown to have warfarin embryopathy. It is characterized by triad of hypoplasia of nasal bones (flat upturned nose), epiphyseal stippling of axial skeleton and resorption of terminal phalanges (Figure 5.4). Additional features of coumarin embryopathy include growth retardation, eye defects, optic atrophy, scoliosis, congenital heart defects and seizures. Heparin is safe as it does not cross the placental barrier except when it is low molecular weight or unfractionated.

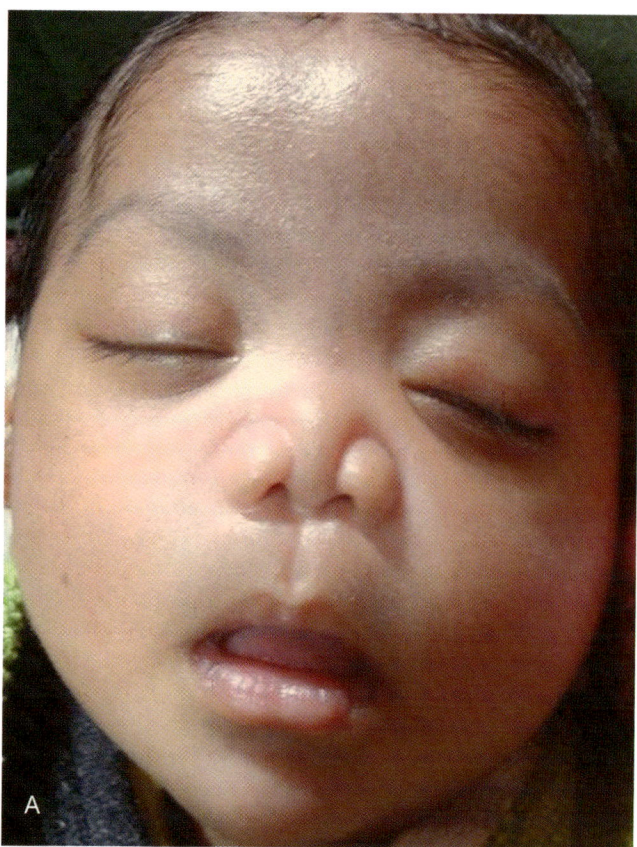

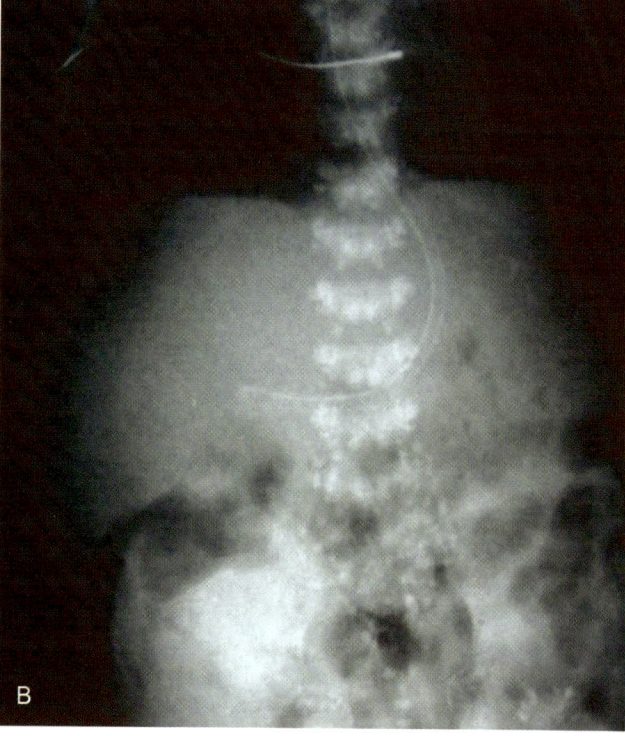

Figure 5.4 (A) Newborn infant with nasal deformity because of hypoplasia of nasal bones due to warfarin embryopathy. (B) X-ray spine shows calcification secondary to epiphyseal stippling.

Anticonvulsants

Phenobarbitone, primidone and phenytoin may cause neonatal hemorrhage due to deficiency of vitamin K-dependent coagulation factors. Phenobarbitone can induce the maturation of UDP-glucuronyl transferase and Y-acceptor protein and thus protects the baby from developing severe jaundice. Infants exposed to phenobarbitone throughout pregnancy may manifest drug-withdrawal symptoms. Infants of epileptic mothers on anticonvulsant therapy have increased risk of developmental defects, such as cleft lip, cleft palate and congenital heart disease as compared with general population. About 10% of infants exposed to diphenyl hydantoin during first trimester of pregnancy may be associated with a variety of developmental defects. Fetal hydantoin syndrome is characterized by intra-uterine growth retardation with slow postnatal growth, microcephaly and mental retardation. They have facial dysmorphism with broad and depressed nasal bridge, ptosis, coloboma, low set ears, ridged metopic suture, wide anterior fontanel, ocular hypertelorism, broad alveolar ridge and short neck with low-set hair line. The nails are hypoplastic with abnormalities in the palmar ridge pattern with digitalization of the thumb and hypoplasia or absence of distal phalanx. Cafe-au-lait spots, hypopigmented nevi and pilonidal dimples are seen at times. Recent evidence has suggested that constellation of these dysmorphic features may be related to genetic constitution of epileptic mothers or anoxic damage to the fetus due to seizures during pregnancy and not necessarily due to specific teratogenicity of phenytoin.

Trimethadione is strongly suspected to be teratogenic with increased incidence of facial dysmorphism (V-shaped eyebrows, low set ears, epicanthal folds), cleft lip or palate, cardiac anomalies, skeletal defects and mental retardation among the offsprings. Women receiving valproic acid during pregnancy have 1 to 2% risk of neural tube defects, craniofacial defects, microcephaly, abnormal digits, hypospadias, cardiac defects, delayed psychomotor development and fetal growth restriction. Carbamazepine crosses the placenta and may cause spina bifida, craniofacial defects, hypoplasia of finger nails, developmental delay and other non-specific malformations in their offsprings. Ethosuximide may cause cleft lip/palate, mongoloid facies, patent ductus arteriosus, altered palmar creases, accessory nipples and hydrocephalus. Topiramate intake during first trimester may cause cleft lip/palate in the offspring. Due to high teratogenic risk of anticonvulsants, it is preferable to taper off anticonvulsants when a woman is seizure-free for two years or more, so that she is off anticonvulsants during pregnancy.

Those women who seek advice later than three months of pregnancy, should be advised to continue their medications. They should be assured that the risk of anticonvulsant to the fetus is rather small. Untreated seizures during pregnancy can lead to fetal death, brain damage because of hypoxia and neurologic sequelae later in life. When use of anticonvulsant is inescapable during early pregnancy, phenobarbitone, carbamazepine, levetiracetam and lamotrigine are relatively safe.

When an epileptic pregnant woman is taking an enzyme-inducing anticonvulsant, the need for administration of vitamin K during late pregnancy is controversial. Some workers recommend administration of vitamin K 10 mg/d PO from 36th week of gestation till the baby is delivered. However, the neonate must be given the mandatory prophylactic dose of vitamin K 0.5–1.0 mg IM at birth.

Antidiabetic Agents

Tolbutamide is potentially teratogenic while sulfonylureas may cause severe intractable hypoglycemia in the neonate which may require exchange transfusion. Insulin is the drug of choice for control of diabetes mellitus during pregnancy.

Antihypertensive Agents

Hydralazine, alpha-methyldopa and calcium channel blockers are effective antihypertensives for the treatment of pregnancy-induced and pregnancy-associated hypertension and are safe for the fetus. Infants born to mothers receiving reserpine during late pregnancy manifest nasal stuffiness, snuffles, respiratory difficulty with intercostal recessions and lethargy. Administration of beta blockers, like propranolol and labetalol during pregnancy, is not recommended because it may be associated with intrauterine growth retardation, maternal and fetal bradycardia, premature labor, resuscitation difficulties, neonatal hypoglycemia and hyperbilirubinemia. There is some evidence to suggest that labetolol may actually enhance lung maturity and reduce the incidence of hyaline membrane disease. Clonidine is an effective antihypertensive but its use is not recommended during pregnancy because sudden cessation of therapy may cause rebound hypertension. Angiotensin-converting enzyme (ACE) inhibitors should be avoided during pregnancy because of the risk of causing congenital malformations including renal dysgenesis, oligohydramnios, reduced ossification, pulmonary hypoplasia and stillbirth. Angiotensin II receptor antagonists (ARAs) should be avoided during pregnancy due to risk of fatal tubular dysgenesis, oligohydramnios, fetal dysmorphism and stillbirth.

Antimalarials

Quinine in high doses may cause abortion. In moderate doses, it may result in deafness and thrombocytopenia. Chloroquine for the treatment of malaria is quite safe but its prolonged administration for conditions, such as rheumatoid arthritis, may cause deafness and retinal pigmentation in the infant. Primaquine during pregnancy should be avoided as it may cause hemolytic anemia in G-6-PD deficient infants.

Antithyroid Agents

Antithyroid agents in high doses may cause fetal goiter and cretinism. It is recommended that lower dose of antithyroid drugs should be used during pregnancy even if it means keeping the mother in a relative hyperthyroid state because thyroxine sparingly crosses the placenta. Propylthiouracil is safe while intake of methimazole during pregnancy is associated with development of focal scalp defects due to aplasia cutis congenita. [131]I is contraindicated during pregnancy as it is likely to damage fetal thyroid gland and produce hypothyroidism and brain damage.

Antitubercular Drugs

In general, most of the antitubercular drugs are safe during pregnancy. Tuberculosis during pregnancy is best treated with isoniazid, rifampicin and ethambutol because they lack any consistent risk of teratogenicity. Fetal hepatotoxicity due to rifampicin and INH may lead to deficiency of vitamin K-dependent coagulation factors at birth. Ethambutol usage during pregnancy has been associated with 19% incidence of minor congenital malformations comprising of supernumerary nipples, midtibial torsion, congenital dislocation of hips, hydrocele, skin tag over fifth digit and strawberry marks. Streptomycin sulfate is well known to cause damage to 8th nerve leading to permanent deafness and vestibular dysfunction. Ethionamide has been documented to produce abortions and congenital malformations in rats and rabbits. There is very little available information regarding the safety of pyrazinamide during pregnancy.

Cholinergic Agents

Edrophonium chloride (tensilon), neostigmine and other related compounds when administered to the mother with myasthenia gravis may result in withdrawal symptoms in the form of transient neonatal

Perinatal Pharmacology

5

myasthenia gravis. However, the myasthenia status of the mother *per se* rather than withdrawal of drugs may be contributing to this symptomatology.

Corticosteroids

The increased risk of prematurity and perinatal mortality is probably related to the severity of underlying maternal disease rather than the direct outcome of cortisone administration. High doses of cortisone in the mice have been shown to result in posterior cleft palate. Prolonged cortisone therapy during pregnancy poses a theoretical risk of adrenal crisis in the infant though no actual cases have been documented.

Diuretics

Maternal electrolyte disturbances by diuretics are mirrored in the fetal blood. Thiazides may directly suppress the megakaryocytes and result in fetal thrombocytopenia. They are also known to cause neonatal liver damage. Their use should be restricted to women with pulmonary edema, acute cardiac or renal failure.

Expectorant Mixtures

Iodide containing expectorant mixtures during pregnancy may cause fetal goiter and hypothyroidism. Large goiters may cause difficulty in delivery and would need immediate therapy with triiodothyronine and subtotal thyroidectomy may prove life-saving for relief of respiratory difficulty.

Intravenous Infusions

Maternal hypo- and hypernatremia may reflect identical dyselectrolytemia in the neonate manifested by hypotonia, lethargy and convulsions.

Sedatives and Tranquilizers

The indiscriminate intake of sedatives and tranquilizers during early pregnancy is fraught with the dangers of induction of congenital defects. Heavy sedation during labor is associated with difficulty in initiating breathing, cerebral depression, inactivity, hypothermia, hypotonia and poor nipple feeding during first 1 to 2 days after birth. The prolonged or addictive intake of barbiturates and diazepam throughout gestation may be associated with withdrawal symptoms in the neonate on the same analogy as morphine and alcohol withdrawal syndrome. Phenothiazines may produce symptoms of extrapyramidal dysfunction in the baby manifested by jitteriness, rigidity and opisthotonos which may persist for few weeks. These are not drug withdrawal symptoms but instead a manifestation of phenothiazine toxicity. Their role in the aggravation of neonatal jaundice is doubtful. Prozac administration is associated with premature delivery, jitteriness and breathing difficulties.

Sex Hormones

The prolonged administration of synthetic progestins during pregnancy in women with habitual abortion is fraught with dangers of masculinization of female fetus and hypospadias in the male offspring. This may be associated with acceleration of fetal bone age and permanent alteration in subsequent sexual behavior. The incidence and severity of the fetal defect is greater with the newer synthetic progestins, such as norlutin (17 α-ethinyl 10 nortestosterone) as compared to non-synthetic progestins. Estrogen and androgen therapy during pregnancy may also induce virilization of female fetus though its occurrence is rare. There is evidence to suggest that administration of diethyl stilbestrol during pregnancy may lead to carcinoma of the vagina in their female offsprings 20 years later. At birth, some of these infants may have evidences of vaginal adenosis, congenital malformations of vagina and cervix. Mothers exposed to progestin-estrogen compounds either due to continued usage of contraceptive pills or hormone withdrawal pregnancy tests, have been shown to give birth to infants with a variety of limb-reduction deformities. These congenital malformations are described with an acronym VACTERL which stands for vertebral, anal, cardiac, tracheoesophageal, renal and limb anomalies. Clomiphene which is an antiestrogen is associated with increased risk of neural tube defects, multiple births and Down syndrome.

Vitamins

Synthetic vitamin K when administered in large doses, during labor for prophylaxis against hemorrhagic disease of the newborn, may cause severe neonatal jaundice as a result of hemolysis and hepatotoxicity. Infantile hypercalcemia with supravalvular aortic stenosis may follow administration of massive doses of vitamin D during pregnancy but evidence is controversial. Administration of pharmacological doses of vitamin B_6 during pregnancy may lead to inhibition of lactation by interfering with release of prolactin and development of pyridoxine dependent seizures in the newborn. High doses of vitamin A may produce kidney malformations, neural tube defects and hydrocephalus. Vitamin A analogues (accutane, isotretinoin, retinoic acid) used for treatment of acne by teenager pregnant girls are associated with increased risk of spontaneous abortion and congenital malformations. The spectrum of malformations includes small, malformed or absent ears, atretic ear canals, cleft palate, anomalies of great vessels, hydrocephalus, microcephaly, abnormalities in neuronal migration, posterior fossa structural abnormalities and cortical blindness.

Immunizations

Live vaccines should not be administered during pregnancy due to potential risk of spontaneous abortion, infection of the fetus and development of congenital malformations. When there is a definite indication, antirabies vaccine should not be denied to the pregnant woman because of universally fatal nature of rabies.

Miscellaneous Drugs

Magnesium sulfate, when administered for the management of severe eclampsia, may cause hypotonia and respiratory failure in the neonate as a result of peripheral neuromuscular block. The baby may need assisted ventilation and exchange transfusion with citrated blood to inactivate magnesium ions by forming citrate complex. There is some evidence that imipramine therapy during pregnancy may induce conduction defects and arrhythmia in the baby. There is increasing evidence to suggest that infants born following oxytocin induction of labor are likely to manifest early and more intense jaundice. Simvastatin and other statins should be avoided during pregnancy as they adversely affect the fetal growth by lowering cholesterol level. Lithium carbonate readily crosses the placenta and can cause fetal goiter. Fetal exposure to lithium during first trimester has been associated with right-sided congenital cardiovascular malformations, like Ebstein's anomaly, VSD, mitral and tricuspid atresia, coarctation of aorta and dextrocardia. Neonates exposed to lithium *in utero* may manifest with persistent pulmonary hypertension, poor tone, hypothyroidism, goiter, reduced activity and sluggish sucking behavior, cardiac dysfunction, atrial flutter and nephrogenic diabetes insipidus. Pregnant women exposed to Bhopal gas disaster had increased incidence of spontaneous abortions and higher perinatal and neonatal mortality in their offsprings. The incidence of congenital malformations was not enhanced. Intake of aspartame (dietary sugar substitute) during pregnancy is safe but should be avoided by women with phenylketonuria because of adverse cognitive effects on the fetus due to excessive elevation of phenylalanine.

The above frightening list of chemotherapeutic agents demands that there is a need for alertness and awareness on the part of physician to recognize and manage the baby who may have received *in utero* medications (Table 5.1). From the fetal stand point, no drug is entirely safe during pregnancy. *A drug which may be apparently safe and well tolerated by the mother may be harmful and damaging to the growing fetus.*

While prescribing any medicines to the pregnant woman, it is mandatory to ask oneself few questions. Is medication indicated? Is the disease more dangerous as regards fetal safety compared to the known hazards of the therapeutic agent? Has the drug withstood the test of time? Whenever feasible, medications should be given and imaging studies conducted during 2 weeks postmenstrual phase when it is certain that the woman is not pregnant. There is an urgent need for health education to discourage self medications by expectant mothers.

MEDICATIONS TO THE LACTATING MOTHER AND NEONATAL HAZARDS

The precise knowledge regarding the excretion of various drugs in breast milk is often lacking but the available evidence suggests that practically all products taken by the mother are excreted in her milk though generally in insignificant (<1.0%) amounts. *By and large, whatever is safely tolerated by the nursing mother, is generally safe for her suckling infant.* At times, the nature of the maternal illness rather than the drug may necessitate weaning from the breast. Drug exposure to the nursing infant may be minimized by asking the mother to take the medication immediately after breastfeeding the infant.

Breastfeeding by a mother receiving anticancer drugs or cytotoxic agents especially amethopterin, methotrexate and cyclophosphamide is contraindicated because of risk of immune suppression, adverse effects on neonatal growth and carcinogenesis. Antithyroid drugs and ^{131}I appear in the milk in a concentration higher than the plasma and can cause damage to the thyroid gland of the baby resulting in hypothyroidism. Therefore, breastfeeding by a thyrotoxic mother receiving these drugs is contraindicated. Propylthiouracil is safe and does not appear in the breast milk. The maternal intake of dicumarol derivatives (phenindione) for long-term anticoagulation following mitral valve replacement, contraindicates breastfeeding

TABLE 5.1 Neonatal disorders due to maternal medications during pregnancy

Neonatal disorders	Maternal medications
■ Anomalies (developmental defects) *Specific:*	
Limb defects	Thalidomide, haloperidol and progestin-estrogen combinations
Hypoplasia of nasal bones and stippling of epiphyses	Warfarin
Virilization of female fetus	Synthetic progestins, estrogens, danazol and androgens
Hypospadias in a male fetus	Diethylstilbestrol, valproic acid, finasteride, dutasteride, loratadine
Neural tube defects	Clomiphene, valproic acid and carbamazepine
Cardiovascular defects	Lithium, imipramine, paroxetine, sulfasalazine, chlorthalidone, quinine, valproic acid, trimethadione, warfarin, alcohol
Cleft palate with or without cleft lip and other non-specific anomalies	Diphenlhydantoin, barbiturates?, trimethadione, diazepam, topiramate, imipramine, cortisone? and trimethoprim
Cataract	Tetracyclines?, warfarin
Non-specific:	
Variety of anomalies	Irradiation, live vaccines, aminopterine, methotrexate, busulfan, trimethadione, isotretinoin, organic mercury, chlorophenyls, ribavirin, tolbutamide, meclizine, cotrimoxazole?, alcohol, LSD, tranquilizers, finasteride, vitamin A, vitamin D, dexamphetamine, salicylates, dicumarol and warfarin and quinine
■ Bleeding Vitamin K-dependent	Phenobarbitone, primidone, phenytoin, carbamazepine, salicylates and dicumarol derivatives
Thrombocytopenia and/or thrombocytopathy	Thiazides, quinine and salicylates
■ Cerebral depression and hypotonia with or without resuscitation difficulties	Pethidine, morphine, anesthetic agents, diazepam, alcohol, barbiturates, magnesium sulfate and tensilon
■ Convulsions	Severe drug withdrawal syndrome, accidental injection of local anesthetic agents into fetal scalp, and chlorpropamide (hypoglycemia)
■ Cretinism with or without goiter	Antithyroid drugs, ^{131}I, iodides and lithium carbonate, povidone-iodine
■ Deafness	Quinine, streptomycin, aminoglycoside, chloroquine and thalidomide
■ Dental abnormalities	Tetracyclines
■ Hyperbilirubinemia and/or predisposition to kernicterus at lower serum bilirubin levels	Vitamin K, long-acting sulfonamides, nitrofurantoin, primaquine, salicylates, oxytocin, bupivacaine and phenothiazines?
■ Intestinal stasis or obstruction (paralytic)	Hexamethonium bromide, succinylcholine and sedatives
■ Intrauterine growth retardation	Various addictions, like smoking, alcohol, LSD, cocaine, caffeine, diazepam, tetracyclines, statins, phenytoin, calcium channel blockers, ACE inhibitors and beta blockers
■ Nasal blockage	Reserpine and antihistamines?
■ Vaginal carcinoma	Diethylstilbestrol
■ 'Withdrawal syndrome' (excessive crying, tremors, jitteriness, vomiting, diarrhea, etc).	Recreational drugs including morphine, pethidine, diazepam, marijuanas, alcohol, and barbiturate addiction

because of potential danger of bleeding in her infant. Excessive intake of salicylates may cause skin rash, platelet abnormalities and bleeding in nursing infants. Tramadol should not be given to the nursing mother as it is excreted in the breast milk. Warfarin is the oral anticoagulant of choice in nursing mothers. Cimetidine appears in high concentrations in the breast milk and may suppress gastric acidity, inhibit drug metabolism and cause stimulation of central nervous system. Acebutolol and atenolol therapy to the mother may cause bradycardia and hypotension in the suckling infant. Maternal intake of gold salts and ergotamine contraindicates breastfeeding. Ergot therapy for involution of uterus and ergotamine taken for migraine may be associated with symptoms of ergotism in the baby in the form of vomiting, diarrhea, vasomotor collapse and convulsions. Amiodarone, retinoids, and tamoxifen are contraindicated in nursing mothers. Bromocriptine is known to suppress lactation and should be avoided by the nursing mother. Lactation may also be suppressed, to a variable extent, by maternal intake of oral contraceptives, thiazides, ergot, pyridoxine and nicotine.

Bromides appear in the milk rather readily and their use may be associated with skin rash and drowsiness. Mothers on lithium carbonate therapy should preferably avoid breastfeeding. Morphine and its derivatives, phenothiazines and other sedatives may produce lethargy and poor feeding in the baby though the effects are variable and unpredictable. Laxatives containing 1, 8 dihydroxy anthraquinone, cascara and aloes when taken by the lactating woman may cause diarrhea in her infant. Aperients, such as milk of magnesia, liquid paraffin, bulk laxatives and glycerin suppository are safe for the nursing mother. Most of the antibiotics appear in the breast milk but their concentration is insufficient for effective treatment of any neonatal infection. It is a common observation that breastfed infants of mothers receiving ampicillin, tetracycline and cephalexin often manifest enhanced motility of gut resulting in frequent passage of small semi-loose stools.

The use of radiopharmaceuticals for diagnostic purposes raises the question of duration of their excretion in the breast milk. Gallium-67 (^{67}Ga), iodine-125 (^{125}I) and iodine-131 (^{131}I) appear in the breast milk for a maximum period of up to two weeks while technetium-99m (^{99m}Tc) and radioactive sodium is excreted in the milk up to 3–4 days after administration. It is desirable that as far as possible those radiopharmaceuticals which have the shortest excretion time in the milk should be used in lactating women and during the period of their excretion, breast milk should be manually expressed and discarded. The milk samples can be screened for radioactivity before resumption of breastfeeding.

Nursing mother should not ingest drugs of abuse because they are hazardous to the breastfed infant and to the health of the mother. Amphetamine, cocaine and heroin may cause irritability, sleeplessness, tremulousness, vomiting, poor feeding and seizures. Maternal intake of cocaine and marijuana is associated with slower motor development of the infant at one year of age. Smoking may suppress milk production and adversely affect the weight gain of the infant. It is associated with increased risk of infantile colic. Nicotine appears in the human milk in concentrations between 1.5 and 3.0 times of maternal plasma concentration. Mothers with silicone breast implants can safely breastfeed their babies. There is evidence to suggest that silicone is present in higher concentrations in cow's milk and formula feeds compared to the milk of mothers with implants.

MEDICATIONS TO THE BABY

The ability of the newborn to deal with drugs depends upon his functional maturity which is related to the conjugatory ability of the liver and excretory capacity of the kidneys. Due to hepatic and renal immaturity, the half life of the drug in the newborn is prolonged so that administration of drugs every 12 or 8 hours is satisfactory. The poor detoxification and clearance of drugs in the newborn predisposes the infant to develop toxic effects unless due caution is exercised during their use. In addition to above factors, absorption handicaps, altered distribution due to membrane permeability, specific protein binding of drugs, deficiency of certain enzymes, such as G-6-PD, pseudocholinesterase and methemoglobin reductase and end organ sensitivity may determine and modify the response of drugs in the newborn.

Table 5.2 outlines the dosage schedule, route of administration, indications and some side effects of commonly used drugs in the newborn. Drugs in the newborn should be used when absolutely indicated and only those agents which have been well tried in the newborn period should be prescribed. As far as possible, oral and intravenous routes should be used because absorption through intramuscular route is erratic. For oral medications, formulation in drops should be preferred over syrups for ease of administration and reduced osmolar load.

TABLE 5.2 Commonly used drugs in the newborn

Agent	Dose/kg/day*	Route of administration	Comments
I. Antibiotics			
■ Amikacin*	10 mg/kg loading dose, 7.5 mg/kg/dose	im, iv (over 20–30 min)	Maintain serum levels between 10 and 25 µg/mL. Furosemide and vancomycin enhance ototoxicity and nephrotoxicity
■ Ampicillin**	25–50 mg/kg/dose	oral, im, iv	Solution is stable only for 4 hours. The dose is doubled in meningitis
■ Aztreonam	90–120 mg q 6–8 hr	im, iv	Crosses blood–brain barrier and is beta-tactamase stable
■ Benzylpenicillin*	25,000 units/kg/dose	im, iv	Use 5 to 10 times this dose for serious infections and meningitis
■ Carbenicillin*	100 mg/kg/dose, 5 mg per intrathecal dose	im, iv	Should not be mixed with gentamicin and watch for hypokalemia
■ Cefazoline sodium*	20 mg/kg/dose	im, iv	Does not penetrate cerebrospinal fluid space
■ Cefepime*	50 mg/kg/dose	iv	Its antipseudomonal activity is similar to ceftazidime
■ Cefotaxime sodium*	50 mg/kg/dose	im, iv	Readily crosses blood–brain barrier
■ Ceftazidime*	50 mg/kg/dose	im, iv	
■ Ceftriaxone sodium	50–75 mg/kg single dose daily	iv	For meningitis, use higher dose twice a day. Avoid in neonates with severe jaundice. Drug of choice for gonococci resistent to penicillin
■ Cefuroxime axetil	100 mg followed by 50 mg after 3 days q 8 hr	im, iv	
■ Chloramphenicol*	25 mg/kg/dose up to 2 weeks q 24 hr, 15–30 d q 12 hr, later q 6–8 hr	oral, im, iv	Gray baby syndrome. Do not exceed 75 mg/kg/day during first week in term and two weeks in preterm babies. Maintain serum levels between 10 and 25 µg/mL
■ Cloxacillin**	25–50 mg/kg/dose	im, iv	
■ Colistimethate sulfate/colistin	50,000–75,000 iu/kg/d, 8 hr	iv	
■ Colistin sodium	2.5–5.0 mg q, 6–8 hr	oral	
■ Erythromycin	25–50 mg q 6–8 hr	oral, im, iv	Antibacterial resistance develops fast.
■ Gentamicin sulfate*	2.5 mg/kg/dose, 4 mg/kg single dose daily, 1.0 mg per intrathecal dose and 1–2 mg/kg per intra-ventricular dose	im, iv	Use pediatric dosage vial (10 mg/mL). For iv use, concentration should not exceed 1.0 mg/mL. Nephro- and ototoxic. Serum levels should be monitored and maintained between 4 and 8 µg/mL
■ Imipenem/cilastin	20 mg/kg/dose	im, iv	im formulation cannot be given iv
■ Kanamycin sulfate*	2.5–5.0 mg/kg/dose	im, iv slow drip	For iv use, concentration should not exceed 2.5 mg/mL. Nephro- and ototoxic. Serum levels should be maintained between 15 and 25 µg/mL
■ Linezolid	20 mg q 12 hr	iv, oral	Useful for vancomycin-resistant enterococci and methicillin-resistant *S. aureus*
■ Meropenem	60 mg q 8 hr	iv slow infusion	Drug of choice for extended spectrum beta lactamase producing micro-organisms
■ Methicillin sodium*	25 mg/kg/dose	im, iv slow infusion	Give double the dose for meningitis
■ Metronidazole	15 mg/kg loading dose followed 24 hours later by 7.5 mg/kg dose every 12 hours	iv, po	Anerobic infections and necrotizing enterocolitis. Reddish-brown discoloration of urine may occur

*The lower dose is used in a preterm baby. Administer every 12 hr for all infants between 0 and 7 days and every 8 hr for infants >7 days.
**Preterm infants up to 7 days administer every 12 hr, term infants up to 7 days and preterm infants >7 days administer every 8 hr, and term infants after 7 days every 6 hr.
Source: Singh M, Deorari AK. Drug Dosages in Children. CBS Publishers & Distributors Pvt. Ltd, New Delhi. 10th Edition, 2019.

(contd.)

TABLE 5.2 Commonly used drugs in the newborn *(contd.)*

Agent	Dose/kg/day*	Route of administration	Comments
Moxalactam Disodium*	50 mg/kg/dose	iv	
Nafcillin	25 mg/kg/dose	iv	Good CSF penetration
Neomycin sulfate*	12.5 mg/kg/dose	oral	
Netilmicin sulfate*	2.5–3.0 mg/kg/dose	im, iv	
Piperacillin sodium with tazobactam	50–75 mg/kg/dose	im, iv	May cause neuromuscular irritability and seizures
Polymyxin B sulfate*	2.5 mg/kg/dose	oral, im, iv	Does not cross blood–brain barrier
Ticarcillin sodium**	75 mg/kg/dose	im, iv	
Tobramycin*	2.5 mg/kg/dose	im, iv	
Teicoplanin	10 mg q 12–24 hr	iv slow infusion	It crosses blood–brain barrier
Trimethoprim sulfamethoxazole (cotrimoxazole)	TMP 2 mg/kg loading dose followed by TMP 1.2 mg/kg every 12 hours	iv, oral	Diluted in 5% dextrose in a ratio of 1:20 and given in 10 minutes. Readily crosses blood–brain barrier
Vancomycin hydrochloride*	15 mg/kg/dose q 8–12 hr Oral dose is 40–50 mg q 6 hr for colitis in a concentration of 5 mg/mL	oral, iv slowly over 30 min	For oral use dilute with water to a concentration of 5 mg/mL. "Red man syndrome" occurs if given as a bolus. Diphenhydramine provides relief

II. Anticonvulsants and sedatives

Agent	Dose/kg/day*	Route of administration	Comments
Chloral hydrate	25–50 mg/kg per dose	oral	Avoid in hepatic and renal impairment
Chlorpromazine	0.5–2.0 mg/kg per dose	oral, im, iv	
Diazepam	0.1–0.3 mg/kg/dose q 15–30 min. Maximum dose 2–5 mg	im, iv, pr	Avoid if infant is jaundiced because it contains sodium benzoate as a preservative
Fentanyl citrate	2–4 µg/kg/dose q 2–4 hr continuous infusion @ 1–5 µg/kg/hr	iv slowly over 3–5 min	Watch for respiratory depression, ileus and muscle rigidity. Naloxone is a useful antidote.
Lorazepam	0.05–0.10 mg/kg/dose q 10–15 min to a maximum of 4 mg	iv over 2–3 min	Dilute with equal volume of normal saline. Flumazenil 5–10 mg/kg/dose iv is effective antidote
Magnesium sulfate	0.2 mL/kg per dose as 50% solution q 6 hr for 4 days	im	Useful for treatment of refractory hypocalcemia
Midazolam	0.1–0.2 mg/kg/dose continuous iv infusion @ 0.4–0.6 µg/kg/min	im, iv over 2–5 min	Give after dilution as it contains 1% benzyl alcohol
Morphine sulfate	0.05 mg/kg/dose Continuous iv infusion 0.01–0.02 mg/kg/hr	sc, iv	Keep watch on respiration
Paraldehyde	0.2 mL/kg/dose	im, per rectum in oil or liquid paraffin	Use ampoules. May decompose into acetic acid and cause necrosis
Pethidine	1 mg/kg/dose	im, iv	

*The lower dose is used in a preterm baby. Administer every 12 hr for all infants between 0 and 7 days and every 8 hr for infants >7 days

**Preterm infants up to 7 days administer every 12 hr, term infants up to 7 days and preterm infants >7 days every 8 hr, and term infants after 7 days every 6 hr.

(contd.)

Perinatal Pharmacology

5

TABLE 5.2 Commonly used drugs in the newborn (contd.)

Agent	Dose/kg/day*	Route of administration	Comments
■ Phenobarbitone sodium	20 mg/kg loading dose followed by 5–8 mg/kg/d q 12 hr	oral, im, iv	Induces maturation of glucuronyl transferase and Y-acceptor protein. Do not give along with diazepam. Optimal serum levels range between 20 and 30 µg/mL
■ Phenytoin sodium	20 mg/kg loading dose followed by 5–8 mg/kg/day q 12 hr	oral, iv	Watch bradycardia, arrhythmia, hypotension. Optimal serum therapeutic level is 10–20 µg/mL
■ Pyridoxine	50–100 mg/dose Maintenance 50–100 mg oral daily	iv	Give under EEG control
■ Triclofos sodium	10–20 mg/kg per dose	oral	
III. Antifungal agents			
■ Amphotericin-B	Initial dose 0.25–0.5 mg/kg. Dose is increased daily by 0.25 mg till the maximum daily dose of 1.0 mg/kg. Total dose 30–35 mg/ kg over 2–4 weeks	iv slow drip over 2 hr	Disseminated fungal infection. Maximum concentration limited to 1.0 mg/10 mL of 5% dextrose. It is incompatible with sodium chloride. Watch renal and hematologic toxicity and hypokalemia. Protect from light
■ Amphotericin-B liposome (ambisome)	5 mg/kg q 24 hr infused over 2 hr in a maximum concentration of 2 mg/ml. Average duration of therapy is 2–4 weeks	iv slow infusion	Avoid concurrent use of corticosteroids and nephrotoxic drugs
■ Fluconazole	Loading dose 12 mg/kg followed by 6 mg/kg/dose q 24–48 hr	oral or iv over 30 minutes	Good CSF penetration, monitor renal and liver functions
■ Flucytocine	25–50 mg/kg/dose q 6 hr	oral, iv	Combined with amphotericin B for severe or CNS fungal infections
■ Ketoconazole	1–2 mg/kg/dose q 12 hr	oral	Avoid in infants with hepatic dysfunction
■ Nystatin	0.5–1.0 mL of 100,000 U/mL q 6 hr	oral and topical	Continue therapy for 3 more days after resolution.
IV. Antiviral agents			
■ Acyclovir	20 mg/kg/dose q 8–12 hr for 10–21 d	iv infusion in a concentration of 5 mg/mL over 1–3 hr	Monitor renal and hepatic function.
■ Ganciclovir	10–15 mg/kg/day q 12 hr for 3–6 weeks. For long-term suppression, 10 mg/kg 3 days in a week for 3 months	iv slow infusion over one hour	Monitor hematologic, renal and hepatic functions Avoid contact with skin and mucous membranes because it is cytotoxic. It has been shown to cause testicular atrophy in experimental animals
■ Vidarabine	15–30 mg in a concentration of 0.5 mg/mL	iv infusion over 12 hr	It has been replaced by acyclovir

*The lower dose is used in a preterm baby. During the first week, parenteral medications are administered 12-hourly in preterm babies and 8-hourly in term babies.

(contd.)

Agent	Dose/kg/day*	Route of administration	Comments
■ Zidovudine	1.5–2.0 mg/kg/dose q 6 hr for 6 weeks	oral, iv infusion over 1 hr	Monitor hematologic, renal and hepatic side effects
V. Corticosteroids			
■ Aldosterone	1 mg per dose	im, iv	Salt-losing adrenal crisis
■ Cortisone acetate	5–10 mg/kg/d	im, iv, oral	Maintenance dose for congenital adrenal hyperplasia.
■ Dexamethasone	0.1–0.25 mg/kg/ dose q 6 hr	oral, im, iv	For cerebral edema, raised intracranial tension, airway edema and BPD. There is increased risk of neuromotor disability and cerebral palsy on long-term follow-up
■ Fludrocortisone	0.1–0.2 mg/day	oral single dose	Adrenogenital syndrome
■ Hydrocortisone	5–10 mg q 8 hr. For shock 50–150 mg q 6 hr	im, iv	Solution is stable for few hours only. Indicated in endotoxic shock, sclerema, adrenal hemorrhage and laryngeal edema following intubation.
VI. Decongestive and cardiotonic drugs			
■ Captopril	0.05–0.5 mg/kg/dose 8–12 hr	oral empty stomach	May cause oliguria, hyperkalemia, renal failure, jaundice
■ Digoxin	0.03–0.05 mg, 1/2 stat, 1/4 after 8 hours and 1/4 after 12–16 hours	oral, im, iv	Intravenous administration should be preferred in seriously sick infants. 1/4 of total digitalizing dose should be given as maintenance dose in two divided doses. Blood levels should be maintained between 3 and 4 ng/mL
■ Dobutamine*	5–25 μg/kg/min	iv through infusion pump	Do not mix with sodium bicarbonate. It does not compromise renal perfusion and is useful alternative, if dopamine administration is associated with tachycardia
■ Dopamine*	2.5–25 μg/kg/min	iv through infusion pump	Low dose infusion is useful to promote renal perfusion. Administration of high dose (>25μg/kg/min) is associated with tachycardia, increase in pulmonary artery pressure and reduction of renal blood flow
■ Epinephrine 1:10,000 (0.1 mg/mL)	0.1–0.3 mL/kg q 3–5 min. Repeat same dose of 1:1000 solution in an unresponsive case. For nebulization, 0.5 ml/kg of 1:1000 soution diluted in 3 mL normal saline	iv push, intratracheal dose is 0.3–1.0 mL/kg	Avoid intracardiac
■ Furosemide	1–2 mg/kg/dose, maximum 6 mg/kg/dose	oral, im, iv	

*mg dobutamine/dopamine per 100 mL solution =
$$\frac{[6 \times \text{infant's weight (kg)} \times \text{desired dose (μg/kg/min)}]}{\text{Desired fluid infusion rate (mL/hr)}}$$

*The lower dose is used in a preterm baby. During the first week, parenteral medications are administered 12-hourly in preterm babies and 8-hourly in term babies.

Perinatal Pharmacology

5

(contd.)

Agent	Dose/kg/day*	Route of administration	Comments
■ Hydralazine	0.15 mg/kg/dose every 6 hourly. Increase by 0.1 mg/kg every 6 hours till desired effect achieved or maximum dose of 2 mg/kg achieved.	oral, iv	
■ Methyldopa	10 mg/kg/dose	iv, oral	
■ Nifedipine	0.2 mg/kg/dose	Sublingual, oral	Sparingly used in neonates
■ Nitroprusside sodium	0.2–6.0 µg/kg/min	iv through infusion pump	Thiocyanate toxicity causes hyperreflexia, seizures and coma
■ Propranolol	0.2–0.4 mg/kg/dose, 2 mg/kg/day q 6–8 hr	iv, oral	Paroxysmal atrial tachycardia, neonatal thyro-toxicosis and asymmetric septal hypertrophy
■ Tolazoline	1–2 mg/kg bolus followed by continuous infusion at 1–2 mg/kg per hr	iv	Persistent fetal circulation

VII. Miscellaneous drugs

Agent	Dose/kg/day*	Route of administration	Comments
■ Acetaminophen	10–15 mg/kg/dose q 6–8 hr	oral	Use formulation dispensed as drops
■ Acetazolamide	10–25 mg/kg/dose q 8 hr	oral	Hydrocephalus unassociated with Arnold-Chiari malformation. Watch for hyper-chloremic metabolic acidosis
■ Acetylcysteine	10 mL of 10% solution every 6 hr	oral, pr	Used for treatment of meconium ileus
■ Albumin-salt free (25%)	0.5 to 1.0 g/kg/dose. Maximum dose 6 g/kg/d	iv slowly over one hour	Half an hour before exchange transfusion. Dilute with saline to 5% solution.
■ Atropine sulfate	0.02 mg/kg/dose q 10–15 min	sc, iv	
■ Caffeine citrate	20 mg/kg stat, 5–10 mg/kg/dose in 1–2 doses daily for maintenance	iv over 30 minutes. Do not give iv bolus push, oral for maintenance therapy	Recurrent apnea of prematurity. Risk of kernicterus and seizures.
■ Calcium gluconate 10%	100–200 mg/kg/dose (1–2 mL/kg/dose) followed by 200–800 mg/kg/day for maintenance	iv slowly over 10 min, stop if heart rate <100 bpm	Do not mix with sodium bicarbonate solution. Dilute with equal volume of distilled water and watch for bradycardia. Avoid in digitalized infants
■ Carbimazole	2.5 mg per dose	Oral	Congenital thyrotoxicosis
■ Cardioversion	0.5 J/kg, double the dose each time for a total of 3 attempts	Administer iv adenosine 0.05–2.0 mg/kg/dose bolus before cardioversion	Correct acidosis

*The lower dose is used in a preterm baby. During the first week, parenteral medications are administered 12-hourly in preterm babies and 8-hourly in term babies.

(contd.)

TABLE 5.2 Commonly used drugs in the newborn *(contd.)*

Agent	Dose/kg/day*	Route of administration	Comments
▪ Carnitine	50–100 mg/kg/d q 24 hr	oral, iv	Diarrhea is a common side effect
▪ Cisapride	0.1–0.3 mg/kg/dose q 8–12 hr	oral	It is contraindicated, if QTC interval is more than 0.44. It should not be co-administered with erythromycin and antifungal drugs which are known to increase QTC interval
▪ Defibrillation	1–2 watt-seconds/kg, double with each successive attempt to a maximum of 10 watt-seconds/kg	local	The paddle diameter should be 4.5 cm. Correct acidosis
▪ Diazoxide	8–15 mg q 8–12 hr	oral, iv	For glucose-refractory hyperinsulinemic hypoglycemia
▪ Doxapram hydrochloride	2.5 mg/kg/stat, infusion rate 1–2 mg/kg/hr	iv	The margin of safety is low. Hypertension, IVH and seizures may occur
▪ Edrophonium bromide (tensilon)	1 mg stat	im, iv	For diagnosis of transient neonatal myasthenia gravis
▪ Ephedrine saline nose drops (0.25%)	One drop 15 minutes before feed for local use		Do not use more than 2–3 times per day. Jitteriness, excessive crying and fever may occur
▪ Ferrous sulfate	Prophylaxis 2 mg q 24 hr. Therapeutic 4–6 mg q 12 hr	oral	Give in-between feeds
▪ Gentian violet (0.5%)	One drop after each feed under the tongue	oral thrush	
▪ Glucagon	0.1–0.3 mg/kg/dose up to maximum of 1 mg	im, iv bolus	Use in macrosomic babies with hypoglycemia
▪ Heparin	100 units/kg/dose every 4 hourly, 10 units/mL for rinsing syringes and catheters	im, iv	To maintain clotting time of 20–30 minutes or 2–3 times of pretherapy clotting time
▪ Hepatitis B immune globulins	0.5 mL/dose (0.16 mL/kg) at birth or alternatively 2.0 mL pooled gamma globulin	im	Given if mother is carrier of hepatitis B virus
▪ Ibuprofen	10 mg/kg stat followed by oral, 5 mg/kg at 24 hr and 48 hr	iv	Pharmacologic closure of ductus arteriosus
▪ Immune gamma globulins	0.15 mL/kg stat for HAV prophylaxis, 500–750 mg/kg iv over 2–6 hr stat for prevention and treatment of sepsis, 400 mg/kg/d for 3–5 days for immune thrombocytopenia	im	The role in prophylaxis and treatment of sepsis is controversial

*The lower dose is used in a preterm baby. During the first week, parenteral medications are administered 12-hourly in preterm babies and 8-hourly in term babies.

Perinatal Pharmacology

5

(contd.)

TABLE 5.2 Commonly used drugs in the newborn (*contd.*)

Agent	Dose/kg/day*	Route of administration	Comments
▪ Indomethacin	0.2 mg/kg/dose q 12 hr for 3 doses	oral, iv over 30 min	Avoid if there is bleeding, renal dysfunction
▪ Isoniazid	5–10 mg q 24 hr	oral	For chemoprophylaxis and congenital tuberculosis Always combine it with pyridoxine
▪ Lomodex (10%)	1–2 g/kg/dose	iv	
▪ Lugol's iodine	One drop q 8 hr	oral	
▪ Magnesium sulfate (50%)	25–50 mg/kg/dose q 6 hr for 4 doses	im	Calcium gluconate 10% is a useful antidote
▪ Mannitol (20%)	1.0 g/kg/dose q 8 hr for 3 doses	iv over 30 min	For relief of raised intracranial tension.
▪ Metoclopramide	0.2–0.3 mg/kg/dose q 6–8 hr	oral	May cause hypertrophy of breast tissue
▪ Methylene blue	0.1–0.2 mg/kg as 1% solution	iv	Given for methemoglobinemia. Blue-green discoloration of urine occurs.
▪ Nalorphine	0.2 mg/kg/dose	iv, im, sc, intratracheal	If mother had received pethidine or morphine 4 to 6 hours before delivery.
▪ Naloxone hydrochloride	0.1 to 0.2 mg/kg/dose q 3–5 min	iv, im, sc, intratracheal	Do not administer to newborns of narcotic-dependent mothers
▪ Neostigmine methyl sulfate	0.05 to 0.1 mg/kg stat	im, iv, oral	Give atropine before administering prostigmine
▪ Omeprazole	0.5–1.5 mg/kg single or two doses daily	oral through NG tube	Monitor hepatic transaminases
▪ Pancuronium bromide	0.05–0.1 mg/kg loading dose q 5–10 min twice. 0.03–0.1 mg/kg/dose q 1–4 hr for maintenance or continuous infusion @ 0.05–0.2 mg/kg/hr	iv bolus or through infusion pump	Neostigmine 0.025 mg/kg iv with atropine (0.02 mg/kg) is an effective antidote
▪ Prostaglandin E$_1$	0.05–0.4 µg/kg/ min	iv infusion @ 0.05 µg/min	Adjust the dose on the basis of improved oxygenation versus side effects. The side effects include apnea, bradycardia, flushing, hypotension, seizure-like activity, hypocalcemia, hypoglycemia, diarrhea and inhibition of platelet aggregation
▪ Protamine sulfate	1 mg for every mg (100 units) of heparin taken during past 4 hours	im, iv	Antidote for heparin
▪ Pyrimethamine	1 mg for 3 days, then 0.5 mg for one month	oral	Folinic acid 5 mg should be given twice weekly.
▪ Ranitidine	1–2 mg/kg/dose q 8–12 hr 0.5–1.0 mg/kg/dose q 6–8 hr	oral iv	Use in VLBW infants is associated with increased risk of NEC
▪ Rifampicin	10 mg/kg/dose q 24 hr	oral	Causes red discoloration of urine and body secretions
▪ Salbutamol	0.1–0.3 mg/kg/dose q 8 hr 0.5 mg/kg/dose with 1.5 mL normal saline q 2–6 hr	oral, nebulization	Stop if heart rate goes >180 bpm. Look for hypokalemia

*The lower dose is used in a preterm baby. During the first week, parenteral medications are administered 12-hourly in preterm babies and 8-hourly in term babies.

(*contd.*)

TABLE 5.2 Commonly used drugs in the newborn (*contd.*)

Agent	Dose/kg/day*	Route of administration	Comments
■ Sodium bicarbonate 7.5%	2–4 mL/kg	iv slowly over 15 min	Never infuse till adequate ventilation is established. Avoid rapid bolus administration due to risk of IVH and pulmonary hemorrhage
■ Sodium polystyrene sulfonate	1g/kg/dose q 6 hr. For rectal administration, use 20–25% sorbitol q 2–6 hr	oral, pr	Constipation and fecal impaction may occur
■ Sulfadiazine	100–150 mg q 8 hr	oral	Toxoplasmosis and urinary tract infection. Avoid during first week
■ Tetanus human immunoglobulins	30–300 units/kg	iv	Neonatal tetanus
■ Theophylline	5 mg/kg stat, 1–2 mg/kg/dose in 3 doses daily for maintenance	iv, oral	For recurrent apneic attacks
■ Thyroxine	10–15 µg/kg/day single dose. Adjust the dose by increments of 12.5 µg every month.	oral empty stomach	Maintain total T_4 between 5.0 to 12.0 µg/dL and TSH less than 10 mU/L
■ Tromethamine (THAM)	Loading dose (mL) of 0.3 M solution = wt (kg) × 1.1 × base deficit (mEq/L). Maintenance 3 mL/kg/hr	iv	Infuse through a peripheral vessel
■ Urokinase	Loading dose 4000 iu/kg followed by constant infusion @ 4000–6000 iu/kg/hr	iv over 20 min as bolus	Watch for bleeding
■ Vitamin E	25 units/day	im, oral	Give to all infants weighing less than 1500 g at birth
■ Vitamin K₁ Prophylactic dose Therapeutic dose	0.5–1.0 mg single 2.0 mg	oral, im, iv	Lower dose is given to infants <1500 g
■ Zinc acetate	0.5–1.0 mg/kg/day	oral	Absorption interfered by concomitant administration of iron

*The lower dose is used in a preterm baby. During the first week, parenteral medications are administered 12-hourly in preterm babies and 8-hourly in term babies.

Over dosage by accidental use of vials (vitamin K and nalorphine) intended for use in the mother must be avoided. It is desirable to use insulin (40 unit marks/mL) or tuberculin syringes for ease and accuracy of administration. The amount of diluent used for administration of intravenous medications should be recorded and subtracted from the recommended daily fluid requirements. The proprietary combinations should be avoided due to risk of inadvertent overdosage of one of the agents.

Chloramphenicol when administered in a dose of 100 mg/kg per day has been shown to result in "gray baby syndrome" which is characterized by abdominal distension, vomiting, hypothermia, shallow and irregular breathing, grayish circumoral cyanosis and circulatory collapse. There is unexplained metabolic acidosis and hyperammonemia. Streptomycin, neomycin, kanamycin and colistin may cause respiratory paralysis by blockage of muscle endplate when applied locally over large raw surface areas or after intraperitoneal instillation. Tetracyclines have been shown to cause growth retardation and brownish staining of teeth by virtue of their chelation with calcium. Hyperbilirubinemia and/or kernicterus may occur at relatively lower serum bilirubin levels during administration of large doses of synthetic vitamin K, long-acting sulfonamides, salicylates, caffeine, lobeline, cedalinid, novobiocin and gentamicin.

It must be remembered that preservatives and vehicles contained in certain drug formulations, which

Perinatal Pharmacology

5

are safe in adults, may be toxic and sometimes dangerous in newborn babies. Sodium benzoate used as a preservative for diazepam is associated with the risk of bilirubin brain damage at relatively lower serum bilirubin levels by blocking bilirubin binding sites in albumin. Propylene glycol (1, 2-propanediol) used as a vehicle in several parenteral drug formulations, such as multivitamins, digoxin, cotrimoxazole, phenobarbitol, phenytoin, diazepam and hydralazine, is fraught with dangers of hyperosmolality. It is desirable that these hyperosmolar medications (including sodium bicarbonate 7.5% and potassium chloride 15%) should be administered slowly after adequate dilution to prevent capillary damage and tissue anoxia. Benzyl alcohol is widely used as a preservative in flush solutions and multiple-dose vials of medications and parenteral electrolyte-containing fluids. It is potentially unsafe in very low birth weight babies and can cause severe metabolic acidosis, encephalopathy and respiratory depression. Benzyl alcohol is oxidized to benzoic acid, conjugated with glycine in the liver and excreted as hippuric acid. This metabolic pathway may not be functional in premature infants and may allow accumulation of benzoic acid and perhaps unmetabolized benzyl alcohol with resultant metabolic acidosis and toxicity.

Hexachlorophene skin applications, without effective rinsing, may result in diarrhea, dehydration, shock, seizures and neuromuscular disturbances. Boric acid applications on large raw areas or accidental oral ingestion may lead to diarrhea, vomiting, generalized skin rash, hepatic necrosis and renal failure. Boric acid must never be stored in the nursery as it is devoid of any therapeutic utility. Lead poisoning may occur following use of lead acetate ointment and lead nipple shields for cracked nipples by the mother.

BIBLIOGRAPHY

American Academy of Pediatrics. Committee on Drugs. Anticonvulsants and pregnancy. *Pediatrics* 1979, 63: 331.

American Academy of Pediatrics. Use of psychoactive medications during pregnancy and possible effects on the fetus and newborn. Committee on Drugs. *Pediatrics* 2000, 105: 880–887.

American Academy of Pediatrics. Committee on Drugs. The transfer of drugs and other chemicals into human milk. *Pediatrics* 2001, 108(3): 776–789.

Anker JV, Allegaert K. Perinatal Pharmacology. *Semin Fetal Neonatal Med.* 2013, 18(1):1–2.

Boyle RJ. Effects of certain prenatal drugs on the fetus and newborn. *Pediatr Rev* 2002, 23: 17–24.

Briggs GG. Drugs in Pregnancy and Lactation, *Lippincott Williams and Wilkins*, Philadelphia 2002.

Cahen RL. Evaluation of teratogenicity of drugs. *Clin Pharm Therap* 1964, 5: 450.

Dean JC, Healey H, Moore SJ, *et al.* Long term health and neurodevelopment in children exposed to antiepileptic drugs before birth. *J Med Genet* 2002, 39: 251–259.

Done AK. Developmental pharmacology. *Clin Pharm and Therap* 1964, 5: 432.

Fulroth R, Phillips B, Durand DJ. Perinatal outcome of infants exposed to cocaine and/or heroin in-utero. *Amer J Dis Child* 1989, 143: 905.

Harmful effects of diagnostic irradiation (leading article). *Lancet* 1963, 1: 255.

Holmes LB, Harvey EA, Coull BA, *et al.* The teratogenicity of anticonvulsant drugs. *N. Engl J Med* 2001, 344: 1132–1138.

Jacqz-Aigrain E, Koren G. Effects of drugs on the fetus. *Semin Fetal Neonat Med* 2005, 10: 139–147.

Janerich DT, Piper JM, Glebatis DM. Oral contraceptives and congenital limb reduction defects. *New Engl J Med* 1974, 291: 697.

Klevit HD. Corticosteroid therapy in the neonatal period. *Pediatr Clin N Amer* 1970, 17: 1003.

Knowles JA. Excretion of drugs in milk. *J Pediatr* 1965, 66:1068.

Koren G, Florescu A, Costei AM, *et al.* Nonsteroidal anti-inflammatory drugs during third trimester and risk of premature closure of the ductus arteriosus. A meta-analysis. *Ann Pharmacother* 2006, 40 (5) : 824–829.

Lucey JF. Hazards to newborn infant from drugs administered to mother. *Pediatr Clin N Amer* 1961, 8: 413.

MacKintosh DA. Drugs in lactation. *Indian J Pediatr* 1986, 53:53.

Moudgil VV, Sobel JD. Antifungl drugs in pregnancy: A review. *Expert Opin Drug Saf* 2003, 2(5): 475–483.

Murray L, Seger D. Drug therapy during pregnancy and lactation. *Emerg Med Clin North Am* 1994, 12: 129–149.

Nyhan WL. Toxicity of drugs in the newborn. *J Pediatr* 1961, 59: 1.

Ramenteria JL (Ed). In: Drug Abuse in Pregnancy and Neonatal Effects. *The CV Mosby Co* 1977.

Sachdeva P, Patel BG, Patel BK. Drug use in pregnancy: a point to ponder! *Indian J Pharmaceut Sciences* 2009, 71(1): 1–7.

Shaikh AK, Kulkarni MD. Drugs in pregnancy and lactation. *Int J Basic Clini Pharmacol* 2013, 2(2): 130–135.

Singh M, Deorari AK. Drug Dosages in Children. *CBS Publishers & Distributors Pvt. Ltd., New Delhi,* 10th edition, 2019.

Smithells RW. Drugs, infections and congenital abnormalities. *Arch Dis Child* 1978, 53 : 93.

Thomas B, Pallivalapila A, El Kassem W, *et al.* Maternal and perinatal outcomes and pharmacological management of Covid-19 infection in pregnancy: a systematic review protocol. *Syst Rev* 2020, 9:161 https://doi.org/10.1186/s13643-020-01418–2.

Tsamantioti ES, Hashmi MF. Teratogenic medications. In: StatPearls (Internet). Treasure Island (FL); StatPearls Publishing; Jan 2020.

Ward RM. Drug therapy of the fetus. *J Clin Pharmacol* 1993, 33: 780–789.

Wildnes SF, Schjott J. Risk perception regarding drug use in pregnancy. *Am J Obstet Gyneocol* 2017, 216(4): 375–8.

Care of the Baby in the Labor Room

Every birth must be considered as a medical emergency. In India alone, we should be prepared to meet the challenge of 26 million medical emergencies every year (75,000 every day!). Perinatal hypoxia is one of the leading causes of perinatal mortality in low and middle income countries (LMICs). Birth asphyxia is an important cause of static developmental and neurologic handicaps both in term and preterm infants. *In utero*, the placenta serves to transfer nutrition and oxygen from the mother and eliminates fetal waste products. After separation from the mother, the baby must breathe immediately to safeguard against anoxic damage to brain and other vital organs. In the labor room, the newly born baby should be helped to establish independent breathing without delay because within two minutes of tying the cord the arterial oxygen tension falls to 1–2 mm Hg. The way in which an asphyxiated baby is managed at birth determines the immediate morbidity and quality of life among survivors. In order to provide optimal care to mothers during delivery and ensure intact survival of newborn babies, it is desirable that the delivery complex should be designated as perinatal intensive care unit (PICU) and provided with necessary physical infrastructure, equipment, staff and facilities. The health professionals working in this area should have adequate knowledge and skills to resuscitate a newborn baby and should be able to work smoothly as a team.

THE 'FIRST' BREATH

Cry after birth is not really the 'first' breath of life because around 20 weeks of gestation, fetus starts making relatively rapid (80 to 120/min) and ineffective respiratory movements. To what extent amniotic fluid bathes the air passages is unknown but there is a considerable quantity of alveolar fluid in the fetal lungs before delivery. The lung fluid appears to be an ultrafiltrate of plasma, it is more acidic and has higher chloride content than amniotic fluid. During vaginal delivery, some amount of lung fluid is squeezed out and the rest is rapidly reabsorbed through lymphatics.

The 'first' functional breath after birth is produced by integrated activity of several stimuli, the most important being hypoxia, acidosis, cord occlusion and thermal changes. From a well cushioned, dark, warm and comfortable aqueous milieu of uterus, the infant emerges out into a hostile physical environment providing a volley of sensory stimuli in the form of light, sound, cold and air currents. It is no wonder that most babies cry and yell! At birth, average value for oxygen saturation of arterial blood is 22%, PCO_2 60 mm Hg and pH 7.28. These biochemical stimuli which are produced as a consequence of physiological hypoxia during delivery, stimulate carotid and aortic chemoreceptors which are functional in the newborn. Clamping of cord is followed by sudden rise in fetal systemic blood pressure and stimulation of aortic baroreceptors and sympathetic nervous system. Sudden cooling after birth, when human newborn baby may lose up to 600 kcal/minute at room temperature, provides respiratory drive by operating through trigeminal cold receptors located in the facial skin. As soon as breathing is established and following lung expansion, pulmonary vascular resistance rapidly falls. This occurs largely by direct effect of rise in arterial oxygen and fall in carbon dioxide tension on the pulmonary arterioles. There is a gradual transition from fetal to adult type of circulation although foramen ovale and ductus arteriosus may remain open for varying period of time. During the first few hours after birth, flow of blood in ductus arteriosus is bidirectional but soon shunt becomes predominantly left-to-right and by 24 hours of age it is functionally insignificant.

Sequence of Events during Respiratory Failure

The induction of experimental hypoxia at birth in the newborn of different animal species shows characteristic sequence of events. The initial strangulation and labored breathing is followed by gasping and primary apnea. Thereafter, there are spontaneous gasps. If animal stays in the hypoxic environment, the heart slows, blood pressure falls and then it lapses into terminal apnea (Figure 6.1). Though the sequence of events in the various species of animals is similar, the duration of different phases is specific. Respiratory failure may be prolonged due to immaturity, hypothermia, drugs and anesthetics administered to the mother during labor. These experimental observations have practical implications in the management of an asphyxiated newborn baby at birth.

The baby with primary apnea starts gasping spontaneously. Since the labor room environment has an oxygen concentration of about 21%, the baby becomes pink after a few gasps and establishes normal breathing. Any method of resuscitation in such a baby would succeed. This explains, why a variety of physical and chemical stimuli have been hailed and recommended for resuscitation of an asphyxiated baby. When faced with an apneic baby at birth, it is difficult to decide whether the baby is having primary or terminal apnea. Absence of evidences of fetal hypoxia, stable or rising heart rate (if it was slow initially) and onset of apnea after initial cry (as in babies born by cesarean section) favor the diagnosis of primary apnea. The improvement in the baby's color, if preceded by gasping or respiratory efforts, confirms the existence of primary apnea in retrospect.

The infant with terminal apnea needs immediate ventilation after endotracheal intubation. No other method of resuscitation succeeds. The baby has severe bradycardia and cardiovascular collapse and may appear pale rather than blue. Prolonged fetal hypoxia is associated with terminal apnea. The babies become pink before they start breathing spontaneously and are prone to develop sequelae of hypoxic brain damage.

It is important to remember that as a result of fetal hypoxia, the infant may go through both primary apnea and secondary apnea while *in utero*. Therefore, when one is faced with an apneic baby at birth, it must be assumed that one is dealing with secondary apnea and active resuscitation must begin without delay.

PHYSIOLOGICAL BASIS OF RESUSCITATION

During intrauterine life, the fetal lungs are filled with fluid and they do not serve any ventilatory purpose since the placenta supplies oxygen to the fetus. The blood flow through the lungs is markedly diminished due to constricted arterioles and right-to-left shunt through the ductus arteriosus during fetal life.

During vaginal delivery, one-third of fetal lung fluid is removed as the chest is squeezed and lung fluid comes out through the nose and mouth. The first few breaths of most newborn babies are extremely powerful to inflate the alveoli and replace the lung fluid with air. Infants who are apneic at birth and those having weak respiratory efforts cannot achieve this function. In order to ensure adequate expansion of lungs and clear the lung fluid, the initial ventilation requires at least two to three times (30–40 cm H_2O) the pressure needed for subsequent breaths (15–20 cm H_2O).

Asphyxia interferes with the transition from fetal to neonatal cardiopulmonary circulation. Due to hypoxemia and acidosis, pulmonary arterioles remain constricted with perpetuation of right-to-left shunt through ductus arteriosus. In this situation, even when the infant is adequately ventilated, satisfactory oxygenation of the tissues of the baby is not possible due to decreased pulmonary perfusion. It must be remembered that oxygenation depends not only on the oxygen reaching the alveoli but also on oxygen entering the bloodstream for delivery to the tissues and organs. In severely asphyxiated babies with metabolic acidosis, ventilation with 100% oxygen alone may not be adequate to enhance pulmonary perfusion. After establishing adequate ventilation, administration of sodium bicarbonate would correct acidosis and enhance pulmonary perfusion and tissue oxygenation by opening up pulmonary arterioles.

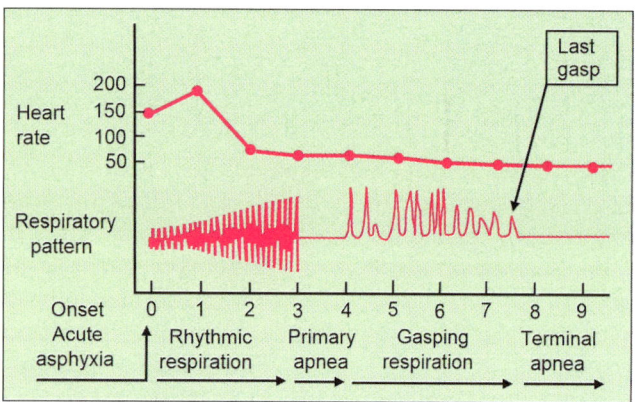

Figure 6.1 Schematic presentation of sequence of events of respiratory failure in experimental animals.

FETAL HYPOXIA

The existence of certain high-risk factors during pregnancy and labor serves to forewarn and alert the labor room staff that they should be fully prepared to meet the challenge of an asphyxiated baby (Table 6.1).

All high-risk pregnancies should be monitored for fetal growth, presence of congenital malformations, adequacy of placental functions and evidences of fetal hypoxia (see Chapter 3 for details). Mother can be advised to maintain fetal activity record by counting the number of fetal 'quickenings' during third trimester of pregnancy. A number of biochemical agents and hormones elaborated by uteroplacental unit have been employed to assess its functional status. Serial measurements of estriol in maternal plasma or 24 hours urinary excretion are useful indicators of integrity of fetoplacental unit. Isolated estriol levels are of no significance but a decline of more than 30% in serial plasma estriol level or in 24-hour urine assay is indicative of placental dysfunction.

During labor, non-stress fetal monitoring, i.e. simultaneous continuous record of fetal heart rate, uterine contractions and fetal movements with a cardiotocometer, provides useful information. Fetus is considered as 'reactive' and without any distress, if he can demonstrate acceleration of his heart beats by 15 or more for 15 seconds in association with fetal movements at least twice in a 20-minute record period. A persistently slow fetal heart rate without any variability in response to fetal movements or uterine contractions is indicative of fetal hypoxia.

If fetus is non-reactive, oxytocin challenge test is used to biologically assess integrity of uteroplacental unit. Uterine contractions are induced with oxytocin and their effect on fetal heart is monitored which simulates exercise tolerance studies in patients with suspected coronary artery disease. When uteroplacental unit is optimal, uterine contractions would not have any adverse effect on the circulation or oxygenation of the fetus. Consistent slowing of fetal heart rate following termination of each uterine contraction (late deceleration) is indicative of uteroplacental insufficiency and is considered as a positive oxytocin challenge test. Uterine contractions can also be induced by stimulation of nipples of the mother.

The biophysical profile of the fetus by ultrasonographic evaluation of Manning score is non-invasive and most reliable parameter of fetal wellbeing. It evaluates neurobehavior of the fetus and status of placenta by observing fetal breathing movements, posture, gross body movements and size of amniotic fluid volume. Fetal scalp blood sample can be obtained transvaginally with the help of an amnioscope in a vertex presenting fetus when membranes are ruptured and cervix is adequately dilated. There is a good correlation between fetal scalp pH of less than 7.15, positive-oxytocin challenge test and severe birth asphyxia.

In order to provide optimal care to high-risk pregnancies, there is a need to establish above referred tests in all centers providing Level II perinatal care for early diagnosis of fetal hypoxia and immediate delivery of a compromised fetus. The high-risk deliveries should be attended by a physician adequately trained in the art of cardiorespiratory resuscitation. At times a baby may manifest severe birth asphyxia without any predisposing warning signals thus emphasizing the need that all personnel concerned with providing perinatal care should be conversant with the basic principles of resuscitation of an asphyxiated newborn.

TABLE 6.1 Conditions demanding resuscitation alert

Antepartum risk factors

1. Maternal age less than 18 years or more than 35 years
2. Previous fetal or neonatal deaths
3. Placental insufficiency: Toxemia, hypertension, diabetes mellitus, postmaturity
4. Malpresentation or abnormal lie
5. Multifetal gestation
6. Poor fetal growth
7. Malformed fetus
8. Rhesus isoimmunization
9. Bad obstetrical history
10. Bleeding in the second or third trimester
11. Maternal systemic disease
12. Poly- or oligohydramnios
13. Drug therapy: Reserpine, lithium carbonate, magnesium sulfate, adrenergic blocking agents, maternal drug abuse, etc.

Intrapartum risk factors

1. Evidences of fetal distress
2. Premature or post-term gestation
3. Antepartum hemorrhage: Placenta previa, abruptio placentae
4. Cord prolapse
5. Tight nuchal cord
6. Meconium-stained liquor
7. Prelabor rupture of membranes (>18 hours) or chorioamnionitis
8. Prolonged labor (>24 hours)
9. Prolonged second stage of labor (>2 hours)
10. Large or macrosomic fetus
11. Non-vertex presentation
12. Assisted delivery or emergency casarean section
13. Use of general anesthesia and narcotics

Apart from availability of several newer techniques for evaluation of fetal wellbeing, the following time honored clinical parameters of fetal distress offer useful guidelines to an experienced obstetrician.

Exaggerated fetal movements The asphyxiated fetus behaves like a strangulated individual and makes desperate physical efforts followed by reduced or absent physical movements terminally.

Fetal heart rate Due to release of catecholamines, initially there is tachycardia followed by bradycardia and slow-irregular heart beats. Bradycardia is a compensatory mechanism that allows longer coronary blood flow and ventricular filling because of prolonged diastole. The heart rate should be assessed during the later phase of uterine contraction.

Visceral overactivity The passage of meconium in a vertex presenting baby is an important and ominous sign of fetal hypoxia. It is fraught with the risk of aspiration of meconium by the gasping fetus. In preterm babies, fetal diarrhea as a result of listeriosis is an uncommon cause of meconium staining of the liquor in the absence of fetal hypoxia.

PATHOPHYSIOLOGY OF ASPHYXIA

Birth asphyxia is associated with reduction in the arterial oxygen tension, accumulation of carbon dioxide and fall in blood pH. Acidosis occurs due to anerobic utilization of glucose, production of lactic acid and accumulation of carbon dioxide. These biochemical changes cause constriction of relatively muscular pulmonary arterioles and raise the pulmonary arterial pressure. This results in reduced filling of the left heart and right-to-left shunts. These physio-chemical changes perpetuate asphyxia, unless corrected by therapy. In asphyxiated term appropriate-for-dates babies, blood glucose is significantly increased during first 90 minutes due to mobilization of glycogen stores as a result of increased release of catecholamines and ACTH. The severe and prolonged hypoxia in preterm and growth-retarded babies is followed by depletion of cardiac glycogen stores and tendency towards hypoglycemia.

Hypothermia and hypoglycemia lead to accumulation of non-esterified fatty acids and glycerol. The cord blood concentration of glycerol, free fatty acids and beta-hydroxybutyrate do not show any correlation with the severity of asphyxial episode. Due to intracellular hypoxia, net catabolism of adenosine triphosphate (ATP) results in release of adenine metabolites, hypoxanthine (>16 mmol/L), xanthine, inosine and uridine in the cord blood. These metabolites are also unreliable predictors of severity of birth asphyxia because of wide variations in their blood levels in normal infants. The asphyxiated term neonates have significantly elevated plasma (>60 mg/dL) and CSF lactate levels. Elevation of creatine kinase brain isoenzymes (CK-BB) in cord blood is a reliable biochemical marker of perinatal hypoxia. Chronic placental insufficiency and fetal hypoxia is associated with elevated erythropoietin levels in blood. Anoxic damage to cells results in failure of energy dependent sodium pump mechanism with release of potassium and phosphates into the extracellular fluid. Petechial hemorrhages due to anoxic capillary damage, intracellular collection of sodium and inappropriate release of antidiuretic hormone are associated with development of cerebral edema.

Safety of Maternal Analgesics and Anesthetics

Most drugs used for relief of apprehension and pain during labor and delivery are capable of passing through the placenta and affecting the infant. As compared to an adult, fetus is about four times more sensitive to depressant and narcotic drugs. Barbiturates, diazepam and opium derivatives including morphine, pethidine (meperidine) can cause serious depression and hypothermia in a newborn baby. They can prolong the duration of various stages of respiratory failure and delay establishment of spontaneous breathing. Pethidine should preferably be administered intravenously for prompt excretion by kidneys and its dose should be restricted to 50 mg in an average Indian woman. The respiratory depressant effect of opium derivatives can be effectively reversed by administration of nalorphine and naloxone to the infant. Pentazocine, a synthetic opiate, is a relatively safe analgesic and has minimal side effects on the fetus. The regional anesthetic drugs are also known to cross the placenta in significant amounts and can cause fetal depression. Bupivacaine is the agent of choice for epidural block. It is safe, effective and long acting with minimal side effects on the neonatal neurobehavior. Epidural analgesia is associated with high incidence of maternal fever due to thermoregulatory changes induced by epidural medication. The combination of thiopental, succinylcholine and light nitrous oxide-oxygen mixture is safe for general anesthesia.

Most mothers do harbor the fear of anticipated pain and discomfort of labor. Some are haunted by the unpleasant experience of witnessing difficult and traumatic deliveries with unfortunate consequences among their relatives. Their anxiety should be relieved and doubts cleared during antenatal visits. The mother should be trained in the art of relaxation and explained the importance of deep breathing during labor. The health personnel working in the delivery room should exude exemplary confidence and provide emotional strength and sympathetic support to the mother during the physical turmoil of labor. The current labor room scene of loud shouts of health care workers to drown the shrieks of laboring mothers should be replaced by more humane and compassionate attitude of genuine concern by providing comforting touch, gentle handling and encouragement during one of the most crucial moments of woman's life. The practice of allowing the husband to provide comfort and emotional support to the wife during birthing has gained popularity in the west and needs to be promoted in India. There is a need to evaluate the utility of acupuncture to provide safe analgesia during labor. The research is also needed to identify the most comfortable posture during labor to ensure prompt, safe and relatively painless delivery.

Cord Clamping

The issue of early versus late clamping of the cord is still unresolved despite availability of several studies. American College of Obstetrics and Gynecology currently recommends delayed cord clamping (at least 30–60 seconds) in term and preterm infants. Early or immediate clamping of cord is associated with increased risk of intraventricular hemorrhage, respiratory distress syndrome, late-onset sepsis, anemia and elevated lead levels. When clamping of cord is delayed beyond one minute, the infant is at an increased risk to develop polycythemia, transient tachypnea of the newborn, jaundice, elevated blood pressure and patent ductus arteriosus. When cord clamping is delayed until breathing is established, placental blood flow through the umbilical venous return continues to fill the right side of the heart ensuring adequate pulmonary vascular filling over several breathing cycles. Recent studies on preterm lambs have documented that delayed clamping of cord after ventilation was established, is associated with smooth maintenance of carotid and cerebral blood flow. It is recommended that the obstetrician should follow a relaxed approach in clamping the cord, neither immediate nor deliberate delay should be adopted. It is recommended to delay clamping of cord for at least 1 minute in all infants not requiring any resuscitation. In situations with cord around the neck, severe fetal hypoxia and Rh-isoimmunization, it is desirable to ensure early clamping of the cord. In normal circumstances, taking cue from nature, it would appear that delayed clamping (as late as the birth of placenta during deliveries in animals) does not lead to any adverse consequences as long as the baby and mother are placed at the same level. In developing countries with high incidence of nutritional anemia among pregnant women, delayed clamping of cord is likely to be beneficial by providing additional hemoglobin to the baby with improved iron status and reduced risk of late-onset physiologic anemia.

WHAT IS BIRTH ASPHYXIA?

There is no consensus regarding the definition of birth asphyxia. There is a need to have different definitions for purposes of defining the incidence of birth asphyxia, for initiating and making decisions for resuscitation and for predicting neuromotor outcome. Asphyxia refers to a combination of hypoxia, hypercarbia and metabolic acidosis. National Neonatology Forum of India has suggested that birth asphyxia should be diagnosed when a "baby is gasping and having inadequate breathing or no breathing at 1-minute". It is a simple and useful definition which can also be used in the community. It corresponds to 1-minute Apgar score of 3 or less. Gasping or no breathing at 1-minute or Apgar score of less than 4 at 1-minute is an acceptable definition for purposes of estimating the incidence of birth asphyxia. However, most of these babies do not need specialised care and they do not have enhanced neonatal morbidity or increased risk of neuromotor disability on follow up if by 5 minutes the infant is stable and breathing normally. Specialised neonatal care and long-term follow-up for developmental assessment are indicated in babies who fail to establish effective breathing at 5 minutes or the 5-minute Apgar score is 3 or less.

The American Academy of Pediatrics has proposed that the diagnostic label of perinatal asphyxia should be reserved to describe an infant who manifests all of the following features:

- Cord umbilical artery pH of <7.0 with a base deficit of >10 mEq/L.
- Neonatal neurologic manifestations suggestive of hypoxic-ischemic encephalopathy (HIE).
- Evidences of multisystem organ dysfunction (e.g. cardiovascular, renal, gastrointestinal, hematologic or pulmonary).

EVALUATION OF THE INFANT AT BIRTH

In 1953, Virginia Apgar, an anesthetist, published a clinical protocol to assess the physical condition of the neonate at birth.

The word APGAR has been used as a mnemonic to express the components of the Apgar score

- **A**ppearance (color)
- **P**ulse (heart rate)
- **G**rimace (reflex irritability)
- **A**ctivity (muscle tone)
- **R**espirations (respiratory effort)

Despite its limitations, Apgar scoring system is conventionally used for assessing the condition of a newborn baby at 60 seconds after birth (Table 6.2). The respiratory efforts and heart beats are the most critical components of Apgar scoring system because muscle tone, response to reflex stimulus and color are dependent upon the cardiorespiratory status of the baby.

Apgar scoring system ignores the time of cry after birth which is important to identify and differentiate between primary and terminal apnea. The peripheral cyanosis is awarded a score of one, although majority of healthy normally breathing babies are never totally pink at 1-minute. Tone and response to reflex stimulus are dependent upon gestational maturity. Moreover, centrally blue (asphyxia livida) and totally pale (asphyxia pallida) babies are given identical score, although latter are more gravely sick due to the combined effect of cardiac as well as respiratory failure. Above all, there is sufficient recent evidence to suggest that there is a poor correlation between Apgar score at birth, cord blood pH and future mental prognosis of asphyxiated babies. However, when 10 minutes Apgar score is 3 or less, or there are no spontaneous breathing efforts by 10 minutes, the baby is likely to develop neuromotor disability during follow-up. In view of the inherent limitations of Apgar scoring system, it is no longer used to make dicisions for

TABLE 6.2 Apgar scoring system			
		Score	
Criteria	*0*	*1*	*2*
▪ Breathing	Absent	Slow, gasping	Crying
▪ Heart rate/min	Absent	Up to 100	More than 100
▪ Muscle tone	Flaccid	In-between	Fully flexed
▪ Reflex response*	Nil	Grimace	Cough, sneeze, cry
▪ Color	Blue or pale	Peripheral cyanosis	Pink

*By inserting a catheter in the nostrils or tactile stimulation by rubbing the back or flicking the soles.

neonatal resuscitation. Nevertheless, it remains a useful tool to predict the neuromotor outcome of an asphyxiated newborn.

Infants born following acute blood loss during or before delivery are often limp, pale and in shock. They must be differentiated from severely asphyxiated babies with circulatory collapse because of life-saving therapeutic implications (Table 6.3). The presence of antepartum hemorrhage and evidence of blood loss from placenta or umbilical cord should alert to the possibility of fetal hemorrhage. The vaginal blood can be tested for the presence of fetal hemoglobin to confirm whether bleeding is maternal or fetal in origin. Initial cord blood hematocrit may be normal but repeat venous hematocrit after 4 to 8 hours may show significant fall due to hemodilution.

Resuscitation Kit

It is a sad fact that most delivery rooms in developing countries are not adequately equipped for resuscitation of an asphyxiated newborn baby. Each delivery

TABLE 6.3 Salient differences between asphyxia pallida and severe anemia with shock at birth		
Features	*Asphyxia pallida*	*Anemia and shock*
Predisposing factors	Placental insufficiency, toxemia, cord prolapse, cord around the neck, traumatic delivery	Amniocentesis, manual removal of placenta, cesarean section and twin pregnancy
Associated features	Evidences of fetal distress	Antepartum hemorrhage, blood loss from fetal surface of placenta or umbilical cord
Cyanosis	May be present	Absent or minimal
Respiration	Absent or gasping	Tachypnea or gasping irregular breathing
Heart rate	Bradycardia	Tachycardia with weak pulses
Venous pressure	Normal	Low with poor tissue perfusion in case of acute fetal hemorrhage and elevated in infants with severe erythroblastosis and chronic fetomaternal hemorrhage
Response to therapy	Dramatic improvement following endotracheal intubation and administration of oxygen	Administration of blood or plasma expander is life saving

room must have a well-lighted and warm micro-environment to receive the newly born infant. Open care system with an overhead radiant warmer and in-built suction and intermittent positive pressure ventilation facility is ideal. The practice of carrying newly born baby from the delivery room to another room for resuscitation is most unsatisfactory. The resuscitation kit must be checked by the staff nurse of every duty shift and rechecked by the physician before each delivery. The pencil-handle laryngoscope with infant (0 and 1) straight blade is preferred. Its light source and batteries should be in working condition. Gamma-irradiated disposable endotracheal tubes with internal diameter of 2.5 mm, 3.0 mm, 3.5 mm and 4.0 mm mounted with adapters should be available. The electrical points and suction should be in working order. Mechanical suction facility with different sized suction catheters (6 Fr, 8 Fr, 10 Fr and 12 Fr) and meconium aspiration device should be available. Press-type rubber bulb or mechanical suction device must be available to meet the exigencies of electrical failure (Figure 6.2). Oxygen cylinder should be checked for its contents. The complete list of equipment and drugs required for neonatal resuscitation is given in Table 6.4.

Ambu bag and mask is extremely useful and handy to resuscitate an apneic baby. The self-inflatable bags are easy to use but provide only 40 to 50% oxygen. The attachment of a corrugated tube provides reservoir for oxygen and can deliver up to 90% oxygen to the infant. The anesthesia bags are more effective because they can provide up to 100% oxygen but they are cumbersome to use and require at least 5 liters of oxygen flow per minute for their inflation. The kit should contain disposable sterile endotracheal and suction catheters, plastic oral airway, syringes and needles, 7.5% sodium bicarbonate, epinephrine 1:10,000, neonatal nalorphine (1.0 mg/mL), naloxone hydrochloride (0.4 mg/mL), ampoules of distilled water, physiological saline, and 10% dextrose. Sterile neonatal delivery packs containing bowl, scissors, cotton swabs and umbilical ties should be available for each delivery. Umbilical vessel catheterization supplies should be available so that venous access is established promptly for administration of medications. The bassinet on which the baby is to be received should be kept warm and provided with an over head radiant heat source and a stopclock to accurately time the sequence of events after birth.

In tertiary centers, availability of a cardiac monitor and a pulse oximeter is useful. T-piece resuscitator is a useful device but can be used only if compressed

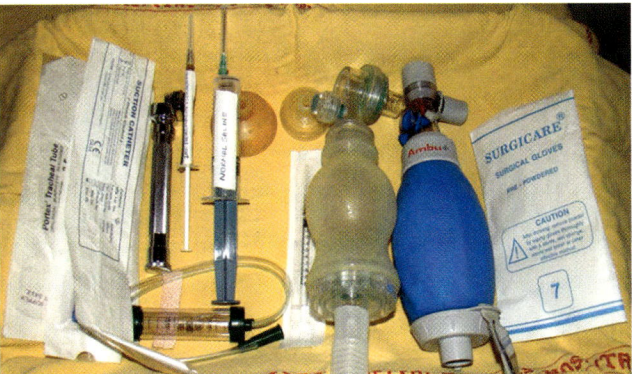

Figure 6.2 Resuscitation kit. The kit should be checked by the nurse on duty in each shift.

TABLE 6.4 Equipment, disposables and drugs needed for neonatal resuscitation

- Radiant warmer
- Warmed linen
- Stop clock or a clock with seconds hand
- Oxygen source
- Stethoscope
- Pulse oximeter
- Suction facilities* (mechanical or electrical) with 10Fr or wider suction catheters, 5–6 Fr catheters for suctioning of the endotracheal tubes, 8 Fr feeding tubes
- *Ventilation devices*: Self-inflating bag (250–750 mL) and masks (size 0 and 1). It must have a safety popoff and oxygen reservoir. T-piece resuscitator with CPAP facility
- Pencil-handle infant laryngoscopes (0 and 1 size) with straight blades with extra set of batteries and bulbs
- Endotracheal tubes with internal diameters of 2.5 mm, 3.0 mm, 3.5 mm and 4.0 mm mounted with adapters
- Scissors and adhesive tape
- Plastic oral airways
- Umbilical catheters 3.5 Fr and 5 Fr with three-way stopcock
- Disposable syringes 1 mL, 2 mL, 5 mL, 10 mL, 20 mL and needles
- Sterile gloves, bowl, umbilical ties or clips, cotton swabs, surgical spirit, etc.
- *Medications*: Epinephrine (1.0 mL of 1:1000 solution is diluted with 9 mL of normal saline to produce 1:10,000 concentration), naloxone hydrochloride (0.4 mg/mL), normal saline, Ringer's lactate, 10% dextrose solution

*Oral suction devices should not be used due to potential risk of transmission of HIV infection

gas with a blender is available. It is provided with controls to fix PIP (40 cm H_2O) and adjust PEEP (4–6 cm H_2O). The ventilation rate is maintained between 40 and 60 breaths per minute by occluding and releasing the outlet aperture (hole in the PEEP valve) with a finger or thumb. T-piece device can be used with a face mask, nasal prongs or endotracheal tube. The setting of T-piece resuscitator should be checked on a test lung before attaching the device to the baby. It is desirable that equipment for resuscitation should be maintained in a sterile condition and baby received in sterile warm sheets with due aseptic precautions. Above all, the physician must be adept in the art of cardiopulmonary resuscitation. The art of endotracheal intubation should be learnt and perfected by regular practice on the simulators or stillborn and dead neonates. Several life support neonatal training simulators and modules are available to learn the skills of external cardiac massage and assisted ventilation. The retention of cardiopulmonary skills is short lived unless they are constantly revised and practised. The resuscitation of an asphyxiated newborn is not cost-intensive but it is highly skill-oriented.

BASIC CARE OF A NORMAL BABY AT BIRTH

Plea of a baby at birth

I have come from an extremely warm, clean, quiet and comfortable abode.
Protect me at birth from microbes and cold.
I am wet and naked, dry me, cover me and place me under a warmer.
I don't know how to smile, let me announce my arrival by a cry.
Don't hurt me but gently clean my windpipe to let me cry.
Don't give me injections but give me a breath to save my life.
I have been swimming all through in the womb, don't be in a hurry to bathe me in the labor room.

Meharban Singh

There is no consensus regarding the ideal time for clamping the umbilical cord. The cord should be clamped as soon as the infant is completely delivered. Early clamping of cord is advocated in babies with severe birth asphyxia, cord around the neck and rhesus isoimmunization. In most cases, a relaxed approach should be followed for clamping the cord, neither immediate nor deliberate delay, should be practiced. Milking of cord is hazardous in infants with cardiovascular anomalies, asphyxia with circulatory failure, intracranial hemorrhage and materno-fetal blood group incompatibility. Holding the infant in an inverted position by the feet and slapping over the buttocks or squeezing the stomach or chest should be avoided. Avoid keeping the head too low and for too long especially in babies suspected to have cerebral trauma. Nearly 90% of newborns are vigorous term babies with no risk factors and clear amniotic fluid. They can

be directly placed on the mother's abdomen or chest, dried effectively and covered with dry linen. Warmth is maintained by direct skin-to-skin contact with the mother which also facilitates early bonding and promotion of breastfeeding. The baby's mouth and nose should be wiped with a gauze piece or suction bulb to clear the upper airways. The baby should be watched for breathing, color and activity or muscle tone. Around 10% of the newborns require some assistance to establish breathing while 1% are likely to need active resuscitation measures including endotracheal intubation.

Initial Steps for Resuscitation

The first minute of life (golden minute) is considered as crucial to ensure the integrity and survival of a newborn infant. The resuscitation kit should be checked before the baby is born. The radiant warmer should be put on and plenty of sterile prewarmed linen should be available. Due to increasing prevalence and risk of AIDS, it is desirable that the pediatrician resuscitating the baby wears the gloves and no oral suction should be done. The baby should be received in a warm sheet and head kept slightly low. The conventional practice of holding the baby upside down from its feet is undesirable (Figure 6.3). The baby should be placed under the radiant warmer and both hypothermia as well as hyperthermia should be prevented. The baby should be placed supine or on one side, with the head in a neutral or slightly extended position. The infant's mouth, oropharynx, hypopharynx and nose are sucked, in that order, using thick 10 Fr suction catheter with gentle intermittent suction. The nose should not be sucked first as it would lead to reflex breathing with the risk of aspiration of secretions contained in the oral cavity. The baby should be dried effectively and wet linen should be removed. Head constitutes a large surface area of the baby and must be effectively dried. In resource poor

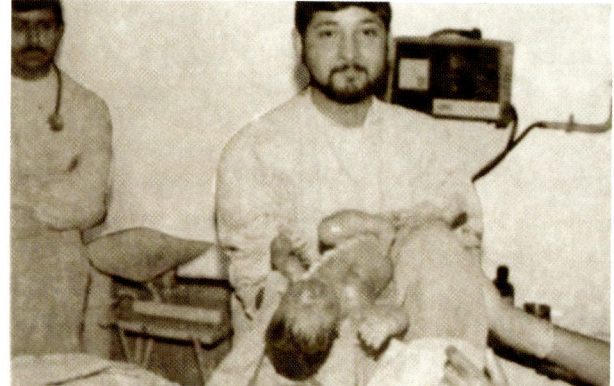

Figure 6.3 The correct method of receiving the baby at birth.

additional risk of respiratory morbidity due to meconium aspiration syndrome. The detection of *in utero* passage of meconium may be delayed, if membranes are intact. Thick meconium staining of liquor (pea-soup appearance) is ominous. Yellow staining of skin, umbilical cord and nails indicates that meconium has been passed at least 4–6 hours before delivery. It is associated with increased risk of birth asphyxia and meconium aspiration syndrome. When amniotic fluid is meconium-stained, the baby should be promptly delivered either by cesarean section or by forceps, if cervix is adequately dilated. Recent multicentric study has shown that intrapartum suctioning does not reduce the risk of meconium aspiration syndrome because babies breathe *in utero* and aspirate meconium before head is delivered. Therefore, suctioning of oropharynx and nasopharynx before delivery of shoulders is no longer recommended. Instead, the baby should be promptly delivered and effectively sucked after birth.

When a meconium-stained baby is crying vigorously and breathing normally, no special initial steps are needed. The baby should be placed on the mother's abdomen and handled as in a case of non-meconium-stained baby. In a meconium-stained baby who is depressed or apneic, the following management protocol should be followed.

1. Oral cavity, oropharynx and glottis area should be promptly and effectively sucked under direct vision with the help of a laryngoscope by using a thick bored (12 or 14 Fr) suction catheter.
2. When a meconium-stained baby is depressed, endotracheal intubation should be done. The endotracheal tube should be attached directly to a gentle intermittent suction source to suck out the meconium. The endotracheal tube is gradually withdrawn while intermittent suction is being applied. The infant may have to be intubated 2–3 times till all the traces of meconium have been sucked out. At times saline lavage may be required to remove thick particulate meconium. It is not possible to suck out the meconium by inserting a suction catheter through the endotracheal tube.
3. The practice of sucking the ET tube with the help of oral negative suction by the resuscitator is not recommended because of potential risk of infection by HIV.
4. After effective suctioning of air passages and when all traces of meconium have been sucked out, the baby should be hand ventilated with a bag to expand the lungs and relieve hypoxia.
5. When infant's heart rate and respirations are severely depressed it is desirable to institute early

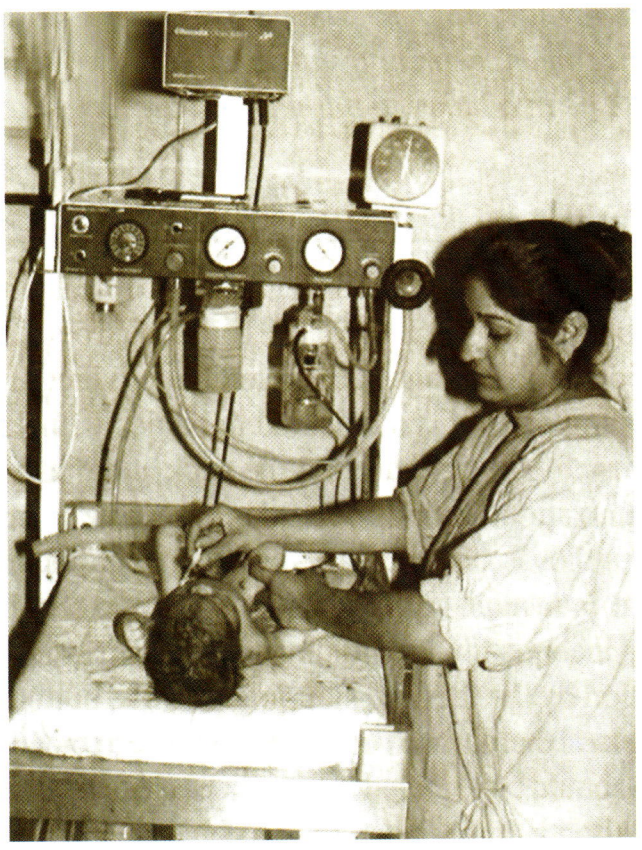

Figure 6.4 Resuscitator with an overhead warmer and in-built facilities for suction, oxygen supply and intermittent positive pressure ventilation. Availability of a stop clock is useful.

settings, when a warm microenvironment cannot be provided to the baby, drying and effectively covering the baby should take precedence over suctioning except when baby is born through meconium-stained amniotic fluid.

The process of drying and suction produce enough stimulation to initiate effective breathing in most newly born babies. If an infant is not breathing or his breathing efforts are sluggish, he should be stimulated by flicking the soles or rubbing the back. The tactile stimulation should not be continued beyond 3 to 4 flicks and when it is ineffective the baby should be promptly ventilated with a bag and mask. Evaluate the infant every 30 sec by simultaneously observing respirations, heart rate and color or SpO_2 to decide the need for further steps in resuscitation. Availability of a stop clock mounted on the resuscitator is essential to accurately time the sequence of events after birth (Figure 6.4).

Approach to a Meconium-stained Baby

About 10–15% pregnancies are complicated by passage of meconium *in utero* during labor. It is a reliable sign of fetal distress in vertex born babies with positive pressure ventilation despite the presence of some meconium in the airways.

6. If a meconium-stained baby is vigorously crying at birth, no attempt should be made to intubate the infant. There is a potential risk of causing injury to the vocal cord while trying to intubate a vigorously crying term infant.

7. After transfer of the baby to NICU, stomach wash with normal saline is recommended to reduce the risk of gastritis and aspiration of meconium-stained gastric contents.

8. Infant should be closely watched for development of respiratory distress due to meconium aspiration syndrome and onset of persistent pulmonary hypertension.

RESUSCITATION OF AN ASPHYXIATED BABY

American Academy of Pediatrics (AAP) and American Heart Association (AHS) along with several other organizations have formalized a partnership with International Liaison Committee on Resuscitation (ILCOR) to update and revise recommendations for neonatal resuscitation program (NRP). The recent Consensus on Science and Treatment Recommendations (COSTR) of ILCOR published in 2010 provides the latest NRP guidelines which are considered as the gold standard.

Most babies have a smooth transition from fetal to neonatal life and establish spontaneous breathing at birth without any active assistance. About 5 to 10% babies are likely to have difficulty in initiating spontaneous breathing at birth and need active resuscitation. Advanced measures for resuscitation including endotracheal intubation, chest compressions and medications are required in less than 1.0% of births. Perinatal asphyxia accounts for almost 20% of neonatal deaths in India. At every delivery, there should be at least one person, who is adequately trained in the art of neonatal resuscitation, to look after the needs of the newly born baby. When the delivery is high risk, at least two trained personnel are required to perform complete resuscitation including bag and mask ventilation, endotracheal intubation, chest compressions and administration of medications. When a mother is having multiple gestations, separate teams of trained personnel and equipment should be available to handle and resuscitate each baby. The procedure of neonatal resuscitation must be carried out by skilled and experienced person with a sense of urgency but without any panic. The revised neonatal resuscitation program (NRP) guidelines of the Technical Committee of National Neonatology Forum of India (7th edition 2016) recommends that the newly born baby should be assessed by asking the following question:

Is baby breathing or crying?

When answer to the above question is YES, the baby needs routine care. But when answer is NO, the baby is provided with initial steps for resuscitation. During the initial steps, the baby is correctly positioned, airway is cleared and he is effectively dried and kept warm. Suctioning and drying the baby provides stimulation and trigger to the baby to take a breath. When a baby is breathing but is cyanosed, he is administered free-flow oxygen at a rate of 5 liters/min till he becomes pink. Free-flow oxygen is administered through an oxygen mask or flow-inflating bag or a hand cupped around the oxygen tubing. If a baby is not breathing or having gasping breaths, he is provided tactile stimulation by giving 1 or 2 flicks or slaps to the soles, or by gently rubbing the back once or twice to promote breathing. The baby is simultaneously assesed for respiration, heart rate and color to take further decisions for resuscitation (Figure 6.5).

During resuscitation of an asphyxiated baby, apart from clinical parameters, routine monitoring includes arterial oxygen saturation (SaO_2), heart rate by pulse oximetry, electrocardiograph and point-of-care (POC) echocardiography. In advanced NICUs of the west, there is increasing interest to monitor oxygenation and perfusion of the brain by near-infrared spectroscopy (NIRS), during immediate transition after resuscitation. Using cerebral NIRS in combination with intervention guidelines have been shown to reduce the burden of cerebral hypoxia in preterm neonates.

Resuscitation with Room Air

Based on a number of research studies conducted during the last 15 years, it has been shown that room air (21% oxygen) is as effective as 100% oxygen for effective resuscitation of an asphyxiated newborn baby. Instead, there is evidence to suggest that resuscitation with 100% oxygen is associated with several hazards including higher neonatal mortality (Table 6.5). It is, therefore, recommended to start

TABLE 6.5 Hazards of resuscitation with 100% oxygen
■ Delayed recovery with a need for prolonged resuscitation.
■ Increased oxidative stress to the baby at 4 weeks of age.
■ Higher risk of myocardial and renal injury.
■ Increased cerebral blood flow with greater risk of IVH.
■ Increased neonatal mortality.
■ Higher potential risk of childhood leukemia and cancer?

Based on Saugstad OD, Ramji S, Soll RF, Vento M. Resuscitation of newborn infants with 21% or 100% oxygen: An updated systematic review and meta-analysis. *Neonatology* 2008, 94:176–182.

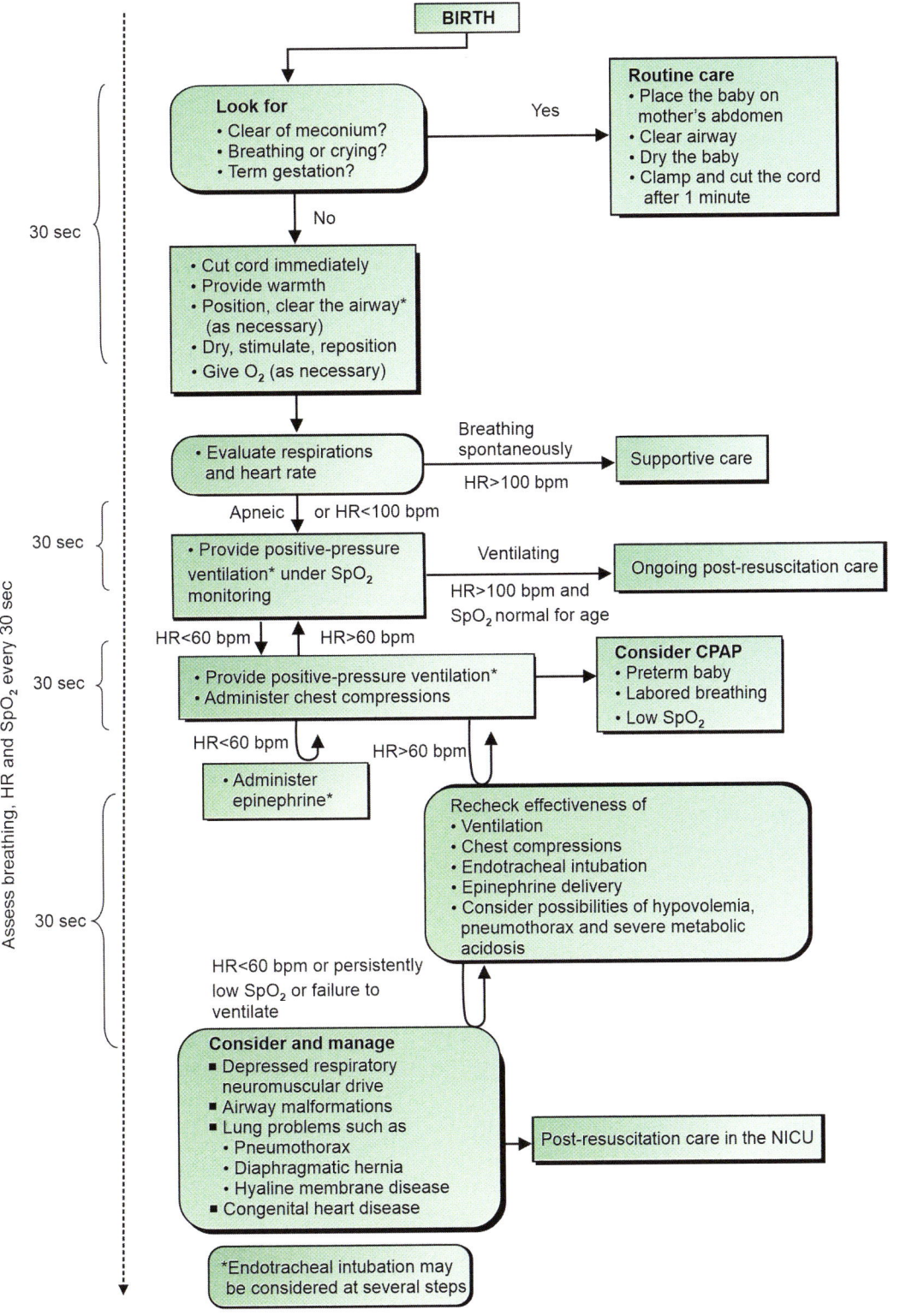

Figure 6.5 Algorithm for resuscitation of an asphyxiated newborn baby (Adapted from NRP–India guidelines).

resuscitation with room air and when it is ineffective, extra oxygen (up to 40%) may be provided after 90 seconds. It is reassuring that in rural settings or when oxygen is not available, it is possible to effectively resuscitate a newborn baby with room air. However, in preterm babies and infants with pulmonary disorders, resuscitation or ventilation with 40% oxygen is desirable to maintain SaO_2 between 85 and 95%.

Bag and Mask Ventilation

If despite stimulation, the baby is still apneic or having ineffective ventilations as evidenced by heart rate of less than 100 per minute, he should be given bag and mask ventilation. Either a flow inflating or self-inflating bag or a T-piece mechanical device designed to regulate pressure are acceptable choices to provide assisted ventilation. Position the infant supine by placing a small roll of towel under the shoulders in order to extend the neck and open the airways. Thorough suctioning of oral cavity, hypopharynx and nose is mandatory before starting bag and mask ventilation. The mask should tightly fit on the face enclosing nose and mouth of the baby. The oxygen reservoir should not be attached to the bag in order to restrict the oxygen concentration to 40% (Figure 6.6). In community setting, when oxygen is not available, the infant can be successfully ventilated with room air (21% oxygen) with the help of a bag and mask or tube and mask. The infant should be ventilated at a rate of 40–60 breaths per minute. To avoid alveolar rupture and pneumothorax, the operator should train himself to deliver 15–20 cm H_2O pressure with the help of a manometer. In order to open up the collapsed alveoli, few initial inflatory pressures of 30–40 cm H_2O pressure are recommended. There should be a noticeable rise and fall of the chest during each ventilation. Naloxone hydrochloride 0.1 mg/kg should be administered intravenously through the umbilical vein, if mother had received pethidine or morphine within 4 hours before delivery. If needed, it can be repeated after every 2–3 minutes. However, effective ventilation should take precedence over administration of naloxone.

During bag and mask ventilation, heart rate should be closely monitored after every 30 seconds. Heart rate is assessed by auscultating the precordium. To save time, heart rate is counted for 6 seconds and multiplied by 10 to get the heart rate per minute. A pulse oximeter probe should be attached to the right hand or wrist of the baby to record preductal oxygen saturations. Target arterial oxygen saturations during first 15 minutes of life are shown in Table 6.6. When there is no improvement by 90 seconds of bag and mask ventilations with room air, oxygen concentration is gradually increased to maintain target preductal oxygen saturations. The sensor of the pulse oximeter should be applied over the right hand or wrist of the baby. In preterm babies with persistent hypoxia or respiratory distress, CPAP through nasal prongs is started in the labor room. If despite effective bag and mask ventilation, heart rate is not coming up or it further slows down and drops below 80 per minute, the infant should be intubated. *A large majority of asphyxiated babies can be effectively revived and resuscitated by using bag and mask ventilation alone and intubation is usually not required.* In Indian setting, the use of laryngeal mask airway is not currently recommended due to the expense involved and lack of training and expertise in this procedure. In preterm neonates, a T-piece resuscitator is more useful as it can provide PEEP (6–8 cm). There is no role of dexamethasone, atropine, calcium and respiratory stimulants, like nikethamide and lobeline during resuscitation. The Apgar scoring system is not taken into consideration while taking management decisions during resuscitation of a newborn baby. The management is guided by the status of breathing, heart rate and oxygen saturation of the baby. Apgar score may be recorded at 1-minute, 5-minute and subsequently (till it is more than 7) to serve as a prognostic indicator of the outcome of an asphyxiated baby. For details of bag and mask ventilation, techniques of tracheal intubation and external cardiac massage, refer to Chapter 27.

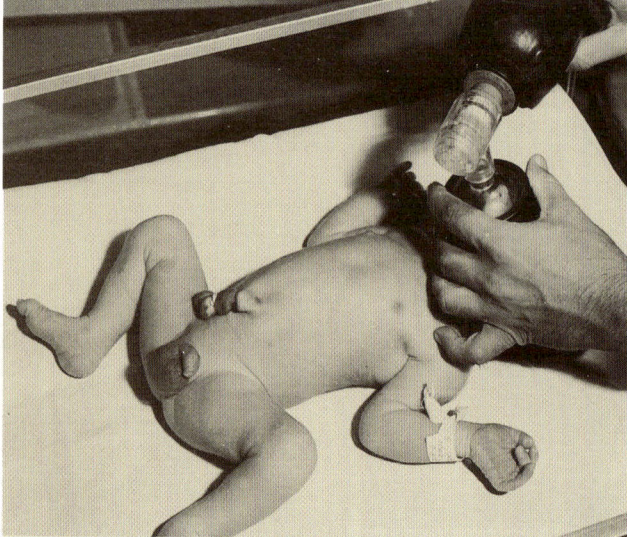

Figure 6.6 Bag and mask resuscitation. Most of the asphyxiated infants can be successfully resuscitated by this technique.

TABLE 6.6 Target preductal oxygen saturations in term and preterm babies at birth	
Time (minutes)	*SpO_2 (%)*
1	60–65
2	65–70
3	70–75
4	75–80
5	80–85
10	85–95
15	95–98

TABLE 6.7 Recommended corrective steps when bag and mask ventilation is ineffective

Corrective steps		Actions
M	Mask adjustment	Ensure good seal of the mask on the face
R	Reposition airway	The head should be in the "sniffing" position
S	Suction of mouth and nose	Check for secretions, suck if present
O	Open mouth	Ventilate with the baby's mouth slightly open and lift the jaw forward (sniffing position)
P	Pressure increase	Gradually increase the pressure every few breaths, until there are adequate bilateral breath sounds and visible chest movements with each breath
A	Airway alternative	Consider endotracheal intubation or laryngeal mask airway

The corrective steps for improvement of ventilation can be remembered by the acronym MR.SOPA.

The best criterion for adequate ventilation is prompt improvement in heart rate. If heart rate and oxygen saturations do not improve quickly (after 5–10 breaths), corrective steps should be taken as listed in Table 6.7. If the corrective steps fail to improve ventilation and oxygenation, the infant should be intubated or ventilated after insertion of laryngeal mask airway.

Endotracheal Intubation

Endotracheal intubation is indicated in following situations:

- When tracheal suctioning is required in a meconium-stained depressed baby.
- When bag and mask ventilation is ineffective (heart rate remains <100/min) or ventilation is required for a prolonged period.
- When chest compressions are performed.
- Extremely preterm babies (<28 weeks or <1000 g) and neonates requiring administration of surfactant.
- Neonates with diaphragmatic hernia.

The art of intubation cannot be taught and must be learnt by practicing on simulators, stillborn babies and neonates dying in the nursery. The appropriate sized (4.0 mm in a term baby and 2.5 mm in a tiny baby) endotracheal tube should be prepared by shortening it to 13 cm and attaching a connector. It is easy to intubate an asphyxiated baby with some practice because of lack of resistance and hypotonia. The intubation should be preceeded by bag and mask ventilation with at least 85% oxygen for 15 seconds. When the operator is experienced, intubation should take no longer than 30 seconds. The endotracheal tube should be suctioned before starting positive pressure ventilation with a bag or ventilator. The ventilation can be stopped as soon as the baby establishes spontaneous breathing and heart rate is maintained above 100 per minute.

Laryngeal mask airway (LMA) that fits over the laryngeal inlet has been shown to be effective for ventilating newborns weighing >2000 g or born after a gestation of 34 weeks. The laryngeal mask airway should be considered, if face mask ventilation is ineffective and tracheal intubation is unsuccessful or not feasible.

External Cardiac Massage

External cardiac massage is indicated in babies in whom heart rate drops below 60 beats per minute despite effective ventilation with supplementary oxygen for 30 seconds. The ventilation should be continued by an assistant and simultaneously heart should be massaged either by using two fingers of one hand or encircling the chest of the baby with both the hands and applying sternal compressions with two thumbs (Figures 6.7 A and B). Available data suggest that the 2 thumb-encircling hand technique is more convenient and effective in generating peak systolic and coronary perfusion pressure.

The lower part of the sternum just above the xiphoid cartilage is pressed to a depth of one-third of the anteroposterior diameter of the chest at a rate of 90 compressions and 30 ventilations (3:1 ratio) per minute. The thumbs and tips of fingers (depending upon the method used) should remain in contact with the sternum all the time and they should not be lifted off after each compression. Check the heart rate after every 30 seconds and chest compressions may be stopped when heart rate goes above 60 bpm.

Medications during Resuscitation

A single dose of theophylline 5 mg/kg in term neonates with perinatal asphyxia within the first hour of life is associated with reduced risk of acute kidney injury. Epinephrine is indicated, if the heart rate remains below 60 bpm despite 30 seconds of assisted ventilation and another 30 seconds of coordinated chest compressions and assisted ventilation. The available epinephrine is 1:1000 solution and it must be diluted 10 times (0.1 mg/mL) before administration. Administer 0.3–1.0 mL/kg of 1:10,000 solution (0.01–0.03 mg/kg) of epinephrine through umbilical vein

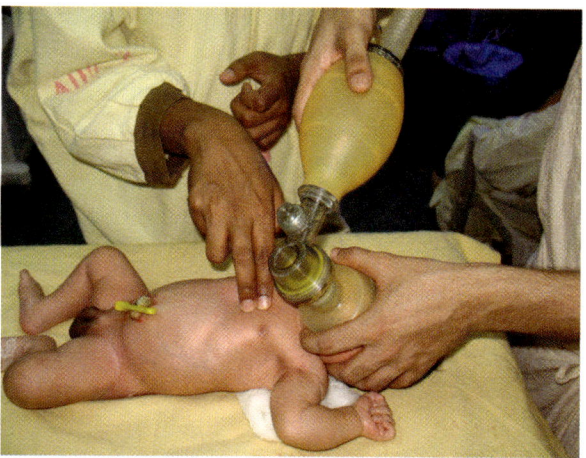

Figure 6.7A Technique of external cardiac massage with two fingers.

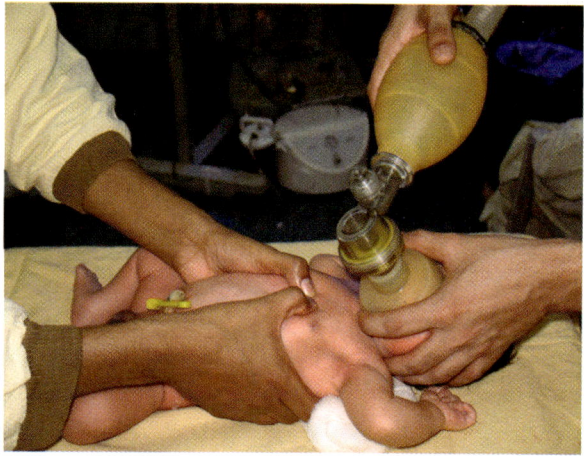

Figure 6.7B External cardiac massage with two thumbs is generally preferred.

or 1.5–5.0 mL/kg (0.05–0.15 mg/kg) through the endotracheal tube. Intracardiac route is dangerous and should be avoided due to risk of damage to the coronary vessels and development of hemopericardium. The dose of epinephrine may be repeated after every 3–5 minutes as indicated. If a baby is in shock, and not responding to resuscitation or there is history of fetal blood loss (placenta previa, abruptio placentae, twin-to-twin transfusion, etc.), consider the use of plasma expander (ORh-negative packed RBCs, normal saline or Ringer's lactate) in a dose of 10 mL/kg slow intravenous push over 5 to 10 minutes. The fluid of choice for volume expansion is an isotonic crystalloid solution, like physiological saline or Ringer's lactate. Effective ventilation is followed by spontaneous correction of acidosis and alkali therapy should be guided by monitoring blood acid–base parameters. When blood gasometry facilities are not available, sodium bicarbonate 5–10 mL of 7.5% solution (adequately diluted with equal volume of distilled water or double volume of 5% dextrose) should be administered intravenously slowly at a rate of 1.0 mL/minute to infants in whom effective ventilation is not established even by 10 minutes or later (Apgar score of less than 7 at 10 minutes). Effective ventilation must be established before administration of sodium bicarbonate. Bolus administration of sodium bicarbonate should be avoided in preterm babies because of risk of development of intraventricular hemorrage.

RESUSCITATION OF PRETERM BABIES

Depending upon the severity of prematurity, they are at an increased risk of problems and complications which are listed below:

1. Difficult transition and adaptation from intrauterine to extrauterine life.
2. Increased risk of hypothermia.
3. Ineffective breathing because of weak chest muscles and poor respiratory drive.
4. Risk of poor ventilation and RDS due to immaturity of lungs and deficiency of pulmonary surfactant.
5. Increased risk of infection.
6. Increased chances of intraventricular bleeding and paraventricular leucomalacia.
7. Hypovolemic shock is more common.

When expecting a preterm delivery, the health team must be well prepared as regards the expertise, equipment and disposables of appropriate size to resuscitate preterm babies. There should be at least two well trained personnel to resuscitate and manage preterm babies. Attempts should be made to prevent hypothermia, hypoxia or oxidative damage, infection, intraventricular hemorrhage and hypovolemic shock. The risk of various complications of immaturity are reduced when preterms are appropriately handled during the initial minutes of life.

Special Considerations

The general principles and algorithm for resuscitation of preterm babies is identical to the protocol described for term babies. The delivery room temperature should be raised to 26°–28°C and radiant warmer switched on 20–30 minutes before the anticipated delivery. The baby should be effectively and promptly dried immediately after birth. The extremely preterm babies with a gestation of 28 weeks or less can be enclosed in food grade polythene plastic bag from neck downwards. A preheated transport incubator should be available for transfer of the baby from labor room to neonatal intensive care unit (NICU). It is desirable to attach a preterm baby to a pulse oximeter for ensuring a delicate balance to prevent hypoxia and oxidative damage. The target oxygen saturations to be achieved during early minutes after birth in preterm babies are similar to that of term babies. It is preferable to use an air-oxygen blender and pulse oximeter to titrate supplemental oxygen concentration while resuscitating preterm neonates. In a gasping or nonbreathing preterm babies, positive pressure ventilation (PPV) with minimal oxygen concentration and ventilation pressures by using self inflating bag or T-piece resuscitator should be provided. It is desirable to provide PEEP of 2–5 cm during resuscitation of preterm babies. In a spontaneously breathing preterm baby who is unable to maintain effective ventilation or develops RDS, CPAP should be provided by T-piece resuscitator by using a mask or nasal prongs. The desired CPAP pressure of 4–6 cm H_2O should be achieved by holding the mask snugly against your palm and adjusting the PEEP or flow control valve. The mask or nasal prongs should snugly fit to the baby's face or nares, so that the effective pressure is transmitted to the airways. In tertiary care neonatal centers, prophylactic or rescue surfactant therapy is instituted to high risk extremely preterm babies in the labor room. The bolus administration of sodium bicarbonate, normal saline or colloids should be avoided in preterm babies to reduce the risk of intraventricular hemorrhage.

When to Deny or Stop CPR at Birth?

Resuscitation at birth may be denied or abandoned when it is considered futile in terms of survival or survival is likely to be associated with gross neuromotor disability with extremely poor quality of life. It is justified and ethical to deny resuscitation to infants with gross non-correctable lethal congenital malformations and micropremies (<26 weeks or <500 g). The resuscitation efforts may be abandoned in fresh stillborn babies (zero Apgar score at one minute), if there are no signs of life at 10 minutes or if spontaneous breathing is not established by 30 minutes.

POST-RESUSCITATION CARE OF AN ASPHYXIATED BABY

Infants with birth asphyxia (Apgar score of <4 at 5 min) should be admitted to the NICU for observation and management during the next 12 to 48 hours. Those babies who require endotracheal intubation, chest compressions or medications should be transferred to the NICU irrespective of the 5-minute Apgar score.

The baby should be attached to a vital sign monitor and pulse oximeter or arterial blood gases should be monitored to assess oxygenation and acid–base status. A stomach wash should be done with normal saline and vitamin K 0.5–1.0 mg should be given intramuscularly. The infant should be nursed in a thermoneutral environment. Intravenous infusion with 10% dextrose (without sodium and potassium) should be started to prevent hypoglycemia. Fluid volume should be restricted to two-thirds of maintenance fluid needs because of syndrome of inappropriate ADH secretion. Infants with prolonged birth asphyxia (infants needing bag and mask ventilation even at 5 minutes) should be given 7.5% sodium bicarbonate 2 to 3 mL/kg diluted with equal volume of distilled water or double volume of 5% dextrose slowly to correct any acidosis. When facilities are available, pH and base deficit should be determined to guide alkaly therapy. Sodium bicarbonate should be administered only when effective respirations have been established otherwise it will lead to further accumulation of carbon dioxide in the blood.

Hypovolemic shock should be corrected by the administration of 10 mL/kg of fresh ORh-negative blood, or physiological saline or Ringer's lactate. As an emergency measure, 20–25 mL of maternal blood can be withdrawn in an heparinized syringe and transfused to the baby without crossmatching. Maintenance of tissue perfusion is the corner stone of therapy of an asphyxiated newborn baby to prevent damage to the vital organs of the baby. Dopamine infusion (6 µg/kg/min) should be started, if tissue perfusion is unsatisfactory because of hypotension as a result of hypoxic cardiomyopathy. Antibiotics are administered, if perinatal high-risk factors for development of early-onset bacterial infection coexist. A skiagram of chest should be taken to exclude pneumothorax and congenital malformations of the respiratory system. The infant should be closely monitored and observed to detect any manifestations of hypoxic damage to various organs. Urine should be checked for RBCs and protein to rule out acute tubular necrosis. Urine output, body weight, serum electrolytes and blood glucose should be monitored frequently during first few days after birth. Seizures should be promptly managed by correction of any metabolic distubances and by administration of phenobarbitone 20 mg/kg intravenously slowly over 10 minutes. The neurological behavior of the infant should be closely watched till he is able to establish self-feeding. Enteral feedings should be delayed for 48 hours and started when ventilation and tissue perfusion are adequte.

Intractable Birth Asphyxia

The conditions listed in Table 6.8 should be suspected, if ventilation remains unsatisfactory even after 10 minutes of birth. Effective and thorough suctioning, endotracheal intubation and assisted ventilation are mandatory in these infants. Skiagram of chest is taken for further management of such an infant. Blood gases, acid–base parameters, electrolytes, glucose, BUN and lactate should be monitored. Drainage of ascites and thoracocentesis would improve respiration in hydropic infants. Removal of air from pleural cavity in an infant with tension pneumothorax is life saving. It can be promptly diagnosed in the labor room with the help of fiberoptic cold light. Oral airway facilitates breathing in infants with choanal atresia. When congenital diaphragmatic hernia is suspected, stomach should be decompressed with an orogastric catheter and infant should be ventilated after endotracheal intubation. Many centers advocate routine elective intubation of extremely preterm babies to support ventilation and administer surfactant. Bolus administration of volume expanders or hyperosmolar solutions should be avoided due to potential risk of causing intraventricular hemorrhage.

TABLE 6.8 Causes of intractable birth asphyxia and failure to initiate spontaneous breathing

- Severe hypoxic ischemic encephalopathy
- Meconium aspiration or tracheal plug
- Congenital malformations of airways namely choanal atresia, laryngeal web, diaphragmatic hernia, esophageal atresia with tracheoesophageal fistula, lobar emphysema or cyst, and asphyxiating thoracic dystrophy
- Pneumothorax and pneumomediastinum
- Intracranial hemorrhage
- Shock (cardiogenic or hypovolemic)
- Profound metabolic alterations
- Congenital pneumonia
- Neuromuscular disorder or malformation of brain
- Maternal sedation with drugs such as narcotics, magnesium sulfate or general anesthetic
- Hydrops fetalis
- Severe immaturity (<28 weeks gestation)
- Paralysis of respiratory muscles or malformation of brain
- Pulmonary hemorrhage
- Excessive maternal sedation

SYSTEMIC MANIFESTATIONS OF SEVERE BIRTH ASPHYXIA

Seeds of neonatal morbidity and neuromotor disability are sown in the labor room. A variety of clinical problems are encountered during early neonatal

TABLE 6.9 Systemic manifestations of severe birth asphyxia

Organ/system	Features
Brain	Hypoxic-ischemic encephalopathy, intracranial hemorrhage, apneic attacks, seizures, long-term neuromotor disability.
Heart	Persistent fetal circulation, dysrhythmias, myocardial damage, tricuspid regurgitation, congestive cardiac failure.
Lungs	Meconium or liquor aspiration, hyaline membrane disease, transient tachypnea, persistent pulmonary hypertension, pulmonary hemorrhage, pneumonia, pneumothorax and shock lung.
Kidneys	Hematuria, renal failure, acute tubular necrosis and renal vein thrombosis.
Hematologic	Coagulopathy (DIC), hyperbilirubinemia and thrombocytopenia.
Gastrointestinal	Necrotizing enterocolitis, GI bleeding, paralytic ileus and stasis and hepatic dysfunction.
Endocrinal	Syndrome of inappropriate secretion of antidiuretic hormone, adrenal hemorrhage and transient hypoparathyroidism.
Immunologic	Septicemia.
Metabolic	Acidosis, hypoglycemia, hypocalcemia, hyponatremia and hyperkalemia.

period among babies who are severely asphyxiated at birth (Table 6.9). Hypoxia can cause damage to almost every tissue and organ of the baby. During hypoxia, series of protective mechanisms collectively called as 'diving sea reflex' attempt to redistribute available blood flow from lesser to more vital organs. The blood flow to brain, heart and adrenal glands of the newborn is preserved at the expense of reduction of perfusion to kidneys, lungs, gastrointestinal tract, liver, spleen and skeletal muscles.

HYPOXIC-ISCHEMIC ENCEPHALOPATHY

Neonatal encephalopathy, following severe birth asphyxia or perinatal hypoxia is referred to hypoxic-ischemic encephalopathy (HIE). Cerebral ischemia occurs as a consequence of cerebral edema (which compresses cerebral vessels) and reduced cerebral perfusion due to myocardial dysfunction as a result of hypoxic cardiomyopathy. Following severe birth asphyxia, 25% infants are likely to develop the syndrome of HIE.

Pathogenesis

Two types of asphyxial damage to the brain have been recognized in the experimental animal models. In acute total asphyxia, which is rare in human clinical setting, there is no time for the compensatory mechanisms to sustain cerebral circulation leading to severe damage to the basal ganglia, thalamus and brainstem. It usually leads to death and an occasional survivor is likely to have severe spastic quadruplegia. In the more common variety of partial asphyxia in the human infant, the homeostatic mechanisms divert the blood from less vital organs to the brain, heart and adrenals. When asphyxial damage is severe and prolonged, the compensatory mechanisms are overwhelmed, leading to neuronal necrosis and ischemic changes in the para-sagittal areas of cerebral cortex. In partial asphyxia, non-brain multiorgan dysfunction (ARF, NEC, RDS, etc.) is common because of preferential vasoconstriction and reduced blood supply to the "non-vital" organs.

Hypoxic damage to neurons may lead to both cytotoxic and vasogenic cerebral edema though brain swelling *per se* is not a prominent feature of HIE in the human newborn. Inappropriate secretion of anti-diuretic hormone (SIADH) may also contribute to development of cerebral edema. Severe hypoxia causes selective neuronal necrosis in hippocampus, thalamus, basal ganglia, brainstem and cerebellum. "Water shed infarcts" due to preferential blood flow to brainstem rather than cerebrum, leads to parasagittal cerebral injury in term and post-term infants. In preterm babies, asphyxial damage on the other hand leads to periventricular leukomalacia. Hemorrhage in the germinal matrix leading to IVH may occur because of rupture of pressure-passive choroidal capillaries due to sudden elevation of systemic blood pressure by crude handling, crying, seizures, bolus administration of sodium bicarbonate or mannitol and CPAP.

Asphyxial damage sets up a cascade of intracellular events which causes neuronal death due to primary and secondary energy failure because of hypoxia and ischemia. During severe asphyxia, energy failure occurs leading to depletion of intracellular high-energy phosphate compounds, such as phosphocreatine and adenosine triphosphate (ATP). During anerobic conditions, one molecule of glucose yields only 2 molecules of ATP as opposed to production of 38 molecules of ATP during aerobic conditions. Failure of ATP-dependent membrane-bound Na^+/K^+ ATPase pump leads to depolarization of cells, allowing influx of Na^+ and Ca^{++} ions with osmotic influx of water causing cytotoxic neuronal edema. Calcium ions inside the cells cause activation of intracellular proteases and lipases with generation of oxygen free radicals causing further damage to the cellular membranes. Calcium also contributes to the formation of oxgen-free radicals by production of xanthine oxidase, nitric oxide and prostaglandins. There is evidence to suggest that brain damage due to HIE is mediated by release of pro-inflammatory cytokines like IL-6, IL-1β, tumor necrosis factor alpha (TNF-α) which are released within 24 hours of brain insult. The studies have shown that blood levels of IL-6 and IL-1β are significantly higher in babies with perinatal asphyxia and correlate well with severity of asphyxia and adverse neurological outcome.

During secondary energy failure, the decline in phosphocreatine and ATP is not accompanied by acidosis of brain. The pathogenesis of secondary energy failure involves contribution of excitotoxic-oxidation cascade, apoptosis, inflammation and altered growth factors and protein synthesis. The interval between primary and secondary energy failure represents a "latent phase" that corresponds to a "therapeutic window". The duration of window is found to be about 6 hours in near-term sheep following timed hypoxic-ischemic injury.

During reperfusion following asphyxial insult, highly reactive oxygen-derived free radicals are generated in many organs including developing brain. Free radicals are produced by several mechanisms during reoxygenation including oxygenation of arachidonic acid and hypoxanthine; and accumulation of nitric oxide. Xanthine oxidase metabolizes molecular oxygen to produce oxygen free radicals. Naturally occurring oxygen free radical scavengers, like cholesterol, ascorbic acid and glutathione, try to limit the production of toxic radicals but these may be overwhelmed by the asphyxial insult. Due to secondary energy failure as a result of damage by oxygen free radicals, there is ongoing neuronal injury in the area of the brain adjacent to infarction. This peri-infarction area is called penumbra which continues to show adverse changes in the form of neuronal necrosis or apoptosis (programmed cell death) during next 24–48 hours.

Glutamate is one of the most ubiquitous endogenous excitatory neurotransmitter in the developing brain. Asphyxia causes excessive release of glutamate from the presynaptic vesicles. The glutamate receptor is stimulated by at least three ligands of which N-methyl-D-aspartate (NMDA) opens a receptor operated channel which allows calcium to enter the neurons causing further neuronal damage.

Clinical Features

The clinical syndrome of HIE must be preceded by at least one of the following three antecedents:

1. Evidences of fetal hypoxia/distress
2. Apgar score of three or less at 5-minute or later
3. Cord arterial blood pH <7.0

The clinical features of HIE are well described in term babies and can be assessed by Sarnat and Sarnat staging system (Table 6.10) and Levene grading system (Table 6.11). In preterm babies, multiorgan dysfunction may dominate the clinical picture leading to high risk of mortality. Seizures occur in approximately 50% of affected infants mostly within 6 to 12 hours after birth and invariably by 36 hours of age. Term babies produce gross seizures while preterm infants usually manifest subtle seizures. There is CNS irritability, jitteriness, excessive crying followed by lethargy, inactivity, apneic spells and stupor. Initially there is generalized hypotonia which is followed by hypertonia. Anterior fontanel may be level or bulging due to cerebral edema and IVH. Brainstem involvement is ominous and is characterized by irregularity of breathing, apneic attacks, changes in pupillary size and dysconjugate eye movements. There may be no attempt at sucking and swallowing with pooling of secretions in the oral cavity. Moro reflex may be hyperreactive initially followed by incomplete or absent Moro response. Persistence of neurologic abnormalities beyond 7 days is usually associated with poor neuromotor outcome on follow-up. Associated metabolic and electrolyte disturbances may produce additional clinical features. A large number of perinatal disorders are known to produce acute neonatal encephalopathy and should be seriously considered in the differential diagnosis of HIE (Table 6.12).

Management

Efforts should be made to prevent further hypoxic damage to the brain and correct any associated acid–base and metabolic abnormalities. If despite active resuscitation efforts, 5-minute Apgar score is less than 5, the infant should be admitted in the neonatal intensive care unit for close monitoring and management.

Clinical Monitoring

Vital signs should be monitored preferably with the help of a multi-channel vital sign monitor. Color of the baby should be closely watched for cyanosis, greyness, pallor (hypotension) and jaundice. Detailed record should be maintained to assess CNS integrity

TABLE 6.10 Sarnat and Sarnat staging of hypoxic-ischemic encephalopathy

Features	Stage I	Stage II	Stage III
Consciousness	Hyperalert	Lethargic	Comatose
Muscle tone	Normal	Hypotonic	Flaccid
Tendon reflexes	Brisk	Exaggerated	Absent
Myoclonus	Present	Present	Absent
Sucking	Slow	Weak or absent	Absent
Moro response	Exaggerated	Incomplete	Absent
Oculocephalic reflex (Doll's eyes)	Normal	Over reactive	Reduced or absent
Pupils	Dilated and reactive	Constricted	Dilated and fixed, unequal in size
Breathing	Regular	Periodic	Apneic attacks
Heart rate	Tachycardia	Bradycardia	Variable
Seizures	Absent	Common	Uncommon but decerebration may occur
EEG	Normal	Low voltage periodic or paroxysmal	Periodic, isoelectric

TABLE 6.11 Levene grading of hypoxic-ischemic encephalopathy

Features	Mild	Moderate	Severe
▪ Consciousness	Irritable	Lethargic	Comatose
▪ Tone	Some hypotonia	Moderate hypotonia	Severe hypotonia
▪ Seizures	Nil	Present	Persistent
▪ Sucking/breathing	Poor suck	Unable to suck	Unable to sustain spontaneous breathing

TABLE 6.12 Causes of neonatal encephalopathy

- Hypoxic-ischemic encephalopathy
- Birth trauma
- Intracranial hemorrhage
- Hypoglycemia
- TORCH-related or bacterial meningitis
- Bilirubin encephalopathy
- Idiopathic cerebral infarction
- Inborn errors of metabolism
- Developmental defects of CNS
- Narcotic withdrawal syndrome
- Intracranial space occupying lesion
- Local anesthetic intoxication (pudendal block)

with the help of Sarnat staging system (Table 6.10). The clinical features of HIE are not well described in preterm babies because Sarnat staging system outlines early neurologic consequences of HIE in term babies. Tissue perfusion should be evaluated by capillary refill time on blanching which should be less than 2 seconds. When gradiant between the core and peripheral body temperature is more than 2.5°C, it is also indicative of poor tissue perfusion. Development of respiratory distress following birth asphyxia may occur due to meconium aspiration syndrome, hyaline membrane disease, congenital malformations (diaphragmatic hernia, tracheoesophageal fistula) and pneumothorax following aggressive ventilation at the time of resuscitation. Abdominal girth should be monitored to identify abdominal distension and look for occult blood and reducing substance in the stools as early markers of necrotizing enterocolitis. Periventricular-intraventricular hemorrhage is best diagnosed with the help of ultrasound examination but can be clinically suspected by features of sudden pallor/jaundice, fall in hematocrit, subtle seizures, bulging anterior fontanel and marked hypotonia. Renal perfusion should be monitored by recording urine output which must be kept above 2 mL/kg/hr. Infants with severe birth asphyxia are predisposed to develop septicemia which should be monitored by undertaking frequent screening tests for sepsis.

Biochemical Monitoring

Acid–base parameters and blood gases should be monitored as soon as the infant is transferred to the NICU. Blood glucose should be frequently monitored to identify hypoglycemia and hyperglycemia. Among all sources of energy, glucose alone is capable of sustaining energy metabolism in the brain under conditions of total cerebral ischemia via anerobic glycolysis. Most infants with prolonged hypoxia, especially when they have associated prematurity or intrauterine growth retardation, are predisposed to develop hypoglycemia and polycythemia which are known to enhance the risk of neuromotor disability. Serum electrolytes should be monitored. Hyponatremia may occur as a consequence of inappropriate secretion of antidiuretic hormone while hypernatremia occurs due to frequent administration of sodium bicarbonate for correction of acidosis. Hyperkalemia is ominous and can occur due to acute renal shut down or tissue catabolism. Tissue injury as a consequence of perinatal hypoxia leads to release of phosphate in the bloodstream and consequent hypocalcemia because of inverse relationship between calcium and phosphate.

Non-oliguric renal failure may occur in infants with profound birth asphyxia and is diagnosed by elevation of BUN and creatinine. Urinary neutrophil gelatinase associated lipocalin (NGAL) on day one of life is a useful marker to predict the severity of acute kidney injury (AKI) due to hypoxic-ischemic encephalopathy. NGAL is a 25-kD protein which is increased in the epithelial cells of renal tubules exposed to stress due to inflammation. Elevation of cardiac troponin-T (CTnT) is a useful marker of myocardial dysfunction which can be confirmed by point-of-care echocardiography. Severe birth asphyxia is also associated with elevation of lactate and pyruvate, brain specific creatine kinase (CK-BB), adenine derivatives (hypoxanthine) and nonesterified free fatty acids which are more often used as research tools. During cerebral hypoxia and ischemia, mitochondrial oxidative phosphorylation is impaired causing degradation of adenosine triphosphate (ATP) and accumulation of hypoxanthine.

Laboratory Investigations

Skiagram of chest should be taken in all cases to exclude pneumothorax, diaphragmatic hernia and congenital pneumonia. Availability of cold light transilluminator is useful for prompt diagnosis of pneumothorax in the labor room. Sepsis screening and blood culture should be taken to make an early diagnosis of bacterial infection. When facilities are available, EEG should preferably be taken during first three days of life to identify any abnormalities, like burst suppression, low voltage or isoelectric pattern. A two channel amplitude-integrated encephalography (aEEG) within few hours after birth can assess the severity of brain injury (Figure 6.8). The presence of wide fluctuations in amplitude, peak amplitudes of <5 mV and seizure spikes are suggestive of poor outcome. Ultrasound of the brain is best done during 4 to 7 days of life for the diagnosis of periventricular-intraventricular hemorrhage and leukomalacia in preterm babies. Hypoechoic areas due to cerebral infarction may be seen in severely asphyxiated term babies. Ultrasound examination of the brain is more rewarding for identification of periventricular-intraventricular hemorrhage, while CT scan is more useful to diagnose parasagittal infarction and ischemic changes and it should preferably be done after the age of 2 weeks. MRI is better than CT scan because of lack of radiation exposure, identification of abnormalities in the thalamus, basal ganglia, white and grey matters which provide more reliable prognostic information. In term infants with HIE, MRI findings typically show involvement of ventrolateral thalamus, posterior putamen, perirolandic cortex and

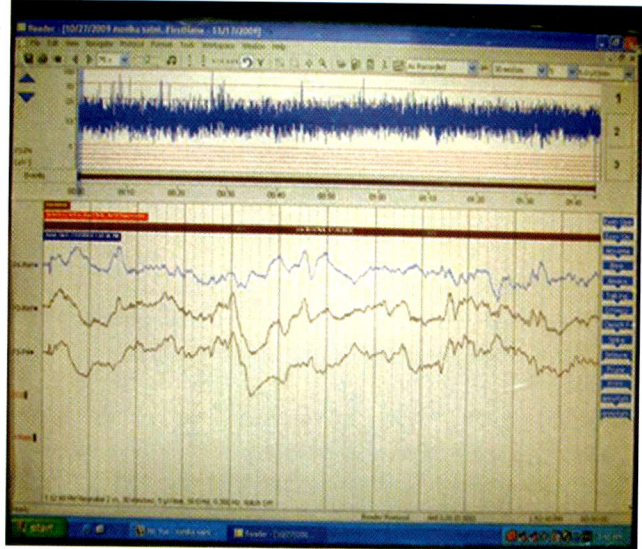

Figure 6.8 Amplitude integrated EEG display showing normal aEEG pattern.

corticospinal tracts. Watershed zones including the parasagittal cortex and subcortical white matter are typically involved in mild-moderate injury. There is relative sparing of the deep gray matter, brainstem and cerebellum. Severe hypoxic-ischemic injury in preterm neonates shows characteristic involvement of the basal ganglia, thalami, dorsal brainstem and anterior vermis. Germinal matrix hemorrhage and periventricular leukomalacia is commonly associated with mild to moderate hypoxic-ischemic insult to the brain of preterm neonates. Brainstem-evoked responses and visual-evoked potentials are of limited prognostic value.

Brain-Oriented Resuscitation

Infants with absence of spontaneous breathing efforts by 10 minutes or those with clinical evidences of hypoxic-ischemic encephalopathy demand urgent measures to reduce cerebral edema, improve cerebral perfusion and prevent further ongoing neuronal damage due to hypoxia, ischemia and metabolic disturbances. Brain-oriented resuscitation demands availability of highly sophisticated supportive and nursing care and assisted ventilatory facilities. The baby should be nursed in a thermoneutral environment with head raised by 30° to prevent further elevation of intracranial pressure. The infant should be intubated and attached to a mechanical ventilator and provided with hyperventilation to maintain PaO_2 between 80 and 100 mm Hg in term babies and 60 and 80 mm Hg in preterm infants, $PaCO_2$ between 25 and 30 mm Hg. Hypocarbia should be maintained

to prevent vasodilatation and is extremely useful to reduce intracranial pressure. When invasive monitoring is not available, oxygen saturation on pulse oximeter should be maintained between 90 and 95% in term babies and 90 and 93% in preterm infants.

During first 48 hours, infuse 10% dextrose solution (two-thirds of maintenance requirements) without sodium and potassium. Acidosis, hypoglycemia, hyperkalemia and hypocalcemia (QoTc >0.2 sec) should be identified and appropriately managed. Blood glucose should preferably be maintained between 60 and 100 mg/dL. Calcium gluconate (150–200 mg/kg/day) should be administered intravenously for initial 48 hours to counteract hypocalcemia due to intracellular flux of calcium, elevated serum potassium and phosphate levels. This may be given as a constant infusion or half-diluted slow boluses of calcium gluconate under cardiac monitoring. Hypotension and poor tissue perfusion should be identified and promptly managed by administration of normal saline or Ringer's lactate and by use of dopamine 5–10 µg/kg/min when myocardial dysfunction is strongly suspected. If blood pressure is low or tissue perfusion is still poor despite administration of dopamine 10 µg/kg/min, dobutamine is started in a dose of 5 µg/kg/min.

The use of mannitol is controversial and must be avoided in preterm babies because of potential risk of causing IVH. Furosemide in a dose of 1.0 mg/kg every 12 hours intravenously for 4 doses is recommended especially when there is oliguria to ensure diuresis and reduce intracranial pressure. Therapeutic utility of oral glycerol and diamox is doubtful while former is also associated with the risk of necrotizing enterocolitis due to hyperosmolality. The use of corticosteroids is not recommended for treatment of cerebral edema. It has been shown that corticosteroids may reduce vasogenic cerebral edema but they are useless for the treatment of cytotoxic brain edema in infants with HIE. In an animal study, it has been shown that high dose steroid therapy was associated with increased mortality as compared to low dose steroid-treated animals or saline treated control animals. *There is enough data to suggest that glucocorticoids administered to perinatal animals may have adverse effects on several aspects of brain development and enhance the risk of cerebral palsy.*

Neonates with moderate and severe HIE may manifest seizure activity within 12 hours after birth. There is controversial evidence that prophylactic administration of phenobarbitone at birth in severely asphyxiated babies may be associated with improved survival and reduced risk of neuromotor disability. It has been shown in rats that phenobarbitone improves CNS metabolism, ensures intergrity of neurons and raises threshold for seizures. It is recommended to administer a loading dose of phenobarbitone 20 mg/kg followed by 5 mg/kg/d as maintenance dose intravenously. It should be administered with the help of an infusion pump at a rate of 1 mg/kg/min. However, prophylactic administration of phenobarbitone is still controversial and should be undertaken only in centers which are equipped to provide assisted ventilation. Therapeutic utility of phenobarbitone in infants who develop seizures following birth asphyxia is unquestionable and it is the anticonvulsant of choice for management of HIE-related seizures once metabolic abnormalities are excluded or appropriately managed. When seizures are unresponsive to a loading dose of phenobarbitone, it is recommended to administer a loading dose of phenytoin 20 mg/kg followed by maintenance dose of 5–7 mg/kg/d intravenously. Topiramate and levetiracetam have been approved for use in neonates with seizures and are credited to be neuroprotective. In majority of neonates with HIE, seizure activity usually disappears within 3 to 10 days. At the time of discharge, all anticonvulsants except phenobarbitone should be stopped. The infant should be re-evaluated at the age of 3 months. If there is no recurrence of seizures and both CNS status and aEEG examination are normal, phenobarbitone should be stopped. When phenobarbitone is continued beyond 3 months, the infant should be re-evaluated at the age of six months to decide whether phenobarbitone therapy should be continued as in a case of epilepsy or terminated at this stage.

Newer Therapeutic Modalities

The understanding of current mechanisms of hypoxic-ischemic injury has resulted in identification of several newer modalities of treatment. They may help in preventing ongoing neuronal cell injury, though most of them are at an experimental stage as yet.

Oxygen-free Radical Inhibitors and Scavengers

Oxygen-free radicals are implicated as pathogenetic mediators in many disease processes including HIE. Free radicals are known to initiate and perpetuate a cascade of chain reactions. Drugs that inhibit the formation of oxygen-free radicals or that rapidly destroy the free radicals or block entry of calcium ions into the cells may be effective in reducing severity of hypoxic-ischemic brain damage. Administration of specific enzymes including superoxide dismutase (SOD), endoperoxidase and catalase to degrade highly reactive radicals to non-reactive compunds and use of scavengers of oxygen-free radicals, like vitamin E, vitamin C and mannitol, have been shown to improve neurologic outcome and decrease biochemical markers of brain injury in animals. Studies of exogenously administered antioxidants have shown promising results and their use will depend on the ability to develop appropriate delivery system that will allow action at the cellular and specific tissue sites.

Drugs that are known to inhibit the biochemical reaction that promotes the production of prostaglandins and xanthine may indirectly lower the formation of oxygen-free radicals. Indomethacin, a cyclooxygenase and phospholipase A_2 inhibitor, N-acetyl cysteine, melatonin and allopurinol, a xanthine oxidase inhibitor, have been shown to be of benefit in ischemic neuronal or myocardial damage in animals. The allopurinol-treated animals demonstrated less severe cerebral edema during the recovery period and milder chronic neuropathologic changes due to birth asphyxia. Melatonin, an antioxidant, has shown encouraging neuroprotective results in animal models and pilot studies in human neonates. The clinical trials are in progress and it may become a potential therapy for HIE in the near future.

Calcium Channel Blockers

Calcium (Ca^{++}), often called as an intracellular second messenger, is a regulator of cellular metabolism. Among the available calcium channel blockers, flunarizine and nimodipine appear most efficacious in adult animals. Using a rat model, two studies have shown an amelioration of neuropathologic alterations in animals pretreated with flunarizine. The results of clinical trials are awaited regarding usefulness of this modality in the treatment of HIE of the newborn.

Erythropoietin

Erythropoietin (Epo), a glycoprotein, is upregulated in babies who suffer from perinatal asphyxia which may be an endogenous repair mechanism. Its neuroprotective mechanism is mediated through different mechanisms including direct neurotropic effect, decreased susceptibility to glutamate toxicity, release of antiapoptotic factors, reduced inflammation, decreased nitric oxide-mediated injury and direct antioxidant effects. The antioxidant effect of Epo may be enhanced by the increased erythropoiesis utilizing the free iron which accumulated during perinatal hypoxia. High (5000 U/kg) and multiple doses of recombinant human Epo (rEpo) have been shown to provide significant neuroprotection and improved outcome. However, its exorbitant cost is a major deterrent for its use in developing countries. It is effective during all phases of HIE.

Excitatory Amino Acid Antagonists

Glutamate has been implicated in the pathogenesis of hypoxic-ischemic injury. Excessive exposure of neurons to glutamate leads to neuronal injury. The damage to neurons due to anoxia can be prevented by the presence of magnesium ions (Mg^{++}) which block glutamate receptors or by specific glutamate antagonists. Pretreatment with magnesium sulfate has been shown to prevent neuronal damage in piglets by reducing lipid peroxidation, decreasing influx of Ca^{++} into neurons and by blocking NMDA receptors. Animal experiments have shown that direct injection of glutamate into the specific regions of brain *in vivo* produces neuronal injury identical with that seen after hypoxia-ischemia. Agents which block glutamate release or block its postsynaptic action may be useful in preventing neuronal injury. Baclofen, an inhibitor of glutamate release has not been evaluated for its therapeutic utility. Other agents, like phencyclidine, dextromethorphan, ketamine, MK-801, and topiramate which affect N-methyl-D-aspartate (NMDA) receptors, have received maximum attention. They work even when administered later when the hypoxic-ischemic insult has already occurred.

The protective role of MK-801 appears greater in immature rats as compared to their adult counterparts. Unfortunately, MK-801 and NMDA receptor antagonists are highly toxic. Magnesium appears to be a naturally occurring antagonist of NMDA which has a receptor site deep within calcium channel. The role of magnesium sulfate as a neuroprotective agent for prevention of brain damage due to hypoxia-ischemia deserves active consideration and evaluation in future.

Prevention of Excess Nitric Oxide Formation

Nitric oxide is a free-radical gas that can be rapidly produced by a nitric oxide synthase enzyme in cerebral endothelial cells and neurons in response to an increase in the intracellular calcium. It has been shown that administration of nitroarginine 15 hours prior to cerebral hypoxia-ischemia in immature rats causes prolonged inhibition of nitric oxide synthesis and reduction in the extent of brain injury.

Opiate Antagonists and Cannabinoids

The elevation in the endogenous opiate levels (endorphins) in term fetus with evidences of asphyxia and in the newborn with hypoxemia support the notion that these compounds may be released in infants with HIE. It is not clear, whether these opiates have any adverse physiological effects that should be blocked by an antagonist, like naloxone or whether they in fact play an important adaptive role. In experimental animals, the use of naloxone for hypoxemic-ischemic injury has not shown consistent benefit.

Whole Body Cooling

There are several publications on the neuroprotective effects of cerebral hypothermia in animal experiments. Multicentric studies are being conducted in human asphyxiated newborns to assess the neuroprotective effects of selective head cooling or total body moderate (core temperature 33.5°C–34.5°C) hypothermia. Hypothermia raises the threshold for seizures by reducing release of excitatory neurotransmitters. It reduces the formation of reactive oxygen-free radicals, decreases brain metabolism, stabilizes the blood–brain barrier, reduces inflammatory response and mitigates apoptotic death of neurons. A fall in core body temperature by 1°C is associated with reduced cerebral metabolism by 7% with concomitant reduced demand for glucose and oxygen. The beneficial effects of hypothermia are highest, if it is provided within 6 hours of hypoxic-ischemic injury and is maintained at least for 3 days. Whole body cooling or therapeutic hypothermia (TH) is recommended in term infants (>36 weeks), if three of the following five inclusion criteria are fulfilled.

i. Apgar score ≤5 at 10 minutes.
ii. pH of cord blood or infant's blood within one hour of age ≤7.0.
iii. Base deficit of cord blood or infant's blood within one hour of age ≥16 mEq/L.
iv. Need for assisted ventilation at birth for at least 10 minutes.
v. History of seizures or CNS abnormalities suggestive of grade 3 or more of HIE.

The exclusion criteria when whole body cooling is denied include (i) inability to initiate cooling by 6 hours of age, (ii) gestation ≤36 weeks, (iii) presence of life-threatening congenital malformations or chromosomal anomaly, (iv) severe intrauterine growth restriction (birth weight <1800 g in a term infant), and (v) infants with multiorgan failure, shock or grade 4 intraventricular hemorrhage.

Infrastructure and Equipment

TH demands the availability of level 3 or tertiary care NICU facilities with adequate staff having high level of expertise and skills. The list of equipment required includes radiant warmer, cooling device, vital sign monitor, thermisters for recording rectal temperature and facility for invasive ventilation. The facility should be readily available or point-of-care facilities should be available for ABG, blood glucose, electrolytes and hematologic monitoring, access to X-rays, ultrasonography, echocardiography, aEEG, CT or MRI facilities.

Procedure

Whole body cooling devices (Blanketrol™) and selective head cooling helmets have been used for therapeutic hypothermia (TH). Head coolers are less popular because they are more expensive, associated with difficulties in rewarming with higher risk of complications and lower dividends of therapeutic benefits. The infant who fulfills the criteria for whole body cooling is admitted in the NICU and placed in the cooling device. *The subject must be more than 36 weeks gestation and less than 6 hr of age and kept in the cooling device no longer than 72 hr (critical window).* During therapeutic hypothermia, the target core temperature is kept around 33.5°C ±0.5°C.

After 72 hr of cooling, rewarming is done by stopping cooling strategies and increasing the temperature of the radiant warmer by 1°C per hour. The final temperature goal of the baby is core temperature of 36.5°C and should be achieved in about 7 hours.

Clinical and Laboratory Monitoring

Vital signs Core body temperature, heart rate, respiratory rate, blood pressure, capillary refill time (CRT), SPO_2 and urine output should be recorded.

Fluids and electrolytes Initial fluid should be 10% dextrose followed by one-fifth 5% glucose-saline as maintenance. Body weight and urine output should be closely monitored to regulate fluid therapy. Syndrome of inappropriate secretion of antidiuretic hormone (SIADH) should be looked for and managed by fluid restriction.

Pain and supportive care Pain and discomfort of cooling should be controlled with narcotic agent like morphine or fentanyl. Provide developmentally supportive care to optimize neuromotor development.

Nutritional support Enteral nutrition should be delayed till rewarming has been completed. During TH, there is decrease in mesenteric circulation with increased risk of NEC. The infant should be kept on total parenteral nutrition (TPN) during the phase of cooling and rewarming. Vitamin K 1.0 mg should be given parenterally. Hematologic abnormalities should be looked for and managed with fresh frozen plasma.

Pharmacological therapy A number of pharmacological agents like allopurinol, glutamate inhibitors, calcium channel blockers and opiate antagonists have been tried in experimental animals with variable results. Among these, multiple high doses (5000 U/kg) of recombinant human EPO (rEPO) have been shown to provide significant neuroprotection with reduced risk of neuromotor sequelae. However, the cost of thus intervention is exorbitant.

Respiratory system Assisted ventilation is required to support breathing and maintain ABG within normal range. Low body temperature may require higher tidal volume due to stiffness of chest. The lung compliance and ventilatory parameters should be closely monitored during initiation of cooling and rewarming phases.

Circulatory system TH leads to bradycardia and decreased cardiac output. Point-of-care or functional echocardiography is useful to monitor superior vena-cava (SVC) flow which is a useful marker of cerebral circulation. Cardiac troponin-T (CTnT) and brain natriuretic peptide (BNP) should be monitored. The dose of inotropes is adjusted to maintain adequate tissue perfusion and prevent multiorgan failure.

Central nervous system Daily CNS ultrasonography for intraventricular hemorrhage, Doppler studies for cerebral blood flow and aEEG are useful to monitor integrity of the brain. Neurological examination and Sarnat staging should be done daily till day 7 after TH. MRI study of brain is done as and when indicated.

Skin Skin should be examined daily for petechial hemorrhages, subcutaneous fat necrosis and sclerema neonatorum.

Biochemistry Complete blood count (CBC), screening markers for infection, hematologic profile, electrolytes, liver and kidney function tests and cardiac enzymes should be monitored on a regular basis.

Complications The common complications of TH include shock, cardiac failure, sepsis, IVH, NEC, persistent pulmonary hypertension, hyperglycemia, consumptive coagulopathy and multiorgan failure.

Cooling Therapy in Developing Countries

There is insufficient evidence to promote the hi-tec modality of therapeutic hypothermia for management of HIE in low and middle income countries (LMICs). It is difficult to recruit suitable candidates within the narrow window of 6 hr. The intervention is cost-intensive

Care of the Baby in the Labor Room

6

and demands high level of facilities and expertise to safely administer it. Various low cost cooling devices like frozen gel, ice packs, cold water bottles and cooling mattresses made of phase changing material (PCM) have been used in LMICs with variable results. The phase change material is a substance which releases/absorbs sufficient energy at phase transition to provide useful heat/cooling. The PCM consists of salt hydrates, fatty acids, and paraffins that melt at a set temperature. The PCM cooling mattresses (Climator™, Criticool™, Tecotherm™, MiraCradle™) have been used with favorable results in studies conducted in Kerala. These devices use the advanced savE® phase change material technology to rapidly induce therapeutic hypothermia.

Key Messages

TH is considered as a gold standard intervention for management of neonates with grade 2 and 3 HIE by the developed nations. When instituted during the critical window period of 6 hr, it is credited to improve the survival and enhance neuromotor quality of life among the survivors. In tertiary NICUs of the west, TH has emerged as a standard of care for neonates having severe hypoxic-ischemic encephalopathy. The feasibility and safety of TH in low-middle income countries (LMICs) is controversial. It is hoped that a large phase III randomized controlled trial (HELIX trial) being conducted in India, Bangladesh and Sri Lanka shall provide guidelines for rational launch of TH in developing countries.

Stem Cell Transplantation

There is evidence to suggest that neonatal brain is endowed with the capability for endogenous neurogenesis following hypoxic-ischemic injury. There is experimental evidence to suggest that stem cell transplantation may repair the damaged neurons in the brain. Several types of stem cells have been used in rodent models including neuronal stem cells, mesenchymal stem cells and hematopoietic stem cells. There is evidence to suggest that genetically modified stem cells may be more effective than native unmodified stem cells. Stem cell transplantation has the potential to become a future neuroprotective and regenerative therapy for hypoxic-ischemic brain injury.

Prognosis

"Seeds of cerebral palsy are sown in the perinatal period".
Meharban Singh

Birth asphyxia is an important cause of neonatal mortality accounting for a case fatality rate of 15–50%

depending upon the definition of birth asphyxia and quality of newborn care facilities. Mortality among preterm asphyxiated babies is much higher as compared to term babies. Among term babies, most deaths are attributed to HIE and systemic effects of asphyxia while in preterm babies majority of deaths are accounted for by prematurity, i.e. hyaline membrane disease, intraventricular hemorrhage, sepsis and multiorgan failure.

Following severe birth asphyxia, 25% infants are likely to develop evidences of HIE. Infants with severe HIE have increased risk of long-term neurological sequelae and it is a better predictor of subsequent handicap than poor Apgar scores or biochemical changes alone. The causal relationship between cerebral palsy (CP) and birth asphyxia is controversial. Most cases of CP occur in infants who have no history of adverse perinatal events and many infants with adverse perinatal history recover without developing CP. Precause of advances in perinatal monitoring and management, newborn survival has improved but the incidence of CP has not shown any significant decline. Are deaths being converted to disability? It is believed that prenatal antecedents, like genetic factors, teratogenic agents and adverse early influences, may cause both birth asphyxia and CP independently.

The commonest neuromotor sequelae following birth asphyxia is CP of varying grades and severity. Isolated mental retardation without CP is usually not attributable to birth asphyxia. The incidence of CP following birth asphyxia varies between 6.5 and 18.5%. Birth asphyxia is an important cause of CP accounting for about 10% of cases but it is not the leading cause. A large number of clinical, biochemical and laboratory parameters are reliable predictors of occurrence of cerebral palsy (Table 6.13).

TABLE 6.13 Clinical correlates of adverse neuromotor outcome following birth asphyxia

- Low birth weight and prematurity (periventricular leukomalacia)
- Apgar score of <4 at 10 minutes or later
- Assisted ventilation for >24 hours
- Severe metabolic acidosis (cord umbilical artery blood pH ≤7.0)
- Hypoglycemia
- Polycythemia
- Intractable seizures or brainstem signs (poor sucking, pooling of oral secretions, pupillary changes, etc.)
- Severity of HIE (Sarnat stage II and above)
- Abnormal neurological behavior for more than 7 days
- Multiorgan failure especially development of acute renal failure

Apgar scores have a poor predictive value but when establishment of spontaneous breathing is delayed beyond 10 minutes or later and Apgar scores remain low, it is associated with adverse long-term outcome. Hypoglycemia, polycythemia and severe metabolic acidosis are associated with increased risk of CP and should be promptly managed. Development of seizures and other clinical and laboratory evidences of HIE are associated with increased risk of CP. Persistence of abnormal neurological behavior, poor tone, pupillary changes, incomplete or absent Moro reflex for more than one week is associated with poor long-term outcome. If following resuscitation of an asphyxiated newborn baby, there are no neurological abnormalities during early neonatal period, it guarantees normal neuromotor development on follow-up. The presence of a CNS or a non-CNS malformation enhances the risk of occurrence of neuromotor disability and must be looked for and excluded.

EEG abnormalities during first 3 days of life in the form of multifocal seizure discharges of >10 sec duration, burst suppression or isoelectric record are associated with poor outcome. Intraventricular hemorrhage of grade II and more on cranial ultrasound and evidences of ischemia or infarction over the parasagittal area on CT scan are associated with adverse outcome. Brainstem auditory, visual or somatosensory evoked responses by and large are of limited prognostic utility. Inferior colliculi which are credited to produce wave V are specfically damaged by hypoxia. In normal infants, wave V obtained during brainstem auditory evoked response is bigger in amplitude as compared to wave I. The ratio of wave V (actually waves IV and V which are often merged) to wave I gets reversed when there is hypoxic damage to the inferior colliculi which is associated with increased mortality and poor late neuromotor outcome among the survivors. During follow-up, detailed neurological and developmental examination should be conducted to identify early clinical markers of CP (Table 6.14).

TABLE 6.14 Early clinical markers of cerebral palsy

- Episodes of inconsolable crying, chewing movements, excessive sensitivity to light or sound, etc.
- Persistent asymmetric neck tonic posture beyond 4 weeks.
- Clenched fists (cortical thumb) beyond 8 weeks.
- Lack of social smile by 6 weeks.
- Abnormalities in tone (hypertonia in lower limbs and hypotonia in neck/upper limbs).
- Paucity or absence of playful or fidgety limb movements during 6–12 weeks of life.
- Persistence of automatic reflexes beyond 4–5 months.
- Slow head growth.

HOME DELIVERY

The detailed care of the baby at birth outlined in this chapter is unfortunately applicable to only about 50% of newborn babies who are born in the hospital. In rural India, 75% of babies are born at home and delivery is attended mostly by traditional untrained *dais*. Moreover, infants born in the hospital return back to their homes within a week of their birth. Therefore, the programs designed to reduce the alarmingly high perinatal mortality, must take these facts into cognizance.

Trained Personnel

From time immemorial, the traditional birth attendants (*dais*) have earned their place and recognition in our sociocultural milieu. Efforts made to popularize supervision of deliveries by auxiliary nurse midwives and other trained paramedical staff have generally failed. It is difficult to replace *dais* because they undertake additional household chores, such as body massage, washing soiled linen, feeding the infant, helping in the kitchen and of course talking about the mother-in-law! In any case, auxiliary nurse midwives are far too insufficient in numbers to cope with the expected births and traditional birth attendants (TBAs) or *dais* must be trained to handle the situation more effectively. It is suggested that initial four weeks of intensive coaching of all prospective *dais* in the art of essential natal care and recognition of high-risk pregnancy should be followed by periodic on-going training. The TBA should be trained to assess the condition of the baby by evaluating cry, breathing movements, cord pulsations and color. The useless and potentially harmful cultural practices for resuscitation of an asphyxiated baby, such as milking the cord towards the baby, roasting the placenta while it is still attached to the baby, throwing cold water on the face of the baby, squeezing onion juice into baby's nostrils, beating drum or metal plate, forcibly flexing limbs on to the abdomen, persistent slapping of the buttocks, etc. should be condemned.

Accredited social health activists (ASHAs) and midwives should be taught the art and skills of resuscitation in a simple and practical manner. Cleaning the oral cavity with a gauze piece wrapped round the finger is adequate for most babies. In a baby, who fails to cry or breathe, oral suction with a thick bored 10 Fr catheter with the help of a DeLee suction trap is desirable. The effective use of mouth-to-mouth breathing, mouth-to-mask or bag and mask ventilation should be taught. The principles of keeping the baby warm by prompt drying, effective clothing, use of cotton wool, close proximity to the mother, keeping the room warm, avoiding bath at birth and preserving vernix should be emphasized. They should be trained to identify high-risk mothers so that they can be referred for delivery to a community health center or district hospital. The use of injections, both for augmentation of uterine contractions and for resuscitation of a newborn baby are condemned.

In 21st century, we must delink ourselves from the concept of *dais* for providing antenatal care and conducting home deliveries. The Ministry of Health and Family Welfare, Government of India is making concerted efforts to train community newborn health workers (CNHW) and ASHAs to ensure that all deliveries are conducted by skilled birth attendants. It is envisaged and hoped that after the launch of National Rural and Urban Health Missions and India Newborn Action Plan (INAP), all pregnant women shall receive good quality antenatal care and all deliveries shall be conducted by skilled health functionaries in well-equipped health care facilities.

Equipment

It is essential that *dais* or expectant mothers should be provided with free disposable sterile delivery packs containing cotton, gauze, razor blade, tie, Tr. iodine or triple dye and soap. Availability of a mucus oral suction trap and a portable spring balance is also desirable. Auxiliary nurse midwife should be provided and trained for active resuscitation of an apneic baby with a bag and mask or mouth and mask.

Essential Care during Delivery

The delivery should be conducted in a clean, well-lighted and warm room. The five cleans should be maintained namely clean surface or sheet for conducting delivery, clean hands, clean razor blade, clean cord tie and by keeping the cord open. The hands should be washed with soap and water. The cord must be cut with a sterile blade and tied with a sterile tie. The infant should be placed on mother's abdomen or chest and head kept lower than the rest of the body to prevent aspiration. The oral cavity should be cleaned gently with a piece of sterile gauze or suction done with a mucus trap. The infant must be promptly dried and effectively covered soon after birth. The cord should be dabbed with an antiseptic lotion. The bath should preferably be deferred to the next day. The mother should be encouraged to feed colostrum to the baby within 1 to 2 hours of birth. The application of cow dung or any "home antiseptics" over the umbilical stump is strongly condemned. The use of *Janam ghutti* and other prelacteal feeds should be discouraged. It is essential to have well-coordinated referral system linked and supported by efficient transport and communication system so that prompt referral can be effected as and when needed.

ROUTINE CARE OF THE BABY IN THE LABOR ROOM

After having ensured that the baby is breathing and he has been adequately protected from becoming hypothermic, the baby should be quickly screened for any evidences of life-threatening congenital anomalies and birth injuries. The eyes should be cleaned with sterile normal saline using one swab for each eye. There is no evidence to support routine chemoprophylaxis for prevention of ophthalmia neonatorum. When indicated, prophylaxis against gonococcal ophthalmia can be achieved by local instillation of either freshly prepared 1.0% silver nitrate drops or 2.5% povidone-iodine solution or 0.5% erythromycin ophthalmic ointment. Erythromycin provides additional protection against conjunctivitis due to *Chlamydia trachomatis*. The skin should be dried and cleaned off any mucus and blood before the baby is shown to the mother. The umbilical cord should be tied using two ligatures, rubber band or a disposable clamp. When the base of the cord is bulbous and it is suspected to contain minor exomphalos, the ligatures should be placed distally to avoid cutting of the gut. The base and tip of umbilical stump should be painted with ethyl alcohol or triple dye. Vitamin K 0.5–1.0 mg is administered intramuscularly to all babies especially those weighing less than 2000 g, traumatic deliveries especially difficult forceps and vacuum extraction, preoperatively and babies in whom mother had received dicoumarol derivatives, salicylates and anticonvulsants.

Stomach wash with normal saline is routinely done in the following situations:
1. Babies born by cesarean section
2. Severely asphyxiated babies
3. Meconium-stained liquor
4. Polyhydramnios
5. Single umbilical artery
6. Hypoplastic small-for-dates babies
7. Infants of diabetic mothers

In situations 4 to 7, stomach wash is done to confirm the patency of esophagus to rule out esophageal atresia and to assess the volume of gastric contents as an aid to the diagnosis of upper intestinal obstruction. The

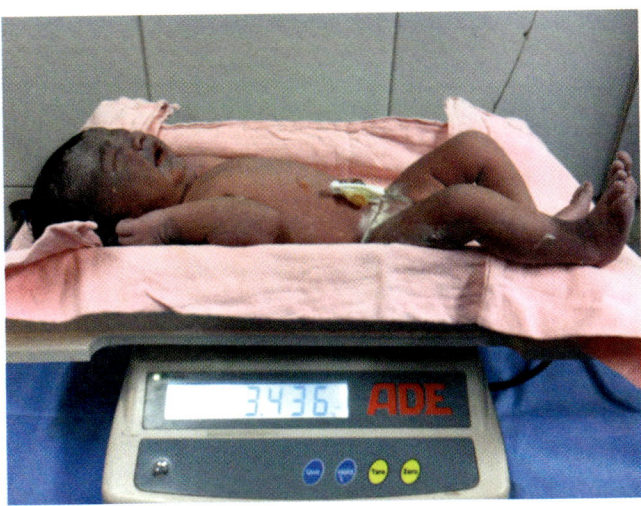

Figure 6.9 Infant being weighed on an electronic weighing scale at birth.

baby should be weighed and identification tag applied before transferring to the special care nursery or to the mother in the lying-in ward (Figure 6.9). The identification band should be affixed on the baby's wrist depicting mother's name, her admission number, baby's sex, date and time of birth and birth weight. Some centers follow the policy of recording baby's foot print as an additional measure of identification. The health care provider responsible for care of the baby at birth must communicate with mother and family members regarding time, weight, gender and well-being of the infant and mother. The infant should be shown to the family members so that they have no misgivings about the gender of the baby. The following babies are transferred by the nurse to the special care nursery or neonatal intensive care unit under the supervision of a neonatologist without unnecessary delay. The practice of asking an *attendant or aya* to take the baby to the nursery is strongly condemned.

1. Birth weight of less than 2000 g
2. Gestation of less than 36 weeks
3. Severe birth asphyxia (5-min Apgar score of 3 or less)
4. Rhesus isoimmunization
5. Gross congenital malformations
6. Maternal diabetes mellitus
7. Respiratory distress or any other systemic problem in the baby
8. Unwell or unwed or unwilling mother

The cord blood should be collected in cases of rhesus isoimmunization, group O mother, maternal diabetes mellitus and small-for-dates babies in whom intra-uterine infection is suspected.

EXAMINATION OF THE PLACENTA

The organ that constituted a vital link between the mother and fetus should not be viewed as a by-product destined for the dustbin but should be accorded due attention because its examination may offer useful clues to anticipate the problems and their outcome in the neonate. The following observations should be made regarding the placenta, its membranes and attached cord.

Weight

The average weight of placenta varies from 400–500 g. The placental weight is about 12–15% of baby's weight. The placenta may be abnormally small in low birth weight babies due to *in utero* malnutrition, trisomy 17–18 and rubella. Large placenta may be associated with polyhydramnios, erythroblastosis, maternal diabetes mellitus, congenital nephrosis, syphilis, toxoplasmosis and cytomegalic inclusion disease.

Surface and Color

Dull and milky appearance of fetal surface of placenta and foul smelling liquor are associated with intra-uterine bacterial infection, while grayish-yellow staining of placenta and membranes is seen in cases of passage of meconium *in utero* and erythroblastosis. The presence of central infarctions on the maternal side of placenta with or without calcification is associated with placental dysfunction and fetal hypoxia. The presence of subchorial thrombi towards fetal side of placenta is of no significance. The oligohydramnios may be suspected by the presence of granular brown nodules of amnion nodosum. The presence of angiomatous malformation in the placenta may result in hydrops fetalis due to protein leakage from angioma.

Retroplacental Hemorrhage

In a baby who is pale and in shock at birth, the presence of retroplacental clots, especially if associated with velamentous insertion of cord, would suggest the possibility of fetal blood loss rather than asphyxia pallida.

Umbilical Cord

The velamentous cord insertion and circumvallate placenta is likely to be associated with antepartum hemorrhage, premature labor and fetal hypoxia. The presence of single umbilical artery may be associated with high incidence of congenital malformations.

Care of the Baby in the Labor Room

6

Zygosity of Twins

It is essential to determine whether twin babies are monozygous or dizygous for several reasons. The presence of vascular anastomoses in monozygous twins may lead to inter-twin transfusion syndrome. They offer useful models to biologists for study of influence of genetic versus environmental factors in various disorders and for transplantation experiments as they have unique tissue compatibility.

If the twin babies are of different sexes, they are obviously dizygous. The twins of identical sex with a monochorionic placenta would support the existence of monozygous twins. In dichorionic placenta with like-sexed twin pairs, the zygosity is doubtful. In such babies determination of blood groups, red blood cells and placental enzyme studies may establish the existence of dizygosity but monozygosity can only be proven with absolute certainty by HLA typing.

Examination of Placenta for the Number of Chorions

Place the placenta on the table with the fetal surface facing you. Try to strip the amnion somewhere between the two umbilical cord insertions. It can be easily stripped off, if chorion is single. In dichorionic placenta, the amnion cannot be stripped off and on lifting the membranes at the place of the junction against light, two layers of vascular chorion would be seen enclosed between the two layers of amniotic membranes (Figure 6.10). In rare instances of monoamniotic monochorionic twins, which can be diagnosed by the absence of junction of membrane between two cord insertions, there is very high incidence of congenital malformations and stillbirths.

Placental Histology

The presence of amnionitis and placentitis has been shown to be poorly correlated with subsequent develop-ment of early-onset neonatal infection. However, in severely hypoplastic babies and whenever there is a suspicion of some intrauterine infection including maternal tuberculosis and malaria, placental tissue should be preserved for histolgical examination.

Umbilical Cord Blood Banking

Stem cell transplantation and cord blood banking has received much popularity among general public and medical professionals in the recent past. Umbilical cord blood (UCB) serves as an important source of hematopoietic stem cells and can be used for treatment of various disorders like blood cancers, hemoglobino-pathies, immunodeficiency disorders and few selected inborn errors of metabolism. Cord blood can be collec-ted easily without any difficulty or complications and it has a relatively lower incidence of graft *vs* host reaction compared to bone marrow cells or peripheral blood cells. It is not uncommon these days to find the representatives of various stem cell banking com-panies (Jeevan®, Reliance®, StemCyte India®) to loiter in the labor rooms to advise and cajole parents for collection of the cord blood of their newly born baby and store it for several years for any future use by the donor or his relatives. The practice should be strongly discouraged since the American Society for Blood and Marrow Transplantation encourages the use of public UCB banking because the probability of using one's own or personal blood for management of a genetic disorder is exceedingly small (<0.04%).

Autologous cord blood, stored privately cannot be used for treating one's own genetic condition in future because the cord stem cells are likely to harbor the same genetic abnormality which is the likely cause of the disease. Private or personal cord blood banking is not a "biological insurance" and its role in regenerative medicine is still hypothetical. Personal cord blood banking is recommended only if there is an existing family member (sibling or biological parent) who is currently suffering from a disease which is known to be benefitted by allogenic stem cell transplantation.

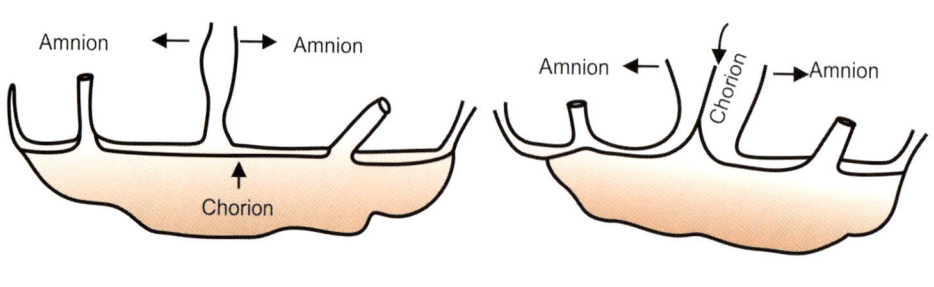

Figure 6.10 Examination of placenta for zygosity of twins. See text for details.

Instead public cord blood banking should be promoted which provides treatment options for management of a host of genetic and malignant disorders. In India, with high birth rate and diverse genetic pool, there is a bright prospect to find HLA-matched hematopoietic stem cells for public cord blood banking for transplant. It is imperative to spread the awareness about myths and facts about personal cord blood banking among the general public and health care professionals. Advertisements for private cord blood banking by companies are often misleading and they exploit parent's emotions for profit during vulnerable period of their lives.

BIBLIOGRAPHY

Ali Z, Khadije D, Elahe A, *et al.* Prophylaxis of ophthalmia neonatorum: comparison of betadine, erythromycin and no prophylaxis. *J Trop Pediatr* 2007, 53 (6): 388–392.

Allwood AC, Madar RJ, Baumer JH, *et al.* Changes in resuscitation practice at birth. *Arch Dis Child Fetal Neonatal Ed.* 2003, 88: F375–F379.

American Academy of Pediatrics, American Heart Association. Textbook of Neonatal Resuscitation. 7th ed. Edited by Gary M Weiner, Jeanette Zaichkin. *Dallas (TX): Elk Grove Village (IL)*, 2016.

American Academy of Pediatrics and American College of Obstetricians and Gynecologists. In: Guidelines for Perinatal Care. Gilstrap LC, Oh W (Eds.) 6th Ed. *Elk Grove Village Ill. American Academy of Pediatrics* 2010, 187.

Azzopardi DV, Strohm B, Edwards AD, *et al.* Moderate hypothermia to treat perinatal asphyxial encephalopathy. *N Engl J Med* 2009, 361: 1349–1358.

Bharathi B, Bhat BV, Negi VS, Adhisivam B. Inflammatory mediators as predictors of outcome in perinatal asphyxia. *Indian J Pediatr* 2015,82(5): 433–38.

Bhatia BD. New NRP guidelines 2010. *J Neonatol 2011,* 25: 9–16.

Bradfor WD. The case for careful examination of the placenta: helpful information from the delivery room. *Clin Pediatr* 1968, 7: 716.

Braly P, Freeman RK. The significance of fetal heart rate reactivity with a positive oxytocin challenge test. *Obstet Gynecol* 1977, 50: 689.

Brann AW, Mantalvo JM. Barbiturates and asphyxia. *Pediatr Clin N Amer 1970,* 17: 851.

Brann AW. Hypoxic ischemic encephalopathy (asphyxia). *Pediatr Clin N Amer* 1986, 33: 451.

Cabal LA, Devaskar U, Siassi B, *et al.* Cardiogenic shock associated with perinatal asphyxia in preterm infants. *J Pediatr* 1980, 96: 705.

Catlin EA, Carpenter MW, Branne BS, Mayfield SR, *et al.* The Apgar score revisited: Influence of gestational age. *J Pediatr* 1986, 109: 865.

Cerio FG, Lara-Celador I, Alvarez A, Hilario E. Neuroprotective therapies after perinatal hypoxic-ischemic brain injury. *Brain Sci* 2013, 3: 191–214.

Deorari AK, Paul VK, Singh M. Birth asphyxia and neurodevelopmental outcome. *Indian Pediatr* 1989, 26: 293.

Donn SM, Grasela TH, Goldstein GW. Safety of a higher loading dose of phenobarbital in the term newborn. *Pediatrics* 1985, 74: 1061.

D'souza SW, Black P, Cadman J, *et al.* Umbilical venous blood pH: a useful aid in the diagnosis of asphyxia at birth. *Arch Dis Child* 1983, 58: 15.

Datta V. Therapeutic hypothermia for birth asphyxia in neonates. *Indian J Pediatr* 2017, 84(3): 219–26.

Eicher DJ, Wagner CL, Katikaneni LP, *et al.* Moderate hypothermia in neonatal encephalopathy: efficacy outcomes. *Pediatr Neurol* 2005, 32(1): 11–17.

Eileen KH, Eman SH. Late versus early clamping of the umbilical cord in full term neonates. Systematic review and meta-analysis of controlled trials. *JAMA* 2007, 297: 1241–1252.

Evans DJ, Levene MJ. Anticonvulsants for preventing mortality and morbidity in full-term newborns with perinatal asphyxia. *Cochrane Database Syst Rev* 2000, CD001240.

Finer NN, Robertson CM, Richards RT, *et al.* Hypoxic-ischemic encephalopathy in term neonates: Perinatal factors and outcome. *J Pediatr* 1981, 98: 112.

Fogarty M, Osborn DA, Askil L, Seidler AL, Hunter K, Lui K, *et al.* Delayed *vs* early clamping for preterm infants: A systematic review and meta-analysis. *Am J Obstet Gynecol* 2018, 218: 1–18.

Freeman JM, Nelson KB. Intrapartum asphyxia and cerebral palsy. *Pediatrics* 1988, 82: 240.

Gluckman PD, Wyatt JS, Azzopardi D, *et al.* Selective head cooling with mild systemic hypothermia after neonatal encephalopathy: multicentre randomized trial. *Lancet* 2005, 365: 663–670.

Goldberg RN, Bloom FL, Bauer CR, *et al.* The use of barbiturate therapy in severe perinatal asphyxia. *Pediatr Res* 1985, 542: 1390.

Goldbeg RN, Moscoso P, Baver CR, *et al.* Use of barbiturate therapy in severe perinatal asphyxia: A randomized controlled trial. *J Pediatr* 1986, 109: 851–856.

Gonzalez FF, Ferriero DM. Therapeutics for neonatal brain injury. *Pharmacol Ther* 2008, 120: 43–53.

Gupta JM, Tizard JPM. The sequence of events in neonatal apnea. *Lancet* 1967, II: 55.

Hall RT, Hall FK, Daily DK. High-dose phenobarbital therapy in term newborn infants with severe perinatal asphyxia: a randomized prospective study with 3-year follow up. *J Pediatr* 1998, 132: 345–348.

Hill A, Volpe JJ. Hypoxic-ischemic brain injury in the newborn. *Semin Perinatol* 1982, 6: 25.

Hill A, Volpe JJ. Pathogenesis and management of hypoxic-ischemic encephalopathy in the term newborn. *Neurol Clin* 1985, 3: 31.

International Guidelines for Neonatal Resuscitation: An Excerpt from the Guidelines 2000 for Cardiopulmonary Resuscitation and Emergency Cardiovascular Care: International Consensus on Science. *Pediatrics* 2000, 106: 1–16.

John S, Wyatt PD, Gluckman PY, *et al*. Gunn for the cool cap study group determinants of outcome after head cooling for neonatal encephalopathy. *Pediatrics* 2007, 119: 912–921.

Joseph S, Kumar S, Ahamed ZM, Lakshmi S. Cardiac troponin T as a marker of myocardial dysfunction in term neonates with perinatal asphyxia. *Indian J Pediatr* 2018, 85(10): 877–84.

Kattwinkel J. Neonatal resuscitation guidelines for ILCOR and NRP: evaluating the evidence and developing a consensus. *J Perinatol* 2008, 28:S27–S29.

Kobli FW, Hon EH, Khazin AF, *et al*. Observations on heart rate and pH in the human fetus during labor. *J Obstet Gynecol* 1969, 104: 1109.

Krishnan P, Shroff M. Neuroimaging in neonatal hypoxic ischemic encephalopathy. *Indian J Pediatr* 2016, 83(9): 995–1002.

Lauener PA, Calame A, Janelek P, *et al*. Systematic pH measurements in the umbilical artery: causes and predictive value of neonatal acidosis. *J Perinatal Med* 1983, 11: 278.

Levene MI, Evans DH. Medical management of raised intracranial pressure after severe birth asphyxia. *Arch Dis Child* 1985, 60: 12.

Levene MI. Management of the asphyxiated full term infant. *Arch Dis Child 1993*, 68: 612–616.

McDonald SJ, Middleton P. Effect of timing of umbilical cord clamping of term infants on maternal and neonatal outcomes. *Cochrane Database Syst Rev* 2008, 16 (2): CD 004074.

Molteno CD, Malan AF, Heese HDV. Neonatal complications and conditions associated with asphyxia neonatorum. *South Africa Med J* 1974, 48: 259.

Narayanan DL, Phadke SR. Concepts, utility, and limitations of cord blood banking: What clinicians need to know. *Indian J Pediatr* 2019, 86(1): 44–48.

Nelson KB, Ellenberg JH. Antecedents of cerebral palsy: Multivariate analysis of risk. *N Engl J Med* 1986, 315: 81–86.

Nemoto EM. Pathogenesis of cerebral ischemia-anoxia. *Crit Care Med* 1978, 6: 203.

Neonatal resuscitation: India. *National Neonatology Forum of India,* 2nd edition, 2014.

Nochimson DJ, Twibeville JS, Terry JE, *et al*. The non-stress test. *Obstet Gynecol* 1978, 51: 419.

Palmer C, Lannucci RC, Toufight J. Reduction of perinatal hypoxic-ischemic brain damage with allopurinol. *Pediatr Res* 1990, 27: 332–336.

Paneth N, Raymond IS. Cerebral palsy and mental retardation in relation to indicators of perinatal asphyxia. *Amer J Obstet Gynecol* 1983, 147–960.

Pasternak JF. Hypoxic-ischemic brain damage in the term infant. *Pediatr Cl N Amer* 1993, 40: 106–1071.

Paul SP, Abdelrhim H, Heep A. Management of hypoxic-ischemic encephalopathy. *Indian J Pediatr* 2015, 82(6): 493–96.

Paul SP, Abdelrhim H, Heep A. Management of hypoxic-ischemic encephalopathy. *Indian J Pediatr* 2015, 82(6): 493–496.

Paul VK, Shankar V, Deorari AK, Singh M. Tracheal suction in meconium-stained neonates. *J Pediatr* 1989, 144: 508.

Paul VK, Singh M, Sundaram KR, Deorari AK. Correlates of mortality among hospital-born neonates with birth asphyxia in Delhi. *Nat Med J India* 1997, 10: 54–57.

Perlman JM, Kattwinkel J. Delivery room resuscitation: past, present and future. *Clin Perinatol* 2006, 100 (10): 899–908.

Perlman JM, Wyllie J, Kattwinkel J, *et al*. Special report on neonatal resuscitation: 2010 international consensus on cardiopulmonary resuscitation and emergency cardiovascular care science with treatment recommendations. *Pediatrics* 2010, 126: e1318–1345.

Pichler G, Schmolzer GM, urlesberger B. Cerebral tissue oxygenation during immediate neonatal transition and resuscitation. *Front Pediatr* 2017, 5:29.

Pleiss AJ, Jhonston MV. Hypoxic-ischemic injury in newborn: cellular mechanism and potential strategies for neuroprotection. *Clinics Perinatol* 1997, 29: 627–654.

Prechtl HFR, Einspieter C, Cioni Giovanni, *et al*. An early marker for neurological deficits after perinatal brain lesions. *Lancet* 1997, 349: 1361–1363.

Raina A, Pandita A, Harish R, Yachha M, Jamwal A. Treating perinatal asphyxia with theophylline at birth helps to reduce the severity of renal dysfunction in term neonates. *Acta Paediatr* 2016, 105(10): e448–51.

Raju TNK, Doshi U, Vidyasagar D. Low cerebral perfusion pressure: An indicator of poor prognosis in asphyxiated term infants. *Brain Dev* 1983, 5: 478.

Robertson NJ, Nakakeeto M, Hagmann C, *et al*. Therapeutic hypothermia for birth asphyxia in low-resource setting: a pilot randomized controlled trial. *Lancet* 2008, 372: 801–803.

Rockoff MA. Brain resuscitation—barbiturates and other anesthetic agents. *Semin Neurol* 1984, 4: 408.

Ruth V, Fyhrquist F, Clemens C, Raivio KO. Cord plasma vasopressin, erythropoietin and hypoxanthine as indices of asphyxia at birth. *Pediatrics* 1988, 24: 490.

Sachdeva A, Gunasekaran V, Malhotra P, Bhurani D, Yadav SP, Radhakrishnan N. *et al*. Umbilical cord blood banking: Concensus statement of the Indian Academy of Pediatrics. *Indian Pediatr* 2018, 55: 489–494.

Saraswat D, Aradhya G, Chaitali R, Guruprasad G. Therapeutic hypothermia in asphyxiated neonates, using phase changing material (MiraCradle): experience from neonatal intensive care unit of tertiary care center south India. *Int J Pediatr Res* 2019, 6(12): 606–612.

Sarnat HB, Sarnat MS. Neonatal encehpalopathy following fetal distress. *Arch Neurol* 1975, 33: 696.

Saugstad OD. Neonatal oxygen radical disease. In: Recent Advances in Pediatrics, 1992 *Churchill Livingstone,* pp 173–187.

Saugstad OD. Practical aspects of resuscitating asphyxiated newborn infants. *Eur J Pediatr* 1998, 157 (suppl 1): S11–S15.

Saugstad OD, Ramji S, Vento M. Resuscitation of depressed newborn infants with ambient air or pure oxygen: a meta-analysis. *Biol Neonate* 2005, 87: 27–34.

Scott H. Outcome of very severe birth asphyxia. *Arch Dis Child* 1976, 51: 712.

Shankaran S. Current status of hypothermia for hypoxemic ischemia of the newborn. *Indian J Pediatr* 2014, 81(6):578–584.

Singh M. Diagnosis and management of perinatal asphyxia: current concepts. *Indian Pediatr* 1994, 31: 1169–1174.

Stockard JE, Stockard JJ, Kleinberg F, Westmoreland BF. Prognostic value of brainstem auditory evoked potentials in neonates. *Arch Neurol* 1983, 40: 360–365.

Svenningsen NW, Blennoth G, Lindroth M, *et al.* Brain-oriented resuscitation. *Arch Dis Child* 1982, 57: 176.

Sykes GS, Johnson P, Ashworth F, *et al.* Do Apgar scores indicate asphyxia? *Lancet* 1982, II, 72: 232.

Tanigasalam V, Bhat BV, Adhisivam B, *et at.* Predicting severity of acute kidney injury in term neonates with perinatal asphyxia using urinary neutrophil gelatinase associated lipocalin. *Indian J Pediatr* 2016, 83(12): 1374–78.

The Apgar score policy statement of AAP/ACOG. *Pediatrics* 2006, 117: 1444–1447.

Thiringer K. Cord plasma hypoxanthine as a measure of foetal asphyxia. *Acta Paediatr Scand* 1983, 72: 232.

Thomas N, Chakrapani Y, Rebekah G, Kareti K, Devasahayam S. Phase changing material: an alternative method for cooling babies with hypoxic ischaemic encephalopathy. *Neonatology* 2015, 107(4):266–70.

Thoresen M, Wyatt J. Keeping a cool head, post-hypoxic hypothermia—an old idea revisited. *Acta Paediatr* 1997, 86: 1029–33.

Vain NE, Szyld EG, Prudent LM, *et al.* Oropharyngeal and nasopharyngeal suctioning of meconium-stained neonates before delivery of their shoulders: multicentric randomized controlled trial. *Lancet* 2004, 364: 597–602.

Van-Rheenen AU, Brabin BJ. Late umbilical cord clamping as an intervention for reducing iron deficiency anemia in term infant in developing and industrialized countries: a systematic review. *Ann Trop Pediatr* 2004, 24: 3–16.

Venucci RC. Current and potentially new management strategies for perinatal hypoxic-ischemic encephalopathy. *Pediatrics* 1990, 85: 961–968.

Wilkinson DJ, Singh M, Wyatt J. Ethical challenges in the use of therapeutic hypothermia in Indian neonatal units. *Indian Pediatr* 2010, 47: 387–393.

Wilson MG. Placental abnormalities and fetal disease. *Amer J Dis Child* 1964, 108: 154.

Wiswell TE. Delivery room management of the meocnium-stained newborn. *J Perinatol* 2008, 28: S19–S26.

Wyckoff MH, Berg RA. Optimizing chest compressions during delivery room resuscitation. *Semin Fetal Neonat Med* 2008, 13: 410–415.

Examination of the Baby

MATERNAL AND PERINATAL HISTORY

Just as children are not mini-adults, the neonates are not mini-children. They have unique health problems and a different clinical approach is followed for their clinical evaluation. It must be remembered that a newborn baby is around 9 months old at birth unless prematurely born. Neonatology is not a system-limited speciality, it deals with all the systems of a newborn baby (up to 28 days of life). A detailed history regarding diseases suffered by the mother and drugs taken during pregnancy should be elicited (Table 7.1).

Basic Indicators

Health and wellbeing of a fetus is dependent upon the health and nutrition of the mother (not the father!) because she is both the seed as well as the soil wherein the baby is nurtured for nine months. Ask whether it was a natural pregnancy or *in vitro* fertilization (IVF) with or without surrogacy. The date of birth, gestational age and birth weight should be recorded. The gestational age is calculated from the first day of the last menstrual period till the date of birth and is expressed in completed weeks and days. For example, gestation of 32 completed week plus 6 days is expressed as 32 6/7 weeks. The education, occupation and economic status of parents should be enquired. Age of the mother is important because young mothers (<18 years) are likely to produce low birth weight babies and have an increased risk of delivery hazards while elderly mothers (>35 years) are at an increased risk to have babies with congenital malformations, inborn errors of metabolism and chromosomal disorders.

Previous Obstetrical History

The gravidity (number of all conceptions including abortions, stillbirths, etc. with possible causes) and

TABLE 7.1 Review of maternal and perinatal history

Family history
History of hereditary, metabolic, chromosomal and developmental disorders, biological child or adopted.

Maternal history
Duration of marriage, or is it child out of wedlock, IVF, and surrogacy. Maternal age, blood group, chronic illnesses like diabetes mellitus, hypertension, renal disease, cardiac disease, lung disease, endocrinal disorder, bleeding disorder, CNS or psychological disorder, sexually transmitted diseases including herpes and HIV, TORCH screening should be recorded.

Previous obstetrical history
Gravidity, parity, abortions, stillbirths, neonatal deaths (with possible causes), prematurity, LBW or growth retarded babies, obstructed labor, cesarean section, congenital malformations and history of blood transfusion.

Current pregnancy
Natural pregnancy or IVF, gestational age, weight gain, excessive vomiting, bleeding, polyhydramnios/oligohydramnios, ultrasound examination, diagnostic and therapeutic procedures done during pregnancy. Ask for history of pregnancy-induced hypertension, pre-eclampsia, infections (UTI, diarrhea/dysentery, malaria and tuberculosis), surgery, drugs of abuse and medications (hormones, glucocorticoids, tocolytic agents and antibiotics).

Labor and delivery
Fetal distress, presentation, mode of delivery, prelabor rupture of membranes, and its duration, duration of labor, amnionitis, amniotic fluid (volume, clear or meconium-stained), anesthesia/analgesia, Apgar score, resuscitation required and examination of placenta.

parity (number of live births) should be recorded. The interval between successive pregnancies and their outcome should be enquired. History of recurrent abortions and stillbirths is suggestive of incompetent cervical os, diabetes mellitus, syphilis and Rh-isoimmunization. Gestational maturity, birth weight, congenital malformations; obstructed labor, and mode of delivery of previous babies should be recorded. The neonatal course, unusual manifestations and outcome of previous babies should be ascertained.

Prepregnancy Health Status

Maternal systemic disorders like heart disease, hypertension, bronchial asthma, chronic renal disease, tuberculosis and anemia, are associated with increased risk of abortions, stillbirths, intrauterine growth retardation, premature births and increased perinatal mortality rate. History of maternal endocrinal disorders, such as diabetes mellitus, thyrotoxicosis, myxedema and hyperparathyroidism should be asked. Systemic lupus erythematosus may be associated with complete heart block in the fetus. Chronic undernutrition of the mother during childhood and adolescence leads to short stature (<145 cm) and low adult weight (<40 kg) which are associated with increased risk of low birth weight babies. History of sexually transmitted diseases including genital herpes, syphilis and HIV should be checked. Rhesus blood group should be identified because of potential risk of Rh-isoimmunization, if Rh-negative mother is carrying an Rh-positive fetus. Tetanus toxoid and rubella vaccination status should be checked.

Course of Pregnancy

The adequacy and quality of antenatal care received should be ascertained. First trimester of pregnancy is characterized by embryogenesis. Diseases suffered and drugs taken during current pregnancy should be recorded. Ask for history suggestive of maternal rubella, cytomegalovirus disease and toxoplasmosis which are manifested by fever, skin rash and posterior cervical lymphadenopathy. Ask history of petechiae or thrombocytopenia during pregnancy. The abnormalities reported on antenatal ultrasound scans should be recorded. In a malformed or sick baby, a detailed history of medications taken during pregnancy should be recorded because they may produce unusual clinical manifestations in the newborn baby.

Maternal ABO and rhesus blood type, indirect Coombs' titer (if mother is Rh-negative), hemogram, VDRL and whenever indicated, carrier status for hepatitis B virus and HIV and TORCH screening should be checked. The diagnostic and therapeutic procedures undertaken during pregnancy should be recorded.

Dietary intake, especially during second half of pregnancy, is crucial to ensure optimal growth of the fetus. During an uncomplicated pregnancy, most Indian mothers gain between 6 and 10 kg body weight.

History of pregnancy-induced hypertension with or without urinary abnormalities is associated with placental dysfunction, intrauterine growth retardation, perinatal hypoxia, and birth asphyxia. Ask for history of bleeding during pregnancy whether it is due to abruptio placentae or placenta previa. The quantity of amniotic fluid should be checked. *Oligohydramnios* may be associated with prolonged rupture of membranes and chorioamnionitis. It is associated with placental dysfunction, postmaturity, renal agenesis, polycystic or multicystic dysplastic kidneys, and obstructive uropathy. It is commonly associated with toxemia of pregnancy and maternal medications with prostaglandin and ACE inhibitors. *Polyhydramnios* (amniotic fluid >2 liters) is associated with maternal diabetes mellitus, syphilis, pre-eclamptic toxemia and fetal congenital malformations, such as open neural tube defects, anencephaly, ectopia vesicae, gastroschisis, esophageal atresia, duodenal/jejunal atresia, diaphragmatic hernia, Down syndrome, twins and hydrops fetalis. Meconium-stained liquor amnii in a vertex presenting baby is indicative of fetal distress or fetal diarrhea due to listeriosis.

Labor and Delivery

History of chorioamnionitis, prolonged rupture of membranes (>24 hours) and unclean or too many vaginal examinations are recognized markers of intrauterine bacterial pneumonia. Chorioamnionitis is diagnosed on the basis of maternal fever plus any two of the five clinical parameters like maternal leukocytosis, fetal and maternal tachycardia, uterine tenderness and foul smelling liquor. Prolonged labor (>18 hr first stage, and >6 hr second stage) and difficult delivery are associated with increased risk of birth asphyxia and birth trauma. Determine whether the baby was delivered vaginally following spontaneous labor or after induction/augmentation with oxytocin. Ask for history of instrumentation (forceps, vacuum), or operative delivery (elective or emergency cesarean section). Check whether any evidences of fetal distress were present during labor. Evidences of cephalopelvic disproportion, cord around the neck or cord prolapse, etc. should be noted. Analgesics and anesthetics used during labor can adversely affect the fetus.

Neonatal History

Ask whether baby cried immediately after birth or was asphyxiated. Details regarding Apgar score should be checked in case of institutionalized delivery. If 1-minute Apgar score is low, it should be checked at 5 minutes and 10 minutes. Determine whether baby was kept in the NICU or roomed-in with the mother. General activity and history of feeding during first week should be asked. Ascertain the time of passage of first urine (upper limit is 48 hours) and stools (upper limit is 24 hours) after birth. Urine may cause discoloration of diaper in certain metabolic disorders. Red diaper syndrome is a benign condition due to excretion of excessive uric acid or overgrowth of *Serratia marcescens*, black staining of diaper on exposure to air due to alkaptonuria and blue diaper because of Hartnup disease and tryptophane gastrointestinal malabsorption syndrome. An occasional vomiting on the first day of life is common and is of no significance. Ask for history of inactivity, severe jaundice, seizures and feeding difficulties during neonatal period.

History of Present Illness

Ask and assess the chief complaints as told by the mother or attendant in a chronological order. The newborn babies manifest non-specific symptoms due to a variety of disorders. They have a limited capacity to produce specific symptoms. Refusal of feeds, lethargy and inactivity are common manifestations due to several neonatal disorders. *The nature of predisposing or associated conditions is more crucial to make a diagnosis in a newborn baby.* Assess the predisposing factors (gestational maturity, birth weight, birth asphyxia, prolonged rupture of membranes, etc.), age of onset, and evolution of symptoms. The common neonatal conditions include birth trauma, asphyxia, respiratory distress syndrome, jaundice, septicemia, bleeding manifestations, inborn errors of metabolism and congenital malformations.

Preterm babies are vulnerable to develop a variety of disorders including hyaline membrane disease, metabolic disorders, hypothermia, infections, necrotizing enterocolitis, intraventricular hemorrhage, patent ductus arteriosus, retinopathy of prematurity, etc. Neonates are known to manifest a large number of minor developmental peculiarities and physiological problems which need to be identified to offer reassurance and advice to the mother. On the other hand, when a neonate is genuinely sick, he cannot be managed on an ambulatory basis and must be admitted in a hospital providing level II or intensive neonatal care.

Family History

Ask for the family history of developmental and metabolic disorders. History of neonatal deaths in sibship or family should be asked. History of a similar disorder in a previous sibling should be ascertained. History of consanguinity among the parents should be asked.

Immunizations

Check whether BCG, hepatitis B and oral polio vaccines have been taken or not. Maternal status of tetanus toxoid vaccination should be enquired.

EXAMINATION AT BIRTH

The examination should be conducted in a warm comfortable room with the baby completely undressed and placed on a flat surface at a height convenient for the physician. A good source of light should be available and examiner's hands should be clean and warm. The detailed examination is conducted routinely at birth, within 24 hours or next day and at the time of discharge.

The aim of examination of the baby at birth is to ensure and assess that lungs have expanded and that air passages are not obstructed, assess Apgar scores at 1 and 5 minutes after birth and to make an early diagnosis of life-threatening congenital malformations and birth injuries. The baby should make a smooth transition from a dependent fetal life to an independent neonatal existence.

SCREENING FOR CONGENITAL MALFORMATIONS

The maternal history should be screened for any ingestion of teratogenic and goiterogenic drugs, irradiation and viral infections during first trimester of pregnancy. The existence of polyhydramnios in the mother should alert the pediatrician to the possibility of obstruction in the upper intestinal tract. About 25% cases of esophageal atresia and 75% cases of obstruction of the duodenum and upper jejunum are associated with polyhydramnios. In fact, one out of every seven cases of polyhydramnios is associated with upper intestinal obstruction. Oligohydramnios, on the other hand, may be associated with bilateral renal agenesis and Potter facies. Family history of any developmental anomalies should be inquired. A quick but complete examination should be conducted with the following scheme in mind.

Birth weight and gestational age The incidence of anomalies in preterm babies is twice compared to term appropriate-for-gestational age babies. In small-for-dates (especially hypoplastic) babies, the incidence of anomalies is 10 to 20 times higher. A thorough clinical examination and observation of these babies is essential for early diagnosis of anomalies.

Single umbilical artery and single palmar crease The cut end of the cord should be inspected for number of the vessels. A single umbilical artery, which has an incidence of around 0.8%, is associated with internal congenital malformations in 15 to 20% of cases. The commonly associated malformations include esophageal atresia, imperforate anus and genitourinary anomalies. Single palmar crease should alert one to make a thorough search for additional anomalies.

Hypoplasia of the depressor anguli oris muscle The asymmetric facies due to congenital hypoplasia of the depressor anguli oris muscle (DAOM) should be looked for because these infants have additional associated anomalies in over 20% of cases. During crying, angle of the mouth and mandible are pulled down with flattening of the nasolabial fold on the normal side due to unopposed action of DAOM. Cardiovascular anomalies and congenital dislocation of hips are most commonly associated.

Orifice counting and their patency The anomalies are concentrated around orifices. Look for cleft palate and ectopic or closed anus. The patency of esophagus should be checked by passing a stiff rubber catheter into the stomach in the situations listed below. Some pediatricians recommend this procedure routinely in all babies.

- Small-for-dates baby
- Single umbilical artery
- Polyhydramnios
- Maternal diabetes mellitus
- Frothiness at mouth and drooling of saliva
- Choking while feeding

When the catheter has reached the stomach, the gastric contents should be aspirated. If gastric aspirate exceeds 20 mL, it is strongly suggestive of high intestinal obstruction.

Midline lesions on the back and front Spina bifida, meningomyelocele, pilonidal sinus, ambiguous genitalia, hypospadias and exomphalos or omphalocele should be looked for.

Evidences of respiratory difficulty The surgical causes of respiratory distress should be excluded and an urgent X-ray chest should be taken when indicated.

Routine systemic examination Abdomen should be palpated for any masses and heart examined for its position and murmurs. 'Dextrocardia', due to pushing of the heart, in association with respiratory difficulty is suggestive of left-sided pneumothorax and diaphragmatic hernia.

FIRST-DAY EXAMINATION

The aim is to record certain measurements, to make sure that no anomalies have been overlooked, to inquire about feeding behavior and to look for onset of jaundice. History of frothiness, choking and vomiting after feeds should be asked and evaluated. Inquiry should be made regarding the time of passage of first meconium and urine.

Vital signs Vital signs should be recorded when baby is quiet and in-between feeds. Respiratory rate varies between 40 and 60 breaths/minute. It is thoraco-abdominal without any retractions and grunting. The breathing is usually periodic and irregular. Heart rate is around 140 ±20 beats/min and can rise sharply following feeding and after a bout of crying. Radial arteries are difficult to palpate in a newborn baby. Average blood pressure in a term baby is around 60/40 mm Hg. Thus, in a term baby, heart rate and breathing rate are double in frequency while blood pressure is one-half of an adult. Skin temperature of a healthy baby is 36.5°C. The nurses and physicians should train themselves to assess the baby's temperature with their hands. The trunk should feel warm while extremities should be reasonably warm and pink. When feet and hands are cold and pale while trunk is warm, it indicates that baby is in cold stress.

General behavior Look for color, respirations, movements of limbs and their posture, general alertness and activity of the child. Routine neurological examination or even elicitation of Moro response is unnecessary, if the baby is active and feeding normally. Onset of jaundice within 24 hours of age is indicative of a serious disorder.

Anthropometry Weight, occipitofrontal head circumference, chest circumference at nipples and crown-heel length are recorded (Figure 7.1). The head circumference should preferably be taken after 24 hours when caput succedaneum and overriding of sutures would have disappeared. The average head circumference in full term babies vary between 34 and 36 cm. The length should be recorded on an infantometer and it varies between 47 and 50 cm in average term babies. Anthropometric measurements should be plotted on an appropriate intrauterine growth chart and interpreted in relation to the gestational age of the baby.

Gestational assessment Assess gestation by physical and neurological examination, if menstrual history is unavailable or uncertain. Refer to page 149 for detailed Assessment of Gestational Age.

Examination of the Baby

7

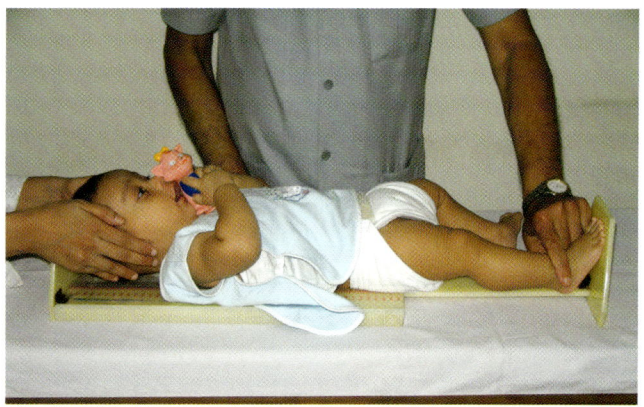

Figure 7.1 Crown-heel length being recorded on an infanto-meter.

Skull Examine for caput succedaneum, cephalhematoma, subgaleal hemorrhage, forceps marks, encephalocele and widely separated or closed sutures. In preterm, small-for-dates and hydrocephalic babies, head circumference is more than 3 cm bigger than the chest circumference. Examine anterior fontanel for size and tension. The fontanel should be flat when baby is examined in a sitting position. Abnormally large anterior fontanel at birth is seen in infants with cretinism, trisomy syndromes, intrauterine growth retardation, rickets, hypophosphatasia and osteogenesis imperfecta. Craniotabes should be looked for away from the anterior fontanel and it is suggestive of congenital rickets and osteogenesis imperfecta. Microcephaly with fused sutures, chinky fontanels or odd shaped skull are suggestive of craniosynostosis.

Face Look for abnormal facies by paying due attention to size, shape and position of ears, distance between two eyes and their alignment, size of the oral opening and tongue, shape of the nose and its bridge, patency of nostrils, size and depth of philtrum, micrognathia or retrognathia when face is assessed in profile. Recheck for cleft palate by examining the oral cavity right up to the uvula. Eyes should be examined for conjunctivitis, subconjunctival hemorrhage, corneal haziness, cataract, coloboma, glaucoma (large and cloudy cornea) and red reflex. The normal cornea in a neonate measures less than 10.5 mm in horizontal diameter.

Neck Examine for goiter, thyroglossal or branchial arch cysts or sinuses, hair line, webbing and range of movements. Look for any torticollis, tightening or "tumor" in the sternocleidomastoid muscle.

Skin Examine for jaundice, cyanosis, petechiae, lanugo hair, birth marks, hemangiomata, rashes and evidences of dysmaturity. Toxic erythema or urticaria neonatorum is common in term babies during first week of life. Erythematous skin rash with central pallor appears on the face on second or third day of life and spreads to the trunk and extremities in next 24 hours. It disappears spontaneously after 2–3 days without any treatment. The rash should be differentiated from pyoderma, transient pustular melanosis and congenital syphilis. Congenital syphilis is characterized by maculopapular exfoliative or vesiculobullous skin eruptions involving palms and soles. Perioral cracks or fissures (rhagades) and perianal condylomata should be looked for. Look for evidences of congenital ichthyosis.

Spine Spina bifida, kyphosis, scoliosis, pilonidal sinus and tuft of hair should be looked for.

Extremities Look for anomalies of digits (oligodactyly, polydactyly, syndactyly), club foot, calcaneo valgus and varus deformities of knees. Mild degrees of forefoot adduction, tibial bowing or torsion are normal.

Abdomen and genitalia A yellow umbilical cord at birth suggests fetal anoxia, meconium staining or severe Rh-isoimmunization. The presence of "scaphoid" or flat abdomen at birth with respiratory distress is suggestive of diaphragmatic hernia. Distended abdomen at birth may be due to meconium peritonitis, large gut obstruction and obstructive uropathy. Look for umbilical and inguinal herniae and palpate for any masses. Liver edge is normally felt 2 cm below the costal margin. Spleen tip and occasionally lower poles of kidneys, especially right, may be palpable with effort. However, if spleen and kidneys are easily palpable, it is abnormal. Abdominal examination in a newborn baby is often unsatisfactory unless the baby is quiet or asleep during feeds, otherwise the abdomen becomes tense during palpation. To relax abdominal wall, the infant is supported with a soft pillow in a semi-reclining position or a supine infant is slightly lifted off the cot by holding at both the ankles. Bimanual palpation for kidneys is attempted with one hand by placing the fingers over the loin while thumb searches for the kidney with gentle, steadily increasing pressure subcostally in a posterior and cephalad direction. Obstructive uropathy is characterized by pressure of three abdominal masses (distended bladder and two kidneys) and overhanging wrinkled skin of the abdominal wall. *The presence of a solitary abdominal mass in a neonate should be considered as malignant unless proved otherwise.*

Genitals should be examined for any anatomical abnormalities, undescended testes and hydrocele. In a term infant, scrotum is large, pendulous, darkly pigmented and testes are easily palpable due to absence of cremasteric reflex at birth. Prepuce is non-retractable in newborn babies. The penile length of less than 2.5 cm is abnormal. Ambiguous genitals with "salt losing syndrome" (vomiting, diarrhea, dehydration and shock) is suggestive of congenital adrenal hyperplasia. Look for opening of urethra to exclude epispadias and hypospadias. The presence of "hooded foreskin" is strongly suggestive of hypospadias and it contraindicates the procedure of circumcision. Inguinal hernia is more common on the right side because processus vaginalis closes earlier on the left side. As opposed to umbilical hernia, inguinal hernia must be operated within 4–6 weeks of diagnosis because of high incidence of incarceration during infancy. Hydrocele should be looked for but its excision should be delayed till 6 months of age because most of them are communicating type and get resorbed spontaneously.

Heart Auscultate for any cardiac murmur when baby is quiet and before doing any painful examination (see Chapter 20 for details). When heart sounds are better heard on the right side, it is suggestive of dextrocardia in a quiet baby and left-sided pneumothorax or diaphragmatic hernia in a distressed baby. Gallop rhythm is ominous while a split S_2 is normal and reassuring. Femorals should be palpated to exclude the possibility of coarctation of aorta. In infants with coarctation, the femoral pulse may be normal in first few days of life while ductus is still open. Babies with structural cardiac malformations may be asympto-matic in the newborn period. It is recommended to measure post-ductal arterial oxygen saturation with a pulse oximeter before the baby is discharged. When fractional oxygen saturation (SaO_2) is below 95% on two occasions in a hemodynamically stable baby, echocardiography should be done to exclude congeni-tal cardiac malformations.

Chest In the absence of respiratory difficulty or any other complaints, such as cough or feeding problem, the routine examination of chest is a waste of time and unnecessary. Look for tachypnea, apnea, dyspnea, grunting and retractions of chest. Cough is an uncommon symptom in newborn babies and may occur due to meconium aspiration syndrome and pneumonia especially due to *Chlamydia trachomatis*.

Central Nervous System

Routine neurological examination in a healthy term baby is unnecessary. The information regarding activity, general behavior and feeding behavior of the baby as reported by the mother, absence of any abnormalities of skull and spine and symmetry of spontaneous movements of limbs on the two sides are enough to rule out any significant neurological abnormality. There is no need to elicit Moro reflex in apparently normal babies. In general, a detailed neonatal neurological examination is usually done for the following purposes.

1. Diagnosis of an acute neurological illness.
2. Prognosis for future neuromotor development following perinatal hazards and neurological illness.
3. Assessment of gestational age.

The common symptoms of neurological disorder in a newborn baby include irritability, frank or subtle seizurs, high-pitched crying, drowsiness, inability to suck (despite gestational maturity of >34 weeks), bulging anterior fontanel, lack of movements of the limb(s) and seizures. Hypoxic-ischemic encephalopathy and metabolic disorders are common causes of seizures in a newborn baby. Age at onset of seizures provides useful clue to the underlying cause of seizures.

Hips The hip joints should be examined in the end for evidences of congenital dislocation in all babies. In dislocation, head of the femur is displaced superiorly and posteriorly. The condition is more common in girls especially first born, breech presentation, post-maturity and oligohydramnios. There may be a family history of the condition and infant may have other associated postural deformities especially in the feet. Place the infant supine on a firm surface and flex both the hips at right angles and look for alignment of the knees. On the side of dislocation, the knee would be at a lower level due to posterior displacement of femoral head (Galeazzi test). The classical signs of dislocation are not seen in the neonatal period. The instability of the hip joint is best detected by a modified Ortolani/Barlow maneuver as described below.

The infant lies on his back with legs towards the examiner. The baby should be undressed from waist downwards. The examination should be performed with care, gentleness and warm hands. The infant should be calm, relaxed and adequately fed. It is preferable to test one hip at a time. The examiner tries to assess whether the hip is dislocated or it is unstable and dislocatable. For examination of the left hip, the examiner steadies the infant's pelvis between the thumb of his left hand placed on the symphysis pubis and the fingers under the sacrum (Figure 7.2). The left thigh is flexed by keeping the knees bent. It is grasped by examiner's right hand by placing index and middle fingers on the outside over the greater trochanter

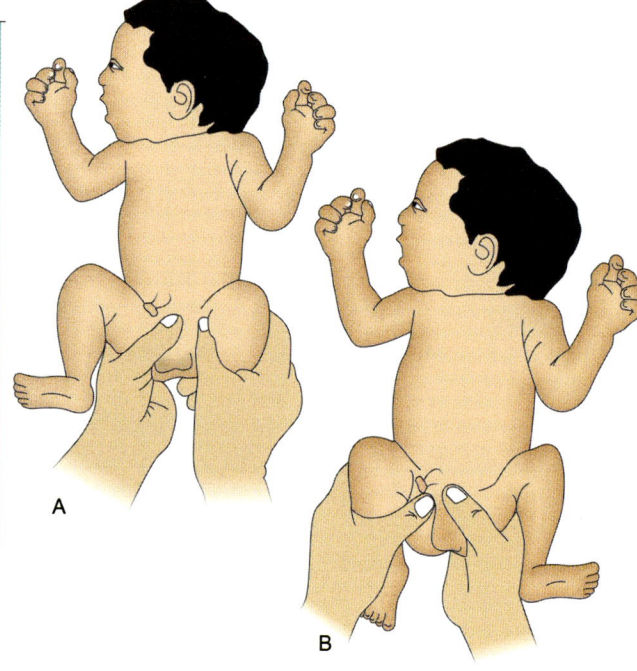

Figure 7.2 Examination for congenital dislocation of hips. Each hip is tested separately. (A) Examination of left hip and (B) shows position for examination of right hip. See text for details.

and thumb on the inner side of the thigh opposite the lesser trochanter. In the first maneuver, the examiner assesses whether the hip is dislocated or not. The pressure is applied over the greater trachanter with the middle finger and hip is abducted in an attempt to relocate the displaced femoral head back into the acetabulum (Ortolani test). If the head is felt to move (usually not more than 0.5 cm) with or without a palpable and/ or audible 'clunk', it confirms the presence of dislocation.

If dislocation is not present, an effort is then made to test for subluxation (dislocatability) of the hip. With the thumb placed on the inner side of the thigh, backward and outward pressure is applied to the head of the femur by adducting the thigh in an attempt to dislocate it. If the femoral head is felt to move backwards over the rim of acetabulum, for a distance of 0.5 cm, with or without a palpable or audible clunk, the hip is said to be dislocatable (Barlow test). The right hip is examined by reversing the role of examiner's hands. The ligamentous clicks without movement of the head of the femur in or out of the acetabulum may be elicited in 5–10% of normal hips and should be disregarded.

Daily "Clinical Screening" of the Baby

Between first-day examination and the day of discharge, detailed examination is unnecessary and

may in fact be harmful for the baby because of potential risk of introducing infection. The baby–mother pair should be approached twice a day to inquire about any feeding problems, vomiting, bowel disorders and to assess and allay the anxiety of the mother regarding various developmental peculiarities which may attract her attention. The baby should "look" healthy, trunk should be warm, and extremities should be warm and pink. The onset and intensity of jaundice should be watched. Any evidences of superficial infections such as conjunctivitis, pyoderma, umbilical sepsis and oral thrush should be looked for.

Examination and Screening at Discharge

A detailed examination of the baby at the time of discharge is essential to make sure that no anomalies and birth injuries have been missed and initial lactational and feeding difficulties have been resolved. Careful auscultation of the heart is essential because previously detected functional murmur may no longer be audible and new murmurs may appear any time during the neonatal period.

Pulse oximetry According to recommendations of American Academy of Pediatrics (AAP), all newborns should undergo pulse oximetry screening before discharge. The screening should be done after 24 hours of age or shortly before discharge, if baby is less than 24 hours of age. The measurement of oxygen saturation should be done in the right hand and either of the foot. The screening is considered 'negative' and the baby is declared 'passed', if the SpO_2 is 95% or greater in both right hand and either foot and the difference between SpO_2 of right hand and foot is ≤3%. The screening is 'positive' and baby is declared 'failed', if the oxygen saturation is less than 90% in any one extremity, or less than 95% in both the extremities, or there is absolute oxygen saturation difference of more than 3% between the right hand and either foot on three consecutive measurements taken one hour apart. The "failed" infants should undergo 2D echocardiography to exclude congenital heart defect.

Hearing Evoked otoacoustic emission (EOAE) testing can be done with a handheld device that produces soft clicks to measure the echoes emitted by the eardrum.

Screening for inborn errors of metabolism Blood samples should be taken on special filter papers for screening of newborns for certain inherited metabolic disorders. There is a lack of uniform policy for routine screening of neonates in various NICUs in India.

The mother should be advised about feeding, vitamins and iron supplements, general cleanliness, immunizations and given an appointment for visit to the Well Baby Clinic. High-risk babies discharged from the NICU should be followed up for developmental assessment and detailed examination of central nervous system and special senses in a Special Developmental Clinic.

Sick Babies in the NICU

Babies are looked after in the neonatal intensive care unit (NICU) when a baby is extremely preterm, critically sick, malformed or when mother is unwell or unwilling to look after the baby. Check perinatal events and nature of resuscitation provided. Look for various life-threatening conditions like RDS, seizures, sepsis, jaundice, bleeding manifestations and shock. Ask for history of procedures, like CPAP, assisted ventilation and its duration, whether received surfactant or not, oxygen dependency, thoracostomy, simple or exchange blood transfusion. The NICU protocol should be followed for routine ultrasound examination of brain and indirect ophthalmoscopy for ROP.

Check the vital signs on the monitor. Assess hemodynamic stability including activity, color, capillary refill time by blanching the sternum. Is the baby having any respiratory distress or apneic attacks? Is the baby tolerating the enteral feeds without any abdominal distension or gastric residuals. The baby should be screened for sepsis, patent ductus arteriosus, necrotizing enterocolitis and intraventricular hemorrhage. Is the daily weight gain velocity of the baby satisfactory? The baby should be screened daily to look for clinical criteria to assess the well-being of the baby in the NICU (Box 7.1).

Box 7.1: Cot-side criteria indicating that a preterm baby is healthy

- Baby is alert, active and pink.
- Vital signs are stable.
- Trunk is warm to touch and extremities are reasonably warm and pink.
- No respiratory distress and apneic attacks.
- Baby is tolerating enteral feeds without any vomiting and abdominal distension.
- Daily weight gain is 1.0–1.5% of the body weight, i.e. 10–15 g/kg per day.

ASSESSMENT OF GESTATIONAL AGE

For classification of babies on the basis of birth weight and gestational age, it is mandatory that accurate gestational age of the baby should be known. The assessment of gestational age on the basis of date of last menstrual period is reliable only if the menstrual cycles are regular and unmodified by oral contraceptives or maternal diseases, and the last menstrual period had been normal for flow and duration. Some mothers may not remember the date of last menstrual period. In these situations, clinical assessment of gestation assumes practical importance.

Antenatal Assessment of Gestational Age

The assessment of gestational maturity of the fetus is required, if induction of labor is being planned or if there is a discrepancy between the size of the fetus and calculated gestation on the basis of last menstrual period.

Clinical The date of last menstrual period, height of uterine fundus during early pregnancy (at 16 weeks uterus is just above the pubic symphysis), date of quickenings (18th week), appearance of fetal heart sounds (16 to 18 weeks), measurement of fetal ovoid and femur length by ultrasonic techniques, maternal weight gain and engagement of head may offer useful guidelines for gestational assessment.

Biochemical Organic constituents in the liquor amnii, creatinine and urea progressively rise with advancing maturity while protein, glucose, lactic and pyruvic acids progressively decline. The rise in creatinine is due to increasing muscle mass as the baby grows and would underestimate the maturity of small-for-dates or growth-retarded babies. Amniotic fluid creatinine level of more than 2 mg/dL is associated with gestational maturity of at least 36 weeks. The lecithin to sphingomyelin ratio of amniotic fluid is a useful criterion of pulmonary maturity and is often taken into consideration when premature induction of labor is planned. Lecithin/sphingomyelin ratio of more than 2 is indicative of satisfactory lung maturity, except in mothers with diabetes mellitus.

Cytological Cytological parameters of gestational assessment include vaginal wall cytology which shows the presence of more superficial cells as term approaches. Amniotic fluid cytology for organophilic squamous cells, which are stained orange with Nile blue sulfate, is a reliable method for prenatal assessment of gestation. These anucleated orange staining cells

Examination of the Baby

7

which are derived from the sebaceous glands of the fetus, considerably increase after 38 weeks of gestation. Between 32 and 37 weeks of gestation, about 10% of amniotic cells show these characteristics. Before 30 weeks of gestation, practically no such cells are seen.

Radiological The ossification centers at the lower femoral and upper tibial epiphyses appear at 36 weeks and 38 weeks, respectively. Intrauterine growth retardation and cretinism delay the ossification. The absence of an ossification center, therefore, does not indicate immaturity, but its presence and size are indicative of maturity.

Assessment of Gestation after Birth

The clinical assessment of gestation at birth by physical and neurological examinations of the baby is more reliable as compared to the methods recommended for assessment of baby *in utero*. As gestation proceeds, the baby grows and matures physically and neurologically. The anthropometric measurements, such as weight, length, head and chest circumference are unreliable parameters of maturity because they may be adversely affected by intrauterine growth retardation. Head circumference and length are relatively spared in a baby with intrauterine malnutrition as compared to weight and chest circumference.

Grouping of Babies into Preterm and Term

In a baby with unknown gestation, assessment of the maturity of the baby on the basis of physical characteristics alone is fairly reliable. This simple approach helps in deciding whether the baby should be roomed-in with the mother or kept in the special care nursery but does not permit classification of the baby on the basis of birth weight and gestational age.

The preterm baby (less than 37 weeks) shows most of the following characteristics:

Sole creases Single deep crease over anterior one-third of sole or no deep crease. The sole may be full of superficial creases (Figures 7.3A and B).

Genitals In male babies, both testes are at or above the external ring and scrotum is small with scanty rugosities (Figure 7.4). In girls, labia majora are widely separated with labia minora fully exposed and clitoris hypertrophied (Figure 7.5).

Breast nodule Breast nodule is less than 5 mm and nipple is small or absent. In small-for-dates babies, breast tissue may be deficient or absent even when they are gestationally fully mature.

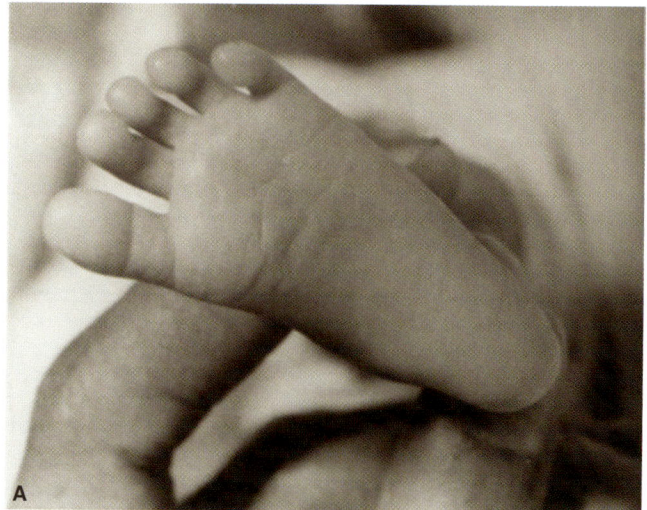

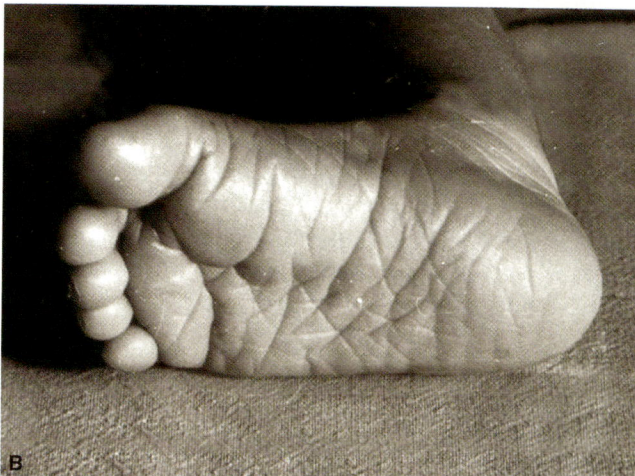

Figure 7.3 Sole creases. (A) Faint sole creases in a preterm baby. (B) The deep sole creases increase as maturity proceeds.

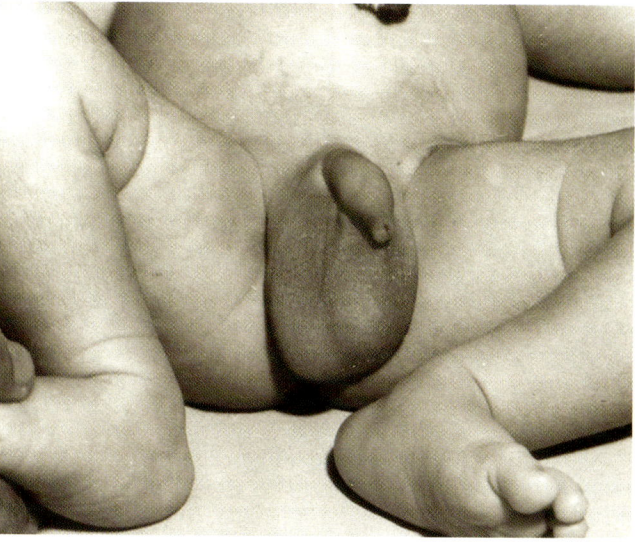

Figure 7.4 Male genitals. Scrotum is fully developed with at least one testis descended in a term infant.

Care of the Newborn

7

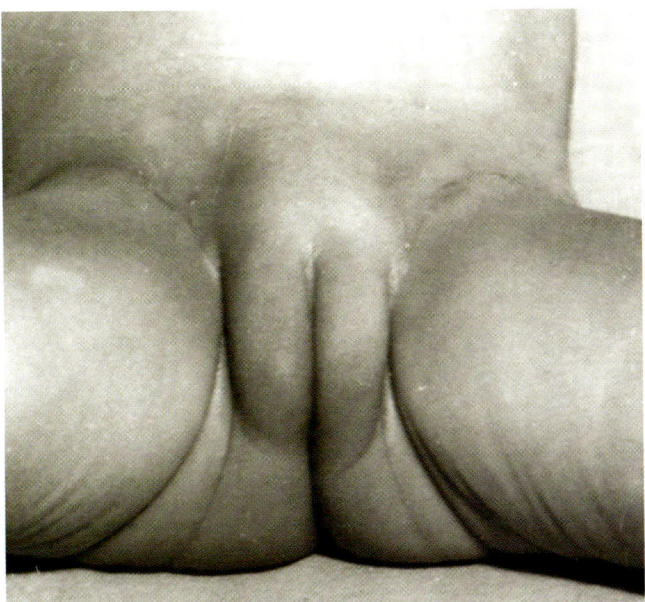

Figure 7.5 Female genitals. Labia majora completely cover the labia minora in a term infant.

Ear cartilage Cartilage is deficient and even absent at places and on folding the external ear, the recoil may be poor (Figures 7.6A and B).

Hair Brownish-black fuzzy or woolly in appearance with no difficulty in identifying the individual hair fibers (Figure 7.7).

Depending upon the degree of immaturity, the preterm babies may have shiny and oily plethoric skin, plenty of lanugo and edema. Neurologically they are less alert, hypotonic and various neonatal reflexes may be absent or incomplete.

Precise Estimation of Gestational Age

The physical characteristics outlined above are very reliable to differentiate between preterm and term babies but are of limited value to assess the precise gestation of babies of less than 36 weeks maturity. On the other hand, neurological parameters are more reliable for precise estimate of gestational maturity of preterm babies, while they are of limited predictive value in relatively mature babies. The neurological assessment is based on four fundamental observations:

1. **Muscle tone** It progressively increases *in utero* as maturity proceeds. The muscle tone in the newborn baby must be assessed by three parameters (Figures 7.8 and 7.9).
   a. Posture or attitude.
   b. Passive tone (popliteal angle and scarf sign).
   c. Active tone (traction response and recoil).

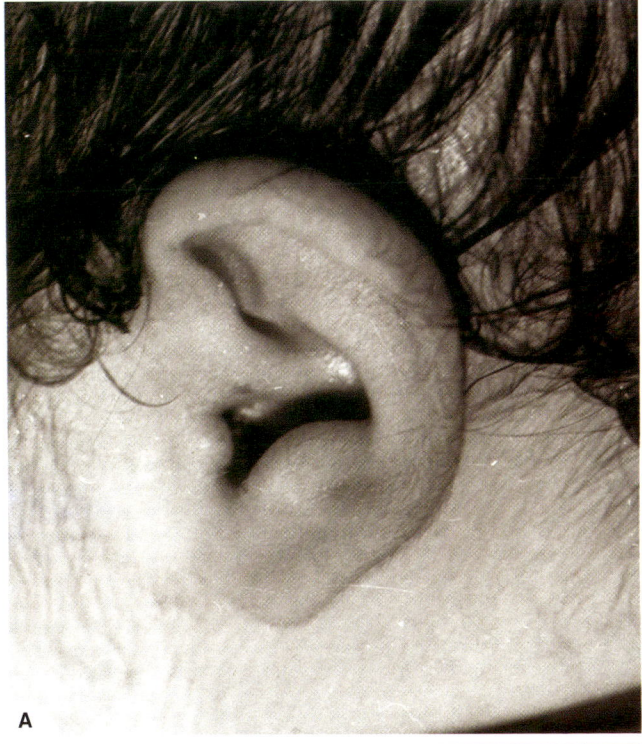

A

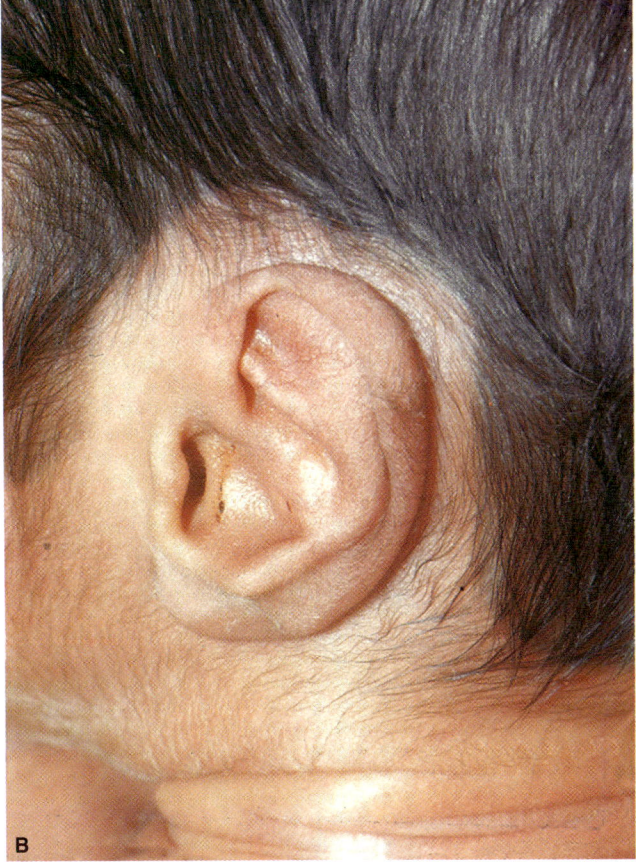

B

Figure 7.6 Ear cartilage. (A) The ear is firm with cartilage and well shaped in a term infant. (B) Ear cartilage is deficient in a preterm baby.

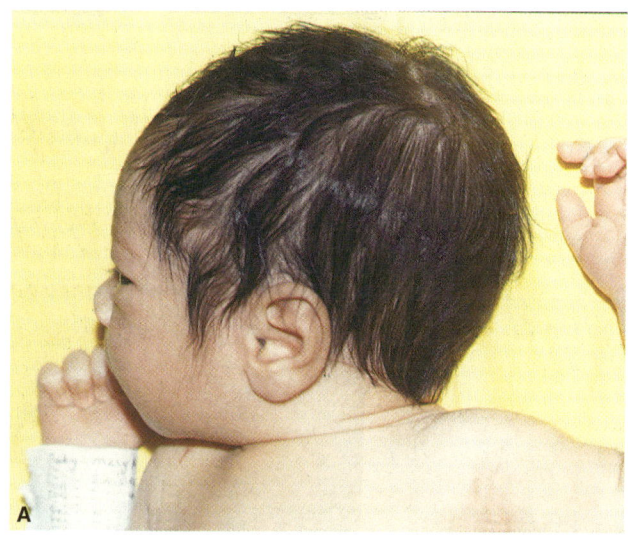
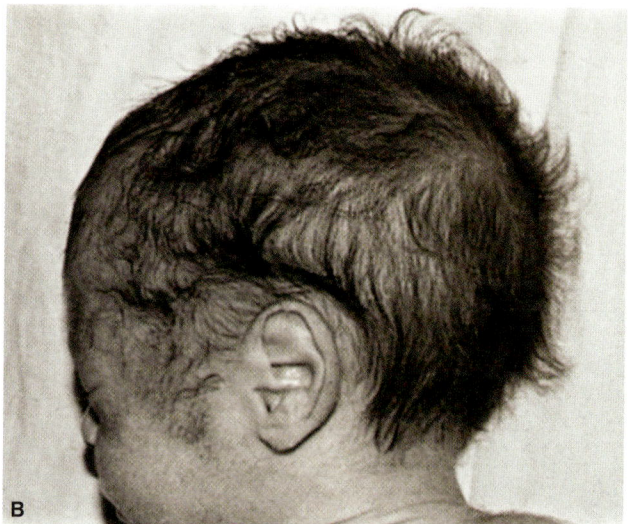

Figure 7.7 (A) The hair are silky and black in appearance in a term infant. (B) Fuzzy and woolly appearance of hair in a preterm baby.

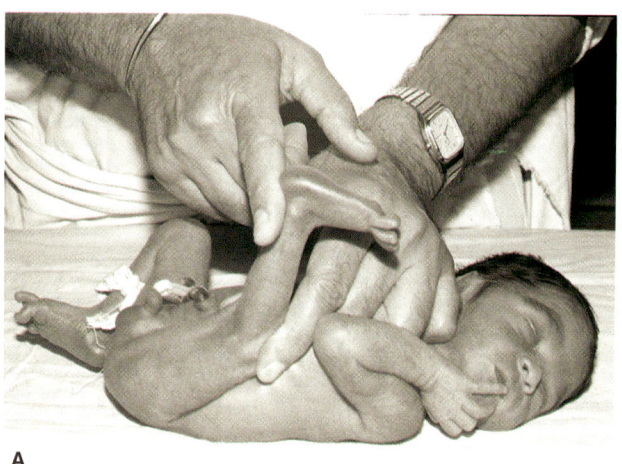
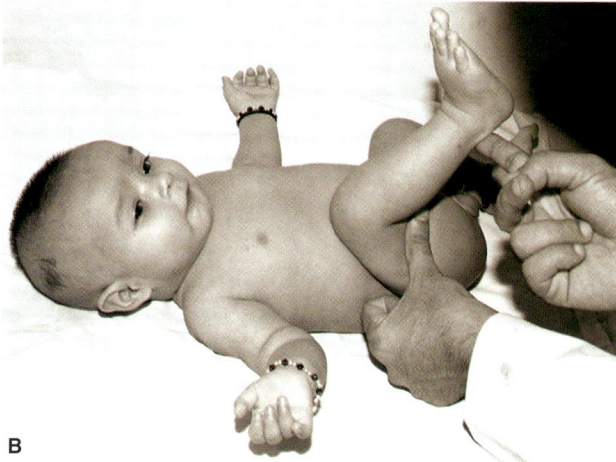

Figure 7.8 Popliteal angle. (A) The angle is almost 180° in an infant less than 32 weeks, 120° among 33–36 weeks and 90° in a term infant (B).

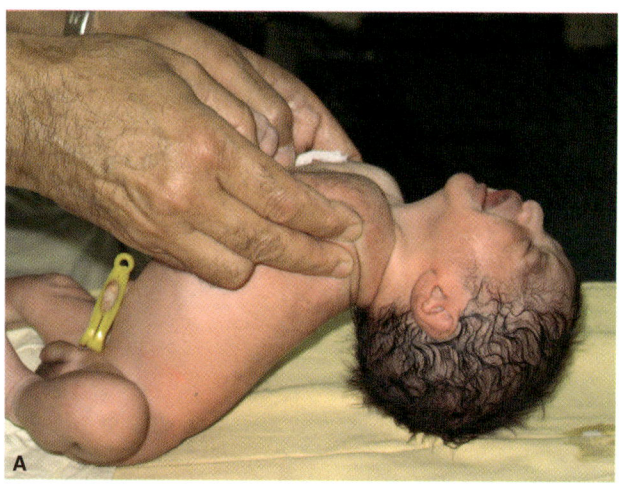
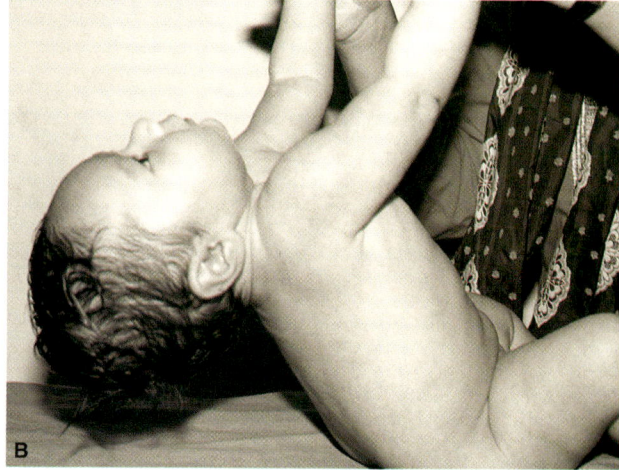

Figure 7.9A and B Traction response. The supine baby is lifted gently by holding at the hands. The term infant is able to maintain his head in line with the trunk.

2. **Joint mobility** The degree of flexion at ankle and wrist (square-window) is limited in preterm babies because of relatively greater stiffness of joints in early gestation. As term approaches, the joints become more flexible and moveable to allow for easy moulding during delivery.

3. **Automatic reflexes** A number of automatic reflexes appear at various specific ages of gestational maturity. Moro reflex appears as early as 28–30 weeks but lacks complete adduction phase till 38 weeks of gestation. Pupillary response to light is present after 30 weeks and infant may turn his head towards diffuse light during 32–36 weeks. Blink response to glabellar tap may appear as early as 29 weeks of gestation. Grasp response makes its appearance around 30 weeks but a strong grasp is elicitable after 36 weeks. Neck flexors are able to contract in response to traction around 33 weeks of maturity. Rooting and coordinated sucking efforts are present around 34 weeks of gestation.

4. **Fundus examination** The disappearance of the anterior vascular capsule of the lens has been used to assess the gestational age of the infant. The anterior capsule is completely vascularized in infants with a gestation of less than 28 weeks. After 34 weeks of maturity, anterior capsular vessels are almost completely atrophied with graded changes in babies between 28 and 34 weeks of gestation. Ophthalmic examination is, however, technically cumbersome in newborn babies due to physiological photophobia and lack of cooperation.

In view of a rather wide overlap in the time of appearance and persistence of various physical and neurological criteria, many workers have evolved scoring systems by using the combined maturity score of physical and neurological criteria for assessment of gestation. Table 7.2 outlines one such simplified scoring system for assessment of gestation. The assessment should be made on babies with normal Moro response, because neurologically damaged and

	TABLE 7.2 Scoring system for assessment of gestational age			
		Score*		
Criteria	0	1	2	3
I. Physical				
a. *Skin texture* Test by inspection and pinching	Very thin and gelatinous	Smooth, medium thickness with superficial peeling	Thick with peeling and cracking over hands and feet	—
b. *Lanugo* Examine on the back	Nil or scanty	Abundant lanugo	Thinning lanugo at places	Scanty lanugo with areas of baldness
c. *Plantar creases* Assess after stretching the skin	Nil	Faint red marks over anterior half of sole	Deep indentations over anterior 1/3rd to 1/2 of sole	Deep indentations throughout the sole
d. *Breast nodule* Test by holding the breast tissue between thumb and index finger	Nil	Breast tissue less than 5 mm on one or both sides	Breast tissue 5–10 mm	Breast tissue more than 10 mm diameter
e. *Ear firmness* Assess by palpation	Pinna feels soft and easily folded into bizarre shapes. No recoil	Soft but some recoil is present	Some cartilage felt along the edge and recoil is instant	Pinna firm with definite cartilage throughout and instant recoil
f. *Genitalia* Male	Neither testis in scrotum	At least one testis in the inguinal canal and can be pulled down into the scrotum	At least one testis present in the scrotum	—
Female	Labia majora widely separated and labia minora protruding	Labia majora partly cover labia minora	Labia majora completely cover the labia minora	—

(contd.)

TABLE 7.2 Scoring system for assessment of gestational age *(contd.)*

Criteria	Score*			
	0	*1*	*2*	*3*
II. Neurological				
a. *Posture*				
Observe with infant quiet and in supine position	Arms and legs extended	Beginning of flexion of hips and knees. Arms extended	Stronger flexion of legs and some flexion of arms	Legs flexed and abducted while arms completely flexed
b. *Arm recoil*				
In a supine infant the flexed forearm is extended by pulling at hands and then released	No recoil or only random movements	Arm returns to incomplete flexion or sluggish response	Arm briskly returns to full flexion	—
c. *Popliteal angle***				
With infant in a supine position, the thigh is held in the knee chest position by supporting the thighs with examiner's left hand. The leg is then extended by gentle pressure with examiner's right hand index finger placed behind the ankle and popliteal angle is measured	180°	180°–150°	150°–120°	120°–90°
d. *Head lag*				
With infant lying in supine position, the baby is grasped at hands and slowly pulled towards sitting position. During the procedure, the position of the head in relation to trunk is observed	Complete head lag	Partial head control	Able to maintain head in line with the body	Brings head anterior to the body
e. *Glabellar tap*				
Tap sharply at glabella (mid-point between eyebrows) and look for closure of the eyes	Absent	Weak response	Brisk response	

Physical score = 0–16;   Neurological score = 0–13;   Combined total score = 0–29

*Whenever, a criterion, physical, or neurological, when tested bilaterally gives a different score on the two sides, the mean score should be taken.

**Popliteal angle may be unreliable in babies born by breech presentation.

(Reproduced from Singh M, Razdan K and Ghai OP. Modified scoring system for clinical assessment of gestational age in the newborn. *Indian Pediatr* 1975; 12(4): 311–16).

severely ill babies would be grossly under scored on neurological assessment. The babies with severe intrauterine growth restriction may also be under scored to some extent due to its adverse effects on the development of breast tissue and muscle tone. On the basis of combined physical and neurological scores, the expected gestational age of the baby can be read from Table 7.3 with a predictive error of ±2 weeks.

In order to assess the gestational age of extremely premature infants and improve the accuracy of assessment of mature infants, new Ballard score is widely used in clinical practice (Table 7.4).

EVALUATION OF A SICK BABY

Stable and Healthy Infant

Term appropriate-for-dates baby without any congenital malformations is likely to have better outcome. The healthy baby looks pink without any pallor, circumoral grayness, cyanosis or jaundice. Tissue perfusion is good as assessed by capillary refill (<2 sec over upper chest), and pink color with warm extremities. There should be no breathing difficulty or apneic attacks. Review of different organ systems should not reveal any abnormalities. The baby should

TABLE 7.3 Relationship between combined total score with gestational age			
Combined total score	Gestation (weeks)	Combined total score	Gestation (weeks)
9	28	18	35
10	29	19	36
11	30	20	37
12	31	23	38
13	32	25	39
15	33	≥26	40
16	34	—	—

TABLE 7.4 New Ballard scoring system for assessment of gestation of extremely premature babies

Physical maturity	Score						
	−1	0	1	2	3	4	5
Skin	Sticky, friable, transparent	Gelatinous, red, translucent	Smooth, pink, visible veins	Superficial peeling and/ or rash, a few veins	Cracking, pale areas, rare veins	Parchment, deep cracking, no vessels	Leathery, cracked, wrinkled
Lanugo	None	Sparse	Abundant	Thinning	Bald areas	Mostly bald	
Plantar surface	Heel–toe 40–50 mm (−1) <40 mm(−2)	<50 mm, no creases	Faint red marks	Anterior transverse crease only	Creases on anterior 2/3rd	Creases over entire sole	
Breast	Imperceptible	Barely perceptible	Flat areola, no bud	Stripped areola, 1–2 mm bud	Raised areola, 3–4 mm bud	Full areola, 5–10 mm bud	
Eyes/ears	Lids fused loosely (−1), tightly (−2)	Lids open, pinna flat, stays folded	Slightly curved pinna; slow recoil	Well-curved pinna, soft but ready recoil	Formed and firm, instant recoil	Thick cartilage, ear stiff	
Genitals							
Male	Scrotum flat, smooth	Scrotum empty, faint rugae	Testes in upper canal, rare rugae	Testes descending, a few rugae	Testes down, good rugae	Testes pendulous, deep rugae	
Female	Clitoris prominent, labia flat	Prominent clitoris, small labia minora	Prominent clitoris, enlarging labia minora	Majora and minora equally prominent	Majora large, minora small	Majora completely cover clitoris and minora	

Maturity rating on Ballard scoring	
Score	Gestation (weeks)
−10	20
−5	22
0	24
5	26
10	28
15	30
20	32
25	34
30	36
35	38
40	40
45	42
50	44

Total physical score

(contd.)

Examination of the Baby

7

TABLE 7.4 New Ballard scoring system for assessment of gestation of extremely premature babies *(Contd.)*

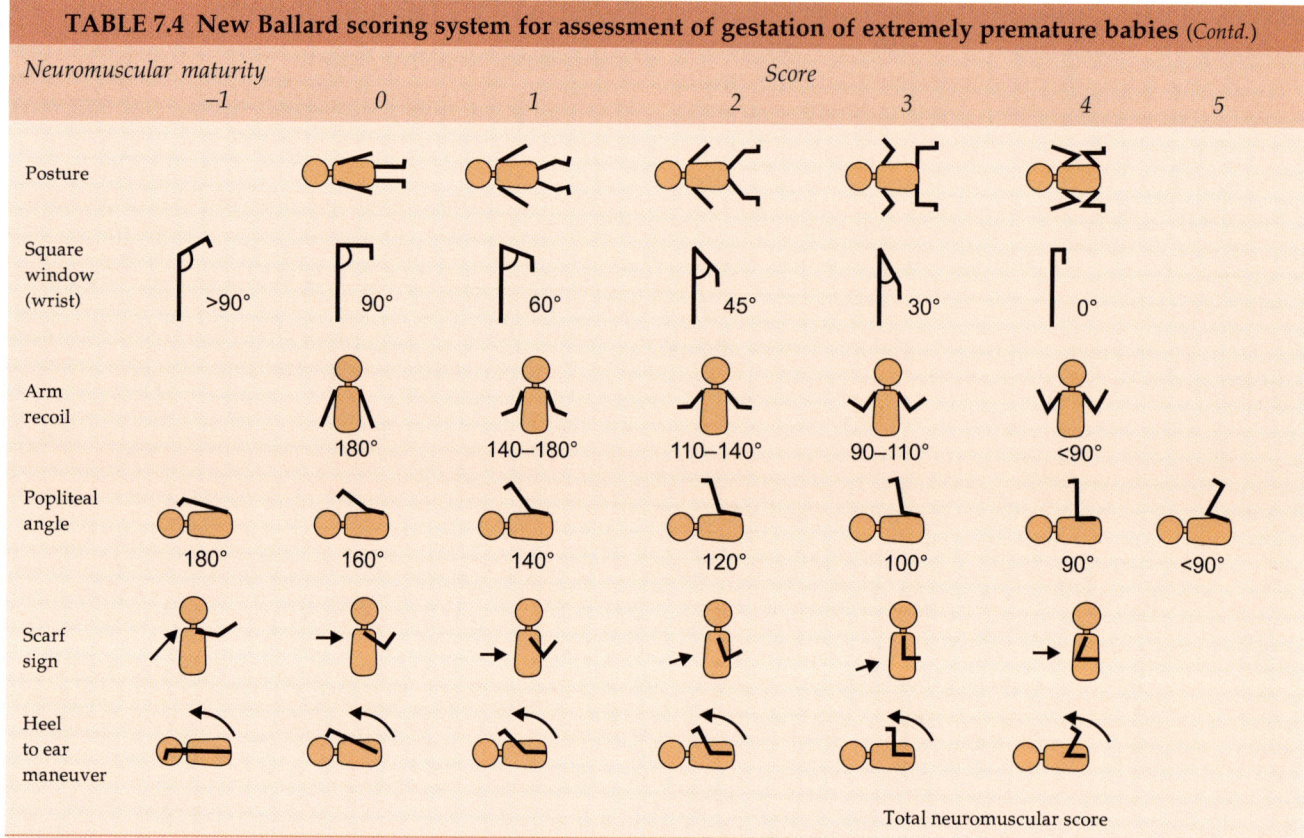

Neuromuscular maturity				Score			
	−1	0	1	2	3	4	5
Posture							
Square window (wrist)	>90°	90°	60°	45°	30°	0°	
Arm recoil		180°	140–180°	110–140°	90–110°	<90°	
Popliteal angle	180°	160°	140°	120°	100°	90°	<90°
Scarf sign							
Heel to ear maneuver							

Total neuromuscular score

Adapted from Ballard JL, Khoury JC, Wedig K, *et al.* New Ballard Score, expanded to include extremely premature infants. *J Pediatr* 1991;119:417–423.

tolerate enteral feeds and gain 1.0–1.5% of body weight everyday.

Acutely Sick Baby

The baby should be attached to a multi-channel vital sign monitor including a sensor for arterial oxygen saturation. Assess the skin color by looking for pallor, jaundice and cyanosis. Exclude presence of sclerema neonatorum. Assess general activity and muscle tone. Assess degree of respiratory distress by evaluating breathing rate/min, severity of retractions and grunting. Look for evidences of respiratory failure clinically and on ABG. Are there any apneic attacks and their response to stimulation? Is the baby maintaining body temperature or having cold stress? Evaluate tissue perfusion by assessing capillary refill time at upper chest and recording blood pressure. Assess CNS integrity by assessing level of consciousness, anterior fontanel, seizures and muscle tone. Evidences of bleeding manifestations due to DIC should be looked for. Look for abdominal distension, bowel sounds and blood in the stools. Strict input, urine output and daily weight should be monitored. Appropriate but simple monitoring chart incorporating

above mentioned information should be developed for use in the NICU by the nurses.

Scoring Systems to Assess Severity of Illness

The physiological status of the baby can be reliably assessed by using an acronym STOPS, i.e. **S**ensorium (lethargic or alert), **T**emperature (cold stress, heater output of the incubator or open care system), **O**xygen (FiO_2 needs to maintain normal arterial oxygen tension or saturation), **P**erfusion (capillary refill time and urine output) and **S**ugar (avoidance of both hypoglycemia and hyperglycemia).

A number of scoring systems have been developed to assess and quantify the severity of illness and predict the morbidity and mortality in critically sick neonates admitted in the NICU.

CRIB (Clinical Risk Index for Babies) Score

The score has been developed in four tertiary care referral centers in UK on a cohort of 812 infants with a birth weight of <1500 g or gestational age of <31 weeks. The assessment of 6 parameters is done during 12 hours period of observation after admission and is shown in Table 7.5.

TABLE 7.5 CRIB score	
Risk factor	*Score*
Birth weight (g)	
1351–1500	0
851–1350	1
701–850	4
≤700	7
Gestation (wk)	
>24	0
≤24	1
Congenital malformations*	
None	0
Not acutely life-threatening	1
Acutely life-threatening	3
Maximum base excess in first 12 hr (mmol/L)	
≤ –7.0	0
–7.0 to –9.9	1
–10.0 to –14.9	2
≥ –15.0	3
Minimum appropriate FiO$_2$ in first 12 hr	
≤0.40	0
0.41–0.60	2
0.61–0.90	3
0.91–1.00	4
Maximum appropriate FiO$_2$ in first 12 hr	
≥0.40	0
0.41–0.80	2
0.81–0.90	3
0.91–1.00	5

*Excluding babies with lethal congenital malformations.
The CRIB score of 0–5 is associated with a mortality of 5%, 6–10 score with 35%, 11–15 score with 70% and >16 score with over 80% mortality.

SNAP (Score for Neonatal Acute Physiology) Score

SNAP score is more complex and developed in USA. It takes into consideration 26 parameters for observation and assessment over a period of 24 hours (Table 7.6). The main limitations of this scoring system include its complexity, long observation period of 24 hours and lack of any weightage to birth weight and gestation. The SNAP score has been further modified to SNAP-PE by including three additional variables of perinatal extension, i.e. LBW, IUGR and low Apgar score. There is a need to develop a simplified scoring system based on a limited number of clinical and biochemical parameters for use in the developing countries.

The next generation variants of these scores have been introduced as SNAP II and SNAP-PE II. They are based on severity of 6 physiological parameters, namely (i) mean arterial pressure (MAP), (ii) ratio of partial pressure of oxygen (PaO$_2$) to fraction of inspired oxygen (FiO$_2$), (iii) core body temperature (°F), (iv) blood pH, (v) occurrence of seizures and (vi) oliguria.

Sick Neonate Score

It is a relatively simple score which can be easily evaluated to assess the severity of sickness of a neonate in resource limited countries. The score is useful to assess the condition of the baby on admission to the NICU and for babies requiring neonatal transport (Table 7.7).

Extended sick neonate score (ESNS) has been proposed with addition of two more parameters, namely Moro reflex and modified Downes' score, and blood pressure values have been expressed in percentiles (Table 7.8). The ESNS can predict the mortality outcome of neonates of all gestations admitted in the NICU with a satisfactory sensitivity and specificity.

TABLE 7.6 Score for neonatal acute physiology (SNAP)			
Parameter	*1-Point range*	*3-Point range*	*5-Point range*
■ Blood pressure			
High	66–80	81–100	>100
Low	30–35	20–29	<20
■ Heart rate			
High	180–200	201–250	>250
Low	80–90	40–79	<40
■ Respiratory rate	60–100	>100	—

(contd.)

TABLE 7.6 Score for neonatal acute physiology (SNAP) (*contd.*)

Parameter	1-Point range	3-Point range	5-Point range
■ Temperature (°F)	95–96	92–94.9	<92
■ PaO_2 (mm Hg)	50–65	30–50	<30
■ PaO_2/FiO_2 ratio	2.5–3.5	0.3–2.49	<0.3
■ $PaCO_2$ (mm Hg)	50–65	66–90	>90
■ Oxygenation index*	0.07–0.20	0.21–0.40	>0.40
■ Hematocrit (%)			
High	66–70	>70	—
Low	30–30	20–29	<2.0
■ White blood cell count (× 1000)	2.0–5.0	<2.0	—
■ Immature to total ratio	>0.21	—	—
■ Absolute neutrophil count	500–999	<500	—
■ Platelet count (× 1000)	30–100	0–29	—
■ Blood urea nitrogen (mg/dL)	40–80	>80	—
■ Creatinine (mg/dL)	1.2–2.4	2.5–4.0	>4.0
■ Urine output (mL/kg/hr)	0.5–0.9	0.1–0.49	<0.1
■ Indirect bilirubin (by birth weight)			
>2 kg: mg/dL	15–20	>20	—
≤2 kg: mg/dL	5–10	>10	—
■ Direct bilirubin (mg/dL)	≥2.0	—	—
■ Sodium (mEq/L)			
High	150–160	161–180	>180
Low	120–130	<120	—
■ Potassium (mEq/L)			
High	6.6–7.5	7.6–9.0	—
Low	2.0–2.9	<2.0	—
■ Calcium (ionized) (mg/dL)			
High	≥1.4	—	—
Low	0.8–1.0	<0.8	—
■ Calcium (total) (mg/dL)			
High	≥12	—	—
Low	5.0–6.9	<5.0	—
■ Glucose (on reagent strip) (mg/dL)			
High	150–250	>250	—
Low	30–40	<30	—
■ Serum bicarbonate (mEq/L)			
High	≥33	—	—
Low	11–15	≤10	—
■ Blood pH	7.20–7.34	7.10–7.19	<7.10
■ Seizures	Single	Multiple	—
■ Apnea	Responsive to stimulation	Unresponsive to stimulation	Complete apnea
■ Stool guaiac	Positive	—	—

*Oxygenation index = $\dfrac{MAP \times FiO_2}{PaO_2} \times 100$

MAP: Main airway pressure, FiO_2: Fractional inspired concentration, PaO_2: Partial pressure of arterial oxygen.

TABLE 7.7 Sick neonate score (SNS)

Parameter	Score		
	0	1	2
Respiratory effort	Apnea or grunting	Tachypnea (>60/min) with or without retractions	Normal (40–60/min)
Heart rate	Bradycardia/asystole	Tachycardia (>160/min)	Normal (100–160/min)
Mean blood pressure (mmHg)	<30	30–39	>39
Axillary temperature (°C)	<36	36–36.5	36.5–37.5
Capillary refill time (s)	>5	3–5	<3
Random blood sugar (mg/dL)	<40	40–60	>60
SpO_2 (in room air)	<85%	85–92%	>92%

SNS of 6 or less is associated with increased risk of mortality.
Adapted from Rathod D, Adhisivam B, Bhat BV. Sick neonate score—A simple clinical score for predicting mortality of sick neonates in resource restricted settings. *Indian J Pediatr* 2016, 83(2): 103–106.

TABLE 7.8 Extended sick newborn score (ESNS)

Parameter	Score		
	0	1	2
Respiratory effort	Apnea	>60/min ± retractions	40–60/min
Heart rate (beats/min)	Bradycardia/asystole	>160	100–160
Axillary temperature (°C)	<36.0	36.0–36.5	36.5–37.5
Mean blood pressure (percentile)	<5th	5th–50th	>50th
Capillary refill time (s)	>5	3–5	<3
Random blood sugar (mg/dL)	<45	45–60	>60
Moro reflex	Absent	Depressed or exaggerated	Normal for gestation
Modified Downes' score*	>6	3–6	0–2

*Modified Downes' score is calculated on the basis of five parameters (respiratory rate, chest retractions, grunt, cyanosis, air entry), each being allocated a score of 0, 1, 2.

BIBLIOGRAPHY

Alexion D, Manolidis C, Pappaevangellon ND, Papadatos C. Frequency of other malformations in congenital hypoplasia of depressor anguli oris muscle syndrome. *Arch Dis Child* 1976, 56:891.

Apgar V. Five-minute diagnosis of hidden congenital anomalies. *Consultant,* June, 1962.

Ballard JL, Khoury JC, Wedig K, *et al.* New Ballard score; expanded to include extremely premature infants. *J Pediatr* 1991; 119: 417–423.

Dubowitz LMS, Dubowitz V, Goldberg C. Clinical assessment of gestational age in the newborn infant. *J Pediatr* 1970; 77:1.

Erhardt P. The CRIB score. *Lancet* 1993; 342: 612–613.

Gordon H, Brosens I. Cytology of amniotic fluid: A new test for fetal maturity. *Obstet and Gynecol* 1967; 30:652.

Hittner HM, Hirsh NJ, Rudolph AJ. Assessment of gestational age by examination of the anterior vascular capsule of the lens. *J Pediatr* 1977; 91:455.

Hope P. CRIB, Son of Apgar, brother to APACHE. *Arch Dis Child* 1995; 72:F81–F83.

Ray S, Mondal R, Chatterjee K, Samanta M, Hazra A, Sabui TK. Extended sick neonate score (ESNS) for clinical assessment and mortality prediction in sick newborns referred to tertiary care. *Indian Pediatr* 2019,56:130–33.

Richardson DK, Tarnow-Mordi W. Measuring illness severity in the newborn intensive care. *J Intensive Care Med* 1994; 9:20–33.

Russel JGB. Radiological assessment of fetal maturity. *J Obstet Gynecol Brit Commonwlth* 1969; 76:208.

Shah P, Wazir S. Assessment of severity of neonatal sickness. In: Neonatal Emergencies. *CBS Publishers and Distributors Pvt Ltd., New Delhi.* Singh M (Ed) 1917, pp179–186.

Singh M, Razdan K, Ghai OP. Modified scoring system for assessment of gestational age in the newborn. *Indian Pediatr* 1975; 12: 311.

Singh M, Sharma NK. Spectrum of congenital malformations in the newborn. *Indian J Pediatr* 1980; 47:239.

Stroud CE, Carne SJ, Dunn PM, *et al.* Screening for the detection of congenital dislocation of the hip. Special report. *Arch Dis Child* 1986; 61:921.

Usher R, Mclean F, Scott KE. Judgement of fetal age. *Pediatr Clin N Amer* 1966; 13:835.

Examination of the Baby

7

8

Care of the Normal Newborns

What is a normal newborn?

The neonate at birth is considered as normal if, (i) birth weight is 2500 g or more, (ii) gestation is 37 weeks or more, (iii) body weight is appropriate-for-dates (between 10th and 90th percentile), (iv) 1-minute Apgar score was 7 or more, (v) infant did not need any active resuscitation, (vi) infant did not suffer from any significant postnatal illness like hypothermia, hypoglycemia, hypocalcemia, polycythemia, respiratory distress and sepsis requiring admission to NICU, and (vii) mother did not suffer from any serious complications like toxemia of pregnancy, Rh-isoimmunization, antepartum hemorrhage and diabetes mellitus.

BASIC CARE OF NORMAL NEWBORN BABIES

At birth baby should be received in a sterile sheet, dressed in a frock with open-back and covered adequately depending upon the environmental temperature. It is desirable to keep the normal term babies with their mothers rather than in a separate nursery. Rooming-in promotes better emotional rapport between the mother and her baby. The mother can participate in the nursing care of her baby. This infuses self-confidence in her and reduces demands on nursing personnel. Cross-infection is prevented and breastfeeding is established easily. The baby's color, respirations, temperature and umbilical stump should be checked on arrival in the lying-in ward. Skin temperature should be recorded twice a day.

MOTHER'S ROLE IN THE CARE OF HER BABY

The health and survival of the newborn baby depends upon the health status of the mother and her awareness, education and skills in mothercraft. *Mother is the best primary health worker.* She has the advantages of instinct, concern and interest to look after her baby. Mother looks after her baby with love, affection and a sense of sacrifice. Early involvement of the mother in the care of her baby is the best way to promote and encourage exclusive breastfeeding. The healthy babies should not be admitted in the nursery. Mother is the best person to identify minor developmental deviations and early evidences of disease process because she is constantly and closely watching her baby. The basic knowledge and skills pertaining to mothercraft, child nutrition, immunizations, environmental sanitation and personal hygiene, and common health problems in children, etc. should be taught to adolescent boys and girls in the schools and colleges. The *Mahila Mandals* and *Anganwadis* should organize regular teaching and training programs in mothercraft. The simple messages for basic care of pregnant women and healthy babies should be widely disseminated through available media including radio and television.

BREASTFEEDING

"Milk is not only species specific, it is baby specific. The milk of a mother is best suited to serve the biological needs of her own baby".

Meharban Singh

All mothers must be emotionally and physically prepared and motivated during pregnancy so that they do not encounter any difficulties to establish successful breastfeeding. The inverted and cracked nipples must be managed during pregnancy so that baby is not faced with any mechanical difficulties during breastfeeding.

Early skin-to-skin contact between infant and mother promotes bonding and breastfeeding. The baby should be put straight to the breast as soon as the mother has recovered from the fatigue of labor. The first feed is usually offered within half to one hour after birth. There is no need to administer any prelacteal feeds in the form of honey, glucose water, tea, etc. The colostrum (milk secreted during the first three days of lactation) must never be discarded and all babies should invariably receive it because it is rich in energy, proteins, protective antibodies and cellular elements. The physiological inadequacy of lactation during first three days of nursing should never be considered as an excuse for supplementing breast-feeding because it does not impose any hazards to a healthy newborn baby. The term neonate has a large pool of extracellular fluid volume and enough quota of glycogen in the liver. There is thus no risk of dehydration or hypoglycemia due to physiologic inadequacy of lactation at this stage. The introduction of supplemental feeds during this period leads to refusal on the part of the baby to suck on the breast resulting in delayed establishment of lactation. The mother must be explained and reassured that the act of sucking is the best stimulus for milk production and the small amount of concentrated milk produced during first two to three days of lactation is adequate to meet the nutritional needs of her healthy term baby.

During first six months of life, the baby should receive exclusive breastfeeding and there is no need to give any water even during summer months because all the fluid requirements of the baby are met through breast milk. The exclusively breastfed babies are likely to have better weight gain because they will drink more milk when thirsty. The baby should be on demand feeding and most babies are satisfied with feeds taken every two to three hours. The mother should sit up comfortably and keep the baby's head slightly raised and supported on her elbow. The baby should not be allowed to merely suck on the nipple but he must grasp the areola and part of the breast tissue into his mouth. The baby should be allowed to suck at the breast till he is satisfied which usually takes 15–20 minutes. Some babies are satisfied by sucking from one breast while others may need to suck at both the breasts during each feeding session. During each feed, one breast must be emptied completely before the baby is put to the other breast. The breast which was partially emptied during the last feed should be offered first at the next feed. The mother should actively interact with the baby while breastfeeding. She should fondly look at the baby and interact with him so that he does not fall asleep half way through the feed. She can tickle her baby by gently stroking the ears or soles to keep him awake. If a baby gets lazy or dopey within 5 minutes, she should try to partially remove her nipple, which is usually followed by vigorous sucking again. The baby is considered to have adequate feeds, if he sleeps well after a feed for at least 2 hours, gains weight regularly on an average of 30 g per day (after the first week of life) and voids urine six or more times in a day.

During first four to six weeks, most babies need to be fed round-the-clock and after that gradually the night feeds can be reduced to one late night feed and one early morning feed. The regurgitation of feeds is often due to faulty technique of feeding and swallowing of air during sucking. The mother must be advised to burp the child after each feed to safeguard against the risk of regurgitation (Figure 8.1). Many babies feel uncomfortable till they eructate out the swallowed air. During lactation, the mother should be advised to take extra liquids and additional 450 kcal per day and supplements of micronutrients in order to maintain her own health and nutrition, and improve the nutritional quality of milk.

Maintenance of Body Temperature

The body temperature in newborn babies is usually unstable and they are particularly vulnerable to develop hypothermia in winter. *The environmental temperature that may feel uncomfortable to an adult may impose serious cold stress to a newborn baby.* The baby bath should not be given at birth and delayed till next day when his temperature has stabilized. The child should be kept dried and adequately clothed. The baby should be nursed in close proximity to the mother so that the baby gains heat from maternal warmth. In winter, the

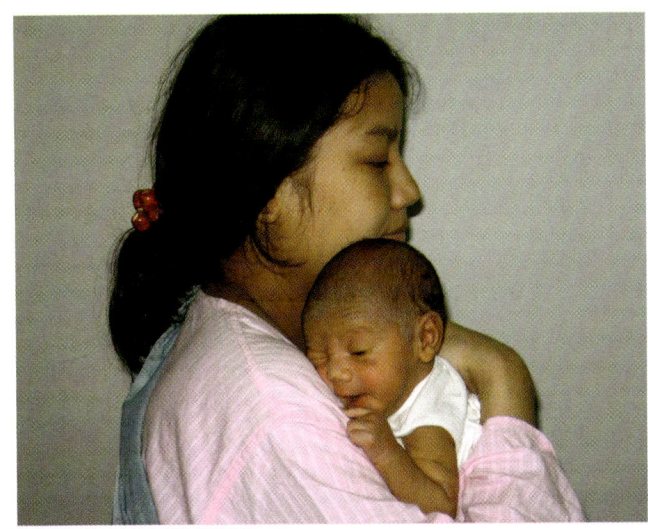

Figure 8.1 Baby is being burped after the feed.

Care of the Normal Newborns

8

linen and clothes of the baby should be prewarmed. He should be provided with a cap, socks and mittens. The room should be kept warm. The mother and health workers should be trained to assess the temperature of the baby by touch alone. When trunk is warm to touch and extremities are warm and pink it is reassuring that the baby is not having any cold stress. The cultural practice of keeping the mother-baby dyad isolated for 40 days is useful and needs to be promoted. It prevents exposure of the baby to cold and safeguards against occurrence of infections. The oil massage is both culturally and scientifically acceptable as it provides insulation against heat and insensible water loss.

BODY MASSAGE

Body massage is culturally accepted in India and South-East Asian and African countries, and has several scientifically proven benefits. It was first introduced in China as early as 200 BC. Oil massage of the baby should be postponed till baby is 3 to 4 weeks old and his body weight is more than 3 kg. Most babies enjoy an oil massage, they cry less and sleep better. It improves the circulation and tone of the muscles, gives comfort to the baby, strengthens infant maternal bonding and provides additional energy to the baby because oil can get absorbed from the thin skin of the baby (Box 8.1). Oil massage is credited to improve weight gain, reduce stress and enhance

Box 8.1: Advantages of body massage

- Promotes bonding between mother and her child.
- It improves blood circulation, muscle tone, bone strength and sense of well-being.
- The massage relaxes the baby, provides a sense of well-being and promotes sleep.
- It makes the baby feel secure and safe and reduces episodes of crying.
- Abdominal massage improves digestion, promotes expulsion of wind and reduces the risk of colic.
- Touching of skin during massage sends salutary massages to CNS for promotion of growth of neurons and dendrites. Touch also produce a cocktail of hormones, the most important being oxytocin which is known as the "love hormone".
- It improves the texture, hydration and functioning of the skin.
- The vegetable oils may get absorbed through the thin skin of the neonate to provide energy, micronutrients and antioxidants.
- Regular body massage is credited to promote weight gain, improves sense of well-being and reduces episodes of crying.

immunological functions of the baby. Oil is used as a lubricant to avoid friction between the hands and body parts being massaged. It prevents dryness and chaffing of skin. It reduces transepidermal water loss and improves thermoregulation. Use a non-irritating vegetable oil like olive oil, sunflower, coconut oil or sesame oil but avoid mustard oil in young infants because it is pungent to the eyes and irritating to the delicate skin of the baby.

What is the best oil for massage?

It is not the nature of the oil but the procedure of massage which is more crucial for harnessing all the virtues of body massage. It is best to use the massage oils which are specially formulated for the babies. The ideal oil for massage depends upon the type of skin, whether normal, dry, sensitive or oily and nature of the season.

Mustard oil It is a popular massage oil in India. Mustard oil is credited to improve thermoregulation, skin texture and skin barrier function. It is rich in oleic acid which makes the skin more permeable and dry. It should be avoided in neonates due to its strong pungent smell and irritant effects on the delicate skin.

Olive oil It is a popular massage oil as it is known to improve skin hydration. The olive oil contains around 55–85% oleic acid which can disrupt the skin barrier leading to dryness. There is increased risk of atopic dermatitis following massage with olive oil.

Coconut oil It is a suitable oil for use during hot and humid climates. It has a light texture and gets absorbed into the skin easily. It contains several nutrients like vitamin E, bioactive compounds like polyphenols, which help nourish the skin. The coconut oil is credited to have antibacterial and antifungal properties that aid in treating eczema, rashes, dermatitis and craddle cap. Both organic copra and virgin coconut oil are equally useful for massaging the babies.

Sesame oil It has antioxidant, anti-inflammatory and antibacterial properties. It may also protect the skin from ultraviolet radiations of sun.

Almond oil It has emollient and sclerosant properties, which have been used to improve complexion and tone of the skin. It is rich in calcium, magnesium and vitamin E. It is also credited to reduce the structural damage to the skin by UV irradiation.

Organic sunflower oil It has a low oleic acid and high linoleum content and is credited to have antibacterial, regenerating, restructuring and moisturising properties. It is a useful massage oil in preterm babies as it provides enhanced skin barrier function. It has virtually no smell, is replete with vitamins and is readily absorbed from skin.

Chamomile oil It is an essential oil which is used for aroma therapy. The FDA has declared chamomile as GRAS (generally recognised as safe). Rarely, allergic reactions may occur, if you are allergic to plants related to chamomile such as daisies, ragweed or marigolds. Essential oils may be used for massage but they should be diluted with a carrier oil to reduce its overloading effects on the olfactory system.

Mineral oil It is a petroleum based product which is not absorbed by the skin, it creates a barrier and does not allow the skin to "breathe". Moreover, it has no nutritional benefits.

Clarified butter (desi ghee) It is a monounsaturated fat and ghee prepared from cow's milk is considered as supreme for all purposes in Indian culture. Its application on the scalp is credited to improve hair growth. It is rich in oleic acid which makes the skin more permeable and dry. It is credited to lighten the tone of skin.

The Procedure of Massage

The baby should be massaged before giving the bath in a room which is kept comfortably warm and free from draughts. In winter, massage is best done by placing the baby in front of a closed window through which sunrays are peeping in the room. The exposure of the skin to sunrays is an important source of endogenous production of vitamin D in the skin.

Make necessary preparations and create a suitable environment before starting the massage. Avoid the procedure, if baby is hungry. Massage is best given 45–60 minutes after a feed to avoid regurgitation. Shut the doors and windows. The room temperature should be maintained between 26°C and 28°C. Keep the pet in another room. Play a soft and relaxing music. The rings should be removed to prevent any scratching of the skin. The massage should be done by using gentle pressure and smooth rhythmical movements by the mother and not by an aggressive nurse-aide or *ayah*. Place the baby supine and start the massage from head, face, chest, abdomen, upper limbs—palms and lower limbs—soles from above downwards (Figure 8.2). Provide gentle but firm rhythmic strokes from above downwards. The procedure is repeated after placing the baby in prone position. The massage is followed by kinesthetic stimulation by performing alternate flexion and extension movements of major joints of upper and lower limbs. Massage is best performed after

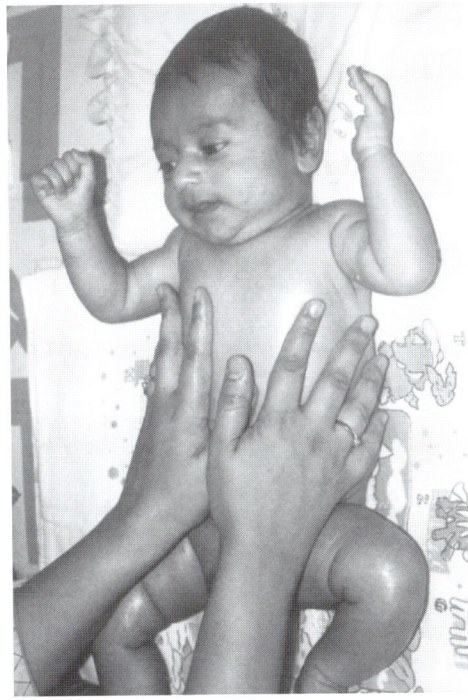

Figure 8.2 The baby is being oil massaged before the bath.

one hour of feed when baby is awake and in good mood. Average massage session should last for about 15–20 minutes. Mother must actively interact and talk with her baby during the massage session. It should be a fun both for the mother and her baby.

SKIN CARE AND BABY BATH

The baby must be cleaned off blood, mucus and meconium before he is presented to the mother. Effective cleaning and drying of skin at birth minimizes the risk of potential infection by micro-organisms such as hepatitis B virus, HIV and herpes simplex virus. Health care worker must wear gloves when skin of a newly born baby is cleaned. When baby is born, skin pH is 7. The acid mantle which protects the baby's delicate skin takes a few weeks to 3 months to develop, when pH of the skin becomes 5.5. It is best to use a mildly acidic (pH 5.5) liquid baby wash or a mild cleanser. When a soap bar is used it should not contain any alkaline detergent that can destroy the skin barrier and cause flaking, scaling and dryness of skin. Liquid cleanser that contains an emollient is particularly useful in infants at high risk of atopic dermatitis. The baby should be bathed or sponged next morning after birth by using unmedicated soap and clean lukewarm water. The useful strategies for care of delicate skin of babies are listed in Box. 8.2. The barrier nursing with separate articles for each baby in their individual lockers is desirable. There should be no centralized

Box 8.2: Skin care mantras for the neonates

- Skin of a neonate is thin and delicate, with excessive insensible water loss.
- Do not rub off the vernix or peel the skin with force.
- Touch, caress and clean the skin gently.
- Avoid using baby skin products containing chemicals, perfumes, detergents and dyes.
- Use those skin products that contain natural ingredients like aloe vera, chamomile, shea butter, clendula, glycerine and panthenol.
- Avoid use of baby skin products containing harsh surfactants which are detrimental to infant's skin.
- The frequency of bathing should be related to weather and ambient temperature. In winter, bathe the baby 2–3 times in a week.
- Avoid exposure of the baby to direct sunlight.*
- Prevent diaper rash by frequent application of protective and soothing cream.
- Avoid use of talcum powder.

*The treatment of neonatal jaundice by exposure of the baby to sunlight is not only useless but also harmful.

bathing facilities for the babies as this often results in cross infection. The nursing toilet of each baby should be carried out by the cot-side because this has the advantage of providing education and ensuring active participation of the mother. Routine use of hexachlorophene is not recommended because of its neurologic toxicity to the newborn babies. In the event of an epidemic of staphylococcal infection, use of chlorhexidine gluconate lotion or medicated soap is recommended, taking care that skin is rinsed thoroughly after its application. It has been shown, that 'no bath' regimen during hospital stay of the baby reduces the incidence of superficial infections.

Baby Bath

During summer months, the baby can be given a bath. The room should be reasonably warm and free of any draught. Take clean, warm water in a plastic basin. Avoid dip baths till the cord has fallen. Use any mild unmedicated soap or baby cleanser. The baby should be held over the forearms or over the thighs. Bathe by wetting and applying soap to small areas of skin beginning from head and proceeding downwards to prevent exposure. Eyes should be cleaned by using a sterile water soaked swab for each eye. The bottom should be washed in the end to avoid contamination of healthy areas of skin. The infant should be promptly dried with a soft towel to prevent damage to the delicate skin of the baby. No vigorous attempts should be made to rub off the vernix caseosa which provides protection to the delicate skin. It should be gently washed off with plain water without using any oil. During winter months, the baby should preferably be sponged rather than bathed to avoid the risk of exposure. The use of talcum powder is unnecessary except for aesthetic purposes. Talcum powder should be taken on the fingers or cotton ball and applied over the axillae and groins taking care that it is not sprinkled over the eyes and nostrils. After the bath, baby should be given a breastfeed. Most babies go to sleep after the ritual of body massage, bath and breastfeeding.

The baby usually wakes up after 2 to 3 hours fully refreshed and ready for the next feed. Body massage and bathing provides a good opportunity to the nurse and mother to identify any developmental peculiarities and superficial skin infections which should be brought to the notice of the physician.

Care of the Umbilical Stump

The umbilical cord is an important site for entry of spores of tetanus. The health care personnel must use sterile instruments to cut and clamp the cord to prevent occurrence of tetanus neonatorum. Even when a new razor blade is used for cutting the cord, it should be sterilized before use by boiling for 5 minutes. The cord must be inspected after 2 to 4 hours of birth. Bleeding commonly occurs at this time because of shrinkage of cord and loosening of ligatures. Ligation of cord with a rubber band or disposable clip safeguards against this hazard. Triple dye, ethyl alcohol, betadine or chlorhexidine should be applied at the tip and around the base of the umbilical stump daily to prevent colonization. The dressing should not be applied. The stump need not be kept moistened in babies with future need for exchange transfusion but precautions should be taken to keep the stump bacteria free by using polybactericidal powder containing neomycin, bacitracin and polymyxin. The cord normally falls after 5 to 10 days but may take longer, if it is dry and shriveled or when infected. The delayed falling of the cord is also a useful marker of immunodeficiency state.

Care of the Eyes

Eyes should be cleaned daily with sterile cotton swabs soaked in normal saline using one swab for each eye. If the eyes are sticky, 10% solution of sulphacetamide should be instilled in the eyes every two to four hours. Prophylactic instillation of human colostrum into the eyes has been shown to reduce the incidence of sticky eyes. The practice of applying *kajal* in the eyes is not recommended because it may transmit infection like trachoma and may even cause lead poisoning.

Dresses for the Baby

The clothes should be loose, soft and preferably made of cotton. They should be open on the front or back for ease of wearing. Avoid the use of large buttons which may hurt the tender skin of the baby. The nappies should be made of thick, soft and absorbant material in order to readily soak the urine and stools. The use of soakable diaper or plastic napkin should be avoided at home because of increased risk of nappy rash. The woollen clothes should not be stored and preserved with moth balls because there is a potential risk of development of severe jaundice in a baby who is deficient in glucose-6-phosphate dehydrogenase enzyme in his red blood cells. When woollens had been protected with moth balls, they should be exposed to bright sunlight for one to two days before being worn.

Early Detection of a Sick Baby

The nurses and pediatricians should be vigilant in the maternity ward to diagnose neonatal abnormalities at the earliest. Most healthy term babies do not pose any serious health problems except appearance of certain developmental peculiarities and minor problems which need identification, reassurance and advice to the mother. However, when a newborn baby is genuinely sick and refuses to take adequate feeds or manifests any other danger signs, he should be considered as seriously ill. The *danger signs* should be closely watched and brought to the notice of the consultant (Box 8.3).

Box 8.3: Danger signs

- Bleeding from any site.
- Appearance of jaundice within 24 hours of age or severe jaundice with yellow staining of palms and soles.
- Failure to pass meconium within 24 hours and urine within 48 hours.
- Vomiting or diarrhea.
- Poor feeding.
- Undue lethargy or excessive crying.
- Excessive frothing or drooling from mouth.
- Choking during feeding.
- Respiratory difficulty.
- Apneic attacks and/or cyanosis.
- Seizures.
- Sudden rise or fall in the body temperature.
- Superficial infection/s (conjunctivitis, pustules, umbilical sepsis and oral thrush, etc.).

Weight Record

The weight should be recorded on an electronic weighing scale with a resolution of ±1.0 or 5.0 g (Figure 8.3). Most babies lose weight during first 2 to 3 days of life. The weight loss varies between 5 and 8% of birth weight. The weight remains stationary during next 1 to 2 days and birth weight is regained by the end of first week. The factors contributing to initial weight loss include removal of vernix, mucus, and blood from skin, passage of meconium and reduction of extra-cellular fluid volume. The transition from *in utero* parenteral nutrition to postnatal oral feeding is associated with transient interruption in the physical growth of babies. Deliberate starvation and delayed feeding is associated with excessive weight loss. Exclusively breastfed babies tend to lose relatively more weight due to inadequacy of lactation during initial 2 to 3 days. Malnourished small-for-dates babies, if fed early and adequately, do not lose weight and start gaining weight within 2 to 3 days after birth. During first year of life, average daily weight gain in healthy term babies is around 30 g, 20 g and 10 g during first, second and third 4-month periods, respectively. Most infants double their birth weight by 4–5 months of age and triple it by their first birth day. It is mandatory that periodic weight record should be taken and charted on Road-to-Health cards during preschool years.

IMMUNIZATIONS

BCG and first dose of OPV and hepatitis B vaccine (HBV) are given at birth or before the baby is discharged from the hospital. The OPV may preferably be given after 3 days because colostrum may interfere

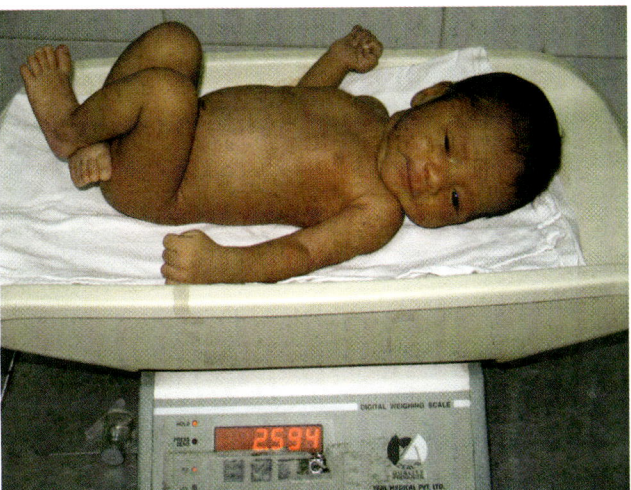

Figure 8.3 Nude infant is being weighed on an electronic weighing scale.

with its uptake. The BCG site should be checked for 'take' response after 4–6 weeks. If there is no "take" response by 6 weeks, repeat BCG vaccine is given. Persistent and recurrent ulceration at the site of vaccination or regional adenitis responds to oral adminis- tration of erythromycin in a dose of 30 mg/kg/day for 14 days or INH 10 mg/kg/day for 3 months. The modified immunization schedule as proposed by Indian Academy of Pediatrics along with optional and additional vaccines is depicted in Table 8.1.

TABLE 8.1 Recommended immunization schedule		
Age	*Vaccine*	
Essential vaccines		
Birth to 2 weeks	BCG	Single dose
	bOPV	1st dose
	HBV	1st dose
6–8 weeks	DTwP or DTaP + Hib+ HBV + IPV	1st dose
	bOPV	2nd dose
		2nd dose
10–12 weeks	DTwP or DTaP + Hib + HBV + IPV	2nd dose
	bOPV	3rd dose
14–16 weeks	DTwP or DTaP + Hib + HBV + IPV	3rd dose
	bOPV	4th dose
9 months	Measles or MMR vaccine	1st dose
	Typhoid conjugate vaccine* (TCV 25 µg)	Singe dose
15–18 months	MMR	2nd dose
	DTwP or DTaP + Hib + HBV + IPV 1st booster	
4 ½–5 years	DTwP or DTaP	2nd booster
	MMR or MR booster	
	HBV booster	
	Typhoid conjugate vaccine (optional)	
10 years	Tdap or Td or TT booster** (every 10 years)	
Optional vaccines (after one-to-one discussion with parents who can afford)		
6–8 weeks	Rotavirus vaccine + PCV 13***	
10–12 weeks	Rotavirus vaccine + PCV 13	
14–16 weeks	Rotavirus vaccine + PCV 13	
12 months	HAV two doses at an interval of 6 months to 1 year.	
15 months	Rotavirus vaccine + PCV 13 booster	
	Chickenpox vaccine (single dose up to 12 years, subsequently two doses 4–8 weeks apart). A booster dose is being recommended after the age of 5 years	
After 9 years	HPV two doses at 0 and 6 months during 9–14 years	
	After 14 years, three doses are given at 0, 1 or 2 and 6 months	
Additional vaccines during special situations		
	IPV (injectable or inactivated polio vaccine) is given to immunocompromised or HIV-positive children. It is being administered routinely as a part of post-polio eradication policy	
	Meningococcal vaccine (during an epidemic, Haj pilgrims, sickle cell disease, CSF rhinorrhea). Polysaccharide vaccine is given in a single dose after 2 years	
	Pneumococcal polysaccharide vaccine, i.e. PPV 23 single dose (chronic lung and heart disease, splenectomy, nephrotic syndrome, immunocompromised child)	

(Contd.)

TABLE 8.1 Recommended immunization schedule (*Contd.*)   **167**

Vaccine

Influenza vaccine (bronchial asthma, immunocompromised child). Initially 2 doses are given 4 weeks apart after the age of 6 months, followed by yearly boosters at the onset of monsoon and winter

Anti-rabies vaccine (high-risk individuals, following animal bites)

Rabies "pre-exposure prophylaxis" is given to high-risk population (children with pets, hostelers), postmen, veterinary doctors, wild life handlers, and technicians. Three primary doses 1.0 mL IM on day 0, 7 and 21 or 28. A booster dose is given after 1 year and then every 5 years. In immunized subjects, for "post-exposure" protection, only two doses are given on days 0 and 3. In these cases, no rabies immune globulins (RIG) is needed.

Cholera vaccine (to control epidemics, visitors to *kumbh mela,* Haj pilgrims)
Two doses are given 2 weeks apart in infants older than one year

Japanese B encephalitis inactivated vaccine (endemic areas, during epidemics) is administered in a single dose
Live attenuated SA-14-14-2 JE vero cell culture vaccine is given in 2 doses (0.5 mL SC) 6 to 8 weeks apart. There is no need for boosters

Yellow fever vaccine (travelers to South Africa). It is given as a single dose after the age of 6 months followed by boosters every 10 years. Avoid during pregnancy

*Vi capsular polysaccharide *S. typhi* Type 2 conjugated to tetanus toxoid (Typbar-TCV) can be given during 9–12 months as a single dose.
**Pregnant woman must receive 2 doses of TT or Td at 4 weeks interval. The second dose should be taken at least 4 weeks before delivery.
***In older children, single or two primary doses are given.

BCG: Bacillus Calmette-Guerin vaccine for TB, HBV: Hepatitis B vaccine, DTP: Triple antigen containing vaccines against diphtheria, tetanus and pertussis (whooping cough), DTwP (whole cell pertussis), DTap (acellular pertussis), WP vaccine is superior to aP vaccine in terms of immunogenicity and duration of protection but is more reactogenic. PCV 7: 7-valent pneumococcal conjugated vaccine, PPV 23: 23-valent pneumococcal polysaccharide vaccine. bOPV: Bivalent oral polio vaccine containing strains 1 and 3. IPV: Inactivated polio vaccine, MMR: Measles, mumps and rubella vaccine, Tdap: Tetanus toxoid with low dose diphtheria and low dose acellular pertussis vaccine, Td: Dual vaccine with low dose diphtheria vaccine (5 Lf or 2 iu) which can be safely given to adults, TT: Tetanus toxoid, Hib: *Haemophilus influenzae* type b, HAV: Hepatitis A vaccine

1. The suggested schedule may be modified by the consultant pediatrician as per the local needs.

2. Breastfeeding can be given after oral polio vaccine and it does not interfere with development of satisfactory immunity.

3. Most immunizations can be given in the presence of a minor illness. Paracetamol can be given following a vaccination for relief of local pain and fever, but it may reduce immunogenicity of the vaccine.

4. There is no need to give Hib vaccine (*Haemophilus influenzae* type b vaccine), if it has not been taken by the age of 1½ years.

5. The need and cost-effectiveness of optional vaccines must be explained to the parents before they are recommended.

6. Live vaccines should be avoided in immunocompromised children and symptomatic HIV-positive infants.

7. A number of vaccines can be administered together simultaneously at two different sites or as a combo formulation without interfering with development of protection against different antigens. A live vaccine can be administered after an inactivated vaccine (or *vice versa*) without any minimum recommended interval. However, a minimum interval of 4 weeks is recommended between administration of two live vaccines.

8. When a dose of a vaccine is missed, the remaining doses should be administered at the earliest opportunity while keeping in mind that the vaccine dose already given is valid.

9. Before giving the next dose of vaccine, ask the mother if the child had any significant reaction to the last dose of the vaccine.

10. OPV-related paralytic poliomyelitis is being increasingly reported from developed countries. These countries have changed their strategy and are giving IPV (injectable or inactivated or killed polio vaccine).

Care of the Normal Newborns

8

Supplements and Follow-up

Human milk of healthy mothers receiving adequate nutrition and supplements of micronutrients is a complete food to look after all the nutritional needs of their healthy normal weight babies. Vitamin K (1.0 mg in term and 0.5 mg in preterm) IM is given to all babies at birth to prevent occurrence of hemorrhagic disease of the newborn. There are recent reports to suggest that some healthy breastfed babies may develop rickets at 3–4 months of age and all exclusively breastfed babies should be provided supplements of vitamin D. Human milk is likely to be deficient in vitamin D, if mother has inadequate exposure to sunlight or is dark skinned. There is enough evidence to recommend routine supplementation of vitamin D in a dose of 400–600 iu/day to all breastfed babies. The infants should be followed up in the Well Baby Clinic for evaluation of their growth and development, immunizations, nutritional advice, early diagnosis of abnormalities and guidance to the parents for the management of day-to-day problems of their children. When complementary weaning foods are started after 6 months of age, supplements of vitamins and minerals should be provided, up to the age of one year.

COMMON NEONATAL PROBLEMS

The knowledge regarding various developmental variations and physiological conditions and their evolution is important for giving proper advice, guidance and assurance to the mother. Most mothers observe their babies carefully and are often worried by minor physical peculiarities, which may be of no consequence. Her complaints, however, must be listened to carefully and should not be ignored lightly without doing proper evaluation of the baby.

Vomiting

A large number of normal babies vomit on the first day due to irritation of stomach by swallowed amniotic fluid. If vomiting is persistent, stomach should be washed with 100 mL normal saline and baby offered 5% solution of glucose in water for the next two feeds. The regurgitation or vomiting soon after feeds is often due to faulty technique of feeding and aerophagy. The regurgitation is non-projectile and adequate weight gain is maintained. The proper advice regarding feeding and burping, whether solicited or not, must be given to all mothers. If the vomiting is persistent, projectile or bile stained, associated with failure to pass meconium during the first 24 hours and/or abdominal distension, the baby should be investigated for intestinal obstruction.

In gastroesophageal reflux and hiatus hernia, vomiting characteristically occurs when the baby is returned to the cot after the feed. It does not occur, if the baby is held upright. Some restless infants may vomit due to pylorospasm. In hypertrophic pyloric stenosis, vomiting characteristically occurs after two weeks of age. It is more likely to occur in a first born male infant and is characterized by non-bilious projectile vomiting, poor weight gain and constipation. Vomiting may be a symptom of raised intracranial tension due to intracranial hemorrhage, birth asphyxia, meningitis, systemic infection, cardiac failure and metabolic disorders such as galactosemia and salt losing variety of congenital adrenal hyperplasia. For blood-tinged vomiting, refer to Chapter 23.

Failure to Pass Meconium and Urine

Some babies may pass meconium *in utero* or soon after birth but all healthy babies must move the bowels within 24 hours of age. The babies pass black tarry stools (meconium) during first 2 to 3 days of life followed by greenish stools (transitional stools) for next 1–2 days. The non-passage of meconium by 24 hours of age is an indication for doing appropriate investigations to exclude intestinal obstruction.

Fetus voids urine regularly *in utero* after 12 weeks of gestation. After birth, most babies void on the first day but all babies must pass urine by 48 hours of age. In most cases of alleged non-passage of urine, usually the baby has actually passed urine which has been overlooked. Infants with genuine delayed passage of urine should be investigated for obstructive uropathy and agenesis of kidneys. The normal neonate voids after each feed, around 6 to 12 times/day. Some babies may cry before passing urine due to discomfort of full bladder, the baby becomes dazed and quiet while passing urine and starts crying again after having passed urine because of wet napkins. The stream of urine should be good and forceful and there should be no straining during micturition or dribbling in the end.

Bowel Disorders

Constipation Babies on cow's milk or formula feeds are often constipated due to hard casein curds. Those receiving breast milk usually pass two to six golden-yellow, sticky, semi-loose stools due to high content of lactose. Constipation is best managed by giving additional glucose water, extra sugar in the milk, honey and orange, tangerine or sweet lemon juice. In United States, honey is avoided in infants below one year of age due to risk of botulism. The usual symptoms of botulism include constipation, weak cry or irritability, floppiness of muscles with inability to control the head, drooping eyelids, drooling and difficulty in sucking. The stimulus of a lubricated rectal thermometer often initiates reflex peristaltic activity of the gut. The laxatives should be avoided. In refractory cases, the possibilities of Hirschsprung's disease, anal stensosis and cretinism should be ruled out.

Diarrhea Change in a baby's established bowel pattern towards greater frequency and looseness should be taken seriously. The transitional stools are passed during the third and fourth day after birth. These are often semi-loose, and greenish-yellow. The frequency of bowel motions is increased which settles spontaneously within 24 to 48 hours. Many babies pass stools while being fed or soon after the feed because of exaggerated gastrocolic reflex which may persist for a couple of weeks. These infants continue to gain weight satisfactorily though their mothers are often worried. The breastfed babies develop increased frequency of stools, if the mother is taking ampicillin, cephalosporins, tetracyclines, certain laxatives and following excessive consumption of foods with high organic acid content such as oranges, tangerines, cherries, tomatoes and chillies. The intake of glucose water and honey by the baby may result in diarrhea. The infective diarrhea is more likely to occur in bottle-fed babies. Stools are watery with mucus and pus cells. Acute infective diarrheal illness in a newborn baby should preferably be treated with parenteral fluid therapy and systemic antibiotics. Diarrhea may also occur due to overfeeding or serious underfeeding, congenital thyrotoxicosis, maternal drug addiction, Hirschsprung's disease, metabolic disorders such as salt-losing variety of adrenal hyperplasia, disaccharidase and enterokinase deficiency.

Physiological Jaundice

In almost two-thirds of term babies, physiological jaundice appears on the second or third day of birth, reaches peak on the 4th or 5th or third day and disappears by 10–14 days. The jaundice is not deep (serum bilirubin <15 mg/dL) and it causes mild yellow staining of the trunk without any staining of palms and soles. The physician attending on the newborn should be alert and look for other causes of jaundice in the neonatal period. For details refer to Chapter 18.

Hiccups, Sneezing and Yawning

These physiological body responses are common in healthy newborn babies. Hiccups are produced by spasmodic contractions of diaphragm and are characterized by sudden, noisy and jerky retractions of suprasternal notch and xiphisternal region. They usually occur immediately after a feed due to distension of stomach and irritation of diaphragm. Sneezing occurs due to irritation of the nostrils by secretions and should not be considered as a sign of upper respiratory infection. Yawning is common before going to sleep or on waking up. The presence of these physiological responses should be viewed as positive attributes of a healthy baby.

Dehydration Fever

During summer months when environmental temperature goes above 39°C, some otherwise healthy newborn babies may develop fever on the second or third day of life. Hyperthermia occurs due to poor heat dissipation mechanisms and inadequate intake of breast milk during the phase of physiologic lactational inadequacy. The fever is transient and usually disappears after 24–48 hours. The baby remains active, alert and cries for feeds. The baby should be dressed with light and loose cotton clothes and his environment kept cool in summer. The newborn babies should never by exposed to direct sunlight during the hot summer months. There is no role of antipyretics in the management of this condition because the set temperature of the thermostat in the hypothalamus is not altered. Hydrotherapy, adequate feeding and nursing in a cool well-ventilated room are enough to manage such a baby.

Superficial Infections

Superficial infections such as skin pustules, conjunctivitis, umbilical sepsis and thrush are common in newborn babies especially during summer months. The opportunity of exposing the baby nude during the procedure of bathing, should be utilized to screen the baby for superficial infections. Refer to Chapter 16 for clinical manifestations and management of superficial infections.

Excessive Crying

During first few days, most babies sleep throughout the day while they are awake, noisy and troublesome during the night. This is due to continuation of *in utero* pattern of their activity. It seems that during waking hours, while mother is walking or working, the baby is rocked in the water-filled amniotic sac. The fetus, therefore, sleeps during the day, while at night when mother goes to bed, the baby wakes up and plays by actively moving his limbs. Moreover, the baby has no perception of day and night and he exhibits identical pattern of activity round-the-clock.

The babies are less likely to be fed at night and they often cry due to hunger. The crying at night, to some extent, may be apparent because episodes of crying sound louder in the solitude of night and they are more disturbing to the tired and sleepy mother and intolerant neighbours. Evening and night crying may occur due to intestinal colic. It usually takes about 6 to 8 weeks before the baby establishes the routine of sleeping more at night and playing during the daytime.

No two babies are alike, some babies cry more readily than others and would scream vigorously without any patience for a minor reason. The babies usually cry when they are hungry or in discomfort. Crying may be due to unpleasant sensation of a full bladder before passing urine, painful evacuation of hard stools or mere soiling by the urine and stools. An experienced mother or physician can distinguish between the cry used as a signal for food and the cry of discomfort. The spells of crying unrelieved either by feeding, changing the soiled napkins or by rocking the baby may be due to abdominal colic. Such a baby may produce audible gurgling sounds and feels comfortable in a prone position which facilitates the expulsion of gas from below and above. The otitis media causes intractable, continuous, uninterrupted crying. Diagnosis may be suspected, if there is associated fever or nasal catarrh. The insect bites should also be kept in mind as an important cause of night crying. The baby may cry due to loneliness and boredom. Night crying with arching of back is a symptom of gastroesophageal reflux. Excessive crying is associated with inflammatory painful conditions, cerebral irritability, narcotic-withdrawal syndrome, thyrotoxicosis and ephedrine toxicity. Most babies are cranky and fussy while dozing off to sleep. The crying baby should be handled with patience, common sense and good humor.

Evening Colic

It is a distinct clinical entity of uncertain etiology. The clinical picture is characterized by sudden bouts of unexplained crying spells in the evening after a few days of birth. The attacks of sudden screaming with flexion of thighs and flushing or frowning of face occur at a precise time in the evening in a clockwise regularity and may last for a couple of minutes or hours. The crying episodes apparently occur due to intestinal colic as evidenced by excessive gurgling or peristaltic sounds on palpation or auscultation of abdomen. Excessive crying due to colic leads to further swallowing of air thus initiating a vicious cycle of colic-crying-colic. The condition is more common among first born wiry and active babies of anxious parents/grandparents. The incidence of disorder is equal among breastfed and formula-fed infants.

Nothing seems to provide relief to the baby who cries with full vigor and the whole family is extremely upset and demoralized by these unexplained shrieking episodes. Holding the baby against skin, rocking, taking him for a drive, cuddling, patting, kissing and prone positioning may provide temporary relief. The crying spell may abate in response to music or lullaby, continuous buzz of a hairdryer, washing machine or a vacuum cleaner. Administration of antispasmodic drops 30 minutes before the anticipated time of colic and placing the baby in a prone position for effective release of wind from above and below provides some relief to most babies. Probiotics have been shown to provide relief to some infants. Local application of asafoetida over the periumbilical area and administration of decoction of *ajwain* and *saunf* are useful and effective home remedies for relief of colic and flatulence in infants. Avoid making unnecessary changes in the feeding regime of the baby. The condition spontaneously resolves after 1 to 2 months. There is a need to conduct follow-up studies to assess the later behavior and personality profile of these colicky infants versus the non-colicky placid babies.

Breath-Holding Spells

Temper tantrums with breath-holding spells are classically seen after the age of six months. Rarely, episodes of crying with holding of breath in expiration and cyanosis may be seen during newborn period. The baby is fussy and temperamental while parents or grandparents are overindulgent and overanxious. The baby is over reactive and lacks patience and demands immediate relief from minor discomfort or inconvenience. The condition must be differentiated from anoxic spells due to tetralogy of Fallot and excessive crying in brain damaged infants.

Excessive Sleepiness

Some babies may keep their eyes closed most of the time during the first 48 hours. This should not be a cause for concern and anxiety. During first few days, many infants go to sleep after taking only few sucks on the bottle or breast. They should be kept aroused during feed by tickling on the soles and behind the ears but it should not be carried to the point of annoyance or discomfort. Heavy maternal sedation during labor may be associated with excessive sleepiness in the baby for first 48 hours. Barbiturates, bromides and opium derivatives when taken by the nursing mother,

may cause sleepiness in her suckling infant. When a baby is floppy, such as in mongolism and cretinism, there is lack of vigour and desire for feeds. *Lethargy and lack of interest in feeds in a baby, who was alert and active previously, is an important sign of serious systemic disease and may be the sole manifestation of septicemia.*

Disorders due to Transplacental Passage of Hormones

Mastitis neonatorum The engorgement of breasts occurs in full-term babies of both sexes on the third or fourth day and may last for a few days or even weeks. Lack of inactivation of progesterone and estrogens after birth due to immaturity of neonatal liver, leads to further rise in their levels thus resulting in hypertrophy of breasts (Figure 8.4). Administration of metoclopramide to the baby may aggravate hypertrophy of breasts. The local massage, fomentation and temptation to express the milk should be curbed and mother reassured regarding benign nature of the condition.

Vaginal bleeding The development of menstrual-like withdrawal bleeding may occur in about one-fourth of female babies after 3 to 5 days of birth. It occurs due to fall in the level of sex hormones after birth when baby is disconnected from the placenta. The bleeding is mild and lasts for 2 to 4 days. The local aseptic cleaning of genitals is advised. Additional vitamin K is unnecessary.

Mucoid vaginal secretions Most female babies have thin grayish-white glairy-mucoid vaginal secretions. These should not be mistaken for purulent discharge. They should be gently cleaned at the time of bathing.

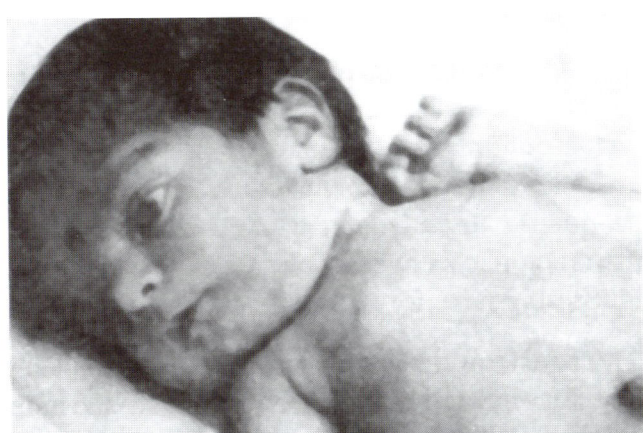

Figure 8.4 Marked hypertrophy of both the breasts in a term baby at the age of 5 days.

Caput Succedaneum

Caput succedaneum is a boggy, diffuse, edematous swelling of soft tissues of scalp over the presenting part. The swelling is present at birth and its size and severity is related to the duration of labor. The swelling is pitting, non-fluctuant and not limited by sutures unlike cephalhematoma. The swelling and ecchymosis may be present over the face in babies born by brow or face presentation. The swelling disappears spontaneously during next few days.

Cephalhematoma

It is subperiosteal collection of blood secondary to injury during delivery. The swelling appears after 2–3 days of birth. It is a fluctuant swelling and does not cross the suture line (Figure 8.5). It may be associated with linear skull fracture in 5–20% cases. Depending upon its size, it resolves spontaneously after a few days or weeks. After recovery, the edge may be elevated and residual calcification is seen in 1% cases. Incision or aspiration is contraindicated unless it gets infected or is associated with critical hyperbilirubinemia.

Subgaleal Hematoma

Following prolonged vacuum extraction, there is massive collection of blood between periosteum of skull and skin of scalp or galea. There is diffuse

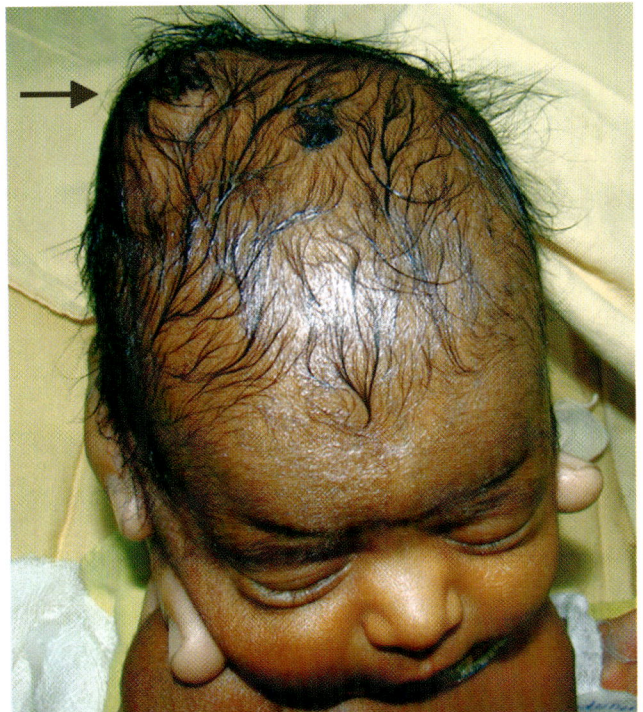

Figure 8.5 Cephalhematoma over right parietal region.

fluctuant swelling over the entire calvarium with periorbital and auricular edema and ecchymosis. The swelling is not limited by suture lines. Massive bleeding may be associated with anemia, shock, jaundice and infection. Management consists of administration of vitamin K, pressure dressing of scalp, blood transfusion and phototherapy.

Cradle Cap

It is characterized by presence of a seborrheic cap with crusting over the scalp. It may lead to development of seborrheic dermatitis during early infancy which is difficult to differentiate from atopic dermatitis. Application of coconut oil or milk scum or *malai*, over the scalp at night followed by shampoo with savlon or cetrimide is usually followed by gradual resolution.

Asymmetric Head Shape

Depending upon *in utero* or postnatal position of head, the baby may develop odd shaped head. Occiput or one of the parietal areas may become flat and bald. If head size is normal, there is no cause for concern. Proper positioning of head with support of soft pillows, to ensure that the prominent part of the head touches the cot, leads to gradual rounding of the head shape.

Craniotabes

Softening of skull bones which can be pressed like a table tennis ball is called craniotabes. It should be looked for away from the sutures and fontanels. Localized craniotabes may be normally seen due to *in utero* pressure of the skull against mother's pubic bone. Craniotabes is suggestive of prematurity, hydrocephalus, congenital rickets, congenital syphilis, osteogenesis imperfecta, lacunar skull, and mandibulofacial dysostosis.

The Setting-Sun Sign

The eyes are rolled down and the sclera becomes visible as it is uncovered by the upper eyelids. Transient and episodic setting-sun sign is seen in normal newborn babies. Persistent and constant setting-sun sign due to paresis of upward gaze is seen in infants with hydrocephalus and kernicterus.

Obstructed Nasolacrimal Duct

It presents as persistent wetness or watering (epiphora) from one or both the eyes which are not congested. There is blockage of nasolacrimal duct which drains tears from the eyes into the nostrils. The condition is common and occurs in 5% of babies. Lacrimal sac areas (between inner canthi of the eyes and nose) are firmly massaged with index finger and thumb and lacrimal duct is massaged by exerting an inward pressure from above downwards along the lateral surfaces of the nose (Crigler massage). The mother must trim her nails before doing this procedure. The massage is done 15–20 times at a time, at least 3 times in a day and is continued for 1–2 months or till watering of eyes disappears. The epithelial debris is often squeezed out and patency of duct is restored. During first week, after the massage, antibacterial drops are instilled in the eyes. If the duct does not open up by 5–6 months, probing and syringing through the punctum is done by an ophthalmologist.

Umbilical Granuloma

It manifests as a small flesh-like pale nodule at the base of umbilicus with persistent discharge. This can be managed by cauterization with silver nitrate or application of common salt. The local applications may be repeated after every 3 to 4 days till the base is dry. Local sepsis should be managed by application of mercurochrome, betadine or antibiotic cream.

Sore Buttocks and Diaper Rashes

Use of nylon or water tight plastic napkins or soakable diaper and delay in changing the diaper causes redness, induration and excoriation due to ammoniacal dermatitis. In boys, foreskin of penis may be affected causing difficulty in passing urine. The bottom should be cleaned gently with wet cotton and kept dry and exposed to air. Baby skin care wipes are convenient to use for cleaning the bottom. Application of soothing ointment containing titanium dioxide and zinc oxide provides relief. When a nappy rash is associated with erythematous papules or vesicles at the periphery, candidal infection should be suspected. The causative factors for monilial infection like vaginal moniliasis or candida infection of the breast nipples of the mother should be looked for. It is treated by local application of skin cream containing clotrimazole or terbinafine.

COMMON DEVELOPMENTAL PECULIARITIES

"Most problems in healthy term newborn babies are minor, physiological, or developmental and without any clinical significance. But when a newborn is "genuinely sick", he is likely to be very sick and cannot be managed on an ambulatory basis".

Meharban Singh

Toxic erythema or urticaria neonatorum It is an erythematous rash with central pallor (wheal-like) appearing on the second or third day in term babies (Figure 8.6). The rash starts on the face and spreads to the trunk and extremities in about 24 hours. It disappears spontaneously after 2 to 3 days without any specific treatment. The exact cause is not known but irritation of delicate vernix-depleted skin of the newborn by various environmental agents, such as toilet articles and clothes have been postulated. This does not explain the self-limiting nature and its rarity in babies below 32 weeks of gestation. The scrapings from skin lesions show eosinophils. Family history of atopy amongst relatives of infants suffering from urticaria neonatorum, further supports the allergic etiology. The rash should be differentiated from pyoderma, transient pustular melanosis and skin lesions of congenital syphilis.

Peeling of skin Dry skin with peeling and exaggerated transverse skin creases is seen in post-term and some term babies. Application of liquid paraffin or coconut oil or glycerine provides relief.

Cutis marmorata It is characterized by an evanescent, lacy, reticulated, red- or blue-marbled cutaneous vascular pattern over the extremities in infants exposed to low environmental temperature. It occurs due to exaggerated physiological vasomotor response to cold and disappears with increasing maturity and postnatal age.

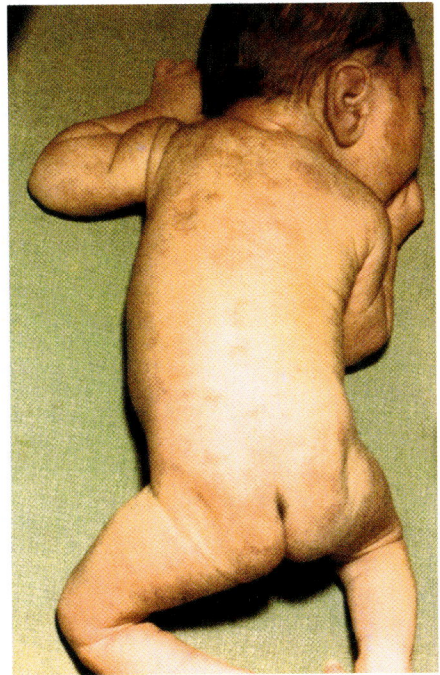

Figure 8.6 Toxic erythema in a 2-day-old term infant.

Harlequin color change The baby suddenly becomes blanched and pale on one half of the body while the other half remains pink. The episodes of color change last for a few minutes and occur in normal babies due to unexplained vasomotor phenomenon.

Subcutaneous fat necrosis (pseudoscleroderma, scleroderma neonatorum) During early newborn period, some babies develop subcutaneous fat necrosis as localized areas of pinkish-blue induration without any inflammatory signs over the buttocks, back, cheeks or limbs. The overlying skin may be blotchy red (but not warm), stretched and non-pinchable. There is no clinical significance and the condition resolves spontaneously.

Milia Pearly-white tiny cysts on the nose and cheeks due to retention of keratin are present in practically all newborn babies and disappear spontaneously.

Acne neonatorum Typical acne-like lesions with comedones may be seen over the forehead, nose and cheeks at birth in term babies. They occur due to transplacental passage of maternal androgens to the fetus. The skin lesions gradually diminish in size and disappear spontaneously within the next couple of days. There is no role of local application of any skin cream.

Stork-bites (salmon patches or nevus simplex) These are discrete pinkish-gray sparse capillary hemangiomata commonly located at nape of the neck, upper eyelids, forehead, and root of the nose. They invariably disappear after a few months.

Mongolian blue spots In babies of African and Asiatic origin, irregular blue patches of skin pigmentation are often present characteristically over the sacral area and buttocks though extremities and rest of the trunk may also be affected. The spots have no relation to Down syndrome and usually disappear by the age of 6 months. They should not be confused with bruising seen in babies delivered by breech presentation.

Subconjunctival hemorrhage Semilunar arcs of subconjunctival hemorrhage located at the outer canthus is a common finding in normal babies. Their presence is brought to the notice of the physician by the observant mother. The blood gets resorbed after a few days without leaving any pigmentation.

Epstein pearls These are whitish-yellow cysts, usually on the gums and either side of the median raphe of the hard palate and are of no significance. They are possibly epithelial inclusion cysts. Epstein pearls may occur over the prepuce or shaft of the penis as pearly white papules. They are benign in nature and invariably disappear within a few weeks.

Care of the Normal Newborns

8

Bohn's nodules These are pearly white papules due to keratin cysts originating from remnants of odontogenic epithelium of dental lamina or minor salivary glands. They occur over the alveolar ridge of gums, more commonly on the maxillary than the mandibular jaw. They should be differentiated from gingival cyst, Epstein pearls and natal teeth. Bohn's nodules are benign and rupture spontaneously and disappear within a few weeks.

Sucking callosities The presence of a button-like cornified plaque over the center of upper lip at birth is suggestive of *in utero* sucking efforts of the baby.

Congenital teeth The eruption of one or more lower incisor teeth before or soon after birth is seen in one in 4000 babies (Figure 8.7). The teeth may become loose and interefere with breastfeeding. There is a risk of spontaneous dislodgement with risk of aspiration. Moreover, culturally they are considered as a bad omen. It is advised to get the natal teeth extracted, if they are loose.

Tongue-tie It may be either in the form of a thin broad membrane or thick fibrous frenulum under the tongue producing a notch at the tip of the tongue due to traction. The tongue cannot be protruded beyond the lip margins. Tongue-tie seldom interferes with sucking or cause any delay in the development of speech. It may affect the clarity of speech. The condition is uncommon and is often overdiagnosed. The genuine tongue-tie may be snipped of excised with a laser by dentist after one year, if it is a source of anxiety to the parents.

Non-retractable prepuce The prepuce is normally non-retractable in all male newborn babies and should not be diagnosed as phimosis. The urethral opening is often pinpoint and is visualized with difficulty. The mother should be advised against forcibly retracting the foreskin during newborn period. After 2 years of age, while bathing, mother should gently retract the prepuce. The diagnosis of phimosis should be cosidered, if prepuce is fibrosed and non-retractable, stream of urine is not forceful and is interrupted and when there is history of recurrent urinary tract infections. Ballooning of foreskin during urination is normal. Circumcision is credited to have a number of health benefits, including ease of maintaining local hygiene, decreased risk of urinary tract infection, sexually transmitted infections and cancer of penis. Circumcision is contraindicated in infants with hooded prepuce, hypospadias, ambiguous genitalia and bleeding disorder.

Congenital hydrocele A small sac containing fluid may be noticed in one of the scrotal sacs at birth or after few weeks of life. It is a small communicating hydrocele of tunica vaginalis and may extend upwards in the spermatic cord. It usually disappears spontaneously during first three months of life.

Hymenal tags Mucosal tags at the margin of hymen are seen in two-thirds of female infants.

Sacral dimple A dimple in the midline over the sacrococcygeal region should not be confused with a pilonidal sinus. It is of no clinical significance.

Prominent xiphisternum Xiphisternal cartilage may stand out rather prominently and is of no significance.

Bowed legs In normal babies, when legs are extended, they form a concavity inwards due to genu varus giving an appearance of bowed legs. It is not suggestive of rickets or bony deformity. After first birth day, bowing of legs is replaced by physiological knock knees.

Umbilical hernia When the cord has fallen off, umbilical hernia may manifest after the age of two weeks or later. It may be associated with divarication of recti (Figure 8.8). Umbilical hernia is more common in infants with hypotonia due to cretinism, rickets and Down syndrome. Most of these usually disappear

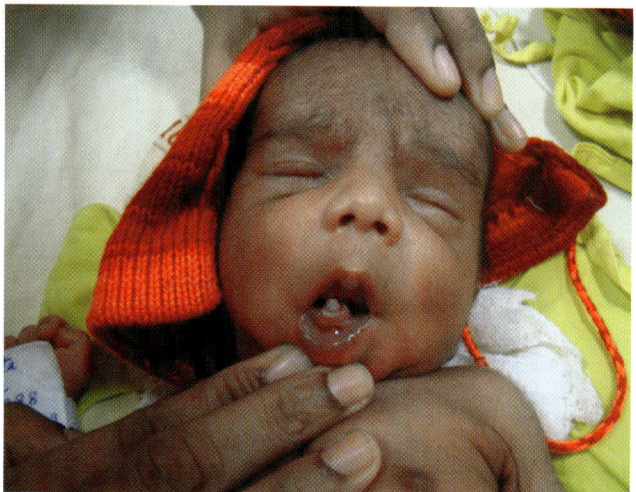

Figure 8.7 Infant born with natal lower incisor.

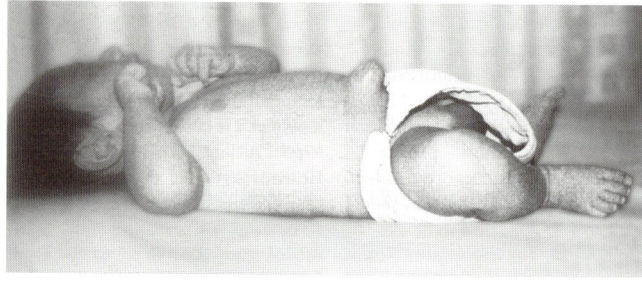

Figure 8.8 Umbilical hernia. No bandage should be applied as hernia spontaneously disappears after a few months.

spontaneously by 6 months to one year. Application of a coin and bandage over the hernia is not recommended, as it may further weaken the anterior abdominal wall. If there are any associated conditions which are recognized to increase the intra-abdominal pressure, like excessive crying, constipation, persistent cough, etc., they should be identified and managed appropriately. When hernia is large or persists beyond 3 years, surgical closure is indicated.

First Ambulatory Visit

The baby should be called for first follow-up visit one week after discharge from the hospital. Ensure that mother is giving exclusive breastfeeding and lactation is well established. The feed should be offered round-the-clock on demand basis. The exclusively breastfed babies should be given supplements of vitamin D 400–600 iu/day during first 6 months of life. Check the temperature of the baby by touching the trunk and extremities. In a stable baby, trunk is warm to touch while hands and feet are warm and pink. Advise the family against risk of nosocomial infection. The visitors should not be allowed to pick or kiss the baby. The family members and visitors must wash their hands with soap and water before touching the baby. The presence of mild yellow staining of trunk is normal. However, if jaundice is significant and baby is two weeks old, ask for the color of urine and stools. If urine is colorless and stools are yellow, the possibilities of breast milk jaundice and congenital hypothyroidism should be considered. When urine is yellow-colored and stools are pale, the infant should be investigated for cholestasis. The exposure of the baby to sunlight for phototherapy is neither effective nor safe and is not recommended. The baby massage is recommended, if there are no health issues and body weight has crossed 3 kg. If the baby has not received any vaccine, administer the first dose of BCG, HBV and bOPV. The mother should be given a Road-to-Health card and advised about further schedule of immunizations. Ask the mother for any problems or issues that may be bothering her and they should be assessed and resolved to her satisfaction. The mother should be advised to record the due dates of various immunizations in her mobile phone so that she can visit the pediatrician for regular follow-up and anthropometry.

BIBLIOGRAPHY

Balasubramanian S. Vitamin D deficiency in breastfed infants and the need for routine vitamin D supplementation. *Indian J Med Res* 2011, 133(3):250–252.

Balasubramanian S, Ganesh R. Vitamin D deficiency in exclusively breastfed infants. *Indian J Med Res* 2008; 127:250–255.

Balasubramanian S, Shah A, Pemde HK; *et al*. Indian Academy of Pediatrics (IAP) Advisory Committee on Vaccines and Immunization practices (ACVIP): recommended immunization schedule (2018-2019) and update on immunizations for children aged 0 through 18 years. *Indian Pediatr* 2018, 55: 1066–74.

Blume-Peytavi U, Cork MJ, Faegermann J, Szczapa J, Vanaclocha F, Gelmettic. Bathing and cleaning in newborns from day 1 to first year of life: recommendations from a European round table meeting. *J Europ Acad Dermatol and Venereol* 2009; 23:751–759.

Blume-Peytavi U, Hanser M, Stamatas GN, *et al*. Skin care practices for newborns and infants: Review of the clinical evidence for best practices. *Pediatr Dermatology* 2012, 29(1):1–14.

Gordon CM, Feldman HA, Sinclair L, *et al*. Prevalence of vitamin D deficiency among healthy infants and toddlers. *Arch Pediatr Adolesc Med* 2008; 162(6):505–512.

Illingworth RS (ed.) The Normal Child. *London, Churchill Livingstone*, 10th edition 1991.

Kulkarni A, Kaushik JS, Gupta P, Sharma H, Agarwal RK. Massage and touch therapy in neonates: The current evidence. *Indian Pediatr* 2010; 47: 771–776.

Mullany LC, Darmstadt GL, Khatry SK, *et al*. Impact of umbilical cord cleansing with 4% chlorhexidine on time to cord separation among newborns in southern Nepal: a cluster-randomized, community-based trial. *Pediatrics* 2006; 118: 1864–1871.

Singh M, Krishnamoorty KS, Sinclair S and Ghai OP. Some developmental characteristics in the newborn. *Indian Pediatr* 1970; 7:378.

Singh M. Common neonatal problems and their management. *Indian Practitioner* 1970; 23:65.

Singh M. Care of normal newborn babies: Some practical points. *Indian J Pract Pediatr* 1993; 1:6–13.

Singh M. The Art and Science of Baby and Child Care. *CBS Publishers and Distributors Pvt. Ltd.*, New Delhi, 4th Edition 2014.

Solanki K, Matnani M, Kale M, *et al*. Transcutaneous absorption of topically massaged oil in neonates. *Indian Pediatr* 2005; 42:998–1005.

Vashishtha VM, Choudhary P, Kalra A, *et al*. Indian Academy of Pediatrics (IAP) recommended immunization schedule for children aged 0 through 18 years: India 2014 and updates on immunization. *Indian Pediatr* 2014; 51: 785–800.

Warren JB, Phillipi CA. Care of the well newborn. *Pediatr Rev* 2012, 33(1): 4–18.

Young Infants Clinical Signs Study Group. Clinical signs that predict severe illness in children under age 2 months: a multicentre study. *Lancet* 2008; 371:135–42.

Ziegler EE, Hollis BW, Nelson JE, Jeter JM. Vitamin D deficiency in breastfed infants in Iowa. *Pediatrics* 2006; 118(2):603–610.

Traditional and Cultural Practices for the Care of Newborn Babies

"Ayurveda literally means a knowledge of life. It is almost 5000 years old art and science of healing, a way of life, happy and healthy living. Ayurveda adds not only years to life but also life to years".

Charaka Samhita

The traditional or indigenous practices are time honored rituals and beliefs which are prevalent in a community and they may pertain to a wide range of activities. According to World Health Organization (WHO), traditional or folk medicine is defined as "sum total of the knowledge, skills and practices based on the theories, beliefs and experiences indigenous to different cultures, whether explicable or not, used in the maintenance of health as well as the prevention, diagnosis, improvement or treatment of physical and mental illness". Every community has its own way of rearing children which is ingrained in the society through traditions established over centuries. The customs and cultural practices pertaining to mother craft and child care are passed on from one generation to another, from grandmother to mother and to their daughters and grandchildren. The ancestral or conventional child care practices, by and large, are based on core knowledge and wisdom although some of them may have emerged purely from intuition, superstitions and unfounded beliefs. The traditional practices are influenced by the educational level, socio-economic status and value system of the family and society. In some Asian and African countries, up to 80% of the population rely on traditional medicine for their primary health care needs. When this approach is adopted in an organized manner it is often called as complementary or alternative medicine.

It is neither possible nor feasible to provide modern medical care to all the people of a huge country like India, which is bogged down by numbers, illiteracy and economic poverty. There is no doubt that a combination of modern and traditional healing is appropriate to serve our health needs. However, the rapidly changing lifestyle and introduction of modern medicine has caused confusion in the minds of tradition-bound people and the promoters of the Indian system of medicine. There is evidence to suggest that the traditional health care practices have a definite link with the science of Ayurveda. The Alma-Ata declaration on primary health care by WHO in 1978 motivated several countries to improve their traditional medicine practices by promoting use of indigenous medicines in their primary health care model. The ancient health care practices and herbal medicine should not be called as "alternative" because they are in fact the "original" medical practices that have been used for thousands of years while modern medicine was discovered about 100 years ago.

IMPORTANCE OF TRADITIONAL HEALTH CARE PRACTICES

"Instead of viewing alternative medicine as a foe to be conquered, a physician would do well to use it to his or her advantage. Even if an alternative treatment hasn't been sufficiently demonstrated to help, it still enables a physician to involve the patient in the healing".

Alan Bryson

Most of our health care practices have their origin in our traditions based on core knowledge and wisdom of our ancestors. The conventional or traditional practices have become part and parcel of our lifestyle. They are available at the doorstep of the people and they are readily acceptable to the society. Above all, they are cheap and affordable and can be utilized by a large segment of our community. The traditional practices and home remedies are promoted by village healers, midwives, physicians, practitioners of Indian system of medicine (Ayurveda, Siddha, Unani), charlatans, quacks and wise old people of the community. The traditional practices are so ingrained in the minds of people that it is difficult to change them easily even when they are identified to be useless or harmful.

TYPES OF TRADITIONAL HEALTH CARE PRACTICES

Traditional health care practices can be categorized into four main sub-groups: Useful, harmful, innocuous and of uncertain utility. The health workers must be conversant with common customs and beliefs pertaining to health care of children in the area or community in which they work.

Useful Traditional Practices

A number of traditional health practices for the care of newborn babies are useful and based on sound scientific knowledge and logic (Table 9.1). They must be promoted and actively encouraged in the society. Their promotion is likely to facilitate the participation of the community and enhance the acceptability of the health care providers of the modern system of medicine. These practices are more appropriate to serve our health needs as they are based on simple technology. A large number of diseases are minor and self-limiting and it is appropriate to treat them with safe and cheap home remedies.

Harmful Traditional Practices

A large number of customs and cultural practices prevalent in our country for mother craft and child rearing are positively harmful (Table 9.2). In certain

TABLE 9.1 List of useful traditional practices

- Drinking milk and avoiding tea or coffee during pregnancy to have a fair-complexioned baby.
- Abstinence during pregnancy.
- Confinement and delivery at mother's place.
- Isolation of the mother-child dyad for 40 days.
- Oil massage and sunbath.
- Universal and prolonged breastfeeding.
- Instillation of colostrum in the eyes.
- Use of cup and spoon or *paladay* for top feeding
- Baby is encouraged to sleep on mother's bed and she avoids to turn her back towards the baby.
- Nursing the babies in supine position which is associated with lower incidence of sudden infant deaths (SIDs).

TABLE 9.2 List of harmful traditional practices and beliefs

- Early marriage of girls.
- Eating less food during pregnancy to reduce the risk of cephalopelvic disproportion.
- Keeping fast even during pregnancy.
- Avoiding iron-folic acid tablets as "they may harm the fetus".
- Avoiding sonography during pregnancy as it may put pressure on the fetus and cause growth retardation.
- Conducting delivery in a dark and ill-ventilated room.
- Use of rags/dirty clothes during delivery.
- Using harmful and ineffective resuscitation practices like holding the baby upside down, sprinkling cold water on the face, instilling onion juice in the nostrils, excessive physical manipulations like, roasting or crushing the placenta, loud beating of a metal plate, blowing into the nose/ears and milking the umbilical cord.
- Use of unsterile knife or blade for cutting the cord.
- Application of ash, mud, cow dung, *ghee,* catechu, *kumkum,* turmeric, etc. on the umbilical cord.
- Bathing the baby at birth.
- Giving prelacteal feeds like honey, sugar or jaggery water, *janam ghutti* or tea.
- Discarding colostrum and delaying breastfeeding for 5 days.
- Giving water to breastfed babies.
- Avoiding certain foods during lactation such as pulses, legumes, vegetables and some fruits.
- Opium for diarrhea/crying child.
- Application of *kajal* in the eyes.
- Use of pacifier or dummy nipple.
- Dilution of milk in a bottle-fed baby.
- Castor oil for constipation and diarrhea.
- Delayed weaning.
- Branding the baby to expel evil spirits.
- Instillation of oil and urine into the ears and nostrils.
- Gender bias in favor of males with suboptimal care or neglect of girls.
- Female genital mutilation (FGM).
- Starving the infant with fever and diarrhea.
- Viewing diseases as personification and wrath of goddesses.

communities, mothers are advised to eat less food during pregnancy as a safeguard against the birth of a big baby with the mistaken belief that it would be associated with difficult delivery. Till recently, tetanus neonatorum accounted for 2,50,000 neonatal deaths every year in our country due to widely prevalent unhygienic practices while cutting the cord and its subsequent care. At birth, the baby should be promptly dried and effectively covered to prevent hypothermia. Bathing the baby at birth is associated with the grave risk of hypothermia. The bath should be delayed till baby's body temperature has stabilized. Colostrum is replete with secretory IgA antibodies and must never by denied to the baby. It provides excellent protection to the baby against bacterial infections during early crucial days of life. Mothers should be encouraged to exclusively breastfeed their babies and even water should not be given during first 6 months of life irrespective of the weather. This is the best safeguard against occurrence of diarrheal disorders during early months of life. Weaning should not be delayed beyond 6 months of age. Infants do tolerate semisolid/semi-liquid cereals like porridge, *khichdi*, yoghurt, *daal*, rice, half-boiled egg, mashed banana, etc. in the absence of teeth. Early administration of adequate quantities of appropriate weaning foods with due precautions against contamination is the best safeguard against development of protein-energy malnutrition and infections in children.

Feeding should not be denied during an episode of fever or illness and instead it should be enhanced and promoted to meet the increased nutritional demands. Application of *kajal* in the eyes is associated with the risk of trachoma and bacterial conjunctivitis and it has been documented as a potential risk for lead poisoning in children. We have confirmed the utility of instillation of colostrum into the eyes for prevention and treatment of sticky eyes but pouring of milk, oil or cow's urine in the ear canal should be avoided as it leads to encrustation, fungal infection and deafness. Instillation of oil into the nostrils is associated with the risk of development of lipoid pneumonia due to aspiration. It is essential that community must be educated so that harmful rituals pertaining to child care can be stopped. There is an urgent need to inform and educate the village healers, rural medical practitioners, midwives, physicians practising Indian system of medicine and quacks regarding the dangers of some of the harmful and dangerous traditional health care practices which are rampant in our country.

Innocuous or Inconsequential Traditional Practices

A large number of traditional health care practices are apparently harmless or innocuous but are widely practiced (Table 9.3). Unless their hazards are recognized, it is best to ignore them because a concerted drive against these practices may actually be counterproductive. Though most of these practices are harmless but due to lack of their utility they may lead to delay in seeking medical aid with resultant deterioration in the condition of the child. Because of

TABLE 9.3 List of innocuous or inconsequential traditional beliefs
■ There is a popular belief that birth weight of the neonate should not be taken as it will cast an evil eye on the baby.
■ Baby bath is given after day 7 or 9 of life by adding gold, silver, hellebore, milk, rice and salt in water.
■ Giving prelacteal feeds like glucose water, honey, jaggery water, tea, cow's urine and ass's milk.
■ Nose and ear piercing, talisman, amulets, removing "*nazar*" or "bad eye" by applying *kala tikka* behind the ears or on the forehead, burning *lahi*, chillies, and alum.
■ Circumcision as a religious ritual.
■ Tying neem leaves on the door of the house.
■ Massage of anterior fontanel.
■ Making or buying clothes only after birth of the baby and not wearing any stitched clothes till day 6.
■ Blowing into the ears of the baby after a bath.
■ Keeping knife under the pillow to protect the infant against harmful spirits.
■ Clipping of nails is delayed till eruption of first tooth or after first birthday.
■ It is believed that if delivery occurs during 8th month of pregnancy, there is no chance of survival of the baby.
■ Baby is covered with a yellow cloth to prevent jaundice.
■ Umbilical cord is buried in the backyard of the home.
■ Blue beads, charm or *tabiz*, and garlic cloves are worn to the baby to keep off the evil spirits.
■ Tying a black thread around the neck and waist.

potential risk of infection, it is preferable to avoid any prelacteal feeds and mother should be encouraged to put the baby straight to the breast as soon as she has recovered from the exhaustion of labor. The physiological inadequacy of lactation during first 2–3 days does not impose any risk to a healthy newborn baby as long as he is not denied the virtues of colostrum. The ritual of circumcision based on religious sanction is safe, if performed by an experienced person and under local anesthesia with due precautions against infection and bleeding.

Traditional Practices of Doubtful or Uncertain Utility

A number of popular child rearing practices are of uncertain or of doubtful utility (Table 9.4). Most of these practices are innocuous but some of them may be harmful. *Janam ghutti* is claimed to cure constipation as well as diarrhea and is advertised on television. We all have enjoyed the taste of gripe water as young kids without realizing that it contains high concentration of alcohol. The currently available gripe waters

TABLE 9.4 Traditional practices of uncertain/doubtful utility

- *Janam ghutti.*
- Gripe water.
- Boiled water containing anisi, cumin seeds, cardamom for the mother after delivery.
- Use of a variety of traditional galactogogues: Garlic, ginger, coconut, jaggery, *jeera, bajra, ghee,* fenugreek, *panjeeri, sonth, khaskhas, harida, hing, peepalamul, sathavari,* pepper, *margosa, jeevanthi,* etc.
- Brandy for cough and cold/pneumonia.
- Application of paste made of egg yolk with rum on the chest for treatment of pneumonia.
- The concept of "Hot" and "Cold" foods.
- Avoiding exposure of pregnant women to eclipse.
- Wearing of copper, steel, and magnetic bracelets.

are, however, free of alcohol. In order to promote universal and effective breastfeeding, there is certainly a need to identify the most effective galactogogue from among the large list of home remedies recommended for promotion of lactation in different communities and regions of the country.

There is an urgent need to systematically study the utility, futility and possible dangers of a large number of traditional health care practices. The blind faith in the traditional health care practices of doubtful utility may lead to non-acceptance of modern system of medicine. All efforts must be made to accord right perspective to the prevalent traditional health care practices in the country in order to derive the maximum benefit for rearing of children and prevent avoidable hazards by launching a crusade against the harmful cultural practices. In order to promote local health traditions and indigenous medicines, the Government of India has provided a kit of medicines containing AYUSH (Ayurvedic, Unani, Siddha and Homeopathy) and allopathic medicines to treat common day-to-day illnesses. There is a need to do further research to ascertain the efficacy and safety of several of the practices and herbal remedies used by practitioners of traditional systems of medicine.

BIBLIOGRAPHY

Bangari A, Thapliyal SK, Ruchi, Aggarwal B, Sharma U. Traditional beliefs and practices in newborn care among mothers in a tertiary care centre in Dehradun, Uttarakhand, India. *Int. J Comm Med Public Hlth.* 2019, 6(6):2600–2604.

Bernard SB, Aurelia R, Sandrine D, Egon J. Evaluation of randomized controlled trials on complementary and alternative medicine. *Internet J Tech Assessment Health Care* 2000; 16(1):13–21.

Bhutta ZA, Darmstadt GL, Hasan BS, Haws RA. Community based intervention for improving perinatal and neonatal health outcomes in developing countries: A review of evidence. *Pediatrics* 2005, 115 (supple 2): 519–617.

Mahadevan S, Anantha Krishanan S, Srinivasan S. Lipoid pneumonia in South Indian infants. *Indian Pediatr* 1991; 28: 1529–1530.

Mathur GP, Kushwaha KP. Superstitions in pediatric practice (Editorial). *Indian Pediatr* 1986; 23:159–161.

Mohapatra SS, Baag RK. Customs and beliefs on neonatal care in a tribal community. *Indian Pediatr* 1982; 19:675–678.

Oliver SJ. The role of traditional medicine practice in primary health care within Aboriginal Australia: a review of the literature. *J Ethnobiology and Ethnomedicine* 2013; 9:46.

Report of a National Seminar on Traditional Practices in Mother and Child Care. *National Institute of Public Cooperation and Child Development,* New Delhi, 1989.

Reshma, Sujatha R. Cultural practices and beliefs on newborn care among mothers in a selected hospital of Mangalore talunk. *Nitte University J Hlth Sc.* 2014, 4(2):21–26.

Singh M, Sugathan PS, Bhujawala RA. Human colostrum for prophylaxis against sticky eyes and conjunctivitis in the newborn. *J Trop Pediatr* 1982; 28:35–37.

Singh M. Traditional health practices for care of children. *Swasth Hind* 1993; 37:50–51.

Tomar BS. Superstitions and child health. *Indian Pediatr* 1980, 17;883–885.

Vani SN. Report of National Workshop on Traditional Practices of Neonatal Care in India. *National Neonatology Forum,* Ahmedabad, 1990.

Wilson K, Richmond C. Indigenous health and medicine in International Encyclopedia of Human Geography. Kitchin R and Thrift NJ (Eds), *Oxford, Elsevier Ltd.,* 2009.

9

Essential Perinatal and Neonatal Care in the Community

Newborn babies constitute the foundation of a nation and no sensible government can afford to neglect their needs and rights. Healthy and sturdy babies are likely to evolve as physically and mentally strong adults with enhanced quality of human resource development. Neonatal deaths account for almost two-thirds of all infant deaths and 40% of all under-5 deaths. In India, optimal perinatal care with improved survival of infants is essential for effective fertility control and stabilization of population dynamics. Neonatal care is highly cost-effective because saving the life of a newborn baby is associated with survival and productivity for over 5 decades as opposed to intensive care of adults with cancer and the degenerative disorders which is associated with an average survival for 2–5 years. The World Bank has estimated that the burden of disease contributed by perinatal causes in India accounts for 25% of the global Disability Adjusted Life Years (DALYs) lost to the society. The Millennium Development Goal (MDG 4) of reducing under-5 mortality by two-thirds or 38 by 2015 cannot be achieved unless there is significant reduction in neonatal mortality.

DEMOGRAPHIC PROFILE

According to 2020 estimates, the current population of India is around 1.37 billion and is distributed in 29 states and 8 union territories which are divided into 739 districts. In a 2.4% of land area, we have 17.7% of the world population which makes India as one of the most densely populated countries. The country has variegated geographical areas, diverse religious and ethnic groups, protean cultures, customs, languages and dialects and heterogeneous socio-economic spectrum. The overall national adult literacy rate is 81.3%, with a male literacy rate of 82% and the female literacy rate of around 65%. The annual per capita Gross National Income (GNI) is only US $ 1530 and human development index is mere 0.702 giving a rank of 135 to our country among 175 nations of the world. The current annual population growth rate is 1.1%. We are thus doubling the population every 50 years. It is amazing that every year we are adding a population which is equivalent to the total population of a number of individual countries such as Canada, Australia, Sri Lanka, Kenya, Algeria, etc. Every minute 50 babies are born in India accounting for 25.6 million births (20% global births) every year. In India, one neonate dies every 40 seconds leading to 0.76 million neonatal deaths every year, thus accounting for 30% of global neonatal deaths.

THE CURRENT PERINATAL SCENE

Despite the fact that in our Ayurvedic system, Obstetrics and Pediatrics were recognized as a different specialty under Kashyap school, the current perinatal services in India are indeed dismal. Women are truly the creators and sustainers of human pogeny. The health and well-being of children is intimately linked with health, nutrition and education of mothers. Unfortunately there is discrimination against their girl children in our society leading to poor health status, illiteracy and lack of empowerment of women. The discrimination against girls begins before birth leading to birth of 17% more boys than girls. According to 2011 census of India, the sex ratio is 940 females per 1000 males. One-third of women are under nourished and have a body weight of <40 kg and height of <145 cm. Due to early marriages, teenage pregnancies are common and account for 25% of all conceptions. Some antenatal care of poor quality is received by 74% of pregnant women and only 47% of deliveries are conducted at health posts and hospitals. Among domiciliary births, only 52% births are attended by skilled birth attendants. The current neonatal and perinatal mortality rates are 22.7 and 35 per 1000 live births. During the last 50 years since independence, the neonatal mortality has almost halved (Figure 10.1). Due to greater reduction of post-neonatal infant deaths, there has been a steady increase in the contribution of neonatal deaths towards infant mortality rate. The current health indices of mothers and children with projected national goals are shown in Table 10.1. It is a sad reality that the lofty goals are still elusive. And we

TABLE 10.2 Selected indices of maternal and child health*

Parameters	China	India
■ Population	1,439,323,776	1,379,196,659
■ Total births per year	18.4 million	25.6 million
■ Antenatal care (at least one contact)	94%	74%
■ Skilled attendants at birth	100%	52%
■ Institutional deliveries	99%	47%
■ LBW babies	5%	20%
■ Neonatal mortality rate per 1000 live births	4	23
■ Infant mortality rate per 1000 live births	7	30
■ Maternal deaths per 100,000 live births	29	122
■ Literacy rate (M/F)	100%/100%	82%/65%

*The State of World's Children, UNICEF, 2018

TABLE 10.1 Current health indices and projected national goals for key child and maternal health indicators

Indicator	Current status* (2014 AD)	Goals
IMR*	30.0	<30.0
NMR**	23.0	<20.0
SBR***	22	<20
MMR****	122	<100
LBW babies	20%	10%
Population growth rate	1.1%	1.2%
Deliveries at health posts	47%	80%
Deliveries by skilled birth attendants	52%	100%

Based on The State of the World's Children, UNICEF, 2018 and State of India's Newborns (SOIN), 2014

*IMR: Infant mortality rate (per 1000 live births)
**NMR: Neonatal mortality rate (per 1000 live births)
***SBR: Stillbirth rate (per 1000 births)
****MMR: Maternal mortality rate (per 100,000 pregnant women)

have a long way to go in improving maternal welfare and perinatal health indices to catch up with an equally populous neighboring country China which has done far better than us (Table 10.2).

INFRASTRUCTURE FOR MCH SERVICES

There is an excellent pyramid of infrastructure for delivery of MCH services through a network of sub-centers, primary health centers, community health centers, district and state hospitals for providing health care services in rural India (Figure 10.2). The provision of health is in the domain of individual states but the federal/central government of the

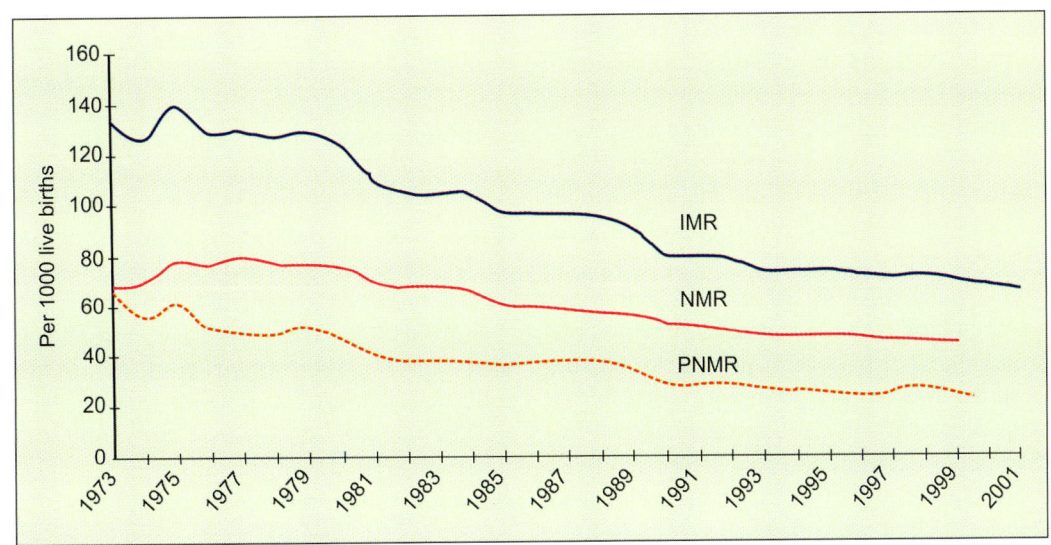

Figure 10.1 Decadal trends in infant mortality rate (IMR), neonatal mortality rate (NMR) and post-neonatal mortality rate (PNMR) in India during 20th century.

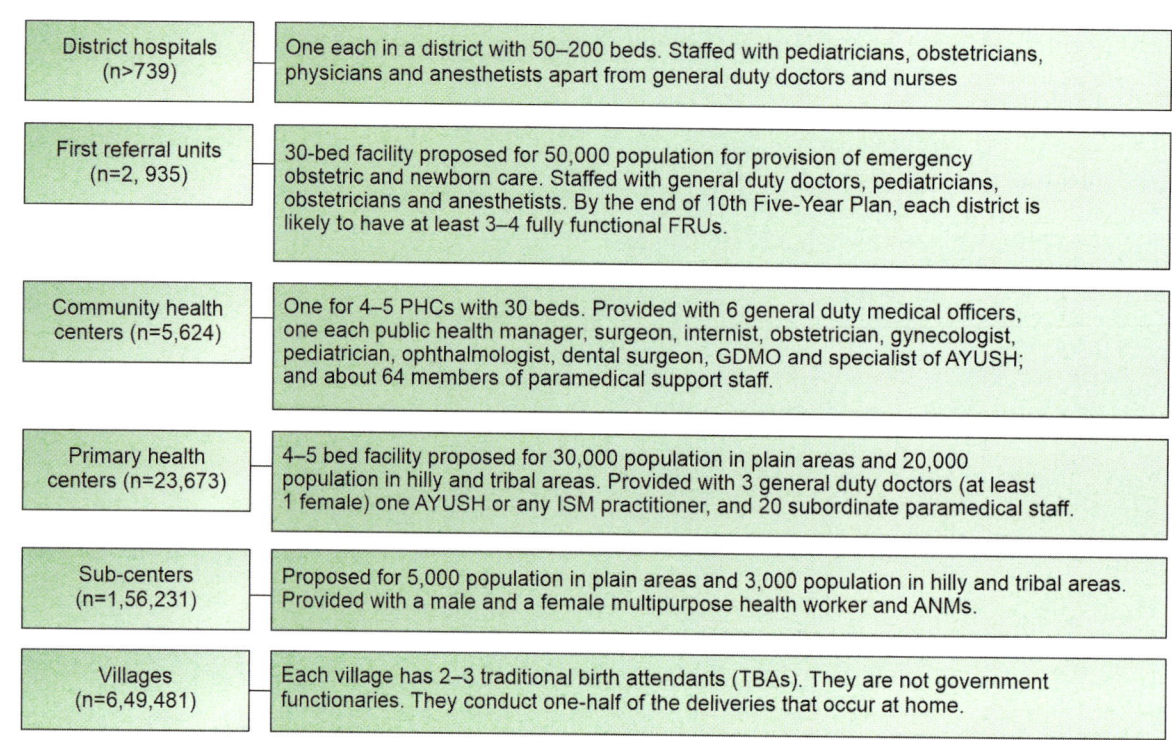

District hospitals (n>739)	One each in a district with 50–200 beds. Staffed with pediatricians, obstetricians, physicians and anesthetists apart from general duty doctors and nurses
First referral units (n=2, 935)	30-bed facility proposed for 50,000 population for provision of emergency obstetric and newborn care. Staffed with general duty doctors, pediatricians, obstetricians and anesthetists. By the end of 10th Five-Year Plan, each district is likely to have at least 3–4 fully functional FRUs.
Community health centers (n=5,624)	One for 4–5 PHCs with 30 beds. Provided with 6 general duty medical officers, one each public health manager, surgeon, internist, obstetrician, gynecologist, pediatrician, ophthalmologist, dental surgeon, GDMO and specialist of AYUSH; and about 64 members of paramedical support staff.
Primary health centers (n=23,673)	4–5 bed facility proposed for 30,000 population in plain areas and 20,000 population in hilly and tribal areas. Provided with 3 general duty doctors (at least 1 female) one AYUSH or any ISM practitioner, and 20 subordinate paramedical staff.
Sub-centers (n=1,56,231)	Proposed for 5,000 population in plain areas and 3,000 population in hilly and tribal areas. Provided with a male and a female multipurpose health worker and ANMs.
Villages (n=6,49,481)	Each village has 2–3 traditional birth attendants (TBAs). They are not government functionaries. They conduct one-half of the deliveries that occur at home.

Figure 10.2 Infrastructural layout for MCH services in rural India.

country provides the policy guidelines and resources especially for the national programs. Most of the deliveries are still conducted at home by traditional birth attendants and relatives. There are 4–5 traditional birth attendants (TBAs) in each village and only one-half of them have been formally trained. Some of the district or subdivisional hospitals and community health centers have been upgraded to serve as First Referral Units (FRUs) for a population of 100,000. They are staffed with specialists like pediatricians, obstetricians, internists and anesthetists who have been provided with basic equipment for newborn care. However, neonatal care facilities are inadequate both at the district hospitals and medical college hospitals. Only 150–180 medical colleges in the country have level II newborn care facilities while 60–80 medical institutions and a few corporate hospitals have level III neonatal intensive care facilities.

The existent health infrastructure has not been effectively utilized due to poor accessibility and low credibility because of lack of communication and poor commitment of the health care professionals (HCPs). There is lack of accountability and supervision of the existent staff which is unwilling to work in rural areas. Above all there is lack of care seeking behavior and fatalistic attitude of the community due to illiteracy and socioeconomic constraints. There is a gender bias with conscious neglect of girl children.

Resource Allocation for Health and Education

Allocation of national financial resources for health and education as a percentage of Gross Domestic Product (GDP) for various countries in South-East Asia and some of the developed countries is shown in Table 10.3. As opposed to the recommended allocation of 5% and 15% of GDP for health and education respectively by WHO, India is able to spare only 4.0 and 3.1% of GDP each for health and education, respectively. It is a pity that India has to earmark and "waste" 14% of GNI for a non-productive sector like defence due to our vulnerable position. Thailand which has made a remarkable progress in all spheres of development including health in the South-East Asia region is providing the most balanced allocation of 11.0% and 20.0% of GNI for health and education, respectively. In India, we are spending a total of 5.5% of GNI annually towards the health of an individual which receives a contribution of 2.0% from public sector and 3.5% from the private sector. Only 15% of the health budget is spent on MCH and family welfare activities. There is a gradual increase in the medical facilities for all age groups in private sector through a network of corporate hospitals in the country. In view of relatively meager GNI of US $ 1,530 per capita per year, the health expenditure works out only US $ 31 (₹ 1250/-) per capita per year or mere 13 cents (₹ 3 Paise 50) per day.

TABLE 10.3 Resource allocation for health, education and defence as % of gross domestic product (GDP)				
Country	GNI* per capita (US $)	Health	Education	Military
India	1,530	4.0	3.1	2.5
Pakistan	1,260	3.1	2.7	3.4
China	5,740	5.4	4.3	2.1
Sri Lanka	2,920	3.1	2.6	2.7
Thailand	5,210	3.9	4.1	1.5
Philippines	2,470	4.6	2.8	1.3
Ghana	1,550	5.2	5.4	0.5
United Kingdom	38,250	9.4	5.5	2.3
USA	50,120	17.9	5.5	3.8

Source: The State of the World's Children, UNICEF, 2018.

*GNI per capita: Gross national income (GNI) is the sum of value added by resident producers plus any product taxes (less subsidies) not included in the valuation of output plus net receipts of primary income (compensation of employees and property income) from abroad. GNI per capita is gross national income divided by mid-year population. GNI per capita in US dollars is converted by using the World Bank Atlas method.

GDP per capita: Gross domestic product (GDP) is the sum of value added by all resident producers plus any product taxes (less subsidies) not included in the valuation of the output. GDP per capita is gross domestic product divided by mid-year population.

In general, there is a good correlation between per capita gross domestic product (GDP) of a country and infant mortality rate. The countries with a higher per capita GDP tend to have a lower infant mortality rate with the exception of Sri Lanka which has done exceedingly well in the health sector despite low GNI. There is excellent interrelationship between health and education. The countries with a higher female literacy rate tend to have lower infant mortality. In Sri Lanka, although the per capita GNI is around US $ 2,920 but infant mortality rate is 8/1000 live births because the female literacy is around 98%. In Kerala, the low infant, neonatal and perinatal mortality (12, 7 and 9 per 1000 live births respectively) is attributed primarily to a high female literacy rate of over 93%, economic independence of women and availability of MCH services within easy reach.

ESSENTIAL PERINATAL/NEONATAL CARE

The components of minimal or essential perinatal/neonatal care have been highlighted by the National Neonatology Forum of India on several occasions and are summarized in Table 10.4. The basic components of perinatal care to prevent neonatal deaths and ensure intact survival should include steps to ensure safe delivery, preferably at the health post, by the trained health care professionals having the knowledge and skills to resuscitate an asphyxiated baby. The maintenance of asepsis, prevention of tetanus neonatorum, provision of warmth and promotion of exclusive breastfeeding are the other key components of basic neonatal care which can be readily provided in the community. The components of essential perinatal services are diagrammatically depicted in Figure 10.3.

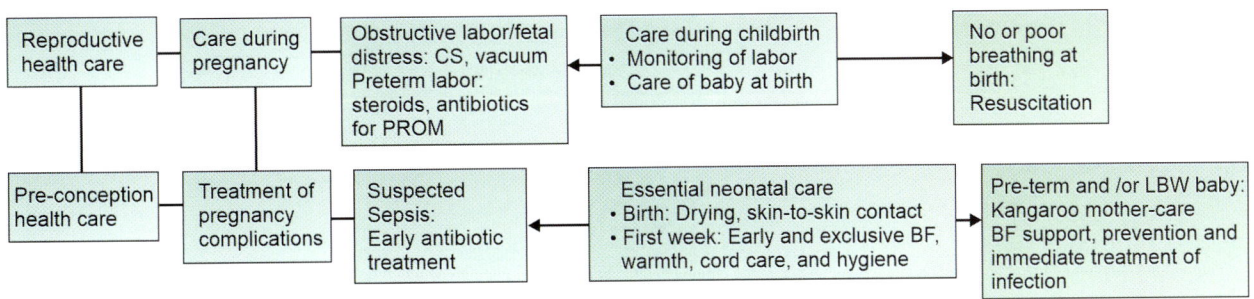

BF: Breastfeeding, CS: Cesarean section, LBW: Low birth weight, PROM: Prolonged rupture of membranes

Figure 10.3 Package of essential interventions to improve newborn survival. The focus should be the critical window of opportunity around childbirth and first day of life.

Essential Perinatal and Neonatal Care in the Community

10

TABLE 10.4 Essential components of perinatal and neonatal care

Care of future mothers

- Provide opportunities for education of girls.
- Improve the nutrition of girls throughout their lifecycle.
- Discourage early marriages and early childbearing.
- Improve the status of women in the society.
- Improve women's health and family planning services.
- Promote safe sexual practices.

Care during pregnancy

- Provide at least four good quality antenatal check-ups and two doses of tetanus toxoid.
- Improve the caloric and protein intake and provide anemia prophylaxis.
- Screen and treat infections, especially syphilis and malaria.
- Improve communication and counseling: Birth preparedness, awareness of danger signs, and immediate and exclusive breastfeeding.
- Ensure facility-based delivery or delivery by skilled birth attendants.
- Ensure five cleans: Clean hands, clean delivery surface, clean blade, clean cord tie, clean undressed cord without application of any home remedies.
- Keep the newborn warm: Dry and wrap the baby immediately, including the head; or provide skin-to-skin contact with mother and dress the baby.
- Avoid bath till cord has fallen.
- Give prophylactic eye care, as appropriate.
- Initiate immediate and exclusive breastfeeding within one hour of birth without any prelacteal feeds.
- Ensure early postnatal contact.
- Promote exclusive breastfeeding for first 6 months of life.
- Maintain hygiene to prevent infections: Ensure clean cord care and counsel the mother on general hygiene practices, such as handwashing and avoidance of unnecessary handling.
- Provide immunizations such as BCG, OPV, and hepatitis B vaccines soon after birth.
- Promote birth spacing.

Special considerations

- Monitor and treat complications, such as anemia, pre-eclampsia, malpresentation, and bleeding.
- Promote voluntary counseling and testing for HIV.
- Reduce the risk of mother-to-child transmission of HIV.
- Early detection of high-risk pregnancy and appropriate referral.
- Recognize danger signs and serious complications in both mother and the baby and avoid delay in seeking care and referral.
- Recognize and resuscitate asphyxiated babies immediately· Pay special attention to warmth, feeding, and hygiene practices for care of preterm and LBW babies.
- Recognize danger signs and serious complications in both mother and newborn, particularly onset of infections, and avoid delay in seeking care and referral.
- Support HIV positive mothers to make appropriate, sustainable choices about feeding the baby.
- Continue to pay special attention to provide warmth, feeding, and hygienic practices for care of LBW babies (>1800 g and >34 weeks).

Adapted from State of the World's Newborns, 2014.

Basic Antenatal Care

During pregnancy, avoidance of unnecessary medications during first trimester of pregnancy, provision of adequate nutrition including supplements of iron and folic acid tablets, immunization with two doses of tetanus toxoid and provision of rest during last trimester of pregnancy are crucial to promote the growth of fetus and prevent developmental malformations.

The concept of identification of high-risk pregnancy should be simplified. The simple methods for assessing the severity of anemia (clinical and with anemiameter) and detection of albuminuria with the help of uristix need to be promoted. There is a need to construct uterine (gravidograms) and abdominal girth charts during pregnancy to serve as simple reckoners for identification of intrauterine growth restriction in the community. Every pregnant woman should receive at least 4 antenatal health check-ups during pregnancy.

Care of the Baby at Birth

The availability of adequately trained birth attendants is most crucial while requirements for equipment are minimal in the community (Table 10.5). Efforts should be made to ensure that all deliveries are conducted at a health post. Every delivery must be considered as a medical emergency. The disposable sterile delivery kits (1/2 blade, cotton, antiseptic lotion, soap and plastic sheet) should be distributed to all pregnant women. The birth attendants should be trained to use simple criteria for assessing the condition of the baby at birth such as cry, breathing efforts and color. They should be provided with reusable de Lee suction traps or readily cleanable transparent suction bulbs. Neonatal masks with attachment for a bag or facility for mouth-to-bag ventilation are useful for resuscitation of asphyxiated newborn babies. Most babies can be effectively resuscitated with room air. However, the oxygen cylinder should be available at the primary health center and health workers should be imparted basic knowledge to give oxygen therapy to newborn babies. Administration of oxygen with the help of a catheter, introduced through the nose for a distance midway between the external naris and lobule of the ear, by maintaining oxygen flow rate at 0.5 L/min has been found to be as effective as a head-box. Twin-holed catheter or nasal cannulae are equally useful and affordable for administration of oxygen. The birth attendants should be provided with cheap and sturdy handy type of spring balance to weigh the babies. Alternatively tricolored measuring tapes (similar to Shakir tapes) should be provided to the health workers to use chest circumference and mid-arm circumference (MAC) as reliable surrogates of birth weight. The

studies have shown that chest circumference of <30.0 cm and <27.5 cm can reliably identify neonates <2500 g and <2000 g respectively with a high degree of specificity and predictive value. The corresponding values for MAC are <9.0 cm and <8.5 cm, respectively.

Provision of Warmth

Adequate maintenance of thermoneutrality is crucial for survival of newborn babies. *The environmental temperature which may be uncomfortable for an adult may impose serious thermal stress to a low birth weight baby.* The health workers should be taught to promptly dry the baby after birth and effectively clothe him with a cap, socks and mittens. The baby bath should be delayed till the cord has fallen. The baby should be nursed in close proximity to the mother so that he gains heat from the maternal warmth. The cot of the mother and infant should be located away from the walls to reduce radiation heat loss. Skin-to-skin contact (kangaroo care) is a useful strategy to keep the babies warm. Skin-to-skin contact at birth for bonding and promotion of lactation and short period intermittent kangaroo mother care are feasible strategies which should be promoted in India.

Mothers and health workers should be explained the technique and art of keeping the babies warm and evaluation of body temperature by touching the trunk and extremities of the baby. When hands and feet of the baby are warm and pink, it indicates that thermal environment of the baby is satisfactory. *It must be remembered that mother is the best primary health worker.* At the home level, baby should be clothed with linen pre-warmed on a *"tawa"* or electric iron. The room can be warmed by using an *"angeethi"* taking care to safeguard against carbon monoxide poisoning. Oil massage is culturally acceptable and provides insulation against heat loss and insensible water loss.

TABLE 10.5 The technology needs for care of newborns in the community

- Birth attendant should be provided with a "disposable delivery kit".
- Mask for providing mouth-to-mask resuscitation at birth.
- Ensuring five cleans (surface, hands, blade, cord tie and cord care)
- Availability of a weighing scale or a tricolored measuring tape.
- Gavage, spoon or *paladay* feeding of LBW babies.
- Simple strategies to prevent hypothermia: No bath at birth, effective clothing with a cap, socks and mittens, close contact with mother, warm room, and external heat source, etc.
- Kangaroo mother care.
- Promotion of hygienic practices: Handwashing, cord care, sun-dried clothes, clean environment.
- Availability of oral and injectable antibiotics.
- Distribution of information, education and communication (IEC) material for care of normal and LBW babies and early identification of sick babies (Danger signs).

At the primary health center, room heater and over-head lamps/electrical bakery bulbs can be effectively used to keep the babies warm. There is a need to fabricate simple incubators which can be warmed either by solar energy or hot water. In the health posts, low-reading thermometers (30°–42°C) should be made available to monitor the temperature of babies.

During transport of high risk or sick babies, there is a considerable risk of hypothermia. It is preferable to transport the baby *in utero* because *mother is the best transport incubator thermostatically maintained at 37°C*. There is no risk of handling and the baby receives parenteral nutrition and oxygen through the placenta. When transport of a baby is desired, he should be effectively clothed and insulated either with a silver foil or cotton padding. He can be transported by keeping him next to the skin of mother/attendant or placing him in a thermocol box or cane-basket. The box or basket can be kept warm by keeping hot-water bottles in hampers affixed on all the sides, while taking due precautions that no part of the baby should come in direct contact with the hot water bottles.

Prevention of Bacterial Infections

The technology for prevention of tetanus neonatorum is readily available and needs universal implementation. All pregnant women should receive two doses of tetanus toxoid 4 weeks apart as soon as they come in contact with the health care worker during pregnancy. The second dose of tetanus toxoid must be received at least 4 weeks before the anticipated date of delivery. The use of disposable sterile delivery kits should be universalized. Even when a new razor blade is purchased from the market for cutting the cord, it must be sterilized by boiling in water for 5 minutes before use. The concept of thorough hand-washing and use of clean, washed and sun-dried linen must be popularized and promoted to prevent bacterial infections. The cultural practice of keeping the mother-baby dyad isolated for 40 days needs to be promoted.

Promotion of Breastfeeding

The health workers and mothers should be educated regarding the importance of colostrum for feeding of newborn babies. All babies should be put straight to the breast, as soon as the mother has recovered from fatigue of labor, without introduction of any prelacteal feeds. During lactation, the mother should be advised to drink extra liquids and take additional 25% calories in order to maintain her own health. The nursing mothers should be given nutritional supplements to improve the quality of breastmilk. The basic physiology of lactation and adverse effects of anxiety, fear and pain on milk output should be explained. The concept of exclusive breastfeeding (even water should not be given) during first 6 months of life should be popularized. Exclusive breastfeeding eliminates the risk of infection and is associated with better weight gain because baby drinks more milk when he feels thirsty. The management of retracted/cracked nipples and engorged breasts with the help of manual expression of milk and use of nipple shield or syringe method should be taught.

HOME CARE OF LOW BIRTH WEIGHT BABIES

Most babies with a birth weight of more than 1800 g or borderline or late preterm babies with a gestational maturity of 34 weeks or more can be managed at home. They account for almost 90% of all LBW babies. Those infants who are too weak to suck, should be given expressed breast milk with a long and narrow spoon or *paladay* (Figure 10.4). These babies are at a greater risk to develop hypothermia and they should be adequately protected against this hazard by indigenous methods outlined *vide supra*. Strict asepsis should be observed to prevent occurrence of bacterial infections. The child should be kept in a room having access to sun and worn clothes which are duly washed and sun dried. The hands must be washed with soap and water before touching or feeding the baby. The handling of the infant by visitors should be restricted to the bare minimum.

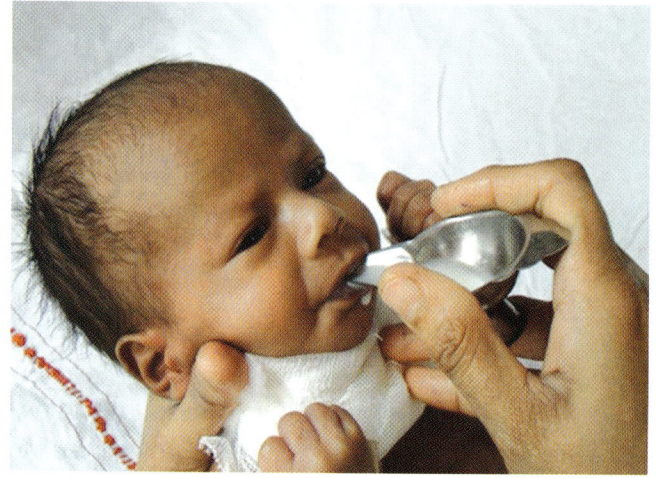

Figure 10.4 Feeding a preterm baby with *paladay*.

Identification and Referral of High-Risk Babies

The health workers should be given instructions to identify sick babies without delay so that they are referred to the health post providing level II neonatal care. The common indications for referral are mentioned in Table 10.6. It is important to demonstrate high-risk signs to the health workers on sick babies so that their clinical judgement can be sharpened. The availability of an icterometer at the Primary Health Center is useful to assess the severity of jaundice.

In view of constraints and difficulties in our referral system and lack of back-up support for specialized newborn care, there is a need to develop innovative modules to manage LBW and sick newborn babies at their homes. Community neonatal health workers (CNHWs) can be trained to identify high risk and sick newborn babies (Figures 10.5 and 10.6). They should be provided with knowledge and skills for assessment

TABLE 10.6 Identification of a high risk and sick baby
1. Birth weight of <1800 g or gestation of <34 weeks.
2. Delayed passage of meconium (>24 hours) and urine (>48 hours).
3. Inability to suck or swallow.
4. Reduced activity or excessive inconsolable crying.
5. Marked changes in color: Pale, blue, yellow.
6. Cold or febrile baby.
7. Rapid breathing (respiratory rate >60 per minute, alae nasi moving, chest retractions).
8. Superficial infections (purulent conjunctivitis, oral thrush, umbilical sepsis, pyoderma, abscess).
9. Persistent vomiting or watery diarrhea.
10. Abdominal distension.
11. Bleeding from any site.
12. Seizures.

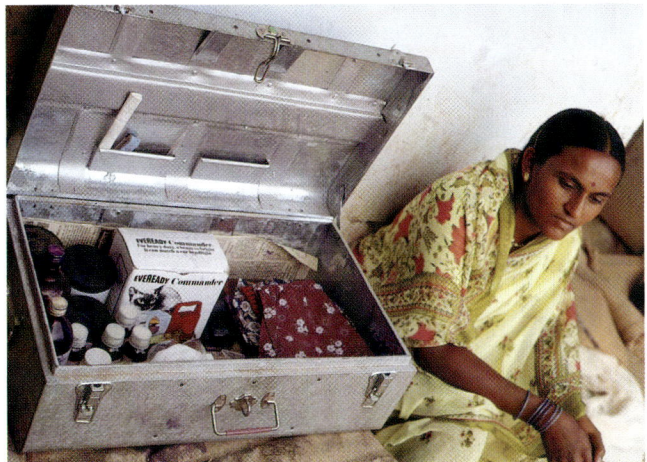

Figure 10.5 Community neonatal health worker with her delivery box at SEARCH, Gadchiroli.

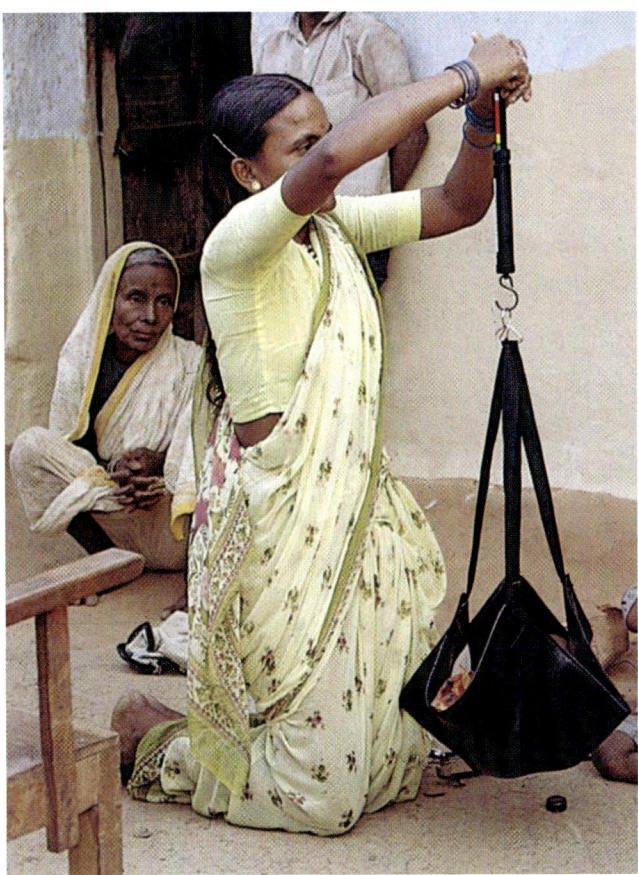

Figure 10.6 Weighing a newborn baby at home with the help of a spring balance.

of a newborn baby, for providing effective resuscitation, ensuring warmth, preventing infections and promoting breastfeeding. They can be trained to give antibiotics through intramuscular injection and administer expressed breast milk to small and sick babies with a spoon or *paladay*. They can also be trained to give gavage feeding with due competence and safety. Attempts are being made by a number of non-government organizations to develop innovative modules for providing newborn care in the rural homes. The pilot observations suggest that this strategy can significantly enhance survival of newborn babies in the community.

NEONATAL MORBIDITY AND MORTALITY

Every fourth baby in India is a low birth weight (<2500 g) baby accounting for a high load of morbidity and mortality. Every year 8 million low birth weight babies, 2.7 million preterm babies (<37 weeks gestation) and over 1 million very low birth weight babies (<1500 g) are born in India. Based on these estimates, it is projected that every year, one million babies each suffer from birth asphyxia, respiratory distress syndrome and hyperbilirubinemia while 0.5 million babies each show evidences of neonatal sepsis and congenital malformations in our country. The National Neonatal-Perinatal Database (NNPD) network of National Neonatology Forum of India is collecting neonatal morbidity and mortality data from 30 major neonatal centers in the country since January 1995. The primary causes of neonatal deaths based on neonatal-perinatal data network are shown in Table 10.7. Birth asphyxia, immaturity (birth weight less than 750 g, hyaline membrane disease, intraventricular hemorrhage) and neonatal infections are leading causes of neonatal mortality in the country. Due to referral nature of AIIMS, the ranking of primary causes of neonatal deaths is different (Table 10.8). The leading causes of neonatal deaths at AIIMS are congenital malformations, immaturity and neonatal infections. Neonatal sepsis, birth asphyxia and prematurity are leading causes of neonatal deaths in home-cared rural neonates (Table 10.9). In rural areas, neonatal tetanus was responsible for 0.35 million deaths per year in early eighties which has been almost eliminated by effective maternal immunization with tetanus toxoid during pregnancy.

The core health problem of newborn babies in India is low birth weight babies which account for over 80% of all neonatal deaths. The high incidence of low birth

TABLE 10.9 Causes of deaths in home-cared rural neonates (n = 763*)

Cause of death	Percent
Sepsis/pneumonia	57.5
Birth asphyxia	20.0
Preterm	15.0
Unknown	7.5

*IMR 76/1000 live births and NMR 52.4/1000 live births in 36 villages, population 36,613 at SEARCH, Gadchiroli

weight babies in India is due to neglect of nutrition, health and education of female children and poor status and empowerment of women in society. Early marriage, frequent teenage pregnancies, maternal malnutrition, anemia, infections and genital colonization are important contributory causes. There is high incidence of pregnancy-induced hypertension among malnourished and socioeconomically deprived women. Excessive physical work during 3rd trimester of pregnancy, wherein energy is diverted for physical labor and denied to the fetus, is an important contributory factor for poor fetal growth.

THE ROLE OF NATIONAL NEONATOLOGY FORUM

During 1980, a group of senior pediatricians got together to create an academic body of National Neonatology Forum of India. The Forum has served as a leading crusader and catalyst to improve newborn health in the country. The current membership of NNF is around 10,000 and comprises pediatricians, obstetricians, community health physicians, nurses and other individuals concerned with perinatal care. During the last 25 years or so, the Forum has made outstanding contributions to improve the infrastructure, facilities and survival of newborn babies in the country. With the help of Task Force Meetings, the Forum has developed recommendations in the form of consensus statements and monographs for a large number of newborn issues including essential newborn care, neonatal nomenclature, definitions and data collection, neonatal monitoring, neonatal biomedical equipment, primary care of the newborn babies, neonatal nursing, human resource development for newborn care, cultural practices for newborn care and education and training in neonatology. The Forum has developed guidelines for accreditation of level II Special Care Neonatal Units (SCNU) in the country. The Forum has organized training programs for district level pediatricians in various accredited neonatal units.

TABLE 10.7 Primary causes of neonatal deaths in India (NNPD data 2002–03) n = 3680

Cause of death	Number	Proportion
Birth asphyxia	1060	28.8%
Immaturity*	968	26.3%
Infections	683	18.6%
Congenital malformations	337	9.2%
Miscellaneous	632	17.2%

*Birth weight <750 g, hyaline membrane disease, intraventricular hemorrhage

TABLE 10.8 Primary causes of neonatal deaths at AIIMS (n = 157)

Cause of death	Number (%)
Congenital malformations	51 (32.5%)
Immaturity*	41 (26.1%)
Infections	29 (18.5%)
Birth asphyxia	15 (9.6%)
Hydrops fetalis	9 (5.7%)
Others	12 (7.6%)

*Birth weight <750 g, hyaline membrane disease, intraventricular hemorrhage

Care of the Newborn

10

The neonatal resuscitation program was launched as a vibrant movement by the Forum in 1985. Till date we have created a certified neonatal resuscitation faculty of over 750 pediatricians and have trained over 50,000 pediatricians, obstetricians, family physicians and nurses in the art of neonatal resuscitation. A number of workshops for training of nurses have been conducted in the country (Figures 10.7 and 10.8). The Forum has established a National Neonatal-Perinatal Data Network. The Forum has conducted regular annual meetings with Indian Society of Perinatology and Reproductive Biology to enhance collaboration with obstetricians for improving newborn survival. There is a regular Indo-US and Indo-Australia Exchange Programs for training of neonatologists. The Forum has developed the competency-based curriculum for newborn care for the benefit of nurses, graduate and postgraduate medical students and for the postdoctoral DM Neonatology Program. The Task Force of the Forum has published evidence-based

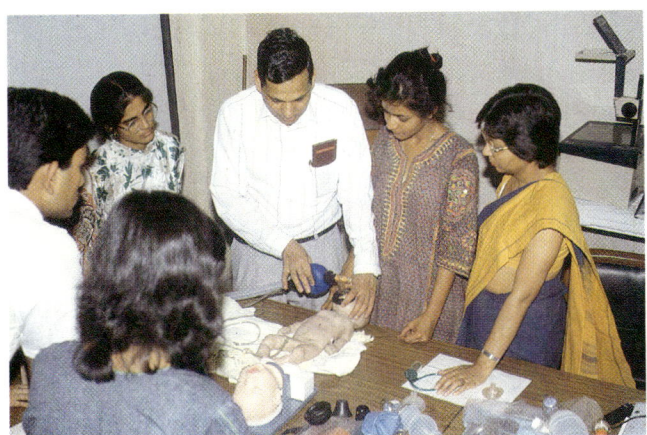

Figure 10.7 NALS workshop to train medical graduates in the art of neonatal resuscitation.

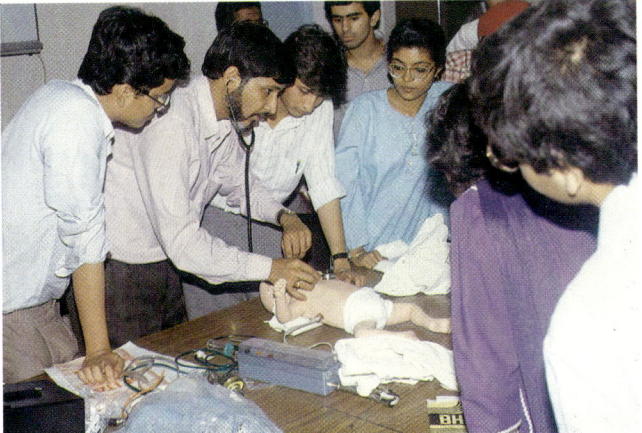

Figure 10.8 NALS workshop in progress to train medical graduates in the art of neonatal resuscitation.

guidelines for care of neonates which have been revised on a regular basis. The Forum has provided expertise to the Ministry of Health and Family Welfare for organization of First Referral Units for newborn care under the CSSM Program. The Forum has regularly published a quarterly Bulletin and a newsletter Chronicle NNF: Health for all Newborns and is now publishing a peer-reviewed Journal of Neonatology. Above all, the Forum has been instrumental in placing newborn care very high among the national health priorities through sustained advocacy, consensus-building and academic contributions. During the year 2000, the efforts of the Forum were rewarded when government of India agreed to celebrate National Newborn Week from 15th through 21st November every year.

INNOVATIVE STRATEGIES FOR NEWBORN CARE IN INDIA

Due to limited resources, financial constraints and lack of expensive equipment, a number of innovative strategies have been developed to improve newborn care in the country. Under the Baby Friendly Hospital Initiative, most neonatal units in the country are feeding preterm and sick newborn babies with expressed breast milk (EBM). The feeding bottles have been by and large eliminated from the NICUs. The feeding of EBM with a spoon or *paladay* (shallow cup with a long snout in the form of a *diya*) is being used as a bridge between gavage feeding and direct breast-feeding for newborn babies between 32 and 34 weeks of gestation. This has eliminated the problem of nipple confusion and risk of enteral infections in the nursery. The preterm babies are being discharged early to prevent overcrowding in the NICU and to bring down the cost of neonatal intensive care. Most babies are being discharged when they have regained their birth weight, are thermostable, free from any disease/infection, achieved a gestational maturity of 34 weeks and are showing a steady weight gain. In view of constraints of resources and technology, most neonatal units are focusing their efforts on babies above the birth weight of 1000 g except a few tertiary care centers who are able to provide satisfactory care to babies up to a birth weight of 750 g.

The warm-chain concept is being closely followed for management of preterm and low birth weight babies by raising the temperature of the nursery and the step-down rooms for care of stable babies. Skin-to-skin contact and kangaroo-mother care is being promoted. Due to shortage of trained nurses in the country (the doctor-nurse ratio in the country is 1:1), some centers have created a cadre of nurse aides to look after the basic nursing needs of newborn babies. Unlike developed countries where the cross training of nurses has revolutionized the newborn care, in India, the resident doctors have been cross trained to undertake several nursing chores to enhance newborn survival. There has been a revolution in the indigenization of neonatal equipment in the country. A large number of monitoring and therapeutic electronic equipment of good quality and acceptable esthetics are being fabricated indigenously with the help and close collaboration between the neonatologists and entrepreneur biomedical engineers. Due to unsatisfactory referral system, the efforts are being made to develop a satisfactory and a sustainable module for identification and management of low birth weight and sick newborn babies in the community.

HOME CARE OF NEWBORN BABIES

About 0.76 million newborn babies die every year in India due to lack of access to medical care. There is a need to provide home-based care to newborn babies because over 65% of births in rural India occur at home. A large number of deaths occur due to potentially preventable disorders like sepsis, hypothermia and birth asphyxia. Majority of parents are unwilling to go to the hospital for delivery or treatment of a sick newborn. In any case, the institutional care is either unsatisfactory, unavailable or inaccessible and is not affordable. Rural medical practitioners (RMPs) have no information or training to manage sick neonates.

A model of home-based newborn care has been developed by Bang *et al* at SEARCH (Society for Education, Action and Research in Community Health) at Gadchiroli, Maharashtra. They have created a cadre of skilled village-level workers to identify sick babies and treat them at home with gentamicin and cotrimoxazole. They have demonstrated significant reduction in the neonatal mortality rate in the intervention villages. The existent cadre of HCPs in the villages (RMPs, ANMs, TBAs and AWWs) should be trained and integrated to create an effective and healthy partnership to provide newborn care in the community.

There is a need to create a cadre of village-based skilled birth attendants (midwife-cum-child health workers and accredited social health activists or ASHAs) to provide care to pregnant women, ensure safe deliveries, look after moderately LBW and sick newborn babies and under-5 children. A beginning has been made by launching pilot projects in those states where newborn health indices are most dismal. Recently, project Ankur has been launched in collaboration with seven local NGOs to cover 100 villages and 6 slums in Maharashtra to provide home-based newborn care through cadre of specially trained barefoot or community newborn workers. Home-based newborn care approach based on SEARCH model needs to be implemented at a larger scale by government of India, state governments, international funding agencies and NGOs to assess its feasibility and reproducibility as a sustainable community-based program. The government of India has already launched a pilot study in five states to test the replicability of this model for incorporating it in the national program. *Nevertheless, home deliveries and home management of sick babies should remain an immediate or interim measure. And as a long-term strategy, we must ensure that every baby is born at a simple but credible consumer-friendly health care facility which should be available to all within a reasonable distance from home.*

RESEARCH ISSUES AND PRIORITIES

It is important that neonatologists working at the tertiary care centers should accept the challenge and responsibility to innovate and adapt available technology for use in the community. They should undertake research to provide answers to a large number of crucial perinatal issues at the grass roots level. Table 10.10 summarizes the key research priorities for care of newborn babies in the community. The cost-effective, evidence-based and useful newborn care practices should be promoted in the community.

NATIONAL MATERNAL AND CHILD HEALTH PROGRAMS

Till recently, none of the national MCH programs provided essential newborn care in the community. The reduction in infant mortality has been achieved by reduction in the post-neonatal mortality by Integrated Child Development Services Scheme, rational case management of diarrhea (promotion of ORT program) and acute respiratory infections, universal immunization program and vitamin A prophylaxis.

India has been at the forefront of global efforts to reduce child mortality and morbidity. The Government of India (GOI) recognizes child survival and development as an important foundation for the overall development of the society and nation. The major child survival and welfare programs launched by GOI are shown in Table 10.11.

TABLE 10.10 Key research issues for care of newborn babies in the community

Neonatal mortality	■ Surveillance of cause-specific neonatal mortality (early and late, urban, rural, tribal) disaggregated by gender and socioeconomic variables.
Newborn care practices and care	■ Care-seeking behavior regarding newborn illness in rural, urban and tribal settings; social autopsy for neonatal sickness and mortality. ■ Traditional newborn care practices in different regions and communities. ■ Evaluation of culturally popular galactagogues. ■ Interventions to improve the care seeking behavior for neonatal illnesses, especially for the girl child.
Integrated management of neonatal and childhood illnesses (IMNCI)	■ Validation of 0–6 days IMNCI algorithms. ■ Evaluation of IMNCI strategy for improving newborn care at the community and facility levels. ■ To design simple pictorial mother and child-linked cards.
LBW babies	■ Trends in the burden of LBW (IUGR and preterm) infants with their distal and proximate determinants. Etiopathogenesis of IUGR; efficacy of maternal supplementation of single and multiple micronutrients in improving birth weight. ■ Role of physical work and indoor pollution during pregnancy on birth weight. ■ Impact of zinc supplementation on morbidity of LBW infants. ■ Utility of tricolored measuring tapes for identification of LBW babies. ■ Home-based management of LBW babies. ■ Can administration of honey prevent hypoglycemia in high-risk neonates? ■ Spoon versus bottle/gavage feeding of LBW babies. ■ Fetal growth standards to identify fetuses with intrauterine growth restriction and classify neonates as appropriate-for-dates and large-for-dates for clinical and epidemiological purposes. ■ Development of modules for home management of LBW and sick newborn babies.
Maternal health	■ Identification of high-risk pregnancy in the community. ■ Prevalence of bacterial vaginosis and its association with prematurity and birth weight.
Neonatal sepsis (NNS)	■ Principal causative organisms of community-acquired NNS, their antimicrobial sensitivity pattern and molecular epidemiology; surveillance studies to provide ongoing information to guide treatment regimens. ■ Simple clinical algorithms for identification of NNS by health workers. ■ Profile of maternal genital tract flora among Indian mothers and its relation with early-onset sepsis. ■ Feasibility of treating NNS with oral and/or injectable antibiotics in the rural and urban slum communities by community-based health workers and private health providers. ■ Simplified regimens for treating neonatal sepsis in the community to avoid or reduce the need for injectable antibiotics.
Birth asphyxia	■ Timing of clamping the cord. ■ Effectiveness of TBAs in the management of birth asphyxia with and without using resuscitation devices (tube-mask, bag-mask). ■ Resuscitation of babies with room air (21% oxygen). ■ Do actively crying babies at birth need any suction?
Kangaroo-mother care (KMC)	■ Effectiveness of KMC in the community for management of LBW infants. ■ Feasibility, acceptability and safety of KMC program in the community implemented by primary care workers/volunteers.
Technology advantages	■ Use of Uniject™ for treatment of neonatal sepsis by health workers. ■ Indigenous designing of low cost transport incubator, warmer cot and other essential equipment.

Adapted from State of India's Newborns, 2004.

TABLE 10.11 Milestones in child survival programs in India

- Child Survival and Safe Motherhood Program (CSSM) 1992.
- Reproductive and Child Health Program I (RCH I) 1997.
- Reproductive and Child Health Program II (RCH II) 2005.
- National Rural Health Mission (NRHM) 2005.
- Reproductive, Maternal, Newborn, Child and Adolescent Health (RMNCH+A) Program 2013.
- India Newborn Action Plan (INAP) 2014.

The Child Survival and Safe Motherhood Program

In order to ensure a substantial improvement in the status of maternal and child health, the Government of India launched the Child Survival and Safe Motherhood Program (CSSM) with the help of World Bank and UNICEF during 1992. The safe motherhood package includes early registration of pregnancy, at least 4 antenatal check-ups, universal coverage with tetanus toxoid and iron-folic acid tablets, early detection and referral of at-risk mothers, deliveries by trained health personnel, facilities to manage obstetrical medical emergencies and birth spacing.

The child survival component of the program comprises universal immunizations, vitamin A prophylaxis, rational case management of acute diarrhea and acute respiratory infections (ARIs) and essential newborn care to ensure safe delivery, neonatal resuscitation and care of low birth weight and sick newborn babies in the community. The CSSM program has for the first time introduced specialized newborn care in the government hospitals at the sub-district and district levels. A concept of a district module for delivery of MCH services through CSSM program has been envisaged. In each district, 4–6 first referral units have been created by upgrading community health centers (CHCs) to cater to a population of 0.5 million each. An integrated training module has been developed for the physicians to provide learning opportunities for essential newborn care, rational case management of acute diarrhea and ARI. Each first referral unit has been provided by the Government of India with resuscitation bags, radiant warmers, suction machines, weighing scales, oxygen hoods and mucus suction traps.

Reproductive and Child Health (RCH) Program

During mid-1997, the National Family Welfare program and CSSM program have been merged into integrated RCH program with enhanced scope of family welfare activities to restrict the population growth and early identification and management of reproductive infections and sexually transmitted diseases. The RCH program provides client-oriented and target-free approach and lays emphasis on the quality of services and satisfaction of the consumers. There is a greater emphasis to provide essential newborn care by strengthening of PCHs, FRUs and district hospitals and training of physicians and TBAs. The additional MCH initiatives included antenatal care, promotion of institutional deliveries and provision of emergency obstetric services at FRUs (Table 10.12). There is a greater emphasis on decentralization of health services at the district level and better quality assurance.

The country launched phase II of RCH program during the next 5-year phase (2004–09). Maternal health interventions in RCH II include antenatal care, institutional deliveries, and operationalization of PCHs for round-the-clock deliveries and CHCs and FRUs for providing emergency obstetric and essential newborn care. *Janani Suraksha Yojana* has been launched to provide incentives to poor families to go for deliveries at government health facilities with the help of TBAs.

Essential newborn care is being provided as a home-based model with the help of *Anganwadi* workers, TBAs, ANMs and link volunteers or village-based newborn workers and ASHAs. They are being trained to provide optimal care at birth, prevent hypothermia and bacterial infections, promote exclusive breast-feeding, provide care to moderately LBW babies (>1800 g), identify sick babies and treat them at home

TABLE 10.12 Package of services under RCH program

Safe motherhood services	*Child survival services*
- Two doses of tetanus toxoid during pregnancy - Prevention and treatment of anemia - Prevention and treatment of RTIs and STDs - Antenatal care and early identification of high-risk pregnancies. Deliveries by trained health care personnel - Management of obstetric emergencies - Birth spacing	- Essential newborn care - Immunizations of under-5 children - Health education for promotion of breastfeeding, nutrition and immunizations - Appropriate case management of acute diarrhea - Appropriate case management of ARI - Vitamin A prophylaxis

ARI; Acute respiratory infections, RTIs; Reproductive tract infections, STDs; Sexually transmitted diseases and refer those babies who cannot be treated at home to a higher level of health facility. The facility-based care of neonates at the PCHs, CHCs, FRUs and district hospitals has been strengthened and upgraded by improving infrastructure and by providing training and skills to the nurses and physicians.

Integrated Management of Neonatal and Childhood Illnesses (IMNCI)

WHO and UNICEF have adopted integrated management of childhood illness (IMCI) approach in Child Health Programs in over 50 countries. In view of the fact that neonatal mortality account for 70% of infant mortality, integrated management of neonatal and childhood illnesses (IMNCI) is being implemented in India under RCH II program. Health workers are trained with hands-on clinical practice for effective management of sick children aged between one week and five years. Algorithms have been developed to diagnose and manage common childhood diseases. Apart from rational management of common diseases, health workers promote breastfeeding, provide immunizations, health and nutrition education. The emphasis has shifted from purely curative services to a package of comprehensive health preventive and promotive services at each contact of the health worker with the consumers. Therefore, IMNCI is not a new program but it is a new approach or a comprehensive health package to provide an holistic approach to harness greater benefits for the welfare and survival of children.

The integrated management of neonatal and childhood illness (IMNCI) strategy is being implemented in a phased manner for teaching of undergraduate medical and nursing students throughout the country. IMNCI program has been implemented in 505 districts in 27 states and 4 union territories, till date.

Rationale

i. Improvements in child health and survival are not necessarily dependent on the use of sophisticated and expensive technologies.
ii. An integrated approach is needed to manage sick children to achieve better outcomes.
iii. A careful and systematic assessment of common symptoms and carefully selected specific signs to provide rational and effective therapy.
iv. Child health programs must go beyond tackling diseases of children and must address overall health and well-being of mothers and children by promotion of breastfeeding, provision of universal immunizations, effective health and nutrition education.

The Components of IMNCI

The IMNCI guidelines for case management of common diseases have been divided into two age categories, i.e. young infants from birth up to 2 months and children above 2 months up to 5 years of age. The salient of guidelines of IMNCI are listed as follows:

1. The frontline workers (ASHAs and AWWs), after completing their IMNCI training, are required to visit newborns at their households, three times, in the first week of life. During the visits, the workers assess the newborns, promote healthy practices, manage simple problems and refer those with serious illnesses.
2. All sick infants up to 2 months of age must be assessed for "possible infection and jaundice" and they must be routinely evaluated for the major symptom of "diarrhea".
3. All sick children between 2 months and 5 years must be examined for "general danger signs" which indicate the need for immediate referral or admission to the hospital. They should be routinely assessed for major symptoms like fever, cough, difficult or rapid breathing, diarrhea and ear problems.
4. All sick under-5 children must be routinely assessed for nutritional and immunization status, feeding problems and other common day-to-day problems.
5. A limited number of carefully selected clinical signs are used, based on their sensitivity and specificity, to diagnose the diseases. These signs were selected considering the conditions and ground realities prevalent at the first-level health facilities.
6. On the basis of a combination of various signs, the child is classified into various groups (instead of a diagnosis) and further divided into color-coded triage as *pink* which requires urgent referral or admission to a hospital, *yellow* when specific treatment is required through the outpatient department and *green* which calls for home management.
7. The IMNCI guidelines address most but not all the major reasons for which a sick infant or child is brought to the clinic. The guidelines do not describe the management of trauma or other acute emergencies due to various accidents or injuries and also do not cover care of the baby at birth.
8. The management procedures outlined in the IMNCI protocols use a limited number of essential drugs and encourage active participation by caretakers in the treatment of sick infants and children.
9. An essential component of the IMNCI guidelines lays emphasis on providing counseling and guidance to caretakers about home care, feeding, administration

Essential Perinatal and Neonatal Care in the Community

10

of fluids, immunizations, and healthy family life and when to return back to health care facility for further management and follow-up.

In order to launch integrated management of neonatal and childhood illnesses (IMNCI) in the country, Government of India established a core group with representatives from Indian Academy of Pediatrics (IAP), National Neonatology Forum (NNF) of India, National Antimalaria Program (NAMP), Department of Women and Child Development (DWCD), Child-in-Need Institute (CINI), WHO, UNICEF, eminent pediatricians and neonatologists and the representatives from Ministry of Health and Family Welfare, Government of India. The core group developed Indian version of IMCI and renamed it as Integrated Management of Neonatal and Childhood Illnesses (IMNCI). The major components of this strategy are discussed below.

   i. Strengthening of skills of health care workers.

   ii. Strengthening of health care infrastructure.

   iii. Involvement of the community.

The first two components are facility-based IMNCI and the third is community-based IMNCI.

The major highlights of the Indian adaptation are listed below.

   i. Incorporation of neonatal care because neonatal deaths account for two-thirds of infant mortality.

   ii. Inclusion of neonates between 0 and 7 days.

   iii. Incorporating national guidelines on malaria, anemia, vitamin A prophylaxis and immunization schedule.

   iv. Training program of health workers reduced from 11 to 8 days.

   v. Training protocol includes sick young infant up to 2 months of age.

   vi. Proportion of training time devoted to sick young infant and sick child is almost identical.

National Rural Health Mission

In view of the fact that 70% population of India lives in villages and existing health services are both unsatisfactory and unavailed by the rural people, the government of India launched National Rural Health Mission (NRHM) in 2005. The goal of NRHM is to improve the availability and accessibility of quality health care to people residing in rural areas with special focus to the most vulnerable segments of population, i.e. economically poor, women and children. The fiscal outlay of NRHM for 2019–2020 is in the range of ₹ 62,398 crores.

Core Strategies

1. The National Rural Health Mission seeks to provide quality health care to rural population throughout the country with special focus on 18 states which have weak public health indicators and poor infrastructure. It is envisaged to raise public spending on health from 0.9 to 4% of GDP with the help of private-public partnerships.

2. The capacity and credibility of Panchayati Raj Institutions (PRIs) shall be enhanced to own, control and manage public health services. Village Health Committee of the Panchayat will over see the Health Plan of each village.

3. It is proposed to create a new cadre of community based female health functionaries, named as Accredited Social Health Activists (ASHAs) to provide health services at the doorstep of people.

4. Home based newborn care (HBNC), newborn care corners (NBCC) and strengthening of facility based newborn care (FBNC) are important components of this program to improve newborn survival. The existent network of rural health services of subcenters, primary health centers (PCHs), community health centers (CHCs), first referral units (FRUs) and district hospitals shall be improved and energized to provide curative health services of a desired standard in accordance with the recommendations of Indian Public Health Standards for adequate personnel, equipment and management protocols.

5. Effective integration and implementation of core public health strategies like environmental sanitation and hygiene, availability of safe drinking water and promotion of optimal nutrition through a District Plan for Health. It is proposed to decentralize health programs and promote the concept of district management of health through the active participation of PRIs.

6. It is proposed to integrate all vertical health and family welfare programs at national, state, block and district levels.

7. It seeks to promote local health traditions and indigenous system of medicines by providing ASHAs a kit of medicines containing AYUSH (Ayurvedic, Unani, Siddha and Homeopathy) and allopathic medicines to treat common day-to-day illnesses.

8. Efforts are being made to strengthen capacities for data collection, assessment and review for evidence-based planning, monitoring and supervision of health interventions.

TABLE 10.13 Goals of NRHM

- Infant mortality rate shall be reduced to 30/1000 live births.
- Maternal mortality ratio to be reduced to 100/100,000 live births.
- Total fertility rate shall be reduced to 2.1.
- Malaria mortality rate reduction by 50% up to 2010 and sustaining that level up to 2012.
- Kala-azar mortality rate reduction by 100% by 2010 and sustaining elimination until 2012.
- Filaria/microfilaria rate reduction by 70% by 2010, 80% by 2012 and elimination by 2015.
- Dengue mortality rate reduction by 50% by 2010 and sustaining at that level until 2012.
- Japanese encephalitis mortality rate reduction by 50% by 2010 and sustaining at that level until 2012.
- Cataract operations to be increased to 46 lakhs per year until 2012.
- Leprosy prevalence rate reduction from 1.8/10,000 in 2005 to less than 1/10,000 thereafter.
- Tuberculosis DOTS services: Maintaining 85% cure rate through entire mission period.
- Upgrading community health centers to the level of Indian Public Health Standards.
- Increase utilization of first referral units from less than 20 to 75%.
- Engaging 2,50,000 female accredited social health activists (ASHAs) in 10 states.

9. Promotion and development of capacities for preventive health care strategies at all levels by promoting healthy lifestyle (controlling consumption of alcohol, tobacco, drug abuse), satisfactory environmental conditions, nutritious diet, universal immunization, etc.

10. It seeks to improve access of rural people, especially poor women and children, to availability of equitable, affordable, accountable and effective primary health care. Presently, over 20,000 ambulances are in operation in the country for transport of high-risk mothers and newborns under NRHM.

The goals of NRHM are listed in Table 10.13.

Accredited Social Health Activists (ASHAs)

ASHAs shall be recruited by the Panchayat in each village from among the married/widowed/divorced women with formal education up to 8th class and having effective communication, caring and leadership skills. She will be given 23 days induction training spread over 12 months along with on the job training and supervision.

1. ASHA is an honorary volunteer and shall receive performance-based compensation for promotion of universal immunizations, referral and escorting pregnant women for delivery at the PHC or CHC, construction of household toilets and participation in various ad hoc health care delivery programs.

2. ASHA shall serve as a bridge between the public health system and the community and shall be accountable to the Panchayat.

3. She will facilitate implementation of the village health plan with the help of *Anganwadi* worker, ANM, functionaries of other departments and self groups, under the leadership of the village health committee of the Panchayat.

4. She will be given a drug kit containing generic AYUSH and allopathic formulations for treatment of common day-to-day illnesses. She will provide directly observed treatment short-course (DOTS) of antitubercular drugs under Revised National Tuberculosis Control Program.

5. Under *Janani Suraksha Yojana* (JSY), ASHA would organize delivery care services at PHC or CHC for the registered expectant mothers, assist in providing immunizations and act as a propagator and motivator for family planning services.

Janani Suraksha Yojana (JSY)

Janani Suraksha Yojana is a 100% centrally sponsored scheme under the overall umbrella of NRHM to promote institutional deliveries of below poverty line (BPL) families. JSY is launched in lieu of national maternity benefit scheme (NMBs) wherein better diet was provided to BPL families. The main philosophy of JSY envisages universal antenated care, institutional deliveries and post-partum care of BPL families with an incentive of cash payment of ₹ 700/-. The main strategic components of JSY are given below:

1. Early registration of all BPL pregnant women by ASHA or an equivalent village health worker.

2. Providing at least 3 antenatal evaluations by ANM and identification of complicated cases.

3. Ensuring institutional delivery by organizing appropriate referral and providing transport to the pregnant BPL women. It is mandatory for ASHA to escort the woman in labor for delivery at the appropriate health care facility. Every year, about 107 lakhs deliveries are conducted in public health facilities.

4. Providing immediate post-partum care and ensuring administration of BCG vaccination within 4–6 weeks.

5. Disbursement of cash assistance to the BPL beneficiary after the institutional delivery. ASHA also gets cash incentive of ₹ 600–1000 for doing her assigned job.

Essential Perinatal and Neonatal Care in the Community

10

Janani-Shishu Suraksha Karyakram (JSSK) The Ministry of Health and Family Welfare, Government of India launched Janani-Shishu Suraksha Karyakram (JSSK) on June 2011 as a national initiative under the ambit of Janani Suraksha Yojana (JSY) for the benefit of pregnant women and newborns. Under this program, every year one crore (10 million) pregnant women and their newborns shall be provided completely free and cashless medical services in government health care facilities both in the rural and urban areas. The program will supplement the cash assistance given to pregnant women under JSY and is aimed at mitigating the burden of out of pocket expenses incurred by pregnant women (both normal deliveries and cesarean sections) and care of their newborns up to 30 days after birth.

National Urban Health Mission (NUHM)

To improve the health status of community living in urban slums and vulnerable populations living in marginalized urban areas, such as homeless, rag-pickers, street children, construction site workers and temporary migrants, the Ministry of Health and Family Welfare, Government of India launched National Urban Health Mission on January 20, 2014. The aims of NUHM include (i) improvement of health status of indigent and disadvantaged urban popula-tion, (ii) strengthening of public health care system, (iii) involvement of the community and urban local bodies in health care delivery and to (iv) complement the National Rural Health Mission under the umbrella of a unified National Health Mission.

Coverage and Commitments

1. To provide health preventive, promotive and essential curative services to estimated 221.3 million urban population including around 77.5 million poor and vulnerable population living in the state capitals, district headquarters and all cities/towns with a population above 50,000.
2. To create 30–100 bedded urban community health centers for cities above 5 lakh population.
3. Creation of network of urban primary health centers for every 50,000 population located within or near slums and shanty settlements.
4. Strengthening of existing First Referral Units (FRUs), Urban Health Centers and Dispensaries in terms of adequate human resources, equipment, medicines and consumables.
5. To provide auxiliary nurse midwife (ANM) for every 10,000–12,000 population and accredited social health activist (ASHA) for every 200–500 slum and urban poor households.
6. Empowerment of communities through *Mahila Arogya Samiti* to look after the health needs of every 50–100 slums and/or urban poor dwellings.

India Newborn Action Plan (INAP)

Children are truly the foundation of a nation and Government of India has launched several programs for welfare of girls (future mothers), women and children. Under the auspices of global Every Newborn Action Plan (ENAP), India envisions a health system that eliminates preventable deaths of newborns and stillbirths, and where every pregnancy is wanted, where every birth is celebrated and where women, babies and children survive, thrive and reach their full potential. The country has witnessed dramatic reduction in maternal and child mortality rates over the past two decades. The child survival has increased in India by virtue of reduction of post-neonatal deaths by promotion of breastfeeding, immunizations, oral rehydration solution (ORS) for treatment of diarrhea and early administration of antibiotics for treatment of acute respiratory tract infections. However, neonatal mortality has not reduced significantly, thereby increasing the contribution of neonatal deaths to mortality of under-5 children from 41% in 1990 to 56% in 2012. Every year about 0.76 million newborns die in India mainly due to preventable causes and an equal number of pregnancies end as stillbirths which are often missed or ignored.

Newborn health has now captured the attention of policy makers at the highest level because further reduction in child deaths can be achieved by improving the survival of newborns. The Ministry of Health and Family Welfare, Government of India has recognised the importance of newborn health (and also their creators, the mothers) as a national priority and development necessity. Two important strategies and commitments in this direction have been the National Rural Health Mission (NRHM) and the Reproductive, Maternal, Newborn, Child and Adolescent Health (RMNCH+A) Strategy. NRHM by virtue of its subsi-diary programs has provided unprecedented attention by allocation of resources for newborn health. While RMNCH+A strategy has provided a paradigm shift to emphasize the need for continuum-of-care from girls-women-mothers-newborns-children and adoles-cents by strengthening the health care system from the grass roots to the tertiary care level. The Ministry of Health and Family Welfare, Government of India launched the India Newborn Action Plan (INAP) on 18th September 2014 as a national commitment towards global Every Newborn Action Plan (ENAP) launched at the 67th World Health Assembly in June 2014. The main focus of the program is to improve the health and welfare of women and launch interventions to reduce maternal deaths, neonatal deaths and stillbirths. The lofty goal of the program is to achieve a target of "single digit neonatal mortality rate (NMR)" and a "single digit stillbirth rate (SBR)" by 2030. It is proposed to improve and scale-up the strategies for interventions and provide clear guidelines for their implementation, monitoring and evaluation. The INAP will be implemented within the existing framework of RMNCH+A and guided by the principles of integration, social and gender equity, quality of care, accountability and partnerships with all the stakeholders. The main focus of intervention packages would be to reduce stillbirths and improve newborn health and survival through a network of home-based newborn care (HBNC), newborn care corners (NBCC) and facility-based newborn care (FBNC) at community health centers or first referral units, special care newborn units (SCNUs) at sub-district and district hospitals, medical colleges and tertiary care centers.

It is proposed to build a strategy of "six pillars" at all levels of health care to provide (i) preconception and antenatal care, (ii) care during labor and child birth, (iii) care of the newborn at birth, (iv) care of healthy newborns, (v) care of small and sick newborns and (vi) care beyond newborn survival. Under the sixth pillar of "care beyond newborn survival", India has taken a vital step toward improving quality of life beyond newborn survival. It is proposed to take necessary steps towards improving the quality of life of survivors with birth defects and those infants who develop neurodevelopmental delay and disabilities due to prematurity and sickness. The strong component of the program is a systematic approach with close monitoring and evaluation to meet pre-set well defined indicators or targets. After the launch of India Newborn Action Plan (INAP), India envisions a health system that eliminates preventable deaths of newborns and stillbirths, and where every pregnancy is wanted, children survive, thrive and they reach there full genetic potential.

INNOVATIVE TRAINING PROGRAMS

The Ministry of Health and Family Welfare, government of India has launched several community based programs to improve the care and survival of newborn babies. No program can succeed unless the health care providers (HCPs), who are expected to oversee the program, are commited, motivated and adequately trained. Apart from formal training of various community based health workers (*Anganwadi* worker, community neonatal health worker, accredited social health activist, auxiliary nurse midwife), their knowledge and skills should be updated by organizing refresher courses and by harnessing innovative tele-education modules. Distance learning modules can be used for teaching and training of nursing and medical students, medical officers and pediatricians. E-learning training programs are available for various aspects of reproductive and child health, like essential care of the newborns, home care of newborns (HCNB), newborns care corners (NBCC), care of sick newborns, or facility based newborn care (FBNC), audio-visual webinars (http://www.newbornwhocc.org/wefinar-essential_newborn htm), "Adobe Connect", online continuous positive airway pressure (CPAP) course and IMCI computerized adaptation and training tool (ICATT) to promote integrated management of neonatal and childhood diseases. The online or digital training efforts can be further augmented by the mentors with the help of SMSs or e-mails and periodic quiz or MCQ interactions and evaluations. There is a need to create a pool of national and state level trainers to take forward the agenda of improving skills and managerial capabilities of HCPs in order to improve the health and wellbeing of mothers and their babies.

STRATEGIES TO IMPROVE NEWBORN HEALTH AND SURVIVAL

"The enhancement of neonatal and infant survival is truly the key to the success of family welfare program and stabilization of population dynamics which is a major public health issue in developing countries".

V. Ramalingaswami

The newborn care is the most urgent key health priority in our country and saving newborn babies should form a national agenda to achieve further reduction in infant mortality rate in order to achieve IMR of less than 10 per 1000 live births. The enhancement of neonatal and infant survival is truly the key to the success of family welfare program and stabilization of population dynamics which is a major public health issue in India. Neonates constitute the foundation of a nation and no sensible government can afford to neglect their needs and rights. The following strategies

Essential Perinatal and Neonatal Care in the Community

10

or *Ten Commandments*, with short- term and long-term goals, have been launched by the Government of India in order to improve newborn health and survival and enhance the quality of life among those who survive.

1. A national movement "India Newborn Action Plan" (INAP) has been launched and is being pursued like a "Mission".

2. Efforts are being made to provide facilities to improve education, nutrition (life cycle approach), health and "status" of girls and women who indeed are the creators and sustainers of progeny.

3. Launch a nationwide socio-political movement to discourage early marriages, teenage and frequent pregnancies.

4. Introduce teaching of mother-craft and family life education to high school boys and girls.

5. Ensure good quality antenatal care to all pregnant women.

6. High-risk pregnant women should be identified and referred to a higher level of care and confinement.

7. All deliveries should be conducted by trained and skilled health care attendants. *And as a long-term policy, infrastructure and facilities should be created to ensure that every baby is born at a nearby health care facility.*

8. There should be a greater focus on preventive rather than curative newborn services. Available health care professionals and a special cadre of community-based skilled birth attendants or village level newborn care workers (accredited social health activists or ASHAs) are being trained and effectively used to provide essential newborn care at the community level.

9. Supervised home care should be provided to moderately low birth weight babies (above 1800 g or >34 weeks gestation) and to all sick and stable babies through sustainable, doable and cost-effective community-based programs.

10. The available infrastructure, facilities and expertise for MCH services should be enhanced to provide good quality level II newborn care at the first referral units and district hospitals under the supervision of well-trained and dedicated health care professionals. There is a need to harness the potential of information technology (IT) to promote innovative interventions, like e-learning, mHealth and change in health-seeking behavior.

BIBLIOGRAPHY

Bang AT, Bang RA, Baitule SB, *et al.* Effect of home-based neonatal care and management of sepsis on neonatal mortality: field trial in rural India. *Lancet* 1999; 354:1955–1961.

Bang AT, Baitule SB, Reddy HM, Deshmukh MD, Bang RA. Low birth weight and preterm neonates: can they be managed at home by mother and trained village health worker? *J Perinatol* 2005 (Suppl 1); 25:S72–81.

Bhutta ZA, Das JK, Bahl R, *et al.* The Lancet Newborn Interventions Review Group and the Lancet Every Newborn Study Group. Can available interventions end preventable deaths in mothers, newborn babies and still births, and at what cost. *Lancet* 2014; 284:347–370.

Deorari AK, Paul VK, Singh M, Vidyasagar D. The national movement of neonatal resuscitation in India. *J Trop Pediatr* 2000; 46:315–317.

Integrated Management of Neonatal and Childhood Illness (IMNCI): Student's Handbook. *Ministry of Health and Family Welfare, Government of India,* 2007.

Kumar P, Nangia S. Research issues in neonatology. *J Neonatol* 2009; 23:279–383.

Kushwaha AS. Newborn care in India: a crying need of the hour. *Med J Armed Forces India.* 2011, 67(2): 104–105.

Lawn JE, Cousens S, Bhutta ZA, *et al.* Why are 4 million babies dying each year? *Lancet* 2004; 364: 399–401.

Lawn JE, Blencowe H, Oza S, *et al.* The Lancet Every Newborn Study Group. Every Newborn: Progress, priorities and potential beyond survival. *Lancet* 2014; 384:189–205.

National Child Survival and Safe Motherhood Program, MCH Division, Department of Family Welfare, *Ministry of Health and Family Welfare,* New Delhi, 1994.

National Family Health Survey NFHS-2, 2005–06, *Ministry of Health and Family Welfare,* Government of India, New Delhi; 2007.

Newborn Health: Key to Child Survival. Child Health Division, Department of Family Welfare, *Ministry of Health and Family Welfare,* Government of India, New Delhi, 2000.

Patel V, Parikh R, Nandraj S, Balasubramaniam P, Naryan K, Paul VK, *et al.* Assuring health coverage for all in India. *The Lancet* 2015, 386(10011):2422–35.

Paul VK. The newborn health agenda: Need for a village level midwife. *Nat Med J India* 2000; 13: 281–283.

Paul VK. Newborn care in India: a promising beginning but a long way to go. *Semin Neonatol* 1999; 4:141–149.

Paul VK, Singh M. Regionalized perinatal care in developing countries. *Semin Neonatol* 2004; 9: 117–24.

Sankar MJ, Neogi SB, Paul VK. State of newborn health in India. *J Perinatol* 2016, 36(suppl 3): S3–S8.

Singh M, Deorari AK, Khajuria RC, Paul VK. A four-year study on neonatal morbidity in a New Delhi hospital. *Indian J Med Res* 1991, 94; 186–192.

Singh M. Strategies to improve the health of mothers and children: Health and non-health approaches, *Reg Hlth Forum* (WHO/SEARO) 1996; 1:57–62.

Singh M, Paul VK. Maternal and child health services in India with special focus on perinatal services. *J Perinatol* 1997; 17:65–69.

Singh M. Care of newborn babies in the community. *Asian J Obstet Gynaec Practice* 1997, 1;21–27.

Singh M. Perinatal services in India; current status and future perspectives. *Natl Med J India* 2003; (Suppl 2); 16:1–4.

Singh M. The challenge of newborn care in India. *Perinatalogy* 2003; 5(6): 255–61.

Singh M. Perinatal care in the community: current perspectives. In: Textbook of Community and Social Pediatrics. SR Banerjee (Ed.) *Jaypee Bros, New Delhi* 2008. pp 14–21.

State of India's Newborns. (SOIN), 2014: A report, Zodpey S and Paul VK (Eds). Public Health Foundation of India, All India Institute of Medical Sciences and Save the Children, New Delhi.

State of the World's Children Report, UNICEF 2018, New York.

Strategic Approach to Reproductive, Maternal, Newborn, Child and Adolescent Health (RMNCH+A) in India. For Healthy Mother and Child. Ministry of Health and Family Welfare, Government of India, January 2013.

10

Humanized Care and Rhythmic Stimulation of Newborn Babies

Nature is supreme the way it looks after all the needs of the baby in the womb. The baby is gently rocked in the warm amniotic fluid and is well protected from infections and effectively shielded against light and sound. The baby is comfortably "nested" in a flexed posture with hands in the midline close to his mouth. The uterine blood flow provides a soothing music akin to a waterfall while tick-tack of the maternal heart beats provides him constant soothing beats of a cuckoo clock. The physiological needs of oxygenation, nutrition and excretion are admirably met by the uteroplacental unit (Table 11.1). Despite several attempts, scientists have failed to fabricate an incubator with all the qualities and characteristics of the womb.

Birthing is a traumatic experience both for the mother and her baby. Apart from the discomfort and trauma associated with the process of delivery, the baby is suddenly thrust into a world of bright lights, loud sounds and cold environment. Healthy term babies are neurologically mature to withstand these environmental onslaughts and they rapidly adjust to the extrauterine environment with minimal assistance without any serious difficulties or hazards. But preterm babies are neurologically immature and physiologically

unstable. They cannot tolerate environmental insults and stresses which may adversely affect their neuromotor development. For example, when a baby is born at 30 weeks of gestation, he is denied the comforts and *in utero* sensory experiences of the womb for 10 weeks because he is born and reared in the hostile environment of the NICU.

Due to advances in technology, the survival of perterm babies has improved but the quality of life among the survivors has not significantly improved. It is believed that differences in cognition, behavior and neuropsychological parameters between preterm and term babies may be explained on the basis of striking dissimilarities between their environments before achieving full maturity.

TECHNOLOGY-ORIENTED NEWBORN CARE

During the last three to four decades, technology has revolutionized the care of preterm babies. The earlier relatively humanized approaches in the care of preterm babies by gentle handling and "masterly inactivity" has been replaced by the use of aggressive and invasive hi-tech modalities to provide life support to tiny babies to improve their survival. The art of newborn care has been sacrificed at the altar of technology. The babies are being handled as "objects" without any concern either for their comfort or for their stimulation. We are lacking in emotional, humane and common sense approach in providing care to preterm babies. The intensive care of the newborn babies has become mechanical or "robotic" and stereotyped instead of being flexible and individualized. We are caring our babies entirely with our brains with total disregard for providing them care with our hearts. It is a pity that technological advances have dehumanized the care of preterm babies. The

TABLE 11.1 The virtues of the womb
■ Cushioned and comfortable aquatic abode
■ Thermal comfort
■ Zero insensible water loss
■ Shielded from light
■ Protected from sound
■ Effective and safe ECMO-like oxygenation
■ Optimal excretion of waste products
■ Isolation and asepsis
■ Parenteral nutrition

widening gap between technology and common sense must be bridged.

We have now realized that there is a need to have synthesis of "art and science" of neonatal care in order to provide holistic care to preterm babies. Hi-tech care should be provided but comfort of the baby should not be ignored. Babies must be given appropriate analgesics and sedatives to relieve pain and discomfort of procedures. The procedures and investigations must be kept at the barest minimum without compromising the quality of care. They should be reared in the neonatal intensive care unit (NICU) which should simulate the ecology of the womb to ensure maximum comfort to the baby. The babies should be handled with gentle touch, love and compassion and the nurses should feel "connected" and "tuned" to the babies under their care.

PRINCIPLES OF HUMANIZED CARE

We should create a baby-friendly womb-like ambience and ecology in the NICU to simulate *in utero* environment. Depending upon the degree of immaturity, graded rhythmic and soothing stimulation should be introduced when baby has achieved physiologic stability. The nurses should be trained to provide individualized developmentally supportive care to preterm babies by adopting a "flexible" approach. All the health care professionals in the NICU should be gentle, considerate and compassionate in providing care to preterm babies. Early and active participation by family members in the care of preterm babies should be encouraged to promote bonding, facilitate physical growth and neuromotor development.

BABY-FRIENDLY AMBIENCE IN THE NICU

It is a common observation that very low birth weight (VLBW) babies are being looked after in an unpleasant, noisy, too bright, and invasive environment without any concern regarding their physiological needs, comfort and periods of rest of individual babies.

Sound

In the uterus, infant is exposed to sound level of about 40–60 decibels. The NICU environment usually provides sound levels between 70 and 80 dB. It has been shown that when sound level exceeds 77 dB it causes discomfort to the baby. The American Academy of Pediatrics recommend that the maximum noise level in the NICU should not exceed 45 dB. The main sources of noise in NICU include telephone rings,

equipment alarms, paging bleeps, air compressor, carting of equipment and loud talking during the rounds. The studies have shown that there are around 4994 peak noises during 48 hours observation period in the NICU and around 90% of loud noises are related to the personnel. It is amazing to realize that babies in the NICU can hardly sleep more than 4–10 minutes at a time. The physiological consequences of loud sound include startle response, apneic attacks, bradycardia or tachycardia and oxygen desaturation. At times, sudden elevation of blood pressure is a risk factor for development of intraventricular hemorrhage. The baby is unable to sleep and is unable to get any rest and thus may remain irritable or cranky. This may lead to depletion of energy reserves with poor weight gain due to constant state of arousal. High noise level may cause damage to the cochlea and even the adverse effects of ototoxic drugs may be enhanced. Preterm babies have 5 times greater risk of development of hearing loss compared to term babies.

The harmful effects of the noise can be minimized by designing an acoustic-friendly nursery. The doors and drawers should be padded and ceilings and walls can be provided with noise-absorbing material. The health personnel should learn the art of speaking softly and walking gracefully in the nursery. Telephone rings should be replaced by blinking lights. Instead of air compressors, centralized sources of compressed air, oxygen and suction should be used. The nurses should anticipate activation of alarms and respond to them promptly or preemptively. The incubator can be covered with a blanket or specially made cover to dampen the noise and light reaching the baby (Figure 11.1). The doors and port holes of incubator should be opened

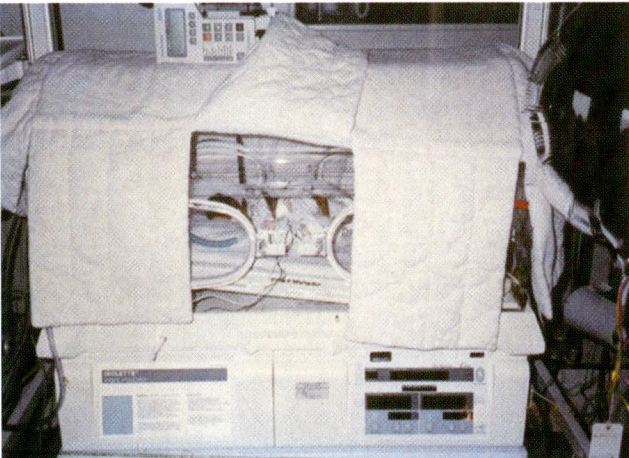

Figure 11.1 The incubator is kept covered to dampen the noise and reduce the light reaching the baby. The baby must be attached to a vital sign monitor.

gently. The incubator top should never be used as a writing surface. Decibel meters should be installed to monitor sound levels in the NICU.

Light

Most NICUs maintain high intensity of day and night illumination ranging between 50 and 150 foot candles for ease of observation. Procedure lights and phototherapy units may provide light intensity between 200 and 400 foot candles resulting in several adverse consequences. Bright light may adversely affect the development of central visual system and may lead to development of squint, "shutting out" behavior with reduced socialization. The duration of rapid eye movements (REM) sleep is increased which may be associated with physiologic lability as manifested by bradycardia and apnea. There is some evidence to suggest that exposure to bright light may predispose the baby to develop retinopathy of prematurity. When nursery illumination is maintained uniformly bright during the day and night, it may adversely affect the circadian biologic rhythm leading to reduced release of growth hormone and poor weight gain.

The illumination in the nursery should be kept dim without compromising ease of observation. The light should be further dimmed off and on to create periods of "quiet time" during each shift and baby should not be disturbed for a procedure unless it is unavoidable. Dim lighting has been shown to improve duration of sleep, decrease motor activity, reduce heart rate, improve tolerance of feeds and increase weight gain of stable preterm babies. The windows of the NICU should be covered with screens and blinds. The light should be dimmed at night to simulate day-night pattern to promote hormonal surge and physical growth. A meta-analysis of effects of cyclic-lighting on preterm infants showed improved weight gain, shorter length of stay in the NICU and reduced incidence of retinopathy of prematurity (ROP) compared with exposure to near darkness or continuous bright light. Bed side lights with dimmer switches should be provided to create specialized microenvironment for each baby. The incubator should be covered with a blanket or specially-designed cover. When incubator is covered, the baby should be attached to a vital sign monitor. Eyes should be covered and protected against exposure to bright light when incubator lid is opened or baby is picked up. The eyes should be shielded or covered with visors while using procedure light or during phototherapy. The lux meter can be used to monitor light intensity in the NICU. According to American Academy of Pediatrics, the ambient lighting level during "quiet period" should be 10–20 foot candles, 60 foot candles for observation and 100 foot candles for precedures.

Gentle Handling and Positioning

The round-the-clock video studies in the NICU have shown that premature infants on an average are disturbed more than 130 times in a day by the nurses. All efforts should be made to handle babies gently and "nestle" them in a comfortable position although it is impossible to achieve *in utero* comfort levels and cushioning. The preemies have poor muscle tone and they lie with their arms and legs straight or extended. Gentle human touch (GHT) and caressing are associated with hemodynamic stability, improved sleep cycle, sucking behavior and cognition. The extended posture for a long period of time may lead to abnormal tone with consequent delay in motor development. It has been shown that preterm babies maintain better oxygenation, temperature control and sleep pattern when they are nursed in a prone or lateral position (Figure 11.2). Body position also affects gastric emptying and neurobehavioural development. When a baby is handled roughly, he feels uncomfortable by squirming, crying and recoiling his arms and legs. There is evidence to suggest that rough handling may lead to hypoxemia and sudden elevation of blood pressure with risk of development of intraventricular hemorrhage.

The infant should be positioned prone or on the side with flexed extremities by providing a "nest" with a rolled blanket. Swaddling, tucking and containment simulates *in utero* feeling of lack of space and it makes the baby less jittery or prone to startle. Swaddling is associated with improved physiological and behavioral state, better sleep, reduced perception of pain and lower risk of hypothermia. Prolonged swaddling

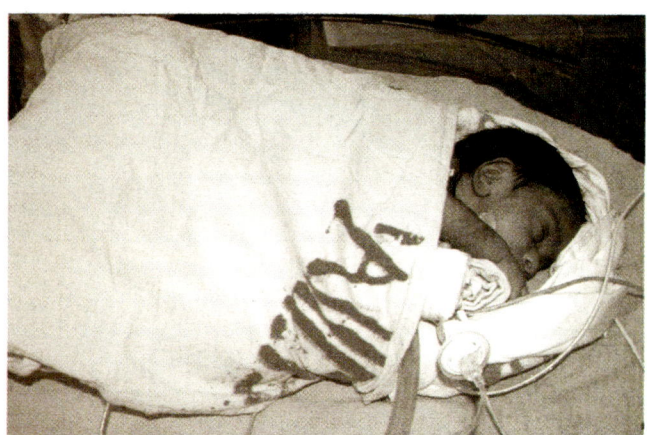

Figure 11.2 Effective nesting of the baby to provide comfort.

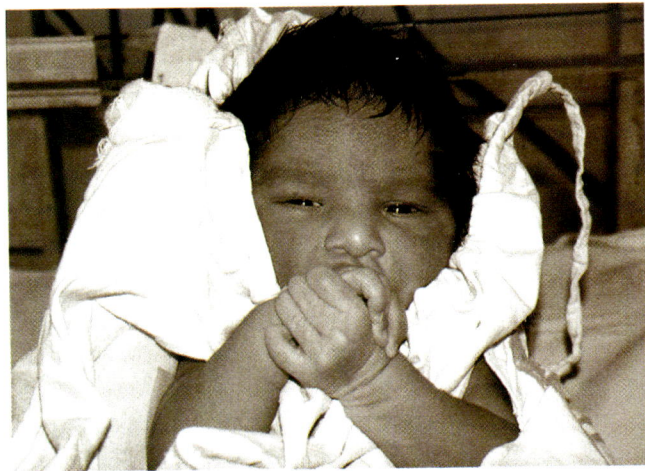

Figure 11.3 The baby enjoys midline orientation and comfort by sucking fingers or hand.

and containment beyond newborn period should be avoided due to increased risk of sudden infant death syndrome (SIDS), dysplasia of hip joint which is kept in extension and adduction and hyperthermia. Babies love to be nursed on a sheepskin, water bed or gloves filled with water. Nursing the baby on a water bed rekindles his memories of *in utero* environment.

Infant should be provided with midline orientation to facilitate hand-to-mouth activities which are self-soothing. The hands of the baby should be left free so that he can get them to his mouth to suck his fingers or just touch his face (Figure 11.3). Putting on a small diaper or placing soft material between the legs provide comfort to the baby. The baby must be handled minimally and gently with clean and warm hands and warm heart. Sudden changes in the position must be avoided. During positioning and moving the infant or while doing procedures such as suctioning, "containment" should be provided. It can be accomplished by holding the arms and legs of the infant close to the midline of the body or by supporting his head and buttocks. When hands of the caretaker are busy in doing the procedure, the flexed legs of the infant can be enclosed in a blanket to provide containment.

Feeding with Human Milk

Nothing is more humanized and natural for a baby than providing feeding with human milk to all babies. The milk of a mother should be given to her baby because milk is not only species specific, it is indeed baby-specific! Extremely preterm babies cannot self feed and they are given expressed breast milk (EBM) through a nasogastric tube. Even when nutritional feeds cannot be provided due to physiologic instabi-

lity, the baby should be provided with minimal enteral feeds to harness its trophic effects on the GI tract. Trophic feeds are credited to enhance maturation and growth of intestinal mucosa and gut musculature. The oxygen uptake and intestinal blood flow are increased. There is early elaboration of a large number of gut endocrines like gastrin, cholecystokinin, motilin and inhibitory peptides. The colonization of the gut with friendly lactobacilli and bifido bacteria prevents entry of pathogenic bacteria.

Physiologic and Autonomic Stability

The hi-tech care to preterm babies should be provided with gentleness and due concern for their comfort and physiologic stability. The major goal of reducing noise, bright light and rough handling is to ensure that babies in the NICU attain physiologic stability. The process of healing and velocity of physical growth and neuro-motor development are enhanced when babies are physiologically stable.

The stable babies are awake, alert and responsive. They are likely to have stable vital signs without undue fluctuations. The baby is pink with satisfactory arterial oxygen saturation and good tissue perfusion as evidenced by capillary refill time of less than 2 seconds. The muscle tone is in accordance with gestational maturity and there are no apneic attacks or subtle seizures. The baby is likely to have satisfactory GI functions and would be able to tolerate enteral feeds.

GENTLE RHYTHMIC STIMULATION

The preemies should be provided with developmentally supportive care to meet their neurobehavioral and physiologic needs in order to foster their normal physical growth and neuropsychological development. It is desirable to assign one or two babies to a nurse and they should follow individualized and flexible approach in their care. Stimulation should be provided when baby is physiologically stable and alert or receptive. The well-organized state of the baby is characterized by well-defined awake and sleep states, robust crying, successful self-consoling and self-quieting. The babies should preferably be left undisturbed during periods of deep sleep. The care in the NICU should not be merely task-oriented but the nurses should feel "connected" or "tuned" with the babies under their care and provide "individualized developmentally supportive care" to promote emotional and neuropsychological development of the babies.

It must be remembered, however, that both lack of stimulation and overstimulation are equally bad for optimal development of preterm babies. Only one stimulus should be introduced at a time while observing infant's physiological and behavioral responses. When baby shows signs of disorganization or hyperalertness, the stimulus should be withdrawn and baby should be provided hand-on-containment and given time for recovery before continuing. The evidences of hyper-alertness include wide-open eyes, a look of fear or panic or the appearance of being "hooked" to the stimulus and baby having difficulty in breaking away. The stimulatory messages to the CNS are transmitted through specially modulated tactile, vestibulokinesthetic, auditory, visual and olfactory sensations.

Tactile-Kinesthetic Stimulation

The tactile stimulation should be provided by gently touching the head or back of the baby while speaking softly in a soothing voice. The baby should be positioned in such a way so that he is able to suck his fingers or hand or is able to touch his face (Figure 11.4). The baby should be encouraged to grasp the finger of the caretaker or edge of the blanket or a small rolled up cloth. The baby should be provided with opportunities for rooting and non-nutritive sucking.

The mother should be encouraged to provide intermittent skin-to-skin contact to her baby. It provides comfort, warmth and "special" smell of the mother to the baby. It improves mother–infant bonding and promotes breastfeeding. When baby is held against mother's heart, he is reminded of the *in utero* soothing music produced by uterine blood flow and maternal heart beats in the womb. During skin-to-skin contact, most babies feel comfortable, stop crying and achieve physiological stability (Figure 11.5). At times intractable apneic attacks may be relieved by skin-to-skin contact. During skin-to-skin contact, there is a possibility of

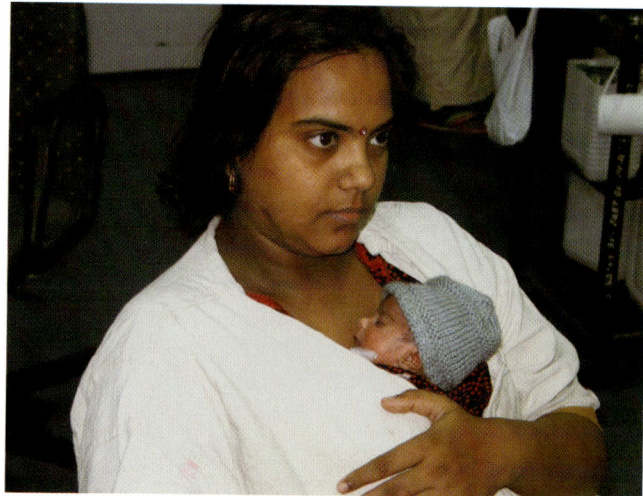

Figure 11.5 Mother providing skin-to-skin care to her preterm baby in the NICU.

transfer of tremendous electromagnetic energy from a compassionate mother to her baby producing calmness, comfort, autonomic stability, promotion of physical growth and augmentation of forces of healing. These virtues of skin-to-skin contact need to be further studied and exploited.

Orobuccal and Gustatory Stimulation

Fetus swallows amniotic fluid and is exposed to oro-motor activity and chemosensory experience early in life. Preterm infants are often denied oromotor and gustatory stimulation because they are usually gavage fed or given parenteral nutrition. During gavage feeding and transition from gavage to cup and spoon or breastfeeding, non-nutritive sucking (NNS) should be encouraged as a part of developmental care intervention. It facilitates the development of sucking behavior of the infant and improves the digestion of enteral feed by elaboration of digestive enzymes mediated by vagal innervation of the oral mucosa. Oromotor stimulation can be provided by sucking at pacifier (dummy nipple) or by putting the baby directly to the breast before expression of breast milk. It promotes mother–infant interaction and bonding and facilitates breastfeeding. Angle of the mouth of the baby can be stimulated with a soft brush or finger of the mother or nurse (digital stroking). NSS is credited to facilitate smooth transition from tube to breast or bottle, earlier intake of full oral feeds and a shorter stay in the NICU.

Body Massage

Body massage is culturally accepted in our society and has scientifically proven benefits. Gentle touch, massage and kinesthetic stimulation should be

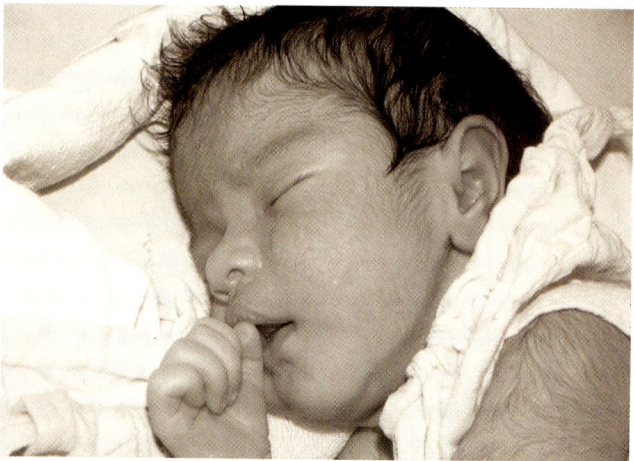

Figure 11.4 The baby enjoys sucking his hand and fingers.

provided when the baby is alert and awake. Massage should be done with a non-irritating and non-scented oil (olive oil, coconut oil, sesame oil and sunflower oil) taking due care to avoid exposure. Application of liquid paraffin or oil to the skin of preterm babies is associated with reduced insensible water loss, better insulation and thermal control. It prevents dryness and chaffing of skin.

Babies enjoy comfort of touch and oil massage. It promotes bonding with the mother and she should talk with her baby while doing the massage, active and passive movements of the limbs. Massage improves circulation and tone of muscles. It provides a sense of well-being and baby cries less and sleeps better after the massage. Because of thin skin of newborn babies, some oil gets absorbed and provides nutrition to the baby. Several studies have shown that massaged babies are more alert and responsive and their weight gain velocity is better due to release of insulin-like growth factor (IGF-1). There is increased mineralization of bones because of increase in circulating leptin levels. It promotes better physiologic and autonomic stability by increasing galvanic skin resistance and vagal tone. Massage has been shown to reduce stress as evidenced by lowering of the cortisol and norepinephrine levels and it may enhance immunological capabilities of the baby by improving the activity of natural killer cells (NK cells).

Auditory and Vestibular Stimulation

Fetus respond to auditory stimuli (especially maternal voice) as early as 20 weeks of gestation. This capability can be exploited to stimulate the baby in the womb and during stay in the NICU.

Music is credited to have numerous qualities and capabilities and it has been shown even to enhance the growth of plants. Studies have shown that soft and soothing music to individual babies enhance their physiologic stability and improve weight gain velocity (Figure 11.6). Babies like and enjoy classical or gentle instrumental music. The baby can be made to listen to the taped voice of his parents and family members on and off. This enhances parent–infant bonding and gives family members the sense of involvement in the care of their baby. Music is credited to ensure autonomic stability, reduce stress and quieten the baby, increase oxygen saturation and reduce heart rate.

Stimulation of the Visual System

Babies should be picked up and encouraged to develop an eye-to-eye contact. Babies often turn to the source of diffuse light. Visual stimuli can be provided

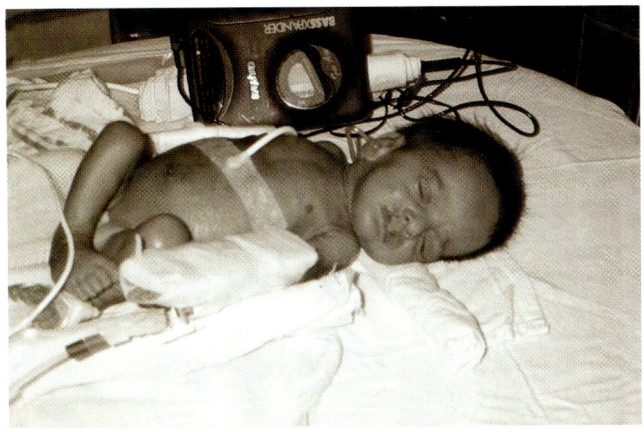

Figure 11.6 Preterm baby is hooked-on to taped music.

with the help of bright toys and pictures. A picture with distinct facial pattern can be placed on the incubator or crib wall in line with the gaze of the baby. Dim-light (10–20 foot candles) encourages babies to open their eyes and look around.

Stimulation of the Olfactory System

The baby should not be exposed to unpleasant or noxious odors. Alcohol, betadine, or other skin scrub bottles should be opened away from the baby. The medicated swabs should be removed from the incubator immediately after their use. The baby should not be dabbed with hair spray or cologne. Skin-to-skin contact provides pleasant and "special" smell of the mother to the baby. Babies are sensitive and attracted to the smell of the mother's milk which is used for rooting the nipple during breastfeeding. The gauze pads or cotton balls soaked in mother's milk can be kept inside the incubator to stimulate olfactory system.

Conclusion and Recommendations

Humanized care is not an alternative to hi-tech care but is complementary in order to provide best or holistic care to preterm babies. We should strive to provide a good mix and balance between technology-based care and humane care to preterm babies. Synthesis of art and science is crucial in every human endevor but much more so in the care of preterm and high-risk newborn babies. The NICU should have womb-like ambience and ecology. The lighting should be kept dimmed with a day–night pattern. The sound level should be low and light kept dimmed to have "quiet periods" during each shift. The baby should be provided with a comfortable "nest" and kept on the side or prone with flexion of limbs. The nurses should be trained to provide an individualized and developmentally supportive care. They should feel connected and tuned with babies under their care. Apart from analgesics and sedatives, caressing; cuddling and containment are useful to provide comfort to the baby during painful procedures. Nothing is more humanized than feeding the baby with milk of her mother because milk is not only species specific; but it is also baby-specific.

Early and intensive family participation in the care of preterm babies is important for their bonding; growth and neuromotor development. We should demystify NICU and actively involve and inform the parents about the care and condition of their baby. Mother should be encouraged to provide the benefits of intermittent skin-to-skin contact to her baby. She should be asked to touch, talk, feed and take care of her baby and provide necessary tactile, visual and auditory stimuli. Mothers are more likely to look after their babies with devotion and compassion and this is likely to augment the forces of healing and promote the process of recovery of high-risk and sick preterm babies. We must handle babies not only with our heads but also with our hearts. Brain is business like but heart brings in harmony and healing. All efforts should be made to enhance the survival of preterm babies but our goal should be to improve the quality of life among those who survive.

BIBLIOGRAPHY

Acolet D, Sleath K, Whitelaw A. Oxygenation, heart rate and temperature in very low birth weight infants during skin-to-skin contact with their mothers. *Acta Paediatr Scand* 1989; 78:189–193.

American Academy of Pediatrics, Committee on Environmental Health; Noise: a hazard for the fetus and newborn. *Pediatrics* 1997; 100:724–732.

Blackburn S. Environmental impact of the NICU on developmental outcomes. *J Pediatr Nurs* 1998; 13(5):279–289.

Chang YJ, Lim LH. Noise and related events in a neonatal intensive care unit. *Acta Paediatr Taiwan* 2001; 42(4):212–216.

Charpak N, Ruis JG, de Calume ZF. Humanizing neonatal care. *Acta Paediatr* 2000; 89:501–502.

Chen CH, Wang TM, Chi CS. Individualized developmental care in the newborn intensive care unit. *Acta Paediatr Taiwan* 2000; 41(3):119–122.

Conde-Agudelo A, Belizan JM, Diaz-Rossello J. Kangaroo mother care to reduce morbidity and mortality in low birth weight infants. *Cochrane Database Syst Rev*, 2011; 3:CD002771.

Depaul D, Chambers S. Environmental noise in the neonatal intensive care unit: Implications for nursing practice. *J Perinatal Neonatal Nurs* 1995; 8:71–76.

Ferronato PAM, Domellof E, Ronnqvist L. Early influence of auditory stimuli on upper limb movements in young human infants: an overview. *Front Psychol.* 2014, 5:1043–67.

Field T, Diego M, Hernandez-Reif M. Potential underlying mechanisms for greater weight gain in massaged preterm infants. *Infant Behav Dev* 2011; 34(3):383–389.

Fleisher BE, Vandenberg K, Constantinou J, et al. Individualized developmental care for very low birth weight premature infants. *Clin Pediatr* 1995; 34(10):523–529.

Khawash P, Banerjee M. Training of NICU staff in early developmental care of newborn: A perspective from India. *EC Paediatrics* 2018, 7:10, 945–955.

Lang JG, Philip AGS, Lucey JF. Excessive handling as a cause of hypoxemia. *Pediatrics* 1980; 65:203–207.

Levin A. Humane neonatal care initiative. *Acta Paediatr* 1999; 88:353–355.

Masterson J, Zucker C, Schalze K. Prone and supine positioning: effect on energy expenditure and behaviour of low birth weight infants. *Pediatrics* 1998; 5:689–693.

Morag I, Ohlsson A. A cycled light in the intensive care unit for preterm and low birth weight infants. *Cochrane Database Syst Rev* 2011; 1:CD006982.

Paul VK, Gupta A, Singh M, Deorari AK, Pandey RM. Effect of Indian classical music on heart rate and oxygen saturation in preterm neonates in the ICU. *Pediatr Res* 1999; 45:16A.

Provasi J, Anderson DI, Barbu-Roth M. Rhythm perception, production and synchronization during the perinatal period. *Front Psychol.* 2014, 5:1048–58.

Ramachandran S, Dutta S. Early developmental care interventions of preterm and low birth weight infants. *Indian Pediatr* 2013; 50:765–770.

Simkiss DE. Kangaroo mother care (Editorial) *J Trop Pediatr* 1999; 45:192–194.

Singh M, Deorari AK. Humanized care of preterm babies *Indian Pediatr* 2003; 40:13–20.

Taquino L, Blackburn S. The effects of containment during suctioning and heel sticks on physiological and behavioural responses of preterm infants. *Neonatal Network* 1994; 13:55–58.

Thomas EB, Ingersoll EW, Acebo C. Premature infants seek rhythmic stimulation and the experience facilitates neurobehavioural development. *J Dev Behav Pediatr* 1991; 12:11–18.

Vickers A, Ohlsson A, Lacy J, Horsley A. Massage for promoting growth and development of preterm and/or low birth weight infants. *Cochrane Database System Rev.* 2011; 3:CD002771.

Ethical, Social and Legal Issues in Perinatal Medicine

"What is not negotiable is that our profession exists to serve the patient, whose interests come first. None but a saint could follow this principle all the time but so many doctors have followed it so much of the time that the profession has been generally held in high regard".

Sir Theodore Fox

Medicine is considered as a noble profession because physicians are charged with the supreme responsibility of maintaining health and preserving life of their fellow human beings. There is an age old trust and respect towards physicians in Indian culture. In our culture especially among the masses, the doctor is viewed as a demigod and his advice and treatment is followed with full confidence without any questions or misgivings. The legendary bond of faith between the patient and doctor is aptly summed up by Charaka:

"No other gift is greater than the gift of life. The patient may doubt his relatives, his sons and even his parents, but he has full faith in his physician. He gives himself up in the doctor's hands and has no misgivings about him. Therefore, it is the physician's duty to look after him as his own...".

To maintain this trust and faith, which is essential to augment the process of healing, it is incumbent upon the physicians to be ethical, honest and up-to-date in their knowledge and skills to effectively and rationally manage the patients under their care. Despite growing commercialism in medical profession, in a survey conducted in UK, 80% people said that they still have faith and trust in their physicians while only 5% had trust in their politicians!

Ethics refers to moral principles or a set of moral values which determine the code of conduct as stipulated by the medical profession. The ethical decisions are based upon a system of moral values

that serve the best interests of society in a humane and caring way. The moral values are governed by the society and they extoll what is correct, righteous, virtuous, noble, desirable and acceptable. The physicians are both morally and legally accountable to the society. Because of tremendous advances in technology, the care of critically ill and tiny preemies has unfolded complex medical, social, ethical, fiscal, philosophical, moral and legal issues. Apart from tremendous financial cost of neonatal intensive care to the parents and society, there is incalculable cost in terms of pain, grief, frustration and guilt with survival of a severely handicapped child.

PRINCIPLES GOVERNING ETHICAL DECISIONS

Ethical decisions are based on the five principles of beneficence, non-maleficence, parental autonomy, correct medical facts and justice. Beneficence bequeaths that we should be the best advocates of our patients and ensure their best interests in accordance with the age old Hippocratic tradition. The physicians should be concerned with saving life and avoid doing any wilful harm to their patients, i.e. they should be non-maleficence in their therapeutic actions. Hippocrates epitomized the principle of *Primum non-nocere*—first do no harm. Florence nightingale also said that the first dictum of patient care is *"Do no harm"*. Almost 1000 years ago, according to Manu's code of conduct for the physicians, it was ordained that *"Dedicate yourself entirely for helping the sick, even though this may be at the cost of your own life. Never harm the sick, not even in thought or dream ...... May the gods help you if you follow this rule. Otherwise may the gods be against you"*. This has been stipulated to maintain the sanctity and dignity of life so that doctor's professional capabilities are not abused which may erode doctor–patient relationship. The parental autonomy should be honored and they should be given the right and taken into confidence while making a decision regarding the medical care of their children. We should assist parents to make an informed decision on the basis of available medical facts. The principle of justice demands that we seek the morally correct distribution of resources at all levels of health care and, ensure cost effectiveness of therapeutic measures by balancing medical benefits and burdens to the family and society. The basic and essential perinatal services must be made available to all irrespective of their habitat, socioeconomic status, religion, caste and creed.

The decisions should be taken jointly after discussion with the concerned consultants and nurses and by taking parents into confidence. The resolutions should be made jointly by weighing all pros and cons. There are several issues which have moral and ethical considerations. Should a newborn baby who is extremely tiny or grossly malformed resuscitated and admitted to the NICU or not? Is there any reasonable chance of survival of the infant with available technology? Whether to continue invasive hi-tech care or replace intensive treatment with palliative care? Would quality of life be worth living if the child survives with aggressive management? Can the family afford expensive management in the NICU? Should we be concerned with the best interests of the patient alone or global interests of the family, society and state? And there are cultural considerations, the issue of fertility of the couple, the concept of destiny or will of God, the doctor-knows-the-best attitude, socioeconomic status, gender of the baby, education of parents, social support system and national priorities. It is unfortunate but true that in a developing country, economic and social realities may outweigh and override ethical considerations.

The sound ethical decisions are based on correct medical facts. The ethical dilemma should be identified and analyzed in depth by all the specialists looking after the baby before a final decision is taken (Figure 12.1). However, whatever the final decision, it must be based on facts and logic and the decision should be justified and recorded in the case file.

The Rights of Fetus and the Indian Law

Nearly 1000 years ago when there was no legal system, as per Manusmriti, fetus was recognized to have the right to live and inherit property. According to Indian Penal Code, way back in 1860, it was recognized that fetus is a living being and any person causing wilful

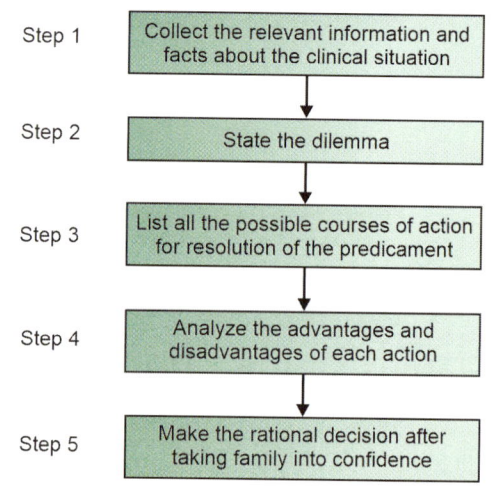

Figure 12.1 The ethical decision-making process.

death of the fetus in the womb shall be accountable. However, if in the opinion of a doctor, termination of pregnancy was considered to be in the interest of the mother, it was legally permitted. The Medical Termination of Pregnancy Act (MTP) was enacted by the Parliament in 1971 further liberalizing abortion for family welfare purposes. According to the provisions of MTP Act, if pregnancy is less than 12 weeks of gestation, it can be terminated on the advice of one registered medical practitioner but if the pregnancy is more than 12 weeks but less than 20 weeks, the opinion of two medical practitioners is mandatory before undertaking abortion. However, selective abortion of female fetuses by antenatal determination of sex is highly unethical which has been legally banned throughout the country. Under section 5 of MTP Act, even if the duration of pregnancy is more than 20 weeks, the physician has the right to terminate pregnancy in order to save the life of mother. The physicians caring for the pregnant women are concerned with the welfare of two lives and of the two, the mother is considered as more precious than the fetus.

Can pregnancy beyond 20 weeks be legally terminated?

According to MTP Act, pregnancy beyond 20 weeks can be terminated for maternal and not for fetal reasons. The cut-off of 20 weeks has been kept possibly because fetus becomes viable at this gestation and the procedure of abortion at this stage is fraught with danger to the life of mother. However, premature induction of labor is routinely done for maternal and fetal indications (unfavorable maternal environment) without raising any ethical or legal issues. It is morally justified though illegal to abort a malformed fetus after 20 weeks, if both of the following conditions are fulfilled:

i. Fetus is afflicted with a condition that is incompatible with postnatal survival beyond a few weeks or survival is likely to be associated with total or virtual absence of cognitive functions later in life.

ii. Prenatal diagnosis of the condition is highly reliable.

These criteria are adequately met by the fetus having anencephaly. The other lethal congenital malformations which can be considered for abortion after 20 weeks are listed in Box 12.1. It must be kept in mind that medical uncertainty regarding correct diagnosis and prognosis in fetal medicine is profound. The decision for termination of pregnancy should, therefore, be taken after due consultations with a group of experts and by informed consent of parents.

There is certainly a need to revise the law to justify and legalize termination of pregnancy after 20 weeks of gestation. Life is life irrespective of gestation and the life is not smaller or lesser on the basis of size of the baby.

Is it Justified to Establish Neonatal Intensive Care Facilities in a Developing Country?

In a developing country like India, a large number of salvageable babies are dying in the community without receiving even basic or essential care. It is logical to ask should we waste our meager resources for a cost-intensive and cost-ineffective intensive care for critically sick and tiny newborn babies? According to the principle of justice and fairness, there is macro-allocation of resources by the society for various activities like defense, agriculture, industry, power and health, etc. Allocation of budget for health shall compete with preventive, promotive and curative services at all levels of health care and for all age groups depending upon the national priorities. The neonatal care becomes one competing component of these multiple areas for "micro" allocation of resources. In view of the fact that about 70% of infant deaths are accounted by neonatal deaths, there is certainly a need to establish special care neonatal units to reduce neonatal mortality. However, the improvements in the neonatal care should not be restricted to specialized neonatal units alone but globally distributed at all levels, i.e. home, sub-center, primary health center, community health center, district hospital, medical college hospital and private nursing homes. It is desirable to ensure equitable development of health care of neonates at all levels, be it at the grass roots level or corps d'elite. There is an urgent need to introduce doable and sustainable strategies to provide essential perinatal services to the community which are highly cost-effective and useful to the society to reduce infant mortality rate.

To ensure effectivity and credibility of the referral system, it is mandatory to establish specialized units of neonatal care where sick and small babies from the community health centers can be referred for optimal management. There is certainly a need to develop and establish NICU facilities in the country in a phased manner. It is unwise to establish intensive care and ventilatory facilities in a district hospital without first strengthening the crucial components of essential newborn care. In order to stabilize the population dynamics, there is a need to reduce infant mortality rate because enhanced survival of babies would discourage parents to produce more children. Moreover, saving the life of the newborn baby is more cost-effective for the society as it is associated with lifelong productivity as opposed to saving a life due to cardiac or cerebral stroke and cancer in the elderly which is followed by survival for a short period of 2–5 years.

Withholding and Withdrawal of Life Support

According to the controversial and historical "Baby Doe" regulations, all newborns should receive maximal life prolonging treatment. However, this policy is not uniformly followed. In an infant who is inevitably destined to die or likely to survive with a profound risk of severe neuromotor disability, "selective non-treatment" is ethically and morally justified. These infants should be provided with a loving tender care comprising of warmth, nutrition and hydration without exploiting any heroic or aggressive therapeutic measures. They should be handled with compassion and provided relief and comfort from pain. This approach of withholding active treatment applies to all those conditions listed for termination of pregnancy after 20 weeks of gestation, infants with gross lethal congenital malformations and extremely tiny babies

---

Box 12.1: Lethal congenital malformations

1. Anencephaly
2. Hydranencephaly
3. Holoprosencephaly
4. Trisomy 13 and 18
5. Triploidy
6. Renal agenesis
7. Sirenomelia
8. Short-limb dwarfing syndromes
9. Miscellaneous conditions: Pterygium syndrome, Meckel-Gruber syndrome, Neu-Laxova syndrome

(<750 g or <26 weeks at our institute). Depending upon the level of expertise and available technology in the special care neonatal unit, different birth weight/gestation cut-offs can be used for providing neonatal intensive care. It is unethical to deny admission to any baby in the NICU but we can specify the type and intensity of care to be provided to different babies. In view of the economic constraints, we should follow the philosophy of utilitarian ethics based on the concept of "value for money" and focus our efforts and resources for the care of salvageable babies. It is generally believed that duodenal atresia or cardiac malformation in an infant with Down syndrome should be operated and only conditions worse than Down syndrome should be considered for non-treatment. However, in clinical practice, the certainty of death (>90% chance of dying) and risk of cognitive or neuromotor disability are extremely difficult to predict with accuracy. The decision for "selective non-treatment" should be recorded in the case file along with clinical justifications and parental consent. Every NICU should clearly define its policies for "selective non-treatment" to avoid guilt feelings and confusion.

The same reasons that justify withholding the treatment, also hold true for stopping the treatment. The withdrawal of life support intervention like assisted ventilation is ethically acceptable, if infant is diagnosed to have brain death, likely to die regardless of any existing medical treatment, and should he live, he would have virtually no chance of leading a normal life. These conditions include extremely preterm baby with massive or grade 4 intraventricular hemorrhage, lethal CNS malformations, severe birth asphyxia with lack of breathing efforts for >30 min or HIE Sarnat stage 4 and persistent vegetative state, etc. In these situations, death is considered as a more humane option than a life filled with suffering and misery. Moreover, in several cases, the daily cost of NICU care may be more than the monthly salary of the family. The financial burden, misery and mental agony of looking after a child with extremely poor quality of life are profound especially in India where there is lack of social support system and inadequate facilities for management of children with serious neuromotor disabilities.

Communication as the Key to Enhance Doctor–Patient Relationship

"What we do say and what we do not say, how we say it and when we say it, makes all the difference between helping and not helping our patients".

John Apley

The all important communication link between a doctor and patient which is crucial to generate faith and trust, is being snapped by the technology boom. Most parental complaints in the NICU originate due to lack of communication or because of abrasive and unsympathetic attitude of the members of the health team rather than due to lack of skills or faulty technical management of the patient. It is an amazing fact that most parents are grateful even when we are unable to save the life of their baby especially if we showed concern, care and compassion and they were made to perceive that whatever was humanly possible was done for the care of their infant. It is crucial to listen and talk with the parents at least twice a day in a relaxed unhurried manner.

Humility, concern, empathy and compassion are crucial to generate faith and provide emotional support to the family. The pediatrician should be careful and tactful not only in deciding "what to tell" to the parents but also "how to tell it". The parents should be told about the condition of the child in a simple language. Try to establish an eye-to-eye contact while communicating and it is better to explain and talk with the family at the cot-side. Efforts should be made to be pragmatic and honest but we should always try to keep the hope alive which has tremendous healing capabilities. Avoid creating confusion in the mind of parents due to conflicting messages given by different physicians. In a critically sick neonate, always give a guarded prognosis which can be tempered or mollified with hope and Godly benevolence. The health team should not only try to do their best, but the family must perceive and appreciate that whatever was humanly possible in the circumstances was actually done for their child. The parents should be encouraged to touch and talk with their critically sick neonate because it transmits healing messages. The benefits of good doctor–parent communication are listed in Box 12.2. The religious faith of the family should be

---

Box 12.2: Benefits of good doctor–parent communication

- Better confidence, trust and faith in the pediatrician.
- Reduced anxiety and greater satisfaction of the parents/attendants.
- Delivery of holistic care rather than mere cure.
- Involvement of parents in decision making process.
- Better compliance of the therapeutic options.
- Better health outcomes and reduced length of stay in the NICU.
- Reduced risk of intolerance and vandalism against health care professionals.
- Reduced risk of malpractice litigations.

honored and if the parents wish they may be allowed to use any *mantras* or *charms* to enhance the process of healing through faith. By and large, efforts should be made to honor all the wishes of the parents of critically sick baby, if they are not obviously harmful or contrary to the recommended therapies in a specific situation.

Ethical Dilemmas

An opinion survey conducted by us among pediatricians and obstetricians revealed that two-thirds of them faced ethical dilemmas during discharge of their professional responsibilities. The common and major ethical issues and dilemmas include management of babies with severe birth asphyxia, lethal congenital malformations, extremely LBW or preterm babies, terminally sick neonates on life support and when parents are unable to afford high-cost intensive care. Due to profound economic disparities, there is lack of social justice and equitable health care in India. In developed countries, where medicare is supported by the social security system of the state or insurance companies, the parents want that everything possible on the earth must be done for their children. They demand initiation and continuation of intensive care with all the conceivable life support measures (including extracorporeal membrane oxygenation) even when the treating health team feels that it is futile to treat. On the other hand, unfortunately in India, at times treatable conditions and salvageable babies are denied essential life sustaining therapies either due to non-availability of technology or because of its non-affordability by the parents.

Maurice King made the controversial ill conceived and immoral statement that to stabilize population dynamics in developing countries, health care activities including immunizations should be withdrawn so that nature is allowed to take its toll to eliminate the "unwanted weaklings and weanlings" from the society. It must be realized that in Indian society children are a source of social security to parents in their old age. When we are unable to provide assurance and confidence to parents that at least two or three children would survive the critical and vulnerable period of infancy, they have no motivation to adopt family planning measures. It is unethical and immoral on the part of any society to accept the Maurice doctrine which recommends "blatant neglect" of its children which constitute an asset and foundation of life.

In perinatal medicine, it is often difficult and at times impossible to correctly prognosticate immediate survival and later neuromotor outcome. The "futility" issue often becomes controversial because as rightly said by Sir William Osler, *"Medicine is a science of uncertainty and an art of probability"*. At times it is difficult to know which interests are "best" for the baby; withholding treatment or treating aggressively. Should we be concerned with the "best interests" of the child, family, society or the state? It is important that our concern should be the global interests of the family and society rather than the narrow interest of the child alone. Should NICU care be denied if family cannot afford it? It is not uncommon to be faced by the critically sick neonate whose parents have been monetarily drained off by the private nursing home and they are then referred to the government hospital when they are at the brink of bankruptcy and their child is at the threshold of death. In view of gloomy prognosis and outcome, both in terms of immediate survival and quality of life after survival, the economic drainage is often unbearable with profound adverse consequences to the family dynamics for many months and years.

There are several other dilemmas. Should a "brain dead" pregnant woman be maintained on the life support system for the sake of her unborn baby? It is morally desirable and ethical to do so if facilities are available and fetus is normal and viable. In view of our limited resources, should a poor risk extremely low birth weight baby be hooked off the ventilator to provide assisted ventilation to a more salvageable baby? I think it is not morally justified to follow this approach. It must be decided beforehand, that based on the benefit-to-burden ratio, which babies should be provided hi-tech care including assisted ventilation. And once that conscious decision has been taken, it is not morally justified to take the baby off the ventilator, irrespective of the fact how appropriate and salvageable the next baby may be. It is desirable to take the family into confidence in the decision making process but the physician should not succumb to the wishes of the family for continued life support facilities when it is felt with certainty and confidence that further treatment is futile. According to Christiaan Bernard, *"The prime goal of a doctor is to alleviate suffering and not to prolong life. And if your treatment does not alleviate suffering, but merely prolongs life, that treatment should be stopped."* Humanistic teachings in general and philosophies of all the major religions of the world recognize that there comes a time in the care of every patient when it is appropriate for the doctor to stop further attempts to prolong unnecessarily the process of dying. *We must accept death as the ultimate truth because medicine can never achieve immortality!*

Ethics of Organ Transplantation

The enaction of Human Organ Transplant Act by the Indian Parliament in 1994 has opened opportunities for cadaveric transplant of organs. It is legally justified to remove organs from brain dead patients. However, the criteria for brain death are not well defined in preterm babies and term neonates less than 7 days of age thus posing difficulties for donation of organs for transplantation (Box 12.3).

However, merely 1% of all perinatal deaths are due to brain death. Anencephalic infants are inevitably destined to die and logically should constitute good source of healthy and intact heart, liver and kidneys for transplantation. In Europe, physicians have removed organs from anencephalic infants without waiting for their death on the ground that these infants are "brain absent". This approach is not generally approved and is illegal at present. If one waits for an anencephalic infant to die, most deaths occur due to cardiorespiratory failure thus compromising the perfusion and viability of organs required for transplantation. They would thus need a life-sustaining support and allowed to die by virtue of cessation of functioning of the brainstem. It is controversial though logical that a legislation should be enacted to consider all anencephalic infants as legally dead for purposes of organ donation. However, medical benefits are likely to be minimal because of low incidence of live born anencephalic infants and even lower incidence of infants whose lives could be prolonged by transplantation. There is a potential fear that such a law may lower the sanctity of life and organs may be surreptitiously removed from patients not fully brain dead.

Assisted Reproductive Techniques

Due to technological advances, the well-to-do infertile couples are seeking parenthood by *in vitro* fertilization with the help of various techniques like GIFT, ZIFT, TOT, etc. When the ovum and sperm of the prospective parents are harnessed it does not raise any ethical or legal issues. In other situations when a donor is used to harness a sperm or ovum, there is a need for maintaining strict confidentiality and there are risks of strained husband–wife relationship, neglect of the child, congenital malformations, issues of paternity, and right to property. Commercial hiring and subletting of a womb (surrogacy) for monetary gains raises ethical and legal issues akin to the sale of body organs and it should be discouraged. Impregnation of a hired womb through a sex act raises additional concerns regarding morality and its acceptability by the law and society. The government of India is considering to introduce an Act in the near future to control the various assisted reproductive techniques (ARTs). The reality of genetic engineering and cloning capabilities in the near future is likely to provide unbelievable medical potentialities which is likely to unfold a variety of ethical concerns and issues.

Perinatal HIV Infection

Physicians are obliged to provide competent and humane care without any discrimination to all patients including those with HIV infection. The denial of appropriate care to any class of patients for any reason is unethical. In view of increasing incidence of HIV, universal precautions should be followed in attending all deliveries. The risk of vertical transmission of HIV infection varies between 15% and 35%. The transmission rate can be reduced by treatment of the mother with antiretroviral therapy and delivering the baby by cesarean section. The definitive diagnosis of HIV infection at birth is difficult due to constraints of culturing the virus and unreliability of IgM antibody assays. Early diagnosis is now feasible with HIV–DNA polymerase chain reaction and antigen detection by P24 analysis. There is a 10–15% chance of transmission of HIV infection through breastfeeding and mother should make an informed decision whether to breastfeed her baby or not. When a decision is made to breastfeed the baby, exclusive breatfeeding (without any complementary formula feeds) is associated with a lower risk of transmission of HIV. There is a need for selective HIV screening of high-risk populations. The infected mother should be told about the risk of vertical transmission of HIV to her offspring and given the option for abortion on medical grounds. The confidentiality should be honored and maintained at all costs.

Handling End-of-Life Situations and Neonatal Deaths

Despite all the technological advances, medicine can never achieve immortality. It is as natural to die, as to be born. According to Bhagavad Gita, *"Death is certain for the born and rebirth is inevitable for the dead. You should*

Box 12.3: Criteria for brain death in the newborn*

- Absent brainstem reflexes for more than 48 hr.
- Two EEGs 48 hr apart showing electrocerebral silence.
- Absence of cerebral blood flow for more than one hour on dynamic scan (133 Xenon isotopic scanning, PET).

*The observation period may be extended up to 72 hr in preterm babies <32 weeks.

not, therefore, grieve over the inevitable". But these philosophical thoughts are very difficult to accept by the bereaved families. When a neonate is destined to die despite our best intentions and efforts or survival is likely to be associated with extremely poor quality of life or vegetative state, the family should be provided with emotional support. The news of adverse outcome should be communicated to both the parents simultaneously in a relaxed atmosphere in a quiet room with due concern and empathy. The family should be encouraged to talk and express their misgivings and doubts. In this session, we should follow the well known dictum "Talk less and listen more" and that is why God has given us two ears and one mouth! The family should be made to understand that whatever was humanely possible has been done for the care of their baby. When a decision is taken to withdraw life support or deny life-saving measures, they should be introduced gradually keeping in mind the acceptance level of the family and comfort of the baby. The process of dying should be made as painless or comfortable for the baby as possible. The permission for autopsy or organ biopsies should be sought with extreme care and diplomacy with the sole objective of helping the family to have normal babies in future and not for advancement of scientific knowledge or for satisfaction of the ago for making an exact or correct diagnosis.

The coping of death of a neonate in the NICU is a challenging and traumatic experience both for the health care professionals and the families. Death deflates our ego and teaches us humility and provides strength to face and accept the greatest reality and truth of life with equanimity, peace and poise. The family's wishes for religious or spiritual support (like amulets, *mantras*, holy water, etc.) and presence of priest at bed side should be allowed. The parents should be encouraged to hold, embrace and cuddle their baby when he is leaving them. They should be allowed to take photographs of the baby with family members for future recollection and remembrance. The family should be emotionally and spiritually prepared before declaration of death. The news of death should be conveyed with utmost compassion but in no unmistakable terms that the baby has died despite our best efforts. The family should be assisted with due compassion and consideration to complete post death formalities without unnecessary delay. When autopsy has been conducted, the family must be provided the autopsy report and given guidance and counseling regarding subsequent pregnancies and newborn babies.

Violence against Health Care Professionals

Intolerance and resentment against doctors is an emerging global phenomenon but India seems to lead the world in violence against doctors. According to World Health Organization, about 8–38% health care workers suffer physical violence at some point in their careers. Many more are verbally abused or threatened. Public is behaving like health sector terrorists and media is exploiting the situation by promoting the mandate. "*A muderer is innocent till proved guilty but a doctor is guilty till proved innocent*". There is a need to arrest the development of further distrust between doctors and their patients and attendants, otherwise it will compromise all achievements of medical science, and adversely affect the healing capabilities of doctors.

Rude and aggressive behavior of the parents or attendants, and arrogant and lackadaisical approach of the physician, is the root cause of intolerance and violence against doctors. Most cases of violence occur in the emergency department and intensive care areas. These areas are the face of medical care and must be provided with adequate staff, infrastructure and life-saving drugs and functional emergency equipment at all times. *There should be no delay in attending to a critically sick patient.* Doctors should handle patients with due empathy and concern. The training of doctors should not focus on writing prescriptions alone, they must be trained in the art of communication, bedside manners and medical ethics. According to our scriptures, physicians should see and visualize God in every human being (*Aham Brahmasmi*) and feel honored that we have been given the supreme responsibility to serve Him.

It is possible to reduce the incidence of intolerance and violance against doctors but difficult to eliminate it completely. The hospitals must have adequate infrastructure, facilities and staff to handle emergencies without delay and with due confidence and skills. The security of health care providers should be improved by having adequate number of security guards, frisking facilities, extensive CCTV network and availability of "Quick Response Team" to handle unruly mob. Laws to prevent violence against doctors do exist but they need to be made more stringent and implemented properly. The government should establish fast track courts to provide justice within 3 months when any incidence of violence and vandalism against health care providers is brought to their notice. In case of any perceived "medical neglect" or genuine grievances, the public should handle the situation in a civilized manner and seek redressal through Medical Protection Act and available legal avenues.

Ethical, Social and Legal Issues in Perinatal Medicine

12

Conclusions and Recommendations

Ethical decisions in perinatal medicine are difficult and often complicated by profound medical uncertainty for making a correct diagnosis and assessment of prognosis in maternal, fetal and neonatal medicine. Ethical issues are indeed complex and often affected by economic and social realities, gender of the child and attitude of 'paternalism' by the pediatricians in a developing country. The narrow principle of 'best interest' of the child should be replaced by global beneficence to the family, society and state. Medicine is enigmatic and many a times it is difficult to be certain which interest is the 'best'—withholding treatment or treating aggressively? Medicine is dynamic and neonatology is far more dynamic and, therefore, ethical perceptions cannot be static. Medical disorders considered lethal in the past can be salvaged by newer technology thus changing ethical perspectives and decisions. One should always put oneself in the situation of parents and ask "Would I want the child to live if it were mine"? We should take joint decisions within the legal framework after due consultations with a group of medical and nursing experts and by taking the family into confidence. Above all, we should avoid dumping decisions to the parents alone and deny unbridled autonomy to them. We should evolve a rational process and sound mechanism to make correct ethical decisions. Bioethics Committees and Grievance Redressal Cells should be constituted in all hospitals who should serve as a watch dog to monitor and maintain the sanctity of all ethical decisions.

It is unfortunate that the physicians are becoming more of technocrats and less of human beings. It is a pity that we are allowing technology to dehumanize neonatology. The revolution in technology is no substitute for trust and communication which indeed is the key for maintaining cordial doctor–parent relationship. When practicing physicians are more considerate, cautious, honest and ethical in their dealings with their patients, there should be no fear of Consumer Fora or "legal eagles". The health personnel should exhibit exemplary humane behavior with compassion, tact and concern towards their patients and serve as role models to their students. The doctors should thus be imbued with the qualities and attributes as extolled in Charak Samhita; ... *"Thou shalt behave and act without arrogance and with undistracted mind, humility and constant reflection, and thou shalt pray for the welfare of all creatures* (not only your patients!) ...". It is timely and mandatory that all medical and nursing schools in the country should initiate regular education programs in the field of behavioral sciences, communication techniques and medical ethics for the graduate and postgraduate medical and nursing students. The physicians should make concerted efforts to resurrect and master the sublime art of medicine and acquire the divine gift of healing. We should not allow the technology to further dehumanize neonatology. We must treat babies not only with our heads but also with our hearts. And the narrow focus on hi-tech medical rescues in NICUs should give way to compassionate acts of social interventions for global benefits for all rather than narrow gains for a few.

BIBLIOGRAPHY

AAP Committee on Fetus and Newborn: Noninitiation or withdrawal of intensive care for high-risk newborns. *Pediatrics* 2007; 19(2):401–403.

American Academy of Pediatrics: Bioethics Committee. Infants with anencephaly as organ sources: Ethical considerations. *Pediatrics* 1992; 89:1116–1119.

American Academy of Pediatrics, Committee on Bioethics. Ethical issues with genetic testing in pediatrics. *Pediatrics* 2009; 123:(5):1421–22, doi: 10–1542/peds. 2009–0405.

American College of Physicians. Ethics Manual, third edition, *Ann Int Med* 1992; 117:947–960.

Ashwal S. Brain death in the newborn. *Clin Perinatol* 1989; 16:501–518.

Berceanu C, Albu SE, Bot M, Ghelase MST. Current principles and practice of ethics and law in perinatal medicine. *Curr Health Sci J.* 2014, 40(3): 162–169.

Bonkovsky FO. Ethical issues in perinatal HIV. *Clin Perinatol* 1994; 21:15–29.

Brewin TB. How much ethics is needed to make a good doctor? *Lancet* 1993; 341:161–163.

Byrne S, Szyld E, Kattwinkel J. The ethics of delivery room resuscitation. *Semin Fetal Neonat Med* 2006; 117 (5):e978-988.

Chervenak FA, Farley MA, Walters LR, *et al*. When is termination of pregnancy during the third trimester morally justifiable? *N Engl J Med* 1984; 310:501–504.

Committee on the Fetus and Newborn. Noninitiation or withdrawal of intensive care for high-risk newborns. *Pediatrics* 2007; 119:401–403.

Critical care decisions in fetal and neonatal medicine: ethical issues; a guide to the report. Nuffield Council on Bioethics 2007. *www.nuffieldbioethics.org*

Doyal L, Wilsher D. Withholding cardiopulmonary resuscitation: Proposals for formal guidelines. *Brit Med J* 1993; 306:1593–1596.

Doyal L, Wilsher D. Towards guidelines for withholding and withdrawal of life prolonging treatment in neonatal medicine. *Arch Dis Child* 1994; 70:66–70.

Fost N. Removing organs from anencephalic infants: Ethical and legal considerations. *Clin Perinatol* 1989; 16:331–337.

Gale G, Brooks A. Implementing a palliative care protocol in a newborn intensive care unit *Adv Neonatal Care* 2006; 6(1): 7–53.

Goldworth A, Silverman W, Stevenson DK, *et al.* Ethics and Perinatalogy. *Oxford University Press New York,* 1995.

Hutti MH. Social and professional support needs of families after perinatal loss. *J Obstet Gynaecol Neonatal Nurs* 2005; 34(5):630–638.

King M. Human entrapment in India. *Natl Med J India* 1991; 4:196–201.

Kopelman LM, Irons TG, Kopelman AE. Neonatologists judge the "Baby Doe" regulations. *N Engl J Med* 1988; 318: 677–683.

Leuthner SR. Decisions regarding resuscitation of the extremely premature infant and models of best interest. *J Perinatol* 2001; 21:1–6.

Meadow W, Lantos J. Moral reflections on neonatal intensive care. *Pediatrics* 2009; 123(2):595–597.

Nolan K. Ethical issues in caring for pregnant women and newborn at risk for human immunodeficiency virus infection. *Semin Perinatol* 1989; 13:55–65.

Paintin D. Ethical issues in maternal-fetal medicine. *J Royal Soc Med* 2002, 95(7): 371–72.

Pellegrino ED, Mc Elbinney TK. The humanities and human values in medical schools: A ten year over view, *Washington DC; Society for Health and Human Values,* 1982.

Pellegrino ED. The metamorphosis of medical ethics. *JAMA* 1993; 269:1158–1162.

Perkins H. Teaching medical ethics during residency programme. *Acad Med* 1989; 64:262–266.

Sauer PJJ. Ethical decisions in neonatal intensive care units: The Dutch experience. *Pediatrics* 1992; 90:729–732.

Singh J, Lantos J, Meadow W. End-of-life after birth: death not dying in a neonatal intensive care unit. *Pediatrics* 2004; 114(6):1620–1626.

Singh M. Behavioral sciences and medical ethics for undergraduate medical students. *Indian J Med Edu* 1994, 33:30–34.

Singh M, Kumar S, Mittal S, *et al*. Ethical issues in perinatology (Panel discussion). *Natl Med J India* 1996; 9:32–37.

Singh M. Ethical considerations in pediatric intensive care unit: Indian perspective (Editorial). *Indian Pediatr* 1996, 33:271–78.

Singh M. Ethical issues and dilemmas in the care of newborn babies in the developing world. *Semin Neonatol* 1999; 4:151–157.

Singh M. Ethical and social issues in the care of newborn babies. *Indian J Pediatr* 2003; 70(5):417–420.

Singh M. Communication as a bridge to build a sound doctor-patient/parent relationship. *Indian J Pediatr* 2016, 83(1):33–37.

Singh M. Intolerance and violence against doctors. *Indian J Pediatr* 2017, 84(10): 768–73.

Stahlamn M. Ethical issues in the nursery: Priorities versus limits. *J Pediatr* 1990; 116:167–170.

Tomlinson T, Brody H. Ethics and communication in do-not-resuscitate orders. *N Engl J Med* 1988; 318:43–46.

Tyson JE, Stoll BJ. Evidence-based ethics and the care and outcome of extremely premature infants. *Clin Perinatol* 2003; 30(2):365–387.

Fluids, Electrolytes and Acid–Base Disorders

FLUIDS AND ELECTROLYTES BALANCE

Infants born at term are well equipped to maintain a slightly positive water and solute balance necessary for growth while preterm infants require several careful considerations. Renal excretory ability is related to gestational maturity. Preterm infants cannot tolerate fluid overload because of reduced glomerular filtration rate. On the other hand, they have excessive insensible fluid losses because of large surface area, thin skin, rapid breathing rates, greater use of radiant heaters, phototherapy units and higher incidence of RDS among them.

Body Water and its Distribution

Next to oxygen, water is the most essential element for life. The relative water content of the body and its distribution between intracellular and extracellular spaces is shown in Figure 13.1. At birth, approximately 75% of body weight is accounted for by water and this percentage is greater in those born before term. There is a gradual decrease in total body water during first year of life due to increase in fat content from 12% of body weight at birth to 30% by one year of age. Moreover, the relative distribution of water between intracellular and extracellular spaces changes during this period. At birth, extracellular fluid compartment is large and accounts for 40% of body weight as compared to intracellular volume accounting for 35%. By 3 months of age, intracellular and extracellular fluid volumes are equal and each represents 35% of body weight. By the age of one year, stability and maturity are achieved as far as the volume and distribution of body fluids are concerned. Around first birth day, total body water contributes towards 60% of infant's weight and intracellular fluid volume is double (40%) of extracellular (20%). Availability

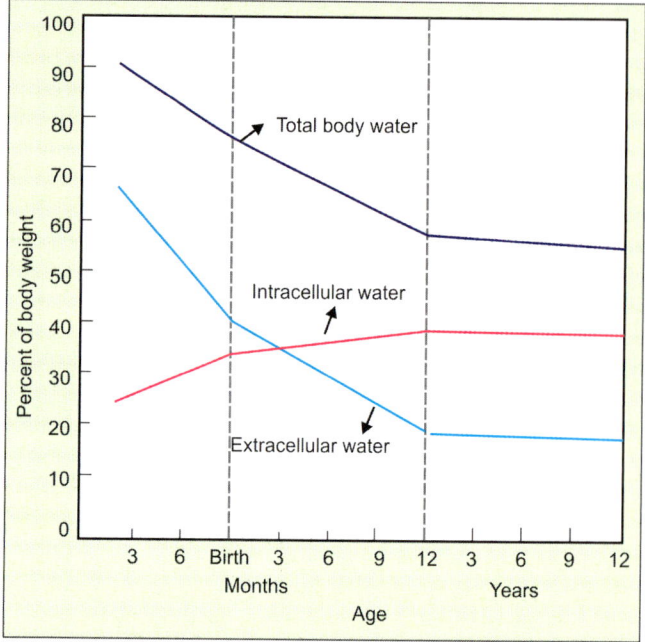

Figure 13.1 Physiological changes in total body water and ratio of intracellular to extracellular water from fetal life to maturity. Refer to text for details.

of relatively large proportion of extracellular fluid volume accounts for greater turn over of water during early infancy.

The major cation in extracellular fluid is sodium as opposed to potassium in the intracellular fluid (Table 13.1). Despite differences in solute composition, osmolal equilibrium between intracellular and extracellular fluid compartments is maintained because cell membrane and vascular membranes are freely permeable to water. Thus, an increase in the sodium concentration of extracellular fluid leads to osmotic movement of water from the intracellular space to the extracellular space. Within the extracellular space, the

TABLE 13.1 Electrolyte composition of body fluids			
Electrolytes	*Intracellular fluid*	*Extracellular fluid*	*Interstitial fluid*
Cations (mEq/L)			
Na^+	9.0	140	147
K^+	158	4.5	4.0
Ca^{++}	3.0	5.0	2.5
Mg^{++}	30	2.0	1.0
Anions (mEq/L)			
Cl^-	4.0	103	114
HCO_3^-	10	25	30
Proteins	65	15	0
Phosphates	95	2.0	2.0
Organic acids	4.0	6.0	7.5
Sulfates	22	–	1.0

relative distribution of water between the intravascular and interstitial compartments is governed by Starling forces. Sodium and its accompanying equimolar anions are major determinants of serum osmolality which can be reliably inferred by doubling the serum sodium concentration (serum osmolality 285–300 mOsm/L). Urea and glucose in normal concentrations contribute very little to the plasma osmolality. In infants with an elevation of blood urea or glucose, a more precise estimate of serum osmolality can be obtained from the following formula:

$$\text{Serum osmolality (mOsm/L)} = 2 \times Na^+ \text{ (mEq/dL)} + \text{BUN (mg/dL)}/2.8 + \text{glucose (mg/dL)}/18$$

PHYSIOLOGICAL REQUIREMENTS OF FLUIDS AND ELECTROLYTES

Fluids

Effective or optimal fluid therapy should maintain a zero balance or slightly positive balance for water and electrolytes to account for growth. During first 3 to 4 days of life, 5 to 15% loss of birth weight is considered as 'physiologic' and is permissible. Lower weight loss occurs in term infants while maximal weight loss occurs in very low birth weight babies. Infants with intrauterine malnutrition lose very little birth weight or none at all. After the first 3 to 4 days of life, therapy should be designed to maintain zero balance so that intake of water and electrolytes must be equal to their output from all sources.

Fluid losses are related most closely to caloric expenditure and this forms the most simple and uniformly acceptable reference for calculation of fluid needs. During the newborn period, non-growing infants (those receiving parenteral fluids or having serious illness) expend about 75 kcal/kg per day. After first week of life, caloric needs of growing newborn babies range between 120 and 150 kcal/kg per day. There are four avenues of water loss, viz. insensible loss, sweat, urine and feces. Insensible loss of water which is not readily appreciated by our senses, takes place from respiratory passages during breathing and evaporation from skin. An average loss of water by this route is 40 mL per 100 calories metabolized by an infant in an environment of moderate humidity (40 to 60%). In infants weighing less than 1,500 g at birth, insensible water loss may be up to three times greater than healthy term infants. The increased insensible water loss in low birth weight babies appears to be due to increased surface area per unit body weight, greater permeability of thin vascular skin and higher breathing rate. Insensible water loss is greatly increased, if infant is reared in a dry ambient environment and placed under overhead radiant heater. Phototherapy is associated with higher evaporative losses through skin due to increased blood flow and from feces due to increase in gastrointestinal transit time and secretory losses from colon. Occurrence of respiratory distress syndrome accounts for higher evaporative losses from the lungs. These abnormal losses of insensible water are proportionately higher among low birth weight babies (Table 13.2). In neonates, the emphasis in fluid and electrolyte therapy should be on prevention of excessive insensible water loss (IWL) rather than replacement of increased IWL. Simple measures like use of transparent plastic barriers, heat shields, cap, socks and mittens are useful to reduce IWL.

The urinary volume is dependent upon water intake, solute load for excretion and the maximal

Fluids, Electrolytes and Acid–Base Disorders

13

TABLE 13.2 Daily physiologic losses of fluids

- **Visible water loss (VWL):** 85 mL/100 kcal
  - Urine: 80 mL/100 kcal
  - Stool: 0–10 mL/100 kcal

- **Insensible water loss (IWL):** 40 mL/100 kcal
  - Skin 70%
  - Breathing 30%

- **Excessive IWL**
  - Preterm or LBW baby
  - Low humidity (open care system)
  - High air currents
  - High ambient temperature or fever
  - Cold stress
  - Use of radiant warmer (up to 50%)
  - Phototherapy (up to 40%)
  - Respiratory distress
  - Seizures
  - Skin defects
  - Naked baby

- **Reduced IWL**
  - High humidity (incubator)
  - Use of plexiglass heat shield
  - Application of paraffin or oil to skin
  - Dressed baby
  - Use of plastic or cellophane cling-wraps
  - Use of humidified gases
  - Covering of skin defects

Note: Efforts should be made to prevent excessive insensible water loss instead of trying to replace it.

recommended that 80 mL of water per 100 calories metabolized, should be provided to enable an infant to produce urine having an osmolality between 100 and 300 mOsm/L so that neither his diluting nor concentrating capabilities are unduly taxed. Water loss through sweat is minimal and often negligible, if infant is nursed in a thermoneutral environment and high humidity. Fecal water losses in normal circumstances vary between 0 and 10 mL per 100 calories, the lower values pertaining to infants receiving parenteral fluids.

In the light of daily physiological losses of water from various sources, it is calculated that for every 100 calories metabolized, a newborn baby should receive about 40 mL of water to replenish insensible loss, 80 mL for urine, and 5 mL for stools adding up to a total of 125 mL per 100 calories metabolized. There is net production of 15 mL of water of oxidation per 100 kcal metabolized. Therefore, maintenance water requirements are around 110 mL/100 kcal metabolized by the baby. Infants receiving lower calories, reduced solute load and having zero or negative growth due to reduced metabolic rate as a result of life-threatening disease or septicemia, would have proportionately lower fluid needs. Fluid requirements of infants with acute renal failure are limited to insensible water losses (25–40 mL/kg/day). Fluid and sodium restriction (negative balance of 30 mL/kg/day) is advocated in infants with congestive heart failure. Fluid retention and hyponatremia due to inappropriate release of ADH occurs in infants with birth asphyxia, RDS, cerebral edema, meningitis and following surgery. The maintenance daily fluid requirements in these situations should be restricted to two-thirds of the usual physiological needs. Insensible water loss through lungs is minimal in infants receiving assisted ventilation with adequately humidified gases.

concentrating and diluting ability of the kidneys. In a term infant, maximal urinary diluting ability of the kidneys is up to 50 mOsm/L while concentration capacity is limited to 700 mOsm/L (up to 600 mOsm/L in a preterm) which is almost half of an older child. An average solute load for an infant on parenteral fluid regimen or oral feeding with human milk or low solute formula is about 20 mOsm. If maximal concentrating ability of the kidneys is limited to 700 mOsm/L, infant must produce at least 30 mL of urine. The maximal urine output would be 400 mL, if he produces maximally dilute urine having osmolality of 50 mOsm/L. Based on these physiological considerations, it is

The daily maintenance fluid requirements depend upon birth weight and postnatal age of the baby (Table 13.3). Due to higher extracellular fluid volume at birth, about 70% of usual maintenance requirements are given during first 2 days. It is gradually increased to an optimal level by 6 to 7 days

TABLE 13.3 Daily maintenance fluid requirements during first week of life (mL/kg/day)						
Birth weight	Day 1	Day 2	Day 3	Day 4	Day 5	Day 6	Day 7
>1500 g or term neonates	60	75	90	105	120	135	150
1000–1500 g	70	90	110	120	130	140	150
<1000 g	80	100	120	130	140	150	160

Note: Fluid needs are higher in preterm and LBW infants.

of life. The fluid requirements of LBW babies is higher due to greater insensible fluid losses because of larger surface area, faster breathing rate, greater use of radiant heaters and phototherapy units and higher incidence of RDS. They have increased metabolic rate and faster growth rate. Fluid requirements are increased during physical activity (seizures), fever, low ambient humidity and cold stress. Gastrointestinal losses due to vomiting or gastric aspiration, ileostomy, diarrhea and "third spacing" (transcellular loss) due to intestinal obstruction and necrotizing enterocolitis must be replaced. However, greater concern for early or aggressive feeding and over infusion of LBW babies during the last decade has brought to light several fluid-related morbidities. *Infants receiving relatively larger volume of fluids have been shown to have higher incidence of patent ductus arteriosus, bronchopulmonary dysplasia and necrotizing enterocolitis.*

Calories

It is preferable to use 10% solution of dextrose to provide for additional calories though caloric needs of 100 kcal/kg per day cannot be met by glucose infusion alone. The rate of glucose infusion should not exceed 0.5 g/kg per hour to prevent hyperglycemia. In extremely low birth weight babies, it is preferable to use 5% dextrose solution as a safeguard against development of hyperglycemia and its consequences. The infusion of hyperosmolar solution can lead to osmotic diuresis and dehydration. In babies in whom intravenous infusion of more than 5 to 7 days is anticipated, intravenous alimentation with proprietary solutions containing amino acids, fructose and fat would be required to sustain growth.

Sodium

Sodium administration is unnecessary during the first 24 hours. After this the usual maintenance needs are 2 to 4 mEq/kg per day in term infants and 4 to 8 mEq/kg per day in preterm infants below 1500 g. This requirement can be met by infusing fifth isotonic saline in 10% or 5% glucose solution. While administering sodium bicarbonate for correction of acidosis, one should guard against overloading with sodium, keeping in mind that 1 mL of 7.5% solution of sodium bicarbonate provides 0.9 mEq of sodium. It is not necessary to give additional isotonic saline when sodium bicarbonate solution is being administered.

Potassium

Potassium supplements are not required for infusion lasting less than 48 hours, unless there is an avenue for excess loss such as diarrhea, vomiting and intestinal fistula. During the first 48 hours of age, potassium is not required because serum potassium and phosphorus levels may be high due to tissue catabolism and reduced glomerular filtration rate. The daily maintenance needs of potassium are 2 to 3 mEq/kg and should be administered only when the baby is passing urine. The concentration of potassium in the infusate should not exceed 40 mEq/L (1 mL of 15% solution of potassium chloride provides 2 mEq of K^+).

Indications for Intravenous Infusion

1. Birth weight of less than 1,200 g. Intravenous infusion is recommended during the first 3 to 4 days to avoid aspiration and to reduce handling.
2. Severe birth asphyxia
3. Respiratory distress syndrome
4. Apneic attacks
5. Hypoglycemia
6. Seizures
7. Intestinal obstruction
8. Dehydration whether impending or existent. Preterm babies with diarrhea must be immediately started on intravenous infusion irrespective of their hydration status.
9. Vehicle for administration of drugs, e.g. neonatal convulsions and septicemia.
10. Total parenteral nutrition

For technique of setting up an intravenous infusion refer to Chapter 29.

ASSESSMENT OF FLUIDS AND ELECTROLYTES STATUS

Physical Examination

The clinical signs of dehydration like loss of skin turgor, sunken anterior fontanel, dry mucous membranes are unreliable and late in newborn babies. Capillary refill time may be delayed (>2 sec) and extremities become cold when there is hypovolemia or shock. Accurate daily weight record on a sensitive electronic weighing scale (resolution ± 1.0 g) is the most sensitive clinical parameter of hydration status. Sudden weight loss (>5% in 24 hr) is suggestive of dehydration while weight gain of more than 3% in a day is a reliable marker of over infusion or congestive heart failure. Tachycardia, puffiness and hepatomegaly are useful clinical markers of over infusion.

Urinary Changes

Urine output should be maintained between 1 and 3 mL/kg/hr, specific gravity between 1005 and 1015 and

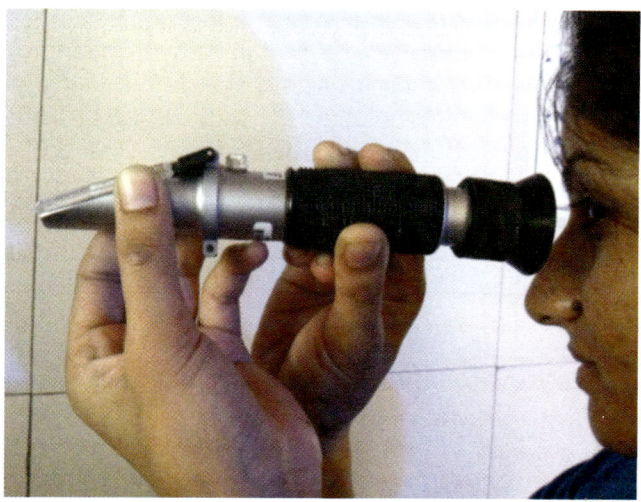

Figure 13.2 Urine specific gravity being examined with the help of a refractometer.

osmolality between 150 and 400 mOsm/L. Specific gravity can be checked by dipstick method or with a hand held refractometer (Figure 13.2) and osmolality with a freezing point osmometer. In a male infant, urine can be collected with ease with a condom or test tube while in a female infant urine collection bag is used but procedure is cumbersome and often unreliable.

Serum Biochemistry

Plasma osmolality should be maintained between 280 and 300 mOsm/L. Dehydration may lead to reduced renal perfusion with alterations in electrolytes and elevation of blood constituents like urea, BUN and bilirubin. Electrolytes and acid–base parameters should be maintained within normal range. Metabolic acidosis is most commonly due to hypoperfusion in newborn babies. Fractional excretion of sodium (Fe–Na) reflects balance between glomerular filtration and tubular reabsorption of sodium. It is calculated as follows:

Fe–Na = (urine Na × plasma creatinine)/(plasma Na × urine creatinine) × 100. Fe–Na of less than 1% is suggestive of reduced renal perfusion due to prerenal factors while a level of more than 2.5% is indicative of intrinsic renal failure. However, it is an unreliable parameter in infants below 32 weeks of gestation.

COMMON FLUIDS AND ELECTROLYTES DISTURBANCES

Dehydration

There is physiological weight loss up to 5–10% in term babies and 10–15% in preterm babies due to efflux of intracellular fluid to the extracellular compartment followed by diuresis. This does not need any correction but early and effective feeding is associated with relatively less weight loss. In primi mothers, lactation insufficiency during initial 3–4 days may be associated with greater weight loss and excessive elevation of serum bilirubin level. During fetal life, insensible water loss (IWL) is zero because the baby floats in amniotic fluid and there is no effective breathing. The fluid needs of the baby rapidly increase after birth due to excessive IWL due to low humidity, thin skin, high breathing rates, use of radiant warmer and photo-therapy. Dehydration commonly occurs due to inade-quate replacement of physiological fluid losses and excessive loss of fluids from gastrointestinal tract due to vomiting, diarrhea, nasogastric drainage, colostomy and third space losses (intestinal obstruction, NEC). Surgical conditions and procedures like gastroschisis, omphalocele, open neural tube defect, thoracostomy, and ventriculostomy are associated with excessive fluid loss. Due to poor concentration capability of kidneys, preterm babies may continue to lose fluids through urine despite dehydration. Excessive diuresis (osmotic or pharmacologic) is an unimportant cause of dehydration.

Clinical and Laboratory Features

Excessive weight loss (>5% in a day) and oliguria (<1 mL/kg/hr) are reliable correlates of dehydration because conventional clinical signs of dehydration like loss of skin turgor, sunken eyes and fontanel, and dry mucosa appear late in newborn babies. Hypotension, cold extremities, delayed capillary refill time (>2 sec) are suggestive of marked hypovolemia. The laboratory parameters include elevation of BUN, alterations in electrolytes, metabolic acidosis or alkalosis, increase in plasma osmolality (>300 mOsm/L), increase in specific gravity (>1015) or osmolality (>400 mOsm/L) of urine.

Management

The severity of weight loss during last 24–48 hours provides reliable estimate of degree of dehydration. If a 3 kg infant has lost 300 g (10%) body weight, he needs replacement of 300 mL fluids. One-half of the deficit is given during first 8 hours along with daily maintenance fluid needs and replacement of any concurrent losses or avenues of excessive IWL (radiant warmer, phototherapy, fever, rapid breathing). When tissue perfusion is compromised or infant is in shock, 10–20 mL/kg of normal saline is given as a bolus over 30 minutes. The fluid deficit is replaced by N/2 saline in 5% dextrose (avoid 10% dextrose during correction of dehydration except when baby has hypoglycemia) while maintenance fluid requirements are provided

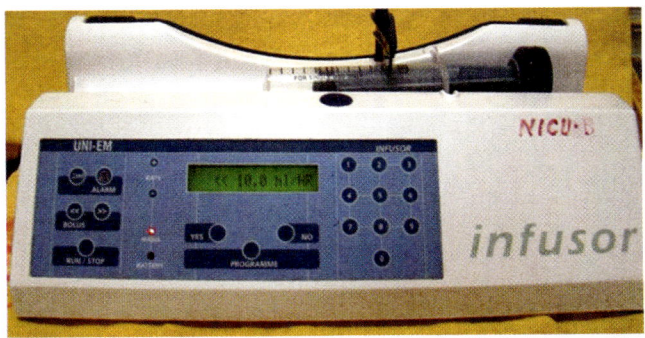
Figure 13.3 Syringe-based infusion pump for accurate administration of intravenous fluids.

as N/5 glucose–saline. The gastric aspirate should be replaced with half-isotonic saline while ileostomy loss should be replaced by isotonic saline. The intravenous infusion should be controlled precisely with a syringe-based infusion pump as a safeguard against under- and over-infusion (Figure 13.3). During rehydration therapy, the baby should be weighed on an accurate electronic weighing scale every 12 hourly. For pre- and postoperative fluid therapy, refer to Chapter 25.

Hyponatremia

The normal serum sodium level varies between 135 and 145 mEq/L. Hyponatremia (serum sodium <130 mEq/L) may occur in association with depleted, normal or excessive extracellular fluid volume (ECF). Factitious hyponatremia may occur due to hyperlipidemia and hyperosmolar or hypertonic hyponatremia may occur due to osmotic diuresis (mannitol therapy, and hyperglycemia).

Hyponatremia with depletion of ECF volume may occur due to use of a diuretic, osmotic diuresis, adrenal or renal tubular salt-losing disorders (congenital adrenal hyperplasia, pseudohypoaldosteronism, Bartter syndrome), gastrointestinal losses (vomiting and diarrhea) and third-space losses of ECF (intestinal obstruction, NEC, burns, skin defects like omphalocele, gastroschisis). The clinical features include weight loss, dehydration, tachycardia, fall in blood pressure, rise in blood urea nitrogen and metabolic acidosis. The on-going losses of sodium are controlled and deficit is replaced by administration of normal saline.

Hyponatremia with normal ECF volume classically occurs due to the syndrome of inappropriate antidiuretic hormone secretion (SIADH). The predisposing factors for SIADH in newborn babies include pain, opiate administration, asphyxia, meningitis, intraventricular hemorrhage, pneumothorax and positive pressure ventilation. The condition is diagnosed by excessive weight gain without edema in association with decreased urine output and increased osmolarity of urine. The condition is managed by water restriction. When serum sodium level is less than 120 mEq/L or there are associated neurological signs, furosemide is given in a dose of 1 mg/kg IV every 6 hr along with administration of 3% sodium chloride 1–3 mL/kg slowly IV.

Hyponatremia in association with excessive ECF volume occurs due to congestive heart failure, sepsis with cardiogenic shock, advanced NEC, abnormal lymphatic drainage and neuromuscular paralysis. There is excessive weight gain with edema, oliguria and azotemia. The condition is managed by treatment of underlying condition and restriction of sodium and water intake.

Hypernatremia

Hypernatremia (serum sodium >150 mEq/L) is relatively uncommon in newborn babies and may occur with normal, deficient, or excessive ECF volume. Hypernatremia with reduced ECF volume usually occur in VLBW babies due to excessive loss of water because of diarrhea, osmotic diuresis, or insensible water loss through skin or lungs. Metabolic acidosis may occur due to reduced renal perfusion because of depletion of ECF volume. The condition is managed by restriction of sodium and infusion of N/5 dextrose–saline solution to replenish excessive water loss. Hypernatremia with excessive ECF volume is rare and may occur if excessive isotonic or hypertonic fluid is administered to infants with reduced cardiac output. The condition is managed by restriction of sodium intake.

Hypokalemia

The normal serum potassium level varies between 3.5 and 5.5 mEq/L. Hypokalemia (serum potassium <3.5 mEq/L) is uncommon in newborn babies. The common causes include acute gastroenteritis, GI losses through gastric aspiration or ileostomy, diuretic therapy, renal tubular defects, prolonged total parenteral nutrition without adequate supplements, amphotericin B, beta adrenergic therapy and increased PGE_2 activity. Due to intracellular shift of K ions, increase in blood pH by 0.1 unit results in fall of serum K by 0.6 mEq/L. The clinical features include muscular weakness, abdominal distension and cardiac arrhythmias. EKG changes include ST depression, T-wave inversion, prolonged QTc and prominent U waves. The deficit should be corrected slowly over 24 to 48 hours by intravenous administration of potassium in a concentration of 40 mEq/L once urine flow is established.

Hyperkalemia

Serm potassium values of more than 5.5 mEq/L are common during first 2 to 3 days of life. Hyperkalemia can occur due to severe birth asphyxia, acute renal failure, adrenal insufficiency (CAH), exchange blood transfusion with an old blood, tissue catabolism due to severe RDS, internal bleeding (IVH), cephalhematoma, hemolysis, major surgery, indomethacin therapy or due to medication error. Severe bradycardia and cardiac arrhythmias may occur. EKG may show wide and bizarre QRS complexes, tall tented T-waves, flat P-waves and increased PR interval. Treatment comprises of administration of 10% calcium gluconate 100 mg/kg 1:1 diluted intravenously slowly over 0.5–1.0 hour while monitoring heart rate followed by infusion of sodium bicarbonate (2 mL/kg of 7.5% solution) in a glucose–insulin drip (500 mg/kg glucose with 0.1 unit/kg insulin) and furosemide 1 mg/kg IV. Nebulization of salbutamol (2.5 mg in two doses 2 hours apart) is useful for prompt reduction of serum potassium level. At times double-volume exchange transfusion with fresh blood may be life saving. Peritoneal dialysis and oral or rectal administration of 1.0 g/kg (0.5 g/mL normal saline) of cation exchange resin (sodium polystyrene-sulfonate) are indicated for management of chronic renal failure. In preterm babies, kayexalate is not administered through NG tube due to risk of hypomotility of gut and NEC. Rectal administration (1.0 g/kg in a concentration of 0.5 g/mL normal saline) as a retention enema for 30 minutes is effective in lowering K level by 1.0 mEq/L.

ACID–BASE DISORDERS

Acid–Base Physiology

Acid–base disorders are common in critically sick neonates. Neonates have a limited ability to compensate the biochemical abnormalities of acid–base disorders and they are susceptible to significant morbidity and mortality because of acid–base imbalance. Arterial blood gas (ABG) analysis is useful to assess oxygenation status, adequacy of ventilation and acid–base status in neonates with various metabolic and respiratory emergencies. The acidity of body fluids is expressed as hydrogen ions (H+). The pH expressed as negative algorithm of H+ ions is used to denote acidity or alkalinity. High H+ concentration is associated with acidity and low pH while low H+ ion concentration lead to alkalinity and raised pH. The pH of the body fluids is expressed by Henderson–Hasselbalch equation:

$$pH = pK + \log \frac{HCO_3^-}{H_2CO_3^+}$$

The value of pK for bicarbonate-carbonic acid buffer is 6.1. In simple term, the pH of blood is a function of ratio of plasma bicarbonate (HCO₃) and carbonic acid (H₂CO₃) concentration, the latter is determined by the level of paCO₂. In healthy subjects, HCO_3^- to $H_2CO_3^+$ ratio in plasma is 20:1. The normal bicarbonate concentration varies between 25 and 27 mEq/L while carbonic acid concentration is around 1.35 mEq/L (paCO₂ in mm Hg × 0.03). The pH of blood is maintained in a narrow range of 7.35–7.45. As a rule of thumb, 1 mm Hg increase in paCO₂ decreases pH by 0.01 while 1 mEq/L decrease in HCO_3^- decreases pH by 0.02.

Buffer Systems

The acid–base balance is regulated mainly by three mechanisms.

Chemical buffering A buffer is a substance that can absorb or donate H+ ions and thereby reduce changes in pH. The four important chemical buffer systems in the body include bicarbonate–carbonic acid buffer, phosphate buffer, hemoglobin buffer and protein buffer. Among these buffers, the bicarbonate–carbonic acid buffer is the most important system that converts strong acids to a weak carbonic acid.

Regulatory respiratory mechanisms These mediate via the central and peripheral chemoreceptors. Respiratory mechanism by virtue of rapid breathing eliminates CO₂ and regulates concentration of carbonic acid. The carbonic acid is a weak acid and it readily dissociates to give CO₂, which is transported in dissolved form to the lungs for excretion as shown in the below mentioned equation:

$$H^+ + HCO_3^- \leftrightarrow H_2CO_3^+ \leftrightarrow CO_2 + H_2O$$

Respiratory mechanism by virtue of rapid breathing eliminates CO₂ and regulates concentration of carbonic acid. The buffering is fast and occurs within minutes to hours.

Renal mechanisms They operate by elimination of excess acids and bases by reabsorption of bicarbonate in the proximal tubules and excretion of H+ ions as phosphate buffer salts and ammonium ions. The buffering occurs slowly over a period of few hours or days.

The various compensatory mechanisms try to bring the blood pH as close as possible to the normal pH. The compensation may be slow or partial and the blood gases that appear to have fully compensated the primary disorder are most likely to display a mixed picture rather than complete correction. The acid–base

Table 13.4 The compensatory changes on the part of the body to maintain acid–base balance

Primary disorders	pH	PaCO$_2$	HCO$_3^-$
Metabolic acidosis	↓	↓	↓
Metabolic alkalosis	↑	↑	↑
Respiratory acidosis	↓	↑	↑
Respiratory alkalosis	↑	↓	↓
Mixed disorders			
Acidosis	↓	↑	↓
Alkalosis	↑	↓	↑

In primary or simple disorders, CO$_2$ and HCO$_3^-$ changes move in same directions, while in mixed disorders, they move in opposite direction.

balance is maintained closely by complex interactions between the respiratory and renal compensatory mechanisms (Table 13.4).

Metabolic Acidosis

Acidosis may occur due to hypoxia, diarrhea, vomiting and starvation or excessive protein intake. It is clinically characterized by deep and rapid breathing (Kussmaul breathing). The blood pH is less than 7.3 and plasma bicarbonate below 18 mEq/L. Acidosis may be associated with normal or increased anion gap. The anion gap is calculated as the difference between serum sodium plus potassium concentration and sum of the chloride and bicarbonate concentration. Anion gap = serum ($Na^+ + K^+$) – ($Cl^- + HCO_3^-$). Acidosis with *increased anion gap (>15 mEq/L)* occurs due to accumulation of organic acids in infants with acute renal failure, inborn errors of metabolism, hypoxia, shock (lactic acidosis), late metabolic acidosis and administration of toxic compounds like benzyl alcohol. Acidosis with *normal anion gap (<15 mEq/L)* indicates excessive loss of buffer due to renal bicarbonate losses (renal tubular acidosis, renal dysplasia, acetazolamide therapy), gastrointestinal bicarbonate loss (diarrhea, small bowel drainage) and hyperalimentation.

In newborn babies, maintenance of adequate tissue perfusion, ventilation and oxygenation are more crucial and desirable therapeutic interventions compared to alkali therapy. Hypovolemia with reduced tissue perfusion is a common cause of metabolic acidosis in sick preterm babies. It is best managed by administration of normal saline 20 mL/kg as IV bolus over 30 minutes. The requirements of sodium bicarbonate can be calculated from pH of the blood and base deficit. Base deficit × weight in kg × 0.4 = mEq or mL of 7.5% solution of sodium bicarbonate needed.

One half of the calculated dose is given immediately as 7.5% sodium bicarbonate solution, half diluted with distilled water or by two volumes of 5% dextrose solution and the rest is administered in the next 4 to 8 hours. In general, total dose of sodium bicarbonate should not exceed 10 to 12 mEq/kg per 24 hour and a close watch should be kept on serum sodium level. Sodium bicarbonate (7.5% solution has an osmolality of 1590 mOsm/L) should never be administered rapidly as a bolus because it may lead to fatal intraventricular or pulmonary hemorrhage.

In dehydrated infants, sodium bicarbonate should preferably be administered in an isotonic concentration (one-sixth dilution). THAM (tris hydroxymethyl aminomethane) may have to be used (2 mL of 3.6% THAM = Approx. 1 mL of 7.5% sodium bicarbonate), if critical hypernatremia is imminent or manifest. The baby should be watched for apneic attacks while injecting Tris-Buffer THAM. The potentially beneficial effects of THAM may be due to its "volume" effects on cardiac output rather than its buffering capacity. There have been no controlled studies demonstrating a beneficial effect of THAM for neonates either with cardiorespiratory arrest or with persistent metabolic acidosis. Calcium gluconate should not be added in an infusion solution containing sodium bicarbonate as the calcium carbonate is precipitated. In the management of acidosis, the correction of predisposing factors, such as tissue hypoxia, shock and starvation are of fundamental importance.

Respiratory Acidosis

It occurs due to decreased elimination of carbon dioxide from the body because of poor ventilation. Accumulation of carbon dioxide in the body leads to generation of carbonic acid without any renal compensation. Acute respiratory acidosis is characterized by primary rise in PaCO$_2$ above 45 mm Hg and mild elevation of carbonic acid (up to 4 mEq/L). When there is sustained elevation of PaCO$_2$ beyond 12 hours, it is associated with increased urinary excretion of ammonium chloride (H$^+$ and Cl$^-$ ions) and increased production of bicarbonate. In chronic respiratory acidosis, hypochloremia is a common feature because of renal chloride excretion.

Respiratory acidosis is relatively common in neonates due to high incidence of birth asphyxia, hyaline membrane disease, congenital malformations, aspiration pneumonia, pneumothorax and bronchopulmonary dysplasia. Hypoventilation may occur because of neuromuscular disorders (Werdnig-Hoffmann disease, diaphragmatic paralysis and myopathies). The clinical manifestations are related to degree of hypercapnia. Initial irritability and restlessness is followed by gradual blunting and loss of consciousness due to elevation of intracranial pressure, tachycardia, fibrillations, fall in blood pressure and shock.

The immediate dangers of respiratory acidosis include carbon dioxide narcosis and anoxic damage to various body organs. Treatment is directed at the underlying cause and improvement of alveolar gas exchange by assisted ventilation. Oxygen administration with high flow rates may help to wash out carbon dioxide. However, breathing with a tight fitting mask or head box may cause dangerous elevation of $PaCO_2$. If hyperkalemia or ventricular fibrillations develop in a child with acute respiratory acidosis, administration of sodium bicarbonate is life saving. It should be administrated only after establishing adequate ventilation. In chronic respiratory acidosis, metabolic alkalosis may develop due to excessive chloride losses in the urine and will need replacement therapy.

Metabolic Alkalosis

Metabolic alkalosis is characterized by increase in the extracellular HCO_3^- concentration sufficient to raise arterial pH above 7.45. In neonates, metabolic alkalosis occurs when there is loss of H^+ ions, gain in HCO_3^- or depletion of extracellular fluid volume with greater loss of chloride compared to HCO_3^-. Chloride loss may occur due to chloride losing diarrhea, Bartter syndrome, loss of chloride through skin in infants with cystic fibrosis.

The common causes of metabolic alkalosis in the newborn period include continuous nasogastric aspiration, persistent vomiting and prolonged diuretic treatment. The commonly encountered clinical scenario of chronic metabolic alkalosis is a mixed acid–base order in a preterm infant with chronic lung disease on long-term diuretic therapy.

Respiratory Alkalosis

When a primary decrease in $PaCO_2$ (due to rapid breathing) results in an increase in the arterial pH beyond 7.45, it is suggestive of respiratory alkalosis. The primary cause of respiratory alkalosis is hyperventilation, which may occur due to fever, sepsis, wet fetal lungs, aspiration pneumonia and central nervous system disorders. In the neonatal intensive care unit, the most common cause of respiratory alkalosis is iatrogenic as a consequence of hyperventilation of the intubated newborn. There is an association between hypocapnia (low $PaCO_2$) and development of periventricular leukomalacia (PVL). It is important to avoid hyperventilation and prevent occurrence of respiratory alkalosis to improve the neurologic outcome of preterm neonates.

BIBLIOGRAPHY

Baumgart S, Costarino AT. Water and electrolyte metabolism of the micropremie. *Clin Perinatol* 2000; 27(1):131.

Bell EF, Acarregui MJ. Restricted versus liberal water intake for preventing morbidity and mortality in preterm infants *Cochrane Database Syst Rev* 2000; 2: CD 000503.

Bhatia J. Fluid and electrolyte management in the very low birth weight neonate. *J Perinatol* 2006; 26:S19–S21.

Chawla D, Agarwal R, Deorari AK, Paul VK. Fluid and electrolyte management in term and preterm neonates. *Indian J Pediatr* 2008; 75(3):255–259.

Dell KR. Fluid, electrolytes, and acid–base homeostasis. In: Neonatal–Perinatal Medicine. Diseases of the Fetus and Infant. Martin RJ, Fanaroff AA, Walsh MC (Eds) *Elsevier Mosby*, St. Louis 2011, 9th Ed, Vol 1, p 669.

Deorari AK, McMillan DD. Alkaly therapy for neonates: where does it stand today? *Indian Pediatr* 1997; 34:613–619.

Dreszen M. Fluid and electrolyte requirements in the newborn infant *Pediatr Clin N Amer* 1977; 24:537.

Flaherman VJ, Schaefer EW, Kuzniewicz MW, *et al*. Early weight loss nomograms for exclusively breastfed newborns. *Pediatrics* 2015, 135: e16.

Lekhwani S, Shanker V, Gathwala G, Vaswani ND. Acid–base disorders in critically ill neonates. *Indian J Crit Care Med* 2010, 14(2): 65–69.

Lian JX. Interpreting and using arterial blood gas analysis. *Nursing Crit Care* 2010, 5(3): 26–36.

Lorcuz JM, Klein LI, Kotagal UR. Water balance in very LBW infants: Relationship to water and sodium intake and effect on outcome. *J Pediatr* 1982; 101:423.

Rahman N, Boineau PG, Lewy JE. Renal failure in the perinatal period. *Clin Perinatol* 1981; 8:241.

Singhi S, Sasidaran K. Fluids, electrolytes and acid–base disorders. In: Medical Emergencies in Children. Singh M (Ed), *New Delhi, CBS Publishers and Distributors Pvt. Ltd.*, 6th edition, 2020.

Temperature Regulation

One of the most critical factors in the survival of low birth weight (LBW) babies is satisfactory maintenance of their body temperature. A newborn baby is physiologically homeothermic and is equipped with a thermostat in the hypothalamus but thermoregulatory efforts are often insufficient in preterm and LBW babies.

Before birth, the baby is warm and well insulated in the aqueous uterine ambience. Fetal temperature is slightly higher than the maternal temperature with a gradient of the heat flow from the fetus to the mother. From this comfortable abode, baby comes out naked, wet and partially asphyxiated in the labor room environment, which is maintained at a temperature geared to ensure the comfort of the mother rather than the biological needs of the baby. Infant loses heat due to evaporation (latent heat of evaporation being 540 kcal/g of water of evaporation) and through other avenues of heat loss (radiation, convection, conduction) when environmental temperature is low (Figure 14.1). After birth, skin and core temperatures of the baby fall by 0.3°C and 0.1°C per minute, respectively. This is equivalent to a heat loss of 200 kcal/kg/minute. Even if an infant were to achieve an heat production

to the extent of double of an adult (per unit body mass) he cannot maintain normal body temperature in these circumstances. It is estimated that almost 15% of newborn babies develop hypothermia at birth in developing countries.

RESPONSE TO COLD

Muscular activity During exposure to cold, baby feels uncomfortable, cries and makes some movements of limbs but the efforts are not sustained. Shivering does occur but is minimal, especially in LBW babies and appears only when the environmental temperature falls below 25°C. Thus muscular activity is not a significant source of heat production.

Metabolic thermogenesis Non-shivering thermogenesis, as a result of metabolism of the brown fat, is the most important source of heat production in the newborn. The fetal brown fat is laid down mostly during the third trimester of pregnancy and is located at the nape of the neck, interscapular region, axillae, groins and around kidneys and adrenals. The quantity of brown fat is directly related to the birth weight of the baby and in a term-AFD baby it accounts for 4% of the total body fat. Brown fat is characterized by a rounded nucleus, granular cytoplasm with a large number of mitochondria (with yellow mitochondrial cytochromes) and fat vacuoles. This fat is metabolically very active in view of a large number of mitcochondria and increased vascularity. Table 14.1 highlights salient differences between brown fat and white fat.

When the skin of the baby becomes cold, afferents convey the message to the heat regulating center located in the preoptic anterior hypothalamic area near the walls of the third ventricle. Neurogenic efferents, on reaching the brown fat, trigger the local release of noradrenaline so that triglycerides are oxidized to

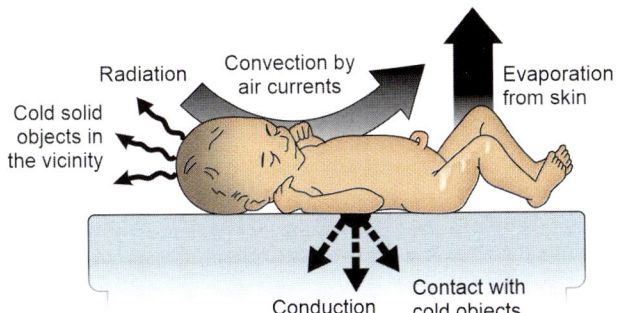

Figure 14.1 Four avenues through which a newborn baby may lose heat to the environment.

TABLE 14.1 Differences between brown and white fat

Features	Brown fat	White fat
▪ Vacuoles/cell	Many	One
▪ Vascularity	Good	Poor
▪ Nerve fibers	Many	Few
▪ Mitochondria	Many	Few
▪ Stimulus for activation	Cold	Starvation
▪ Function	Heat production	Nutrition

glycerol and fatty acids. The blood level of glycerol rises but fatty acids are locally consumed for the generation of heat. About 30% of non-esterified fatty acids are oxidized to generate heat, 60% are re-esterified and 10% are released in the circulation. The areas of brown fat become warm and heat is distributed to various parts of the body through bloodstream. It is obvious that the baby would need extra oxygen and glucose for this metabolic effort in order to keep itself warm. Effective metabolic thermogenesis demands integrity of central nervous system pathways, adequacy of brown fat and availability of glucose and oxygen (Figure 14.2).

THERMONEUTRAL ENVIRONMENT

The narrow range of environmental temperature at which a given baby can maintain normal body temperature with minimal oxygen consumption (and possibly minimal glucose consumption) is called *thermoneutral temperature or zone of thermal comfort*. This is the ideal temperature at which the babies should be nursed to achieve optimal somatic and brain growth. The baby is most comfortable and sleeps better when nursed in this ambient temperature. This is also called the zone of thermal comfort. An isolated measurement of body temperature may fail to indicate whether a baby is being subjected to a thermal stress or not. Even when the environmental temperature deviates beyond the thermoneutral range, the infant tries to maintain his body temperature by increasing oxygen consumption, glucose utilization and heat production. A fall in the environmental temperature merely by 2°C below the neutral range, triggers infant's metabolic machinery to generate 25% additional heat. The environmental temperature at which the metabolic response becomes necessary is called the *critical temperature* (Figure 14.3). In a clinical setting, thermoneutral temperature can also be defined as that narrow range of environmental temperature in which a baby can maintain core temperature between 36.7°C

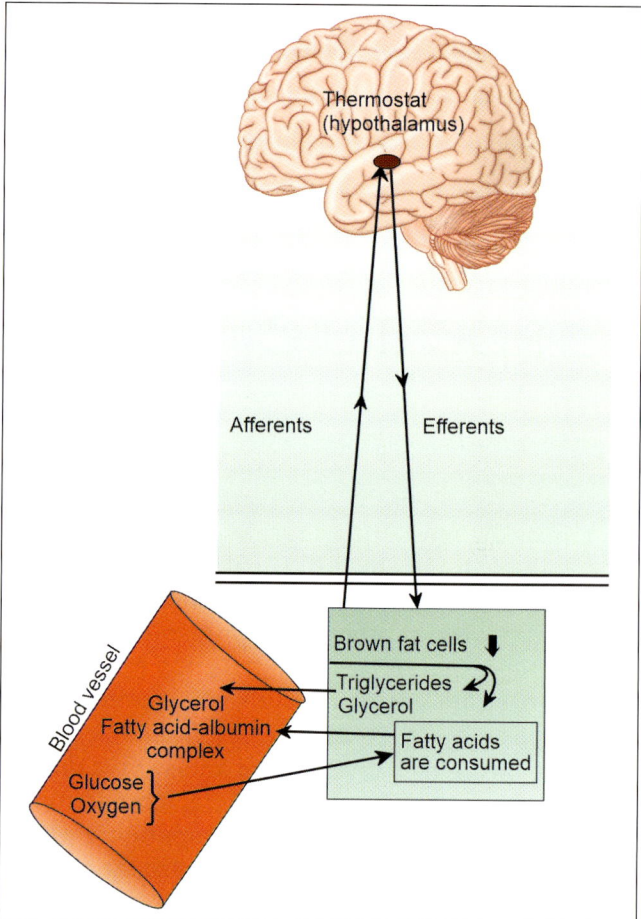

Figure 14.2 Schematic presentation of pathways for metabolic thermogenesis. The optimal functioning of 'heat generating system' is dependent upon integrity of central nervous system, adequacy of brown fat and availability of glucose and oxygen.

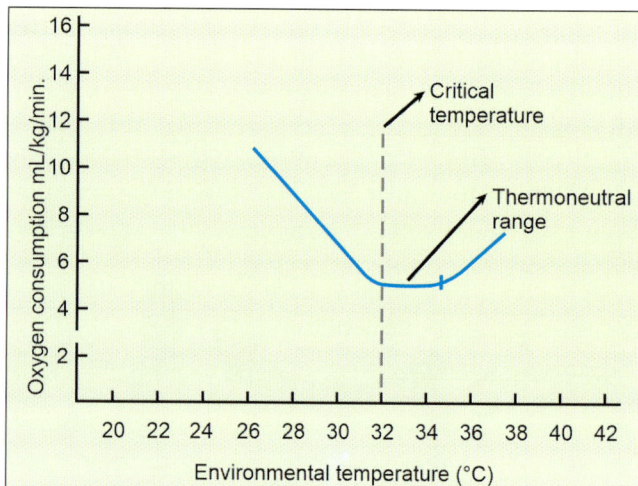

Figure 14.3 The lowest oxygen consumption of approximately 5 mL/kg/minute is observed when an infant is reared in the thermoneutral range of ambient temperature. Elevation or fall in ambient temperature is associated with increase in oxygen consumption and glucose utilization.

and 37.3°C and his mean core and skin temperature does not change more than 0.2°C and 0.3°C per hour respectively when recorded continuously by an electronic thermister probe.

HYPOTHERMIA

Hypothermia in a newborn baby is defined as a skin temperature of <35.5°C or core temperature of <36.0°C.

Causes

Situations contributing to excessive heat loss Cold environment, wet or naked baby, cold linen, during transport and various procedures, such as bath, blood sampling, infusion and surgery predispose to hypothermia. Infants with open neural tube defects like omphalocele, gastroschisis are prone to develop hypothermia. Increased airflow currents coupled with low humidity leads to greater convective and evaporative heat losses.

Poor ability to conserve heat Relatively large surface area, poor insulation, paucity of fat, inability to reduce the effective surface area by assuming flexed posture and poor muscle tone contribute to a greater heat loss in preterm and growth retarded babies. Newborn babies have a large surface area per unit body mass. For example, body mass of a newborn baby is 5% of an adult whereas his surface area is about 15% of an adult. In a newborn baby, heat loss is at least four times per unit body mass as compared to an adult.

Inadequate metabolic heat production Several factors interfere with metabolic heat production.

- Deficiency of brown fat, e.g. preterm and small-for-dates babies.
- Central nervous system damage due to anoxia, intracranial hemorrhage and malformations interferes with the integrity of neurogenic pathways for stimulation of brown fat
- Hypoxia
- Hypoglycemia.

Severity of Hypothermia

According to WHO, babies with *cold stress* have a core temperature between 36.0 and 36.5°C. The difference between the core and peripheral temperature is likely to be more than 1.5°C and extremities are cold and pale. Despite adequate feeding and freedom from any infection, these babies have poor growth velocity because glucose is wasted for metabolic thermogenesis. Moderate hypothermia is diagnosed when core temperature ranges between 32.0 and 35.9°C

while a core temperature of <32.0°C is designated as severe hypothermia. Infants with moderate and severe hypothermia develop a number of clinical manifestations and biochemical consequences.

Clinical Manifestations

When the thermal environment is below the neutral range of environmental temperature of the baby, a number of clinical manifestations are seen. The baby is uncomfortable, restless and cries to generate heat by muscular activity. If unattended at this stage, he becomes sluggish and inactive. Skin becomes cold and mottled due to vasoconstriction. All the vital functions are depressed. There is bradycardia, slow breathing with episodes of apnea and fall in blood pressure. The weight gain is unsatisfactory because food is wasted for heat production rather than for tissue growth. Even brain growth may be adversely affected as evidenced by slow increase in head size. The immunologic system is depressed with enhanced susceptibility to develop septicemia, sclerema and disseminated intravascular coagulation. *It must be remembered that hypothermia is an important symptom of septicemia in preterm babies and hypothermia per se can predispose the baby to develop serious bacterial infection.* Hypothermic babies are more vulnerable to develop bilirubin encephalopathy because of acidemia and elevation of non-esterified free fatty acids in the blood. Preterm babies nursed in a cold environment have a significantly increased risk of morbidity and mortality compared to those nursed in a thermoneutral environment.

Biochemical Consequences

Exposure to cold or nursing the baby in an environmental temperature which is below the neutral range of ambient temperature for his maturity and postnatal age, leads to hypoxia and hypoglycemia because both oxygen and glucose are consumed during metabolic thermogenesis. Hypoxia is further aggravated by right-to-left shunting of blood due to acidemia and release of norepinephrine. There is elevation of glycerol and non-esterified free fatty acids in the blood following oxidation of triglycerides in the brown fat. Metabolic acidosis occurs due to anerobic tissue metabolism and hypoglycemia. There is rise in serum potassium and NPN levels following tissue catabolism.

HOW TO KEEP THE BABIES WARM?

The "warm chain" or thermoregulation protocol is a set of interlinked interventions which should be taken

14

during first few days after birth in order to minimize heat loss. Failure to implement any of these measures is likely to expose the neonate at risk of developing hypothermia. The ten commandments of the "warm chain" are listed in Box 14.1.

Box 14.1: The components of warm chain

1. Warm delivery room or preferably warm microenvironment for the baby.
2. Immediate drying of the newly born baby.
3. Resuscitation under radiant heat source.
4. Early skin-to-skin contact with the mother.
5. Promotion of breastfeeding.
6. Delaying bathing and weighing of the baby.
7. Keeping the mother and baby dyad together on a single bed.
8. Effective clothing of the baby including provision of cap, mittens and socks.
9. Warm intrahospital transportation of the baby for laboratory investigations.
10. Training and awareness of the health care personnel.

Labor room The baby should be received on a prewarmed bassinet having a radiant heat source. After suctioning of the upper airway, he should be immediately dried and effectively covered with a prewarmed blanket. The bath should be given after 12 to 24 hours when the baby has stabilized its temperature. The LBW baby must be immediately transferred to the warm environment of the nursery and housed in the incubator or open care system as per indications.

Lying-in ward Most of the normal lusty term babies can triple their heat production and maintain their body temperature. During winter months, the baby should lie next to the mother rather than in a separate cot. The warm body of the mother serves as a useful biologically controlled incubator. The baby should be adequately clothed and head (which constitutes a very large surface area in the newborn), hands and feet should be covered with a cap, mittens and socks (Figure 14.4). The bath should be replaced by alternate day sponging taking care not to expose the whole baby at a time. If the winter is severe, use of heater or hot air blower is essential to raise the environmental temperature above 25°C and humidity should be maintained at an appropriate level (>60%).

Nursery The ambient temperature should be maintained around 28°C ±2°C although this may be felt as excessively warm by the personnel working in the NICU. Temperature of the baby should be recorded

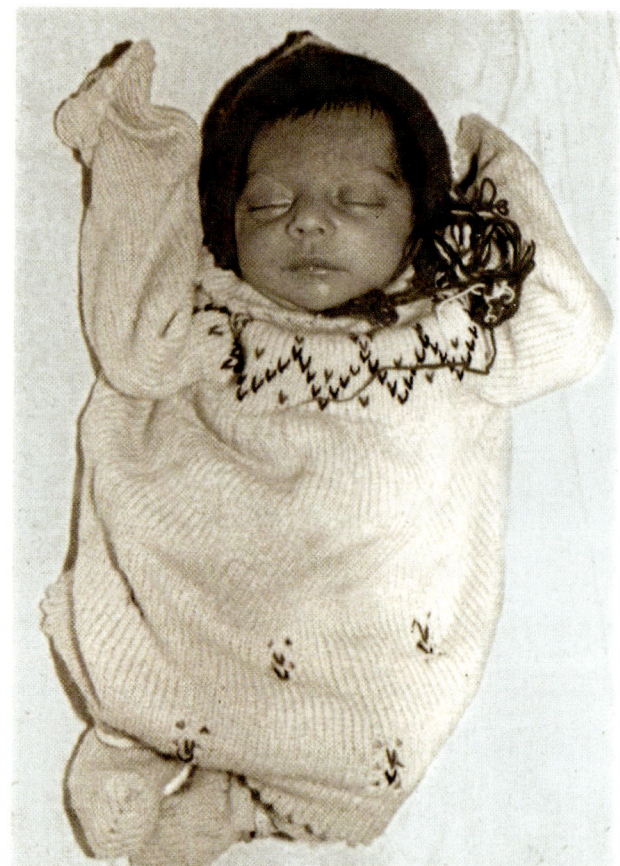

Figure 14.4 Effectively clothed baby to prevent hypothermia.

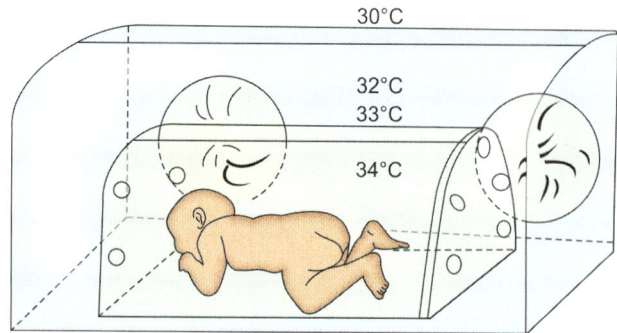

Perspex heat shield

Figure 14.5 The baby in the incubator or open care system should be enclosed in a perspex heat shield to reduce radiant heat loss.

as soon as he is admitted to the nursery. The baby should be placed in the servo-controlled open care system, if the birth weight is less than 1,800 g, gestation below 35 weeks or the rectal temperature is less than 36°C.

In the open care system or incubator, the baby should either be enclosed in a perspex heat shield or should be clothed and provided with a cap to reduce the radiant heat loss (Figure 14.5). Application of oil

TABLE 14.2 Neutral range of environmental temperatures (celsius) for low birth weight babies (mean ±2SD)

Postnatal age	Birth weight (g)			
	<1,200	1,201–1,500	1,501–2,500	>2,500
1st day	35.0 ±0.5	34.3 ±0.5	33.4 ±1.0	33.0 ±1.0
2nd day	34.5 ±0.5	33.7 ±0.5	32.7 ±1.0	32.2 ±1.0
3rd day	34.0 ±0.5	33.5 ±0.5	33.0 ±1.0	32.0 ±1.0
4th day and later	33.5 ±0.5	32.8 ±0.5	32.2 ±1.0	31.5 ±1.0

Adapted from Standards and Recommendations for Hospital Care of Newborn Infants. Ed. 5; 1971; *Evanston, Illinois, American Academy of Pediatrics.*

or liquid paraffin to the skin reduces both heat and evaporative losses. When using the manual mode the temperature of the incubator or open care system should be adjusted to the neutral range of environmental temperature depending upon the birth weight of the baby (Table 14.2). There is no single environmental temperature that is appropriate for all sizes and conditions of the babies. The range of thermoneutral ambient temperature depends upon a number of factors, such as gestational maturity, birth weight, postnatal age, clothing, air currents, humidity and baby's health. The ambient temperature that feels uncomfortable or 'hot' to an adult may impose dangerous cold stress to the newborn baby. A prewarmed incubator should always be kept ready in the nursery to receive an hypothermic baby.

The adjustment of the environmental or incubator temperature should be made in order to maintain the baby's rectal temperature between 36.5°C and 37.0°C or better still, the skin of his exposed abdomen should register a temperature of 36.5°C. It is important that the incubator should be equipped with an efficient thermostat because sudden fluctuations in the ambient temperature are harmful to the baby.

For recording the rectal temperature, a low-reading clinical thermometer (range of 30°C to 40°C) is mandatory, because otherwise severity of hypothermia may be over looked. To avoid rectal perforation, thermometer should be directed slightly posteriorly and should not be inserted beyond 2 cm. The thermometer should be left *in situ* for at least 2 minutes before reading the temperature. Axillary temperature may be erroneously high and unrepresentative of core temperature in a newborn baby due to regional heat production in the brown fat of axilla. The monitoring of the temperature of the exposed skin of abdomen above the umbilicus, with the help of a thermister probe, is preferred. The probe should be shielded from direct heat source. The surface or skin temperature falls sooner than the core temperature, if the environment is too cold and thus an adjustment to the environmental temperature can be made before the baby's deep body temperature falls. In intensive care incubator, the drop in the skin temperature automatically raises the incubator temperature, when it is equipped with a servo-control system, thus eliminating the need for frequent temperature settings of the incubator. The thermister probe must remain in close contact with the skin otherwise the baby would get inadvertently overheated. The heated water filled mattress is a good and relatively cheap alternative to air-heated incubators to keep low birth weight babies warm. The mattress consists of a polyvinyl bag filled with 10 liters of water which is heated by an electrical coil to maintain water temperature between 35°C and 38°C. The bag has a high thermal capacity and continues to provide warmth, even if the power source fails. It is safe to nurse a preterm baby in a cot on a heated water mattress, if the baby in stable and does not need to be undressed for observation.

Infant open care systems with overhead radiant warmer and servo-control are becoming increasingly popular because of ease of observation and handling of the baby (Figure 14.6). When the condition of the baby is stabilized, he should be adequately clothed and provided with a cap, mittens and socks to reduce insensible water and heat loss. The tiny unstable babies nursed in an open care system should be covered with a plastic sheet to reduce heat and evaporative losses (Figure 14.7). EMBRACE™ is an innovative low cost warmer for use in neonates. It is fabricated with phase change material which stays at a constant temperature for 6 hours. It is useful for short distance or intrahospital transport. Infants nursed under radiant warmers should receive additional 45–90 mL/kg/day of maintenance fluids to replenish the increased evaporative loss of water from skin.

The incubator babies should not be bathed. The linen for daily use should be kept in the nursery so that it is reasonably warm. During various diagnostic,

Temperature Regulation

14

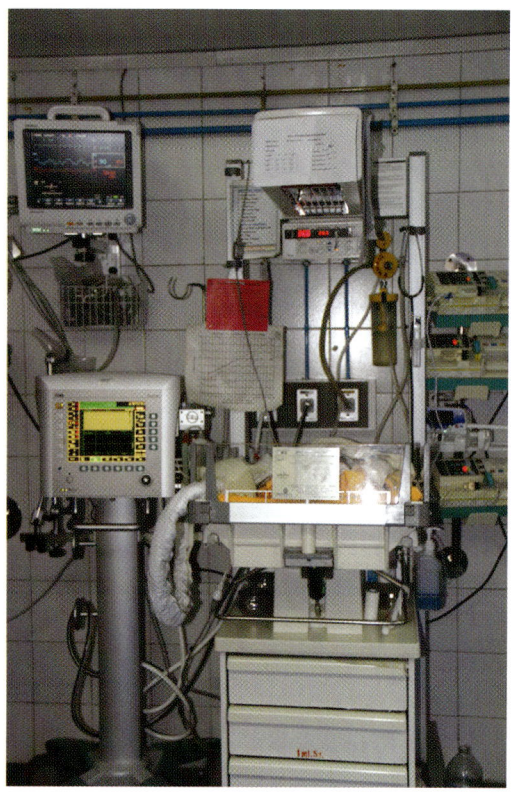

Figure 14.6 Open care system is ideal to nurse preterm and sick infants who need frequent handling and therapeutic interventions.

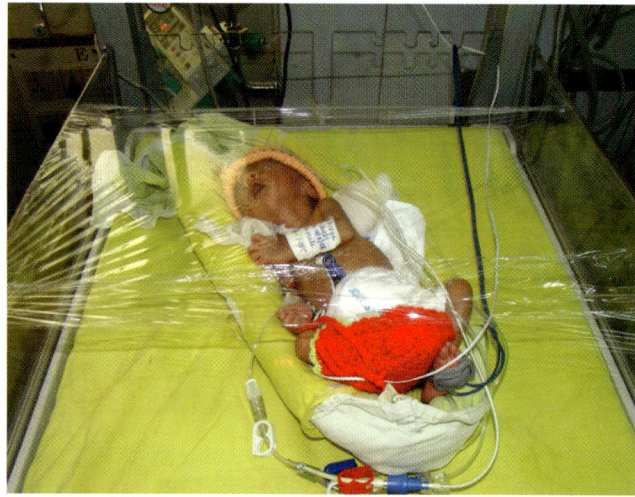

Figure 14.7 Preterm infant enclosed under a plastic cling wrap to reduce heat and evaporative losses.

therapeutic and surgical procedures, radiant heat source should be used to keep them warm. The hot water bottles or electric blankets should never come in direct contact with the skin of the baby and their use should preferably be avoided.

Operation theater Infants are at grave risk to develop severe hypothermia during surgery because of low ambient temperature of operation theater, prolonged exposure, evaporative losses following skin preparation and administration of cold anesthetic gases, intravenous fluids and blood. Rectal temperature of the infant should be monitored with the help of a telethermometer. Infant should be placed on a circulating warm water mattress and infrared overhead warmer should be affixed at a height of 45 cm above the infant to maintain an ambient temperature of around 34°C near the skin. Fiberoptic 'hot pipe' system can be used to effectively enclose the baby with a warm microenvironment during surgery. Anesthetic gases, fluids and biological products should be prewarmed to 37°C before administration.

Transport Whenever feasible, the high-risk mother should be transported to a center equipped to provide intensive care services to the mothers and babies because *"uterus is an ideal transport incubator"*. Transport of sick and premature babies within the hospital or from one hospital to another is associated with several hazards including risk of development of hypothermia. Availability of a transport incubator is ideal but not affordable in low and middle income countries (LMICs). The baby should be effectively covered in woollens (cap, socks, mittens) or wrapped in cotton or tin foil. Skin-to-skin contact during transport is useful to keep the baby warm in resource-limited countries. A padded cane basket with handle and hot water bottles kept in the side hampers can be improvised. *The hot water bottle should never come in direct contact with the baby due to risk of burns.* A thermocole box with a transparent plastic lid can be used as a cheap, safe and effective transport incubator in LMICs. A thermocole box can be warmed with hot water bottles before the start of the journey (Figure 14.8).

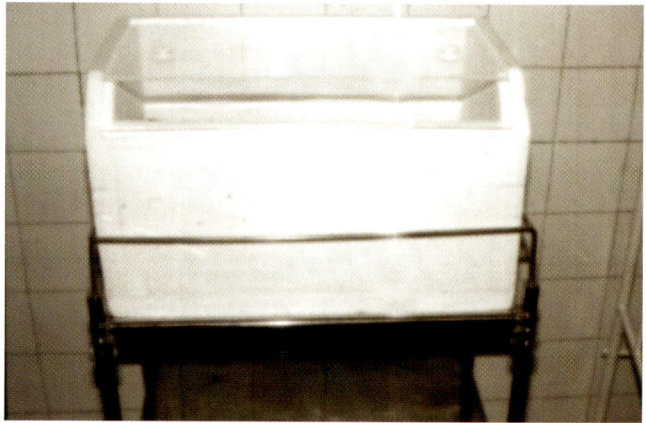

Figure 14.8 Thermocole box for transport of babies in resource-limited countries.

Home care The mother must be explained the risks of changes in the environmental temperature to the health and wellbeing of her newborn baby. The baby should be kept dried, effectively clothed and provided with a woollen cap, socks and mittens. The clothes should be pre-warmed infront of a heater or on a *'tawa'*. The cot of the mother should be kept away from the walls and baby should lie next to the mother to receive maternal warmth. The room can be kept warm with a room heater or *'angeethi'* taking due precautions to safeguard against accumulation of carbon monoxide. The culturally accepted practice of giving oil massage to the babies is useful as it reduces both heat as well as insensible water loss. Exposure should be avoided during the procedure of bathing the baby. In winter, daily sponging with warm water and bathing once a week is recommended. The mother should be trained to assess the temperature of the baby with her hands. *Trunk should feel warm to touch and hands and feet should be reasonably warm and pink.* The parents and health care workers should be provided with knowledge and skills to prevent hypothermia. It must be remembered that lack of awareness is more important cause of hypothermia than lack of equipment.

KANGAROO-MOTHER CARE (SKIN-TO-SKIN CONTACT)

Direct contact with the skin of mother (or even father or any other family member) provides biologically controlled heat source to keep stable LBW babies warm. Kangaroo-mother care (KMC) is based on marsupial care-giving concept of keeping the babies in a maternal pouch, which was introduced in 1978 by Edgar Rey in Bogota, Colombia. It is a cost-effective and useful strategy to enhance the survival of LBW babies in LMIC countries having constraints of financial and human resources.

Kangaroo-mother care may be continuous (round-the-clock) or intermittent. In India, short-term or intermittent KMC has been used with several benefits to the baby but round-the-clock KMC has not been exploited due to following reasons.

- There is poor cultural acceptability of KMC in our society.
- There is a lack of soakable napkin concept and suitable garment design for easy ambulation of mother practicing KMC.
- There are problems and logistic difficulties and disconnection of the baby during sleep, toilet and bathing routines of mother.

- It is uncomfortable for the mother to remain constantly stuck with the baby throughout the day and night during the hot summer months.

There is a need to evolve ways and means to provide protracted or continuous KMC especially to preterm babies of mothers belonging to low socio-economic status. The procedure is most suitable for stable infants with a birth weight between 1500 and 1800 g or gestation 32–34 weeks. A large number of physiological, biochemical and clinical benefits of KMC have been documented though some of them are either doubtful or presumptive (Table 14.3).

The KMC Procedure

KMC is started when baby is stable and receiving oral feeds. Short-term or intermittent KMC can be started in the NICU in babies receiving intravenous or orogastric feeds and low concentration of oxygen. The NICU should have a free-access and an open door policy for the parents. Mother and family members should be motivated and mentally prepared by the health care professionals who have been specially trained to provide KMC. Mother should be free from any infection and explained about importance of daily bath, maintenance of personal hygiene and handwashing. Mother should wear a front-open gown or suitable dress which is culturally acceptable. She should be provided with some privacy and her sensitivities due to some exposure of breasts should be respected.

The baby should be dressed with a front-open sleeveless shirt, cap, socks, mittens and a soakable napkin. The baby is placed between the mother's breasts in

TABLE 14.3 Physiologic and clinical benefits of KMC

- Infant–mother bonding.
- Promotion of breastfeeding with improved yield of milk.
- Stability of vital signs with effective thermal control and reduced risk of apneic attacks.
- Reduced risk of infections.
- Babies cry less, sleep better and show satisfactory neurobehavioral development.
- Better weight gain and early discharge from the hospital.
- Mother may transmit electromagnetic vibrations of healing, love and compassion to her baby.
- There is evidence to suggest that KMC may provide long lasting social and behavioral protective effects including reduced risk of ADHD.

an upright position. The head is turned to one side and kept in a slightly extended position to keep the airway open and enable the mother to maintain an eye-to-eye contact with her baby. The hips and arms should be kept flexed and abducted to maintain frog-like position (Figure 14.9). This enables a large surface area of the nude skin of the baby to maintain a close contact with the chest and abdomen of the mother. The bottom of the baby should be supported with a sling or binder. The back of the baby should be covered with a woollen shawl (Figure 14.10).

Depending upon the maturity of the baby, mother can give breastfeeding or express the breast milk and feed with a cup and spoon or *paladay*. During KMC, mother should sleep in a supine position at an angle of 15° from horizontal. She should be explained and given simple guidelines for monitoring her baby. When mother is bathing or attending to her toilet needs or attending to some household chores, the baby should be effectively covered and kept warm or KMC should be provided by a relative or father. Alternatively, a low cost warmer fabricated with phase change material (EMBRACE™) is useful to tide over these exigencies. When a baby is discharged from the hospital on KMC, the baby should be monitored by a public health nurse by weekly home visits. KMC is continued till baby achieves body weight of around 2500 g. The baby is weaned from KMC when baby feels uncomfortable, tries to show discomfort or wriggling movements, or there is visible sweating. It is important to remember that KMC is labor-intensive procedure and uncomfortable

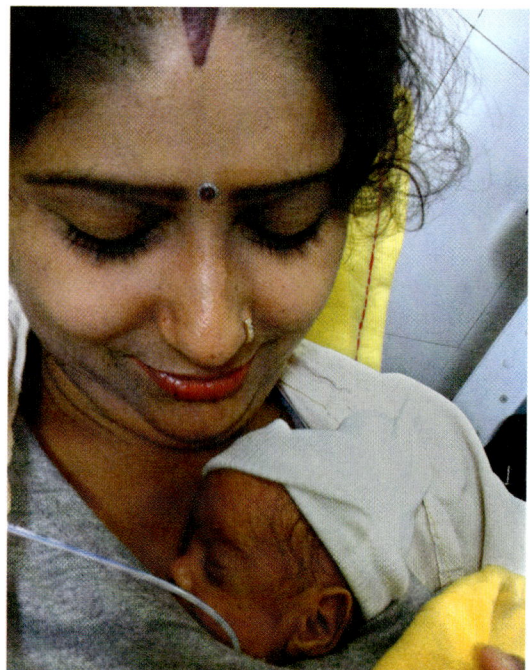

Figure 14.10 Kangaroo-mother care. It is highly cost-effective method to prevent hypothermia and promote bonding and breastfeeding.

to the mother, and she needs emotional support and guidance from health care professionals (HCPs) and family members for its success.

PREVENTION OF HYPOTHERMIA

The goal of good thermal care is to achieve a core temperature between 36.8°C and 37.3°C. The following guidelines and recommendations should be implemented to prevent hypothermia which is associated with reduced morbidity and improved survival of newborn babies.

- High-risk mother should be identified during antenatal period and referred to a center equipped to provide good quality obstetrical and neonatal care services.
- At birth, create a warm microenvironment to provide a warm welcome to the baby. Dry the baby promptly (including head) and cover him effectively with warm linen.
- Do not give bath to the baby at birth or to the babies reared in the NICU.
- The ambient temperature should be maintained around 28°C ±2°C. A standby incubator should be kept warm and ready at all times to receive a sick or cold baby.
- The baby should be nursed in an open care system and skin temperature maintained around 36.5°C with the help of servo mode.

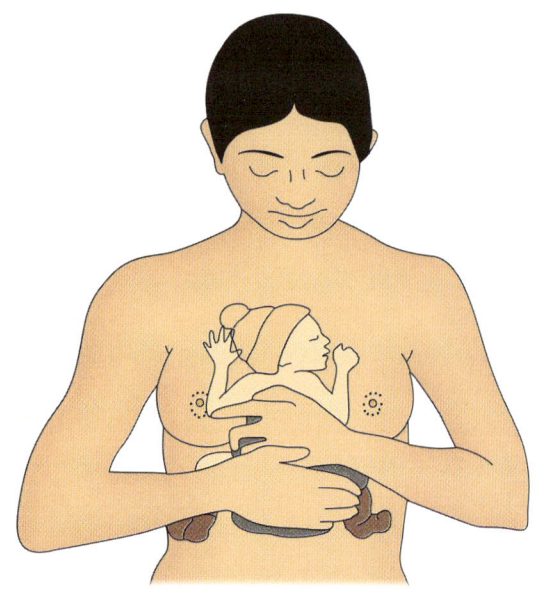

Figure 14.9 Diagrammatic depiction of positioning of the baby for effective kangaroo-mother care.

- The babies should be effectively clothed and provided with a cap, socks and mittens.
- Whatever comes in direct contact with the baby should be prewarmed, viz. cot, linen, clothes, infusates, X-ray plate, etc.
- Take special care to prevent hypothermia during procedures and transport.
- Application of oil and liquid paraffin can reduce evaporation and heat loss from skin.
- Skin-to-skin contact provides an excellent source of biologically controlled heat. Apart from providing warmth, it promotes bonding and breastfeeding.
- The mothers and health care workers should be provided with knowledge and skills for assessment of baby's temperature and prevention of hypothermia. They should be guided and encouraged to develop their skills to assess the body temperature of babies with their hands and use simple ways and means to keep the babies warm. *The use of common sense is more important than the availability of expensive equipment to keep the babies warm.*

NEONATAL COLD INJURY

The LBW babies when exposed to various heat losing situations for prolonged period of time, without due attention to their biological needs, may develop grave manifestations of cold injury. Preterm infants with birth asphyxia and damage to central nervous system are particularly vulnerable to develop cold injury. After initial restlessness, the baby becomes sluggish, inactive and refuses feeds. The skin of trunk is cold to touch. Facial erythema, due to failure of dissociation of oxyhemoglobin at low temperature, gives an erroneous impression of wellbeing. Vital functions are depressed as evidenced by bradycardia, slow breathing and fall in blood pressure. Sclerema and/ or subcutaneous fat necrosis occur in advanced cases. Hemorrhagic manifestations including massive pulmonary hemorrhage may occur as a result of disseminated intravascular coagulation. Septicemia and hypoglycemia may complicate the clinical picture.

Management

The baby should be immediately transferred to an incubator and slowly warmed to achieve normal skin or core temperature in 4 to 6 hours. The ambient environmental temperature and abdominal skin temperature should not differ by greater than 1.5°C to safeguard against apneic attacks. Radiant warmers are useful for treating hypothermic babies by maintaining temperature at 37°C with the help of servo-controlled sensors. Oxygen and glucose solution should be administered intravenously to meet the increased demands and to correct hypoxia and hypoglycemia, which are commonly associated. Antibiotics should be administered after taking blood sample for culture. In the event of hemorrhagic manifestations, 0.5 to 1.0 mg of vitamin K is given intramuscularly. Exchange blood transfusion is recommended when disseminated intravascular coagulation is suspected. Hydrocortisone is indicated in babies with sclerema.

Prognosis is generally poor with a case fatality rate of 25 to 50%. The presence of sclerema and hemorrhagic manifestations herald poor outcome.

HYPERTHERMIA

Hyperthermia is defined as increase in body temperature (>37.5°C) that exceeds the body's capacity to lose heat while fever is caused by release of endogenous pyrogens secondary to an inflammatory disorder or infection. In a tropical country, raised environmental temperature during hot summer months may produce a febrile response in the neonate although the situation is never life-threatening. In addition to the raised environmental temperature, infections, dehydration, disturbances of central nervous system, administration of certain drugs, such as belladonna preparations and ephedrine nose drops may cause hyperthermia. Exposure of the baby to sunlight for phototherapy is hazardous and may lead to severe hyperthermia. Iatrogenic hyperthermia can occur due to strong overhead heat source or inadvertent dislodgment of skin thermister in a baby nursed in a servo-controlled incubator or open care system.

Newborn babies lack effective sweating mechanism and preterm babies below 32 weeks of gestation cannot sweat. In infants with hyperthermia due to increase in environmental temperature, both trunk and extremities are warm because of vasodilatation. In contrast, infants with sepsis are often vasoconstricted and extremities are usually 2–3°C colder than the trunk. It is important to differentiate between a healthy neonate who is over heated (hyperthermia) and a sick neonate who has fever, because they have different prognoses and therapeutic implications. The salient differences between an overheated healthy neonate and a sick neonate with fever are summarized in Table 14.4. Many a times, a sick preterm neonate is likely to be hypothermic and cold rather than febrile. It has already been emphasized that in LBW babies, infections more often produce hypothermia rather than fever.

Temperature Regulation

14

TABLE 14.4 Differences between a healthy neonate who is over heated and a febrile sick neonate

Over heated neonate	Febrile neonate
▪ Irritability and restlessness	▪ Lethargic and lazy
▪ Keen to feed	▪ Refusal to feed
▪ Hands and feet are warm and pink	▪ Hands and feet may be cold and pale
▪ The difference between abdominal skin temperature and peripheral skin temperature is less than 2°C	▪ Abdominal skin temperature exceeds peripheral temperature by more than 2°C
▪ Tachycardia	▪ Tachycardia
▪ Healthy flushed appearance	▪ Looks unwell with circumoral cyanosis
▪ No shock with capillary refill time <2 s	▪ Shock may occur with capillary refill time >2 s

Transient Fever of the Newborn

During the summer months in tropical countries when environmental temperature goes above 38.5°C about 10% of the term babies develop fever on the second or third day of life. The rectal temperature ranges between 37.5°C and 39.5°C and the condition is self-limiting. The baby remains active, alert and craves for feeding. Its higher incidence in breastfed babies and onset on second or third day of life suggest that the fever may be due to dehydration though studies have failed to demonstrate any clinical or biochemical evidences of dehydration in these babies. It appears that raised environmental temperature in association with immaturity of heat regulating center and inefficiency of sweating mechanism in the newborn are most probable explanations. The infant is best managed by cooling the environment rather than provision of extra fluids alone. There is no therapeutic utility of an antipyretic agent because there is no alteration in the setting of the thermostat. Hydrotherapy is required at times for prompt reduction of body temperature.

BIBLIOGRAPHY

Charpak N, Tessier R, Ruiz JG et al. Twenty-year follow-up of kangaroo mother care versus traditional care. Pediatrics 2017, 139(1):e2016–e2063.

Conde-Agudelo A, Diaz Rosello JL. Kangaroo mother care to reduce morbidity and mortality in low birth weight infants. Cochrane Database Syst Rev 2016, 20:5–36.

Hey E. Thermal neutrality. Brit Med Bull 1975, 31: 69.

Hull D. The structure and function of brown adipose tissue. Brit Med Bull 1966, 22: 92.

Knoble RB, Vohra S, Lehman CU. Heat loss prevention in the delivery room for preterm infants: a national survey of newborn intensive care units. J Perinatol 2005, 25: 514–518.

Lawn JE, Mwansa-Kambafwile J, Cousens S. Kangaroo mother care to prevent neonatal deaths due to preterm birth complications. Int J Epidemiol 2010, 39 (suppl 1): 144–154.

Lunze K, Hamer DH. Thermal protection of the newborn in resource-limited environments. J Perinatol 2012, 32:317–24.

Malhotra AK, Deorari AK, Paul VK, Bagga A, Singh M. A new transport incubator for primary care of low birth weight babies. Indian Pediatr 1992, 29: 587–593.

McCall EM, Alderdice FA, Halliday HL, et al. Interventions to prevent hypothermia at birth in preterm and/or low birth weight babies. Cochrane Database Syst Rev 2008, 1: CD004210.

Mullany LC. Neonatal hypothermia in low-resource settings. Semin Perinatol 2010, 34(6):426–33.

Nimbalkar S, Sadhvani N. Implementation of kangaroo mother care: Challenges and solutions. Indian Pediatr 2019, 56:725–9.

Ramanathan K, Paul VK, Deorari AK, et al. Kangaroo mother care in very low birth weight infants. Indian J Pediatr 2001, 68: 1019–1023.

Rao PN, Udani R, Nanavati R. Kangaroo mother care for the low birth weight infants: a randomized controlled trial. Indian Pediatr 2008, 45: 17–23.

Sarman I, Can G, Tunnel R. Rewarming preterm infants on a heated water filled mattress. Arch Dis Child 1989, 64: 687.

Sauer PJJ, Dane HJ, Visser HKA. New standards for neutral thermal environment of healthy very low birth weight infants in week one of life. Arch Dis Child 1984, 59: 18.

Scopes JW. Metabolic rate and temperature control in human baby. Brit Med Bull 1965, 32: 88.

Scopes JW. Thermoregulation in the newborn. In: Neonatology Avery GB (Ed.) Lippincott, Company Philadelphia 1975, p.99.

Sherman T. Optimizing the neonatal thermal environment. Neonatal Netw 2006, 25 (4): 251–258.

Shim WKT, Halford P. Method for maintaining neonates intraoperative core temperature. Surgery 1974, 75: 416.

Silverman WA, Sinclair JC. Temperature regulation in the newborn infant. N Eng J Med 1966, 274: 92.

Sinclair JC. Servo-control for maintaining abdominal skin temperature at 36°C in LBW infants. Cochrane Database System Rev 2002, (I) CD001074.

Singh M, Chowdhry VP, Vasuki K. Pathogenesis of so called 'dehydration fever'. Indian Pediatr 1985, 12: 465.

Singh M, Rao G, Malhotra AK, Deorari AK. Assessment of newborn baby's temperature by human touch: A potentially useful primary care strategy. Indian Pediatr 1992, 29: 449–452.

Thukral A, Chawla D, Agarwal R, et al. Kangaroo mother care: an alternative to conventional care. In: AIIMS Protocols in Neonatology. Paul VK, Deorari AK (Eds.) Indian Journal of Pediatrics, New Delhi 2008, pp 244–256.

World Health Organization (WHO). Kangaroo mother care: A practical guide. Geneva, WHO, 2003.

Care of the Newborn

14

Feeding and Nutrition

After meeting the fundamental needs of establishing breathing and maintenance of body temperature, the subsequent efforts in the care of the newborn babies are directed towards the provision of adequate nutrition and prevention of infections.

FEEDING OF NORMAL BABIES

After birth, a term vigorously crying baby, should be kept on mother's tummy to provide skin-to-skin contact for warmth, promotion of bonding and breastfeeding. The first feed should be offered as soon as the baby is keen to suck and the mother is well enough to suckle. This is generally possible within half an hour of birth. There is no need to offer first feed of plain or glucose water or any other prelacteal feed, and the baby should be straight put on to the breast.

BREASTFEEDING

The human baby, like the offsprings of other mammals, is born with a ready-made food supply of its own and therefore breastfeeding is natural and instinctive. The milk of different animals is uniquely species specific and its composition is adapted to the nutritional needs of the baby. The lowest protein content of human milk is in keeping with the slowest rate of growth of human infant. Milk of different animals is specific to serve the nutritional needs of their offsprings by virtue of its unique biological and the biochemical composition. For example, milk of a cow or buffalo is meant for her calf, milk of mare is meant for her colt, milk of an ass is best for the pony, so on and so

> The nature has designed the provision that infants be fed upon their mother's milk. They find their food and mother at the same time. It is a complete nourishment for them both for their body and soul.
> **Rabindranath Tagore**

forth. The breast milk is not only species specific, it is baby specific. *The milk of a mother is best suited to serve the nutritional and biological needs of her baby!* Breastfeeding is natural and instinctive. The act of sucking promotes bonding and is associated with release of oxytocin, which is a feel good hormone. Every mother wants to breastfeed her baby and she must be provided with necessary guidance, support and encouragement by her husband, family members and health care professionals. And, every mother can successfully breastfeed and provide a best start in life to her baby. *Like mother's love, there is no substitute for mother's milk.*

Virtues of Breast Milk

Breastfeeding provides unique health benefits both to the baby as well as her mother.

Benefits to the Baby

1. Breast milk is a complete food and it provides all the nutrients a baby needs during first 6 months of life. Breast milk is more easily digestible because of presence of special enzyme lipase and high quality of whey proteins. Healthy term breastfed babies do not need any supplements of vitamins and iron during first 6 months of life (except vitamin K and vitamin D).

2. Breast milk contains a number of anti-infective substances, protective antibodies and friendly lactobacilli, which protect the baby against development of diarrhea, respiratory illnesses (cough and cold) and other infections (especially ear infection). Breastfeeding has been shown to reduce the risk of death due to diarrhea by 14 times, acute respiratory infections by 4 times and other infections by 3 times. There is reduced risk of acute

otitis media and necrotizing enterocolitis in breastfed babies.

3. Breastfed babies are less likely to suffer from allergic disorders like asthma and eczema. Rarely breastfed babies may develop an allergic disorder, if mother consumes allergenic foods like cow's milk, eggs, nuts and citrus fruits.

4. Breastfeeding provides immunological benefits to the baby throughout the lifetime. Breastfed babies have been shown to develop better protective response to various vaccines compared to bottle fed babies.

5. Breastfeeding provides emotional security and promotes close bonding between mother and her baby. Breastfeeding provides maternal warmth, physical closeness and comfort to the baby.

6. Breastfeeding stimulates all the five special senses of the baby, i.e. touch, sight, smell, hearing and taste.

7. Breastfed babies are smarter and have been shown to have 8 points higher intelligence quotient (IQ) and enhanced visual development. High concentrations of two key long chain fatty acids (arachidonic acid and docosahexaenoic acid), lactose and sialic acid promote brain growth.

8. Breastfed babies are less likely to suffer from caries teeth, type 2 diabetes mellitus, obesity, high blood pressure, heart attacks and certain cancers during adult life.

9. There is no risk of adulteration, dilution, contamination and infection of breast milk.

10. The risk of cot deaths or sudden infant death syndrome (SIDS) is less in breastfed babies.

Benefits to the Mother

1. During breastfeeding, there is a release of oxytocin to eject the milk. Oxytocin promotes involution of the uterus so that there is reduced risk of bleeding and anemia after delivery. Oxytocin is also a feel good hormone and provides a sense of wellbeing to the mother.

2. Breastfeeding delays ovulation and onset of menstruation which provides natural means to ensure spacing of children. It has been estimated that in India universal and prolonged breastfeeding prevents more pregnancies than all other reversible methods of contraception currently practiced. But the protection is not fool proof and mothers who are breastfeeding must seek proper contraceptive advice.

3. Breastfeeding is convenient and less time consuming. Breast milk is readily available all the time at the desired temperature. There is no need to buy feeding bottles and animal or powdered milk and no time is wasted for sterilization of bottles and preparation of feeds.

4. Breastfeeding mothers have a sense of accomplishment, bonding, indispensability and motherliness and they feel more relaxed and calm in discharging their mothercraft skills with joy.

5. There is a misconception among several women that breastfeeding spoils the figure and shape of the breasts. On the contrary, breastfeeding helps to maintain and regain the pre-pregnancy body weight earlier because energy stores laid down during pregnancy are consumed faster during lactation. As far as the shape of the breasts is concerned, there is no difference whether a mother breastfeeds or gives formula feeds to her baby.

6. Mothers who breastfeed their babies have a reduced risk of development of breast and ovarian cancer and osteoporosis.

7. There is economic saving to the family and society because money and resources are not wasted for purchase of feeding bottles, bottle sterilizer, bottle warmer, animal milk or formula and there is reduction in medical costs because of lower incidence of various infections in breastfed babies. It has been estimated that universal promotion of breastfeeding leads to national cost saving to the tune of US $ 2023 million (₹ 15,780 crores) per annum in India alone.

Breastfeeding and Brain Growth

There is epidemiological evidence to suggest that breastfed babies have 8 IQ points higher congnition and enhanced visual development than formula fed babies. Breastfeeding enhances bonding, sensory stimulation and emotional satisfaction both to the mother and her baby. Human milk contains about 30 times more DHA (about 10 mg/100 mL) than cow's milk which is a predominant structural fatty acid in our brain, neuronal membranes and retina. Human milk is rich in lactose, choline, taurine, iodine, sialic acid and zinc which are brain friendly. Human milk has highest concentration of lactose compared to milk of other animals and lactose is credited to facilitate synthesis of cerebrosides and myelination of central nervous system. Human milk is rich in oligosaccharides especially sialic acid (40 ±10 mg/dL) which is a key component of gangliosides and is mandatory for formation of neuronal synapses.

COMPOSITION OF HUMAN MILK

The composition of human milk is best suited to serve the nutritional and biological needs of human baby. Breast milk has perfect combination of nutrients for steady growth and development of babies. The composition varies depending upon the genetic background or ethnic factors, age, parity, nutritional status and dietary intake of the mother. It also varies depending upon timing of delivery (term or preterm), phase of lactation (colostrum, transitional, mature and weaning milk), time of the day (diurnal variations), frequency of feeding and whether it is foremilk, hindmilk or drip milk. Breast milk of malnourished women may be suboptimal in quantity and quality with lower concentration of fat, water soluble vitamins, vitamin A, vitamin D, and calcium. In a healthy well nourished nursing mother taking a balanced diet, exclusive breastfeeding can serve all the nutritional needs of the baby, except vitamin K and vitamin D which are relatively deficient.

Carbohydrates

Human milk has the highest concentration of lactose (7.2 g/dL) compared to all other mammals. Human milk is sweeter and thinner compared to animal milk because of higher concentration of lactose and lower content of solids. The baby breaks lactose into two simple sugars glucose and galactose. The latter is credited to enhance the production of cerebrosides and growth of neurons. There is evidence to suggest that more intelligent species of mammals are endowed with a higher concentration of lactose in their milk. Lactose is converted to lactic acid by Lactobacilli which makes baby's stomach more acidic thus preventing growth of harmful bacteria. The lowest concentration of lactose is found in reindeer milk while there is no lactose in the milk of pinnipeds (sea lions, walruses). Oligosaccharides are unique to human milk and are present in high concentration (0.7–1.2 g/dL). The most common sugars making up these short chain oligosaccharides include N-acetyl-D-glucosamine, sialic acid and fucose. They work like "fiber" of human milk because infant lacks the enzyme to break or digest them. Human milk oligosaccharides (HMO) produce short chain fatty acids which promote the growth of "friendly" bifidobacteria (probiotics) in the gut. HMO also strengthen the baby's immune system and protect against food allergies and asthma. Sialic acid (N-acetylneuraminic acid or NANA) in human milk is found as sialyllactose (130 ±32.2 mg/dL) which is an oligosaccharide. It is an essential component of mucins, glycoproteins and gangliosides. It is required for proper functioning of cell membranes, membrane receptors and development of brain. In humans, the highest concentration of sialic acid is found in the brain.

Proteins

Human milk has the lowest concentration of protein (1.3 g/dL) among all mammals because of relatively slower physical growth of human babies. Proteins account for 75% of the nitrogen-containing compounds in breast milk. The proteins of breast milk primarily include aqueous whey proteins and micellar casein which exist in a ratio of 60:40. Whey proteins are easy to digest and have high bioavailability. The major whey proteins are α-lactalbumin, lactoferrin, secretory IgA and serum albumin. The predominant casein is β-casein, which forms micelles of relatively small volume to produce soft flocculent curd in the infants' stomach. About 25% of milk's nitrogen is contributed by non-protein nitrogen-containing compounds like urea, uric acid, creatine, creatinine, amino acids and nucleotides. Nucleotides, the building blocks of nucleic acids, are useful for numerous intracellular biochemical processes including development of healthy gut, sturdy immune system, greater tolerance to dietary antigens and promotion of sound sleep. They are one of the most important nonprotein nitrogen constituents of human milk. Human milk DNA and RNA levels are estimated to range between 1 and 12 mg/dL and 10 to 60 mg/dL, respectively. The TPAN (total potentially available nucleotides) level of breast milk is about 72 mg/L and is constant throughout geographic regions.

Fats

Fat content of human milk is relatively lower (4.0 g/dL) compared to milk of other animals but nevertheless it provides 50% calories from lipids. About 98% of lipids in milk are triglycerides and small amounts as di- and monoglycerols, cholesterol, fatty acids and phospholipids. Unlike carbohydrates and proteins, the fat composition of milk varies widely by genetic, lactational and nutritional factors. Human milk is loaded with saturated fatty acids and cholesterol (10–15 mg/dL) which are essential to promote physical growth and brain development. The fatty acid composition of human milk comprises 65% saturated fatty acids, 30% monounsaturated fatty acids and 5% of polyunsaturated fatty acids. The highest concentration of docosahexaenoic acid or

DHA (10 mg/dL) is found in human milk. High levels of cholesterol in breast milk provides "metabolic adaptation" to babies to handle cholesterol in adult life where mantra of "low cholesterol diet" is followed to promote sound cardiovascular health. About 167 fatty acids have been identified in human milk but major fatty acids include palmitic, stearic, oleic and linoleic acids. High levels of antimicrobial lauric acid and capric acid are useful to prevent infections.

Biochemical and Physiological Differences between Human and Cow's Milk

There are several biochemical, nutritional and physiological differences between the human and cow's milk (Table 15.1). The cow's milk is most suited for the biological needs of the calf while breast milk is ideal for the human baby. The lower content of protein and fat in the human milk is in consonance with the slow postnatal growth of human baby. The whey protein in human milk is easily digestible and human milk lipase promotes fat digestion. Higher content of certain amino acids (cystine and taurine), choline, iodine, zinc, long chain fatty acids like arachidonic acid and docosahexaenoic acid (DHA), lactose and oligosaccharides (sialic acid) in the human milk promotes faster development, maturation, myelination and synaptogenesis of human brain which is most highly evolved as compared to other mammals. The nutrients available in the human milk are more readily absorbed and better utilized due to higher biological efficiency. Iron present in breast milk is most efficiently absorbed and levels of serum iron, serum ferritin and red cell folate are significantly higher in breastfed infants compared with those fed on cow's milk. The presence of epidermal growth factor, insulin-like growth factor 1, transforming growth factor alpha and peptides in human milk enhance physical growth.

Immunobiology of Breast Milk

Human milk is not only best suited and specific to serve the nutritional needs of the baby, it also boosts the host defenses of the newborn. It is replete with immunoglobulins, cellular viable elements (macrophages, polymorphonuclear leukocytes, T and B lymphocytes) and non-specific humoral protective factors (Box 15.1). Breast milk contains large quantities of secretory IgA and IgM antibodies which are not otherwise available to the newborn baby because they do not cross the placenta. Some IgG immunoglobulins are also present in breast milk. *The highest concentration*

Box 15.1: Anti-infective agents in human milk

- Immunoglobulins: Secretory IgA, IgG, IgM.
- Cellular elements*: Lymphoid cells, polymorphs, macrophages, plasma cells.
- Probiotics: Over 600 species of friendly bacteria including *Lactobacillus fermentum, L. reuteri, L. rhamnosus, L. paracasei, Bifidobacterium bifidum, B. breve, B. adolescentis, B. longum* and *B. dentium*.
- Opsonic and chemotactic activities of C3 and C4 complement system.
- Unsaturated lactoferrin and transferrin.
- Lysozyme.
- Lactoperoxidase.
- Oligosaccharides.
- Specific inhibitors (non-immunoglobulins): Antiviral and anti-staphylococcal factors.
- Growth factors for *Lactobacillus bifidus*.
- Para-aminobenzoic acid may afford some protection against malaria.

*Colostrum contains 8 million cells/mL

of secretory IgA in any body fluid is found in colostrum. Quantitative and qualitative differences exist between different classes of antibodies in the serum and breast milk of the mother. The immunoglobulin characteristics of breast milk resemble those of surface or secretory antibodies which operate at mucosal sites in the intestinal and respiratory tract. High titers of antibodies present in the colostrum drop sharply over the next few days.

By virtue of its composition, colostrum is best suited to serve the nutritional and immunological needs of the baby and it should not be denied. Milk immunoglobulins are not absorbed in sufficient quantities and do not significantly contribute to serum immunoglobulin level of suckling infant. Secretory IgA binds microorganisms and prevent their penetration into intestinal mucosa. IgA can also lyse certain enteric bacteria in the presence of complement and lysozyme. In addition to specific antibodies, human milk also contains non-specific humoral factors such as lysozyme, oligosaccharides, lactoferrin, complement, fibronectin, mucin, xanthine oxidase and lactoperoxidase. Breast milk contains higher concentration of vitamin B_{12} binding protein, which competes with bacteria requiring vitamin B_{12} for their growth. Oligosaccharides provide protection against infections because of their structural similarity with bacterial antigen receptors. Glycoprotein and oligosaccharides present in human milk promote the growth of bifidus bacteria which prevent the entry of pathogenic bacteria through the gut.

TABLE 15.1 Biochemical and physiological differences between human and cow's milk (composition per 100 mL)

Nutrients	Human milk	Cow's milk
Water	90.0 mL	87.8 mL
Protein	1.3 g	3.5 g
Casein	40%	80%
Whey	60%	20%
	Lactalbumin and whey protein content is high. It is easily digestible. It is rich in cystine and sulfurylated taurine, an apparent neurotransmitter essential for brain growth. It contains abundant anti-infective agents	β-lactoglobulin content is high which is responsible for milk allergy and intestinal colic. Casein curds are formed. Gultamic acid, tyrosine, phenylalanine and tryptophan content is high
Lactose*	7.2 g	5.0 g
	Calcium and iron retention is enhanced by high lactose content. It promotes synthesis of cerebrosides in the brain. Higher content of N-acetylneuraminic acid (NANA) or sialic acid (30–150 mg) is useful for formation of gangliosides and synapses	
Fat	4.0 g	4.0 g
	Essential fatty acids especially linoleic acid and docosahexaenoic acid (10 mg/dL) in high concentrations. They are similar to lipids of human CNS. High content of galactolipids promotes rapid brain growth of human infant. Lipase in milk improves digestion by supplying readily available free fatty acids to the infant. May protect against future atherosclerosis?	Digestibility is poor. Mostly saturated fatty acids with less quantity of essential fatty acids and DHA
Solute load		
Ash content	0.2 g	0.7 g
Electrolytes (mEq/L)		
Sodium	6.5	25
Chloride	12	29
Potassium	14	35
Osmolarity (mOsm/L)	280–300	350–400
		High sodium and low fluoride content. High solute load may aggravate dehydration
Calcium/phosphorus ratio	35 mg/15 mg	140 mg/90 mg
	Ratio of more than 2 promotes calcium deposition	Ratio of less than 2. Tetany may occur
Hematinic factors		
Iron	0.29–0.45 mg	0.01–0.38 mg
Folic acid	0.14–0.36 μg	0.01–0.06 μg
Vitamin B_{12}	0.0008–0.4 μg	0.07–1.15 μg
Vitamin C	1.2–10.0 mg	1.2–1.5 mg
Vitamin A	0.5–10.0 i.u.	70–220 i.u.
Vitamin D	0.5–10.0 i.u.	0.5-4.5 i.u.
Vitamin K	1.5 μg	6.0 μg
	The concentration of hematinic factors is slightly higher and they are better utilized due to increased bioavailability. The incidence of nutritional anemia is lower, if weaning is not delayed.	Thermolabile factors are destroyed by heating. Higher vitamin K content protects against hemorrhagic disease of the newborn.
Contaminants	Pesticides, pollutants, organic mercury, lead, DDT and radioactive compounds.	Strontium, pesticides, antibiotics, adulteration, and bacterial pathogens.

(contd.)

TABLE 15.1 Biochemical and physiological differences between human and cow's milk (composition per 100 mL) (contd.)		
Nutrients	Human milk	Cow's milk
Diseases related to the type of feeding	Hemorrhagic disease of the newborn, breast-milk jaundice, rickets, transmission of viral infections like CMV, HBV and HIV, maternal medications and allergens	Tetany, late-onset metabolic acidosis, milk allergy, iron deficiency anemia, acroderma-titis enteropathica (zinc deficiency), copper deficiency, sucrose intolerance, dental caries, infantile obesity, insulin-dependent diabetes mellitus, hypertension, obesity, and lymphoma.
Calories	65	67 Caloric content can be improved by addition of sugar.

*The highest concentrations of secretory IgA, DHA, lactose and sialic acid are found in human milk (especially colostrum) compared to any other milk. Zebra milk is closest in composition to human milk. Donkey's milk is also similar to human milk in composition but is most expensive compared to any premium brand of dairy milk. Goat's milk composition is also similar to human milk but it is deficient in folic acid. Infant milk formula is similar to cow's milk in composition except some newer formulae have been humanized by matching the composition of macronutrients and by adding essential fatty acids and DHA. They are expensive and do not contain anti-infective agents and cellular elements.

Human milk contains live cells to the extent of $1–2 \times 10^6$ leukocytes/mL. Macrophages make up to 90% of these white cells while 10% are lymphocytes with equal distribution of B and T cells. Macrophages offer primary line of defense against many pathogens. Recent evidence suggests the existence of entero-mammary and bronchomammary immunologic axes in the breast milk. Majority of B cells in the colostrum differentiate into IgA secreting plasma cells similar to B cells at mucosal sites and most of the antibodies elaborated by them are directed against enteric and respiratory pathogens in the environment of mother–infant dyad. Probiotics in human milk provide protection against enteric pathogens. There is evidence to suggest that cell-mediated immune response following BCG vaccination is better in breastfed babies as compared to top fed infants. In general, breastfed babies have better serum and secretory responses to oral and parenteral vaccines. Breastfed babies have also been shown to have reduced risk of lympho-reticular malignancy in later life.

Non-Nutritional Components

Apart from antimicrobial factors and immune modulators, breast milk contains digestive enzymes (especially lipase), hormones, trophic factors (to enhance maturity of gut) and growth modulators. Breast milk lipase breaks down fat into small globules for better digestion and assimilation. There is evidence to suggest that presence of trans-palmitic acid in human milk may reduce the risk of type 2 diabetes mellitus. Breast milk contains endocannabinoids which control the appetite of the baby to prevent under and overfeeding of the baby. Breast milk is loaded with a large number of anti-infective agents as a safeguard against development of infections. In the acidic environment of stomach, α-lactalbumin binds with oleic acid to form a complex called HAMLET (Human α-lactalbumin Made LEthal to Tumor cells) that kills tumor cells and provides protection against cancer to breastfed babies. The presence of epidermal growth factor, insulin-like growth factor 1 and peptides in human milk promotes physical growth.

Preparation for Breastfeeding

The preparation and motivation for breastfeeding should begin during antenatal visits. The cleaning of nipples, their eversion if retracted and treatment for cracked nipples must be instituted well in advance during pregnancy so that the baby should not face any mechanical difficulties. The absence of these problems during early nursing is of fundamental importance to establish a cordial mother–child bonding and to reduce the incidence of lactation failure. There is no correlation between the size of breasts and adequacy of lactation. Milk is produced in special glands in the breasts which are present in adequate number in all women irrespective of the size of breasts. The adequacy or insufficiency of lactation may have genetic basis.

Establishment of Lactation

The motivation and preparation for breastfeeding should begin during antenatal period. Awareness, willingness, keenness and confidence on the part of mother are crucial for successful establishment of lactation. Early bonding soon after delivery promotes breastfeeding. Healthy infant should be roomed-in with the mother and should never be separated from the mother by keeping him in the nursery. Early breastfeeding to all babies, irrespective of the mode of delivery, and avoidance of prelacteal and prolacteal feeds is essential to establish successful breastfeeding. Active support to the mother, use of proper technique and good attachment or latching of the baby to the breast facilitates breastfeeding.

Some women may fail to establish satisfactory lactation because of constitutional or genetic reasons but the condition is uncommon. Malnutrition does not significantly affect the adequacy of lactation but milk produced may be deficient in fat, vitamins and minerals. Mother must take additional food, supplements of micronutrients and drink plenty of liquids during nursing. The milk is produced as a result of interaction between hormones and neuropsychologic reflexes. Prolactin, a hormone produced by the anterior pituitary, stimulates glandular tissue of breast to produce milk. When baby sucks, the nerve endings in the nipple carry messages to the anterior pituitary which in turn releases prolactin in the blood. The more the baby sucks at the breast, greater is the stimulus for milk production by release of prolactin. The earlier the baby is put to the breast, sooner this reflex is initiated. The greater is the demand for milk, higher is the quantity of milk produced.

The release or ejection of milk is facilitated by let down reflex which is mediated through release of oxytocin from posterior pituitary. Oxytocin is released in response to stimulation of the nerve endings in the nipple by sucking as well as by thought, sight, smell or cry of the baby. It is responsible for the contraction of myoepithelium around the glands leading to ejection of milk from the glands into the lacteal sinuses and lacteal ducts located behind the areola. Since this reflex is affected by mother's emotions, a relaxed, comfortable and tension free atmosphere promotes the milk ejection reflex. On the other hand, a tense, apprehensive, worried mother or occurrence pain and discomfort during breastfeeding hinders the milk flow. Effective attachment and emptying of breast during each feeding is associated with enhanced milk production (Figure 15.1). The practice of introducing

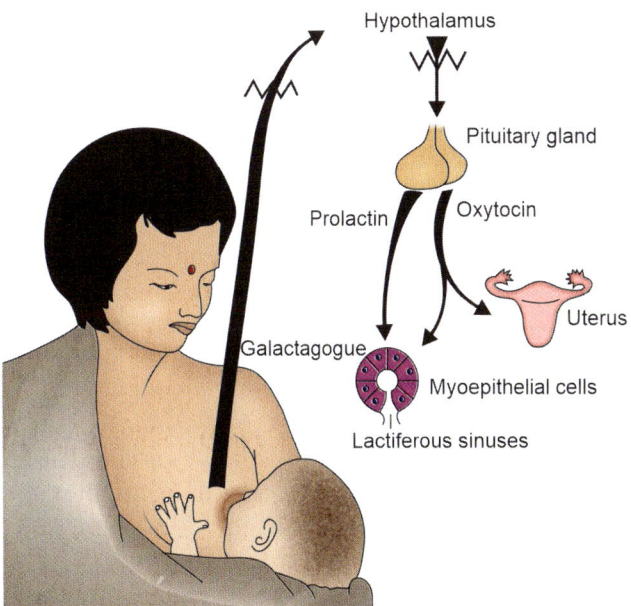

Figure 15.1 The let-down reflex. See the text for details. The release of oxytocin during sucking also causes involution or contractions of uterus so that it rapidly shrinks to pre-pregnancy size. The release of prolactin inhibits ovulation so that there is a state of relative infertility during breast-feeding.

bottle feeds (especially to cesarean born babies) during first 1–2 days is the most important cause of lactation failure.

Adequate nutrition during lactation is crucial to improve the quantity and quality of breast milk. Nutritional supplements are essential to meet the nutritional cost of lactation and enable the nursing mother to preserve her own nutrition and health. It has been documented that undernourished women produce poor quality of milk with marginally lower fat content but significantly reduced levels of essential micronutrients. It is desirable to supplement the diet of nursing mothers with micronutrients to enhance the concentration of vitamins and trace minerals in her milk. Maternal intake of ergometrine, estrogens, or estrogen-containing contraceptives, bromocriptine, thiazides and pyridoxine are known to suppress lactation. There is no ideal galactagogue but administration of domperidone or metoclopramide (10 mg 3 times/day for 7–10 days) to a nursing mother has been shown to increase milk production. Self-confidence in her ability to successfully breastfeed, freedom from anxiety, adequate rest, emotional support, and vigorous sucking by an active baby are the most effective prerequisites for successful establishment of lactation.

Feeding and Nutrition

15

Diet during Lactation

It must be remembered that nutritional cost of lactation is higher than the nutritional cost of pregnancy. The nursing mother must take at least 25% additional calories and nutrients compared to her pre-pregnancy food intake. She should have a well-balanced diet with sufficient proteins in the form of milk and milk products, pulses, legumes, eggs and poultry. She should have sufficient intake of fresh green leafy vegetables and seasonal fruits. It is recommended that a nursing mother should take 2.6 g omega-3 fatty acids and 300 mg DHA everyday from dietary sources or nutritional supplements. Fish and seafood are excellent sources of omega-3 fatty acids and DHA. The diet should be supplemented with commercially available micronutrients to enhance the concentration of vitamins and trace minerals in the breast milk. Mother should drink plenty of water and liquids to replenish the fluids lost through breast milk. Intake of nutritious balanced diet by the nursing mother is associated with improved nutritional quality of her breast milk. Healthy breastfed infants do not need any supplements of vitamins and minerals except vitamin K and vitamin D.

Role of Galactagogues

The substances which are credited to enhance milk production are called galactagogues or lactagogues. In Ayurvedic system, a large number of food items are recommended to promote lactation. Home remedies for improving milk yield include intake of fenugreek (*methi*) seeds, tulsi seeds, pupali, fennel (*saunf*), cumin seeds (*jeera*), cinnamon (*dalchini*), poppy seeds (*khaskhas*), garlic, ajwain, ginger, gum, coriander seeds (*dhania*), alfalfa, unripe papaya, oats, etc. virtually anything in the kitchen. The very fact that the list of galactagogues is so large, it suggests that there is no fool proof remedy and they are all based on folklore, faith and figment of imagination. The aforementioned food items are usually consumed in the form of *laddoos, kheer* or porridge, *burfi, halwa, mukhwas,* sprinklers or decoctions like herbal tea. In modern system of medicine, there is no potent or effective galactagogue. Metaclopramide has been tried with a variable efficacy for promotion of lactation.

Types of Breast Milk

The composition of breast milk varies at different stages of lactation to suit the needs of the baby. Milk of a mother who has delivered a preterm baby is different from milk of a mother who has given birth to a full term baby. *Therefore, the milk is not only species specific, it is baby specific!*

Colostrum It is a thin and golden-yellow milk secreted during the first three days after delivery. It is secreted in small quantities and it is low in carbohydrates (5.3 g/dL) and fats (2.9 g/dL) providing 53 calories per 100 mL. It is rich in protein (3.7 g/dL) and is loaded with protective secretory immunoglobulins, oligosaccharides (sialic acid), beta carotene (imparting yellow color) and sodium. The whey to casein ratio is 90:10 in colostrum. By virtue of its high content of secretory IgA, it virtually works like a "first vaccine shot" for the baby by blocking the entry of pathogenic bacteria through the gut. Colostrum is also credited with laxative effect facilitating the passage of meconium and preventing bilirubin build-up by promoting enterohepatic circulation.

Transitional milk is the milk secreted during the following two weeks, before lactation is established.

Mature milk follows transitional milk. It is thinner and watery but contains all the nutrients essential for optimal growth of the baby.

Weaning milk the breast milk during weaning is characterized by reduced volume, higher concentration of protein, sodium, iron, and reduced concentration of lactose.

Preterm milk The milk of a mother who delivers prematurely contains more calories, higher concentration of fat, protein and sodium which are needed by her preterm baby. The concentration of lactose, calcium and phosphorus are lower as compared to milk produced by mothers of term infants. During next 2–3 weeks, the composition of milk gradually changes and assumes composition akin to mature milk.

The composition of milk also varies during the phase of feeding.

Foremilk is the milk secreted at the start of a feed. It is thin, and sweet and is rich in proteins, sugar, vitamins, minerals and water.

Hindmilk is released towards the end of a feed and it is thicker and richer in fat content and provides more energy and satiety.

For optimum growth, the baby needs both foremilk as well as the hindmilk to satisfy his thirst as well as hunger. The baby should, therefore, be allowed to empty one breast completely before being put on to the other breast.

Drip milk The milk that drips from the opposite breast during breastfeeding is called drip milk. It is mainly foremilk with relatively low energy and fat content.

The Art and Technique of Breastfeeding

Immediately after delivery, the baby should be placed on mother's abdomen which enhances bonding and promotes lactation. The baby should be put on the breast as soon as the mother has recovered from labor preferably within half an hour after birth. Most babies born by cesarean section can be put to the breast within 4 hours of birth. No prelacteal feeds like glucose water, honey or tea should be offered. The feeds should be offered on a semi-demand schedule, keeping in mind that most babies would need to be fed after every 2 to 3 hours. The mother should sit up comfortably and keep the baby's head slightly raised and offer alternate breast at each feed (Figure 15.2). The baby's head and neck are comfortably placed on the hollow of the elbow while back and buttock of the baby are supported by the forearm and hand of the mother. The mother touches the baby's cheek or side of the mouth to her breast to stimulate the rooting reflex and the baby opens the mouth and turns toward the

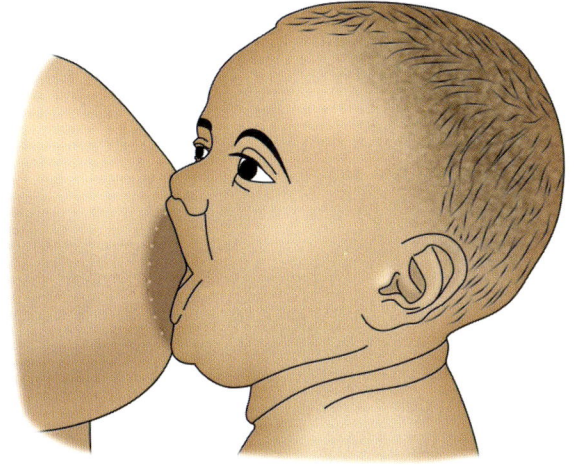

Figure 15.3 Correct technique of breastfeeding. The baby forms an effective seal around the nipple and areola to ensure "attachment" for ejection of milk from lactiferous sinuses.

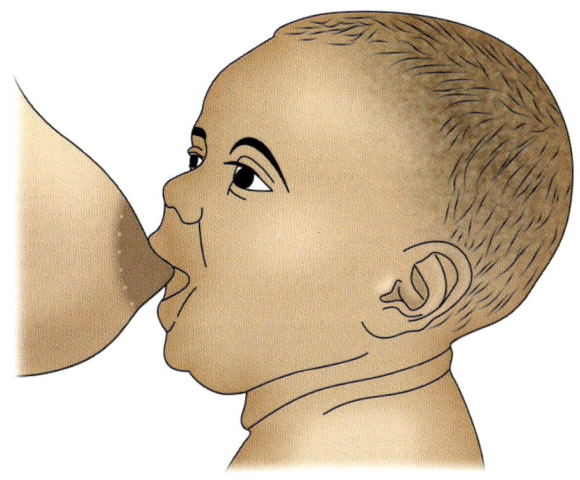

Figure 15.4 Wrong technique of breastfeeding. The baby is merely sucking at the nipple which may lead to soreness of nipple and poor ejection of milk with engorgement of breast.

nipple. She can help position the nipple and areola into the baby's mouth. For effective sucking, the baby must form an effective seal around the nipple and areola to eject the milk from lacteal sinuses. Proper "attachment" or "latchment" is indeed the key for successful breastfeeding and both the nipple and areola must be effectively grasped by the baby (Figure 15.3). If the baby sucks only at the nipple, the milk is not ejected. When baby does not get sufficient milk, he sucks more vigorously resulting in sore nipples (Figure 15.4).

During the first few days, most of the babies fall asleep after taking a few sucks. They should be kept aroused by gentle tickling behind the ears or on the

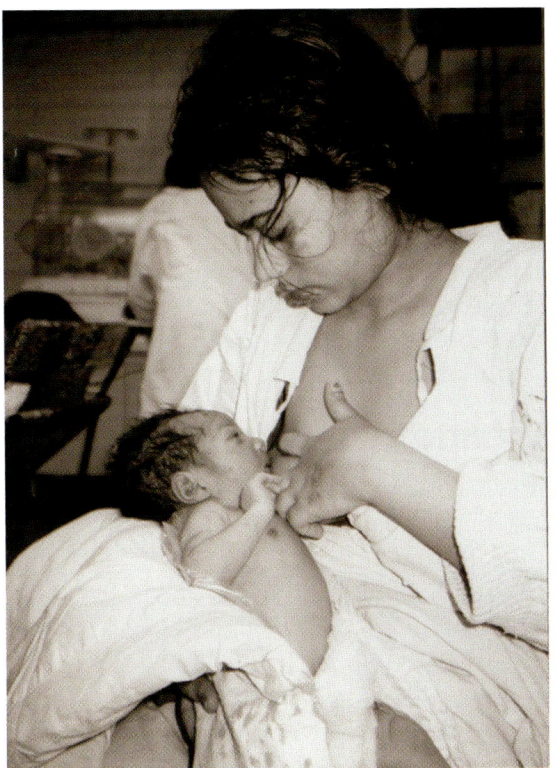

Figure 15.2 Baby is being breastfed soon after birth. Note the position of the infant, support to the breast and 'active' involvement of the mother.

soles during feeds but the ritual should not be unpleasant or annoying to the baby. The mother must actively interact and intently look towards the child during breastfeeding. She should avoid watching the television or talking to somebody while breastfeeding.

The breastfeeding is not a passive ritual, the baby enjoys the maternal warmth, contact and cuddling during the procedure. When mother perceives that baby is getting lazy and sleepy, as evidenced by the reduced force and frequency of sucks, she should try to partially remove the nipple when baby would wake up and start sucking again with renewed vigour. Most babies take 15 to 20 minutes to take an adequate feed. The baby should be allowed to completely empty one breast before offering the other breast. Some babies are satisfied with feeding from one breast, others may need to suck at the second breast as well. The baby should be allowed to take his time at each breast because premature breast-switching may rob babies of "hindmilk" which has a higher fat content. Alternate breast should be offered first at the next feed. The contented baby is playful, sleeps well, gains weight regularly (after first week of life) and voids urine at least six or more times during the day. The baby must be satisfied for at least two hours before he starts crying for the next feed. The mother must be explained the art of burping the baby after each feed to safeguard against regurgitation (Figure 15.5).

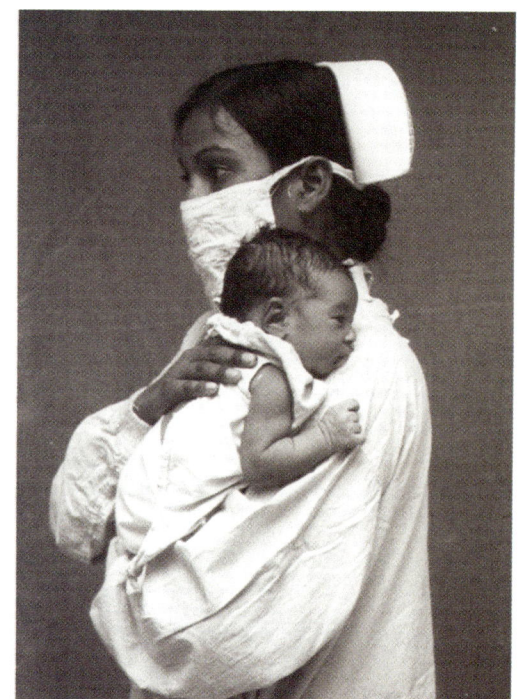

Figure 15.5 The infant should be held upright against the shoulder after every feed to facilitate burping.

During the first 2 to 3 days, when lactation is not fully established, the mother is often anxious that her baby is not getting adequate nourishment. It must be explained to her that the act of sucking establishes lactation and whatever little colostrum the baby receives during the first few days, it is enough to meet the nutritional needs of a normal baby. Healthy babies do have enough stores of glycogen and they do not need any complementary feeds. It is desirable to avoid the introduction of bottle for the fear of contamination and development of diarrhea. The introduction of bottle-feeding would lead to "nipple confusion" and the baby would refuse breastfeeding because mechanism of sucking at bottle teat and breast are totally different. Most babies demand a mid-night feed during the first 6–8 weeks of life, after which their feeding schedule is established satisfactorily and they are satisfied with one late night feed and an early morning feed.

During first 6 months, exclusive breastfeeding (no water should be offered even in hot summer months) is advocated. The exclusively breastfed babies are likely to drink more milk when thirsty and, therefore, have a better weight gain. It is generally agreed that adequate breastfeeding alone is sufficient to support the growth of infants up to 6 months of age. The working mother should try to provide exclusive breastfeeding for at least 6 months by availing most of the maternity leave after the delivery. The duration of maternity leave varies between 12 and 20 weeks in different states in India. There is a need to enhance duration of maternity leave up to 6 months at least to those mothers who maintain the two-baby norm. Availability of creches at the working places should be encouraged both in public and private sectors to promote breastfeeding. The strategies to promote successful breastfeeding are summarized in **Box 15.2**.

BABY-FRIENDLY HOSPITAL INITIATIVE

In order to encourage and promote exclusive breastfeeding to enhance child survival, the Baby-Friendly Hospital Initiative (BFHI) was launched jointly by WHO and UNICEF in 1991, following the Innocenti Declaration of 1990. Bottle being the biggest killer of babies in developing countries, a mission approach has been launched globally to resurrect the dwindling practice of breastfeeding. Efforts are being made to improve the knowledge, attitude and practices of health care workers by providing them with information, scientific facts and skills to promote exclusive breastfeeding during first 6 months of life. Mother–baby

---

Box 15.2: Recommendations for promotion of successful breastfeeding

- Education and advice must be given to every mother in the antenatal clinic. Retracted and cracked nipples must be managed before delivery.
- The first feed should be breast milk. No prelacteal feeds like water, honey, glucose water, and tea should be offered.
- Breastfeeding should preferably be started within first hour of life.
- The baby should be held in the correct position to ensure proper "attachment" to the breast by grasping both the nipple as well as areola.
- Mother can feed in any position that is comfortable both for herself and her baby.
- Rooming-in is a must for bonding and successful breast-feeding.
- Baby should be fed on demand and not by clock.
- Bottle feeds should not be introduced.
- A healthy breastfed baby of a healthy mother does not require any nutritional supplements except vitamin K and vitamin D.
- Frequent suckling, skin-to-skin contact, complete emptying of the breast, correct positioning, supportive care and encouragement are the cornerstones of successful lactation.

---

bonding at birth, avoidance of pre-lacteal feeds, early breastfeeding and practice of keeping the mother and her baby together in the rooming-in ward are encouraged. The representatives of infant food manufacturers are strictly forbidden to contact mothers or health care staff for distribution of low cost or free infant formula, feeding bottles and any literature pertaining to formula feedings. The advertisement and promotion of breast milk substitutes in media and distribution of pamphlets, calendars and growth charts, etc. is against the code of conduct and can attract penalty. The medical and nursing graduates, family physicians, pediatricians and obstetricians should be provided with adequate information, knowledge and skills during their formal training and subsequently by continuing medical education programs to ensure the sustainability of the BFHI program.

Ten Steps for Successful Breastfeeding

The following ten steps are recognized as minimum global criteria for attaining the status of a Baby Friendly Hospital.

Step 1. Have a written breastfeeding policy that is routinely communicated to all health staff The policy guidelines incorporating ten steps for successful breastfeeding should be prominently displayed in the antenatal clinic, delivery room, special care baby unit and maternity ward so that mothers and health care staff are constantly reminded of its importance and implementation. The hospital authorities should clearly state their commitment of not accepting any free or low cost samples of infant formula or any promotional material by the manufacturers of infant formula. The policy statements should be available both in English and local language which is readily understood by the mother and health care staff.

Step 2. Train health care staff in skills necessary to implement this policy The health care staff should be trained in the art and science of breastfeeding. The practical training to implement ten steps for successful breastfeeding should be taught as a part of ongoing in-service training program. They should be provided with practical information and skills to assist the nursing mothers for manual and mechanical expression of breast milk, correct positioning and attachment of the baby during breastfeeding, causes and management of lactation failure and promotion of exclusive breastfeeding.

Step 3. Inform all pregnant women about the benefits and management of breastfeeding During antenatal period, the mothers should be informed and educated regarding the nutritional, biological and emotional advantages of breastfeeding not only to their babies but to the nursing mothers as well. They should be motivated and assisted for promotion of exclusive breastfeeding. The problems like retracted, flat, small or cracked nipples should be managed during the antenatal period. The principles and factors known to promote lactation should be explained. They should be made aware of dangers of bottle feeding.

Step 4. Help mothers to initiate breastfeeding within half-hour of birth Establish mother–baby bonding soon after delivery and encourage all mothers to put the baby on the breast within half-hour of birth. They should be advised not to administer any pre-lacteal feeds. Babies born by cesarean section should be put to the breast as soon as the mother has recovered from the effect of anesthesia.

Step 5. Show mothers how to breastfeed and how to maintain lactation, even if they are separated from their infants The mothers should be taught the art of breastfeeding. When their baby is small or sick, they should be taught the correct technique of expressing the breast milk manually or with the help of breast pump to maintain adequate lactation.

Step 6. Give newborn infants no food or drink other than breast milk, unless medically indicated Ensure, as far are possible, exclusive feeding of all newborn babies with human milk. The staff should know the indications and options when supplementation is required.

Step 7. Practice rooming-in and allow mothers and infants to remain together round-the-clock The policy of keeping healthy normal babies or babies born by cesarean section in a nursery is strongly condemned because it is detrimental for the success of breastfeeding.

Step 8. Encourage breastfeeding on demand The mothers should be encouraged to breastfeed their babies whenever they are hungry and as often and as long as the baby wants.

Step 9. Give no artificial feeds or pacifiers (also called dummies and soothers) to breastfeeding babies No pacifiers should be promoted in the hospital due to their potential risk of causing infection and compromising nutrition. Expressed breast milk or any other medically indicated fluids should be administered either through an orogastric tube or spoon/*paladay* (depending upon the vigor and maturity of the infant) and the use of feeding bottles should be avoided.

Step 10. Foster the establishment of breastfeeding support groups and refer mothers to them on discharge from the hospital or clinic The breastfeeding women's support group should be established in the community for the promotion of breastfeeding. There should be an effective system of follow-up support for all breastfeeding mothers after they are discharged from the hospital or nursing home. The key family members should be sensitized and motivated to support the breastfeeding mother. The nursing mother should be encouraged to take a nutritious diet to sustain her health and to ensure good quality of milk output.

The Procedure for Recognition of a Hospital as Baby-friendly

The BFHI movement is active in India under a national task force comprising of government of India, UNICEF, WHO and a large number of professional bodies and voluntary organizations. A number of regional workshops have been organized on lactation management and for training of BFHI assessors. The

following three steps are mandatory for recognition of a hospital as baby-friendly.

1. A hospital that conducts a minimum of 250 deliveries per year can seek the recognition. After implementation of ten global steps for promotion of breastfeeding, a duly completed self-assessment form and registration form are sent to the BFHI secretariat.

2. The hospital/nursing home meeting all the ten criteria is visited by an assessor for on-the-spot checks and to interview the mothers and health care staff. The assessor sends his report and observations to the BFHI secretariat which is reviewed by the Review Committee for final recommendation.

3. The hospital/s fulfilling the national BFHI requirements are recognized as "baby-friendly". The National Task Force organizes a public ceremony for presentation of BFHI recognition certificate and a logo-plaque. The hospitals who are unable to fulfill the required criteria for certification are informed regarding their shortcomings. They can reapply for certification at a later date after correction of all the shortcomings.

Contraindications to Breastfeeding

There are a few genuine contraindications to breastfeeding. During acute febrile maternal illness and development of breast abscess, the breastfeeding should be withheld temporarily and breast milk expressed manually and discarded. By and large, medications which are safely tolerated by the nursing mother, are generally safe for her suckling infant. The mother receiving anithyroid drugs (except propylthiouracil), ^{131}I, and anticancer agents should not breastfeed her baby. The presence of serious debilitating chronic illness in the mother contraindicates breastfeeding especially when help of some other person can be secured to bottle feed the baby. Infant of a mother with active tuberculosis should be administered INH 10 mg/kg per day for 3 months followed by BCG vaccination. Breastfeeding can be given unless mother is critically ill. Isolation is often impractical and bottle feeding hazardous in the socio-economic milieu in which tuberculosis occurs. Breastfeeding is associated with 10–15% risk of transmission of HIV infection. The decision for advising or withholding breastfeeding should be individualized on the basis of socioeconomic status, education, awareness and risk of bottle feeding (*see* Chapter 16 for details). Following administration of radiopharmaceuticals, breastfeeding should be temporarily withheld till radioactive agent is eliminated from the breast milk. The complete list of medications to the nursing mothers and their hazards to the breastfeeding infants are given in Chapter 5.

ADEQUACY OF LACTATION

The commonest excuse for starting bottle feeding is inadequacy of lactation. The problem of genuine lactation failure does exist but is rare. The condition appears to be genetically determined but is aggravated by poor motivation on the part of mother and lack of social support system and proper guidance to her. The common causes of insufficient lactation include maternal malnutrition or acute illness, poor latching or slow sucking by the baby (preterm, sick or malformed baby), intake of estrogen-containing hormonal contraceptives and rarely postpartum hypopituitarism (Sheehan syndrome). The following conditions and parameters should be evaluated which are indicative of satisfactory lactation.

1. There are no anatomical problems in the breast or nipple and baby is mature and healthy and without any oral abnormalities like cleft lip, cleft palate, and thrush.
2. During feeding, the milk drips from the contra-lateral breast.
3. The mother should actively interact with the baby during breastfeeding to ensure effective feeding for at least 10–15 minutes.
4. The baby is satisfied, happy and playful and sleeps for at least 2 hours before crying for the next feed.
5. The sodium content of breast milk is less than 16 mmol/L.
6. The baby voids urine at least 6 times or more during daytime.
7. The weight gain of the baby is satisfactory.

The best guide to adequate feeding is a satisfactory weight gain. Most term babies lose up to 5 to 8% of their body weight during the first 2 to 3 days and loss is relatively higher in exclusively breastfed babies. The birth weight is regained by 5 to 7 days of age and subsequently they gain on an average of 30 g per day during the first 4 months of life.

COMMON FEEDING PROBLEMS

Primigravida mother problems The primigravida mother, though equipped with instinctive information, may face initial difficulties in breastfeeding because of anxiety, worry and lack of confidence. The poor milk output during the first few days further aggravates

the situation and she may be disheartened unless sympathetic advice, encouragement and moral support are offered to her. The role of sucking for establishment of satisfactory lactation should be emphasized. The primigravida mothers also have a greater incidence of retracted nipples.

Mechanical difficulties Feeding difficulties due to mechanical reasons may occur in certain neonatal conditions such as cleft lip, cleft palate, macroglossia, thrush and incoordinated sucking and swallowing by premature babies. Abnormalities such as retracted nipples and engorgement of the breasts interfere with satisfactory feeding. Antenatal supervision and care of the breasts should reduce these problems. If nipples are retracted, mother should be advised to evert and pull the nipples out and roll them between her index and middle fingers. Syringe method should be used for evertion of nipples because nipple shield is not very effective (Figure 15.6). The mother should wear breast shell under her bra to avoid compression of nipples. The baby should be given EBM with a cup and spoon. Attempts at breastfeeding should be continued and mother should try to ensure proper attachment of the baby to the breast by holding the nipple and areola in her fingers.

Sore or cracked nipples Avoid frequent washing of nipples with soap and water. Do not offer complementary feeds with a bottle (instead give with a cup and spoon/*paladay*) because it leads to nipple confusion. The baby should not suck on the nipple and instead he should grasp the breast tissue along with areola. Pulling the baby forcefully from the nipple without de-latching may cause damage to the nipple. The mother should wear loose clothes and avoid the use of bra. The plastic breast shields or plastic-lined nursing pads should not be worn because they hold the moisture. The breastfeeding should be continued and an emollient cream or hindmilk applied over the nipples in-between the feeds.

Engorged breasts Some mothers develop engorgement of the breasts after the third day of delivery. The breasts become heavy, swollen, hard and painful. This may lead to infection, formation of breast abscess and lactation failure, if not tackled promptly. This is best prevented by early feeding of the baby and frequent suckling. If engorgement continues, the milk must be expressed and collected in a sterile container. If the baby is not in a position to suck, the expressed milk can be fed to the infant with a cup and spoon. Alternatively, a healthy and hungry baby may be put to the breast after expressing the milk and relieving the

- Take a 10 mL plastic syringe and remove its piston.
- After cutting the barrel half a centimeter from the nozzle, insert the piston from the cut end of the barrel.
- Place the other non-ragged end of the barrel around the nipple and withdraw the piston gently. The nipple will slowly protrude into the barrel. After 30–60 seconds, push the piston back gently to release the hold of the syringe on the nipple.
- Repeat this procedure 5–8 times before each breastfeeding.
- As soon as the nipple becomes prominent, the nipple and areola should be held between index finger and thumb to form a teat and the baby is put to the breast.
- Avoid use of a nipple shield which is ineffective and may be harmful.
- Mother should wear a breast shell under her bra to avoid compression of nipples.

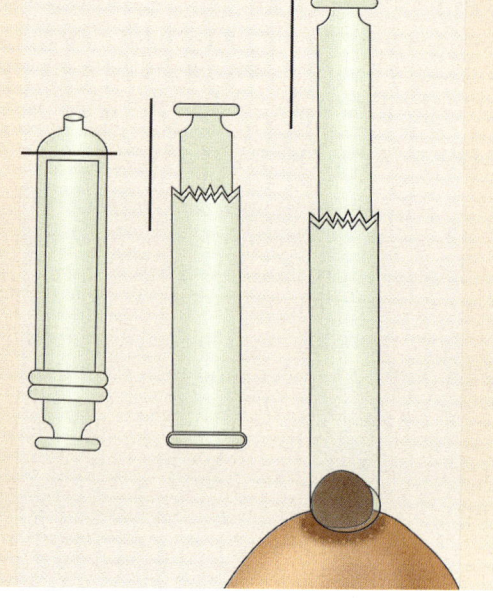

Figure15.6 Syringe method for treatment of retracted nipples.

engorgement. Demand feeding helps to prevent engorgement and frequent sucking keeps the breasts soft and non-tender. Hot fomentation provides relief to the engorged breasts. At times hot fomentation may aggravate engorgement due to increase in blood flow. In this case, cold compresses with chilled cabbage leaves with a hole in the center, is more beneficial. A safe analgesic like paracetamol can be given to the mother for relief of pain.

Regurgitation Most healthy babies regurgitate some feeds off and on but they continue to gain weight satisfactorily. The condition resolves by advising the mother to prop the baby on her lap or hold him against the shoulder to help him eructate the swallowed air (Figure 15.5). After this, the baby should be put to bed in the left lateral position with head end slightly raised.

Alterations of bowel movements The breastfed babies tend to pass frequent semi-loose, golden-yellow sticky stools due to high lactose content. Babies on cow's milk or formula feeding are often constipated and pass hard non-sticky stools due to formation of casein curds. The constipation can be relieved by giving glucose water, extra sugar in the milk or formula, honey and fruit juice to the baby.

Underfeeding and overfeeding Overfeeding is uncommon in the newborn period but underfeeding and starvation due to feeding with diluted milk may adversely affect the growth of the baby. Many a times, dilution is done purely for economic reasons and rationalized explanations are given, particularly so in

case of babies receiving feeds made up from dried milk powders. After about 3 months of age, the cost of feeding full strength powdered milk formula becomes exorbitant and unaffordable.

FAQs REGARDING BREASTFEEDING

How to ensure that baby is having good "Attachment" during breastfeeding?

The following features suggest that the baby has learnt to ensure good "attachment" or "latching" for proper feeding:

1. Baby's mouth is wide open.
2. Chin of the baby touches the breast.
3. Nipple and most of the areola is inside the baby's mouth.
4. Lower lip is turned outwards.
5. Mother feels no pain or discomfort while breast-feeding.

How to delatch the baby from the breast?

When baby is satisfied or falls asleep while feeding, he automatically releases the breast. But when the baby has stopped sucking but is still maintaining strong suction, do not pull him off the nipple. Instead, mother should slide her index finger into the corner of the baby's mouth to break the suction and delatch the baby.

How frequently the baby should be put to the breast?

There should be no fixed timing for feeding. The baby should be fed on demand, day and night, whenever baby appears to be hungry. The more a baby sucks on the mother's breast, more milk is produced. Most babies would like to be fed every 2–3 hours. The night feeds are required for initial 4–6 weeks or even longer in healthy normal weight babies.

What should be the duration of each breastfeed?

It is variable, but most active healthy babies take 10–15 minutes to finish a feed. Many babies fall asleep after a few sucks and then demand a feed after half to one hour. Mother should play and interact with her baby while breastfeeding by caressing the ear lobes or stroking the soles. When baby gets lazy, mother should try to partially remove her nipple; the baby will wake up again and start sucking vigorously. While feeding, mother should look at her baby intently and interact with him during the process of feeding. *Breastfeeding is an active process and mother must pay her full attention to the baby while feeding.* During breastfeeding, mother provides warmth, skin-to-skin contact, love, affectionate look and tender touch and music of her heart beats to her baby thus stimulating all the five special senses of her baby! *Apart from wholesome nutrition, breastfeeding provides global sensory stimulation to the baby.*

The foremilk or first part of milk which flows when a baby starts to breastfeed is thin and rich in protein and lactose while the latter or hindmilk is thick and rich in fat. The baby should be allowed to completely empty one breast so that both his thirst and hunger are satisfied by taking foremilk and hindmilk. Baby should be allowed to feed as long as he wants at one breast before offering the other breast. During the next feed, partially emptied breast should be offered first to ensure complete emptying of each breast.

How long to continue breastfeeding?

During initial 6 months, exclusive breastfeeding is advised, no water should be given to the baby even in hot summer months. The baby will drink more milk when thirsty and would have better weight gain. *Exclusively breastfed babies do not develop infective diarrhea and they have adequate weight gain during first 6 months.* Breast milk is a complete food for the baby and there is no need to give any supplements of vitamins (except vitamin D) and minerals to healthy full term babies of healthy mothers during first 6 months. If mother is malnourished or baby has intrauterine growth retardation, zinc-containing multivitamin drops may be given to the baby. There is no role of giving *janam ghutti, jaiphal* (nutmeg) and gripe water to babies. Semi-solid home-made weaning foods should be offered after 6 months of age but breastfeeding should be continued as long as feasible;

at least for a minimum period of 1–2 years. Breast-feeding is continued as long as feasible or desired but it is important to ensure that the baby gets adequate nutrition by taking enough complementary semisolid weaning foods of cereals, pulses, vegetables and fruits.

What is nipple confusion?

Some mothers start 1 to 2 bottle feeds along with breast-feeds with the mistaken belief that otherwise it will not be possible to wean the baby off the breast. It is unwise and strongly discouraged because firstly the mechanisms for sucking from the breast and rubber teat of the feeding bottle are different and secondly according to current recommendations there is no place for bottle-feeding in the care of babies. Bottle-feeding is easier for the baby because he can readily get the milk by pressing the soft rubber teat while in case of breastfeeding the baby has to firmly take a big bite of the breast tissue under the areola and suck with a considerable effort with coordinated movements of lips, gums and tongue. Breastfeeding demands more effort and is usually tiring. *Once a baby gets used to the easier option of taking milk from the bottle, he refuses to accept the breast because we are all lazy and so are the babies.* Moreover, baby may start sucking or biting at the nipple (like he does to the rubber teat of the bottle) due to "nipple confusion" with unsatisfactory sucking efforts and development of cracked nipples.

How to know that the baby is getting enough milk?

During breastfeeding when milk drips from the other breast, it suggests mother has satisfactory lactation. As a safeguard against the mess and embarrassment of leaking breasts, mother can use absorbent breast pads under the bra. When a baby is adequately fed he is satisfied, happy and playful or sleeps after a feed for 2–3 hours. Most babies pass urine after every feed. When a baby passes dilute water-like urine at least 6–8 times in a day, it suggests that baby is having enough feeds. Some babies enjoy sucking their fingers and it is not suggestive of inadequacy of breast milk. *The best criterion that the baby is getting enough milk is the satisfactory weight gain.* During first 4 months, most babies gain on an average 30 g weight everyday (750–900 g/month). The baby must be weighed on a reliable weighing scale during each visit to the hospital for vaccination and routine check-up. "Test weighing" (weight record before and after giving a breastfeed) is unnecessary and not recommended to assess the adequacy of lactation. Excessive crying alone should not be taken as an evidence of poor feeding because babies cry due to a variety of reasons like discomfort of wet napkins, intestinal colic, gastroesophageal reflux, exposure to cold or being over clothed, insect or mosquito bites, and boredom, etc.

What is the usual stool frequency during breast-feeding?

Most normal healthy breastfed babies pass 4–6 golden-yellow sticky stools. Babies fed on cow's milk or formula feeds tend to be constipated but are more vulnerable to develop infective diarrhea. Some babies may pass a stool during or soon after a feed because they have an overactive gastrocolic reflex. Mother should not be worried about this problem because baby would continue to have satisfactory weight gain.

Should a sick baby be given breastfeeding?

Breastfeeding is an ideal food for a sick baby. Many a times, a sick baby refuses to accept any other food but continues to take breastfeeds. When a sick baby is active and able to suck, he must be given breast-feeding. A critically sick baby can be given expressed breast milk (EBM) through a nasogastric tube.

Should breastfeeding be continued when mother is ill?

Most illnesses in the mother do not contraindicate breastfeeding. The mother produces antibodies against the infective organisms and these antibodies cross-over through the breast milk and protect the baby. Breast milk does not transmit disease causing germs. The baby cannot catch cold through the breast-milk but baby can get infected by close contact with her mother through hands and droplets thrown by her while talking, coughing and sneezing. When a mother is critically sick or suffering from cancer (and receiving anti-cancer medicines) or AIDS, she is advised to bottle feed her baby. Mother with jaundice can safely breastfeed her baby but she should observe strict aseptic precautions to prevent transmission of hepatitis A and E viruses through hands and fomites.

What medicines should be avoided by the nursing mother?

In general what is safely tolerated by the nursing mother is safe for her suckling infant. Mother should avoid intake of sedatives as they can make her baby lazy and inactive. Intake of medicated laxative can cause diarrhea in the suckling infant. It is safe for nursing mother to take milk of magnesia, liquid paraffin and glycerin suppository for relief of constipation. Intake of antibiotics by nursing mother may cause diarrhea in her suckling infant. Intake of anticancer, antithyroid drugs (except propylthiouracil), anticoagulants and certain antidepressant drugs contraindicate breast-feeding.

Can twins be reared on breastfeeding alone?

Many mothers can rear twin babies on exclusive breastfeeding without any complementary feeds. Many lower mammals are endowed with several breasts (and nipples) depending upon their average litter size. It would appear that two breasts should be sufficient to effectively suckle two babies before they are able to accept weaning foods. Mother can offer alternate breast for feeding each twin baby. If weight gain is unsatisfactory with exclusive breastfeeding, complementary feeds should be given alternating with breastfeeds. However, mother of twin babies must receive tremendous support, encouragement and assistance by family members because it is an herculean task to simultaneously nurture and look after two babies. She should take additional calories, proteins and micronutrients to produce enough milk of satisfactory nutritional quality to sustain the growth of two babies.

What foods should be avoided during nursing?

Mother who is breastfeeding should take a normal diet without too much chillies and condiments. Excessive indulgence in any particular food or fruit should be avoided. It is well known that intake of lentils with their covering, black *urad dal,* kidney beans, Bengal gram and *kabli channa* by the nursing mother may cause wind, discomfort and loose motions in her suckling infant. Cruciferous vegetables like cabbage, cauliflower, broccoli sprouts, turnips, radish, beans, mustard leaves (*sarson ka saag*) may also cause distension and gas both in the mother and her suckling infant. When a mother feels that intake of a particular food item consistently upsets her baby by causing colic or loose motions, she should avoid it or take it in moderation.

How can a working mother breastfeed her baby?

Mother should take most of her maternity leave after the delivery of her baby. She should extend her leave as much as she can so that she can ensure exclusive breastfeeding as long as possible. If she has to get back to work, she can follow any one of the following alternatives.

1. Availability of a crèche near the vicinity of work-place is useful so that she can visit her baby for breastfeeding during office hours and lunch break.
2. If a baby is more than 4 months old, he can be fed with a pre-cooked cereal, soft rice-*dal* gruel (*khichdi*), curd and mashed banana. Thus, a working mother can start weaning foods earlier, than the current recommendation of 6 months.

3. Mother can express her milk and store it in a container having a tight-fitting lid. The milk can be safely stored for 8 hours at room temperature and up to 24 hours in a refrigerator. She can breastfeed her baby before going to work and on returning back. When she is away, expressed breast milk can be fed to the baby with a spoon or *paladay. It is desirable not to introduce bottle-feeding to avoid nipple confusion and reduce the risk of infective diarrhea.*

Should cesarean born babies be given formula feeds during initial few days?

In most cases of elective cesarean section, mother can breastfeed her baby as soon as she has recovered from general anesthesia. In case of subdural or spinal anesthesia, she can breastfeed soon after delivery. Nevertheless, when a mother has undergone cesarean section, she needs more support and encouragement to breastfeed. She needs to identify the posture of comfort and should be provided with assistance in holding or supporting the baby. During initial one or two days, she can breastfeed while lying down in bed.

However, in a case of emergency cesarean section, when a mother is critically sick, the baby may be fed with a cup and spoon or *paladay* till she is well enough to breastfeed. Introduction of bottle feeds should be avoided because it may lead to "nipple confusion" thus causing difficulties in subsequent breastfeeding. It is important to remember, that ability to breastfeed depends upon will power and keenness or commitment to breastfeed rather than the mode of delivery or comfort level of the mother.

Should breast and nipple be washed with soap and water before each feed?

There is no need to wash the breasts and nipples with soap and water before each feed as it may lead to dryness and cracking of nipples. Daily bath and maintenance of personal hygiene is all that is needed by the nursing mother. Mother should wear nursing pads to prevent ugly patches on her clothes due to leakage of milk.

Should a baby be fed every 2 hours by clock?

Baby should be fed on demand (and not by clock) as and when he is hungry. There is no need to un-necessarily disturb or wake up a sleeping baby to give him a feed. Whenever baby cries because of hunger (check that he is not crying because of wet diaper or discomfort) mother should offer him a feed whether it is day or night. When a baby is sleeping excessively during daytime and the last feed was taken more than 4 hours ago, he can be woken up for the feed.

Can a mother with small breasts produce enough milk to feed her baby?

Just like other body attributes, breasts come in different shapes and sizes. Irrespective of the size of breasts, every woman is endowed with enough glandular tissue to effectively breastfeed her baby. Adequacy of lactation depends more on the keenness, and confidence of the mother, freedom from pain or discomfort, sucking stimulation provided by an active and healthy baby rather than the size and shape of breasts or nipples. Nevertheless, there may be genetic or constitutional factors which may determine that mothers in certain families are better milk producers than in others.

Should one or two bottle feeds be started along with breastfeeding so that there are no difficulties during weaning?

Nothing is more detrimental to the success of breastfeeding than early introduction of bottle feeding because it leads to "nipple confusion" and the baby would be more keen to feed from the bottle rather than the breast. Moreover, when a bottle is introduced, there is the potential risk of introduction of infection thus compromising the virtues of exclusive breastfeeding. Complementary semisolid weaning foods should be started after 6 months including milk products like yoghurt, *khichdi*, porridge, custard, *kheer* and cheese. The liquid milk should be started after one year directly with a glass or a cup. There is thus no place of bottle feeding to meet the nutritional demands of infants. The use of a sipper should be avoided because like a feeding bottle, it is also difficult to clean and may serve as a source of infection with a potential risk of development of diarrhea.

Why do breast fed babies look rather lean unlike formula fed babies, who are usually "chubby"?

It is true that formula fed babies gain weight faster and look "chubby" but they are "unhealthy" and at an increased risk to develop obesity, Type 2 diabetes mellitus and coronary artery disease later in life. The composition of human milk is ideal and best suited for optimal physical and mental growth of human babies. Nature has profound biological wisdom and milk of an animal is best suited to serve the biological needs of its offsprings and is not meant or is suitable to serve the nutritional needs of babies of other species.

Can a mother successfully breastfeed her second baby if she was unable to breastfeed her first baby?

Mother can successfully breastfeed her second baby if she has the necessary desire, motivation, will power and positive frame of mind. When a mother starts thinking that she cannot successfully breastfeed, it is unlikely that she would succeed. Positive thinking is a well-known mantra for success.

Is excessive crying a useful marker of inadequate lactation?

Apart from hunger, the babies cry due to a variety of other reasons like discomfort because of wet napkins, wind or colic, exposure or over clothing, over-stimulated or bored baby, nappy rash, and insect bites. When milk drips on the mere sight of the baby, baby passes urine at least 8 times or more in a day and is having satisfactory weight gain, it suggests that mother is having satisfactory lactation. Starting one or two bottle feeds on the mistaken belief that there is insufficient lactation, is the commonest cause of lactation failure and its unfortunate consequences.

Is breastfeeding more demanding and troublesome to the mother as opposed to bottle-feeding?

Bottle-feeding demands more effort on the part of the mother for sterilizing the bottles, preparing the formula, ensuring right temperature of the milk before feeding, maintaining strict asepsis especially if all this needs to be done by mother herself without the help of husband or other family members or a maid. Breastfeeding is certainly more convenient and less bothersome especially during night.

Is breastfeeding likely to make the breasts more saggy and unattractive?

The fact is that it is not the act of breastfeeding but pregnancy *per se* that affects the shape, size or firmness of the breasts. During pregnancy, the breasts go through various anatomical changes for promotion of lactation and even if a mother decides to bottle feed, the breasts are likely to sag unless a strong support is provided with a bra. Regular exercise of chest muscles (pectoralis) maintains the shape and contour of breasts. Excessive weight gain during pregnancy, hereditary factors and increasing age are other factors which may make the breasts less globular, loose and soft. Breastfeeding should not be blamed for something which is expected to happen sooner or later.

Should a mother avoid breastfeeding her second baby, when it caused jaundice in her first baby?

It is true that some breastfed babies may develop what is known as "breast milk jaundice". Jaundice may occur again in subsequent babies. There is nothing wrong with the mother's milk and she can safely breastfeed her subsequent babies. There is no need to interrupt breastfeedings for 2–3 days which some

pediatricians recommend as a treatment of "breast milk jaundice". Jaundice may last 6–8 weeks and disappears without any adverse effects to the baby. Infact it would appear that some jaundice is beneficial for the baby because bilirubin is an antioxidant and it is useful to prevent damage to various tissues due to reactive oxygen free radicals.

Should breastfeeding be continued when mother is having an infection or fever?

Unless mother is critically sick, fever due to common day-to-day infections should not be considered as an indication to stop breastfeeding. There is no risk of passage of infective microbes through the breast milk and instead protective antibodies produced in response to infection will get transferred to the baby through breast milk. Mother should continue to breastfeed her baby but take strict precautions like frequent hand washing, wearing a mask (if having cough and cold), not sharing towel or handkerchief, etc. with the baby to reduce the risk of transmission of infection to her baby due to close proximity with the baby.

Should breastfeeding be stopped when mother becomes pregnant?

It is desirable that parents should adopt family planning measures to prevent next pregnancy till the elder sibling is at least 2–3 years old. The next child should be born when the elder sibling is at least 3 years old and relatively independent and attending a play school. However, when a mother gets pregnant early, breastfeeding can be continued till mid-pregnancy. In this scenario, the weaning can be started at 4 months of age instead of the conventional recommendation of 6 months. Prolonged breastfeeding by the pregnant mother may adversely affect the nutritional status of the infant and imposes profound nutritional demands on the mother which may adversely affect the growth of the fetus.

Should breastfeeding be stopped when baby has cut his teeth?

Most babies cut their first tooth around 6–7 months but breastfeeding is continued till at least one year or even longer when all the milk teeth are in place. Most babies are smart and do not bite the nipple and they know how sacred is the breast because it is their life line. An occasional angry fellow may create mischief by biting the nipple either to relieve irritation of the gums or due to frustration of not getting enough milk. Mother should not laugh or approve this prank but should firmly say "no biting" and calmly disconnect the prankster from the breast and divert his attention by talking or distracting him.

Care of the Newborn

15

Should a nursing mother avoid exercise, because it may sour the milk due to elevation of lactic acid?

There is no evidence to suggest that exercise leads to souring of the milk unless exercise is indulged to the point of exhaustion. Aerobic exercises and yoga in moderation are the best. Mother should be advised to wear a firm sports bra and do the exercise immediately after having given the feed to the baby. Mother should drink extra glass of water before and after the exercise especially during summer in order to maintain good hydration status.

BOTTLE FEEDING

Most babies can be fed with exclusive breastfeeding up to 6 months of age. Subsequently when semisolid foods are started, breastfeeding should be continued and there is no need to start bottle or formula feeds. At a later date, generally after first birthday, when breast milk supply wanes off, milk feeds can be started directly from a cup or a glass. Therefore, in the care of healthy term babies, there is no place for bottle feeding.

Despite sincere efforts and because of certain medical or social conditions in the mother, complementary or sometimes total feeding with a formula or animal milk may be required in the following situations:

- Adopted baby
- HIV positive mother
- Inadequate lactation
- Twin or triplet babies
- Mother receiving anti-cancer drugs
- Seriously or critically sick mother
- Working mother who is unwilling to breastfeed
- Social constraints

When for a genuine personal or medical reasons, bottle feeding needs to be given, the mother should not feel guilty or unnecessarily upset. Babies can be fed satisfactorily with formula feeds when due precautions are taken to ensure proper cleanliness and sterility of feeding utensils and bottles.

The Choice of Milk

Any liquid milk which is procured by the family for household use can be given to the baby without dilution. Children should be given full-cream milk except when overweight. Dried milk powders are often preferred because of less chances of contamination and adulteration and ease of storage but they are expensive. Most infant formulas are fortified with iron and vitamins. In order to make their composition as close to human milk as possible, most baby formulas are now fortified with docosahexaenoic acid (DHA) and arachidonic acid (AA). Most commercial formulas are low in saturated fats and soy-based formulas are completely devoid of cholesterol and lactose. Milk powders should be reconstituted as per the instructions printed on the container. In general, one level (not heaped) measure is dissolved in one ounce (30 mL) of pre-boiled warm or RO water to obtain full-strength milk. Reconstitution of milk powder into a larger volume of water is the commonest cause of poor weight gain by the baby. The hands should be washed thoroughly with soap and water before preparing a feed. The powdered milk can be directly taken in the feeding bottle instead of using another container for reconstitution. It is more convenient and there is lesser risk of bacterial contamination. In order to promote breastfeeding, the production, marketing and promotion of breast milk substitutes are governed by Infants Milk Substitutes Act-1992. The Act does not allow advertisement of infant milk substitutes, infant foods or feeding bottles. According to the Act, no baby food (even cereal-based) can be promoted for children below the age of 2 years.

Fresh liquid milk is suitable for feeding babies but it is difficult to store during summer months without an ice box or refrigerator. The milk should be boiled every time before use. During first 2 months, pure cow's or buffaloes milk may be diluted in a ratio of 3 parts of milk and one part of water to reduce protein load to the kidneys. When milk is delivered home by the milkman, the dilution should be left to him! Animal milks have a greater quantity of proteins which are of different kind (casein which is difficult to digest compared to easily digestible lactalbumin or whey protein of breast milk) and are less sweet due to lower content of lactose. Mother can add sugar to sweeten the milk according to baby's liking. The milk should be strained before pouring into the feeding bottle otherwise the cream may block the hole in the teat. After 2 months of age, most babies can be fed with a full strength liquid milk.

How much Milk to Offer?

Breastfed babies regulate their feed intake depending upon their needs and mother does no need to worry about any guidelines or calculations. During bottle feeding, offer 30–45 mL of milk during first weeks of life. Whenever baby completely empties the bottle, additional 15 mL of milk should be offered during the next feed. The volume of feeds should be gradually increased by 15–30 mL after every month or so. The best guide that the baby has taken a full feed is when some milk is left in the bottle after the feed. The left over milk must be immediately discarded (or consumed by an adult) and feeding bottle should be rinsed with water to prevent bacterial growth. The maximum that baby drinks at one feed is a full bottle of 8 ounces (approximately 240 mL). After one year, baby should be given maximum of three bottles of milk feeds and rest of his nutritional requirements should be met by giving cereal-based semisolid foods, lentils, eggs, vegetables and soft fruits like banana, cheekoo, papaya, etc.

Technique of Bottle Feeding

A straight wide-mouthed feeding bottle should be used because of ease of cleaning. The hole in the rubber teat should be created with a red hot sewing needle. It will burn the rubber to make a hole. When a feeding bottle with milk is inverted, there should be a fine spray of milk for 1–2 seconds and then milk should flow in regular drops and not as a stream. When milk flows as a constant stream, the hole in the teat is too big and if the drops fall too slowly, it is too small. In both situations, the baby is likely to swallow too much air while feeding and develop colic or regurgitation of feeds. Mother should check the temperature of milk by pouring a few drops on the back of her hand to make sure it is not too hot. Use pre-boiled safe and potable warm water (which can be stored in a flask) for reconstitution of powdered milk. Feeds should be offered on self-demand as in case of breastfeeding. A common sense approach should be followed instead of any strict ritual or routine. The baby should be fed when he is hungry and allowed to sleep as long as he wants. After some time, baby would establish his own routine and mother can adjust her routine accordingly.

The child should preferably be taken in the lap and offered the bottle. Mother must pay full attention and interact with her baby while bottle feeding. She should provide close skin-to-skin contact and eye contact to the baby while bottle feeding. The bottle should be tilted enough so that nipple is completely filled with milk to avoid swallowing of air by the baby. The nipple may have to be removed from the baby's mouth when it gets collapsed to relieve negative pressure or vacuum in the bottle. After the feed, baby should be made to sit or put on the shoulder to eructate the swallowed air. After burping, the baby may be placed on his back or left lateral position with head end slightly raised. *It is dangerous to support the feeding bottle with a cushion or pillow and leave the baby and bottle alone for self-feeding. There is a potential risk of choking and aspiration or the baby may suck lot of air when bottle rolls down.* During bottle feeding, baby's head should be kept slightly raised, otherwise milk may enter the Eustachian tube and lead to middle ear infection. After the age of 9 months, most babies can hold the bottle and self-feed without any risk of choking. After first birthday, attempts should be made to feed the baby with a cup or a glass. Use of distinctive and decorative cup or a baby glass with motifs may motivate babies to accept this method of self-feeding. Most babies accept water from a cup or a glass as early as 6–9 months but refuse to take milk from a cup because they identify milk with a feeding bottle. The use of a sipper for administration of either water or milk is condemned due to potential risk of infection.

Feeding during Sleep

It is not a good practice to offer a bottle feed during sleep. It may lead to development of dental caries as milk remains in contact with teeth while the baby is asleep. Feeding during sleep is also associated with the risk of development of ear infection as the milk may trickle into the Eustachian tube and cause infection of the middle ear. Occasional bottle feeding during sleep may be given if baby had been fussy, irritable and unwell due to teething or minor illness but it should not lead to development of a bad habit with adverse consequences.

Care of Feeding Bottles and Teats

Bottle feeding is a potential source of infection (especially diarrhea) unless care is taken to maintain sterility. Mother should have at least 4 feeding bottles and enough teats. The left over milk must be discarded (or consumed by an adult) and bottle should be cleaned with a detergent or soap and water by using a brush. The left over milk is the potential breeding ground for bacteria and should not be left in the bottle till next feed. Teat should be cleaned with a small brush and common salt to remove milk curds or cream from the teat's hole. The mother should keep a separate sauce pan or container for boiling bottles. Bottles and teats must completely dip in water and should be boiled for a minimum of 10 minutes. After boiling and cooling, water should be drained and the vessel with bottles and teats should be kept covered for next use. Electrical bottle sterilizers are available and are convenient to use. The bottles and teats can be sterilized by immersing them in a solution of sodium hypochlorite (Milton). One table spoon (15 mL) of Milton is added to a liter of water and bottles are soaked for 3–4 hours. The bottle and teat should be drained and rinsed with RO or boiled water before use. The liquid milk must be boiled before each use. The water used for reconstitution of powdered milk must be boiled for at least 5 minutes to ensure that it is sterile and safe. After taking the feed in the bottle, teat must be kept covered with a plastic lid to prevent contamination by flies unless baby is given the feed immediately. The responsibility of washing, cleaning and sterilization of feeding bottles and teats should not be given to a maid or *ayah* and mother should personally look after this most important aspect of bottle feeding.

Feeding with a Cup and a Spoon or *Paladay*

Because of potential risk of infection and "nipple confusion" with bottle feeding, it is recommended to give complementary feeds to babies with a spoon or *paladay* (small cup with a rounded snout which is normally used as a *diya*). Most babies (even preterm babies) accept feeding with a spoon or *paladay* without any difficulty (Figures 15.7 and 15.8). The baby should be held in the lap, head slightly raised and edge of the spoon or *paladay* is touched to the lips of the baby. As soon as the milk touches the lips and tongue, the baby makes swallowing efforts to drink the milk. When baby is satisfied, he will turn his head away or stop swallowing the milk which collects in the throat. The procedure is safe but time consuming. Mother needs to use lot of patience to feed the baby with a spoon or *paladay* but effort is well rewarded because risk of bacterial contamination is extremely low by this method and it is easier for the baby to accept breastfeeding concurrently or subsequently because there is no "nipple confusion". The feeding cup and spoon/*paladay* should be washed with soap and water immediately after each use and kept effectively covered.

Hazards and Benefits of Bottle Feeding

Bottle feeding is unnatural and animal milks or milk formulas are not suitable to serve the nutritional and biological needs of the human babies. Bottle fed babies are more vulnerable to develop gastrointestinal infections, respiratory infections, allergic disorders, and ear infections. Due to frequent infections and over dilution of formula, the child may have poor weight gain and undernutrition. In well to do families, aggressive bottle feeding with a formula is associated with excessive weight gain, increased risk of obesity, metabolic syndrome X, type 2 diabetes mellitus, high blood pressure and coronary artery disease later in life.

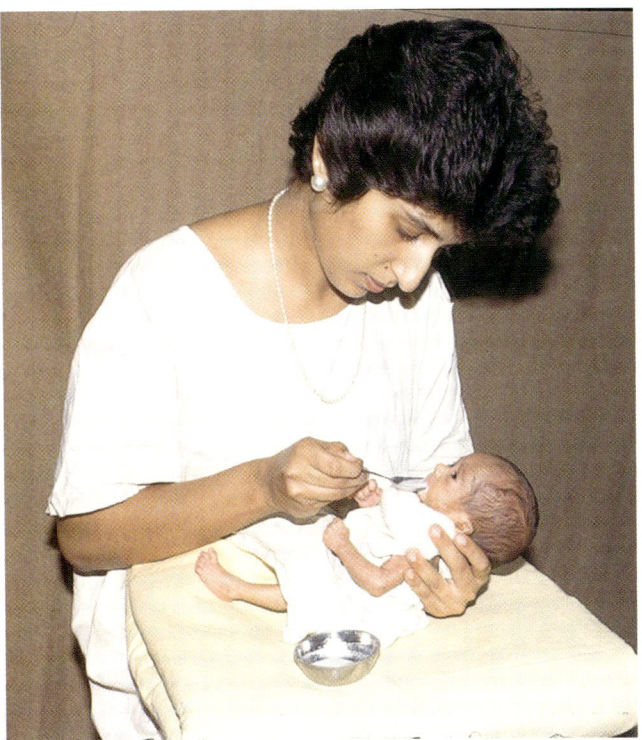

Figure 15.7 Feeding a premature baby with a cup and spoon to avoid nipple confusion.

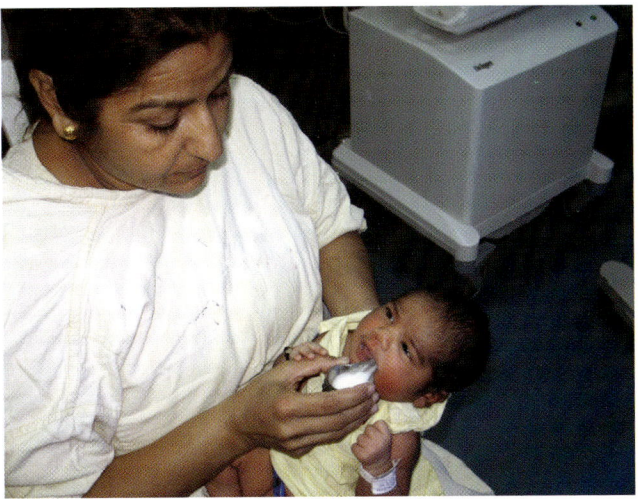

Figure 15.8 Feeding with a *paladay*. It is a small cup or *diya* with a rounded snout and is more convenient compared to spoon feeding. The baby turns his face away or stops swallowing when satisfied.

In well off families, especially when help of a maid is available to look after and feed the baby, bottle feeding does provide greater respite, freedom and option to the mother for joining her job, better social life, lack of need for any dietary restrictions or nutritional demands and greater freedom for resumption of normal sexual activity.

Feeding and Nutrition

15

FEEDING OF PRETERM AND LOW BIRTH WEIGHT BABIES

Physiological and Biochemical Handicaps

By 10 weeks of gestation, the gut is formed and has completed its rotation back into the abdominal cavity. The fetus can swallow the amniotic fluid by 16 weeks of gestation. Gastrointestinal motor activity is present around 24 weeks and effective peristalsis is established by 29–30 weeks and is promoted by antenatal administration of corticosteroids. At term, fetus swallows about 150 mL/day of amniotic fluid which has osmolarity of 275 mOsm/L and contains carbohydrates, proteins, fats, electrolytes, immunoglobulins and growth factors which are credited to promote maturation of lungs and gastrointestinal tract. Preterm birth interrupts the anatomical and functional development of gut.

Depending upon the gestational maturity and vigor of the child, there may be difficulties in self-feeding. The baby may not be able to suck or there may be incoordination between sucking and swallowing. Coordinated sucking and swallowing develops during 32–34 weeks of maturity. Low birth weight babies are prone to develop abdominal distension because of small capacity of stomach and sluggish motility of gut due to autonomic immaturity. They are liable to regurgitate and aspirate the feeds because of lax cardioesophageal sphincter and a poor cough reflex. They have enhanced vulnerability to develop necrotizing enterocolitis due to stasis of gut. There is some evidence that administration of probiotics to VLBW babies is associated with reduced risk of NEC. Their digestive ability is by and large normal except that the animal fat is poorly tolerated because of deficiency of pancreatic lipase and poor quality of bile. The unsaturated fatty acids contained in vegetable oils such as olive oil, coconut oil, corn oil and peanut oil are tolerated better. Preterm babies have relative lactase deficiency.

Caloric and Fluid Requirements

The fluid needs of extremely LBW babies are relatively higher compared to neonates with higher body weight (Table 15.4). Their insensible water loss is more due to large surface area, thin vascular skin and raised metabolic rate. Higher breathing rates, reduced tubular concentration ability, frequent occurrence of hyaline membrane disease and cold stress demand higher fluid intake. Exposure under phototherapy and radiant heat warmer is associated with excessive

TABLE 15.4 Fluid requirements of low birth weight babies (mL/kg/day)

Day	<1000 g	1000–1500 g	>1500 g
1st and 2nd	100–120	80–100	60–80
3rd and 4th	130–140	110–120	90–100
5th and 6th	150–160	130–140	110–120
7th and 8th	170–180	150–160	130–140
9th day onwards	190–200	170-180	150-160

Note: Fluid needs are higher for infants with lower birth weight. Additional allowances for phototherapy (20–40 mL/kg/day) and radiant warmer (40–80 mL/kg/day) should be provided. The higher side of the range refer to larger infants due to greater insensible transepidermal water loss because of exposure of larger surface area.

transepidermal insensible water loss. The newborn kidney is half as effective in concentrating urine with its maximum concentrating ability of 600–700 mOsm/kg (c.f. 1200 mOsm/kg in adults). Therefore, high solute (protein) load results in increased urine flow demanding higher fluid intake to maintain fluid balance. Lack of humidity and exposure to strong air currents also augments insensible water loss. After first week of life, the average maintenance fluid needs during early infancy vary from 150–200 mL/kg per day to maintain positive water balance.

The caloric needs of non-growing preterm babies during first week of life are 70–80 kcal/kg/day. Additional calories are needed for growth (25 kcal/kg/day), activity (15 kcal/kg/day), cold stress (10 kcal/kg/day), specific dynamic action of food (8 kcal/kg/day) and fecal loss (about 12 kcal/kg/day). After first 1 to 2 weeks of life, most preterm babies require 120–150 kcal/kg/day to maintain satisfactory growth velocity. After postconceptional maturity of 40 weeks, the caloric needs decrease to 100–120 kcal/kg/day.

Proteins

Protein digestion and absorption are well developed even in the small preterm infants. Nitrogen is assimilated with avidity and in proportion to the intake provided the protein contains adequate amounts of essential amino acids. However, the metabolism of threonine, sulfur and aromatic amino acids is impaired whereas that of branched chain amino acids is enhanced in preterm infants. Due to incompletely developed amino acid pathways, cysteine, taurine, glycine and histidine are also considered as essential amino acids in preterm babies.

Protein intake must provide adequate amino acids for normal growth and maintenance. Protein requirement for new tissue synthesis between 26 and 36 weeks of gestation is about 300 mg/kg/day. This corresponds to intake of about 1.8 g protein/kg/day to achieve a weight gain of at least 15 g/kg/day. The normal rates of protein turnover are 3 to 4 times greater in LBW infants compared to older children and about 12 g of protein/kg are broken down and resynthesized each day. This leads to a nitrogen loss of approximately 600 mg/kg/day or 1 mg nitrogen/kcal. Taking both these factors into account, the optimal protein intake for preterm infants is about 3.0–3.5 g/kg/day from the second week of life till gestational maturity of 40 weeks when it decreases to about 2.0 g/kg/day. Essential amino acids should constitute 53% of nitrogen intake.

The amount of protein to be given to LBW infants to achieve a nitrogen retention similar to the *in utero* depends on the digestibility and utilization of the protein intake. It appears that a significant advantage accrues by the use of whey predominat formulae with whey to casein ratio similar to that of breast milk (i.e. 60:40). Infants fed with a milk formula containing high casein content show higher serum levels of tyrosine, phenylalanine and ammonia but display similar growth rates suggesting that the higher levels of these metabolites are due to inadequate handling of casein. High protein intake may lead to hazardous accumulation of amino acids, urea, ammonia and hydrogen ions (causing metabolic acidosis) in LBW infants because of the immaturity of several enzymatic pathways and a low glomerular filtration rate.

Carbohydrates

The LBW infant has low levels of intestinal brush border lactase during the first few days of life. If the feed contains large amounts of lactose, undigested lactose may accumulate in high concentration in the distal intestinal tract and serve as a substrate for proliferation of potentially pathogenic bacteria. Additionally, the lactose may cause intestinal distention due to its osmotic effect. Moderate amount of lactose, however, is believed to aid in calcium absorption and allows colonization of the gut by beneficial fermentative flora. Human milk provides 75% of carbohydrates in the form of lactose and remaining as oligosaccharides. Sialated oligosaccharides (sialic acid) are present in a concentration of 40 mg/dL in human milk and they serve as a key component to the gangliosides and are required for synaptogenesis.

Starch digestion in the preterm infants is limited since pancreatic alpha amylase activity becomes significant

only several months after birth. Glycosidase enzymes are well developed even in preterm infants. Thus, sucrose, maltose and glucose oligosaccharides are well tolerated. Maltodextrins have the additional benefit of imposing less osmotic load to the formula as compared to lactose or monosaccharides. From a practical viewpoint, the carbohydrate portions of various special formulas for the LBW infants should contain approximately 40 to 50% lactose and 50 to 60% glucose polymers (maltodextrin, polycose).

Fats

Fats provide the major source of energy for the growing premature infants. Fat absorption is poor in the LBW infants because of low levels of pancreatic lipase and bile salts. The bile in a premature infant is qualitatively inferior because of predominance of taurine conjugates and absence of deoxycholate. Nevertheless, medium chain triglycerides are well absorbed presumably because their digestion and absorption are not dependent on intraluminal bile salt levels. The recently developed special formulas for preterm infants contain a mixture of medium chain triglycerides and predominantly unsaturated long chain triglycerides. The gain in energy through improved absorption of medium chain triglycerides may, however, be offset by an increased frequency of intestinal disturbances (abdominal distension, loose stools, vomiting) attributable to medium chain tri-glycerides.

Fat absorption in LBW infants can be improved by feeding raw instead of pasteurized human milk. Fresh milk contains a very active bile salt-stimulated lipase which can contribute up to half of the total lipase and esterase activity in the duodenum of preterm infants. The addition of raw breast milk to the formula or pooled pasteurized human milk can improve fat absorption in LBW infants. Another reason for the relatively efficient absorption of human milk fat is the distribution of fatty acids in the triglyceride molecule. Palmitic acid in the beta position in human milk leads to a better absorption of fat compared to cow's milk fat, which has stearic acid in the beta position. The lingual lipase starts acting in the stomach while bile salt-activated lipase in the milk continues the digestion in the duodenum.

Preterm babies have higher requirements of essential fatty acids to sustain retinal maturation and myelination of CNS. Essential fatty acid deficiency, presenting with an erythematous scaling rash is a well recognized clinical entity in LBW infants. This may be prevented by adding linoleic acid to all formulae

Feeding and Nutrition

15

in sufficient concentration to supply at least 1.0% of energy intake. Most baby formulae available in developed countries are fortified with docosahexaenoic acid (DHA) and arachidonic acid (AA) to harness its benefits during the crucial phase of brain development. The recommended dietary intakes of macronutrients and micronutrients in preterm babies are summarized in Table 15.5.

TABLE 15.5 Recommended daily nutrient intakes for preterm infants >1000 g at birth till one year of age

Nutrient	Birth to 7 days	8 days to postconceptional age of 40 weeks	Term to 1 year of age
Macronutrients			
Energy (kcal/kg)	70–80	105–135	100–120
Protein (g/kg)	1.0–3.0	3.0-3.6	2.2
Fat (g/kg)	0.5–3.6	4.5–6.8	4.4–7.3
Carbohydrate (g/kg)	5.0–20.0	7.5–15.5	7.5–15.5
Micronutrients			
Minerals			
Calcium (mmol/kg)	1.5–2.0	4.0–6.0	6.3 mmol/d (breastfed) 9.4 mmol/d (formula fed)
Phosphorus (mmol/kg)	1.0–1.5	2.53.8	3.4 mmol/d (breastfed) 8.8 mmol/d (formula fed)
Magnesium (mmol/kg)[a]	0.20–0.25	0.20–0.40	0.20–0.60
Sodium (mmol/kg)[b]	1.0–3.0	2.5–4.0	2.0–3.0
Chloride (mmol/kg)[b]	1.0–3.0	2.5–4.0	2.0–3.0
Potassium (mmol/kg)	2.5–3.5	2.5–3.5	2.5–3.5
Iron (mg/kg)[c]	0	2.0–3.0	2.0–3.0
Zinc (μmol/kg)[d]	6.5	7.7–12.3	15.0 (estimate)
Copper (μmol/kg)	1.1–1.9	1.1–1.9	1.1–1.9
Selenium (μmol/kg)	0.04–0.06	0.04–0.06	0.04–0.06
Chromium (nmol/kg)	1.0–1.9	1.0–1.9	1.0–1.9
Manganese (nmol/kg)	10.20	10–20	10–20
Molybdenum (nmol/kg)	2.0–4.0	2.0–4.0	2.0–4.0
Iodine (μmol/kg)	0.20	0.25–0.50	0.25–0.50
Vitamins			
Vitamin A (IU/kg)	700–1500	700–1500	700–1500
Vitamin E (IU/kg)	6–12	6–12	6–12
Vitamin K (μg/kg)	8–10	8–10	8–10
Vitamin D (IU)	40–260	400–800	400
Vitamin C (mg/kg)	6–10	6–10	20
Vitamin B_1 (mg/kg)	0.04–0.05	0.04–0.05	0.05
Vitamin B_2 (mg/kg)	0.36–0.46	0.36–0.46	0.05
Vitamin B_6 (mg/g of protein intake)	0.015	0.015	0.015
Vitamin B_{12} (μg)	0.15	0.15	0.15
Niacin (NE/5000 IU)[e]	8.6	8.6	8.6
Folate (μg)	50	50	25
Biotin (μg/kg)	1.5	1.5	1.5
Pantothenic acid (mg/kg)	0.8–1.3	0.8–1.3	0.8–1.3

a. Amount required is higher if milk from the premature infant's mother is fortified with other minerals that may diminish the bioavailability and absorption of magnesium.

b. In specific clinical situations, sodium and chloride may need to be omitted for short periods.

c. From 6 weeks after birth.

d. Amount may be increased in specific clinical syndromes.

e. NE = niacin equivalents.

Adapted from: Canadian Pediatric Society Nutrition Committee. Nutrient needs and feeding of premature infants. *Canad Med Assoc J* 1995; 152:1765–85.

Minerals

Preterm infants are prone to develop hyponatremia because of obligatory renal losses secondary to an inadequately developed renal conservation mechanism. Recent studies have suggested that the gut absorption of sodium in these infants is also inefficient. The special formulas for premature infants should provide 2.5 to 3.5 mEq/kg/day of sodium. Very LBW (<1500 g) infants require even higher amounts of sodium (4 to 8 mEq/kg/day). The potassium requirement of 2 to 3 mEq/kg/day is similar to that of term infants. Preterm infants often develop signs of osteopenia or even overt rickets. This is because human milk and most formulas do not contain enough calcium and phosphorus to allow their accumulation at fetal accretion rates. The recommended daily intakes of calcium and phosphorus are 250 mg and 125 mg per kilogram body weight respectively. In practical terms, this means that a breastfed infant requires a supplementation of 220 mg/kg/day of calcium and 100 mg/kg/day of phosphorus.

Iron supplementation in LBW infants is controversial because although their stores and absorption of the mineral are poor, supplemental iron may precipitate vitamin E deficiency and cause hemolytic anemia. Iron also binds lactoferrin, a powerful inhibitor of *E. coli* present in the milk and thus favors overgrowth of that bacterium. Iron supplements may also reduce the absorption of zinc. Iron supplementation (2 to 3 mg/kg/day) is recommended once full enteral feeds are established and baby is gaining weight. Zinc deficiency causes acrodermatitis enteropathica and copper deficiency is associated with later psychomotor retardation, hypotonia, osteoporosis and sideroblastic anemia. Deficiency states can be prevented by supplying 0.5 mg of zinc and 90 µg of copper per 100 kcal. The importance and requirements of other trace elements is not known.

Vitamins

All vitamins are essential for optimal nutrition of LBW infants. The recommended oral intakes for vitamin A, vitamin K, thiamin, riboflavin, niacin, pyridoxine, pantothenic acid, vitamin B_{12} and biotin are similar to those recommended for full term infants. Folate supplementation is controversial as it is difficult to demonstrate differences in hemoglobin concentration or red cell morphology in infants on supplements despite higher serum levels. However, as mucosal lesions may occur in older children with folate deficiency in the absence of hematological abnormalities,

daily supplement of 150 µg is recommended. Some workers have emphasized the need for high ascorbic acid intakes in premature infants to enhance the activity of hepatic hydroxyphenylpyruvic acid oxidase in order to lower blood tyrosine and urinary tyrosine metabolite levels but these studies remain unsubstantiated. In any case, no detrimental effects of transient neonatal tyrosinemia have been shown. Oral intakes of 35 mg of ascorbic acid daily are probably adequate.

The vitamin D metabolism is inadequately developed in the premature infant. This is an important contributing factor for development of osteopenia of prematurity. The prevention of severe bone disease in these infants necessitates high oral intakes of both calcium and phosphorus and at least 600 iu of vitamin D per day. The latter can be achieved by giving 400 iu of vitamin D per day in a multivitamin supplement in addition to the vitamin D in the breast milk or formula. Recent work has suggested that even these intakes may be low, and probably amounts as high as 800 iu per day are required.

The requirement of vitamin E in the small premature infant is higher than that of the term infant because the fat malabsorption of the premature infant also limits the absorption of vitamin E. Vitamin E deficiency may cause a mild hemolytic anemia and generalized edema. The symptoms are exacerbated by a high intake of iron and polyunsaturated fatty acids because they are known to increase the requirement of vitamin E. It has been suggested that vitamin E supplements may decrease the severity of retinopathy of prematurity. Vitamin E has also been used for prevention of bronchopulmonary dysplasia and intraventricular hemorrhage but this remains to be confirmed. The dietary intakes of 0.7 iu of vitamin E per 100 kcal and at least 1.0 iu per gram of linoleic acid are recommended.

Probiotics

There is evidence to suggest that probiotics enhance the tolerance of enteral feeds and reduce the risk of necrotizing enterocolitis in preterm infants. However, the most effective probiotic or combination of probiotics, their dosage and timing of administration are not known. Their safety and long-term effect on gut microbiota of immunologically immature VLBW babies has not been established. The presently available data do not permit recommending the routine use of prebiotics or probiotics as food supplements in preterm infants.

Feeding with Human Milk

The previous concept that preterm babies thrive better on artificial milk formula fortified with higher protein and fat content is replaced by the universal recommendation that breast milk is best for all newborn babies irrespective of their birth weight and gestation. The milk of mothers delivering prematurely provides more calories and have a higher concentration of fat, protein, sodium and secretory IgA during initial 2–3 weeks. *The nature is thus unique because milk is not only species specific, it is indeed baby specific.* It is recommended that preterm babies should preferably be fed with unboiled expressed breast milk (EBM) obtained from their mothers. Besides the biochemical advantages, human milk protects against infections, decreases the risk of necrotizing enterocolitis, retinopathy of prematurity and strengthens mother–infant bonding. The breast milk should be collected in a sterile stainless steel bowl and fed immediately after collection to avoid contamination. The glass container is unsatisfactory because macrophages and lymphocytes tend to stick to its surface walls and boiling kills the cellular elements. The caloric density of EBM can be enhanced by glucose polymers, vegetable oil or medium chain triglycerides. The supplementation with vegetable oil has not been found to be useful to enhance growth velocity of LBW babies due to its poor absorption.

Human Milk Fortifier

Human milk fortifier (HMF) is a milk-based multicomponent supplement to increase the energy, protein, calcium, phosphorus and other nutrients of EBM to meet the nutritional needs of rapidly growing premature infants. Routine use of multicomponent milk fortifier is not recommended. Its use should be restricted to infants <32 weeks of gestation or <1500 g birth weight who fail to gain weight despite adequate breast milk intake. Lactodex-HMF (2 g sachets to be dissolved in 50 mL EBM) has a composition comparable to Enfamil-HMF except that its protein content is almost one-half of Enfamil-HMF and it lacks iron. The fortification of EBM is started in infants <32 weeks gestation after 2 weeks of age when baby is growing. The fortification should be done with due aseptic precautions under laminar flow. The fortified EBM cannot be stored and should be consumed within 2–4 hours. There are potential hazards of increased osmolar load, hypercalcemia, sepsis or NEC. When using a standard formulation of HMF, there is no need to administer additional nutritional supplements to the baby. There is evidence to suggest that initial growth of preterm babies is enhanced by giving fortified EBM but advantage is lost during follow-up.

In clinical practice, despite concerted efforts, it is not possible to meet the total milk requirements of a preterm baby by EBM obtained from his mother. The pooled human milk can be used for supplementation as long it is certified that there is no risk of HIV and CMV infections. Most babies in the NICU do need supplementation of their EBM feedings with a few feeds of "premature baby formula" which is credited to provide additional calories, proteins and nutrients. This practice appears to be more convenient and further limits the need for using a human milk fortifier.

Milk Formula for Premature Babies

Human milk has served as the gold standard in research and development of infant formula. The composition of an ideal formula for LBW babies is shown in Table 15.6. It should be humanized to provide 60:40 ratio of whey protein to casein and fortified with glucose polymers, medium chain triglycerides, DHA, nucleotides, calcium, phosphorus and vitamins. In order to prevent osmolar damage to the intestinal mucosa, the osmolarity should be maintained around 300 mOsm/L to safeguard against necrotizing enterocolitis. The renal solute load should not exceed 100 mOsm/L. Even when the chemical composition of the formula is made similar to human milk, it cannot match the biological characteristics of human milk. The commercial baby formulae lack in immunoglobulins, lipase, lactoferrin, epidermal

TABLE 15.6 Composition of an ideal commercial formula for LBW babies

Constituents	Grams per 100 mL of formula
Protein	2.0 (whey protein to casein ratio 60:40)
Fat	4.0
Butter fat	2.0
PUFA, DHA and medium chain triglycerides	2.0
Carbohydrate	10–12
Lactose	5–6
Maltodextrin	5–6
Osmolarity	Around 300 mOsm/L
Renal solute load	Up to 100 mOsm/L
Calories	80 kcalories
Vitamins and minerals	As per RDA requirements

PUFA; polyunsaturated fatty acid, DHA; docosahexaenoic acid

growth factor, peptides, hormones, probiotics and cellular elements which provide unique advantages to babies fed on human milk. The breast milk substitutes also have an increased risk of contamination and infection when handled incorrectly. It is technically not feasible to produce a commercial milk formula having all the attributes of human milk and if one were to achieve near complete humanization of milk formula, its cost would indeed be prohibitive and unbelievable. It is amazing that nature provides an excellent baby-specific ready made drink, as soon as the baby is born, almost free of cost except the increased nutritional cost of lactation to the nursing mother to maintain her optimal health.

Expression of Breast Milk

It is ideal that preterm babies should be fed with unboiled milk obtained from their mothers. There are logistic difficulties to ensure feeding of babies with human milk every 2 hourly round-the-clock. To circumvent this difficulty, the neonatal unit should establish facilities to store the expressed breast milk (EBM) obtained from mothers whose babies are admitted in the NICU. A public health nurse or lactation management nurse should be available to motivate the mothers for donation of milk and its storage. A refrigerator, deep freeze (–20°C), breast pumps, collection utensils and dispensing bottles is all that is required.

A comfortable, clean, and warm room adjacent to the growing nursery is ideal for promotion of breastfeeding of nursery babies and expression of breast milk. The milk can be collected straight into a sterile polycarbonate or polypropylene or stainless steel bowl. Avoid the use of glass container because cellular elements may stick to the surface. Secretory IgA and some vitamins are lost when milk is stored in a polyethylene bag. The 'drip milk' can be collected from the other breast while mother is feeding the baby. The foremilk obtained by drip method, however, has a much lower fat content.

The milk can be expressed manually or with the help of mechanical or electrical pumps (Figures 15.9 and 15.10). During first 2 to 3 days, most mothers prefer the use of breast pumps because breasts are often engorged and painful to touch. Subsequently manual expression of milk with hands is convenient, more acceptable and provides better yield of milk once lactation is established. The hands must be thoroughly washed with soap and water. The mother encircles the breast with her both hands. By gentle pressure, the breast is massaged by moving hands towards the

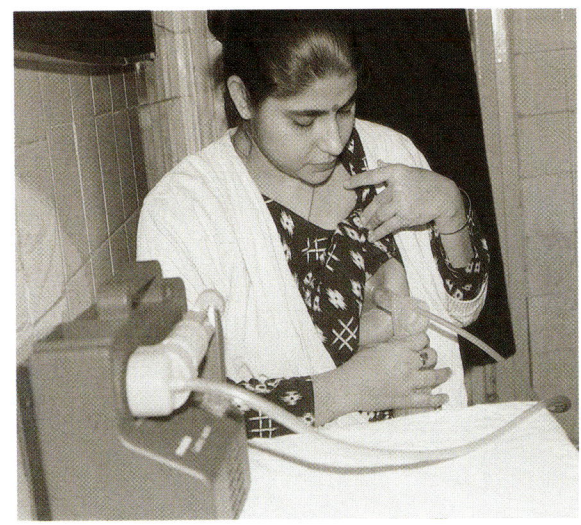
Figure 15.9 Expression of breast milk with an electrical breast pump.

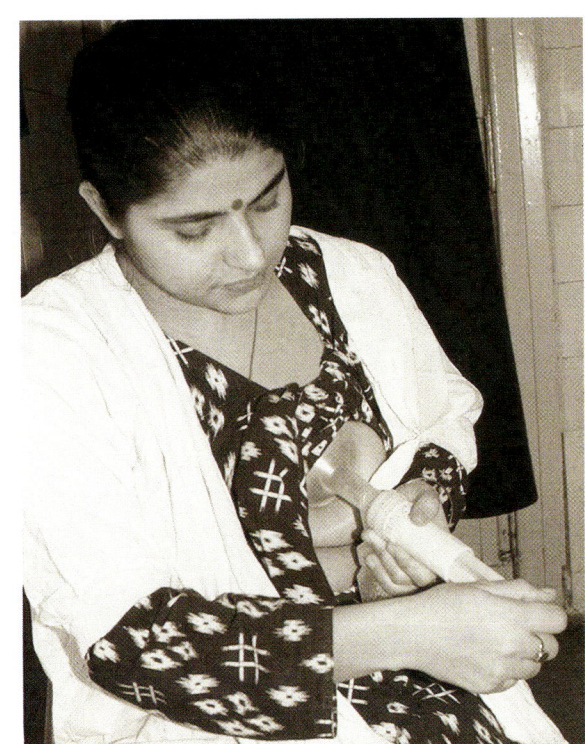
Figure 15.10 Expression of breast milk with a syringe-type mechanical pump.

areola. The procedure is continued for 2 to 3 minutes to transport the milk into lactiferous ducts. The index finger and thumb are then placed on either side of the nipple over the areola. The fingers are pressed backwards towards the ribs, then pinched together and pulled forwards to express the milk (Figures 15.11 and 15.12). The mother can be trained for effective expression of breast milk in one or two sittings. The

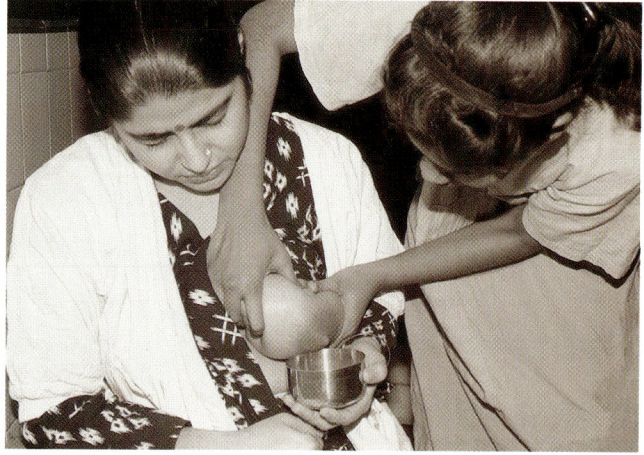

Figure 15.11 Manual expression of breast milk. The breast is massaged from the base towards the areola to transport milk into lactiferous ducts.

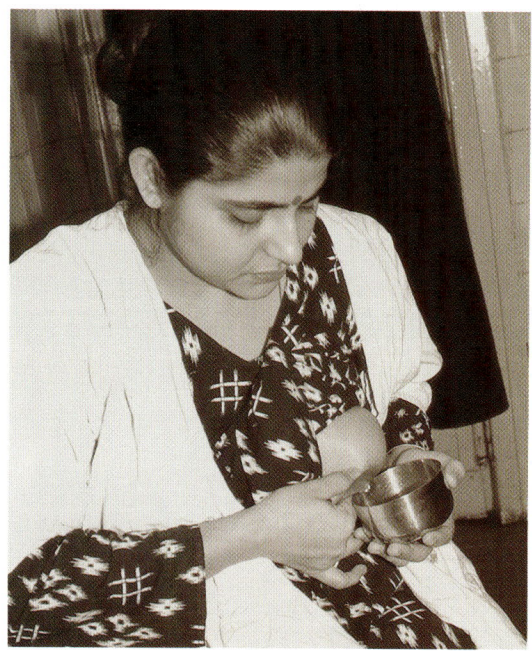

Figure 15.12 Manual expression of breast milk. Areola is pinched and pressed backwards with thumb and index finger to empty lactiferous ducts.

milk should be collected in a wide-mouthed stainless steel or polypropylene bowl. The container with EBM should be covered with a tight lid. It can be kept at room temperature (25°C) for 6–8 hours or stored in a refrigerator (4°C) up to 24 hours. Milk can be stored in a freezer compartment (–15°C) up to 2 weeks and deep freezer (–18°C) up to 3–6 months and can be used by thawing. The deep freezer must be provided with uninterrupted power supply by attaching it to a stand by generator. Freezing and thawing of milk causes disruption of fat globules. Pasteurization is better for

ensuring sterility but is expensive and inactivates milk lipase and immune components. If the milk is being pooled from different mothers, it raises the ethical issues of ensuring that milk is free from infective agents like HIV, HTLV 1 and 2, CMV, hepatitis B and C and syphilis.

HUMAN MILK BANKING

Human milk banking is a service for screening, collecting, processing, storing and distributing the donated human milk. According to a joint statement by WHO and UNICEF, when it is not possible for the biological mother to breastfeed, the first alternative, if available, should be the use of human milk from other sources. Human milk banks should be made available in appropriate situations. Banked or pooled human milk is regarded as "the next best option" for feeding the babies, if biological mother is unable to breastfeed. It is most suitable for feeding preterm and sick babies in the neonatal intensive care units (NICUs). The main indications for use of pasteurised donor human milk (PDHM) are given in Box 15.3. Other indications for use of human milk include malabsorption, short-gut syndrome, intractable diarrhea, intolerance to formula feeds, immune deficiencies (IgA), HIV-positive mother and adopted child. It is not difficult to start a human milk bank (HMB) but sustaining voluntary milk donation and maintaining quality of donor human milk (DHM) are arduous tasks. Currently nearly 50 HMBs are operational in India.

Screening

One of the major issues and concerns regarding milk banking is the transmission of infections via the milk. A detailed medical history of the donor should be taken to exclude infectious diseases which can be transmitted through breast milk. Her blood should be screened for HIV-1 and 2, HTLV-1 and 2 (potential risk for causing T cell leukemia), CMV, hepatitis B and

Box 15.3: Indications for use of donor human milk

- Inadequate lactation, flat or inverted nipples and mother with multiple babies.
- Abandoned or orphaned neonates.
- Sick neonates transferred to a referral NICU without mother.
- Infant at health risk from breast milk of the biological mother.
- Temporary interruption of breastfeeding.

C and syphilis. A consent form is filled by the donor mother and her doctor stating that neither the donor nor her infant will suffer, if she donates milk.

Collection and Quality Control

Strict aseptic precautions should be taken while collecting milk. The milk can be expressed either manually or with the help of a manual or an electric pump. Drip milk, i.e. the milk that drips from the other breast while baby is being breastfed is suitable for collection but it has lower caloric content and is more susceptible to contamination. The milk is usually pooled from 4 to 6 donors and best collected in stainless steel containers because leukocytes and macrophages may stick to the surface of glass container while poly-ethylene bags are likely to decrease the IgA content of milk. The bacterial count of each donor's milk before pasteurization should be $<10^3$ colony forming units because pasteurization may be ineffective to sterilize the milk, if it is heavily contaminated. The measurement of pH of DHM is a simple parameter to assess the quality of milk compared to Dornic acid test which is cumbersome and associated with wastage of precious milk. A pH value of >6.57 suggests that DHM is suitable for further processing. The pooled milk is pasteurized by heating it to 56°C for 30 minutes because most viruses and bacteria are killed at this temperature without compromising the nutritional and immunological properties of the milk. After pasteurization, the milk is again checked for bacterial growth and it should be sterile.

Storage

Fresh-raw milk or pasteurized milk can be stored at 4°C up to 72 hours after expression. Pasteurized culture-negative donor human milk collected in tightly sealed containers can be stored at –20°C for 3–6 months. The frozen milk is thawed by keeping the container in a water bath at a temperature not exceeding 37°C or under running lukewarm water. It should never be thawed in microwave as it results in reduction of IgA content of milk. Some centers lyophilize the milk (fresh-frozen milk is dried under vacuum) which can be stored at room temperature up to 18 months but this method is expensive and associated with inaccuracies in its reconstitution and loss of calcium and phosphorus during processing.

Funding

Most milk banks are run by non-profit voluntary organizations or funded through hospital budget. Most donors do not receive any payment (except incidental expenses) but recepients may have to pay a nominal charge to cover the cost of screening tests and storage. Apart from tertiary hospitals, milk banks can be established within the blood banks because they are equipped with technology and trained staff which can collect, screen, pasteurize and store the milk in a cost-effective manner.

In conclusion, WHO recommends that when a baby is unable to receive the milk of her biological mother, milk of another mother is next best option compared to a formula milk or milk from another animal. Human milk is ideal to serve the nutritional and immunological needs of babies especially when a baby is preterm or sick. It has been shown that the stored and pasteurized milk is also credited to reduce the risk of necrotizing enterocolitis (NEC). The guidelines published by North American Milk Bank (NAMB) are ideal and should be followed to reduce the risk of transmission of infections through pooled human milk. Apart from infrastructural and logistic issues, there is a need to educate and inspire lactating mothers to donate breast milk (akin to blood donation!) and explain benefits and safety of breast milk over commercially available formulae to the parents and treating doctors. You can obtain further information on human milk banking in India at info@breastfeedingindia.org and www.iycfchapteriap.org

The First Feed

The old concept of deliberate starvation of babies for 48 to 72 hours has been replaced by the recommendations of early feeding to permit growth continuity as early as possible and to lessen the incidence of hypoglycemia, hyperbilirubinemia and metabolic acidosis. Early and aggressive feeding is associated with dangers of regurgitation and aspiration. All low birth weight and small-for-dates babies must be fed within half an hour of birth. The first feed should be EBM and there is no need to give a trial feed with distilled water or glucose water.

The term LBW babies or IUGR babies They do not pose any serious difficulties because they are mature and have no problems in self-feeding. To prevent hypoglycemia, they should be fed early and put to breast soon after birth. The breastfeeding can be supplemented with sugar-fortified formula feeds with a cup and spoon/*paladay* every 2 hourly during first 72 hours till lactation is established and risk of hypoglycemia is minimized. The mother should not be asked to purchase the formula or feeding bottle, and it should be provided from the hospital. The baby should be receiving exclusive breastfeeding after

Feeding and Nutrition

15

3 to 4 days. When adequately fed, term-IUGR babies do not lose any weight and they start gaining weight after 1 to 3 days of life.

Trophic Feeds

It is recommended that preterm babies, with a gestation of <32 weeks, or birth weight <1500 g should receive minimal or sub-nutritional amount (5–10 mL/kg/d q 4–6 hr) of EBM to harness its trophic benefits on the immature gastrointestinal tract of the baby. In view of its outstanding biological virtues, EBM is indeed used like a "medicine" in extremely premature babies. "Gut priming" promotes the growth of intestinal mucosa and maturation of intestinal musculature by virtue of free nucleotides and hormones contained in human milk. There is enhanced oxygen uptake due to increase in the intestinal blood flow. There is early elaboration of gut endocrines like gastrin, motilin and inhibitory peptides. Early colonization of gut with *Lactobacillus acidophilus* and *bifidus* is associated with reduced risk of development of necrotizing enterocolitis. Trophic feeds are contraindicated in babies with hemodynamic instability, necrotizing enterocolitis, intestinal obstruction, perforation and paralytic ileus.

Methods of Feeding

The mode of initial feeding depends upon the gestational maturity, birth weight and hemodynamic stability of the baby (Table 15.7). Babies with a birth weight of less than 1,200 g or gestation of <30 weeks should be started on intravenous infusion (10% dextrose in babies >1000 g and 5% dextrose in babies <1000 g) and kept on a drip for 3 to 4 days. Infants with severe birth asphyxia, respiratory distress, apneic attacks, seizures, sepsis, NEC and hemodynamically unstable babies should be maintained on intravenous infusion till their clinical condition stabilizes. Strict asepsis and use of medicaths is desirable to reduce chances of nosocomial infections. Over infusion through parenteral route is associated with risk of congestive cardiac failure, patent ductus arteriosus and bronchopulmonary dysplasia.

Gastrostomy feeding for very low birth weight babies has not received general acceptance due to high incidence of local leaks and infections. The decision whether a baby is to be fed on a bottle or through an intragastric catheter is guided by the maturity, birth weight, vigor, general condition of the baby and experience of the nurses. Nasogastric gavage feeding should be started in stable infants between 30 and 34 weeks gestation. Weaning from gavage feeding to cup

TABLE 15.7 Mode of initial feeding depending upon the gestational maturity

Gestational age (birth weight)	Mode of feeding	Caution
<30 weeks (<1200 g)	Intravenous fluids	Use infusion pump and avoid over infusion. TPN is usually required in infants <28 weeks
30–32 weeks (1200–1500 g)	Orogastric or nasogastric feeds	Watch for feed intolerance and NEC
32–34 weeks (1500–1800 g)	Spoon, *paladay* or cup feeding	Avoid aspiration
>34 weeks (>1800 g)	Breastfeeding	Monitor weight gain to assess adequacy of breastfeeding

- Infant should be encouraged to practice non-nutritive sucking directly on the breast of the mother before expression of breast milk.
- Kangaroo-mother care is a useful adjunct to maintain and enhance output of breast milk.
- There is no need to burp tube fed babies.
- The infant is promoted to the next level or mode of feeding depending upon his post conceptional maturity and hemodynamic stability.

and spoon/*paladay* feeding is attempted in babies with a gestational maturity of 32 weeks or above. The use of bottle should be avoided due to potential risk of infection and "nipple confusion" leading to failure of breastfeeding. Direct breastfeeding should be tried once infant achieves a gestational maturity of 34 weeks. Preparation for breastfeeding should begin in all babies irrespective of their gestation by promoting development of rooting reflex by stimulation of corners of mouth with a soft brush and by putting them to breast for non-nutritive sucking before expressing the breast milk. There is evidence to suggest that 5-minute premature infant oromotor intervention (PIOMI) three times daily for 7 days in stable preterm infants between 28 and 32 weeks of gestational age significantly improves their oromotor skills. It is effective in reducing transition time from gavage to oral feeds and infants had increased weight gain with shorter duration of hospital stay. Apart from promoting the sucking capability of the baby, it is likely to enhance lactation of the mother. If a baby takes more than 20 minutes to finish the recommended amount of feed during a trial of bottle feeding, he should preferably be fed through a nasogastric tube. The muscular exertion involved in sucking may tire and exhaust such a baby and result in poor weight gain.

Technique of Gavage Feeding

The length of the polyurethane or silicone nasogastric catheter (size Fr. 6, each Fr. unit equals 0.33 mm) to be inserted should be measured from the external nares to the lobe of the ear and from lobe of the ear to the ensiform cartilage and marked. The head is slightly raised and a wet (not lubricated) catheter is gently passed through the nose down into the esophagus and stomach. Its position should be verified by aspirating gastric contents and checking that its pH is 5.5 or less. The "whoosh test", i.e. auscultation of epigastric region during insufflation of air through the tube, is not reliable. The outer end of the tube is attached to a 20 mL syringe and feed is allowed to trickle by gravity (Figure 15.13). After conclusion of the feeding, about 2 mL of distilled water should be injected to rinse the tube. The baby should be placed in the left lateral position for another 15 to 20 minutes to avoid regurgitation. There is no need to burp the tube fed babies. Bolus feedings are preferable compared to continuous NG feeds. The polythene nasogastric tube may be left *in situ* for 2 to 3 days and while removing the tube, it must be kept pinched or pulled out gently while applying constant negative pressure with a syringe to avoid trickling of gastric mucus into the trachea.

In some NICUs, orogastric tubes are used for feeding because infants are obligatory nose breathers and they feel uncomfortable when one nostril is occluded with an NG tube. Nasogastric tube may cause inflammation and blockage of nostril. Orogastric tube is difficult to fix and may need to be inserted frequently (even before each feed) and hence is labor-intensive and difficult to practice when there are constraints in the availability of adequate number of nurses.

Amount and Frequency of Feeds

The concentration and volume of the feeds administered should be gradually increased during the first week of life (Table 15.4). The introduction of enteral feeds should be slow and gradual in very LBW babies (<1500 g). When baby is stable, start NG feeds at a rate of 20–30 mL/kg/d on the first day and provide the balance amount (say 50 mL/kg/d) of fluids as 10% dextrose intravenously. The feeds should be given as a slow bolus by gravity every 2 hourly. Depending upon the tolerance by the baby, increase the quantity of enteral feeds everyday by 20–30 mL/kg/d and reduce the intravenous infusion volume and rate accordingly. Recently, higher advancement of feed volumes of 30–40 mL/kg/d in stable preterm babies have been recommended with good results. After 7–

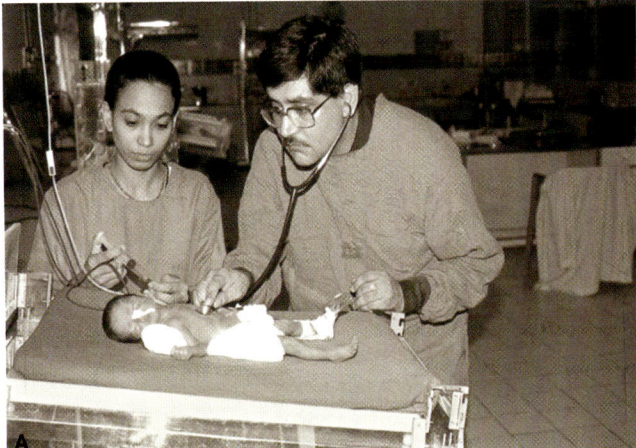

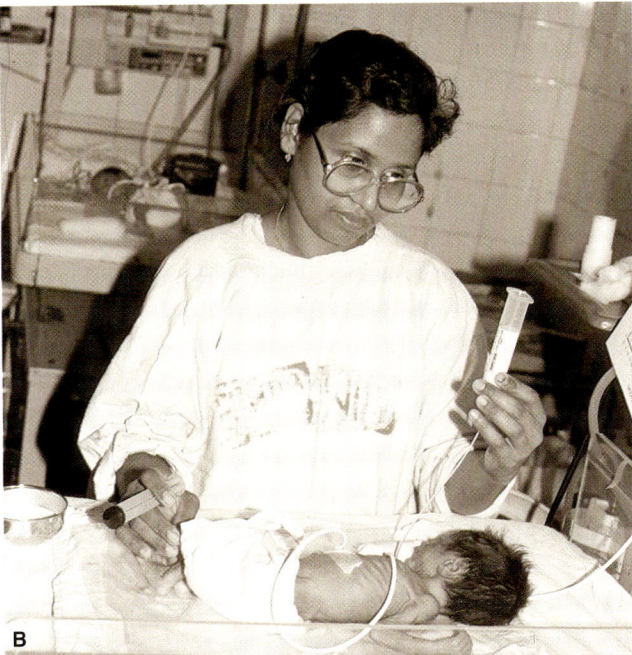

Figure 15.13 (A) Gavage feeding. The position of the catheter is verified by auscultating over the stomach while injecting air. (B) The feed is allowed to flow slowly by gravity. There is not need to burp the gavage fed infant.

10 days, most preterm babies should receive enteral feeds at a rate of 120–150 mL/kg/d providing 150 kcal/kg/d. When EBM is not supplemented by a milk fortifier, most babies would need and tolerate 180 mL/kg/d of human milk to ensure satisfactory growth velocity. Nutritional supplements are added once full enteral feeds are established. The oral cavity must be inspected before and after each feed to detect any thrush and pooling of milk in the oropharynx.

Tolerance of Feeds

There is a need for vigilance and awareness by experienced nurses to safeguard against the risk of aspiration. Abdominal girth should be monitored and abdominal distension should be looked for as an early marker of feed intolerance and necrotizing enterocolitis. Whenever gastric aspirate exceeds 50% of the last feed volume or abdominal girth has increased by 2 cm, stools should be screened for presence of occult blood and reducing substance. Forceful gastric aspiration may lead to iatrogenic bleeding and it should be avoided. Bilious residuals are ominous and a reliable marker of NEC. Gastric stasis at times responds to evacuation of meconium by glycerin suppository or low enema (1–2 mL glycerine) and cautious use of metoclopramide or domperidone. Erythromycin has been used as a prokinetic agent in a dose of 20 mg/kg/d in 3–4 divided oral doses 30 minutes before feeds. There is controversial evidence to suggest that it may lead to development of hypertrophic pyloric stenosis.

NASOJEJUNAL FEEDING

Several developments in feeding techniques have been introduced to reduce the risk of aspiration of feeds and at the same time ensure adequate intake of calories and nutrients by offering increased amounts of feeds. Nasoduodenal or nasojejunal feeding provides a simple, non-invasive means of delivering adequate amount of enteral feeds in low birth weight or ill infants. The objective of this technique of feeding is to deliver the feeds beyond pylorus so that chances of regurgitation are minimized while absorption of nutrients is facilitated because of relatively large surface area of the jejunal wall.

Technique

Nasojejunal feeding is indicated in babies weighing less than 1,500 g and sick neonates having respiratory distress syndrome, sepsis, asphyxia and seizures. Radio-opaque polyvinyl or silastic feeding tube Fr. 5 (length 30 inches) with a weighted-end is used. The length of the tube to be inserted is estimated by measuring the distance between the glabella to the heel and marked on the tube. The tube is inserted through the nostril into the stomach as already described under gavage feeding. The infant is turned towards left lateral position. The tube is further inserted gradually till the measured mark is reached. The aspirate would show the presence of bile (pH of 5 to 7) when the tube lies in the duodenum or beyond. Before feeding is started, posteroanterior and lateral roentgenograms of abdomen are taken to check that the tube tip lies at the level of ligament of Treitz. The

outer end of the tube is secured to the nose and face with an adhesive tape. The infant is restrained by wearing mittens over the hands to prevent dislodging of tube. The milk formula is suspended in a sterile glass burette and connected with an infusion pump for continuous slow infusion. The reservoir for milk is changed daily but nasojejunal tube may be kept *in situ* for several weeks. The feeding formula should preferably be iso- or hypo-osmolar to safeguard against osmotic diarrhea or 'dumping syndrome'.

Advantages

Nasojejunal feeding reduces handling of the baby and time taken for feeding. Risk of aspiration is minimized while effective caloric intake can be ensured without causing gastric distension. There are less chances of reflex bradycardia due to vagal stimulation unlike gastric gavage feeding. It is safer and less expensive than parenteral alimentation.

Complications

The procedure is relatively safe but it does compromise the airway which may be critical to an infant with respiratory distress syndrome. Local irritation, congestion and infection of nasal passages with increased airway impedance may occur. Blockage due to clogging of feeding tubes may necessitate flushing or reinsertion. The fat may separate and stick to the walls of syringe and tube. The risk of perforation of gut is minimized by the use of a silastic tube. The procedure has not gained popularity because of the need for frequent supervision, change of infusion sets every 4 to 6 hours and risk of complications.

Nutritional Supplements

All low birth weight babies should receive vitamin K 0.5–1.0 mg intramuscularly or orally at birth to prevent hemorrhagic disease of the newborn. Water soluble preparations of vitamins are administered to VLBW babies (<1500 g) after 2 weeks of age and continued till the post conceptional maturity of 38 weeks or body weight of 2000 g. In babies fed with EBM, calcium (160 mg/kg/d) and phosphorus (80 mg/kg/d) supplements are given to prevent osteopenia of prematurity. There is no need to administer nutritional supplements when human milk fortifier is used to supplement EBM. Iron (2–3 mg/kg/d) supplements are provided when full enteral feeds are established and baby is gaining weight. The timing of giving iron supplements is controversial and is often delayed to 6–8 weeks by some neonatologists. Iron and vitamin D supplements are continued up to one year of age. Infants born early (<32 weeks) are likely to have low quota of docosahexaenoic acid (DHA) because substantial amount of DHA is transferred from mother to fetus during the last trimester of pregnancy. Human milk is a good source of DHA, but when a baby is given formula feed, he should receive supplements of DHA (4–5 mg/kg/d) which is likely to improve his visual perception, stereopsis and cognition.

Criteria for Adequacy of Feeding

In clinical practice, satisfactory weight gain is the most useful criterion of adequacy of feeding, because it is simple and less liable to error as compared to the measurement of length. The optimal feeding regime is associated with prompt postnatal resumption of growth at a rate approximating intrauterine growth velocity. It should be achieved without imposing any stress on the developing metabolic or excretory systems of the LBW babies. Accurate daily weight record of LBW babies is essential to assess the adequacy of feeding (Figure 15.14). After initial weight loss of up to maximum of 15%, the birth weight is regained by the end of second week. Subsequently, the baby normally gains at a rate of 10–15 g/kg (1.0–1.5% of body weight) per day and should be able to maintain his growth rate above the 10th percentile on the intrauterine growth chart. Postnatal weight charts of healthy preterm babies are available which can be used for recording the anthropometric measurements. They are representative of postnatal growth and also show the initial weight loss that occurs in the first 2 weeks of life. The average linear growth is around 1.0 cm per week but it is difficult to assess it reliably. The urinary osmolality should vary

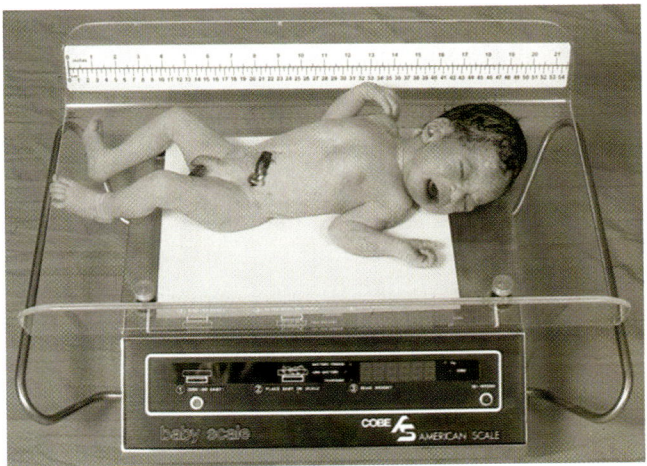

Figure 15.14 Weighing of a baby on an electronic weighing scale having an accuracy of ±1.0 g.

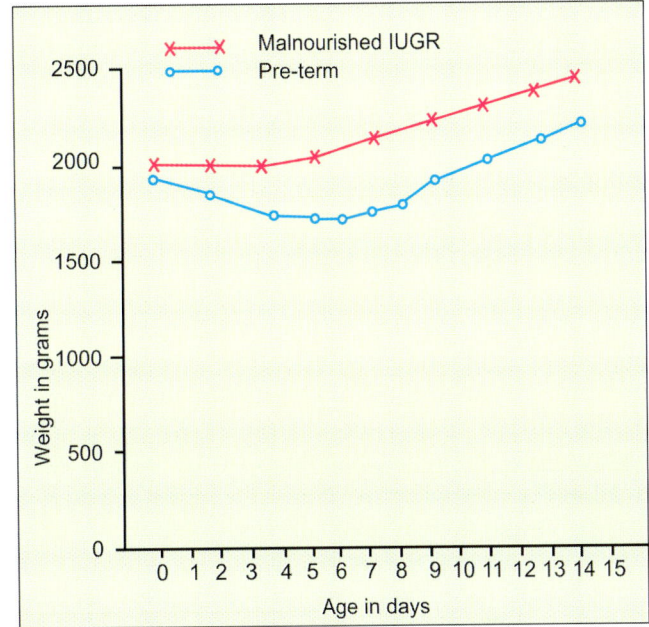

Figure 15.15 Early postnatal growth of preterm and term-SFD infants of identical birth weights.

between 150 and 300 mOsm/kg and baby should void at least 1 mL/kg/hr of urine. Hematocrit should be maintained above 40%. When adequately fed, the malnourished small-for-dates baby does not lose any weight and starts gaining weight by 2 to 3 days of age (Figure 15.15).

Unsatisfactory early postnatal growth pattern of LBW baby, who is not sick, is suggestive of subtle illness, inadequate feeding due to less than adequate number of nurses, unfortified EBM feeds and cold stress or excessive evaporative losses. The baby should be screened for any latent infection especially urinary tract infection, late metabolic acidosis, anemia and bronchopulmonary dysplasia. The nurses should be encouraged to chart the timing of feeds when they are actually given (and not on the basis of recommendation), without any guilt and fear, even if they are unable to meet the requirements of feeding schedule recommended by the neonatologist so that unnecessary work up of the infant is avoided. In addition to steady weight gain, a satisfactory feeding regimen should be associated with freedom from morbidity, improved survival, enhanced functional maturation and optimal future prognosis regarding physical and mental development.

Criteria for Discharge from the Hospital

The infant can be discharged from the hospital when (i) there is no evidence of any clinical illness, (ii) infant can breastfeed, (iii) maintain body temperature in an

Feeding and Nutrition

15

open crib, (iv) infant is having steady weight gain and (v) mother is able to demonstrate satisfactory care giving skills. Several RCTs have shown that there are no adverse outcomes of early discharge of a preterm baby from NICU, if aforementioned criteria are met.

PARENTERAL NUTRITION

Intravenous alimentation or parenteral nutrition (PN) is considered in the treatment of critically sick or tiny newborn babies when it is impossible to provide nutrition through gastrointestinal route due to immaturity of the gut or clinical condition of the baby. The technique is, however, handicapped by lack of easy availability of satisfactory infusates which are rather expensive and there is relatively high incidence of side effects and complications. Satisfactory growth velocity comparable to intrauterine growth pattern can be achieved by parenteral alimentation. Unfortunately administration of parenteral nutrition has not kept pace with development of other high-tech neonatal interventions in India. Adequacy of nutrition is crucial to enhance linear growth, neuromotor development and ensure optimal functioning of various body organs.

Indications

1. Birth weight less than 1000 g or gestation <28 weeks.
2. Sick LBW babies requiring prolonged intravenous infusion exceeding 4–5 days, e.g. RDS, apneic attacks, sepsis, seizures, bronchopulmonary dysplasia, and necrotizing enterocolitis.
3. Chronic intractable diarrhea.
4. Neonates born with major anomalies of gastrointestinal tract requiring extensive surgical procedures. They include gastroschisis, omphalocele, tracheoesophageal fistula, intestinal atresia, meconium ileus, malrotation of gut, and short bowel syndrome.
5. Partial parenteral nutrition to supplement gavage feeding is recommended in infants weighing less than 1,200 g.
6. All neonates with catabolic states where enteral feeding is limited, not feasible or not tolerated.

Contraindications

1. Hypoxia, acidemia and shock
2. Hyperbilirubinemia (serum bilirubin >12 mg/dL)
3. Azotemia (blood urea >48 mg/dL)
4. Thrombocytopenia

Infrastructural needs to set up PN Facility

Parenteral nutrition (PN) or intravenous alimentation is a mandatory requirement for critical care of preemies with life-threatening disorders. Every tertiary care NICU must have facilities for providing PN. The basic requirement for setting up PN facilities are listed in Box 15.4.

Box 15.4: Basic requirements for setting up parenteral nutrition in the NICU

- Availability of dedicated trained personnel like neonatologist, nutritionist, pharmacist, nurse, perfusionist and resident staff.
- TPN cabin 150–200 sq feet.
- Laminar flow system for preparation of PN solutions.
- Refrigerator.
- Computer with a printer.
- Kimaya NICU software™ for calculation of parenteral nutrients.
- Infusion pumps (at least two per patient).
- Nutrient solutions (macro- and micronutrients).
- Provision of central venous access.
- Disposable (infusion sets, connectors, filters).
- Scrub linen, gowning, mask, gloves, antiseptics.
- Laboratory support with microchemistry facilities.

The Composition of Infusates

Energy Preterm infants should not be starved as they have low energy reserves because of poor fat content as well as low reserves of glycogen. The parenterally nourished infants need about 100–120 kcal/kg/day (as opposed to 120–150 kcal/kg/day for enterally fed) for satisfactory weight gain because there are no losses due to digestion, specific dynamic action of food or wastage in stools. The ideal distribution for availability of calories from different sources include 50–55% from carbohydrates, 10–15% from proteins and 30–35% from fats.

Carbohydrates Glucose is the most suitable source of carbohydrate because of its immediate bioavailability to the central nervous system. Carbohydrates from other sources like fructose, galactose, sorbitol, glycerol and ethanol may produce serious complications in premature infants. Due to its osmolarity (18 mg/dL of glucose contributes osmolarity of about 1.0 mOsm/L) and sclerosing effect, concentrations in excess of 12.5% (125 mg glucose per mL) should not be infused through a peripheral vein. Higher concentrations up to a maximum of 20% may be infused

Care of the Newborn

through a silastic or silicone catheter placed in a central vein. To reduce intolerance, it is recommended that dextrose infusion should be started at a rate of 6 mg/kg/minute and gradually increased to a maximum of 12–14 mg/kg per minute in increments of 2 mg/kg/minute everyday over next couple of days. Insulin is given (0.05 units/kg/hr) to manage hyperglycemia (>120 mg/dL) when despite lowering glucose infusion rate to 4–6 mg/kg/min it is not possible to achieve euglycemia.

Proteins Amino acids are building blocks of the body. Protein requirements are inversely related to gestational age or birth weight because of rapid growth velocity and greater protein losses in ELBW babies. Solutions containing crystalline amino acids are satisfactory to provide nitrogen during parenteral nutrition. Protein hydrolysates carry greater risk of infection and hyperammonemia. In addition to eight amino acids which are essential in the older infants, histidine, cysteine, tyrosine, glutamine, arginine, proline, and glycine are probably essential for premature and possibly full term infants. The commonly used formulations include Aminoven Infant 6% and 10% (Fresenius Kabi India Pvt Ltd) and Primene 10% (Baxter Healthcare Ltd). Amino acid solutions are administered in a starting dose of 0.5 g protein equivalent per kilogram per day and increased daily by 0.5 g/kg and maintained between 3.0 and 3.5 g/kg per day. To prevent hyperchloremic acidosis, amino acid mixture should be buffered with sodium bicarbonate or hydrochloride salts of arginine, lysine and histidine should be replaced by acetate equivalents. Administration of fresh frozen plasma is also useful to provide opsonins and immune antibodies in addition to proteins.

Fats In order to provide sufficient calories without enhancing osmolar load, availability and administration of fat emulsions is mandatory. Apart from high energy density, they are required for supply of essential fatty acids and delivery of fat-soluble vitamins. Intralipid (10% or 20% emulsion of soya bean oil stabilized with 1–2% egg phospholipid) and Liposyn (derived from safflower oil) are commercially available and provide all the essential fatty acids. Linoleic fatty acids are provided directly in the emulsion while arachidonic acid is derived by *in vivo* conversion of linoleic acid. Intralipid is infused in a dose of 1.0 g/kg day which is gradually increased by 0.5–1.0 g/kg eveyday till maximum of 3.0 g/kg/day is achieved. The daily requirement of essential fatty acid can be met by infusion of 0.5–1.0 g/kg of intralipid per day. Higher quantities of intralipid can be infused by slow infusion spread over a period of 24 hours with an infusion pump. The rate of intralipid infusion should be maintained below 0.25 g/kg per hour and a concentration of 10–20% can be used in the newborn.

Lipids do not impose any osmolar load. The use of 20% intralipid emulsion is preferred due to lower risk of hypertriglyceridemia, hypercholesterolemia and hyperphospholipidemia. Lipids should be infused through a separate infusion syringe which can be used as a vehicle for administration of vitamins to prevent their photodegradation and adhesion to the infusion tubing. When lipids are exposed to light, they can form potentially toxic lipid hydroperoxides. Photoprotection of PN solution reduces the peroxide load and is credited to reduce the risk of BPD. Therefore, the lipid syringe and tubing should be wrapped with an aluminum foil. Lipids should be avoided or used with caution in low doses in critically sick ELBW babies on assisted ventilation, disseminated intravascular coagulation, hyperbilirubinemia and thrombocytopenia. Lipids can adversely affect the gas exchange. Lipids and free fatty acids compete with binding sites in the albumin and thus predispose to development of bilirubin encephalopathy at lower serum bilirubin levels. A free fatty acid to albumin ratio (FFA: albumin) should be kept below 6:1 in high-risk situations. Lipids are administered in minimum doses to meet the nutritional needs of essential fatty acids.

Minerals and Vitamins

Prolonged and exclusive intravenous alimentation must be supplemented with electrolytes, minerals, trace elements and vitamins. Daily sodium and potassium needs of the newborn baby are 2–3 mEq/kg. Preterm babies especially those below 1500 g require higher sodium intake of 4–6 mEq/kg/day. The estimated intravenous requirements of both elemental calcium and phosphorus are 20–40 mg/kg/day. Magnesium should be supplemented in a dose of 0.25–0.50 mEq/kg/day. Except phosphates, all the minerals are available for intravenous use. The precise parenteral requirements of trace elements are uncertain. Zinc (150–400 µg/kg/d) should be started from day one of TPN while other trace elements are gradually introduced. MVI adult is the most suitable preparation for providing daily requirements of vitamins to newborn babies on TPN. Daily administration of 0.5 mL/kg of intravenous multivitamin preparation is satisfactory though it provides higher than recommended concentrations of certain vitamins. Folic acid (100 µg), vitamin B_{12} (100 µg) and vitamin K (500 µg) should be administered weekly through intramuscular route. Carnitine is a conditionally essential nutrient for neonates as it facilitates beta oxidation of long chain fatty acids. It should be supplemented in a dose of 5 mg/kg/d in infants receiving TPN. The available PN solutions in Indian market are shown in Table 15.8.

Fluids

Fluids serve as the carrying medium for parenteral nutrients. They are started at a rate of 60–80 mL/kg/d and gradually increased by 10–20 mL/kg/d to maximum of 150 mL/kg/d by the end of first week of life. Fluid therapy is fine tuned by monitoring hydration status of the infant by daily weight changes, urine output, serum sodium/osmolality and urinary specific gravity and osmolality. The evidence-based recommendations for administration of various nutrient-solutions for parenteral nutrition are listed in Table 15.9. A computer software (Kimaya NICU software™) is available which can be used for calculation of various components of PN solution because manual calculation is time consuming and cumbersome.

Technique of Administration

It is preferable to use a peripheral vein by inserting a polyvinyl catheter. Thorough asepsis must be ensured during the procedure. Intralipid emulsion with

TABLE 15.8 Available parenteral solutions in Indian market

Component	Source	Concentration
Glucose	Dextrose	5%, 10%, 25%, 50%
Protein	Aminoven	6% and 10%
	Primene[a]	10%
Lipids	Intralipids[b]	10%, 10% PLR, 20%
	Linoleic[c]	PLR, i.e. phospho-lipids reduced 20%
Sodium and chloride	NaCl	0.9% and 3%
Potassium and chloride	KCl	15%
Calcium	Calcium gluconate	10%
Magnesium	Magnesium sulfate	50%
Multivitamins	Adult MVI	—
Trace elements	Celecel[d] 4, 5 TMA	—

[a]Fresenius Kabi India Pvt Ltd.
[b]Baxter Healthcare Ltd.
[c]Drugs and Pharmaceuticals Pvt Ltd.
[d]Claris Life Sciences Ltd.

TABLE 15.9 Summary of salient recommendations for administration of various nutrient solutions for parenteral nutrition

Component	Recommendations
Fluids	60–80 mL/kg/d on day 1, gradually increased up to 120–150 mL/kg/d by the end of first week. Postnatal weight loss up to 10–15% is acceptable.
Energy	50 kcal/kg/d on day 1, gradually increased up to 100–120 kcal/kg/d by the end of first week.
Glucose	6 mg/kg/min on day 1, gradually increased by 2 mg/kg/min daily up to maximum of 12 mg/kg/min to maintain euglycemia (glucose 50–120 mg/dL). When hyperglycemia (and glycosuria) occurs even when glucose infusion rate is reduced to 6 mg/kg/min, insulin is infused @ 0.05 units/kg/hr to maintain euglycemia.
Protein	Amino acid infusion is started @ 1.5 g/kg/d on day 1 and gradually increased by 0.5–1.0 g/kg/d up to maximum of 3.5 g/kg/d. Glucose and amino acid solution are mixed together and administered through one syringe.
Fat	Intralipid infusion is started @ 1.0 g/kg/d on day 1, gradually increased by 0.5–1.0 g/kg/d up to maximum of 3.0 g/kg/day. It is administered as 20% intralipid through a separate syringe which is shielded from light with an aluminum foil. It should be infused continuously over 24 hours.
Minerals and trace elements	Essential minerals include sodium, chloride, potassium, calcium, phosphorus and magnesium. Essential trace elements should include zinc, copper, selenium, manganese, iodine, chromium and molybdenum.
Vitamins	Vitamins are added to the syringe containing fat emulsion to minimize the risk of peroxidation, photodegradation and adhesion to infusion tubing.

vitamins on one hand and protein–carbohydrate mixture with electrolytes and trace elements on the other, are suspended through separate infusion sets and connected with a Y-connector just proximal to the catheter or micropore filter (Figure 15.16). It is also feasible to administer TPN solution through a single bottle. A Y-connector or triple lumen connector can be used for administration of amino acid solution and intralipid through a single line. A short-term PN can be provided through a peripheral venous line by

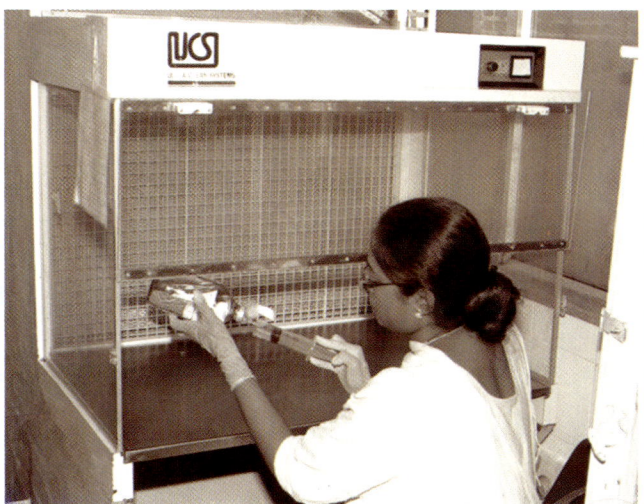

Figure 15.17 The preparation of TPN solution under laminar flow.

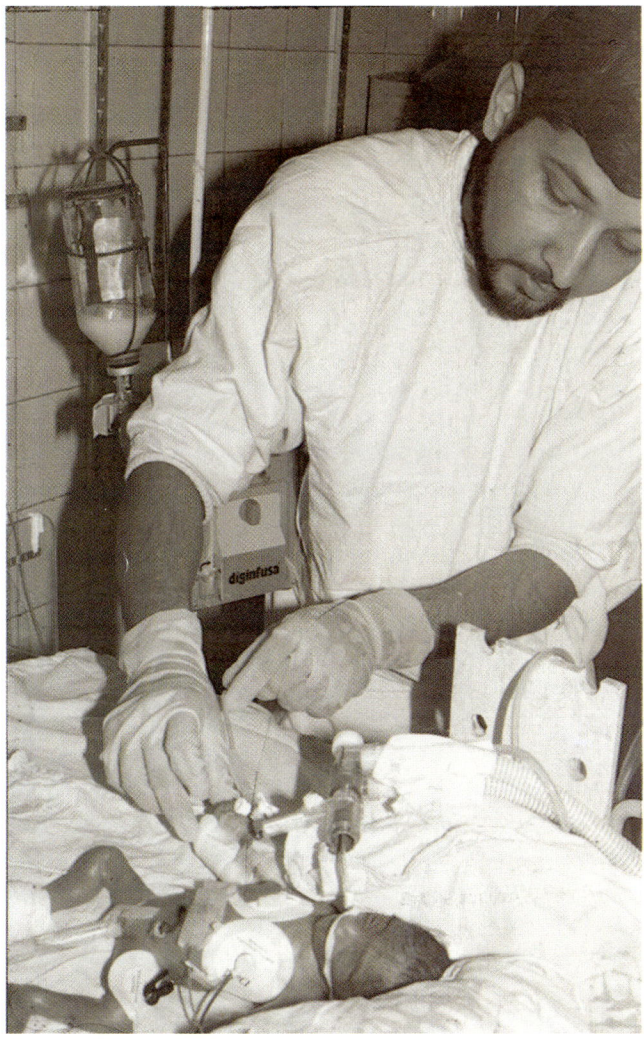

Figure 15.16 Setting up 3-way stopcock for administration of TPN with strict aseptic precautions.

restricting dextrose concentration up to 12.5%. When prolonged PN is anticipated it should be delivered through peripherally inserted central catheter (PICC). Single lumen catheter is inserted to ensure that its tip lies in the superior or inferior vena cava which should be confirmed by an ultrasound or X-ray examination. In neonates, a central line can be established through umbilical vein. Silicone or polyvinyl catheter should be used to establish central venous line. Carbohydrates and amino acid solutions are mixed first. Fat emulsion is added subsequently by gently shaking the bottle during mixing. Mixed TPN solution must contain heparin (1 unit/mL) and is stable up to 36 hours. The amino acid and lipid solutions should be protected against light to reduce the risk of peroxide load to the baby.

It is essential that precise infusion rate is maintained by regulating its flow through a constant infusion pump. It is desirable to use bacterial filters (0.2 μ) which are now available in India. Infusion bottles and sets must be changed everyday to reduce chances of contamination. Infusion site should be promptly changed at the first sign of reddening or devitalization of the skin. Strict asepsis and local application of antimicrobial cream at the site of exit wound of catheter are essential to prevent septic complications. Most infusates are marketed in large-volume packs entailing considerable wastage unless mini-bagged. The formulation or sub-packing of commercial infusates into small packs should be undertaken under a laminar flow with meticulous aseptic precautions by using sterile plastic bags (Figure 15.17). The osmolarity of various infusates should be restricted to 300–900 mOsm/L when PN is administered through a peripheral venous line. The volume and concentration of various nutrients should be increased gradually. The venous access used for PN should not be exploited for administration of antibiotics and medications. A separate intravenous line should be established for this purpose. As soon as clinical condition of the patient permits, oral feeding should be started and infant gradually weaned off from intravenous feeding over a period of 3 to 4 days.

Monitoring during TPN

A flowchart should be maintained to record daily changes in weight, status of hydration, urine output and intake of fluids, calories and its sources. Serum electrolytes, BUN, glucose, hematocrit, blood pH, plasma and urinary osmolality should be checked daily. Plasma osmolality should be maintained between 285 and 300 mOsm/L. Plasma should be

Feeding and Nutrition

15

TABLE 15.10 Monitoring schedule for neonates receiving parenteral nutrition

Parameter	Frequency
Anthropometry*	
Weight (g)	Daily (same time each day) Length (cm) weekly
Head circumference (cm)	Weekly
Biochemistry	
Urine glucose and specific gravity	8 hourly first week, then once daily
Inspection of plasma sample for lipemia	Once daily
Blood glucose	6 hourly initially, 12 hourly when glucose infusion rate is static
Serum sodium and potassium	Daily initial 3–4 days, then twice weekly
BUN, creatinine	Daily initial 3–4 days, then twice weekly once protein intake becomes static
Blood pH	Daily initial 3–4 days, then twice a week once protein intake becomes static
Hemogram	Weekly
Serum calcium, phosphorus, magnesium, proteins, triglycerides, liver function tests	Weekly

*The target anthropometric gains during TPN include weight gain 15–18 g/d (1.0% of body weight/d), increase in length 0.75–1.0 cm/week, and head circumference gain 0.75 cm/week.
Note: Daily intake of fluids (mL/kg/d), urine output (mL/kg/hr), energy intake (kcal/kg/d), glucose infusion rate (mg/kg/min), protein intake (g/kg/d) and lipids (g/kg/d) should be recorded. Catheter-related complications including hospital acquired infection (HAI) should be looked for. Eosinophilia is a useful marker of allergy to intralipid. Blood transfusion is mandatory as soon as 10% of blood volume has been removed by sampling.

inspected daily to look for turbidity due to fat emulsion. Liver function tests, serum proteins and fatty acids should be checked once every week (Table 15.10). An accurate record of amount of blood removed for biochemical monitoring should be maintained.

Complications

They may be related to the catheter or to the infusate. Inflammation and sloughing of skin at infusion site is alarming. Hospital-acquired infection (HAI) is a common life-threatening complication and should be prevented by use of effective aseptic precautions like use of laminar flow for mixing of PN solutions, use of

bacterial filter in amino acid-glucose line and daily change of infusion sets. The metabolic complications include competitive displacement of albumin-bound bilirubin by free fatty acids, and alterations in the concentration of a variety of blood constituents such as glucose, acid–base status, sodium, potassium, chloride, calcium, magnesium, phosphorus, BUN, essential amino acids, vitamins and trace elements. Hyperglycemia with osmotic diuresis and dehydration can occur among ELBW babies receiving hyperosmolar infusates. A constant clinical and chemical monitoring with the aid of a micro chemistry laboratory support is essential for early diagnosis and prompt management of metabolic alterations.

Hepatomegaly with cholestasis and jaundice is a frequent complication of TPN in very LBW babies. TPN-associated hepatic dysfunction is possibly related to disorder in bile secretion because of toxic effect of certain amino acids, deficiency of essential fatty acids or associated sepsis. The deficiency of essential fatty acids is managed by cutaneous application of sunflower oil, oral administration of sunflower oil 2.5–5.0 mL/day and intermittent plasma transfusion. Intralipid administration is contraindicated in infants with jaundice and bleeding manifestations. Rapid infusion of intralipid in tiny preterm babies may cause reduction in pulmonary diffusion capacity producing dyspnea and cyanosis. Thrombocytopenia and hypercoagulability of blood are rare complications.

BIBLIOGRAPHY

Agastoni C, Buonocare G, Carnielli VP, et al. Enteral nutrient supply for preterm infants. Commentary from the European society for Paediatric Gastroenterology, Hepatology and Nutrition Committee on Nutrition. *J Pediatr Gastroenterol and Nutr* 2010; 50(1):1–9.

American Academy of Pediatrics. Working Group on Breastfeeding. Breastfeeding and use of human milk. *Pediatrics* 2005; 115(2):496–506.

American Dietetic Association. Robbins ST, Beker LT (eds.) Infant Feeding: Guidelines for Preparation of Formula and Breast milk in Health Care Facilities. *Chicago Ill: American Dietetic Association* 2004:91.

Anderson J, Johnstone BM, Remley DT. Breast-feeding and cognitive development: a meta-analysis. *Am J Clin Nutr* 1999; 70:525–535.

Arora K, Goel S, Manerkar S, et al. Prefeeding oromotor stimulation program for improving oromotor functions in preterm infants: A randomized controlled trial. *Indian Pediatr* 2018; 55:675–8.

Atkins SA. Human milk feeding of the micropremies. *Clin Perinatol* 2000; 27: 235–247.

Banapurmath CR, Banapurmath S, Kesaree N. Developing brain and breastfeeding. *Indian Pediatr* 1996; 33:35–38.

Berseth CL, Van Aerde JE, Gross S, *et al*. Growth, efficacy and safety of feeding an iron-fortified human milk fortifier. *Pediatrics* 2004; 114:e699–706.

Bharadva K, Tiwari S, Mishra S, *et al*. Human Milk Banking Guidelines: Infant and Young Child Feeding Chapter, Indian Academy of Pediatrics. *Indian Pediatr* 2014; 51:469–474.

Bhat BV, Adhisivam B. Human milk banking in quality control. *Indian J Pediatr* 2018; 85(4):255–6.

Brake FW, Van den Akker CH, Rvedijk MA, *et al*. Parenteral aminoacid and energy administration to premature infants in early life. *Semin Fetal Neonatal Med* 2007; 12:11–18.

Brans YW. Parenteral nutrition of the very low birth weight neonate: A critical view. *Clin Perinatol* 1977; 4:367.

Breastfeeding promotion network of India (2006). Joint statement on infant and young child feeding. www.bpni.org accessed on October 20th, 2009.

Cashore WJ, Sedaghatian M and Usher RH. Nutritional supplement with intravenously administered lipid, protein hydrolysate and glucose in premature infants. *Pediatrics* 1975; 82:955.

Chawla D, Thukral A, Agarwal R, *et al*. Parenteral Nutrition. In: AIIMS protocols in Neonatology. VK Paul and AK Deorari (Ed); *Indian Journal of Pediatrics, New Delhi* 2008; p 128–40.

Check JA and Staub GF. Nasojejunal alimentation for premature and full-term newborn infants. *J Pediatr* 1973; 82:955.

Davidson M, Levine SZ, Bauer CH and Dann M. Feeding studies in low birth weight infants. *J Pediatr* 1967, 70: 695.

Davies DP. The first feed of low birth weight infants. *Arch Dis Child* 1978; 53:187.

Deshpande G, Rao S, Patole S. Probiotics for prevention of necrotizing entrocolitis in preterm neonates with very low birth weight. A systematic review of randomized controlled trials. *Lancet* 2007; 369:1614–1620.

Easton LB, Halata MA and Dweck HS. Parenteral nutrition in the newborn. A practical guide. *Pediatr Clin N Amer* 1982; 29:1171.

Edmond K, Bahl R. Optimal feeding of low birth weight infants. Technical review. *World Health Organization* 2006.

Ehrenkranz RA. Growth outcomes of very low birth weight infants in the newborn intensive care unit. *Clin Perinatol* 2000; 27(2):325–345.

Filler RM, Eraklis AJ, Rublin VG and Das JB. Long-term total parenteral nutrition in infants. *N Engl J Med* 1969; 281:589.

Georgieff MK, Sasanow SR. Nutritional assessment of the neonate. *Clin Perinatol* 1986; 13:73.

Greer FR. Vitamin metabolism and requirements in the micropremie *Clin Perinatol* 1995; 22:95–110.

Greer FR. Do breastfed infants need supplemental vitamins? *Pediatr Clin N Am* 2001; 48:415–423.

Grover A, Khashu M, Mukherjee A, *et al*. Iatrogenic malnutrition in neonatal intensive care units: urgent need to modify practice. *J Parent Enteral Nutr* 2008; 32:140–144.

Hanson LA, Carlsson B, Ahlstedt S, Svanborg EC and Kaijser B. Immune defence factors in human milk. In: Breastfeeding. *Annales Nestle* No. 39 Switzerland, 1977.

Hartman BT, Pang WW, Keil AD, *et al*. Best practice guidelines for the operation of a donor human milk bank in an Australian NICU. *Early Human Dev* 2007; 83:667–673.

Hay WW, Lucas A. Nutrition of the extremely low birth weight. *Pediatrics* 2000, 12: 58–66.

Heird WC and Anderson TL. Nutritional requirements and methods of feeding low birth weight infants. Current problems in Pediatrics. Gluck L (Ed). *Year Book Medical Publishers Inc. Chicago,* Vol. VII, June, 1977.

Heird WC, Driscoll J. Total parenteral nutrition. *Neonatal Rev* 2003; 4:e137–139.

Joy R, Krishnamurthy S, Bethou A, *et al*. Early versus late enteral prophylactic iron supplementation in preterm very low birth weight infants: a randomized controlled trial. *Arch Dis Child Fetal Neonatal Ed* 2014, 99(2): F105–109.

Klein CJ. Nutrient requirements for preterm infant formulas *J Nutr* 2002; 132:S1395–577.

Lang S, Lawrence CJ, Orme RLE. Cup feeding: an alternative method of infant feeding. *Arch Dis Child* 1994; 71:365–369.

Lucas A, Fewtrell MS, Morley S. Randomized outcome trial of human milk fortification and developmental outcome in preterm infants. *Am J Clin Nutr* 1996; 64:142–151.

Malhotra AK, Deorari AK, Paul VK, Bagga A, Singh M. Gastric residuals in preterm babies. *J Trop Pediatr* 1992; 38:262–264.

Modi M, Ramji S, Jain A, Kumar P, Gupta N. Early aggressive enteral feeding in neonates weighing 750–1250 g: A randomized controlled trial. *Indian Pediatr* 2019; 56:294–8.

Molloy C, Doyle LW, Makrides M, Anderson PJ. Docaso-hexaenoic acid and visual functioning in preterm infants: A review. *Neuropsychol Rev* 2012; 22:425–437.

O'Connor DL, *et al*. Growth and development of premature infants fed predominantly human milk, predominantly preterm infant formula or a combination of human milk and premature formula. *J Pediatr Gastroenterol Nutr* 2003; 37(4):437–446.

Paul VK, Singh M, Deorari AK, Pacheco J, Taneja U. Manual and pump methods of expression of breast milk. *Indian J Pediatr* 1996; 63:87–382.

Paul VK, Singh M, Srivastava LM, *et al*. Macronutrients and energy content of breast milk of mothers delivering prematurely. *Indian J Pediatr* 1997; 64:379–382.

Rigo J, Senterre J. Nutritional needs of premature infants: current issues. *J Pediater* 2006; 149(suppl):580–588.

Singh M. Breastfeeding. In: The Art and Science of Baby and Child Care. *CBS Publishers & Distributors Pvt. Ltd., New Delhi,* fourth edition 2014; p78–94.

Feeding and Nutrition

15

Singh M. Feeding and nutrition. In: Essential Pediatrics for Nurses. *CBS Publishers & Distributors Pvt. Ltd., New Delhi,* third edition 2014; p141.

Singh M. Feeding and nutrition. In: A Manual of Essential Pediatrics. *Thieme Medical and Scientific Publishers Pvt. Ltd., New Delhi,* second edition 2013; p 60–89.

Stern L. Early postnatal growth of low birth weight infants: what is optimal? *Acta Pediatr Scand* (suppl.) 1982; 296:6.

Tagare A, Vaidya U. Parenteral nutrition: current guidelines. *J Neonatol* 2007; 21:186–188.

Vaidya U. Falak K. Parenteral nutrition. In; Neonatal Emergencies. Singh M (Ed), *New Delhi, CBS Publishers & Distributors Pvt Ltd* 2017; pp 304–311.

Victoria CG, Bahl R, Barros AJD, Franca GVA, Horton S, Krasevec J, *et al.* Breastfeeding in the 21st century: epidemiology, mechanisms, and lifelong effect. *The Lancet* 2016, 387(10017): 475–490.

Wang H-J, Hua C-Z, Hong L-Q *et al.* Sialic acid and iron content of breast milk in Chinese lactating women. *Indian Pediatr* 2017; 54:1029–31.

Williamson MT, Murti PK. Effects of storage time, temperature and compostion of containers on biological components of human milk. *J Hum Lact* 1996; 12(1):31–35.

Wright K, Dawson JP, Fallis D, *et al.* New postnatal growth grids for very low birth weight infants. *Pediatrics* 1993; 91:922–926.

Yu Vuh. Scientific rationale and benefits of nucleotide supplementation of infant formula. *J Paediatr Child Hlth.* 2002; 38:543–549.

Ziegler E, Carlson S. Early nutrition of VLBW infants. *J Maternal-Fetal Neonat Med* 2009; 22:191–197.

Perinatal Infections

Perinatal infections especially neonatal bacterial sepsis is one of the leading causes of neonatal mortality in India. The fetus may get infected *in utero* and during passage through the birth canal or neonate may develop nosocomial infection any time after birth.

INTRAUTERINE INFECTIONS

The intrauterine infections may occur due to viruses, *Toxoplasma gondii* a protozoan, spirochetes and occasionally by bacteria including *Mycobacterium tuberculosis*. They are popularly described with an acronym of TORCH wherein T stands for toxoplasmosis, O for others (syphilis, gonococcal ophthalmia, tuberculosis, malaria, varicella, hepatitis type B, coxsackie B, echo, parvovirus B19, HIV, zika, COVID-19, etc.), R for rubella, C for cytomegalovirus and H for herpes simplex hominis. Due to relatively large basket of "Others", TORCH acronym has become obsolete and is not commonly used. The fetal infection occurs either as a result of direct transplacental passage of infecting agents or following infection of the placenta. Ascending infection with contamination of liquor amnii and amnionitis may also result in *in utero* bacterial infection of the fetus.

Clinical Features

The baby may be normal at birth and manifestations may be delayed for a few days to several weeks. Some infants may show evidences of infection at birth. Viral infections during early pregnancy may lead to fetal death, congenital malformations or severe systemic manifestations of the disease. Incidence of these complications, as a result of maternal infection, is uncertain but available evidence suggests that viruses do not play a major role in neonatal morbidity or mortality. The combined overall incidence of intrauterine infections appears to be about 0.5–2.0% of all births. Cytomegalovirus infection and rubella appear to be the commonest. The incidence of HIV infection is gradually rising over the years.

The presence of any three of the following clinical features should alert the pediatrician to the possibility of intrauterine infection (Table 16.1).

Maternal history of infection The clinical manifestations of maternal infection are either absent or mild to attract attention. History of fever, skin rash, painful cervical lymphadenopathy during the first trimester of pregnancy suggest the possibility of maternal rubella and toxoplasmosis. Primary CMV infection may manifest with a clinical picture similar to infectious mononucleosis with mild hepatitis. Genital herpes may be detected on physical examination of the mother. Pleurodynia may be caused by Coxsackie B group of viruses. High-risk sexual behavior and drug abuse are associated with STDs including HIV and HBV. Routine estimation of isolated titers of antibodies against TORCH antigens during pregnancy are useless and confusing.

Intrauterine growth retardation (IUGR) About two-thirds of infants with cytomegalic inclusion disease and rubella and about one-third of infants with congenital toxoplasmosis may manifest with intrauterine growth restriction. Such babies appear hypoplastic rather than malnourished.

Hepatosplenomegaly The incidence of hepatosplenomegaly is similar to that of intrauterine growth retardation. The enlargement of liver and spleen may persist for weeks or months. In infants with no evidence of hepatitis, extramedullary hematopoiesis appears to be responsible for hepatosplenomegaly.

TABLE 16.1 Characteristic clinical features of intrauterine infections

Infection	IUGR	Hepato-splenomegaly and jaundice	Petechiae and bleeding	Ophthalmic signs	Neurological features	Others
Cytomegalic inclusion disease	60–70%	About two-thirds of the patients	About two-thirds of the patients. "Blue-berry muffin spots" on skin due to extra-medullary hematopoiesis	Diffuse white perivascular infiltrates with hemorrhages and necrosis giving an appearance of "cottage cheese with ketchup" type of peripheral chorioretinitis with sparing of macula, microophthalmia, uveitis and optic atrophy. They develop strabismus and roving eyes in infancy.	Microcephaly, periventricular calcification (15%) and psycho-motor retardation. CNS manifestations may appear later.	Anemia, interstitial pneumonia and sensori-neural deafness.
Rubella	About 60%	60–70%	50–60%	Cataracts, micro-ophthalmia, corneal opacity and glaucoma. Salt and pepper type of chorioretinitis.	Meningo-encephalitis, psychomotor retardation; and deafness; micro-cephaly is rare.	Congenital cardiac defects, namely PDA, pulmonary artery stenosis, valvular pulmonic stenosis, aberrant subclavian vessels and VSD. Meta-physeal lesions characterized by linear areas of radio-lucency and increased bone density in the longitudinal axis.
Toxo-plasmosis	About 20–30%	40–50%	30–40%	Central destructive chorio-retinitis characterized by white or yellow foci with edematous elevated margins with involvement of macula, may be recurrent. Optic atrophy and cataracts following uveitis.	Hydrocephaly or sometimes microcephaly. Diffuse nodular cerebral calcifi-cation in one-third of cases.	Strabismus, nystagmus and visual impairment during infancy.
Congenital syphilis	Uncommon, may develop hydrops fetalis	30–40%	Uncommon	Interstitial keratitis and chorioretinitis later in life	Meningo-encephalitis.	Rashes and snuffles; flat or depressed nasal bridge; periostitis and chondritis. Deafness.

(Contd.)

TABLE 16.1 Characteristic clinical features of intrauterine infections *(contd.)*

Infection	IUGR	Hepato-splenomegaly and jaundice	Petechiae and bleeding	Ophthalmic signs	Neurological features	Others
Herpes virus hominis type 2	None	About 50%	Uncommon	Keratitis, conjunctivitis and chorioretinitis and cataracts.	Meningo-encephalitis and microcephaly. Intracranial calcification may occur rarely.	Vesicles, muco-cutaneous lesions, pneumonia, hepatitis and neuromotor sequelae. Herpes genitalis in the mother.
Coxsackie B infection	None	About 50%	Uncommon	None	Meningo-encephalitis	Respiratory distress due to carditis. History of pleurodynia in the mother.

IUGR, Intrauterine growth restriction, VSD; ventriculoseptal defect, PDA; patent ductus arteriosus.

Jaundice may occur any time during the neonatal period. There is rise of both indirect and direct reacting bilirubin with elevation of serum alkaline phosphatase and transaminase enzymes. Jaundice is relatively uncommon with rubella infection but is frequent with toxoplasmosis and cytomegalic inclusion disease.

Petechiae and purpura Thrombocytopenia is common with rubella and cytomegalic inclusion disease. It is relatively infrequent in infants with congenital toxoplasmosis.

Meningoencephalitis Microcephaly (rubella, CMV), hydrocephaly (toxoplasmosis), cerebral calcification, retinopathy, cataracts (rubella) and abnormal neurologic signs occur in various combinations (Figure 16.1).

Radiological abnormalities Intracranial calcification (rubella, toxoplasmosis, CMV), osteochondritis, metaphysitis and periosteal reaction may be seen (Figure 16.2).

Raised IgM in cord blood Cord blood IgM level of more than 20 mg/dL is indicative of fetal infection because IgM is not transferred transplacentally from the mother to the fetus. Both false positive and false negative results may be encountered. False positive elevation of IgM in cord blood may occur due to contamination with maternal blood, cross-reaction between viruses and presence of rheumatoid factor. Delayed hormonal antibody response on the part of fetus may lead to false negative test. The presence of specific IgM fluorescent antibody is diagnostic of the specific fetal infection.

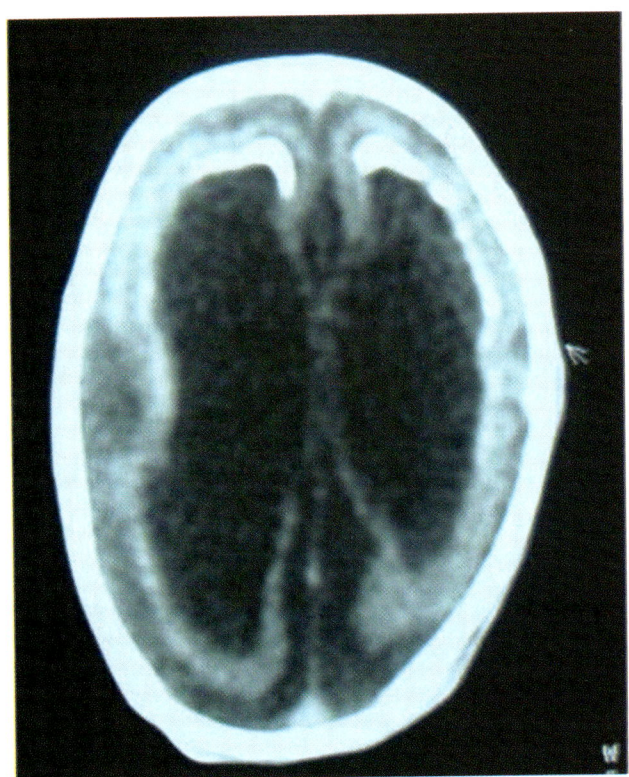

Figure 16.1 NCCT head in a neonate showing diffuse periventricular calcification with dilated ventricles due to congenital CMV infection.

Perinatal Infections

16

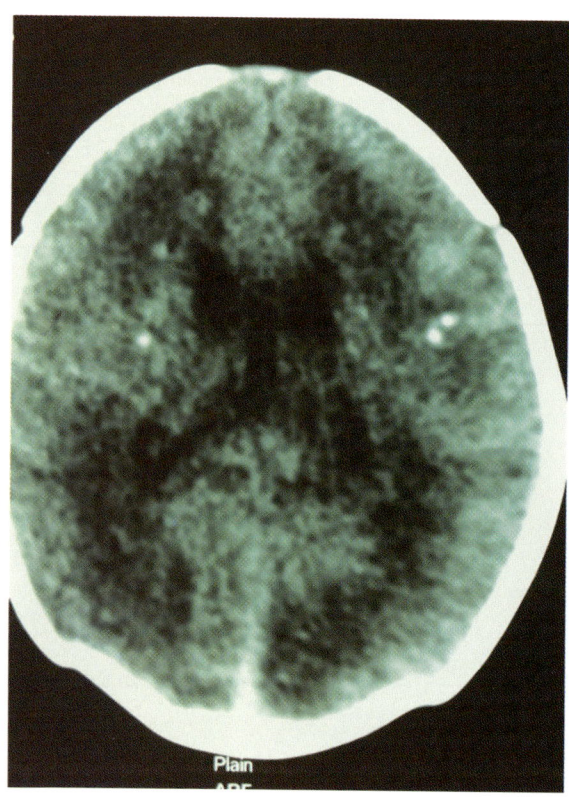

Figure 16.2 Diffuse nodular calcification due to congenital toxoplasmosis.

Screening of Pregnant Women for TORCH Infections

There is widespread practice of one time screening of pregnant women for TORCH infections in our country. This practice is of doubtful utility and leads to considerable confusion and unnecessary tension among obstetricians and pregnant women. Routine one time screening of pregnant women for TORCH infections is not recommended due to the following reasons.

1. It is difficult to differentiate between primary infection and reinfection which has different implications for fetal involvement. Reinfection of the mother is relatively safe for the fetus except in an occasional case of CMV infection and when woman is immunodeficient (SLE, HIV, cancer, etc.).
2. The sensitivity and specificity of available serological tests in different laboratories are of doubtful reliability and reproducibility. There is a need to use standard and reliable diagnostic kits for serological tests.
3. The risk of fetal morbidity following intrauterine infection is low. TORCH infections are not associated with recurrent abortions, stillbirths or congenital malformations.
4. Unfortunately, there are neither good therapeutic options nor a satisfactory outcome for most

TORCH-affected infants except congenital syphilis and gonococcal infection.

Ideally, the mother should be screened for TORCH serology just before pregnancy or soon after conception to assess whether she has had any of the TORCH infections in the past and is thus protected or she is susceptible to develop them during the course of pregnancy due to lack of any protective IgG antibodies. During the course of pregnancy, she needs to be closely watched and followed up for those infections to which she is susceptible. The TORCH serology (for susceptible infections) should be rechecked around 20 weeks of gestation or earlier, if there are any clinical evidences of infection. If there is any evidence of active primary infection by any of the TORCH agents in the mother, ultrasound examination and cordocentesis is recommended to confirm the fetal diagnosis. Mother should be treated with appropriate therapeutic agents as per standard recommendations. The family needs to be counseled and given the option of medical termination of pregnancy, if fetus is seriously affected and postnatal treatment of affected baby is associated with poor immediate and later outcome.

Diagnosis

The main clinical features and laboratory procedures essential for the diagnosis of intrauterine infections are summarized in Table 16.2. Majority of infants with TORCH infection are asymptomatic at birth. Infants with perinatal transfer of Au antigen and HIV are invariably normal. The isolation of the infecting agent and demonstration of the specific IgM fluorescent antibody on ELISA are useful for prompt confirmation of the diagnosis. The virus neutralizing, hemagglutination inhibition and complement fixing antibodies are predominantly IgG (except during the early stages of the infection) and are passed transplacentally from the mother to the fetus. Thus, any antibodies present in the maternal blood will be found approximately in the same titer in the infant. The titer of passively transmitted antibodies shows a significant fall when the infant's blood is retested at 3 to 4 months of age. The repeat titer should remain the same or become elevated, if the infant was infected *in utero* and had started producing his own antibodies.

Management

Specific treatment of some of the TORCH-affected newborn babies is given below. In severely affected infant, specific therapy may offer limited therapeutic benefit because most of the damage has already occurred in fetal life.

TABLE 16.2 Main clinical features and investigations for the diagnosis of intrauterine infections

Maternal infection	Chief clinical manifestations	Site for isolation of infecting organisms	Additional tests
Bacterial			
Non-specific pyogenic	Pneumonia, septicemia and meningitis	Blood, umbilical cord, CSF, feces, ear and throat swab	Gastric aspirate for polymorphs and placental histology
Listeria monocytogenes	Meconium-stained liquor, pneumonia, maculopapular rash at birth, apneic attacks	Liquor amnii, blood, ear swab, meconium and CSF	
Mycobacterium tuberculosis	Miliary tuberculosis	Gastric washings	Placental histology and X-ray chest
Neisseria gonorrhoeae	Ophthalmia	Eye swab	
Fungal			
Candida	Oral and perineal moniliasis, pneumonia	Oral swab and feces	—
Protozoal			
Pasmodium (Vivax and falciparum)	Congenital malaria	Blood smear	Placental histology and specific IgM fluorescent antibody
Toxoplasma gondii	Choroidoretinitis and meningoencephalitis (hydrocephalus and intracerebral calcification), hearing and visual impairment, mental deficiency, hepatitis and thrombocytopenia. Blueberry muffin rash due to dermal erythropoiesis	CSF	Specific IgM and IgA fluorescent antibodies by ELISA and ISAGA techniques. Paired maternal and cord sera for complement fixation, Sabin-Feldman dye and hemagglutination inhibition tests. Repeat at 3–4 months of age.
Treponema pallidum	Rashes, snuffles, hepatitis and periostitis. Hutchinson triad refers to the combination of eighth cranial nerve deafness. Hutchinson teeth (peg-shaped, notched upper central permanent incisors) and interstitial keratitis	—	Specific IgM fluorescent antibody. Paired maternal and cord sera for VDRL or RPR, repeat at 3–4 months of age. Placental histology.
Viral			
Cytomegalovirus	Small-for-dates, meningoencephalitis, choroidoretinitis, microcephaly, sensorineural hearing loss, periventricular calcification, hepatitis and thrombocytopenia	Freshly voided urine, throat swab and leukocytes by spin-enhanced culture or "shell vial"	CMV-DNA for PCR, specific IgM fluorescent antibody by RIA or Elisa. Cytomegalic inclusion cells in baby's urine. Paired maternal and cord sera for complement fixing antibody. Repeat at 3–4 months of age.
Herpes virus hominis Type 2	Meningoencephalitis, hepatitis, and vesicles. Neutropenia, thrombocytopenia and coagulopathy, EEG and CT/MRI brain	New vesicular lesions, throat swab and CSF	Virus can be isolated from vesicular fluid or CSF by culture techniques or PCR. Viral particles can be identified directly when tissue samples are swabbed on a glass slide and evaluated by direct fluorescent antibody technique. Specific fluorescent IgM antibody is delayed up to 3 weeks. Cytological examination of vesicular fluid for multinucleated giant cells and intranuclear inclusions with margination of nuclear chromatin (Tzanck test)

Perinatal Infections

16

(Contd.)

TABLE 16.2 Main clinical features and investigations for the diagnosis of intrauterine infections (*contd.*)

Maternal infection	Chief clinical manifestations	Site for isolation of infecting organisms	Additional tests
Vericella zoster (chickenpox, herpes zoster)	Congenital varicella, and congenital herpes zoster	Vesicles	Multinucleated giant cells and/or intranuclear inclusions from vesicular fluid in vesicles
Myxoviruses			
Influenza	Abortion	—	—
Measles	Abortion and congenital measles	Throat swab	—
Mumps	Abortion and endocardial fibroelastosis	Feces and throat swab	
Picornaviruses			
Coxsackie	Carditis and systemic viremia	Feces and throat swab	Cord serum for specific IgM, paired sera for complement fixing, neutralizing and hemagglutination inhibition antibodies titers. Repeat at 3–4 months of age.
Echoviruses	Meningitis and enteritis	Feces and throat swab	As above
Poliovirus	Abortion and congential polioencephalitis	Feces and throat swab	As above
Poxviruses			
Vaccinia virus	Abortion and congenital vaccinia	Vesicles	Vesicular fluid for intracytoplasmic inclusions
Others			
Hepatitis (HBsAg/Au antigen)	Hepatitis	Blood for Au antigen	Maternal blood for hepatitis e-antigen
Rubella	Small-for-dates, cardiac malformations, cataract, deafness, hepatitis, thrombocytopenia, anemia and metaphyseal lesions in bones.	Throat swab, CSF and urine	Isolation of rubella virus. Cord serum for IgM and specific IgM fluorescent antibodies. Paired maternal and cord sera for complement fixing, neutralizing and hemagglutination inhibition titers. Repeat after 3–4 months.
Mycoplasma hominis	Ophthalmia and pneumonia	Eye swabs	
HIV (AIDS)	Asymptomatic during early life. The common opportunistic infections include *P. jirovecii* (previously known as *pneumocystis carinii*), lymphocytic interstitial pneumonitis, recurrent bacterial infection, candida esophagitis, encephalopathy, cytomegalovirus infection, *Mycobacterium avium* infection, herpes simplex viral infection, cryptosporidiosis	Blood	Viral detection by *in vitro* cell culture, p 24 antigen detection, PCR or HIV-specific DNA in infected cells, ELISA for detection of specific IgM and IgA antibodies.

Maternal Toxoplasmosis

The available drugs act on tachyzoite forms and they do not eradicate the encysted forms of *T. gondii*. Spiramycin 2 g/d in 4 divided doses should be given throughout pregnancy. After 20 weeks gestation, add sulfadiazine (75 mg/kg or maximum 4 g loading dose followed by 75–100 mg/kg/d or maximum of 6 g is given in 2 divided doses everyday) and pyrimethamine (15 mg/m^2 or 1 mg/kg up to maximum of 50 mg twice a day for 2 days followed by 25 mg once daily for 7 days and then twice a week subsequently). Give folinic acid (calcium leucovorin) 5 mg twice a week along with pyrimethamine.

Congenital Toxoplasmosis

In cases of overt congenital toxoplasmosis, treatment is given for one year. Pyrimethamine (1 mg/kg/d single dose) and sulfadiazine (100 mg/kg/d in 2 divided doses) are given for 6 months. Sulfadiazine should not be used during the first week of life due to danger of displacement of bilirubin from protein binding sites. Subsequently, pyrimethamine and sulfadiazine therapy for one month is alternated with spiramycin (100 mg/kg/d in 2 divided doses) for one month during next 6 months. Folinic acid should be given along with pyrimethamine therapy. When overt toxoplasmosis is associated with acute inflammatory response (chorioretinitis, raised CSF proteins, jaundice; etc.), corticosteroids are given for 8–12 weeks. Eyes should be examined every 3 months till the age of 18 months and then yearly.

In subclinical (IgM-ELISA and IgA-ELISA positive with no clinical abnormalities) cases of congenital toxoplasmosis, give pyrimethamine and sulfadiazine for 6 weeks. Subsequently, alternate pyrimethamine with spiramycin and sulfadiazine with spiramycin for every 4 weeks for a period of one year. To a healthy neonate (negative serology) of a mother who had definite primary toxoplasmosis during pregnancy, pyrimethamine and sulfadiazine or spiramycin are given for one month.

Prevention

Toxoplasmosis is endemic in cat-friendly populations unlike Indians. Cats should be handled with gloves, kept indoors and fed with dry cooked or canned food. Meat should be eaten after thorough cooking. Gardening should be done with gloves on and vegetables should be washed thoroughly especially when eaten raw. Hands should be thoroughly washed with soap and water before eating food.

Cytomegalovirus Disease

Worldwide, CMV is the most common intrauterine infection. Indications for specific antiviral therapy are not well defined. Apart from chorioretinitis which forms a definitive indication for specific therapy , other relative indications include colitis, esophagitis, hepatitis, pneumonitis and meningoencephalitis. Therapeutic utility is doubtful in acquired CMV pneumonia in recepients of blood transfusion or bone marrow. Ganciclovir (9-1,3-dihydroxy-2-proproxy-methyl guanine or DHPG) is given IV 5 mg/kg/dose twice daily for 2–3 weeks of induction phase. Maintenance therapy is continued with 5 mg /kg/d IV single dose for 5–7 days in a week for 8–12 weeks. The drug is very toxic and demands daily or every other day monitoring of blood counts and platelets and weekly assessment of renal function parameters. Therapy should be stopped, if neutrophil count falls below 500/mm^3 or platelet count drops to 25,000/mm^3. The hematological side effects are reversible within 5–7 days on cessation of therapy. Testicular atrophy is another recognized serious side effect. Recently oral valganciclovir has been used for prophylaxis and treatment of CMV infection.

Prevention

Prevention of CMV disease with a vaccine may provide limited benefit because reinfections are known to occur in partially immune subjects. Two live-attenuated vaccines (Towne strain, AD-169) have demonstrated safety and effectiveness among healthy adults and renal transplant patients on limited trials. A more attractive option appears to be a sub-unit vaccine that contains surface glycoproteins of CMV (qB). Perinatal transmission of CMV infection to premature babies can be curtailed by avoidance of unncessary blood transfusions and use of CMV-negative or leukocyte-depleted blood. Avoid use of donor breast milk due to potential risk of transmission of CMV. It has been documented that 3–50% of lactating women may excrete CMV. In extremely preterm babies, CMV infection acquired through breast milk may cause a serious disease. It is possible to remove CMV from breast milk but the process may damage other important constituents of the milk.

Herpes Simplex Virus (HSV)

Several trials have shown efficacy and safety of treating pregnant women with clinically symptomatic primary HSV infection with a 10 days course of acyclovir. In a woman with genital herpes, infant should be delivered by elective cesarean section preferably within 4 hours of rupture of membranes. Acyclovir is now preferred over vidarabine due to ease of administration and minimal side effects. In infants with localized skin, eye and mouth disease, acyclovir 20 mg/kg/dose is given IV every 8 hr for 10–14 days. Infants with disseminated or CNS infection with HSV should receive 20 mg/kg/dose IV every 8 hr for at least 21 days or longer, if CSF PCR remains positive. There are no serious side effects.

SARS-COV-2 or COVID-19

Corona viruses are RNS viruses with glycoprotein spikes that give an appearance of a crown. There are four species of corona viruses which cause life-threatening respiratory disease with generalized thrombosis and a storm of inflammatory markers in critical patients. There are reports of vertical transmission of COVID infection from infected mother or horizontal infection from the mother, relatives or health care providers. Most cases in neonates are mild with fever, flu- like illness and diarrhea. Encephalopathy and severe respiratory illness has occurred in an occasional infant. Among 707 neonates born to COVID-19 positive women, 20 developed pneumonia and three died. The diagnosis can be screened by an antigen-based test and confirmed by RT-PCR on nasopharyngeal swab. There is no specific therapy and neonates with severe respiratory difficulty are managed with non-invasive ventilation.

During delivery of COVID-19 positive mother, standard universal precautions should be followed to prevent horizontal transmission of infection to the neonate and health care workers. Neonates with COVID-19 should be isolated. The mother should be advised to practice respiratory hygiene and wear a mask while breastfeeding. Silver hydrogen peroxide (100 mL H_2O_2 10% V/V solution diluted with 900 mL distilled water) is used for sanitization of equipment and fomites because new COV-2 viruses are highly contagious. Sodium hypochlorite 2% solution is useful for decontamination of floors.

CONGENITAL MALARIA

Malaria during neonatal period most commonly occurs due to administration of infected blood. In endemic areas, it is difficult to differentiate between congenitally acquired malaria from postnatal infection acquired through mosquito bites or blood transfusion. It appears that placenta acts as a barrier to the malarial parasite and its transplacental transmission is further blocked, if mother is immune. The incidence of placental malaria in endemic areas may be as high as 30% while incidence of congenital malaria in infants of immune mothers is estimated to be as low as 0.3% (up to 10% in the non-immune mothers). Placental malaria is asymptomatic and it silently causes fetal wasting. Among firstborn, it can significantly affect the birth weight, the differences between the birth weight of an infant born with a negative and positive placenta for malarial parasites is usually around 150 to 300 g. The blood film of the mother is often negative. It is recommended that in endemic areas routine administration of chloroquine to all mothers during third trimester of pregnancy is desirable and is associated with improvement in the birth weight of the offspring.

Maternal malaria during pregnancy may cause serious anemia and adversely affect the placental circulation interfering with oxygenation and nutrition of the fetus. It is associated with abortion, stillbirth, prematurity, fetal growth retardation and neonatal deaths. Fetal infection may occur due to direct penetration of parasites through chorionic villi, premature separation of placenta, and maternofetal transfusion at delivery. The relative resistance of red blood cells containing fetal hemoglobin against malarial parasites and passively transferred IgG from immune mothers may explain relatively low incidence of congenital malaria. The disease manifests around 2 to 8 weeks of age with fever, jaundice, hemolytic anemia, reticulocytosis, thrombocytopenia and hepatosplenomegaly. The delay in clinical manifestations is attributed to transplacental passage of maternal antimalarial antibodies. Congenital malaria in preterm babies is rare but manifests with clinical features at birth or within first week of life. Maternal history of fever with rigors and positive smear for malarial parasites during late pregnancy is often available. The condition should be differentiated from other intrauterine infections. Treatment consists of oral administration of chloroquine phosphate in a dose of 10 mg base/kg followed by 5 mg base/kg at 6, 24 and 48 hours. Intramuscular chloroquine therapy is unsafe during neonatal period due to risk of seizures. Radical therapy with primaquine is unnecessary because congenital malaria is a form of transfusion malaria and it has no exoerythrocytic (hepatic) phase. In cases of chloroquine-resistant congenital malaria due to *P. falciparum*, oral quinine sulfate (25 mg/kg/d q 8 hr for 3 to 5 days) is recommended.

CONGENITAL TUBERCULOSIS

Despite adoption of several national strategies, tuberculosis continues to be a disease of public health relevance in India. It has assumed more sinister severity due to increasing incidence of HIV infection and emergence of multi-drug resistant strains of *M. tuberculosis* due to non-compliance of therapy. Fortunately, congenital tuberculosis is relatively uncommon. Women with pulmonary tuberculosis do not pose any threat to the fetus but may infect the baby after birth. Congenital tuberculosis may occur, if mother is having tubercular endometriosis, miliary tuberculosis or placenta is infected by tubercular bacilli. The infection may be transmitted to the fetus through umbilical vein or infant may aspirate infected secretions at the time of birth. Postnatal exposure from an infected mother or other family member and an infected health care worker is far more common.

Infant with congenital tuberculosis may be born with active disease or symptoms may appear anytime during the first 8 weeks of life. History of disseminated or genital tuberculosis in the mother and involvement of placenta by tuberculosis are essential for the diagnosis of congenital tuberculosis. The infant may present with classical features of miliary tuberculosis with hepatosplenomegaly, lymphadenopathy and tachypnea. There may be fever, lethargy, poor feeding, skin papules and jaundice. Mantoux test is usually negative. Skiagram of chest may show evidences of miliary tuberculosis. CSF should be examined to exclude CNS involvement. Acid-fast stains and cultures should be performed on gastric and tracheal aspirate and spinal fluid.

Treatment should be started with INH (5 mg/kg/d), rifampicin (10 mg/kg/d) and pyrazinamide (30–40 mg/kg/d). Pyrazinamide is given for 2 months, while INH and rifampicin are continued for 9–12 months. INH should be supplemented with pyridoxine owing to low levels of this vitamin in breast milk. Corticosteroids should be given for 8 weeks, if there is CNS involvement. HIV-infected newborn babies with congenital tuberculosis need more intensive management including use of streptomycin (20–40 mg/kg/day single dose IM) or amikacin for initial 2 months.

Infant of a Mother with Active Tuberculosis

Isolation of the baby is neither feasible nor desirable as it would compromise breastfeeding. Isolation is recommended, if mother is non-adherent to therapy or suffering from MDR-TB. Mother should receive appropriate and aggressive treatment for her disease. She should be advised to breastfeed her baby by using a surgical mask and should follow strict hand-washing routines. Infant should be given BCG vaccination and administered oral INH 10 mg/kg/d single dose for 3 to 6 months. Infant should be assessed for any clinical or radiological abnormalities in the chest. If Mantoux test is negative, repeat BCG vaccination should be given.

PERINATAL HIV INFECTION (AIDS)

Around 80% of HIV infections in children occur during perinatal period. There is 20–45% risk of mother-to-child transmission (MTCT) of HIV infection during perinatal period. It is believed that 30% of vertical transmission of HIV occurs during pregnancy while 70% occurs during labor and delivery. The risk of infection through breast milk is well documented and varies between 10 and 15%. The risk of mother-to-child transmission can be reduced to 5%, if proper maternal and infant prophylaxis measures are taken.

Abbreviations

▪ Abacavir	ABC
▪ Antiretroviral therapy	ART
▪ Didanosine	ddI
▪ Efavirenz	EFV
▪ Indinavir	IDV
▪ Lamivudine	3TC
▪ Lopinavir/ritonavir	LPV/r
▪ Nelfinavir	NFV
▪ Nevirapine	NVP
▪ Ribavirin	RBV
▪ Stavudine	d4T
▪ Single dose nevirapine	SdNVP
▪ Tenofovir	TDF
▪ Zidovudine	AZT

Risk Factors for Perinatal HIV Transmission

The risk of transmission is increased, if mother has advanced disease, high viral load, HIV-1 disease, low CD4 count, symptoms of AIDS, P_{24} antigenemia and when mother has not received any antiretroviral therapy. Vaginal delivery, chorioamnionitis, antepartum hemorrhage, prolonged rupture of membranes and prematurity are associated with higher risk of perinatal transmission of HIV infection. The risk of transmission is higher in developing countries.

Transmammary transmission of HIV during breastfeeding is higher, if breast milk viral load is high, presence of cracked nipples or mastitis and when baby is given mixed feeding (breast plus formula feeds) instead of exclusive breastfeeding.

Prevention of Mother-to-Child Transmission (PMTCT) of HIV

The national strategies for prevention of parent-to-child transmission (PPTCT) of HIV are listed below.

- Primary prevention of HIV, especially among women in childbearing age.
- Integration of PPTCT interventions with general health services such as basic antenatal care (ANC), sexual reproductive health and family planning, early infant diagnosis (EID), pediatric ART and adolescent reproductive and sexual health (ARSH), TB and STI/RTI services.
- Strengthening postnatal care of the HIV-infected mother and her exposed infant.
- Providing essential package of PPTCT services.

The vertical transmission of HIV from mother to her baby can be reduced to less than 2% by administration of antiretroviral therapy (ART) to the mother during pregnancy and labor, and to the infant after birth (Figure 16.3). The baby should be delivered prior to onset of labor and before rupture of membranes by elective cesarean section. The revised national guidelines recommend that cesarean section in HIV positive pregnant women should be performed only on the basis of obstetric indications. Avoidance of multiple vaginal examinations, artificial rupture of membranes and episiotomy are associated with reduced risk of mother-to-child transmission of HIV. Invasive procedures, like amniocentesis, chorionic villus sampling, fetal scalp electrodes or blood sampling, should be avoided. There is no convincing evidence that vaginal douches with betadine or administration of vitamin A to the mother reduces the risk of infection. Hyperimmune gamma globulins,

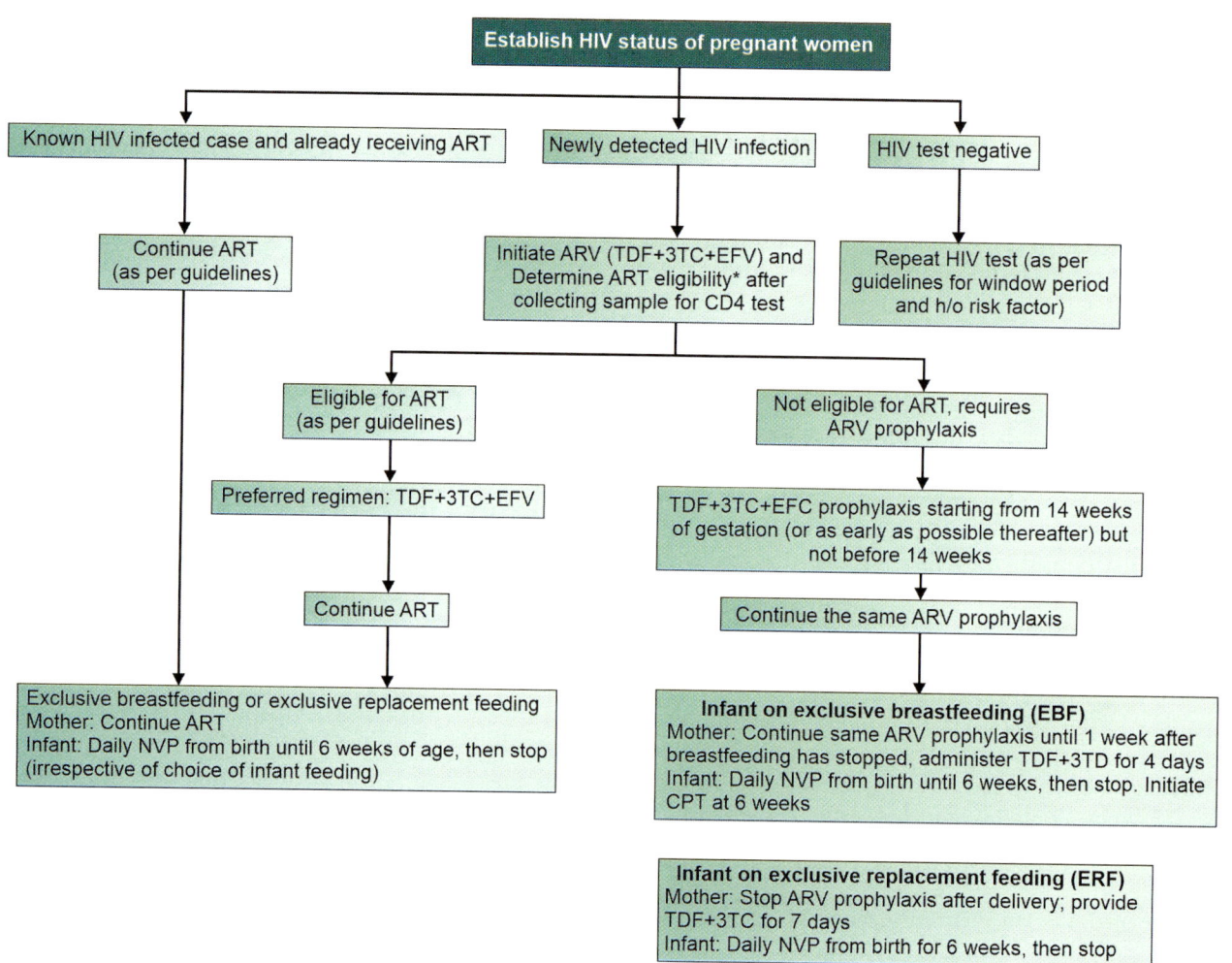

*Determine ART eligibility—the regimen will be the same for ARV prophylaxis/ART and initiated for all irrespective of CD4 count or WHO clinical stage at baseline. However, CD4 count is necessary to guide duration of ART or during breastfeeding (ARV prophylaxis)

Abbreviations: ART: antiretroviral therapy, ARV: antiretroviral, TDF: Tenofovir, 3TC: lamivudine, EFV: efavirenz NVP: nevirapine, CPT: cotrimoxazole prophylactic therapy

Figure 16.3 National guidelines for prevention of mother-to-child transmission (MTCT) of HIV (NACO 2013).

prepared from healthy HIV-infected volunteers, is being tried to reduce the risk of infection. A number of research centers are actively pursuing efforts to produce a vaccine against surface glycoprotein of HIV (gp120).

Breastfeeding

Breastfeeding is associated with 10–15% risk of transmission of HIV infection. There is increased risk of HIV transmission through breastfeeding when (i) maternal CD4 count is low, (ii) high maternal viral load, (iii) mastitis and (iv) whether exclusive breastfeeding or bottle cum breastfeeding and (v) duration of breastfeeding. The decision for advising or withholding breastfeeding should be individualized on the basis of education, awareness, socioeconomic status and risk of bottle feeding. According to current WHO recommendations, breastfeeding should be avoided by HIV-positive mother, if formula feeding is acceptable, feasible, affordable, sustainable and safe (AFASS). In order to reduce the risk of formula feeds in mothers belonging to poor socioeconomic status, it is preferable to give the feeds with a cup and spoon or *paladay*. When a mother opts to breastfeed her baby, exclusive breastfeeding for 6 months poses less risk of transmammary transmission of HIV compared to a combination of breastfeeding and formula feeds. After 6 months, breastfeeding should be "abruptly stopped" and infant weaned to formula feeds or animal milk with a cup and spoon, milk products and cereal-based complementary feeds.

Delivery of an HIV-positive Mother

In order to reduce the intrapartum risk of transmission of HIV, it is recommended to deliver the baby around 38 weeks of gestation by elective cesarean section before rupture of membranes or onset of labor. It is unethical on the part of health care professionals to deny care to HIV-positive patients due to concerns of their own personal safety. However, it is mandatory to follow universal precautions in all deliveries with the premise that any pregnant woman may be a potential carrier of HIV or HBV infection. It must be remembered that hepatitis B virus (HBV) is a tougher and 100 times more contagious than HIV. The latter is a relatively fragile virus and can be easily killed by drying, heating to 50°C–60°C, bleaching solutions like 10% sodium hypochlorite, 5% formaldehyde, 3% hydrogen peroxide, 0.5% lysol, glutaraldehyde (cidex) and 35% isopropyle alcohol. Gloves must be worn while conducting all deliveries and when handling products of conception and the baby. During resuscitation of a newborn baby, mouth-to-mouth breathing and oral suction of endotracheal tube should not be done.

When it is known before delivery that mother is HIV-positive, additional precautions, like wearing occlusive gown and goggles are recommended as a safeguard against splashes of blood. The baby should be given bath with warm water in the labor room to wash off any traces of blood and amniotic fluid. The baby can be nursed along with other babies in the NICU because there is no risk to other babies and health care personnel who are likely to touch, cuddle, kiss or feed the baby. Universal precautions should be followed for taking and handling specimens of blood, splashes of blood and disposal of used needles and syringes.

Clinical Spectrum

Perinatal HIV infection is associated with abortion, prematurity, intrauterine growth retardation and perinatal wastage. Fetal malnutrition may occur due to maternal malnutrition and drug abuse. The occurrence of embryopathy is controversial and may be associated with microcephaly, box-like forehead, hypertelorism, flat nasal bridge, oblique slant of eyes, long palpebral fissures with patulous lips.

The incubation period of perinatal AIDS is shorter and disease is more severe and runs a fulminant course. The normal and infected infants are indistinguishable at birth. The symptoms usually appear between 6 months and 18 months and most children succumb to the disease within 5 years of onset of symptoms. HIV causes profound and irreversible damage to T cell immunological system, making the child vulnerable to suffer from recurrent infections by a variety of common and unusual pathogens. The disease is characterized by failure to thrive, protein-energy malnutrition, persistent and recurrent gastrointestinal and respiratory infections (intractable cough), unexplained fever or recurrent bacterial infections, generalized lymphadenopathy and hepatosplenomegaly. AIDS-associated diarrhea is caused by conventional organisms and unusual pathogens like Cryptosporidium, Isospora, *Campylobacter jejuni*, Microsporidia and Giardia.

The clinical features which should alert to the possibility of AIDS include lymphoid interstitial pneumonitis with nodular opacities in the lungs, recurrent oroesophageal candidiasis (recalcitrant thrush and swallowing difficulties), parotitis and clubbing. These children are susceptible to develop a variety of opportunistic infections like Pneumocystis pneumonia (PCP) due to *Pneumocystis jirovecii*, cytomegalovirus (CMV), Herpes simplex and *Mycobacterium tuberculosis*. The risk of opportunistic infections has considerably reduced after introduction of highly active antiretroviral therapy (HAART).

Diagnosis

The ELISA and Western Blot tests may be positive in the neonate in the absence of actual infection because maternal HIV-IgG antibodies are passively transferred from the mother to the fetus through the placenta. These antibodies gradually wane off and disappear by 15 months of age. Their persistence beyond 15 months is indicative of active HIV infection of the infant. Early diagnosis of active HIV infection can be made by demonstration of HIV-specific IgM antibodies, p24 core antigen, ultrasensitive p24 Ag assays, plasma RNA, viral culture, demonstration of HIV DNA with polymerase chain reaction (PCR) technology and branched DNA for assessing viral load (Figure 16.4).

The immunological abnormalities which can be identified in infants with AIDS include lymphopenia, reduced CD4 counts ($<4000/mm^3$) with reduction of CD4/CD8 ratio and elevated serum immunoglobulins. Primary immunodeficiency disorders and secondary immunodeficiency states due to other causes should be ruled out by appropriate laboratory tests and clinical findings.

Management

Care at Birth

1. All health care professionals attending the delivery should wear gloves, gown, goggles and mask and maintain universal precautions.

2. The baby's mouth and nose should be wiped as soon as head is delivered. Avoid routine oropharyngeal suctioning and if liquor is meconium stained, suctioning is done with an electrical device.

3. The cord should be clamped immediately after delivery and no "milking" should be done. Cover the cord with a gloved hand and a gauze piece at the time of cutting the cord to avoid splashing of blood.

4. The baby should be bathed immediately soon after birth to wash off all traces of blood, secretions and meconium.

5. The mother should be provided information and counseled during pregnancy regarding the choices for feeding. When mother decides to breastfeed the baby, the baby should be put to the breast within one hour of birth and should be given exclusive breastfeeding.

The National AIDS Control Organization (NACO) guidelines for prevention of Parent-to-Child Transmission 2013 (PPTCT) of HIV are summarized in Table 16.3.

Supportive Therapy

The mainstay of therapy is supportive and palliative. Efforts should be made to provide high caloric nutritious diet to prevent malnutrition. The risk of breastfeeding for transmission of HIV infection should be explained to the mother so that she can make an informed decision regarding the mode of feeding. Cotrimoxazole (trimethoprim 20 mg and sulfamethoxazole 100 mg single daily dose) prophylaxis against *Pneumocystis jirovecii* is started at 4–6 weeks of age and continued till HIV infection is excluded. Early topical application of ketoconazole and ensuring oral hygiene

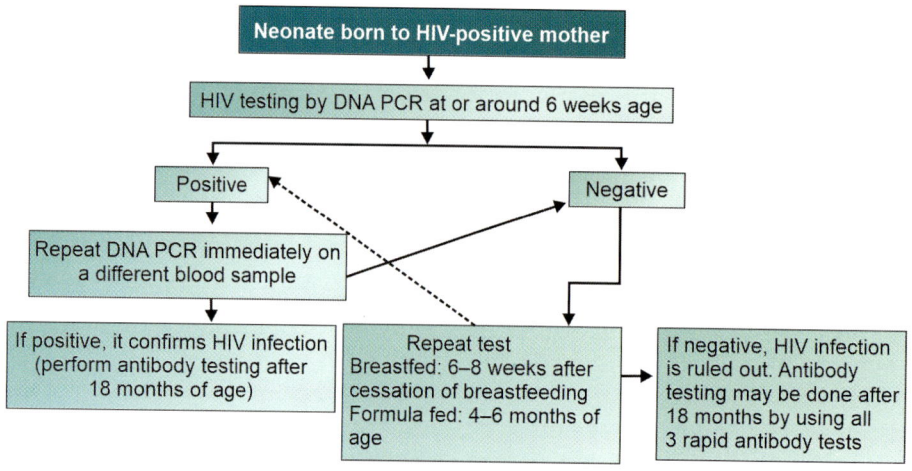

Figure 16.4 Algorithm for diagnosis of HIV infection in a newborn baby

TABLE 16.3 The NACO guidelines for prevention of mother-to-child transmission (PMTCT) of HIV

- Routine HIV counseling and testing of all pregnant women attending antenatal care services with "opt-out" option (medical termination of pregnancy).
- Ensure involvement of spouse and other family members and move from an "ANC Centric" to a "Family Centric" approach.
- Provide antiretroviral therapy (ART) to all HIV-infected pregnant women regardless of WHO staging and CD4 count. The preferred drug regimen is TDF + 3TC + EFV.
- Promote institutional deliveries of all HIV-infected pregnant women. ANMs, ASHAs and community workers should accompany the pregnant women to institutions and try to reduce stigma and discrimination among health care providers through sensitization and capacity building.
- Provision of care and treatment for associated conditions (STI/RTI, TB and opportunistic infections).
- Provide nutrition counseling and psychosocial support to HIV-infected pregnant women with the help of ANMs, ASHAs and community outreach workers.
- Provide counseling and support for initiation of exclusive breastfeeding within one hour of delivery as the preferred option and continue it for 6 months. After 6 months, give complementary or weaning foods along with breastfeeding. A small number of babies born to HIV-infected mothers who have serious illness (or have died) and a few reluctant mothers (at their own risk despite counseling) may decide not to breastfeed but give exclusive replacement feeding (ERF).
- Provide antiretroviral prophylaxis to infants from birth up to a minimum period of 6 weeks. Nevirapine (NVP) in a single oral dose (5 mg or 0.5 mL <2.0 kg, 10 mg or 1.0 mL, 2.0–2.5 kg and 15 mg or 1.5 mL >2.5 kg) is started within 6–12 hours of birth and continued for 6 weeks. If an HIV-positive mother presents in labor without having received any ART, NVP prophylaxis is continued up to 12 weeks. The dose of NVP is increased to 20 mg (2.0 mL) once daily after 6 weeks.
- Integrate follow-up of HIV-exposed infants into routine health care services including immunizations.
- Ensure initiation of cotrimoxazole prophylactic therapy (CPT) and early infant diagnosis (EID) using HIV DNA PCR at 6 weeks of age onwards as per EID guidelines.
- Strengthen follow-up and outreach through ANMs, ASHAs and other outreach workers to support HIV infected pregnant women and their families.

can provide safeguard against development of thrush and candidal esophagitis. Intravenous polyvalent immunoglobulins are recommended for long-term administration at intervals of every 3 weeks for boosting humoral immunity. Intercurrent infections should be recognized early and managed aggressively in accordance with the protocol followed for other immunocompromised children. The children with AIDS and their families should be given comfort and provided holistic care with due compassion.

Specific Therapy

Antiretroviral therapy is indicated in most HIV-infected infants younger than 12 months of age. Therapy is also recommended when HIV RNA load is more than 100,000/mL of plasma or there is marked suppression of CD_4 lymphocyte counts irrespective of the age of the child. Therapy is not curative but reduces the risk of opportunistic infections by 50%. The therapy is highly cost-intensive and it is recommended to give a combination therapy with at least 3 antiretroviral drugs. A combination of zidovudine + lamivudine or zidovudine + didanosine and one protease inhibitor (nelfinavir or indinavir or ritonavir) is given. The use of minimum of 3 drugs in combination is referred to HAART (highly active antiretroviral therapy) and is mandatory to prevent drug resistance.

Immunizations

Live vaccines should be given before the disease becomes symptomatic (ARC, AIDS). BCG, oral polio, MMR, yellow fever and chickenpox vaccines should be avoided in children with manifest AIDS. Affected children and siblings should be given killed or inactivated polio vaccine. Pneumococcal and influenza vaccines should be given to all children with HIV infection whether manifest or asymptomatic. When HIV-infected children develop serious viral infections, like chickenpox and measles, specific immune globulins are life-saving.

CONGENITAL SYPHILIS

Syphilis is common in many low and middle income countries (LMICs) and venereal disease research laboratory (VDRL) test is routinely performed in all mothers during antenatal visits. In high-risk populations, a repeat VDRL test should be performed at 28 weeks gestation and at delivery. Contrary to conventional opinion, transplacental infection by *Treponema pallidum* can occur during first trimester of pregnancy. If mother has untreated primary or secondary syphilis, the risk of fetal infection is almost 100%, whereas in late maternal syphilis (of more than 2 years duration) risk of infection is minimal. When one of the non-treponemal tests (VDRL), rapid plasma reagin (RPR) or automated reagin test (ART) is positive during pregnancy, the expectant mother should be interviewed by taking a detailed history and examined thoroughly for any clinical evidences of the disease or its stigmata. The diagnosis should be confirmed by *Treponema pallidum* hemagglutination assay or by fluorescent treponemal antibody absorption test. The treatment of syphilis during pregnancy, at any stage, is similar to the drug schedule used in non-pregnant patients.

Most infants are normal at birth when adequate treatment has been taken during pregnancy. In untreated cases, congenital infection may result in still-birth, hydrops fetalis or premature delivery. The infant should be examined and followed for snuffles (noisy breathing due to blood-tinged nasal discharge), depressed nasal bridge, maculopapular exfoliative or vesiculobullous skin eruptions involving palms and soles, hematological (jaundice, petechiae, anemia, hepatosplenomegaly, lymphadenopathy), skeletal (osteochondritis and periostitis) and CNS manifestations. Perioral ulcerations, perianal fissures and condylomata should be looked for.

The diagnosis can be confirmed either by higher than maternal titer or rising titer of VDRL or RPR (rapid plasma reagin) or preferably by fluorescent treponemal antibody absorption (FTA-ABS) IgM test or *Treponema pallidum* particle agglutination (TP-PA) test. Examination of blood (for normocytic normo-chromic anemia, thrombocytopenia, reticulocytosis, autoimmune hemolysis and liver dysfunction), bones (osteochondritis, periostitis) and CSF is indicated in all cases. A positive VDRL test on CSF is diagnostic of neurosyphilis. The blood or CSF titers of non-treponemal tests (VDRL, RPR, ART) are useful to assess disease activity and response to therapy.

In infants without any evidences of CNS infection, aqueous crystalline penicillin G 100,000–150,000 units/kg/d IM or IV q 12 hours is administered for 10–14 days. Infants with neurosyphilis should be treated with crystalline penicillin G 150,000 units/kg/d IV or IM q 12 hours for one week and q 8 hours for next 2 weeks. The patient becomes non-infectious after 24 hours of penicillin therapy. The infant should be closely monitored clinically and by serological tests. Non-treponemal (VDRL or RPR) antibody titers should decline by 3 months and become negative by 6 months of age. If antibody titers are still raised at 3 months or are positive at 6 months, retreatment should be given. Infant with neurosyphilis should be followed with CSF examination every 6 months for 3 years or until cell count is normal. If spinal fluid cell count is still elevated at 6 months or VDRL in the CSF is positive, the infant should be retreated. Treponemal tests are not useful to assess the activity of the disease process because they remain positive for life.

CHLAMYDIAL INFECTIONS

During the last decade, genital venereal infection with *Chlamydia trachomatis* has come to be recognized as an important STD with a high infectivity to the new-born baby. Chlamydial cervicitis has been implicated to cause premature rupture of membranes, premature labor, high incidence of LBW babies and increased perinatal mortality rate. Several population surveys have reported 5 to 20% genital colonization rate with *Chlamydia trachomatis* in pregnant women with extremely high rate of vertical transmission of the infection to the newborn baby during delivery. Conjunctiva and respiratory passages are most vulnerable to infection by this organism. The usual incubation period varies between 5 and 14 days.

Conjunctivitis is usually mild to moderate in severity and has onset after the 5th day of life. There is edema of lids, chemosis, congestion of palpebral conjunctiva and copious yellow exudates. The diagnosis can be suspected by demonstration of intra-cytoplasmic inclusion of chlamydiae in the epithelial scrapings of conjunctiva stained with Giemsa. Smear examination is useful to exclude any associated gonococcal infection. A direct immunofluorescent monoclonal antibody stain technique has been developed for rapid diagnosis. The condition is treated with local instillation of 10% sulfacetamide eyedrops for 10 to 14 days. Tetracycline or erythromycin 0.5% ophthalmic ointment is equally effective. A 2-week course of oral therapy with erythromycin 50 mg/kg/d in 3 divided doses is mandatory for effective resolution of conjunctivitis and for prevention of chlamydial pneumonia.

Chlamydial pneumonia usually occurs during 2 to 12 weeks of age. There may be preceding history suggestive of inclusion blenorrhea (mucous discharge from urethra or vagina) in 50% of infants. The onset is insidious and clinical picture is characterized by nasal congestion, mild tachypnea with intractable paroxysmal cough (akin to pertussis) for several weeks. Examination of chest may reveal bilateral rales and rhonchi. Infant is usually afebrile. Middle ear infection with bulging tympanic membrane is commonly associated. Skiagram of chest reveals diffuse interstitial infiltrates with hyperinflation and patchy areas of density. Peripheral blood may show eosinophilia and elevation of IgA and IgM immuno-globulins. The diagnosis can be confirmed by identification of etiologic agent by Giemsa stain of nasopharyngeal secretions, rise in antibody titer or by culture from lung biopsy.

Management consists of administration of erythromycin 50 mg/kg/day q 8 hr or sulfisoxazole 150 mg/kg/day q 8 hr orally for 14 days. Supportive management in the form of fluid therapy, oxygen and chest physiotherapy is essential.

BACTERIAL INFECTIONS

Next to prematurity and perinatal asphyxia, septicemia in the newborn is a leading cause of neonatal morbidity and mortality. Damage by infective agents during this period of rapid growth may leave lasting effects on the ultimate size and function of various body organs in the survivors.

Colonization

The fetus is well protected *in utero*. Most of the babies at birth are uninfected except in situations, such as acute febrile illness in the mother before labor, delay in the birth of the baby after rupture of the membranes and infected birth canal. After birth, the baby is exposed to the environment contaminated with microorganisms which start settling or colonizing at various places. Feeding initiates colonization in the gut. Within 2 to 7 days of birth, most of the sites, such as rectum, umbilicus, nasopharynx and skin of the baby get colonized in that order. Therefore, the isolation of bacteria from these sites should not be interpreted as evidence of infection, unless pus cells are demonstrated. Heavy colonization with one group of microorganisms may predispose to development of local and systemic infection.

DEFENSE MECHANISMS OF THE FETUS AND NEWBORN

The fetus is not "immunologically null" and newborn baby has a well-developed and functional immune system but with certain limitations. During intrauterine period, fetus generally lacks antigenic challenge but has the ability to respond. There are, however, maturational deficiencies in complement activity, immunoglobulin content and defective phagocytic response leading to diminished inflammatory response in the newborn. During first 8 to 12 weeks of embryonic phase, fetus is immunologically incompetent. Agents such as rubella, cytomegalovirus, and toxoplasma which produce minimal or no disease in an adult, can be lethal or devastating to the unborn child. With such an early immunologic encounter, host defenses are so altered, that fetus is unable to eliminate

the infecting agent thus resulting in shedding of pathogens for several months and years after birth.

Humoral Immune Response

Passive maternal transfer Humoral immunity to the newborn is provided by passive transfer of maternal antibodies through placenta during fetal life. Immunoglobulins of IgG class (7S) are passively transferred to the fetus beginning at about third month of gestation. At term, IgG concentration in the cord blood exceeds that in the maternal serum but prematurely born infants have lower quota of passively transferred antibodies and their level is directly related to gestational maturity. Adequate IgG levels (except IgG 2-subtype) at term, afford protection against several Gram-positive bacteria and viruses during first six months of life. The process of transplacental transfer is an active one by virtue of pinocytosis. The level of passively transferred IgG antibodies gradually falls reaching lowest level around 3 to 4 months of age, when they start to rise again by virtue of synthesis of antibodies by the infant. Passively acquired IgG antibodies have been shown to interfere with humoral response of the infant against live vaccines especially measles during early infancy. The macromolecular (19S) immunoglobulins of other classes, viz. IgM, IgA, IgD and IgE, do not cross the placental barrier and are generally absent at birth. The increased susceptibility of the neonate to Gram-negative bacteria may be explained by the fact that the antibodies against these microorganisms are primarily IgM type.

Active humoral antibody responses Immunocompetent B lymphocytes are seen in the fetal liver at 12 weeks and in the peripheral blood subsequently. They elaborate immunoglobulins and the sequence of their appearance is IgM first followed by IgG and IgA. The immunoglobulins first appear within the cytoplasm of B cells which subsequently appear on their surface and are released in the blood. The fetal B cells are capable of synthesizing immunoglobulins after 10 to 12 weeks of gestation in response to antigenic stimulation. At birth most newborns have only small amounts of self-derived or actively produced immunoglobulins because of lack of antigenic challenge. Infants born following intrauterine exposure of infectious agents may have increased levels of IgM and sometimes IgA antibodies. *Elevated level of IgM (>20 mg/dL) in cord blood is thus indicative of intrauterine infection and is useful for screening purposes.*

After birth, infant is exposed to a variety of antigens and noxious agents which provoke an antibody

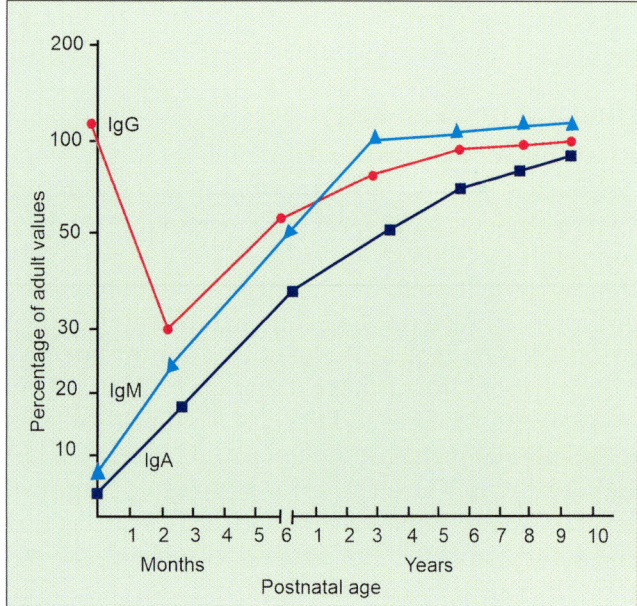

Figure 16.5 Immunoglobulin levels in blood at birth and its dynamics till maturity.

response. The neonate has higher percentage of B cells than an adult. Antibody producing plasma cells are not seen during first 3 to 4 weeks of life suggesting that antibody production in the neonate is limited to the spleen rather than the lymph nodes. Like older children and adults, following exposure to an antigen, the neonate responds by production of first IgM and then IgG antibodies. However, the transition from IgM to IgG takes longer time in the newborn. An adult starts to produce IgG after 1 to 2 weeks of an infection, whereas infant may elaborate IgM only after 3 to 4 weeks. This delayed transition from IgM to IgG is present up to first 6 months of life. The postnatal rise of various immunoglobulins proceeds at varying rates. IgM rises rapidly in the first 3 to 4 weeks of life and slowly thereafter, reaching adult levels by 2 years of life. The IgG immunoglobulins after reaching their nadir around 3 to 4 months, gradually increase in concentration, attaining adult values by 5–6 years of age (Figure 16.5). Secretory IgA on mucosal surfaces develops rapidly after antigenic exposure and can be detected as early as 10 to 20 days after birth but adult levels of plasma IgA antibodies are attained around 10 years of age.

Cellular Immune Response

Unlike humoral immunity, there is no passive or transplacental transfer of markers of cell-mediated immunity. Lymphocytes are seen in the yolk sac as early as 3 to 6 weeks of fetal life. Thymus-dependent lymphocytes precede the appearance of antibody bearing lymphocytes in the fetus. By the end of first trimester, functional cellular immunity is well developed as evidenced by formation of T lymphocyte rosettes with sheep red blood cells and their response to mitogen stimulation. The absolute number of T cells in the cord blood is greater as compared to adults but percentage of T lymphocytes is lower due to relative lymphocytosis in the newborn. There is increased number of T suppressor cells in newborn babies. It would appear that cell-mediated immunity is satisfactory in a healthy term infant including production of lymphotoxin and interferon. The diminished delayed hypersensitivity responses in the newborn are now being explained on the basis of decreased inflammatory responses in the neonates, rather than defective cell-mediated immunity. Like postnatal malnutrition, it is well documented that cell-mediated immunity is deficient in infants born with intrauterine malnutrition.

Humoral Mediators

The inflammatory response is governed by a number of plasma and tissue-derived humoral mediators. The production of complement precedes immunoglobulin synthesis and there is no passive transplacental transfer of complement. At birth, total hemolytic activity of complement system is around 50–60% of the maternal levels. The levels of complement proteins increase rapidly after birth, reaching adult values by 3 to 6 months of age. Due to deficiency of complement at birth, opsonic activity is markedly deficient, especially against Gram-negative compared to Gram-positive organisms. Deficiency of opsonic activity coupled with IgM deficiency at birth is responsible for greater susceptibility and vulnerability of newborn babies to infections caused by Gram-negative bacteria. These quantitative and qualitative complement deficiencies resulting in opsonic handicaps may well be partly responsible for the rapid and often fulminant course of neonatal infections. The production of other mediators, like interferon and fibronectin, is poor in newborn babies.

Phagocytes

The various phagocytes, microphages (neutrophils, eosinophils) and macrophages (histiocytes, monocytes, reticuloendothelial cells in spleen, liver and bone marrow) are functionally active by the end of first trimester. Granulocytopoiesis begins around the second month, but there are a few circulating granulocytes during first half of gestation when their number is limited to 1000/mm^3. Tissue macrophages begin to appear in a 3 to 4 weeks embryo and circulating monocytes are seen by 10 to 20 weeks. The process of phagocytosis comprises distinct stages of cell movement or chemotaxis, ingestion and intracellular killing. Polymorphonuclear leukocytes in the newborn have deficient chemotaxis and defective phagocytic activity thus producing ineffective inflammatory response. During neonatal period, eosinophilic or monocytic response is predominant at the site of inflammation. The chemotactic and phagocytic activities of monocytic cells are normal. However, maturational deficiencies in complement activity and immunoglobulin content coupled with serious defects in phagocytic function, result in a diminished inflammatory response.

Immunological Status of LBW Babies

Low birth weight babies, whether preterm or small-for-dates, are more handicapped and vulnerable to develop infections. They are more likely to succumb to them due to ineffective immunobiological responses. Preterm babies have lower levels of IgG because it is passively transferred to the baby during third trimester of pregnancy. They have poor mucosal defences and low levels of various components of complement system. The storage reserve of neutrophils is low.

Neonates with severe intrauterine growth retardation suffer from poor cell-mediated immune response. Thymus is atrophic and relative as well as absolute number of T cells is markedly diminished. Delayed hypersensitivity response to BCG and other antigens is impaired. Even maternal transfer of immunoglobulins is adversely affected as a result of placental changes associated with intrauterine growth retardation. Levels of C3, C4, factor B, lysozyme and interferon are lower than normal. Small-for-dates babies exhibit poorer neutrophil function in terms of chemotaxis, phagocytosis and intracellular killing.

Factors Predisposing to the Development of Neonatal Infections

Low birth weight Preterm babies are more susceptible to develop infection due to deficient humoral and cellular immune mechanisms. Their exposure to warm and humid atmosphere of potentially infected incubators, respirators, resuscitators and catheters is conducive to the development of infections.

Contaminated *in utero* environment Prolonged rupture of membranes, unhygienic and multiple vaginal examinations, prolonged labor and poor personal hygiene lead to ascending infection of the amniotic fluid which is good culture medium for bacterial growth especially when it is contaminated with meconium.

Infected birth passages A number of bacterial and non-bacterial infections are contracted by the baby during its passage through the birth canal, e.g. *Neissera gonorrhoeae*, *Listeria monocytogenes*, *Escherichia coli*, *Streptococcus hemolyticus*, *Candida albicans* and *Herpes virus hominis*. Nearly 90% of pregnant women harbor potentially pathogenic organisms in their genital tract. Chorioamnionitis is characterized by maternal fever, pain and tenderness in the uterus, foul smelling liquor, leukocytosis and positive CRP.

Infection at birth The neonates not only have enhanced vulnerability to infections but they also have greater opportunities to get infected in the labor room and NICU. Hands of personnel are a potent source of microbes unless due precautions are taken. The high-risk neonates are exposed to a variety of fomites which are potential sources of pathogens, such as open care systems, incubators, cots, linen, suction and oxygen catheters, thermometers, endotracheal tubes and resuscitation equipment. The congestion and overcrowding in the nursery are associated with increased risk of nosocomial infections. The lack of enough disposables (small-vein infusion sets, catheters, endotracheal tubes, syringes, needles, etc.), use of stock solutions (heparinized saline for establishing IV line) and multi-dose drug vials are potent sources of infection. Maintenance of absolute asepsis while feeding (whether bottle, gavage or parenteral) is mandatory to prevent exposure of neonates to microbes. Neonates requiring advanced life support (assisted ventilation), parenteral nutrition and exchange blood transfusion are at an increased risk to develop infection. The type and density of nursery flora depends on the practice of aseptic routines like hand-washing, housekeeping, asepsis protocols, fumigation, spectrum of antibiotics being used, colonization pattern of the personnel and type of neonatal admissions (intramural or extramural). Most neonatal units harbor *E. coli*, *Klebsiella pneumoniae*, *Acinetobacter baumannii*, *S. aureus*, *Pseudomonas aeruginosa* and drug-resistant Gram-positive organisms (methicillin resistant *Staphylococcus aureus* and vancomycin-resistant enterococci) from time-to-time.

Congenital anomalies The babies with exposed meningomyelocele, esophageal atresia and tracheoesophageal fistula, cleft palate and thymic aplasia are particularly susceptible to infections.

Top feeding It is associated with risk of contamination and infant is denied humoral, cellular and other anti-infective factors available in the breast milk. Excessive administration of vitamin E and early supplementation of iron to preterm babies is also associated with increased risk of bacterial infection.

Procedures Endotracheal intubation, assisted ventilation, umbilical catheterization and exchange blood transfusion, when carried out without due regard to asepsis, constitute important portals for entry of microorganisms.

Gender Neonatal sepsis is twice as frequent in the male infants as compared to female infants, though the exact explanation is uncertain. The possible locus of gene for synthesis of immunoglobulins at X-chromosome probably accounts for relative resistance of the female infants to infections. The sex difference in the leukocyte counts, present in later life, has not been studied in the neonatal period.

Types of Infections

The infection may remain superficial and localized or the baby may develop fulminant and disseminated systemic infection. Due to inability on the part of the neonate to develop sufficient inflammatory response to localize the infection, it gets readily disseminated especially in the low birth weight and preterm babies.

SUPERFICIAL BACTERIAL INFECTIONS

Superficial infections are common and their incidence is related to the standard of hygiene and attitude of the personnel working in the maternity units. Majority of these infections are caused by Gram-positive organisms, *Staphylococcus aureus* and *albus*. The infection is conveyed to the baby through contaminated hands of nurses, doctors and relatives who may be nasal carriers of staphylococci.

Pyoderma

Pustules are commonly seen on scalp, neck, groin and axillae. These are more common during the summer months. Their frequency can be reduced considerably by routine application of triple dye to the umbilical cord and hexachlorophene skin prophylaxis during epidemics. The spread of infection may lead to formation of abscess, parotitis, osteomyelitis and septicemia. Life-threatening staphylococcal infection may lead to manifestations of pemphigus neonatorum which is characterized by marked erythema, bullous lesions and exfoliation giving an appearance of scalded skin syndrome.

The isolated lesions should be punctured and pus sent for Gram staining of smear and culture. Hexachlorophene skin care and application of triple dye over the punctured lesions is enough in most cases to prevent the spread of infection. In case the lesions are spreading, erythromycin 40 mg/kg per day orally in 3 divided doses should be administered for 7 days. The baby must be examined thoroughly everyday for detection of abscess, osteomyelitis and/or septicemia which would require parenteral anti-staphylococcal therapy.

Conjunctivitis

The sticky eyes without purulent discharge are common during first 2 to 3 days after birth. They should be washed with sterile cotton swabs soaked in physiologic saline or by instilling 10% sulfacetamide eye drops. Unilateral conjunctivitis having onset after 5 days of life, is often due to *Chlamydia trachomatis* and is best treated with local instillation of sulfacetamide drops or 0.5% erythromycin ointment and oral administration of erythromycin. Purulent conjunctivitis is generally due to Gram-positive cocci and should be managed with local instillation of penicillin (2,500 units per mL), framycetine sulfate or chloramphenicol eye drops depending upon the sensitivity of the organisms to the antibiotic. It is desirable to instil the drops every half to one-hourly during the first 12 to 24 hours and increase the interval gradually. Gonococcal ophthalmia should be suspected, if profuse purulent discharge occurs in one or both the eyes, within 48 hours of age. After obtaining specimens for smear and culture, local and parenteral penicillin therapy should be initiated promptly. Intracellular Gram-negative diplococci are characteristically seen on a Gram stain. Eyes should be washed frequently with normal saline irrigations. Topical appplication of 1.0% tetracycline or 0.5% erythromycin ophthalmic ointment every 2–4 hourly is recommended but is of doubtful utility. When gonococci are sensitive to penicillin, aqueous crystalline penicillin G 100,000 units/kg/d q 12 hr IM or IV is administered for 7–10 days. If organisms are resistant to penicillin, ceftriaxone 25–50 mg/kg (up to maximum of 125 mg) single dose IV or IM is the drug of choice. Mother should be treated as per standard recommendations to eliminate gonococci from her genital tract.

The presence of dacrocystitis and orbital cellulitis in association with purulent conjunctivitis should be managed with parenteral therapy and drainage. The baby should be watched for development of osteomyelitis of the neighboring bones. Persistence of the watery discharge should arouse the suspicion of blocked nasolacrimal duct. The mother should be instructed to massage the duct area before instilling eye drops. If the blockage is not relieved by the age of five to six months, probing and dilatation of the nasolacrimal duct may have to be done.

Umbilical Sepsis

The routine application of triple dye, ethyl alcohol or betadine has considerably reduced the incidence of umbilical infection. The pathological evidence of acute omphalitis at birth may be obtained in some babies but its correlation with subsequent neonatal infection cannot be predicted. Umbilical sepsis may follow umbilical catheterization and exchange blood transfusion. Catheterization through umbilical vessels should never be done, if stump is already infected. The presence of white slimy discharge should not be mistaken for umbilical sepsis. Purulent discharge, red and inflamed periumbilical area and foul smell are indicative of umbilical sepsis. The positive bacterial growth from the umbilical swab, in the absence of pus cells, suggests colonization rather than umbilical sepsis.

In mild cases, frequent cleaning with surgical spirit or alcohol and application of antibiotic powder (containing neomycin, bacitracin and polymyxin) are enough. If periumbilical inflammation is marked or systemic infection is present, parenteral therapy should be started. Spread of infection along the umbilical vein may lead to pyelophlebitis with formation of microhepatic abscesses. This may be followed by development of portal hypertension later in life. The incidence of this complication is low.

Oral Thrush

Candida albicans infection generally does not establish in healthy individuals except in the newborn period. The infection most commonly occurs during passage of the baby through infected birth canal. Infected feeding bottles, candidiasis of breast nipples or vagina and prolonged antibiotic therapy may result in thrush and/or perianal candidiasis. The oral lesions are characterized by adherent discrete white patches or spots over the buccal mucosa and gums. The baby may be able to suck normally but swallowing may be difficult due to posterior oropharyngeal or esophageal white patches. Monilial diarrhea may be associated with perineal moniliasis. Oral application of 0.5% aqueous solution of gentian violet after each feed gives prompt response in most cases. Nystatin (100,000 units/mL of glycerine), and clotrimazole 1% or miconazole 2% lotion are equally effective and less messy. Topical

therapy should be continued for a minimum of 10–14 days. Intractable or severe moniliasis in association with neonatal tetany, trismus and failure to thrive, should alert to the possibility of thymic hypoplasia (DiGeorge syndrome) and HIV infection.

Candidal Diaper Rash

The predisposing factors include maternal infection (breast nipple or vaginal), bottle feeding, chronic diarrhea and prolonged use of broad spectrum antibiotics. It is characterized by marked erythema, maceration, and erythematous papules or vesicles at the periphery. Oral thrush may be associated. It is treated with topical application of 2% nystatin ointment, 2% miconazole ointment, 1% terbinafine or 1% clotrimazole cream for 2 weeks. In refractory cases, oral administration of nystatin or fluconazole is recommended for 2 weeks.

NEONATAL SEPTICEMIA

Neonatal sepsis is the leading cause of morbidity and mortality especially among LBW and preterm babies in developing countries. Neonatal sepsis is diagnosed when generalized systemic features of sepsis are associated with pure growth of bacteria from one or more sites. When clinical and laboratory findings are consistet with bacterial infection but blood culture is sterile, infant is labeled to have "probable sepsis". According to pooled hospital data based on neonatal–perinatal data (NNPD), the incidence of neonatal sepsis is around 30 per 1000 live births. Neonatal sepsis can be divided into two main subtypes depending on whether the onset is during the first 72 hours of life or later. In our experience, there is almost equal distribution of early-onset and late-onset cases.

Definition

An international consensus conference on pediatric sepsis in 2005 defined sepsis as systemic inflammatory response syndrome (SIRS) due to suspected or proven sepsis. The diagnosis of SIRS is made, if two of the following 4 criteria are met and at least one of the criterion is abnormal temperature or leukocyte count. This definition is applicable to term neonates alone.

1. Core body temperature of >38.5°C or <36°C.
2. Unexplained heart rate >180/min or <100/min for more than 30 min duration.
3. Mean respiratory rate of >50/min (0–7 days) or >40/min (8–28 days), or when there is a need for mechanical ventilation for an acute illness which is not due to neuromuscular problem or because of general anesthesia.

4. Leukocyte count elevated or depressed for age or >10% immature neutrophils.

Early-onset septicemia (EOS) is caused by organisms prevalent in the genital tract or in the labor room and maternity operation theater. In the west, early-onset infections are mostly caused by *Group B streptococci* (GBS) and *E. coli* while in our set-up most cases are due to Gram-negative organisms especially *E. coli*, Klebsiella, and Enterobacter sp. Majority of neonates with early-onset sepsis manifest as respiratory distress due to intrauterine pneumonia. The onus for prevention of early-onset septicemia rests with the obstetricians.

Early-onset bacterial infections occur either due to ascending infection following rupture of membranes or during the passage of baby through infected birth canal or at the time of resuscitation in the labor room. When at least three of the following high-risk factors are present, the baby is considered to be infected and should be treated with appropriate antibiotics. The presence of foul smelling liquor alone warrants initiation of antibiotic therapy.

1. Very low birth weight (<2000 g) or a preterm baby. The incidence of early-onset sepsis is nearly 10 times higher in infants with birth weight <1000 g compared to infants with normal birth weight.
2. Febrile illness in the mother during or within two weeks of delivery.
3. Foul smelling and/or meconium-stained liquor amnii
4. Prolonged rupture of membranes (>18 hr).
5. Single unclean or more than three vaginal examinations during labor.
6. Prolonged labor (>24 hours both stages) and difficult delivery with instrumentation.
7. Birth asphyxia and difficult resuscitation.
8. Pathological evidences of funisitis (inflammation of the connective tissue of the umbilical cord that occurs with chorioamnionitis), omphalitis, or presence of polymorphs (>5/HPF) in the gastric aspirate.

Late-onset septicemia (LOS) is acquired as nosocomial infection from the nursery or lying-in ward. The onset is delayed for 72 hours after birth. In most cases, symptoms appear by the end of first week or during the second week of life. About two-thirds cases of late-onset septicemia are caused by Gram-negative bacilli, viz. *Klebsiella pneumoniae,* Enterobacteria, *Escherichia coli, Pseudomonas aeruginosa, Alkaligenese fecalis, Salmonella typhimurium,* Proteus, Citrobacter and Serratia spp. while the rest are contributed by Gram-positive organisms including coagulase-positive *Staphylococcus aureus* and coagulase-negative staphylococci (CONS).

It is improtant to remember that bacterial flora is dynamic, different from one place as compared to the other and it changes in the same place over a period of time. It is essential to closely monitor the bacterial flora of the NICU and the antibiotic sensitivity pattern of pathogens to evolve rational antibiotic policy which is most suitable and specific for a particular NICU. The usual sources of infection include incubators (especially humidity tank), resuscitators, ventilators, solutions for cold sterilization, feeding bottles, catheters, endotracheal tubes, face masks and infusion sets and sites of venipunctures.

Clinical Features

Early-onset neonatal sepsis is characterized by prolonged rupture of membranes, perinatal hypoxia, resuscitation difficulties and evidences of congenital pneumonia in the form of respiratory distress. The response may be modified by the birth weight and maturity of the infant. The clinical presentation of late-onset neonatal sepsis may be silent in a very small baby who may suddenly die without exhibiting any signs and symptoms. *The ability of the newborn baby to respond to an infection is limited to identical stereotyped responses to a wide range of insults, thus producing an identical clinical picture in a variety of conditions.* The alteration in the behavior and established feeding pattern of the child are characteristic early features. The baby who had been sucking normally, gradually or suddenly becomes lethargic, inactive, unresponsive and refuses to suck. The previously alert and well baby appears pale, lethargic with grayish-blue circumoral cyanosis and vacant stare. The baby just "does not look well" may sound vague but is the most useful clue to an experienced physician and nurse. Therefore, a high index of suspicion and frequent evaluation of laboratory markers of neonatal infection is mandatory to make an early diagnosis of neonatal septicemia. Hypothermia is a common manifestation of sepsis in preterm babies, while term babies may manifest with fever, especially in association with Gram-positive infections and meningitis. Diarrhea, vomiting and abdominal distension may precede or occur during the course of illness. Onset of jaundice after 72 hours of age and elevation of direct reacting bilirubin to more than 2 mg/dL is suggestive of associated hepatitis. Hepatosplenomegaly may or may not be present. Episodes of apneic spells with cyanosis may be the sole manifestation of sepsis in preterm babies. In some babies, failure to gain weight or unexplained loss of weight may be the only manifestation. In addition to the above features of disseminated infection, localizing features may appear depending upon the predominant involvement of different systems of the baby, as discussed below.

Meningitis

About 5–15% of the neonates with septicemia may have coexistent meningitis. The evidences of meningeal irritation are generally absent in newborn babies. Therefore, a high index of suspicion and frequent resort to lumbar puncture are essential to make an early diagnosis. In a baby with a clinical profile of septicemia, presence of fever, onset of convulsions or twitchings, staring look, bulging anterior fontanel and high pitched cry or excessive crying should arouse the suspicion of meningitis. Meningitis is more common in late-onset septicemia and must be ruled out in all cases by doing a lumbar puncture. The presence of meningitis modifies the management and is associated with adverse outcome.

Ventriculitis should be suspected when there are associated congenital anomalies, like meningomyelocele and intraventricular shunt and there is poor clinical or laboratory response to antibiotic therapy. Recurrent convulsions, persistently bulging anterior fontanel, increasing head size and neck retraction are suggestive of ventriculitis. Cranial ultrasound examination would show ventricular dilatation, increased echogenicity and formation of septations. Ventricular tap reveals >100 WBCs/mm^3 and Gram smear or culture is positive for microorganisms.

Pneumonia

Early-onset sepsis due to GBS is characterized by life-threatening respiratory distress and must be differentiated from hyaline membrane disease. The baby may die of fulminant hemorrhagic pneumonia without producing any localizing signs and symptoms, thus emphasizing the need for taking the skiagram of chest in all babies with septicemia. Apneic spells with cyanosis, tachypnea and rales are suggestive of pulmonary involvement. Cough is usually absent in newborn babies.

Diarrhea

Sudden appearance of watery diarrhea in a neonate, who is not exclusively breastfed, is suggestive of bacterial infection. The presence of mucus and/or blood in stools is suggestive of invasive diarrhea. Neonates with "definite diarrhea" should be treated with intravenous fluids and parenteral antibiotics, like sepsis. Infants with passage of motions after each feed or semi-loose "transitional stools" should not be confused with infective diarrhea. Passage of loose stools with obvious or occult blood, abdominal distension and ileus are suggestive of necrotizing enterocolitis.

Pyelonephritis

The incidence of urinary tract infection in newborn babies is reported to range between 0.1 and 1%. Like sepsis, UTI is more common in preterm and male babies. There are generally no suggestive clues for the clinical diagnosis of pyelonephritis. Occasionally infant may have prolonged jaundice and kidneys may be enlarged and palpable. In all neonates with poor weight gain, in spite of adequate intake of feeds, urinalysis and culture must be done to exclude urinary tract infection.

Osteomyelitis and Septic Arthritis

The involvement of bone and joint is uncommon and may occur through hematogenous seeding or direct extension from the overlying skin following venipuncture or skin abscess. The infection may occur with any bacterial pathogen but is more common with *S. aureus* and *N. gonorrhoeae*. There are classical signs of inflammation, like redness, swelling, pain and limitation of movements. The hip, knee and wrist are commonly involved in septic arthritis while osteomyelitis may involve any bone. Plain skiagram, ultrasound examination and needle aspiration of pus for Gram staining and culture are diagnostic. Surgical drainage, local rest and prolonged parenteral antibiotic therapy for 4–6 weeks (at least 4 weeks of parenteral antibiotics) are advocated. There is significant risk of disability and damage to the growth plate of the affected bone.

The additional clinical features of sepsis may appear depending upon the development of following complications.

Shock

The baby would appear markedly pale (in the absence of bleeding), ashen-gray, with cold extremities and absent peripheral pulsations and fall in blood pressure. The capillary refill time (CRT) is delayed for more than two seconds. The fall in serum sodium and rise in potassium may suggest the possibility of adrenal insufficiency due to adrenal hemorrhage.

Sclerema

In advanced moribund cases, the skin assumes hidebound characteristics and is stretched out over the underlying structures. The change begins over the skin of the face and legs which becomes unpinchable and subsequently skin change advances centripetally. When skin of the chest is affected, the breathing movements are interfered resulting in shallow rapid breathing and cyanosis.

Necrotizing Enterocolitis

There is marked abdominal distension, bilious vomiting and passage of blood and mucus per rectum. The bowel sounds are diminished or absent with evidences of peritonitis and free air may be seen under the diaphragm with obliteration of hepatic dullness in terminal stages. A vague ill-defined inflammatory mass may be palpable in the right iliac fossa. Stools are likely be positive for occult blood and reducing substance.

Disseminated Intravascular Coagulation (DIC)

In severely ill babies with prolonged hypothermia and acidosis, bleeding manifestations may appear due to consumptive coagulopathy as a result of disseminated intravascular coagulation. There is excessive bleeding from venipuncture sites, spontaneous ecchymoses, massive pulmonary hemorrhage and hemorrhagic cerebral infarcts.

Clinical Suspicion of Etiologic Agent

It is desirable to identify the possible infective agent on clinical grounds alone in order to guide the initial therapy, pending blood culture report. Different etiologic agents produce identical clinical manifestations with certain exceptions.

In staphylococcal infections, the onset of symptoms is usually after 72 hours of age. Evidences of superficial infections, such as conjunctivitis, pyoderma, umbilical sepsis, abscess, parotid swelling, arthritis and osteomyelitis, favor the diagnosis of staphylococcal infection. Even coagulase negative staphylococci (CONS) are pathogenic in the newborn baby. These infections often cause fever in term babies. Staphylococcal septicemia may produce characteristic exfoliative dermatitis with formation of bullae giving an appearance of scalded skin.

Early-onset *group-B streptococcal* (GBS) infection is characterized by history of maternal fever during labor or prolonged rupture of membranes and development of respiratory distress within two hours of birth.

Apneic attacks and shock occur rather early during the course of disease which runs a fulminant course. Unlike hyaline membrane disease, the lung compliance is normal. The condition is relatively uncommon in our setting as compared to the west.

Listeria monocytogenes is a Gram-positive motile bacterium that causes infections mainly at the extreme ends of life, i.e. neonates or elderly. Peripartal flu-like maternal illness, fever or gastroenteritis are commonly associated with neonatal listeriosis. The liquor is often meconium-stained or greenish in color due to fetal diarrhea. Infant is moderately depressed, limp and unwell at birth. Respiratory difficulties in the form of shallow breathing or respiratory distress, skin rash, apneic attacks and hepatosplenomegaly are common on the first day. Gram staining of meconium smear may be diagnostic, if it shows Gram-positive rods.

The development of grayish-black gangrenous patches on the skin is suggestive of septicemia due to Pseudomonas and Klebsiella. The clinical utility of this sign is limited because the patches appear rather late during the course of the disease and the baby is often in a moribund state by that time. The knowledge of the prevailing bacterial flora in the humidity tanks of the incubators, incidence of various pathogens causing septicemia during a particular period of time and their antibiotic sensitivity pattern offer useful diagnostic and therapeutic clues.

Diagnosis

There is no rapid and reliable test for confirmation of etiologic diagnosis. The treatment is generally started when clinical picture is supported by indirect early markers of neonatal infection. The appropriate culture specimens must be obtained before initiating antibiotic therapy which is modified subsequently on the basis of the laboratory reports and response of the patient to the presumptive treatment.

Complete blood counts (CBC) The total leukocyte count has a low predictive value for the diagnosis of sepsis because of the wide range of normal counts from 8000 to 20,000/mm^3. Leukopenia (<5000/mm^3) or absolute neutropenia (<1000/mm^3) is usually associated with neonatal sepsis. The cut off values for absolute neutrophil count (ANC) can be checked from Manroe chart in term and Mouzinho chart in case of preterm babies. A band neutrophil is an immature neutrophil, wherein the width of the narrowest segment of its nucleus is more than one-third of the broadest segment (Figures 16.6 and 16.7). The band

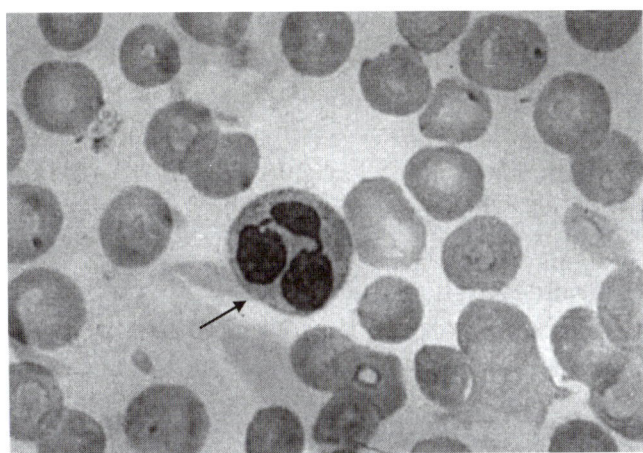

Figure 16.6 Typical appearances of mature multi-lobed polymorphonuclear leukocyte.

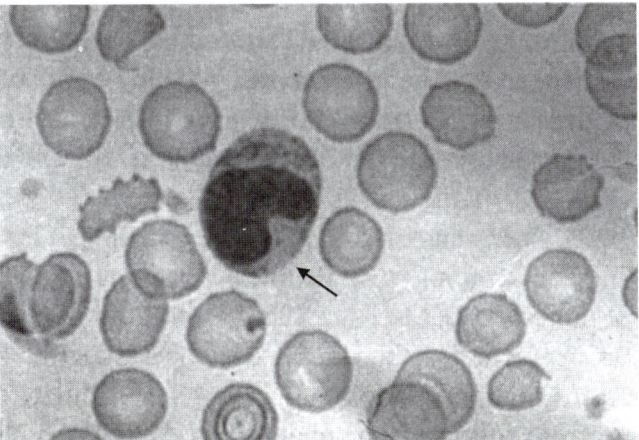

Figure 16.7 Typical band cell or immature leukocyte.

cell count of more than 20% and band count to total neutrophil ratio of equal to or more than 0.2 has a reported sensitivity of 82 to 90% for the diagnosis of septicemia. In addition, the neutrophils may show abnormal morphology with the appearance of Dohle bodies (aggregates of rough endoplasmic reticulum which stain light blue with Giemsa stain), toxic granulations (eosinophilic granules in the cytoplasm of neutrophils) and vacuolization.

Microerythrocyte sedimentation rate Micro-ESR (M-ESR) is a simple and inexpensive test but it is not very reliable marker of neonatal infection. Normal value is up to 6 mm in the first hour during the first 3 days of life. During the neonatal period, a value of more than 15 is considered as suggestive of infection. Micro-ESR is obtained by collecting capillary blood in a standard preheparinized microhematocrit tube (75 mm length, internal diameter of 1.1 mm and outer diameter 1.5 mm) and by reading the fall of erythrocyte column after one hour.

Acute phase proteins A number of acute phase proteins serve as useful indicators of infection in the neonates (Table 16.4). The best studied among them is the C-reactive protein (CRP). Two proteins, namely, prealbumin and transferrin, are negative reactants because their levels fall with inflammation and increase with recovery. CRP has been found useful in differentiating pneumonia from other causes of neonatal respiratory distress syndrome. Serial decline in CRP levels with therapy is suggestive of adequate response to antibiotics and recovery. Elevation of CRP level may precede relapse of infection.

C-reactive protein is synthesized in the liver. Levels rise following any inflammation and it is the most reliable indicator of neonatal infection. A level of more than 1.0 mg/dL is considered as abnormal in the neonate. When CRP is negative at the onset of disease, it must be repeated after 12 hours. Accurate measurement of CRP can be made by laser nephelometry or single radio-immunodiffusion assay. A semi-quantitative bedside latex agglutination technique gives results within 15 minutes by using capillary blood sample. CRP levels have a sensitivity and specificity of 87% and 83%, respectively.

Procalcitonin (PCT) is a precursor protein of the hormone calcitonin which is produced in the plasma of patients suffering from bacterial and fungal infections. It is physiologically elevated during first 3 days of life. It has been found to be a reliable marker of late-onset sepsis in newborn babies with a sensitivity and specificity of nearly 100%. The comparative studies have shown that PCT is a more reliable marker of sepsis compared to CRP. Quantitive measurement of PCT is performed, using an immuno-luminometric assay (ILMA) with two monoclonal antibodies. After the initial surge of PCT during first 3 days of life, the mean normal serum PCT level is

TABLE 16.4 Acute phase proteins
Those increasing with inflammation
■ C-reactive protein
■ Procalcitonin
■ Cytokines (IL-6, IL-10 and IL-1ra)
■ Alpha-1 acid glycoprotein (orosomucoid)
■ Haptoglobin (alpha-2 glycoprotein)
■ Alpha-1 antitrypsin
■ Presepsin
Those decreasing with inflammation
■ Elastase-alpha-1-proteinase inhibitor
■ Fibrinogen
■ Prealbumin
■ Transferrin

Perinatal Infections

16

around 0.5 µg/L. The test is not readily available and is cost-intensive. Elevation of serum interleukin 10 (IL-10 >14 pg/mL) is a useful marker of onset and severity of neonatal sepsis.

Presepsin The cleavage of soluble CD14 generates a fragment called presepsin. It is generated as a part of body's response to bacterial infection. A recent study demonstrated that umbilical cord blood presepsin is a predictor of early onset neonatal sepsis (EONS) in preterm infants with premature rupture of membranes (PROM). There is evidence to suggest that presepsin has a better sensitivity and negative predictive value compared to CRP and PCT.

Nitroblue-tetrazolium test (NBT) This test is unreliable in the neonates because of the normally high rates of reduction in the neonatal leukocytes.

Limulus amoebocyte lysate assay The assay detects the endotoxins released by Gram-negative bacteria. Its usefulness in the diagnosis of neonatal sepsis is limited.

Broad based PCR A broad based PCR with amplification of bacterial DNA, i.e. 16 Sr DNA has been used for identification of bacteria but its cost is prohibitive.

The 'Sepsis Screen'

A battery of above indirect markers of infection when collectively studied provide an extremely reliable index of neonatal sepsis and serve as a useful guide for initiating antibiotic therapy. When at least two of the indirect markers of infection are positive, it gives the sensitivity and specificity of 93% and 88%, respectively (Table 16.5).

Sepsis screen has a limited utility to support the diagnosis of early-onset sepsis, instead high-risk factors and gastric aspirate polymorphs are looked for to make the diagnosis. The septic screen is indicated at birth, if an infant is born following prolonged rupture of membranes, foul smelling liquor, peripartal maternal fever and severe birth asphyxia with active resuscitation. After birth, if a baby develops RDS or non-specific features of neonatal sepsis, septic screen is checked to support or refute the clinical suspicion so that unnecessary antibiotic usage is curtailed during neonatal period.

Flow Cytometry

Flow cytometry allows measurement of several inflammatory parameters which are useful for the diagnosis of neonatal sepsis. A combination of CRP,

TABLE 16.5 The sepsis screen*

Parameter	Abnormal value
■ Total leukocyte count	<5000/mm^3 or >20,000/mm^3
■ Absolute neutrophil count	Low count as per Manroe chart for term infants and Mouzinho chart for VLBW babies
■ Immature or band cells to total neutrophil ratio	>0.2
■ Micro-ESR	>15 mm 1st hour
■ C-reactive protein (CRP)	>1 mg/dL

*• Sepsis screen is considered as positive when 2 or more parameters are positive.
• When initial screen is negative, it should be repeated after 12–24 hours when clinical suspicion of infection is strong. When repeat sepsis screen is also negative, the diagnosis of sepsis can be excluded with reasonable certainty.
• In early-onset sepsis, polymorphs in the gastric aspirate as a marker of chorioamnionitis, can be used as an additional parameter of sepsis screen.

IL-6, CD64 and CD11b are useful markers of sepsis. CD64 is also known as FC gamma receptor 1 (FCγR1) and binds monomeric IgG antibodies with high affinity in the process of phagocytosis and intracellular killing of opsonized microbes. CD11b, which is also known as integrin alpha M (ITGAM) or complement receptor 3A (CR3A), mediates inflammation by regulating leukocyte adhesion and migration. These tests can be done on 150 µL sample of blood in EDTA vial and report is available in 2 hours.

Gram's Stain and Culture Studies

Culture of blood should be taken before starting anti-microbial therapy. The venipuncture site overlying a peripheral vein should be thoroughly sterilized before obtaining specimen of blood for culture. Alcohol-povidone iodine-alcohol should be applied in three consecutive steps. Povidone-iodine should be applied in concentric circles moving outwards from the center and allowed to dry for at least 30 seconds. It is recommended to take 1 mL of blood in a 10–20 mL broth (or 0.5 mL blood in 5–10 mL broth) for blood culture, so that the inoculated blood sample constitutes 5–10% of the amount of liquid broth medium. Automated BACTEC and BACT/ALERT method of blood culture is superior because of faster result (12–24 hr) and greater yield. Blood culture is considered as the gold standard for the diagnosis of sepsis but it is positive in only 60% of cases.

Lumbar puncture should always be done in a suspected case of late-onset neonatal sepsis except when the infant is too sick to undergo the procedure. Cerebrospinal fluid should be promptly inoculated for culture and its smear subjected to thorough search for organisms after Gram staining. When LP is traumatic, CSF must be sent for Gram staining and culture studies. The interpretation of CSF cytology and biochemistry is often difficult (Table 16.6). CSF cytology showing >10 cells with more than 60% polymorphs, glucose less than 50% of blood glucose, protein more than 120 mg/dL in term babies and 170 mg/dL in preterm babies are suggestive of meningitis. Urinalysis and culture are done, if there is clinical suspicion of urinary tract infection, evidences of urinary tract anomalies, history of bladder catheterization or turbid urine. Suprapubic specimen of urine is ideal (especially in girl infants) for cytology and culture studies. In the presence of evidences of superficial infection (abscess, pustules, vesicles), pus smear should be stained and swab cultured to identify pathogens. Diarrheal stools should also be cultured to identify enteropathogenic microorganisms.

It is generally believed that cultures of superficial healthy sites, such as throat, umbilicus, skin and perianal area, do not help in the diagnosis and are unnecessary. However, it has been documented that pathogens cultured from maternal genital tract and baby's throat and/or ear canal correlate well with the etiological diagnosis in neonates with early-onset septicemia which usually presents as pneumonia. Examination of a stained smear (methylene blue) of gastric aspirate also helps in the diagnosis of early-onset sepsis, if more than 5 neutrophils per high power field are documented.

The culture studies are time consuming, but the bacterial antigens (even if the organisms are killed) can be identified by a simple and quick bedside procedure by using counterimmunoelectrophoresis (CIE). Buffy coat smear examination involves Gram staining of buffy layer of the blood obtained after centrifugation

and separation of plasma. If carefully done, bacterial pathogens can be identified in 57 to 70% cases of neonatal sepsis.

Evaluation of Extent of the Disease

The infection may localize in any system of the baby. Lumbar puncture should be done in all LOS cases and most septic neonates withstand the procedure well. It is safer to do the procedure in either sitting position or lateral decubitus without neck flexion. Suprapubic puncture should be done to obtain a clean specimen of urine for microscopic examination and culture. More than 10 leukocytes/mm^3 in uncentrifuged urine and colony count of more than 10^4 organisms/mL of clean catch or catheter urine sample are suggestive of pyelonephritis. In case of a urine sample obtained by suprapubic puncture, any cell or organism count is considered as suggestive of infection. Skiagram of chest should be taken in all cases to document pneumonia while abdominal film will show presence of ileus and changes of necrotizing enterocolitis (NEC). Stools should be examined for occult blood and reducing substance to exclude impending NEC. Neurosonogram and computed tomography (CT scan) of brain should be performed in all neonates diagnosed to have meningitis. Radionuclide bone and liver scan may be done, if there is suspicion of osteomyelitis and pyemic liver abscesses.

Biochemical Abnormalities

Blood should be examined for glucose (to detect hypo- and hyperglycemia), bilirubin, urea and creatinine (to detect renal failure due to disease or aminoglycosides) and electrolytes. Hyponatremia is suggestive of syndrome of inappropriate secretion of antidiuretic hormone (SIADH) and adrenal insufficiency especially when potassium is raised. Acid–base parameters and arterial blood gases should be monitored in infants with pneumonia.

Management

Early recognition, prompt administration of effective and appropriate antibiotic therapy with optimal supportive management are mandatory to improve their intact survival. In view of very high morbidity and mortality due to neonatal sepsis, prevention must be accorded highest priority (see Chapter 3 for details).

Specific Antimicrobial Therapy

Antibacterial agents are greatly over prescribed in the neonatal period because of non-specific clinical

TABLE 16.6 Cerebrospinal fluid findings in newborn babies	
Components	Values mean (range)
Total cells (mm^3)	8 (0–30)
Polymorphonuclear cells (%)	60
Protein (mg/dL)	90 (20–170)
Glucose (mg/dL)	52 (34–119)
CSF to blood glucose ratio (%)	51 (44–248)

Adapted from Sariff LD, Platt LH, McCracken GH Jr. Cerebrospinal fluid evaluation in neonates. J Pediatr 1976, 88: 473–477

Perinatal Infections

16

features of sepsis and delay in laboratory confirmation of diagnosis. Nevertheless, early therapy based on high index of suspicion and support by 'sepsis screen' is mandatory for improved salvage. The rational use of antimicrobial agents in neonatal sepsis is governed by the knowledge of the prevalent bacterial flora of a particular newborn nursery and their sensitivity pattern against available antibiotics. The initial regimen must cover the most common pathogens. It should be borne in mind that there can be no single universal recommendation for the antimicrobial regimen. Each treating unit should adopt a suitable protocol on the basis of considerations highlighted vide supra. Based on changes in the spectrum of etiologic agents and the antibiotic sensitivity pattern, the choice of antibiotics must be constantly reviewed and modified. Periodic changes in antibiotic schedule is associated with delayed emergence of antibiotic-resistant bacteria. In community setting where antimicrobial resistance is less likely to be a problem, rational choice of antibiotics would include a combination of kanamycin or gentamicin (an aminoglycoside) with benzyle penicillin or ampicillin. Gentamicin 4 mg/kg single dose per day intramuscularly is effective for ambulatory management of neonatal sepsis in the community.

Since common organisms causing neonatal sepsis in most neonatal units in our country are Klebsiella, E.coli, Enterobacter, Acinetobacter, and Staphylococcus aureus, the initial antibiotic regimen must cover these pathogens. The logical initial choice would be a combination of an aminoglycoside (gentamicin or amikacin) and ampicillin or cefazoline or cloxacillin. The newer antibiotic preparations, like tobramycin, netilmicin, vancomycin, cefotaxime, ceftriaxone, ceftazidime, cefoperazone, cefepime and imipenem should be kept in reserve for treatment of meningitis and life-threatening infections. In centers with high incidence of resistance to third generation cephalosporins and emergence of extended spectrum beta lactamase (ESBL) positive organisms, piperacillin-tazobactam or methicillin-vancomycin are drugs of choice. Ciprofloxacin should be used as a last resort in critically sick neonates when bacterial isolates are resistant to all other antibiotics.

In desperate situations, newer antibiotics, like aztreonam and meropenem, may be used. Aztreonam has excellent activity against Gram-negative organisms while meropenem is effective against most bacterial pathogens except methicillin-resistant Staphylococcus aureus (MRSA) and enterococci. Imipenem is generally avoided in newborn babies due to risk of seizures.

Indiscriminate use of 'shot gun' antibiotic therapy is not only unscientific but it is also unethical and fraught with risks of emergence of resistant strains of bacteria. The empirical use of newer antibiotics should be avoided and their use should be reserved in situations when sensitivity of the isolated organisms warrants their use.

When etiological agent is identified or suspected on the basis of characteristic clinical picture, antimicrobial therapy can be made highly specific. Benzyle penicillin (250,000–450,000 iu/kg/d) or ampicillin (200–300 mg/kg/d) is most suitable for the treatment of infections due to Group B streptococci. Septicemia due to Pseudomonas aeruginosa carries a poor prognosis and is best managed with ceftazidime or cefepime. Beta lactamase-resistant penicillins and vancomycin are indicated for the treatment of infections caused by Staphylococcus aureus. Ampicillin and gentamicin are given for treatment of an occasional case of listeriosis.

The presence of bacterial meningitis in association with septicemia modifies the choice, duration and mode of administration of antibiotics. Aminoglycosides, polymyxin and first generation cephalosporins do not effectively cross the blood–brain barrier. Cefotaxime and moxalactam, the third-generation cephalosporins, are not only highly active against Gram-negative enteric organisms but also attain excellent CSF levels. A combination of amikacin and cefotaxime or ceftazidime is ideal for treatment of neonatal meningitis. Cefuroxime, the only second-generation cephalosporin with good CSF penetration, may also be used, though enough data regarding its use among neonates is not available as yet. Chloramphenicol has superb penetration across all body cavities including blood–brain barrier. For susceptible organisms or when organisms are unknown, its use should be considered. When administered in recommended doses there is no risk of gray-baby syndrome. Cotrimoxazole, an antimicrobial drug combination with excellent diffusibility into the CSF, has not been studied well in neonates because of the possible ill effects of sulphamethoxazole on bilirubin–albumin binding. It should theoretically have a useful place in the management of neonatal meningitis after first week of life. Ciprofloxacin does not penetrate blood–brain barrier and is not recommended for treatment of meningitis.

Intraventricular administration of antibiotics for treatment of ventriculitis is controversial and not recommended because of the risk of development of porencephalic cysts with repeated needle punctures. Serial cranial ultrasound examination should be conducted to exclude development of septa and loculations. CECT head is indicated when there is rapid increase in head circumference or presence of focal seizures or neurological signs. Bilateral intraventricular shunts with fenestration of septa is indicated for management of ventriculitis complicated by loculations and hydrocephalus.

Mode of Administration and Duration of Therapy

Antibiotics should be administered intravenously at least in the initial phase of management and as long as intravenous fluids are being administered. Subsequently, except for the more fulminant infections (e.g. meningitis, osteomyelitis), it is acceptable to give antibiotics intramuscularly. Maintaining intravenous lines for the full duration of therapy is difficult and fraught with the risk of extravasation, swelling and infection in most neonatal set-ups in our country. Duration of antimicrobial therapy should be individualized depending upon the severity and site of infection (Table 16.7).

Supportive Care and Treatment of Complications

The neonate must be nursed in the thermoneutral zone of ambient temperature. If possible, servo-controlled incubator or an open care system should be used. Intravenous fluids are started and enteral feeding is stopped in a sick infant for a couple of days. In case of documented hypoglycemia and when facilities to check blood sugar are not readily available, it is prudent to give a mini-bolus of 2 mL/kg of 10% glucose (200 mg/kg). Injection vitamin K 0.5–1.0 mg is given intravenously at admission and twice a week till enteral feeds are re-established. Metabolic acidosis is corrected by using appropriately diluted sodium bicarbonate. Peripheral perfusion is supported with transfusion(s) of fresh blood or fresh frozen plasma.

Anemia is corrected with aliquotes of packed cells. Fresh blood or FFP is useful to improve defense mechanisms by providing opsonins and polymorphonucelar leukocytes.

Shock is managed by careful volume expansion (preferably with central venous pressure monitoring), dopamine and high doses of dexamethasone. Corticosteroids are indicated in gravely sick neonates with endotoxic shock, sclerema and adrenal insufficiency. A number of therapeutic products, like monoclonal antibodies, tumor necrosis factor (TNF) and interleukin-1 (IL-1), have been tried with success for treatment of shock in experimental models. In addition, pentoxifylline, a phosphodiesterase inhibitor, has been tried to decrease the production of TNF. The role of prostaglandins, ibuprofen, ketoconazole and inhibitors of nitric oxide synthase is under evaluation and holds promise.

Hyperbilirubinemia should be managed more aggressively with phototherapy and exchange blood transfusion. Bilirubin encephalopathy is likely to occur at a lower serum bilirubin level in the setting of septicemia. Oxygen and ventilatory therapy should be instituted in the event of respiratory failure as per the standard indications. Bleeding tendency is managed by judicious administration of fresh blood, fresh plasma, platelet concentrates and vitamin K. Efforts should be made to identify collection of pus (in the joint, bone, parotid, liver, etc.) which must be drained.

In meningitis, fluids are restricted because of risk of syndrome of inappropriate secretion of antidiuretic hormone. Seizures are treated with diazepam and phenobarbitone. In the presence of manifestations of raised intracranial pressure, mannitol can be used.

Immunotherapy

Exchange blood transfusion in infected neonates can theoretically help achieve improved peripheral and pulmonary perfusion, correction of coagulation abnormalities and removal of toxins; and provides specific antibodies, complement and phagocytic cells. The procedure is recommended in critically sick neonates with sclerema, DIC and hyperbilirubinemia. Controlled studies are, however, needed to further evaluate the therapeutic utility of exchange blood transfusion.

Granulocyte transfusion (1×10^9 granulocytes/kg) is recommended as an adjunct to immunologic therapy for septic newborn infants with neutropenia and has been used successfully in a limited number of infected babies to decrease mortality. Granulocyte transfusions may be associated with serious graft-versus-host disease. It is not established whether it is desirable to

TABLE 16.7 Duration of antibiotic therapy in neonatal sepsis*

Diagnosis	Duration
■ Culture and sepsis screen negative but clinical picture is suggestive of sepsis	5–7 days
■ Sepsis screen positive but blood/CSF culture negative	7–10 days
■ Blood culture positive but no meningitis	10–14 days
■ Meningitis (irrespective of culture report)	21 days
■ Arthritis, osteomyelitis and endocarditis	4–6 weeks
■ Ventriculitis	6 weeks

*Efforts should be made to administer antibiotics intravenously as long as feasible.

irradiate white cells before transfusion. Precise indications to institute this therapy are not documented.

Immunoglobulin preparations containing type-specific monoclonal antibodies to *Group B streptococci* have been shown to be beneficial. Data regarding Gram-negative organisms is not available. There is no evidence to suggest that administration of a single dose of non-specific IVIG is associated with improved survival. In future, specific immune globulins harnessed in donors or produced by monoclonal antibody technique are likely to be used.

Fibronectin therapy in a septicemic neonate is experimental at present. No randomized controlled trial is available and the present evidence is anecdotal. Fibronectin, a large molecular weight glycoprotein, influences neutrophil and macrophage response to infection.

There is some evidence to suggest that zinc sulfate given in a dose of 3 mg/kg twice a day for 10 days is credited to reduce neonatal mortality and improve neurodevelopment outcome at one year of age.

Colony stimulating factors (rh G-CSF and rh GM-CSF) are endogenous proteins which can enhance the production and functional capabilities of granulocytes. They have been shown to increase the bone marrow granulocyte pool by proliferation of progenitor cells and improve neutrophil functions, macrophage chemotaxis, phagocytosis and neutrophil oxidative metabolism. Recombinant technology has now made available the human G-CSF and GM-CSF for commercial use. There is insufficient evidence to suggest that G-CSF may lower the mortality among neutropenic septic VLBW babies. There is a need to conduct multicentric trials to assess the utility of colony stimulating factors in the management of neonatal sepsis.

Prognosis

The outcome depends upon weight and maturity of the infant, type of etiologic agent and its antibiotic sensitivity pattern; and adequacy of specific and supportive therapy. Associated congenital malformations, like meningomyelocele, tracheoesophageal fistula and surgical procedure, adversely affect the prognosis. The early-onset septicemia due to *Group B streptococci* and nosocomial infections due to Klebsiella and *Pseudomonas aeruginosa* are associated with adverse outcome. Early and aggressive therapy is mandatory for improved salvage because extension of infection into various body organs and development of complications such as endotoxic shock, sclerema, NEC and DIC is associated with extremely high mortality. The reported mortality rates in neonatal sepsis in various studies from India range between 15 and 50%. Early institution of specific antimicrobial therapy with the aid of 'sepsis screen', excellent supportive care, close monitoring of vital signs, and judicious use of fresh blood, FFP and immunotherapy is likely to improve the outcome of neonates with septicemia.

SYSTEMIC CANDIDIASIS

Systemic infections due to pathogenic fungi are assuming increasing importance in the neonatal intensive care units. Most infections are caused by Candida species *C. albicans and C. parapsilosis.* All Candida species form pseudohyphae which are responsible for invasive desease. Other species that are known to cause fungemia include Malassezia, Mucorales, Zygomycetes and Aspergillus. Fungal infections in the neonates are essentially nosocomial and a known hazard of intensive care techniques. Preterm babies below 1500 g especially those requiring prolonged advanced life support management, like ventilation, venous catheterization, exchange blood transfusion and total parenteral nutrition are susceptible to develop candidemia. Intralipids, especially when efforts are made to divide them into small aliquotes, are potent source of infection. Other risk factors include birth asphyxia, use of systemic steroids and H_2-blockers. Many cases are preceded by bacterial sepsis and prolonged administration of broad-spectrum antibiotics. Gastrointestinal mucormycosis (GIM) is a rare potentially lethal fungal infection in term neonates with birth asphyxia. The clinical picture is similar to NEC. The diagnosis is confirmed on histopathological examination of intestinal tissue obtained on laparotomy. The slides are stained with hematoxylin and Eosin, Periodic acid-Schiff, and Gomori. Methamine-silver nitrate staining shows characteristic angioinvasive, broad, branching and nonseptate hyphae.

Clinical Features

The clinical manifestations of candidemia are nonspecific and similar to stereotyped features of neonatal sepsis. The onset of fungal infection is usually delayed beyond 2 to 8 weeks of age. When an infectious process is suspected, but bacterial pathogens are not identified and there is no response to antibiotic therapy, candidemia should be considered. The evidences of superficial fungal infection in the form of thrush, perineal or dermal candidiasis are usually absent. Initial symptomatology simulates features of NEC though pneumatosis intestinalis and candida peritonitis are rare. Intolerance of feeds, hyperthermia, hyperglycemia and thrombocytopenia are commonly associated. The infection readily gets disseminated and microabscesses may form in any organ of the body especially lungs, heart, liver, kidneys, GI tract and CNS. Candida species have special predilection to involve the urinary tract. Renal manifestations include hematuria, proteinuria, pyuria, renal microabscesses and acute renal failure.

Diagnosis

The diagnosis is readily confirmed by blood culture but presence of budding yeasts or hyphae in the urine is a strong evidence of candidemia. In high-risk very low birth weight babies, urine should be routinely examined for hyphae once a week after two weeks of age. Persistently elevated C-reactive protein and thrombocytopenia are useful markers of systemic fungal infection. Selective culture media with low pH (Sabouraud dextrose agar) or culture media containing antibacterial agents should be used for fungal culture. Fundus examination, brain and renal ultrasonography and echocardiography of heart provide useful supportive information. Ocular manifestations like chorioretinitis and endophthalmitis with visual loss may occur in 3.2% cases. Before starting antifungal therapy, CSF should be examined for cell count and fungal culture.

Treatment

The condition carries ominous prognosis but early specific antifungal therapy may salvage some infants. The indwelling catheters should be removed. Amphotericin B is the drug of choice. Therapy is started with 250 µg/kg/day and gradually increased to 1 mg/kg/day dissolved in 5% dextrose and infused intravenously over a period of 4 hours for a duration of 3 to 4 weeks. The drug should be protected against exposure to light and serum potassium levels and renal functions should be monitored. The liposomal preparations of amphotericin B (5 mg/kg/d) are preferred because of lower risk of toxicity, shorter duration of administration over 2 hours, lesser risk of thrombophlebitis and better efficacy (except renal candidiasis). There is *in vitro* synergism between amphotericin B and fluorocytosine and therefore, combination therapy is recommended especially when there is meningeal involvement. Fluorocytosine is given orally in a dose of 100–150 mg/kg/day in four divided doses. It has good CNS penetration but is available only as an oral formulation thus limiting its use in sick VLBW infants. Fluconazole 5 mg/kg/d IV or oral once daily is an effective and safer alternative to amphotericin B but more trials are needed for its universal acceptance. In recurrent or intractable cases of candidemia, endocardial vegetations should be ruled out by echocardiography. In chronic disseminated candidiasis, endocarditis and endophthalmitis, antifungal therapy is continued for at least 6 weeks. GIM carries poor prognosis and is best treated with a combination of liposomal amphotericin B and posaconazole.

Prevention

In view of the fulminant course and high mortality of candidemia, attempts should be made to prevent fungal infection. Minimizing use of cephalosporins, H_2-blockers, and use of laminar flow system for preparing infusates and changing lipid infusion sets every 12 hours are useful strategies. Strict aseptic protocols in NICU, restricted use of central venous lines, avoidance of prophylactic antibiotics and early trophic feeds with breast milk are associated with reduced risk of fungal infections. The meta-analysis of randomized controlled trials suggests that biweekly prophylactic administration of oral ketoconazole is associated with reduced risk of colonization and candidemia in VLBW babies but there is potential risk of emergence of resistant strains of *C. albicans*.

TETANUS NEONATORUM

In India, tetanus is endemic and remains an important health problem. The annual incidence of neonatal tetanus is 1.74/1000 live births. Tetanus is the only vaccine preventable disease that is not contagious. The disease is caused by infection of the umbilical stump by *Clostridium tetani*. Effective implementation of public health measures has reduced the incidence of tetanus neonatorum. Contamination and infection of the umbilical stump at the time of cutting the cord is an important cause. The condition is limited to domiciliary midwifery, as untrained *dais* use unclean sharp weapons to cut the umbilical cord. They even paint the stump with cowdung with the mistaken belief of its purifying properties. Lack of active immunization of adult population with tetanus toxoid also contributes to the high incidence of this highly fatal though entirely preventable disease.

Clinical Features

The common age of onset of symptoms is 5 to 15 days. Neonatal tetanus does not manifest during the first two days of life and is rare after the age of two weeks. Initial symptoms include excessive unexplained crying, followed by refusal of feeds and apathy. The infant keeps the mouth slightly open due to pull as a result of spasm of the muscles of the neck but reflex spasm of the masseters is invoked on trying to open the mouth during feeds. Reflex spasms of pharyngeal muscles lead to dysphagia and choking during feeds. During handling and touching, lock-jaw or trismus is followed by spasms of the limbs. The usual flexed posture of the baby is replaced by generalized rigidity and opisthotonos in extension. The spasm of larynx and respiratory muscles is associated with apnea and cyanosis. The spasms are characteristically induced by stimuli of touch, noise and bright light. Due to lack of inhibiting impulses from the higher centers in newborn babies, the anterior horn cells react more violently resulting in more severe spasms. The spasms or rigidity are less marked in preterm babies. Frequent muscular spasms lead to fever, tachycardia and tachypnea. Constipation persists till the spasms are relieved. Umbilical stump does not show any characteristic appearance except for evidences of omphalitis in some infants. Intercurrent infections, dehydration and acidosis often complicate the clinical picture.

Differential Diagnosis

The diagnosis is based on the presence of predisposing factors and characteristic clinical picture which is well known to physicians working in developing countries. Rarely, severe isolated trismus due to sustained contractions of jaw-closing muscles may occur because of certain developmental defects and metabolic disorders. The syndrome of brainstem dysfunction is characterized by trismus during 1–12 days of age, facial dysmorphism, strabismus, apneic attacks, gastroesophageal reflux and vagal reactivity. Trismus may also occur during early neonatal period in infants with maple syrup urine disease (MSUD), infantile Gaucher's, encephalitis, brainstem dysfunction and hypoparathyroidism (DiGeorge's syndrome). When predisposing factors for tetanus neonatorum are absent and trismus is an isolated symptom without any associated stimulus-provoked spasms of skeletal muscles, the aforementioned conditions should be ruled out. They require specialized investigations and carry a poor prognosis.

Management

Active immunization of the pregnant women against tetanus during the last trimester of pregnancy with two injections of tetanus toxoid at monthly interval

and public health education regarding the need for asepsis while cutting the umbilical cord, have effectively reduced the incidence of tetanus neonatorum.

General measures The infant should be nursed in a quiet room. Handling should be reduced to the barest minimum. Intramuscular injections must be avoided. Temperature should be watched and controlled. Oral secretions should be sucked periodically.

Intravenous infusion Oral feeding should be stopped and an intravenous line should be established, preferably with a medicath. Apart from its utility to provide adequate fluids, calories and electrolytes, it offers a convenient route for administration of various drugs. After two to three days, milk feeding through nasogastric tube may be started.

Antitoxin serum Its main utility lies in neutralizing the circulating toxins but it has no role in dislodging the toxin already fixed to the nerve roots. Human tetanus specific immunoglobulin in a single dose of 250 iu/kg intravenously is generally sufficient because higher doses have not been shown to be of any additional benefit. The use of intrathecal anti-tetanus serum (250 units of human tetanus specific immunoglobulin) appears to confer additional therapeutic benefit by bathing and traversing along the nerve roots to inactivate the toxin. It is not associated with any serious side effects.

Sedation Diazepam 2 to 5 mg (maximum of 2 mg/kg/dose) and chlorpromazine 2 mg/kg/dose should be administered slowly intravenously every 2 to 4 hours, alternating with each other, so that a sedative dose is being given every 1 to 2 hours. In intractable cases, intravenous administration of paralydehyde (0.2 ml/kg) is generally effective. Phenobarbitone should preferably be avoided during diazepam therapy to safeguard against apneic attacks. The dosages and frequency of administration of sedatives need to be delicately titrated by clinical observations to achieve maximum sedation and relaxation with minimal side effects.

Muscle relaxants They are of limited use. Methocarbamol (50–75 mg/kg/day IV in 2 divided doses) or mephenesin (30–120 mg/kg/dose every one hourly orally) may be tried.

Antibiotics In addition to penicillin, gentamicin or amikacin and cefotaxime should be given intravenously to treat associated or intercurrent infection.

Tracheostomy and assisted ventilation Early resort to assisted ventilation along with muscle relaxants has significantly improved the outcome in tetanus neonatorum. It is indicated whenever the infant gets frequent episodes of laryngeal spasms, apneic attacks with cyanosis or central respiratory failure.

Prognosis

The overall mortality varies from 50–75% but those who survive do not manifest any mental sequelae except when apneic episodes are unduly prolonged and unattended. Neonatal tetanus does not produce prolonged immunity and survivors require routine tetanus immunization shots. The prognosis is poor in the following situations.

1. Onset of symptoms within first week of life.
2. Interval between lock-jaw and onset of spasms of less than 48 hours.
3. Presence and intensity of fever.
4. Severity of tachycardia.
5. High frequency and greater severity and duration of muscular spasms especially of larynx.
6. Frequent and prolonged duration of apneic episodes.

BIBLIOGRAPHY

Abadie V, Cheron G, Madjiidi A, Couly G. Neonatal trismus. *Arch Pediatr* 1994, 1(6): 568–572.

Ahmed A, Cerilli LA, Sanchez PJ. Congenital malaria in a preterm neonate: case report and review of literature. *Amer J Perinatol* 1998, 15:38–42

Athavale VB, Pai PN. Tetanus neonatorum: Clinical manifestations. *J Pediatr* 1965, 67: 649.

Benjamin DK, Stoll BJ, Fanaroff AA, *et al*. Neonatal candidiasis among extremely low birth weight infants: Risk factors, mortality rates, and neurodevelopmental outcomes at 18–22 months. *Pediatrics* 2006, 117(1): 84–92.

Center for Disease Control. Sexually transmitted disease treatment guidelines. *MMWR* 1993, 42:1

Chawla D, Chirla D, Dalwai S, Deorari AK, Ganatra A, Ghandhi A, *et al*. Perinatal-neonatal management of COVID-19 infection: Guidelines of the Federation of Obstetrics and Gynecological Society of India (FOGSI), National Neonatology Forum of India and Indian Academy of Pediatrics. *Indian Pediatr* 2020, 536–48.

Cooper ER, Charurat M, Mofenson L, *et al*. Combination antiretroviral strategies for the treatment of HIV-1 infected women and prevention of perinatal HIV-1 transmission. *J Acquir Immune Defic Syndr* 2002, 29 (5): 484–494.

Davies PA. Bacterial infections in the fetus and newborn. *Arch Dis Child* 1971, 46: 1.

Davies PA. Neonatal bacterial meningitis. *J Appl Med* 1978, 4: 435.

Fanaroff AA. Fluconazol for the prevention of fungal infections: get ready, get set, caution. *Pediatrics* 2006, 117(1): 214–215.

Fierro JL, Priya BA, Prasad A, Zaontis TE. Ocular manifestations of cadidemia in children. *Pediatr Infect Dis J* 2013, 32(1):84–86.

Gendrel D, Assicot M, Raymond J, *et al*. Procalcitonin as a marker for the early diagnosis of neonatal infection. *J Pediatr* 1996, 128: 570–573.

Goldman DA, Durban WA, Freeman J. Nosocomial infections in a neonatal intensive care unit. *J Infect Dis* 1981, 144: 449.

Harris MC, Palin RA. Neonatal septicemia. *Pediatr Clin N Amer* 1983, 30: 2.

International Neonatal Immunotherapy Study: Non-specific intravenous immunoglobulin therapy for suspected or proven neonatal sepsis: An international placebo controlled multicentre randomized trial. *BMC Pregnancy Childbirth* 2008, 8:52.

Kishore K, Deorari AK, Singh M, Bhujwala RA. Early-onset neonatal sepsis: Vertical transmission from maternal genital tract. *Indian Pediatr* 1987, 24: 45.

Kumar A, Paul VK, Singh M. Neonatal systemic candidiasis. *Indian Pediatr* 1986, 23: 643.

Kumar N, Dayal R, Singh P, *et al*. A comparative evaluation of presepsin with procalcitonin and CRP in diagnosing neonatal sepsis. *Indian J Pediatr* 2019, 86(2):177–9.

Labib ZA, Mahmoud AB, Eissa NA, *et al*. Early diagnosis of neonatal sepsis: A molecular approach and detection of diagnostic markers versus conventional blood culture. *Int J Microbiol Res* 2013, 4(1):77–85.

Leddy MA, Gonik B, Schulkin J. Obstetrician-Gynecologists and perinatal infections: A review of studies of the Collaborative Ambulatory Research Network (2005–2009). *Infect Dis Obstet Gynecol* 2010, 2010:583950.

Manroe BL, Weinberg AG, Rosenfeld CR, Browne R. The neonatal blood count in health and disease I Reference values for neutrophil cells. *J Pediatr* 1979, 95: 89–98.

McCracken GH, Nelson JD. Antimicrobial therapy for newborn. 2nd ed; *Grune and Stratton, Orlando* 1983, 7–104.

Meisner M, Tschaikowsky K, Palmaers T, Schmidt J. Comparison of procalcitonin (PCT) and C-reactive protein (CRP) plasma concentrations at different SOFA scores during the course of sepsis and MODS. *Crit care 1999*, 3: 45–50.

Mok JO, De Rossi A, Ades AE, *et al*. Infants born to mothers seropositive for HIV. *Lancet* 1987, 1:1164.

Moore MR, Schrag SJ, Schuchat A. Effects of intrapartum antimicrobial prophylaxis for prevention of Group-B streptococcal disease. *Lancet Infect Dis* 2003, 3:201–213.

306 Mouzinho A, Rosenfeld CR, Sanchez PJ, Risser R. Revised reference ranges for circulating neutrophils in very low birth weight neonates. *Pediatrics* 1994, 94:76–82.

National guidelines for prevention of parent-to-child transmission (PPTC T) of HIV. NACO, Ministry of Health and Family Welfare, Government of India, 2013.

Overall JC, Glasgow LA. Virus infections of the fetus and the newborn infant. *J Pediatr* 1970, 77 : 315.

Paul VK, Singh M. Diagnosis and treatment of neonatal sepsis. *Indian Pediatr* 1986, 23 : 1023.

Rhae JW, Akhnoukh F, Parthew CT, Elhassani SB. Convulsions scoring in treatment of neonatal tetanus. *J Pediatr* 1970, 76, 949.

Rosenberg RE, Ahmed AN, Saha SK, *et al*. Nosocomial sepsis risk score for preterm infants in low-resource settings. *J Trop Pediatr* 2009, epub July 21.

Singh M, Sugathan PS, Bhujwala RA. Human colostrum for prophylaxis against sticky eyes and conjunctivitis in the newborn. *J Trop Pediatr* 1982, 28:35.

Singh M, Deorari AK. Pneumonias in newborn babies. *Indian J Pediatr* 1995, 62:293–306

Singhal TA. A review of corona virus disease-2019 (COVID-19). *Indian J Pediatr* 2020, 87:281–6.

Starr SE. Antimicrobial therapy of bacterial sepsis in the newborn. *J Pediatr* 1985, 65:542.

Stoll BJ, Hanson N, Fanaroff AA, *et al*. Late-onset sepsis in very low birth weight neonates. The experience of the NICHD Neonatal Research Network. *Pediatrics* 2002, 110 (2 part I):285–291.

Vasikeri J, Janeas M, Gronroos P, *et al*. Neonatal septicemia. *Arch Dis Child* 1985, 65:542.

Wilson RD. Acute perinatal infection and the evidence-based risk of intrauterine diagnostic testing: a structured review. *Fetal Diagn Ther* 2020, 47:653–64.

Wolach B. Neonatal sepsis: pathogenesis and supportive therapy. *Semin Perinatol* 1997, 21:28–38.

Yoder MC, Polin RA. Immunotherapy of neonatal septicemia. *Pediatr Clin N Amer* 1987, 33:481.

Zaidi AK, Huskins WC, Thaver D, *et al*. Hospital-acquired neonatal infections in developing countries. *Lancet* 2005, 365:1175–1188.

Disorders of Weight and Gestation

LOW BIRTH WEIGHT BABIES

Babies with a birth weight of less than 2,500 g, irrespective of the period of their gestation, are classified as low birth weight (LBW) babies. Nearly 15% of babies worldwide are LBW. These include both preterm and term small-for-dates babies. Their clinical problems and prognoses are quite different from each other. About 18% of babies in India are LBW as opposed to about 5 to 7% of newborns in the West. In India alone, 4 to 5 million LBW infants are born annually. After Pakistan and Bangladesh, India has the dubious distinction of having the highest incidence of LBW babies in the South-East Asia region (Table 17.1). High incidence of LBW babies in our country is accounted for by a higher number of babies with intrauterine growth retardation (small-for-dates) rather than the preterm babies. In the present circumstances, it is not possible to offer special care to all LBW babies. As babies with a birth weight of less than 2,000 g are more vulnerable, they deserve priority in admission to the special care nursery. By this criterion alone, 10% of the babies in India qualify for admission to the special care nursery.

There is no indicator in human biology, which tells us so much about the past events and the future trajectory of life, as the weight of infant at birth.

V. Ramalingaswami

Birth weight is the single most important marker of adverse perinatal and neonatal outcome. Over 80% of all neonatal deaths, in both the developed and developing countries, occur among the LBW babies. Low birth weight is also a major determinant of malnutrition during infancy because over 40% of LBW babies are malnourished at one year of age. Birth weight is an important determinant of success and duration of breastfeeding, which is a well known protective asset against infant deaths in the developing

TABLE 17.1 Incidence of low birth weight babies in SEAR	
Pakistan*	31.6%
Bangladesh	21.6%
India	18.6%
Sri Lanka	16.6%
Thailand	11.3%
Indonesia	11.1%
Myanmar	8.6%
China	5.1%

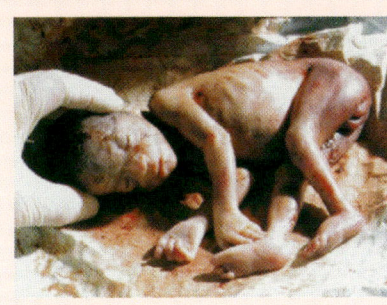

*2014 data
The State of the World's Children, UNICEF, 2015.

world. It is estimated that in a developing country, LBW infants have 2.3 times increased risk of mortality due to infections compared to normal birth weight babies after controlling for all the confounding variables. The neurodevelopmental sequelae of birth asphyxia are three times in LBW babies compared to their normal weight counterparts. Small-for-dates babies may remain stunted throughout life leading to impaired physical work capacity. They are more vulnerable to develop atherosclerotic coronary artery disease, hypertension and Type 2 diabetes mellitus during adult life.

PRETERM BABIES
(Immature, Truly Premature, Born Early)

About 10 to 12% of Indian babies are born preterm (less than 37 completed weeks) as compared to 5 to 7% incidence in the west. These infants are anatomically and functionally immature and therefore, their neonatal mortality is high.

Causes of 'Prematurity'

The mechanisms initiating normal labor are not clearly understood and much less is known about the triggers that initiate labor before term. There may be spontaneous onset of premature labor or it may be induced by the obstetrician to safeguard the interests of the mother or baby.

Spontaneous The cause of premature onset of labor is uncertain in most instances. The known causes include poor socioeconomic status, low maternal weight, chronic and acute systemic maternal disease, antepartum hemorrhage, cervical incompetence, maternal genital colonization and acute infections, cigarette smoking during pregnancy, threatened abortion, acute emotional stress, physical exertion, sexual activity, trauma, bicornuate uterus, multiple pregnancy and congenital malformations. Premature births are relatively common among very young and unmarried mothers. Past history of preterm birth(s) is associated with 3 to 4 times increased risk of prematurity in the subsequent pregnancies. There is genetic predisposition to preterm birth as suggested by increased risk of preterm birth with (i) previous preterm birth, (ii) sister of the mother having delivered a preterm baby, (iii) mother herself was born preterm, (iv) there is a risk of preterm birth even when mother changes the partner, and (v) African race. There is evidence to suggest that maternal genotype, fetal genotype and epigenetic mechanisms may operate through anti-inflammatory cytokine pathways (IL-6, IL-10, TNF-α) leading to enhanced risk of preterm birth.

Induced The labor is often induced before term when there is impending danger to mother or fetal life *in utero,* e.g. maternal diabetes mellitus, placental dysfunction as indicated by unsatisfactory fetal growth, eclampsia, fetal hypoxia, antepartum hemorrhage and severe rhesus isoimmunization.

Clinical Features

Measurements Their body size is small with a relatively large head. Crown-heel length is less than 47 cm, head circumference is usually less than 33 cm but exceeds the chest circumference by more than 3 cm (Figure 17.1).

Activity and posture The general activity is poor and their automatic reflex responses, such as Moro response, sucking and swallowing are sluggish or incomplete. The baby assumes an extended posture due to poor tone.

Face and head Face appears small for the disproportionately large head size, sutures are widely

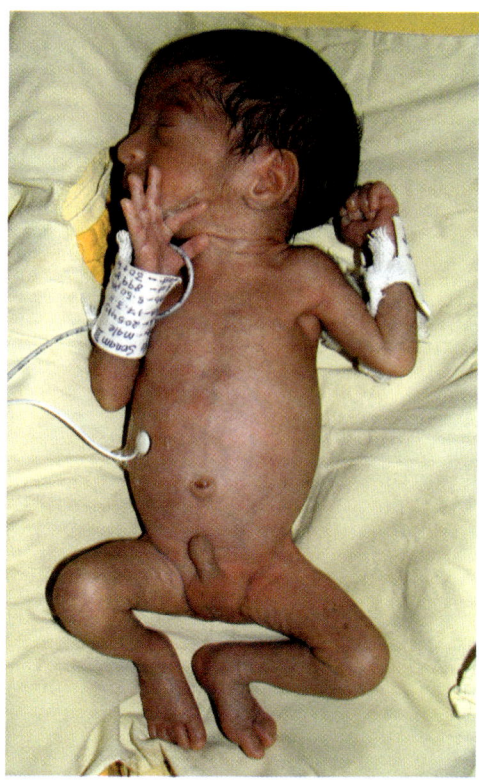

Figure 17.1 Preterm infant with a gestation of 34 weeks and birth weight of 1800 g.

separated and the fontanels are large. Other characteristic features include small chin, protruding eyes due to shallow orbits and absent buccal pad of fat. Optic nerve is often unmyelinated but presence of pupillary membrane makes its visualization difficult. Ear cartilage is deficient or absent with poor recoil. Hair appear woolly and fuzzy and individual hair fibers can be seen separately.

Skin and subcutaneous tissues Skin is thin, gelatinous, shiny and excessively pink with abundant lanugo and very little vernix caseosa. Edema may be present. Subcutaneous fat is deficient and breast nodule is small or absent. The sole creases are faint and shallow.

Genitals In males, testes are undescended and scrotum is poorly developed. In female infants, labia majora are widely separated exposing labia minora and hypertrophied clitoris.

Physiological Handicaps

The functional immaturity of various body systems result in several clinical problems and their knowledge is essential for the satisfactory management of these babies.

Central nervous system The immaturity of central nervous system is expressed as inactivity and lethargy, poor cough reflex and incoordinated sucking and swallowing in babies weighing less than 1,800 g or born before 34 weeks of gestation. Resuscitation difficulties at birth and recurrent apneic attacks are common. Retinopathy of prematurity due to oxygen toxicity is limited to babies with a gestation of less than 35 weeks. On the other hand, they are more resistant to toxic effects of hypoxia as compared to the term babies. They are extremely vulnerable to develop intraventricular-periventricular hemorrhage and periventricular leukomalacia due to relative deficiency of vitamin K dependent coagulation factors and increased capillary fragility. The blood–brain barrier, which is possibly a function of available serum proteins, is inefficient in preterm babies, thus brain damage may occur at lower serum bilirubin levels.

Respiratory system The cuboidal alveolar lining in babies with a gestational age of less than 26 weeks results in poor alveolar diffusion of gases, and therefore, the infant may not be viable. They pose resuscitation difficulties at birth, often followed by hyaline membrane disease, if associated with deficiency of pulmonary surfactant. The breathing is mostly diaphragmatic, periodic and associated with intercostal recessions due to soft ribs. Pulmonary aspiration, recurrent apneic attacks and atelectasis are common. They are vulnerable to develop chronic pulmonary insufficiency due to bronchopulmonary dysplasia.

Cardiovascular system The closure of ductus arteriosus is delayed among preterm infants. About one-third infants with gestational age of 34 weeks or less manifest clinical evidences of patent ductus arteriosus with or without congestive heart failure. Its incidence is much higher among preterm infants with hyaline membrane disease or protracted hypoxia due to any cause. In grossly immature infants (less than 32 weeks), EKG shows left ventricular preponderance. They are at risk to develop thromboembolic complications and hypertension due to indwelling venous and arterial catheters.

Gastrointestinal system Due to poor or incoordinated sucking and swallowing, there are difficulties in self-feeding, although their digestive ability is generally good. Animal fat is not tolerated as well as the vegetable fat. Regurgitation and aspiration are common because of incoordinated sucking, small capacity of stomach, incompetence of cardioesophageal junction and poor cough reflex. Gastroesophagal reflux and its consequences are common. Abdominal distension and functional intestinal obstruction are common due to hypotonia. Necrotizing enterocolitis occurs when other predisposing factors are present. Immaturity of glucuronyl transferase system in the liver leads to hyperbilirubinemia, which may be aggravated by dehydration, delayed feeding and hypoglycemia. Relatively low serum albumin, acidosis and hypoxia in these babies predispose to the development of bilirubin brain damage at lower serum bilirubin levels. The poor hepatic glycogen stores, delayed feeding, birth asphyxia and respiratory distress syndrome contribute to the development of hypoglycemia.

Thermoregulation Hypothermia is invariable and life-threatening unless environmental temperature is monitored. Excessive heat loss occurs due to relatively large surface area and poor generation of heat because of paucity of brown fat in a baby who is equipped with an inefficient thermostat.

Infections Infections are an important cause of neonatal mortality in low birth weight babies. The low levels of IgG antibodies and inefficient cellular immunity predispose them to infections. Excessive handling, humid and warm atmosphere, contaminated incubators and resuscitators expose them to infecting organisms, thus contributing to high incidence of nosocomial or hospital-acquired infections.

Renal immaturity The blood urea nitrogen is high due to low glomerular filtration rate. The renal tubular ammonia mechanism is poorly developed thus acidosis occurs early. They are vulnerable to develop late metabolic acidosis especially when fed with a high protein milk formula. The maximum tubular diluting ability in the newborn is satisfactory but ability to concentrate urine is very poor. Preterm baby has to pass 4 to 5 mL of urine to excrete one milliosmole of solute as compared to 0.7 mL by an adult for the same purpose. Therefore, the baby cannot conserve water and gets dehydrated readily. The solute retention and low serum proteins explain occurrence of edema in some preterm infants.

Toxicity of drugs Poor hepatic detoxification and reduced renal clearance make a preterm baby vulnerable to toxic effects of drugs unless caution is exercised during administration of medications.

Nutritional handicaps Low birth weight babies are prone to develop anemia around 6 to 8 weeks of age. This is due to diminished stores of iron because of short gestation. They may also manifest deficiencies of folic acid and vitamin E. Vitamin E deficiency occurs among infants weighing less than 1,500 g, particularly those fed on iron fortified milk formula. These infants are prone to develop hemolytic anemia, thrombocytopenia, and edema at 6 to 10 weeks of age. Vitamin E being an antioxidant, its deficiency state may be associated with oxygen toxicity to the vulnerable tissues in the form of retinopathy of prematurity (ROP) and bronchopulmonary dysplasia. Rapid growth following adequate feeding may result in osteopenia and rickets unless calcium, phosphorus and vitamin D are administered.

Biochemical disturbances These babies are prone to develop hypoglycemia, hypocalcemia, hypoproteinemia, acidosis and hypoxia.

Management

High-risk mother should be identified early during the course of pregnancy and referred for confinement to an appropriate health care facility which is equipped with good quality obstetrical and neonatal care facilities. *Mother is indeed an ideal transport incubator!*

Arrest of Premature Labor

Advances in perinatal care including fabrication of a variety of electronic gadgets cannot compete with the unique security and optimal care provided to the fetus by the uteroplacental unit. Efforts should always be made to arrest the progress of premature labor especially when fetus is normal. The onset of 'true' labor is suspected by occurrence of two or more uterine contractions lasting at least 30 seconds during a 15-minute period in association with dilatation and effacement of cervix. Apart from bed rest and sedation, a variety of tocolytic agents are available but none is entirely safe or effective. Tocolytic agents prolong gestation for a short period, which may be sufficient to harness beneficial effects of antenatal steroids. Ethanol though popular at one stage is rarely used now due to its dangers of inebriation, vomiting, headache, flushing, restlessness, disorientation and diuresis. Magnesium sulfate is effective and is being increasingly used though there is a potential risk of respiratory depression in the newborn. It is given in a loading dose of 4 g followed by continued infusion at a rate of 1 g/min. The observational studies have shown that maternal treatment with magnesium sulfate is associated with reduced risk of IVH, cerebral palsy and neuromotor disability in their preterm babies.

Sympathomimetic agents specifically mediating via β_2-adrenergic receptors are powerful tocolytic agents and currently used. Isoxsuprine (duvadilan) is useful but its effect is mediated both through β_1 and β_2

receptors. Its use is associated with untoward β_1 receptor side effects such as apprehension, palpitation, hypotension, fetal tachycardia and neonatal hypoglycemia. Therapy is initiated by intravenous infusion of 40 mg isoxsuprine diluted in 200 mL of 5% dextrose at a rate of 3 mL/kg/minute. This is followed by intramuscular administration of 10 mg isoxsuprine every 4 hours for 24 and 48 hours. Oral therapy is continued for at least 2 weeks with maintenance doses of 10 mg every 6 hours. Therapy is continued till the time of delivery or 37 completed weeks of pregnancy. Ritodrine has been approved by the US Food and Drug Administration for treatment of premature labor and is more effective than ethanol. The common side effects are maternal and fetal tachycardia. The usual dose is 100–400 µg/minute intravenously through an infusion pump for a period of 12 hours followed by oral ritodrine 10 mg every 2 hours. Salbutamol and terbutaline are selective β_2 receptor stimulators and are very effective tocolytic agents. They are generally safe but an occasional patient may develop tachycardia and pulmonary edema. Terbutaline is administered as an intravenous bolus of 0.25 mg followed by constant infusion of 10–80 µg/minute for 1–2 hours. After control of uterine contractions, maintenance therapy is continued by administration of 0.25 mg of terbutaline subcutaneously (or 2.5 µg orally) every 4 hours. Indomethacin, an inhibitor of prostaglandin-synthetase, has also offered some hope in arresting premature uterine contractions. It must be used with caution because it may also block production of prostaglandin E thus markedly decreasing uteroplacental perfusion and may cause premature closure of ductus arteriosus.

Induction of Premature Labor

When induction of labor is contemplated before term, either in the interest of mother or the fetus, maturity of fetus should be ascertained by examination of amniotic fluid for phosphatidyl glycerol or L:S ratio. As far as possible, delivery should be postponed till fetal pulmonary maturity is assured. When delivery can be safely delayed for 36 to 48 hours, corticosteroids should be administered to the mother to enhance fetal lung maturity.

Antenatal Corticosteroids

Antenatal administration of corticosteroids is one of the most cost-effective perinatal strategies which must be universally exploited. It is associated with 50% reduction in the incidence of RDS due to surfactant deficiency. It provides additional benefits by reducing the incidence of intraventricular hemorrhage and necrotizing enterocolitis. The over all neonatal mortality is reduced by 40% by this simple and cheap intervention. Injection betamethasone 12 mg IM every 24 hours for 2 doses or dexamethasone 6 mg IM every 12 hours for 4 doses should be administered to the mother, if labor starts or is induced before 34 weeks of gestation. Betamethasone is more potent and is associated with reduced risk of side effects. The optimal effect is seen, if delivery occurs after 24 hours of the initiation of therapy and its therapeutic effect lasts for 7 days. Weekly "booster" doses of corticosteroids are no longer recommended. A repeat single dose of betamethasone may be given, if labor becomes active again after 7–10 days of successful tocolysis. Antenatal corticosteroids should be administered even when delivery is imminent because of several health benefits and reduced mortality of preterm babies. The beneficial effects are better in female babies compared to the male. The need and safety of repeat courses of antenatal steroids is controversial and is under investigation by multicentric clinical trials. Tocolytic therapy should be continued concomitantly. Corticosteroids can be given even in the presence of maternal hypertension or diabetes mellitus but should preferably be avoided, if preterm premature rupture of membranes (PPROMs) is associated with definitive clinical evidences of acute febrile chorioamnionitis.

Care of Preterm Babies

Optimal Management at Birth

When a preterm baby is anticipated, the delivery should be attended by a senior pediatrician, fully prepared to resuscitate the baby. The cord should be clamped after 1 min or it should be milked towards the baby before being clamped. The delayed clamping of cord helps in improving the iron stores of the baby. It may also reduce the incidence and severity of hyaline membrane disease. Other benefits include better hemodynamic stability at birth, reduced need for blood transfusion and inotropic support, lower risk of intraventricular hemorrhage, necrotizing enterocolitis and sepsis. Elective intubation of extremely LBW babies (<1000 g) is practiced in some centers to support breathing and for prophylactic administration of exogenous surfactant. The baby should be promptly dried, kept effectively covered and warm. Vitamin K 1.0 mg (0.5 mg in babies <1500 g) should be given intramuscularly. The baby should be transferred by the doctor or nurse (not by an *Ayah* or nursing orderly!) to the NICU as soon as breathing is established.

Monitoring

The following clinical parameters should be monitored by specially trained nurses. The frequency of monitoring depends upon the gestational maturity and clinical status of the baby.

- Vital signs with the help of a multi-channel vital sign monitor (non-invasive with alarms).
- Activity and behavior.
- Color: Pink, pale, grey, blue, yellow.
- Tissue perfusion (Figure 17.2). Adequate tissue perfusion is suggested by pink color, capillary refill over upper chest of <2 sec, warm and pink extremities, normal blood pressure, urine output of >1.5 mL/kg/hr, absence of metabolic acidosis and lack of any disparity between PaO_2 and SaO_2.
- Fluids, electrolytes and ABGs.
- Tolerance of feeds by monitoring vomiting, gastric residuals, and abdominal girth.
- The baby should be watched for development of RDS, apneic attacks, sepsis, PDA, NEC, and IVH.
- Weight gain velocity.

Criteria for a Healthy Preterm Baby

During daily clinical evaluation of a preterm baby, the following clinical characteristics should be looked for because they suggest that the baby is healthy. The vital signs and arterial oxygen saturation should be stable. The healthy baby is alert and active, looks pink without circumoral cyanosis (smells good too!), trunk is warm to touch and extremities are reasonably warm and pink. The baby is able to tolerate enteral feeds and there is no abdominal distension, respiratory distress or apneic attacks and baby is having a

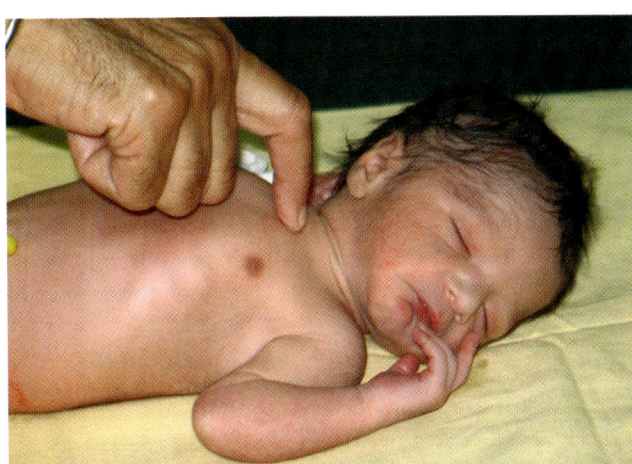

Figure 17.2 Testing for tissue perfusion. The blanching on the upper chest should disappear within 2 seconds in healthy preterm babies.

17

steady weight gain of 1.0–1.5% of his body weight (10–15 g/kg/d) everyday.

Provide In Utero Milieu

Uterus provides ideal ambient conditions to the baby. All attempts should be made to create uterus-like baby-friendly ambience in the nursery. *Womb is our gold standard for care of preterm babies.*

- Create a soft, comfortable, "nestled" and cushioned bed.
- Avoid excessive light, loud sound, rough handling and painful procedures. Use effective analgesia and sedation for conducting procedures.
- Provide warmth.
- Ensure asepsis.
- Prevent evaporative skin losses by effectively covering the baby, application of oil or liquid paraffin to the skin and increasing humidity to near 100%.
- Provide effective and safe oxygenation.
- Uterus provides optimal parenteral nutrition, if there is no placental dysfunction. Efforts should be made to provide at least partial parenteral nutrition and give trophic feeds with expressed breast milk (EBM).
- Provide rhythmic gentle tactile and kinesthetic stimulation like passive movements of limbs, skin-to-skin contact, interaction, music, caressing and cuddling.

Position of the Baby

Most babies love to lie in a prone position, they cry less and feel more comfortable. It relieves abdominal discomfort by passage of flatus and reduces risk of aspiration. Prone posture improves ventilation, increases dynamic lung compliance and enhances arterial oxygenation. Unsupervised prone positioning, beyond neonatal period, has been recognized as a risk factor for sudden infant death syndrome (SIDS).

Thermal Comfort

A pre-warmed open care system or incubator should be available at all times to receive any baby with hypothermia or with a birth weight of less than 2000 g. The baby should be nursed in a thermoneutral environment with a servo sensor geared to maintain skin temperature of mid-epigastric region at 36.5 °C so that there is virtually no or minimal metabolic thermogenesis (Figure 17.3). Application of oil or liquid paraffin on the skin reduces convective heat loss and evaporative water losses. The extremely LBW baby should be covered with a cellophane or thin transparent plastic sheet to prevent convective heat loss and evaporative losses of water from skin (Figure 17.4).

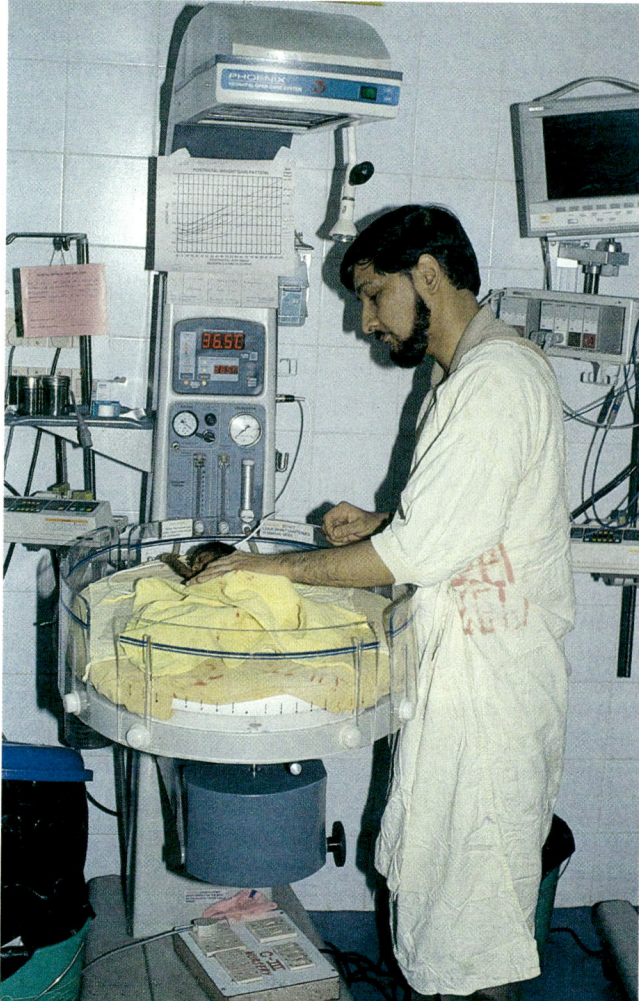

Figure 17.3 Baby being nursed in an open care system. After initial stabilization, the baby should be effectively clothed to prevent evaporative water losses.

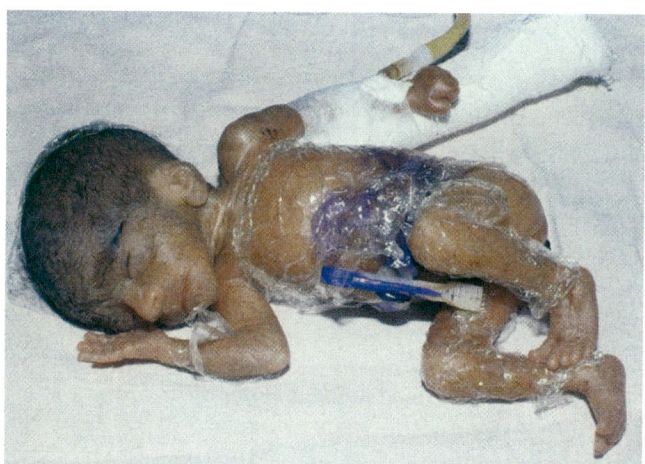

Figure 17.4 The extremely LBW baby covered with a cellophane sheet to prevent convective heat loss and evaporative losses of water from skin.

Care of the Newborn

17

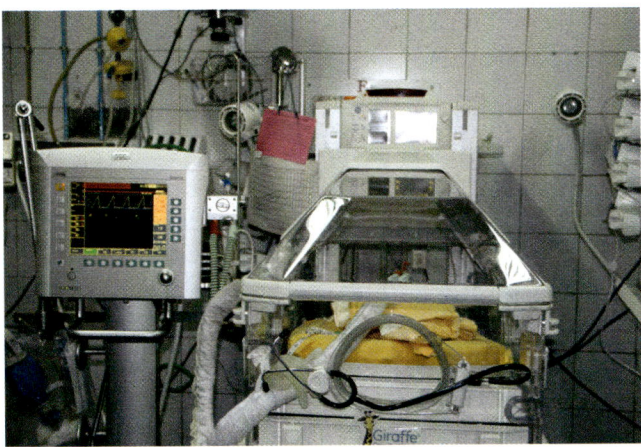

Figure 17.5 Extremely low birth weight infant being nursed in an intensive care incubation and is attached to various electronic monitors.

As soon as baby's condition stabilizes, he should be covered with a perspex shield or effectively clothed with a frock, cap, socks and mittens. After one week or so, stable babies with a birth weight of <1200 g should preferably be nursed in an intensive care incubator (Figure 17.5). It is associated with reduced chances of handling, better temperature control, reduced evaporative losses from skin and better weight gain velocity. The mother should be encouraged to provide partial kangaroo-mother-care to prevent hypothermia, to promote bonding and breastfeeding and to transmit healing electromagnetic vibrations of love and compassion to her baby. For further details regarding prevention of hypothermia refer to Chapter 14.

Oxygen Therapy

Oxygen should be administered only when indicated, given in the lowest ambient concentration and stopped as soon as its use is considered unnecessary. It is difficult to judge the need for oxygen therapy on clinical grounds in preterm babies. The oxygen should be administered with a head box when SaO_2 falls below 85% and it should be gradually withdrawn when SaO_2 goes above 90%. The lowest ambient concentration and flow rates should be used to maintain SaO_2 between 85 and 95% and PaO_2 between 60 and 90 mm Hg.

Phototherapy

Jaundice is common in preterm babies due to hepatic immaturity, hypoxia, hypoglycemia, infections and hypothermia. Due to immaturity of blood–brain barrier, hypoproteinemia and perinatal distress factors, bilirubin brain damage may occur at relatively lower serum bilirubin levels. Early phototherapy is advised to keep the serum bilirubin level within safe limits in order to obviate the need for exchange blood transfusion. Refer to Chapter 18 for details of phototherapy.

Prevention of Nosocomial Infections

A preterm baby, who survives the initial stormy and unstable period of one week, is likely to do well, if protected against infections and provided with adequate nutrition. The handling should be reduced to bare minimum. Vigilance should be maintained on all procedures recommended for reduction of hospital-acquired infections in the NICU. High index of suspicion, early diagnosis and effective treatment of infections are essential for improved survival. For further details regarding prevention of nosocomial infections, refer to Chapter 3.

Feeding and Nutrition

Starvation should be avoided and early enteral feeding should be established as soon as the baby is stable. Babies weighing less than 1200 g or gestation of <30 weeks and sick babies (severe birth asphyxia, RDS, sepsis, seizures, apneic attacks, assisted ventilation, etc.) should be started on intravenous dextrose solution (10% dextrose in babies >1000 g and 5% dextrose in babies <1000 g). Trophic feeds with EBM (1–2 mL 4 times/day) through a nasogastric tube can be started in all babies irrespective of their birth weight or clinical condition to harness its unique benefits. When baby's condition is stabilized, enteral feeds are begun with EBM starting with a volume of 30 mL/kg/d on the first day and depending upon the tolerance, the enteral feeds are increased by 10–20 mL/kg/d everyday and intravenous fluids are reduced accordingly. For complete details regarding the type of enteral feeding, volume and frequency of feeds, mode of feeding and monitoring, refer to Chapter 15.

Nutritional Supplements

After two weeks when baby is stable and tolerating enteral feeds, EBM can be fortified with human milk fortifier (HMF). The fortification of EBM with formula feeds (especially during night) also provides additional calories and protein to the baby. Multivitamin drops containing folic acid should be started at two weeks of age. Iron supplementation (2–3 mg/kg elemental iron) should be started after 2–3 weeks when baby is having steady weight gain. Free radical lipid peroxidation in cell membranes is catalyzed by iron and polyunsaturated fatty acids (PUFA) thus increasing the requirements of vitamin E in very low birth weight babies. The requirements of vitamin E are, therefore, related to linoleic acid content of the formula. It is recommended that vitamin E to linoleic acid ratio should be greater than 1.0 iu/gram of linoleic acid (vitamin E 1.0 iu = 1.0 mg) in the feeding formula for LBW babies. The α-tocopherol/linoleic acid ratios are 6.23, 1.43 and 0.78 mg/g in human colostrum, transitional and mature milk, respectively. Vitamin E is a powerful antioxidant and prevents the hemolytic anemia and edema of prematurity. In infants weighing less than 1500 g at birth, milk formula should provide at least 1.0 iu of vitamin E per gram of linoleic acid and supplemented with daily adminis-tration of 15 iu of vitamin E. Metabolic bone disease (MBD) or osteopenia of prematurity occurs in 16% of VLBW babies and 40% of ELBW neonates. The key etiological factors include inadequate calcium and phosphorus stores, accelerated skeletal growth, medications (steroids, caffein), prolonged parenteral nutriton and poor physical activity. Supplements of calcium (220 mg/d) and phosphorus (100 mg/d) are essential to prevent osteopenia of prematurity. When EBM feeds are fortified with human milk fortifier (HMF), no additional supplements are required. The supplements are continued till the baby achieves post-conceptional maturity of 38 weeks or weight of 2000 g.

Gentle Rhythmic Stimulation

Availability of sophisticated high technology has revolutionized the care of preterm and sick newborn babies. But the technology should not be allowed to become a barrier between communication, compassion and concern of the treating team and the family. Gentle touch, massage, cuddling, stroking and flexing of limbs by the nurse or preferably by the mother provide useful tactile stimuli to the baby. Rocking bed or placing a preterm baby on inflated gloves rhythmi-cally rocked by a ventilator provide useful vestibular-kinesthetic stimuli for prevention of apneic attacks of prematurity. Soothing auditory stimuli can be given to the preterm baby in the form of taped heart beats, family voices or music. Music has been shown to reduce the stress of procedure and enhance weight gain velocity of preterm babies. Visual inputs can be provided with the help of colored objects, diffuse light and eye-to-eye contact.

Utility of Corticosteroids

Unnecessary administration of corticosteroids should be avoided because of its potential side effects. Antenatal administration of betamethasone or dexamethasone is universally recommended, if labor starts before 34 weeks of gestation. A single dose of dexamethasone 0.2 mg/kg IV at 4 hours of age may be given to very LBW babies (<1500 g) to reduce the incidence and severity of HMD, IVH and NEC but its use is contro-versial. Corticosteroids are also indicated to assist the process of difficult weaning following prolonged assisted ventilation and for attenuation of inflamma-tory changes in infants with bronchopulmonary dysplasia. Hydrocortisone is safer with fewer adverse effects on central nervous system. In infants with chronic lung disease (CLD), it is given in a dose of 5 mg/kg/d in divided doses over a period of 2–3 weeks. Inhaled steroids are safer but have not been found to be useful to reduce the risk of CLD. Corticosteroids have some therapeutic utility in the management of sclerema neonatorum. They have no role in the management of hypoxic-ischemic encephalopathy, sepsis, meningitis and meconium aspiration syndrome. There is increasing evidence to suggest that prolonged use of corticosteroid therapy should be avoided in newborn babies because of serious concerns for short-term (hypertension, hyperglycemia, GI bleeding, infections) and long-term (cerebral palsy and neuromotor disability) side effects.

Transient Hypothyroxinemia of Prematurity

In preterm babies below 30 weeks gestation, total T_4 levels may be low but free T_4, T_3 and TSH levels are usually normal. The condition is transient and is attri-buted to a normal adaptive response of an immature hypothalamic-pituitary axis or because of sick euthyroid syndrome. Its clinical significance is contro-versial. The current Cochrane Neonatal Collaborative Review does not recommend routine T_4 supplementa-tion in preterm babies.

Prevention, Early Diagnosis and Prompt Management of Common Problems

In the best pediatric tradition, neonatology provides the maximum scope for the practice of preventive medicine. Refer to the appropriate chapters regarding details for prevention, early diagnosis and management of specific disorders which are common in preterm babies.

Nosocomial infections Housekeeping rituals, strict housekeeping routines and high index of suspicion should be maintained to prevent and make an early diagnosis of nosocomial infections. Early treatment with an appropriate antibiotic is the key for survival of sick and septic preemies.

Hypothermia Preterm infants must be nursed in a thermoneutral environment.

Respiratory distress syndrome Antenatal administration of corticosteroids, prevention and effective treatment of perinatal distress, prophylactic administration of exogenous surfactant and early administration of CPAP are useful strategies to reduce the incidence and severity of hyaline membrane disease (HMD).

Aspiration Availability of trained nurses is essential for safe administration of enteral feeds and prevention of aspiration of feeds.

Patent ductus arteriosus Avoid over infusion and manage HMD effectively to reduce the risk of PDA.

Chronic lung disease During assisted ventilation, airway pressure should be kept at the bare minimum without compromising gas exchange. In infants <1000 g, administration of vitamin A 5000 units IM 3 times in a week for 4 weeks has been shown to reduce the risk of CLD by 10%. Corticosteroids should preferably be avoided or only short courses of hydrocortisone (5 mg/kg/d q 8 hourly) should be used because of potential risk of causing neuromotor disability.

Necrotizing enterocolitis Ensure feeding with human milk, trophic feeds, avoidance of hyperosmolar feeds and over infusion to reduce the risk of NEC.

Intraventricular hemorrhage Antenatal corticosteroids, avoidance of rough handling, excessive CPAP and bolus administration of sodium bicarbonate may reduce the incidence of IVH.

Retinopathy of prematurity Maintain PaO_2 below 90 mm Hg, avoid excessive light, blood transfusions and ensure feeding with human milk.

Late metabolic acidosis Protein intake should be restricted to 3 g/kg/d and avoid use of formula feeds.

Nutritional disorders Provide supplements with calcium, phosphorus, vitamin K, vitamin D, vitamin E, iron and folic acid.

Drug toxicity Side effects of drugs can be reduced by giving lower doses at 12 hourly intervals.

Weight Record

Accurate weighing of babies is a sensitive index of their well-being. The weight is routinely recorded everyday but in sick babies twice daily weight record is recommended. Most preterm babies lose weight during the first 3 to 4 days of life and loss is up to a maximum of 10 to 15% of the birth weight. The weight remains stationary for the next 3 to 4 days and then the babies start gaining at a rate of 1.0 to 1.5% of body weight (10–15 g/kg/d) per day. The preterm babies regain their birth weight by the end of second week of life. Excessive weight loss, delay in regaining the birth weight or slow weight gain suggest that either the baby is not being fed adequately or he is unwell and needs immediate attention. Sudden weight loss in a baby who had been gaining weight satisfactorily would suggest the possibility of dehydration. Excessive weight gain of 100 g or more per day may occur in babies with cardiac failure though sometimes healthy babies may also gain weight more rapidly.

What therapeutic interventions should be avoided in the care of preterm babies?

In the care of preterm babies, at times greater harm is done by unnecessary therapeutic interventions which may lead to iatrogenic disorders. The following interventions should be avoided because they are unnecessary, useless and often associated with serious side effects.

- Routine oxygen administration without monitoring.
- Intravenous immunoglobulins for prevention of neonatal sepsis.
- Prophylactic antibiotics (except during assisted ventilation).
- Unnecessary use of corticosteroids.
- Prophylactic administration of indomethacin or high doses of vitamin E.
- Unnecessary blood transfusions (definite indications include hematocrit of <40% in a sick neonate, <30% in a symptomatic neonate and <25% in an asymptomatic neonate).
- Formula feeds and dummy nipple or pacifier.
- Rough handling, excessive light, loud sound, pungent odors, painful procedures without proper sedation and analgesia.

Immunizations

Preterm babies are able to mount a satisfactory immune response and they can be vaccinated at the usual chronological age like term babies. The dose of vaccine is not reduced in preterm babies. However, there is some evidence to suggest that administration of hepatitis B vaccine in preterm infants is associated with low seroconversion rate. Because during their stay in the NICU, there is no risk of contracting vaccine-preventable diseases, it is desirable to administer 0-day vaccines (BCG, OPV, HBV) on the day of discharge from the NICU. This policy seems more logical and appropriate to ensure satisfactory immune response against various vaccines. However, if mother is HBV carrier and is e-antigen positive, baby should be given hepatitis B vaccine and hepatitis B specific immunoglobulins within 72 hours of age. Live vaccines should be avoided in symptomatic HIV positive babies. WHO recommends that BCG and oral polio vaccine can be given to asymptomatic HIV positive infants.

Family Support

The prolonged stay of preterm and sick newborn babies in the NICU is associated with emotional trauma, uncertainty, anxiety and lack of bonding with the baby on the part of parents. The family dynamics are greatly disturbed apart from tremendous physical stress and financial implications because of high cost of neonatal intensive care. These issues and problems should be handled with equanimity, compassion, concern and caring attitude of the health team. The frightening scene of NICU should be demystified and family should be constantly informed and involved in the care of their baby. The mother should be encouraged to touch and talk with her baby and provide routine care under the guidance of nurses. She should be assisted to provide partial kangaroo-mother care to her baby in the NICU which would enhance bonding and promote breastfeeding. She should provide visual and auditory stimuli to her baby and try to establish eye-to-eye contact. The anxiety and concern of the family should be cushioned by providing necessary emotional support and guidance.

Transfer from Incubator to Cot

A baby who is feeding from the bottle or cup and spoon or *paladay,* and is reasonably active with a stable body temperature, irrespective of his weight, qualifies for transfer to the open cot. The baby should be observed for another 12 hours after putting the incubator off to see whether he can maintain his body temperature. The infant should stay in the incubator for as short a period as possible because incubators are a potent source of nosocomial infection.

Discharge Policy

The mother should be mentally prepared and provided with essential training and skills for handling a preterm baby before she is discharged from the hospital. The mother-baby dyad should be kept in a step-down nursery where she is able to independently look after the essential needs of her baby like kangaroo-mother care, maintenance of body temperature, ensuring asepsis, feeding with a cup and spoon/*paladay* or breastfeeding and toilet needs. The baby should be stable, maintaining his body temperature and should not have any evidences of cold stress. At the time of discharge, the baby should be having daily steady weight gain velocity of at least 10 g/kg per day. The home conditions should be satisfactory before the baby is discharged. The public health nurse should assess the home conditions and visit the family at home every week for a month or so.

Follow-up Protocol

After discharge from the hospital, babies should be regularly followed up for assessment of the following parameters. The specialized perinatal follow-up services demand a close collaboration and interaction with a large number of specialists like pediatrician, developmental physician, dietetian, ophthalmologist, audiologist, child psychologist, physio-occupational therapist and social worker. The following parameters should be closely monitored and followed.

- Common infective illnesses, reactive airway disease, hypertension, renal dysfunction, gastro-esophageal reflux.
- Feeding and nutrition.
- Immunizations.
- Physical growth, nutritional status, anemia and osteopenia/rickets.
- Neuromotor development, cognition and seizures
- Eyes: Retinopathy of prematurity, vision, strabismus
- Hearing.
- Behavior problems, language disorders and learning disabilities.

Home Care of Preterm Babies

In view of rather marked disparity between the available facilities for special care of low birth weight babies versus number of such babies requiring care in LMIC countries, it is essential that general principles of home care are explained to the mother. Most healthy near term or borderline preterm infants with a birth weight of 1,800 g or more and gestational maturity of 34 weeks or more can be managed at home. The policy of early discharge from the hospital in an effort to decongest the NICU, has imposed additional responsibilities that their care should be extended to their homes. It is, however, essential that a low birth weight infant should not be discharged unless he has regained his birth weight, is self-feeding from the bottle, cup and spoon, *paladay* or breast and is showing a steady weight gain. Before discharge, the mother should be encouraged to breastfeed her baby and look after his toilet needs. She must be explained about the need and importance of maintaining asepsis, keeping the baby warm and ensuring satisfactory feeding routine. It is true, though unfortunate, that many a low birth weight babies after discharge from the hospital, do come back or succumb to diarrhea, sepsis and exposure to cold. The services of postpartum program, public health nurse and social worker can be utilized to provide home care after discharge. It is essential that proper appraisal of available physical facilities, resources and environmental conditions be made by a predischarge home visit by a health visitor or a public health nurse before the baby is discharged. It should be followed by periodic home visits to assess the progress of the child.

Environmental control It must be remembered that the desirable environmental temperature to safeguard the biological needs of the low birth weight infant, is likely to be uncomfortable for an adult. Skin-to-skin contact or kangaroo-mother care can be provided till a body weight of 1800 g or gestations of 34 weeks is achieved. The infant should be effectively clothed taking care to avoid smothering. Woolen cap, socks and mittens should be worn. The infant should preferably lie next to the mother to serve as a useful biologically controlled heat source. In winter, the room can be warmed with a radiant heater or *angeethi*. A table lamp having a 100 watt bulb can be used to provide direct radiant heat. Hot water bottle, if ever used, should never come in direct contact with the baby. The cot of the mother and infant should be located away from the walls to reduce radiation heat loss. The mother and health workers should be trained to assess the temperature of a newborn baby by touch and advised to ensure that the extremities are kept warm and pink. Low birth weight babies do relatively much better in summer than in winter.

The visitors and handling of the infant should be restricted to the bare minimum. The hands must be washed before touching or feeding the baby. The emotional urge for kissing the baby should be curbed. The linen should be clean and sun-dried.

Feeding Whenever feasible, breastfeeding is ideal and must be encouraged. When infant is unable to suck from the breast, expressed breast milk should be given with a bottle, spoon or *paladay* depending upon his maturity. In case formula feeding is unavoidable, specially designed formula for premature babies is recommended. If cow's or buffalo's milk is unavoidable, it should be given after 3:1 dilution. Mother must be given detailed instructions and practical demonstration for maintenance of bottle hygiene to prevent contamination of feeds.

Prognosis

The outcome of uncomplicated premature babies is comparable to the babies born after full maturity. In fact, several renowned and famous people, who were born premature, grew up to become world leaders and intellectuals. Sir Isaac Newton, the greatest mathematician genius, weighed merely 3 lbs at birth. Sir Winston Churchill, the legendary Prime Minister of Britain, was born after 7 months of pregnancy when his mother was participating in a royal dance. The world renowned artists Pablo Picasso and Anna Pavlova, Victor Hugo, the French dramatist, Napolean Bonaparte, Charles Darwin, the British naturalist and the famous writer Mark Twain came into this world a bit too early and left their mark for succeeding generations. The parents of premature children, therefore, should not feel despondent because there is enough historical evidence that their infant has a bright future and he may grow up to become an intellectual giant or a leader.

Prognosis for survival is directly related to the gestation and birth weight of the child and quality of the neonatal care. Over three-fourths of neonatal deaths occur among low birth weight babies. Therefore, in countries with high incidence of LBW babies, neonatal mortality is likely to be higher. The risk of neurodevelopmental handicaps is increased 3-fold for LBW babies and 10-fold for very LBW babies (<1500 g). The prognosis for mental development is good, if the baby had not suffered from birth asphyxia, apneic attacks, respiratory distress syndrome, hypoglycemia or hyperbilirubinemia.

Their physical growth correlates better with their conceptional age rather than the age calculated from the date of birth. Preterm AFD babies catch up in their physical growth with term counterparts by the age of 1 to 2 years. Long-term follow-up studies of infants with a birth weight of 1500 g and less have revealed 15 to 20% incidence of neurological handicaps in the form of cerebral palsy, seizures, hydrocephalus, microcephaly, blindness (due to ROP), deafness and mental retardation. There is high incidence of minor neurologic disabilities in the form of language disorder, learning disabilities, behavior problems, attention deficit hyperactivity disorder requiring specialized support for education. The incidence of neurological handicaps is related to the quality of obstetrical and neonatal services. Neurological prognosis is adversely affected by degree of immaturity, intrauterine growth restriction, severity of perinatal hypoxia, intraventricular hemorrhage, periventricular leukomalacia and severity of respiratory failure demanding assisted ventilation.

Disorders of Weight and Gestation

17

SMALL-FOR-DATES BABIES
(Light-for-dates, Small-for-gestational Age, Intrauterine Growth Retardation)

There is lack of consensus regarding the definition of small-for-dates babies. Some pediatricians classify a baby as small-for-dates, if its birth weight falls below 10th percentile for the period of gestation, while others accept the dividing line of –2SD or 3rd percentile (Figure 17.6). The choice of intrauterine growth charts for classification of babies is also not agreed upon. Ideally, local growth curves should be obtained from babies of healthy mothers belonging to the high socio-economic group after exclusion of maternal and fetal conditions which are known to affect the growth of the fetus. They would, probably, represent the true growth potential of the babies.

FETAL GROWTH

Life begins when ovum is fertilized by the sperm and a microscopic monocellular zygote is formed. It receives X-chromosome from the mother and X or Y chromosome from the father and shares the genetic material of both the parents. It is endowed with a

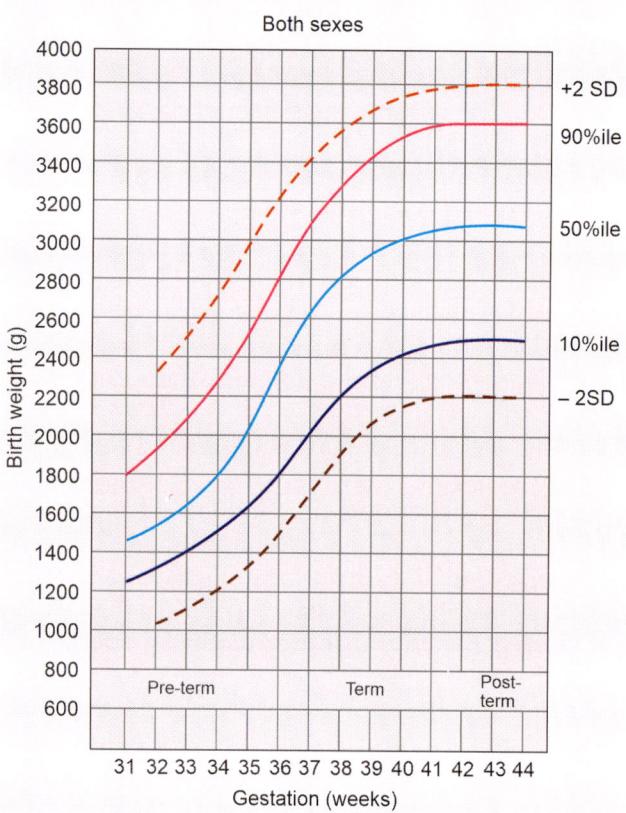

Figure 17.6 Intrauterine weight chart of infants of both sexes (AIIMS).

tremendous growth potential. From a weight of about 0.005 mg at conception, zygote grows rapidly to achieve an average weight of 3000 g at term accounting for almost 65 million% increase in size. During first trimester, growth is characterized by differentiation of various organs. Organogenesis is complete by 12 to 20 weeks of gestation. During this critical embryonic period when organs are differentiating and evolving there is a little increase in size. At about 8 weeks, embryo weighs approximately 1.0 g and measures 2.5 cm and by the end of 12 weeks it weighs 14 g and measures 7.5 g. By this time, all body organs are differentiated and start assuming their functions. Subsequently there is rapid increase in the weight and dimensions of the fetus accompanied by increasing functional maturity of various body organs.

During second trimester of pregnancy, increase in the length of the fetus is proportionately greater as compared to increase in weight. By the end of 28 weeks, fetal weight is about 1000 g and crown-heel length is 35 cm. During last trimester, there is rapid increase in the weight and size of the fetus imposing considerable nutritional demands on the mother. At 40 weeks, an average Indian baby weighs 3000 g and has crown-heel length of 48 cm and head circumference of 34 cm. The brain growth is much faster during fetal life compared to somatic growth. The birth weight of a baby is about 5% of an adult but his brain weight is 60% of the adult. Boys grow faster than girls though differences are marginal and combined intrauterine growth curves of infants of both sexes are satisfactory for clinical purposes.

During early fetal or embryonic life, virtually all growth is due to increase in cell number. Subsequently, there is both increase in cell number and size including increase in intercellular material. After 20 weeks of gestation and during postnatal period, growth occurs virtually by increase in cell size. The impact and outcome of a growth-impairing insult depends upon its timing in relation to specific phase of growth. Interference with the growth of fetus during the embryonic period is associated with permanent retardation of growth potential of the fetus because of less number of body cells. When an insult operates during the period of growth which is characterized by increase in size of the cells, the affected fetus would have normal number of small-sized cells. These infants with malnourished or small-sized cells can be rehabilitated effectively by providing optimal nutrition after birth. They grow fast and catch up with their growth deficit in due course of time. However, if an intra-uterine constraint operates over a longer period of time, when increase in both cell number and cell size is taking place, the organism would have relatively less number of small-sized cells. On nutritional rehabilitation, these infants do grow but they are unable to catch up with their peers who did not encounter any intrauterine growth constraints.

Intrauterine malnutrition which operates mostly during second half of pregnancy produces profound effects on somatic and visceral growth. Body weight is significantly reduced because of lack of subcutaneous fat and muscle mass. Skeletal growth is less affected but there may be delay in the appearance of epiphyseal centers at the distal ends of femur and proximal end of tibia. Brain, heart and lungs are least affected by intrauterine malnutrition. Brain growth may not be spared, if malnutrition is severe and prolonged. Other viscera such as liver, spleen, thymus and adrenals are severely reduced in size during states of under nutrition.

Classification of Small-for-dates Babies

The babies with intrauterine growth failure do not constitute a homogeneous group and are composed of at least three types of babies.

Malnourished small-for-dates babies (asymmetric IUGR) The fetus gets malnourished during the latter part of gestation due to placental dysfunction and appears long, thin and marasmic (Figure 17.7). Head circumference and brain weight are unaffected or show minimal reduction while internal organs, such as liver is grossly shrunken, so that brain/liver weight ratio is more than five. Head circumference is generally more than 3 cm bigger than chest circumference. Double-skinfold thickness is reduced. Due to loss of subcutaneous fat, skin is loose and often hangs in folds at buttocks (Figure 17.8). The ponderal index can be calculated as follows:

$$PI = Weight\ in\ grams/(Length\ in\ cm)^3 \times 100$$

The index is usually less than 2 in infants with a symmetric IUGR (as compared to ponderal index of more than 2.5 in term-AGA infant). In asymmetric IUGR, the growth retardation is mainly due to reduction in the size of cells whereas the number of cells are unaffected. Thus, they retain the potentiality for normal growth on nutritional rehabilitation.

Hypoplastic small-for-dates babies (symmetric IUGR) Intrauterine infections and certain genetic and chromosomal disorders exert their adverse influence from early embryonic life and result in reduced growth potential of the fetus. The baby is proportionately small in all parameters including the head size. The

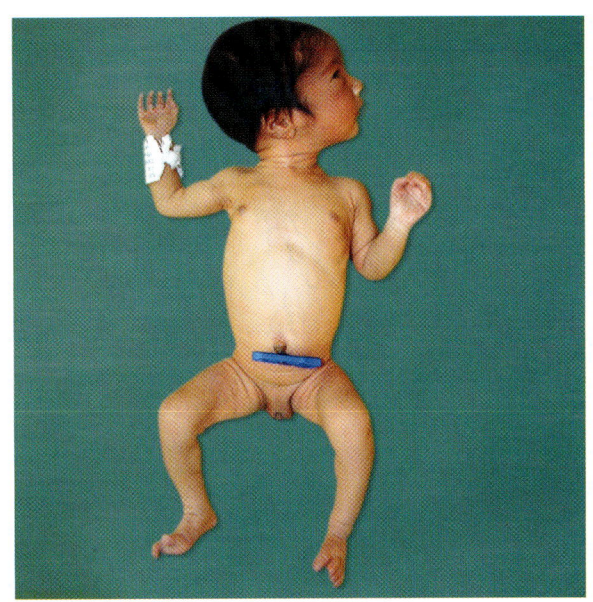

Figure 17.7 Malnourished small-for-dates infant of a toxemic mother (gestation 39 weeks, birth weight 1800 g).

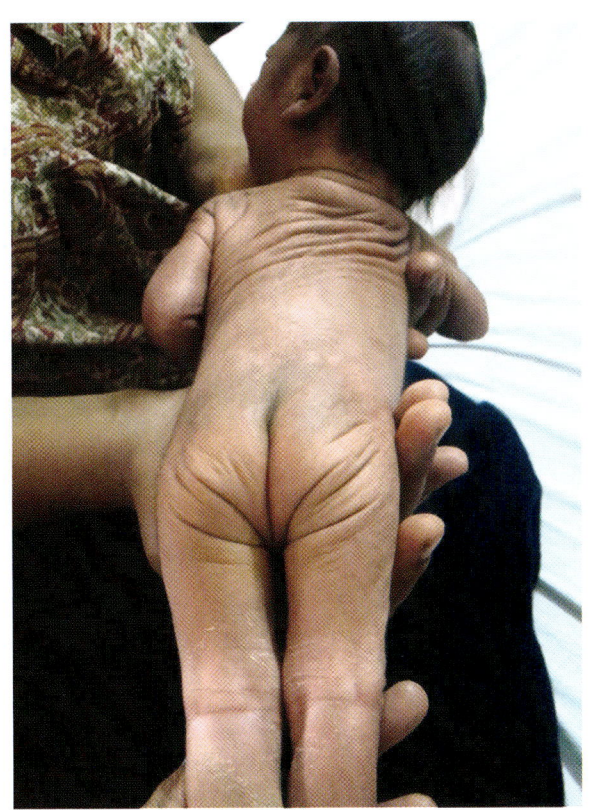

Figure 17.8 Gluteal and truncal folds of skin in a baby with intrauterine growth retardation.

ponderal index is usually more than 2. They have a high incidence of congenital anomalies including abnormal palmar creases and dermatoglyphics. Their cell population is also reduced, resulting in permanent mental and physical growth retardation.

Disorders of Weight and Gestation

17

Mixed small-for-dates babies They are the outcome of adverse intrauterine environmental influences operating from early or mid-pregnancy. These infants, though small for the period of their gestation, neither look obviously malnourished nor grossly hypoplastic. They show varying degrees of reduction in cell population and their size. The constitutionally small babies of small mothers also fall into this category.

Common Determinants of Intrauterine Growth Retardation

In view of the above clinical description of growth retarded babies, it is obvious that the cause of IUGR may rest with the mother and placenta or the fetus itself (Table 17.2). Infant with IUGR is likely to have a small placenta but fetoplacental ratio is unaffected and it varies between 6.0 and 1.0. The salient causes of intrauterine growth restriction are discussed below.

TABLE 17.2 Common correlates of intrauterine growth restriction

- **Fetal**
  - Multiple gestation
  - Sex of the baby (girls are lighter by 100 g)
  - Congenital malformations
  - TORCH infections

- **Placental**
  - Placental dysfunction (PIH, pre-eclampsia)
  - Placental mosaicism
  - Placental embolization with microspheres
  - Abnormal cord insertion
  - Placental infections
  - Chorioangiomata
  - Abruptio placentae

- **Maternal**
  - Genetic, familial and racial factors
  - Low socioeconomic status
  - Primigravida mother
  - Teenage pregnancy
  - Maternal undernutrition
  - Poor dietary intake during pregnancy
  - Inter-pregnancy interval of less than one year
  - Maternal infection: Malaria, tuberculosis, urinary tract infection, diarrhea/dysentery, periodontal disease, vaginal colonization, bacterial vaginosis
  - Pregnancy-induced hypertension and toxemia of pregnancy
  - Maternal systemic diseases
  - Uterine anomalies and fibroids
  - Smoking, tobacco chewing and substance abuse
  - Excessive physical workload
  - Mental tension and stress

Epidemiologic Correlates

Socioeconomic status Socioeconomic status encompasses family income, occupation, maternal education and size of dwelling. Interestingly, available global information indicates that socioeconomic factors do not have an independent effect on gestation or birth weight.

Racial and ethnic differences There is some evidence to suggest that there is genetic or constitutional predisposition for giving birth to LBW babies. In USA, the caucasian child at birth weighs more than the child of negroid origin. As compared to the caucasians, Indian or Pakistani mothers in UK give birth to infants with a relatively lower weight. It has been shown that babies born to mothers of Indian origin had lower mean birth weight than those born to Malaysian or Chinese mothers. However, these studies are not well controlled for confounders such as maternal stature, weight-for-height, and gestational weight gain. It has been shown by case control studies in India that Muslim women had significantly reduced risk of giving birth to term LBW babies compared to their Hindu counterparts.

Previous obstetrical history Primipara mothers are at a distinctly higher risk of producing a LBW baby especially due to IUGR. On the other hand, birth weight is also adversely affected in grand multipara women (i.e. para 3 and more). Previous history of spontaneous abortions, stillbirths or neonatal deaths are important risk factors for delivery of a LBW baby. Interpregnancy interval of <13 months is associated with increased risk of giving birth to a LBW baby.

Antenatal care It is not the number of antenatal visits but the quality of antenatal care that has been shown to improve birth weight and survival of newborn babies.

Maternal Factors

Maternal weight and height They are determined not only by nutritional status but also by genetic, ethnic and constitutional factors. Healthy well nourished tall mother is likely to give birth to a healthy normal weight baby. The health and growth of the fetus is mostly dependent upon the health and well-being of the mother (not the father!) because she is both the seed as well as the soil where the baby is nurtured for 9 months. Pre-pregnancy maternal weight of <40 kg and maternal height of <145 cm are associated with significant risk of LBW. In India, we are faced with a large number of malnourished, small and short

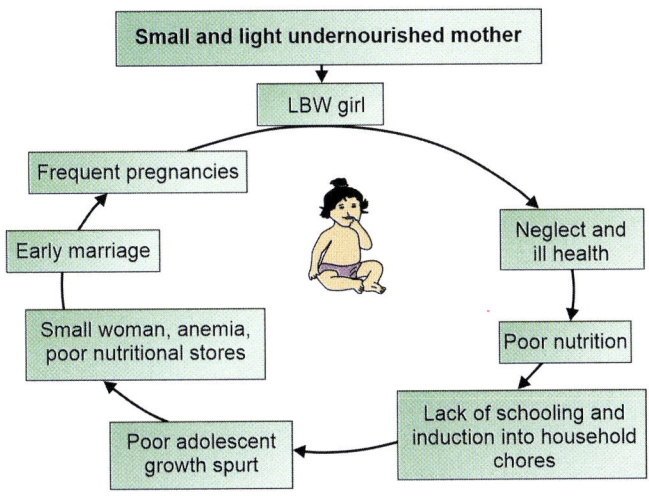

Figure 17.9 Vicious cycle of low birth weight babies.

mothers who tend to produce small babies because of maternal ill health, frequent pregnancies and malnutrition. If a baby happens to be a girl, she grows up in neglect and discrimination during infancy, develops frequent infections, is fed poorly and is likely to have a poor adolescent growth spurt. She will grow to become a small woman who will perpetuate the cycle of producing LBW babies in the next generation (Figure 17.9). It appears that adverse environmental factors may become genetic and constitutional when they operate over several generations and this trend cannot be reversed by merely giving nutritional supplements during current pregnancy alone. It is important to adopt long-term measures to improve the status of women in our society, reduce neglect of girls and provide them with adequate nutrition during infancy, adolescence, pregnancy and lactation.

Weight gain during pregnancy Gestational weight gain represents laying down of maternal fat stores, growth of breasts and uterus, increased plasma volume and growth of the fetus, placenta and amniotic fluid. The relative risk of gestational weight gain of less than 7 kg for causing IUGR is 1.98 among well nourished women. It is estimated that population attributable risk for IUGR may be as high as 40% or more in women of developing countries who gain less than 7 kg of weight during pregnancy.

Energy and protein intake The effects of low caloric intake or food deprivation during pregnancy are less profound because of relatively slow growth of human fetus as compared to certain experimental animals like rats. For example, at term, weight of the litter in mice approximates 30% of mother's body weight as compared to the weight of human infant at birth which

is 5% of the maternal weight. Moreover, fetus is a true parasite and in situations of food deprivation, maternal tissues are catabolized or sacrificed to cater to the metabolic and nutritional demands of the fetus. During states of acute starvation or food deprivation as a consequence of nutritional calamities or during war, the birth weight is reduced by about 200 g of the expected weight at birth when compared to mean birth weight of infants born before and after the disaster. The adverse effects of food deprivation are most marked when it operates during last weeks of pregnancy. Intervention studies have also shown that when mothers are provided additional 200 kcal and 20 g proteins per day during the last 6–8 weeks of pregnancy, their offsprings on an average weigh 110 g more as compared to the non-supplemented controls. There is evidence to suggest that balanced energy and protein supplements (up to 25% calories from protein) is associated with enhanced fetal growth. Excessive protein intake has no additional benefit and may infact adversely affect the fetal growth and perinatal outcome. The incidence of LBW babies is reduced to half by food supplementation during pregnancy. It is understandable that salutary effects of food supplements during pregnancy would be even greater in populations with lower nutritional status and higher incidence of LBW babies.

> There is a mistaken cultural belief that good nutritional intake during pregnancy should be avoided because it would lead to the birth of a large baby with attendant risks of obstructed labor and birth trauma!

Essential fatty acids and docosahexaenoic acid WHO and FAO recommend intake of 2.6 g/day omega-3 fatty acids and 300 mg/day DHA during pregnancy and lactation. There is evidence to suggest that adequate intake of omega-3 fatty acids and DHA is associated with enhanced uteroplacental circulation and reduced risk of toxemia of pregnancy. DHA is credited to reduce the level of thromboxane (TXA_2) and increase the blood level of prostacyclin (PGI_2) leading to thinning of blood and vasodilatation akin to benefits of low dose aspirin. The risk of preterm delivery is reduced by one-fourth and birth weight is significantly improved.

Energy expenditure and physical activity Strenuous physical activity during third trimester of pregnancy may adversely affect fetal growth because energy is consumed by the mother for physical labor and denied for fetal growth. Physical activity entails energy expenditure, may reduce uterine blood flow when physical work is conducted in an upright posture and may cause psychological stress. The continued physical labor throughout pregnancy is more often undertaken in economically deprived, nutritionally compromised and illiterate women who work as labor force in the fields and for civil construction work.

The role of micronutrients There is enough evidence to suggest that nutritional anemia during pregnancy is associated with compromised fetal growth. Supplements of iron (60 mg/d of elemental iron) and folic acid (500 µg/d) during second half of pregnancy is associated with mean improvment in birth weight by 300 g. There is some evidence to suggest that zinc deficiency during pregnancy may affect fetal growth though more well-controlled prospective studies are needed. The effects of various micronutrients within the body are interrelated. Supplementing iron and folic acid without zinc has questionable utility. Zinc administration without copper is suspected to cause hypercholesterolemia and immunodeficiency. Concomitant administration of magnesium helps in better absorption of calcium. There is some evidence to suggest that supplements of DHA, calcium, riboflavin, vitamin C and vitamin E during pregnancy may reduce the risk of pregnancy-induced hypertension.

Placental dysfunction and fetal disorders Pregnancy-induced hypertension, toxemia of pregnancy and postmaturity are important causes of fetal growth retardation. Toxemia of pregnancy is more common among primigravida mothers belonging to low socio-economic status. Multiple pregnancy is associated with fetal growth retardation because two fetuses can be nourished statisfactorily only up to 35 weeks of gestation. Beyond this period, single placenta is unable to sustain the normal growth of two fetuses. Placental mosaicism, embolization, abnormal cord insertion, chorioangiomata and abruptio placentae are recognized to cause fetal growth restriction.

Chronic systemic diseases Hypertension, chronic heart disease, especially when associated with congestive heart failure or cyanosis, renal disease, bronchial asthma, collagen vascular disease, diabetes mellitus (class D, E, F, R) and sickle cell disease are associated with poor fetal growth because of impaired energy availability due to increased maternal catabolism or poor nutrient transfer to the fetus across the placenta or both.

Maternal infections Malaria, tuberculosis, urinary tract infection and recurrent diarrhea/dysentery during pregnancy are recognized correlates of fetal growth retardation. In endemic areas, prophylaxis against malaria during pregnancy has been shown to improve birth weight on an average by 170 g. The infections during pregnancy should be promptly identified and adequately treated with appropriate antibiotics.

Colonization of maternal genital tract by *Chlamydia trachomatis, Mycoplasma hominis, Ureaplasma urealyticum* and bacterial vaginosis have been found to be associated with birth of relatively smaller babies both by virtue of prematurity and IUGR though the impact is not of great clinical relevance.

Maternal substance abuse Drug abuse during pregnancy is associated with several adverse effects on the fetus including developmental defects and compromised fetal growth. The incidence of LBW babies doubles, if the pregnant woman smokes more than 20 cigarettes per day. Tobacco chewing which is common among rural and tribal women in several states in India, is also associated with IUGR. There is evidence to suggest that if a pregnant woman chews 400 mg of tobacco everyday, the birth weight of her baby is reduced by up to 542 g compared to control women. If a mother consumes two alcoholic drinks everyday during pregnancy, the birth weight of the baby is reduced on an average by 155 g. Effect of marijuana and LSD addiction of the pregnant woman on the birth weight of her baby is not conclusive and is controversial. In many women who are addicted to various drugs, the socioeconomic status of the mother, family background, neglect of nutrition, conception out of wedlock, and occurrence of sexually-transmitted diseases may have the adverse effects on the birth weight rather than the addictive drugs *per se*.

Environment pollutants Insecticides and pollutants may adversely affect the birth weight of the babies. It has been shown that women living in Love Canal, New York, a waste dump site, had high incidence of LBW babies. In Japan, women living near the airport gave birth to babies with a lower birth weight due to increased noise pollution caused by the aircraft. But a Dutch study did not support the association between noise pollution and fetal growth retardation.

Fetal Conditions

Sex The female infants are lighter at birth compared to male babies. However, the differences are not significant and combined (computing birth weight data of boys and girls together) intrauterine growth charts are used in clinical practice.

Chromosomal and genetic disorders Trisomy syndromes, Turner syndrome and various types of short-limbed dwarfism are associated with hypoplastic babies. Some babies are classified as primordial dwarfs due to genetic or constitutional factors.

Intrauterine infections Rubella, cytomegalovirus inclusion disease and toxoplasmosis are classical examples in this group. These infants are hypoplastic at birth and suffer from physical growth retardation and neuromotor sequelae during childhood.

THERAPEUTIC INTERVENTIONS

Early-onset Fetal Growth Restriction

When life-threatening congenital malformations are identified during first trimester, medical termination of pregnancy is recommended. Identification of TORCH infections during early pregnancy does not have any therapeutic implications. However, when maternal toxoplasmosis is diagnosed, treatment of the mother with spiramycin, sulfadiazine and pyrimethamine have been shown to reduce the risk of congenital toxoplasmosis.

Late-onset Fetal Growth Restriction

When fetal growth restriction is identified after 28 weeks of gestation, abnormalities in the uteroplacental unit and placental dysfunction are common incriminating factors. There is no consensus in the literature regarding the most effective management strategy. The following interventions have been tried mostly in experimental animals with variable results.

Bed rest Bed rest is usually recommended to conserve energy and improve circulation of blood in the uteroplacental unit. No consistent benefits of bed rest have been demonstrated and results of various studies are variable. Moreover, there is increased risk of deep vein thrombosis and pulmonary embolism during bed rest.

Parenteral nutrition to the mother There are sporadic reports that intravenous hyperalimentation with 10% glucose and 12% amino acids to women with fetal growth restriction may improve the birth weight. It has not received universal acceptance due to lack of convincing evidence for its benefits.

Nutritional supplements to the fetus It has been estimated that ingestion of amniotic fluid provides the fetus with 10–13 calories/day and 0.2–0.3 g protein/kg/day in the third trimester. Transamniotic fetal feeding (TAFF) with 10% dextrose, amino acids, lipids and epidermal growth factor has been shown to improve fetal growth in rabbits. There are no controlled clinical trials of TAFF in human pregnancy. Direct intragastric and intravenous administration of nutritional supplements have been shown to improve fetal growth in experimental sheep model. The relevance of these experimental studies to clinical practice remains to be determined.

Oxygen therapy Chronic hypoxia due to placental insufficiency, maternal cyanotic heart disease and living at high altitudes is associated with compromised fetal growth. It has been found that umbilical venous oxygen tension is significantly lower in growth retarded fetuses. Therapeutic utility of continuously administered oxygen to the mother (55% oxygen at a rate of 8 L/min round-the-clock) has been evaluated. There was no significant improvement in birth weight but perinatal mortality rate is significantly lower in babies born to mothers who received oxygen supplementation.

Antibiotic therapy It has been incriminated that genital colonization with Mycoplasma and Chlamydia may be associated with both prematurity and intrauterine growth retardation. Prophylactic therapy with erythromycin during third trimester of pregnancy is associated with variable results and is not recommended in clinical practice.

Pharmacologic therapy It has been shown that low-dose aspirin (1–2 mg/kg/day single dose) inactivates platelet cyclooxygenase enzyme and results in decreased synthesis of thromboxane (TXA_2) while it has no effect on prostacyclin (PGI_2) which is a vasodilator. The results of various therapeutic trials for prevention and treatment of intrauterine fetal growth restriction are conflicting. Low-dose aspirin has been shown to cause a modest reduction in the incidence of pre-eclampsia but its use may be associated with increased incidence of abruptio placentae. Some obstetric anesthetists consider low-dose aspirin use as a relative contraindication for regional anesthesia for cesarean section. Based on current data from large randomized controlled trials, one can conclude that the efficacy of aspirin is not yet proven in the prevention and treatment of IUGR. Dipyridamole, a phosphodiesterase inhibitor causes delay in the degradation of cyclic adenosine monophosphate (cAMP) which renders platelets more sensitive to degradation and enhances synthesis of prostacyclin. However, most clinical trials have not demonstrated any additional therapeutic benefits by adding dipyridamole to low-dose (60 mg/day) aspirin regime.

β-adrenergic agonists are credited to cause myometrial relaxation with decreased resistance to uterine blood flow. They are also known to have direct vasodilatory effect on uterine perfusion. But clinical trials with β-agonists have failed to demonstrate consistent benefits to enhance fetal growth.

Atrial natriuretic peptide (ANP) is an endogenous peptide synthesized in the right atrium that has direct diuretic, natriuretic and vasodilator effects. The role of ANP in the pathogenesis of IUGR resulting from uteroplacental insufficiency has been studied recently. Studies have shown that plasma ANP levels are significantly higher while there is 80% reduction in the number of ANP receptors in pregnancies complicated by IUGR. It has been shown that continuous low-dose infusion of ANP to pregnant guinea pigs in whom uterine artery is ligated, is associated with 26% increase in blood flow to the placenta. Further research is needed to elucidate the role of ANP in the pathogenesis of IUGR before human trials are conducted.

Recent advances in the understanding of somatotrophic axis has unfolded the role of insulin-like growth factors (especially IGF-1) in various experimental animal models of IUGR. It has been shown that there is a decrease in the level of circulating IGF-1 and increase in IGF binding proteins (IGFBP) when IUGR is induced in experimental animals. IGF-1 molecules have structural similarity to proinsulin and is bound to at least six specific IGF-binding proteins that regulate its effect. It has been recently documented that cord blood IGF-1 levels are significantly decreased in IUGR babies. The therapeutic utility of exogenous IGF-1 to improve fetal growth has been studied in experimental animals with positive results. Because maternal IGF-1 does not cross the placenta, the mechanism for beneficial effect of exogenous IGF-1 on fetal growth is unclear. There is a need to study stomatotrophic axis in human pregnancies complicated by IUGR before clinical trials can be launched for administration of IGF-1 through the mother or to the fetus directly.

Nitric oxide donors L-arginine, a potent NO donor, has been found to improve uteroplacental blood flow. Those pregnant women who demonstrate increased uterine blood flow on Doppler velocimetry after sublingual intake of 0.3 mg glyceryl nitrate, are likely to show benefit after administration of NO donor. There is some evidence that oral intake of L-arginine 3 g daily for 20 days is associated with enhanced fetal growth. There is a need to undertake controlled randomized clinical trials before this modality is recommended in clinical practice.

Intermittent abdominal decompression It has been shown that intermittent abdominal decompression is associated with improvement in uteroplacental blood flow and fetal oxygenation. The abdominal decompression is produced by wearing a plastic suit over a rigid frame in which pressure can be reduced with a vacuum. A negative pressure (70 mm Hg) is applied for 30 seconds every minute for 30 minutes twice a day. The method is cumbersome and no controlled trials have been conducted till date. The meta-analysis of three studies of this treatment modality has documented significant reduction in perinatal mortality without any improvement in birth weight.

Common Problems in Small-for-dates Babies

The clinical problems and outcome of small-for-dates babies are very different as compared to preterm babies (Table 17.3). By and large most clinical problems and biochemical abnormalities are limited to severely growth retarded babies with a birth weight of less than minus two standard deviations below the mean for gestational age or less than 3rd percentile. They need to be screened and watched for the following clinical problems:

1. Fetal hypoxia and intrapartum death due to placental dysfunction
2. Severe birth asphyxia
3. Aspiration of meconium before birth
4. Symptomatic hypoglycemia and hypocalcemia
5. Congenital malformations
6. Pulmonary hemorrhage due to unknown cause
7. Polycythemia because of chronic hypoxia
8. Thermoregulation may be unsatisfactory due to scanty brown fat
9. Hyperbilirubinemia
10. Vulnerability to infections
11. Poor growth potential on follow-up
12. Increased risk of development of metabolic syndrome X, diabetes mellitus, hypertension and coronary artery disease in adult life.

In preterm small-for-dates babies, combined hazards of immaturity and intrauterine growth retardation are likely to manifest.

Management

Timing of Delivery

The timing of delivery of a baby with intrauterine growth restriction poses a great challenge to the obstetrician. Early delivery is indicated to ensure intact survival of the baby whenever there is late-onset fetal growth restriction with uteroplacental dysfunction. The indications for delivery include severe oligohydramnios or lack of fetal growth over a period of two weeks especially when fetal well-being is at stake

TABLE 17.3 Differences between preterm and term small-for-dates babies

Clinical problems	Preterm	Term small-for-dates
▪ Intrauterine hypoxia	+	+++
▪ Respiratory difficulties		
a. Birth asphyxia	+	+++
b. Aspiration *in utero*	+	+++
c. Hyaline membrane disease	+++	0
d. Apneic attacks	+++	0
▪ Feeding difficulties		
a. Inability to suck and swallow	+++	0
b. Aspiration of feeds	++	0
c. Functional obstruction and enterocolitis	++	+
▪ Symptomatic hypoglycemia	+	+++
▪ Hypothermia	+++	+
▪ Polycythemia	+	+++
▪ Hyperbilirubinemia	+++	+
▪ Susceptibility to infections	+++	++
▪ Congenital malformations	++	+++
▪ Hemorrhage		
a. Intraventricular	+++	0
b. Pulmonary	+	+++
▪ Prognosis		
a. Immediate	High mortality	Better prognosis but increased mortality when compared with normally grown term babies.
b. Future physical and mental development	Good if there are no perinatal complications except in extremely preterm babies.	Poor especially in hypoplastic and severe IUGR babies. There is increased risk of development of hypertension, coronary artery disease and diabetes mellitus later in life.

as assessed by biophysical profile, NST and Doppler velocimetry studies (Figure 17.10). During labor, up to 50% of growth-restricted fetuses are likely to exhibit evidences of fetal distress. Delay in delivery may lead to *in utero* death of the fetus, fetal distress, birth asphyxia and adverse neuromotor consequences. When a baby is delivered prematurely, he is likely to suffer from consequences of immaturity (like RDS, IVH, NEC, etc.) although there is some evidence that chronic stress in IUGR babies may be associated with elaboration of endogenous corticosteroids that may enhance pulmonary maturity. Nevertheless, antenatal administration of corticosteroids are recommended whenever delivery is being contemplated before 34 weeks of gestation in a growth retarded fetus. Administration of antenatal corticosteroids are associated with significant decrease in the incidence of RDS, necrotizing enterocolitis, and periventricular hemorrhage.

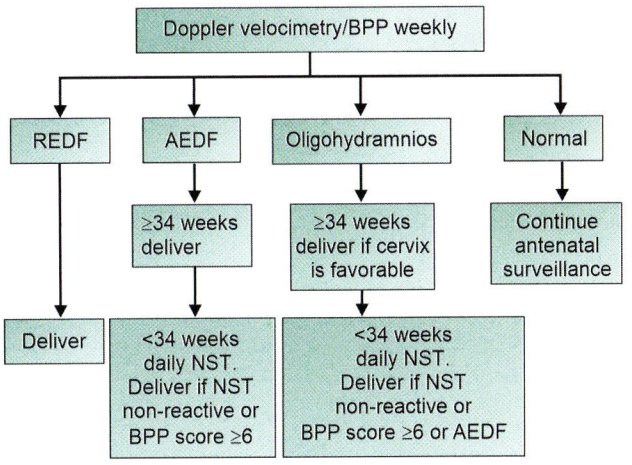

BPP: biophysical profile   NST: non-stress test
AEDF: absent end-diastolic umbilical artery blood flow
REDF: reversal of end-diastolic umbilical artery blood flow

Figure 17.10 Algorithm for management of a fetus with late-onset growth restriction.

Care of the Baby

Fetal hypoxia may necessitate emergency cesarean section and the pediatrician should be prepared to receive an asphyxiated baby. The suctioning of glottic area under direct vision is essential, if baby is meconium stained. The baby should be screened for any congenital malformations. Early and adequate feeding must be ensured to prevent hypoglycemia. Breastfeeding should be initiated immediately after birth. Babies weighing less than 3rd percentile should receive supplementary feeds fortified with sugar during first 3 to 4 days. Sugar-fortified formula feeds should be provided from the nursery and given with a cup and spoon/*paladay*. The mother should not be asked to purchase any formula or feeding bottle. Symptomatic polycythemia should be managed with partial exchange with plasma or physiological saline. The blood glucose and hematocrit should be monitored during first three days of life. When adequately fed, they do not lose weight and start gaining weight after 2 to 3 days of age. Their initial weight gain is rapid which subsequently slows down after three months of age.

Prognosis

The immediate outlook for small-for-dates babies is better than the preterm babies of identical weight but their mortality is 2 to 3 times higher compared to appropriately grown babies of identical maturity. Depending upon the duration and severity of intrauterine environmental constraints, postnatal physical growth may be retarded. It has been shown that body weight of SGA infant at 2 years of age is about 10% lower compared to AGA infant of identical maturity. The hypoplastic babies remain permanently physically and mentally handicapped. Malnourished small-for-dates babies with symptomatic hypoglycemia and polycythemia during neonatal period are also likely to manifest evidences of brain damage later in life. Long-term follow-up studies of uncomplicated malnourished small-for-dates babies have also shown higher incidence of clinical manifestations of minimal brain dysfunction, learning disability and suboptimal physical growth.

Prevention

The relatively high incidence of perinatal mortality in developing countries directly correlates with the higher incidence of LBW babies. Over 80% of all neonatal deaths and 50% of all infant deaths are limited to LBW babies. Prevention and reduction in the incidence of LBW babies is the most important strategy to reduce perinatal and infant mortality rates and improve the quality of life among those who survive. The important long-term and short-term strategies for prevention of LBW babies are listed in Chapter 3.

LARGE-FOR-DATES BABIES
(Heavy-for-dates, Overgrown Babies, Macrosomia)

These babies need to be observed closely as they have a higher neonatal mortality as compared to normally grown babies of identical gestation. The criteria for diagnosis include a birth weight of more than 90th percentile for the period of gestation. Infants with a birth weight of more than 2 standard deviations from the mean weight for gestation or more than 97th percentile are likely to pose clinical problems.

Causes

1. **Genetic or constitutional** Tall and heavy mother is likely to produce a big baby. There is no relationship between size of the father and birth weight of the offspring.

2. **Maternal diabetes mellitus and prediabetes** It is the commonest cause of large-for-dates (LFD) babies. Utilization of large quantities of transplacentally transmitted glucose appears to be the basic mechanism producing islet cell hyperplasia and overgrowth of the fetus. Human placental lactogen, a growth-hormone like substance is increased in infants of diabetic mothers (*see* Chapter 4 for details).

3. **Transposition of great vessels** The large fetal size appears to be related to hyperinsulinemia. Arteriolized blood containing more glucose and oxygen is shunted from the heart towards the viscera, thus leading to hyperplasia of islet cells.

4. **Hydrops fetalis** The large size is usually due to generalized anasarca rather than exaggerated somatic growth. There is some evidence to suggest that breakdown products of hemolyzed red blood cells (glutathione) inactivates circulating insulin leading to hyperplasia of islet cells to maintain adequate insulin levels in infants with erythroblastosis fetalis.

5. **Cretinism** The mean birth weight is higher in babies with congenital hypothyroidism.

6. **Overgrown syndromes with advanced skeletal maturation** In a number of babies with fetal macrosomia due to endocrinal or developmental disorders, advanced skeletal maturation provides a useful diagnostic marker. Overgrowth syndrome is

diagnosed when at least two of the three growth parameters (weight, length and heard circumference) are 2 SD or >97th centile above the mean for age and sex.

i. Administration of progestins during pregnancy or virilizing ovarian tumor in the mother.

ii. Congenital adrenal hyperplasia

iii. Thyrotoxicosis

iv. *Wiedemann-Beckwith syndrome* The syndrome occurs due to epigenetic abnormalities of 11p15.5 region. These babies have characteristic grooves in the ear lobes, macroglossia, exomphalos, visceromegaly and somatic overgrowth (Figure 17.11). They are prone to develop hypoglycemia due to hyperplasia of islet cells. Hypospadias, cleft palate, coloboma of the iris and capillary hemangiomata may be associated. They are at increased risk to develop Wilms' tumor, hepatoblastoma and neuroblastoma in the first seven years of life. There is higher incidence of mental sequelae during childhood. In some patients, partial duplication of chromosome 11 has been demonstrated on karyotyping studies with banding technique.

v. *Marshall-Smith syndrome* The craniofacial characteristics include broad forehead with hypertelorism, large ears, micrognathia, long philtrum and mild microstomia. The joints cannot be extended due to hypertonia. These babies also manifest disproportionately advanced maturation of carpal bones but can be distinguished from infants with cerebral gigantism by the presence of large punctate epiphyses, broadened ends of long bones and continuation of excessive growth postnatally as well. The developmental retardation is absent or minimal.

vi. *Sotos syndrome (cerebral gigantism)* It is possibly a single gene defect due to NSD1 mutation and deletion. These children have large anthropometric measurements at birth with relatively large hands and feet. The cardinal features include facial dysmorphism, physical overgrowth and advanced bone age, neuromotor retardation and learning, difficulties. The face is long and narrow with dolichocephaly, hypertelorism with anti-mongoloid slant of eyes, bossing of forehead, prominent chin and thinning of hair over forehead and temples (Figure 17.12). They are likely to have neuromotor retardation, seizures, mental subnormality, learning disability, behavior disorders and autistic features. Hypotonia and laxity of joints are common. They are vulnerable to develop sacrococcygeal teratoma and lymphoreticular malignancy. About 20% of patients are likely to have cardiac abnormalities like PDA, ASD and VSD. Bone age is advanced without any hormonal abnormalities. Neurosonography and CT scan shows ventriculomegaly, hypoplasia or agenesis of corpus callosum, cerebral atrophy and small cerebellar vermis. EEG abnormalities are common. A number of genetic deletions and duplications can cause overgrowth. Multi-gene next-generation sequencing (NGS) panels can be sequenced from a single test for a definitive diagnosis.

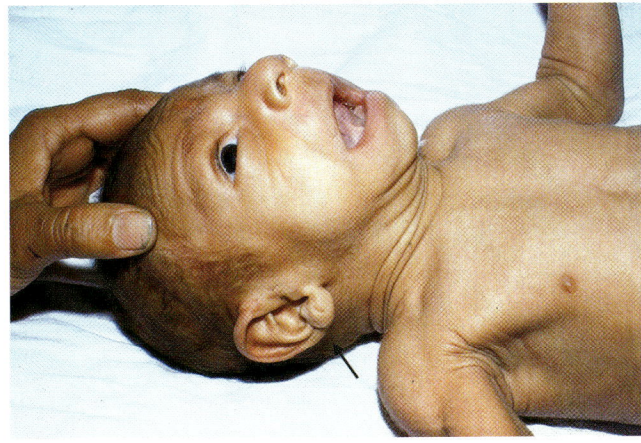

Figure 17.11 Wiedemann-Beckwith syndrome. Arrow points to the characteristic groove on the lower part of helix.

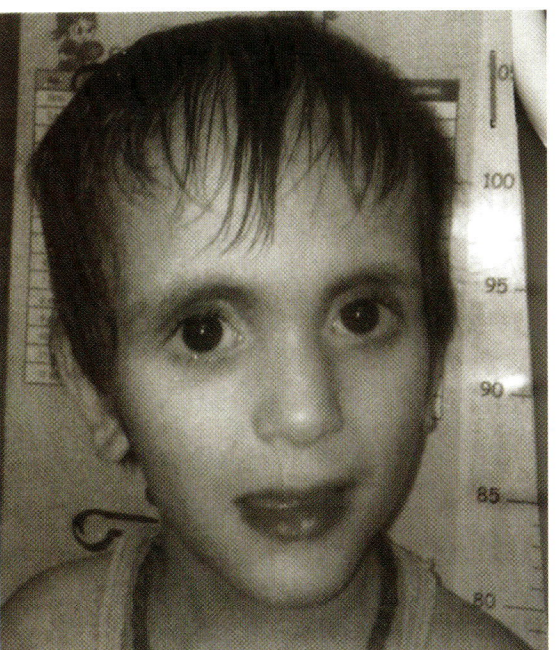

Figure 17.12 A 2-year-old boy with Sotos syndrome. Note long narrow face, frontal bossing, hypertelorism, prominent chin and sparse hair.

Management

The large-for-dates infant should be accorded special care depending upon his gestational maturity and etiology of somatic overgrowth. They must be fed early with sugar-fortified feeds and blood glucose should be monitored during first 72 hours of life because most overgrown infants are associated with hypertrophy of islet cells of pancreas. Hematocrit should be monitored to identify polycythemia and managed appropriately. Most overgrowth syndromes have facial dysmorphism, developmental delay, congenital anomalies, neurological problem and increased risk of neoplasia. For clinical problems and management of infants of diabetic mothers, refer to Chapter 4.

POST-TERM BABIES (Postmature, Post-dated)

Infants born at a gestation of 42 weeks or later are called post-term. In majority of instances, the cause of postmaturity remains uncertain. Post-dating of labor is common among primiparous women. Fetus with anencephaly fails to initiate labor at term because of failure of pelvic engagement of the head and lack of pituitary-adrenal axis. Infants with trisomy 16–18 or Seckel's syndrome (bird-headed dwarfism) are generally several weeks post-term.

Clinical Features

Human placenta can sustain the growth of the fetus up to 42 weeks, beyond which it becomes too senile or dysfunctional to support the growth. In developing countries, due to nutritional constraints, plateau in intrauterine growth is reached around 38 weeks. Postmaturity is an important cause of placental dysfunction, fetal malnutrition and stillbirth. The fetus is at an increased risk to suffer from hypoxia and birth asphyxia. The *in utero* passage of meconium poses grave hazards of respiratory distress due to aspiration of meconium. Vernix caseosa and quantity of liquor begins to decrease around 36 weeks and almost disappears by 41 weeks of gestation. Lack of vernix in post-term infants is associated with maceration of unprotected skin leading to its desquamation and formation of deep sole creases. Infant may appear long, thin and wasted (dysmature). Skin, umbilical cord and nails may be stained yellow because of passage of meconium *in utero*. The presence of long nails is an unreliable sign of postmaturity because many term babies have rather long nails. Skull bones are usually hard. The infant is alert at birth and shows advanced neurological development.

The common clinical problems in post-term babies include congenital malformations, perinatal hypoxia, meconium aspiration, persistent pulmonary hypertension, hypoglycemia, hypocalcemia and polycythemia.

Management

Placental functions must be monitored to assess fetal well-being whenever pregnancy advances beyond 41 weeks. The fetus should be watched for any signs of fetal distress. In the event of *in utero* passage of meconium, thorough oropharyngeal suction as soon as the head is delivered, followed by meticulous suction of glottic area under direct vision, must be undertaken. Early feeding and screening for blood glucose is recommended for dysmature infants. Application of oil or moisturizing cream prevents dryness of skin due to desquamation.

BIBLIOGRAPHY

Allen MC. Developmental outcome and follow up of the small-for-gestational age infant. *Semin Perinatol* 1984; 8:123.

Altman DG, Hytten FE. Intrauterine growth retardation: Let's be clear about it. *Brit J Obstet Gynecol* 1989; 96:1127.

Arora NK, Paul VK, Singh M. Morbidity and mortality in term infants with intrauterine growth retardation. *J Trop Pediatr* 1987; 33:186.

Arora NK, Singh M, Paul VK, Bhargava VL. Etiology of fetal growth retardation in hospital born infants. *Indian J Med Res* 1987; 85:395–400.

Aylward GP, Pfeiffer SI, Wright A, Verhulst SJ. Outcome studies of low birth weight infants published in the last decade: A meta-analysis. *J Pediatr* 1989; 115:515.

Barker DJ. Fetal origins of cardiovascular disease. *Ann Med* 1999; (31 Suppl.) 1:3–6.

Behrman RE. Preventing low birth weight: A pediatric perspective. *J Pediatr* 1985; 107:842.

Bergner L and Susser MW. Low birth weight and prenatal nutrition. An interpretative review. *Pediatrics* 1970; 46:946.

Chacham S, Pasi R. Assisted physical exercise for preterm neonates. *Indian Pediatr* 2018, 55:111–12.

Chawla D. Genetic polymorphism and preterm birth. *Indian J Pediatr* 2018, 85(2):83–84.

Chawla D. Placental transfusion in preterm neonates. *Indian J Pediatr* 2018, 85(3):165.

Bortholomsew J, Kovacs L, Papaglorgiou A. Review of the antenatal and postnatal use of steroids. *Indian J Pediatr* 2014; 81(5):466–472.

Chiswick ML. Intrauterine growth retardation. *Brit Med J* 1985; 291:845.

Clasp Collaborative Group. CLASP: A randomized trial of low-dose aspirin for the prevention and treatment of pre-eclampsia among 9364 pregnant women. *Lancet* 1994; 343:619–629.

De Boer L, Le Cessie S, Wit JM. Auxologic data in patients clinically suspected of Sotos syndrome with NSD1 gene alterations. *Acta Paediatr* 2005; 94:1142–1144.

Dorling J, Kempley S, Leaf A. Feeding growth restricted preterm infants with abnormal antenatal Doppler results. *Arch Dis Child Fetal Neonatal Ed* 2005; 90:F359–363.

Heinonen KM. Assessing the effectiveness of care of very low birth weight infants: Do we really need population-based data? *Pediatrics* 1990; 2: 91.

Kitchen WH, Ford GW, Doyle LW. Growth and very low birth weight. *Arch Dis Child* 1989; 64:379.

Kramer MS. Determinants of low birth weight. *Bull WHO* 1987; 65:663–735.

Kramer WB, Weiner CP. Management of intrauterine growth restriction. *Clin Obstet Gynecol* 1997; 40:814–823.

Low JA, Galbraith RS and Muir D, *et al*. Intrauterine growth retardation : A study of long-term morbidity. *Amer J Obstet and Gynecol* 1982; 142:670.

McAnarney ER, Stevens-Simon C. Maternal psychological stress/depression and low birth weight. *Amer J Dis Child* 1990; 144:789.

Paul VK, Radhika S, Deorari AK, Singh M. Neurodevelopmental outcome of at-risk nursery graduates. *Indian J Pediatr* 1998; 65:857–862.

Paul VK, Singh M, Buckshee K. Erythromycin treatment of pregnant women to reduce incidence of low birth weight and preterm deliveries. *Internat J Gynec Obstet* 1998; 62:87–88.

Paul VK. Singh M, Gupta U, *et al*. Chlamydia trachomatis infection among pregnant women. Prevalence and prenatal importance. *Nat Med J India* 1999; 12:11–14.

Pollack RN, Yaffe H, Divon MY. Therapy for intrauterine growth restriction: Current options and future directions. *Clinical Obstet Gynecol* 1997; 40:824–842.

Saigal S, Rosenbaum P, Stoskopf B and Milner R. Follow-up of infants 501–1500 g birth weight delivered to residents of a geographically defined region with perinatal intensive care facilities. *J Pediatr* 1982; 100:606.

Silverman WA and Sinclair JC. Infants of low birth weight. *N Engl J Med* 1966; 274:448.

Singh M, Giri SK and Ramachandran K. Intrauterine growth curves of live-born babies. *Indian Pediatr* 1974; 11:475.

Singhi S and Singh M. 'Birth weight to birth weight' postnatal weight pattern of preterm infants. *Indian J Pediatr* 1979; 46:223.

Suri M. Approach to the diagnosis of overgrowth syndromes. *Indian J Pediatr* 2016, 83(10):1175–87.

Tipton RE, Wilroy RS and Summitt RK. Accelerated skeletal maturation in infancy syndrome. *J Pediatr* 1973; 83:829.

Walker JJ, Smith G, Dekkar GA. Prevention and treatment of IUGR. In: Intrauterine Growth Retardation. Kingdom J, Baker P (Eds.) *Springer NY* 2000.

Disorders of Weight and Gestation

17

Jaundice

INTRODUCTION

Jaundice is the commonest abnormal physical finding during the first week of life. Over two-thirds of newborn babies develop clinical jaundice and by adult standards almost all newborn babies are 'jaundiced' during early days of life. Yellow discoloration is first manifest on the skin of face, nasolabial folds and tip of the nose. It is masked by physiological plethora of the newborn and is best seen by blanching the skin so that underlying yellowness of subcutaneous tissues and blood vessels can be visualized. The yellow staining of sclera is difficult to evaluate because of physiological photophobia. Eyes and sclera are best examined by holding the infant against diffuse light and without trying to forcibly open the eyelids. The jaundice must be looked for in good daylight and there should be no yellow clothes or curtains in the background which can lead to an error of over estimation. As the intensity of jaundice increases, there is cephalopedal progression of yellow discoloration of skin from face to trunk, palms and soles. The clinical jaundice manifests as yellowness on the face at a serum bilirubin level of 5 mg/dL (1 mg/dL = 17 μmoles/L). The yellow staining of trunk indicates serum bilirubin of 10–15 mg/dL but when soles or palms are distinctly yellow stained, the serum bilirubin is expected to be more than 15 mg/dL. The cephalopedal progression of jaundice is apparently related to the relative thickness of skin at various parts, skin being thinnest on the face and extremely thick over the palms and soles. The skin of premature babies is relatively thinner and, therefore, jaundice shows through more readily even at lower serum bilirubin levels. Cephalopedal color difference may also be related to differences in blood flow or lipid content of skin and because of conformational changes in the newly formed bilirubin-albumin complexes. The cephalocaudal color difference decreases with increasing gestational maturity and postnatal age. There is no difficulty in clinically recognizing jaundice among Indian babies because increased skin pigmentation generally appears after two weeks of age. It is essential that all newborn babies must be clinically screened twice a day in good daylight to detect the onset and severity of jaundice.

BILIRUBIN TURNOVER

Several physiological handicaps lead to increased frequency and severity of jaundice among newborn babies. Bilirubin is produced in the reticuloendothelial system by biotransformation of heme released from hemolyzing red blood cells. The heme ring is oxidized in reticuloendothelial cells to biliverdin by the microsomal enzyme heme oxygenase. During this reaction, carbon monoxide (CO) and iron (which is reutilized) are released. Biliverdin is then reduced to bilirubin by the enzyme biliverdin reductase. Catabolism of one mole of hemoglobin produces one mole each of carbon monoxide and bilirubin. The expired CO concentration is a good marker of bilirubin production.

Physiological polycythemia and shorter lifespan of fetal red blood cells (90 days vs 120 days in adults) result in release of 0.15 g/kg of hemoglobin everyday because 1.0 mL/kg (approximately 1%) of blood hemolyze everyday. One gram of hemoglobin yields about 35 mg of bilirubin, so that in a 3 kg infant about 15 mg of bilirubin is produced daily from hemoglobin sources. Additional 1 mg/kg bilirubin is produced from non-hemoglobin sources, viz. myoglobin, cytochromes and catalases thus resulting in net daily load of about 20 mg of bilirubin to the liver in a healthy term infant (Figure 18.1). Hepatic uptake, conjugation

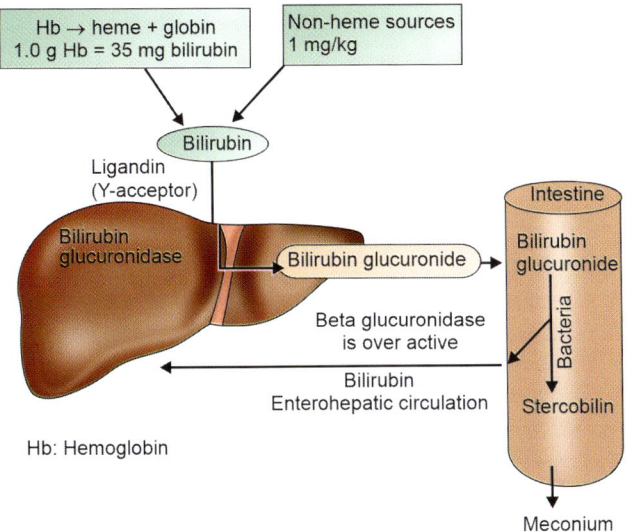

Figure 18.1 Schematic presentation of bilirubin turnover in the newborn.

and excretion of bilirubin is limited due to transient deficiency of Y and Z-acceptor proteins and UDP glucuronyl transferase enzyme in newborn babies especially those born prematurely. Because of relative lack of hepatic conjugatory enzyme, hyperbilirubinemia is mostly limited to unconjugated fraction of bilirubin during early days of life. On an average, 100–200 mg of bilirubin is present in the gut in a concentration of 1.0 mg of bilirubin per gram of meconium. Due to paucity of bacterial flora in the gut of a newborn baby and overactivity of intestinal beta-glucuronidase enzyme, the conjugated bilirubin entering the duodenum is rapidly deconjugated and recirculated in the blood and delivered to the liver for reconjugation through enterohepatic circulation. Thus increased production of bilirubin, reduced hepatic clearance and enhanced enterohepatic circulation contribute to increased prevalence of jaundice among newborn babies. The rate of bilirubin production (6–8 mg/kg/day) is at least twice in magnitude in the normal newborn population compared to older children. These biophysiological handicaps are worse among prematurely born infants thus resulting in greater incidence and severity of jaundice among them.

ASSESSMENT OF SEVERITY OF JAUNDICE

The severity of jaundice is assessed in natural daylight by observing cephalocaudal progression of jaundice *vide supra*. By experience and with concerted efforts, the observational skills can be sharpened and the accuracy of clinical assessment of severity of jaundice can be enhanced to within ±2 mg/dL of serum bilirubin. After phototherapy, the skin gets bleached and clinical assessment of severity of jaundice becomes unreliable. Icterometer can be used for assessment of jaundice by inexperienced health workers by matching the skin color with the color codes depicted on the plastic strips. Transcutaneous bilimeter works on the principle of computerized spectrophotometry to provide digital display of total bilirubin. The photoprobe is pressed against the forehead or sternum to take the bilirubin reading (Figure 18.2). During first week of life, total serum bilirubin (TSB) is by and large equivalent to unconjugated bilirubin for practical purposes. Bilimeter which takes a microcentrifuged sample of blood in a capillary tube provides an instant digital read-out of total bilirubin. Bilimeter, a bedside spectrophotometer, is one of the most useful and desirable equipment to have in the NICU for proper monitoring and management of neonatal jaundice (Figure 18.3). It takes into account the effect of hemoglobin and other solutes in the serum while giving the test result. Bilirubin estimations are conducted by the conventional van den Bergh test (Diazo method) in most neonatal units. Its limitations include the need for a large blood sample size, lack of accuracy, reliability and reproducibility of test result. Interlaboratory variations in the levels of serum bilirubin estimated by van den Bergh reaction range between 10 and 20% for total bilirubin and up to 24% for conjugated bilirubin. High performance liquid chromatography (HPLC) is a reliable method to assess total serum bilirubin (TSB) level. The catabolism of heme for bilirubin production is associated with production of carbon monoxide.

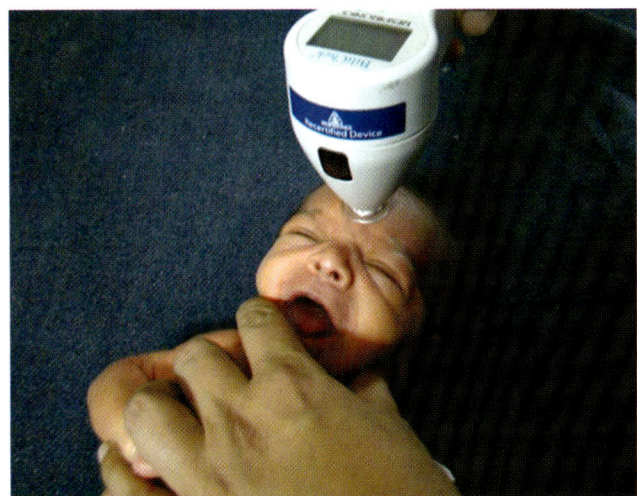

Figure 18.2 Transcutaneous bilirubinometer being used to assess the severity of jaundice. The device takes into account the skin color of the infant while giving the read-out for TSB.

Jaundice

18

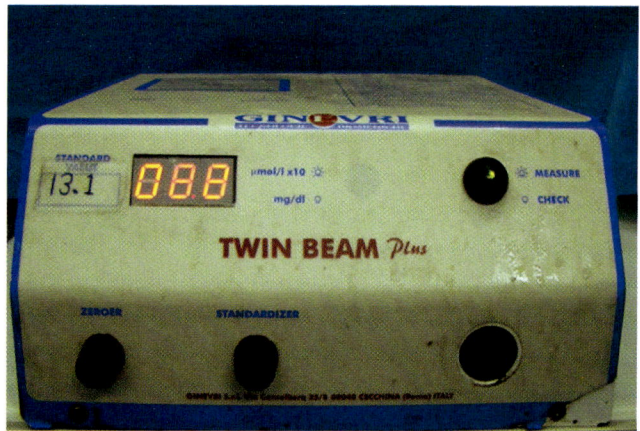

Figure 18.3 Bilimeter with a microcentrifuge. It is an essential equipment for rational management of hyperbilirubinemia.

Measurment of carboxyhemoglobin, pulmonary excretion rate of carbon monoxide or end-tidal carbon monoxide (EtCO) breath level are reliable correlates of total bilirubin production. They are harnessed as useful research tools to observe the effects of various therapeutic interventions on bilirubin production.

CAUSES OF JAUNDICE

The age at onset of jaundice gives an important clue to the possible etiology (Table 18.1). The appearance of jaundice on the first day of life is always suggestive of a serious disease process and such a baby should preferably be transferred to a center where adequate facilities for neonatal care are available. The common causes of jaundice in order of their frequency include physiological jaundice, immaturity, blood group incompatibility between the mother and fetus, infections both intrauterine and postnatal, G6PD deficiency, subcutaneous bruising and cephalhematoma, drugs and breast milk jaundice. Even after detailed investigations, the cause of neonatal hyperbilirubinemia remains uncertain in about one-third of cases. This is due to the fact that currently there are no available laboratory methods to assess the adequacy of hepatic clearance of bilirubin and extent of enterohepatic circulation. Many a times neonatal hyperbilirubinemia is multifactorial in origin.

PHYSIOLOGICAL JAUNDICE

Jaundice due to physiological immaturity of newborn babies is seen in nearly 60% of term and 80% of preterm babies. Nature has supreme biological wisdom and it appears that physiological jaundice provides useful protection to the baby against oxygen free radical triggered neonatal disorders because bilirubin

TABLE 18.1 Causes of jaundice on the basis of age of onset

- **Within 24 hours of birth**
  - Hemolytic disease of the newborn due to feto-maternal blood group incompatibility in the Rhesus, ABO and minor blood group systems.
  - Intrauterine infections,* such as toxoplasmosis, cytomegalic inclusion disease, syphilis, rubella, Au antigen-hepatitis, herpes simplex and bacterial infections.
  - Deficiency of red cell enzymes, such as glucose-6-phosphate dehydrogenase, pyruvate kinase, hexokinase, phosphoglucose isomerase and unstable hemoglobins.
  - Administration of large amounts of certain drugs, such as vitamin K, salicylates, sulfisoxazole, etc. to the mother.
  - Hereditary spherocytosis
  - Crigler-Najjar syndrome
  - Lucey-Driscoll syndrome
  - Homozygous alpha-thalassemia

- **Between 24 and 72 hours of age**
  - Physiological jaundice appears during this period but may be aggravated and prolonged by immaturity, birth asphyxia, acidosis, hypothermia, hypoglycemia, drugs, cephalhematoma or concealed hemorrhage and bruising, polycythemia, high altitude, cretinism, breastfeeding, infections and mild hemolytic states due to fetomaternal blood group incompatibility, spherocytosis and deficiency of red cell enzymes

- **After 72 hours of age (and within first 2 weeks)**
  - Septicemia
  - Neonatal hepatitis including other causes of intrauterine infections
  - Extrahepatic biliary atresia
  - Breast milk jaundice
  - Metabolic diseases, such as hypothyroidism, galactosemia, tyrosinemia, hereditary fructosemia, organic acidemias, Gilbert syndrome, cystic fibrosis and intestinal obstruction.

*Intrauterine infections should be considered in the differential diagnosis of jaundice having onset any time during the neonatal period.

is a potent antioxidant. In term babies, the physiological jaundice appears between 36 and 72 hours of age. Maximum intensity of jaundice is seen on the 4th day, serum bilirubin does not exceed 15 mg/dL and jaundice disappears by 10 days of life (Figure 18.4). There are no characteristic clinical features of physiological jaundice and its diagnosis cannot be made by examining the baby at one point of time. Instead, diagnosis is made retrospectively by taking

 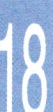

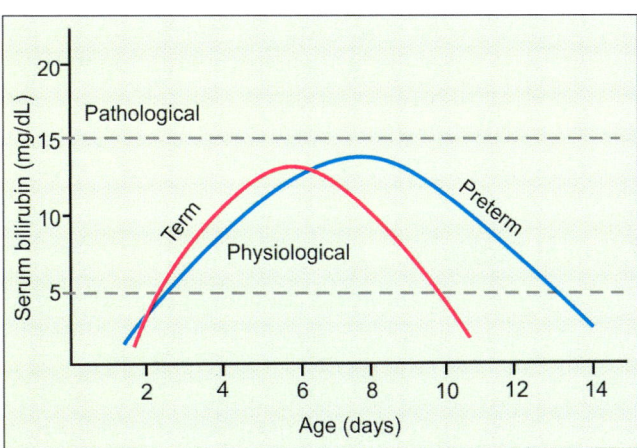

Figure 18.4 Time table of physiologic jaundice.

into consideration the onset of jaundice, maximal limits of intensity and age of disappearance besides the exclusion of pathologic causes. Among preterm babies, the age of onset of physiologic jaundice is similar to the term babies. It may manifest earlier but never before 24 hours of age. The maximum intensity of jaundice is reached on the 5th or 6th day, serum bilirubin may go up to 15 mg/dL and it may persist up to 14 days (Figure 18.4). The designation of "physiological" jaundice in the preterm may appear as a misnomer because jaundice due to physiologic handicaps of immaturity often requires phototherapy and may even cause brain damage.

The etiology of physiologic jaundice appears to be multifactorial. There is over production of bilirubin due to polycythemia and reduced lifespan of fetal red blood cells. There is increased production of bilirubin from non-hemoglobin sources in the newborn. There is reduced uptake of bilirubin by the liver because of deficiency of ligandin or Y-acceptor protein in the hepatocytes. There is deficiency of UDP glucose dehydrogenase during first few days of life and, therefore, substrate UDP glucuronic acid is not available for glucuronidation. There is thus poor hepatic uptake, conjugation and excretion of bilirubin. These hepatic functions may be further depressed by maternal factors transmitted through the placenta or breast milk and certain perinatal distress factors that are common in the neonatal period, viz. hypoxia, hypothermia, acidosis, and hypoglycemia.

The conjugated bilirubin entering the gut through bile cannot be converted to stercobilin because of relative lack of bacteria in the gut during the first week of life. Due to over activity of beta-glucuronidase enzyme in the sterile gut of the newborn, bilirubin is deconjugated in the gut and recirculated to the liver through enterohepatic circulation. After feeding, when gut is colonized, bacteria destroy beta-glucuronidase enzyme thus blocking enterohepatic circulation. Exclusively breastfed babies are likely to have higher bilirubin levels due to inadequacy of lactation during first three days of life. The upper limit of serum bilirubin among exclusively breastfed babies is considered as 18 mg/dL. These physiologic handicaps are worse among prematurely born infants, resulting in higher incidence and greater severity of jaundice among preterm babies. The physiological jaundice does not need any therapy but the baby must be watched closely for the severity of jaundice and mother should be instructed to give adequate feeds to the baby. She should be reassured about the benign nature of the physiologic jaundice and her fears regarding infection or hepatitis should be allayed. When jaundice becomes severe or persists beyond 2 weeks, the conditions enumerated in Table 18.1 should be reviewed and infant investigated accordingly.

PATHOLOGICAL JAUNDICE

When jaundice in the newborn does not conform to the time table described for physiological jaundice *vide supra*, it is designated as pathological and demands investigative work up. In our experience, about 5% of newborn babies develop pathological jaundice or hyperbilirubinemia. Occurrence of jaundice within 24 hours of age is always pathological. Whenever trunk is distinctly yellow-stained or palms and soles are tinged yellow, it calls for biochemical estimation of bilirubin levels and additional investigations should be undertaken to identify the cause of hyperbilirubinemia (Table 18.2). The persistence of clinical jaundice beyond 14 days due to elevation of unconjugated bilirubin should alert the pediatrician to the possibilities listed in Table 18.3.

TABLE 18.2 Criteria for the diagnosis of pathological jaundice

- Onset of jaundice withing 24 hours or after 72 hours of age.
- Distinct yellow staining of palms and soles with total serum bilirubin >15 mg/dL.
- Persistence of jaundice beyond 2 weeks of age.
- Jaundice with hepatosplenomegaly and/or edema.
- Elevation of direct reacting bilirubin by >2.0 mg/dL (yellow-colored urine and/or clay colored stools).
- Jaundice in association with clinical evidences of bilirubin-induced neurologic dysfunction (BIND).

Jaundice

18

TABLE 18.3 Causes of prolonged unconjugated hyperbilirubinemia in the newborn

1. Immaturity
2. Hemolytic disease of the newborn due to fetomaternal blood group incompatibility
3. Breast milk jaundice
4. Hypothyroidism
5. Pyloric stenosis and conditions associated with functional and organic intestinal stasis
6. Crigler-Najjar syndrome
7. Gilbert syndrome
8. Concealed hemorrhage
9. Malaria
10. Urinary tract infection

HEMOLYTIC DISEASE OF THE NEWBORN (HDN)

Hemolytic disease of the newborn due to blood group incompatibility between the mother and fetus is the commonest cause of hyperbilirubinemia in the newborn. The incompatibility may occur between Rhesus, ABO or minor blood group systems (C, E, M and Kell). Any RBC antigen which is inherited by the fetus from father and is not present in the mother, can cause hemolysis in the fetus due to maternal sensitization.

Rhesus Hemolytic Disease of the Newborn (Rh-HDN)

Erythroblastosis due to Rhesus incompatibility between the mother and fetus, though entirely preventable, is still an important cause of hyperbilirubinemia requiring exchange blood transfusion in low and middle income countries (LMICs). The prevalence of Rh negative blood group (dd) is 5% in Indian population compared to 15% in Europeans. There are no inborn antibodies in the Rhesus blood group system. During pregnancy, especially after the first 3 months, when placental circulation is well established, fetal red blood cells may seep into maternal circulation. When an Rh-negative mother is carrying an Rh-positive fetus, the antigen of the fetal red blood cells may invoke antibody response by the maternal immunologic system. Enough antibodies are not produced during the first pregnancy but each subsequent pregnancy with an Rh-positive fetus leads to increasing antibody response. The anti-D antibodies being IgG in type, crossover to the fetus and destroy D-positive fetal red blood cells. If there is concomitant fetomaternal ABO incompatibility, some protection is achieved against Rh-HDN because fetal Rh-positive cells get destroyed by maternal antibodies of ABO system before they get a chance to stimulate anti-D antibody production.

Rh-HDN can be suspected prenatally by knowing the blood group of the mother and estimating the titer of anti-D antibodies by indirect Coomb's test. The severity of the *in utero* disease can be assessed by amniotic fluid bilirubin and optical density measurements.

Clinical Features

Many Rh-negative mothers do not get isoimmunized for several reasons. The husband may also be Rh-negative or heterozygous positive which offers a 25% chance of having an Rh-negative baby. The coexistent fetomaternal ABO incompatibility and inability on the part of the mother to respond by producing antibodies (non-reactors) also offer protection against Rh-HDN. The clinical picture is characterized by increasing severity of the disease with each subsequent pregnancy. There is a wide spectrum of clinical manifestations ranging from normal to stillborn baby with hydrops fetalis. The baby may be anemic and has hepatosplenomegaly. Jaundice appears within 24 hours of age and rapidly increases in intensity. Despite deep jaundice, the urine remains colorless and does not stain the diaper because unconjugated bilirubin is lipid-soluble (not water-soluble) and is not filtered in the urine. In severely affected babies, the clinical picture is characterized by severe anemia, gross hepatosplenomegaly and generalized anasarca (hydrops fetalis) and the baby may die *in utero*. The severely affected infants suffer from birth asphyxia, acidosis and hypothermia which predispose to development of disseminated intravascular coagulation. It has recently been shown that infants with severe Rh-HDN are also likely to have leukopenia and thrombocytopenia due to marked erythropoiesis. Hypoglycemia may occur during the first 24 hours because of hyperplasia of islet cells. There are some evidence to suggest that breakdown products of hemolyzed red blood cells (glutathion) inactivate circulating insulin and cause hyperplasia of islet-cells in infants with erythroblastosis fetalis as a compensatory response to maintain adequate levels of insulin.

Diagnosis

The cord blood should be collected in all babies of Rh negative mothers for Rh and ABO typing, direct Coomb's test, hemoglobin, reticulocyte count, red blood cells morphology and serum bilirubin. Positive direct Coomb's test in an Rh-positive baby clinches the diagnosis of Rh-HDN. False negative Coomb's test may be obtained, if blood sample is contaminated with Wharton's jelly or due to laboratory error. In the affected baby, serum bilirubin should be monitored every 6 to 12 hours depending upon the rate of rise of bilirubin. There is no need to keep the cord moist but it should be maintained sterile by dusting it with antiseptic powder to avoid the risk of infection during the procedure of umbilical catheterization.

Management

For prevention of Rh-HDN refer to Chapter 3. For exchange blood transfusion and other measures for reducing serum bilirubin refer to Chapter 29.

Intrauterine Transfusion

In severe Rh-isoimmunization with past history of stillbirth and hydrops fetalis, it is mandatory to determine the level of anti-D antibodies and optical density of amniotic fluid from 24 weeks of gestation onwards every fortnightly in order to assess the severity of Rh-HDN. The optical density difference (ODD) at 450 nm between the baseline of amniotic fluid and the peak which occurs in the affected infant should be determined. In general, ODD of greater than 0.1 or a rising ODD suggests a severely affected baby (Figure 18.5). The severely affected baby may die *in utero* due to severe anemia. Hemoglobin or hematocrit of the fetus can be checked by taking a percutaneous umbilical blood sample (PUBS). Elevated peak systolic velocity of middle cerebral artery of the fetus on Doppler is a useful non-invasive correlate of fetal hematocrit and has been effectively used for timing intrauterine fetal transfusions. When fetal hematocrit falls below 30%, 50 mL of O Rh-negative packed red blood cells are infused trans-uterine into the fetus by cordocentesis. The blood is obtained from a CMV-negative donor and irradiated to kill lymphocytes to avoid graft vs host disease. The procedure may be repeated every 3 to 4 weeks till the baby is mature enough for extrauterine survival. The same sample of amniotic fluid can also be analyzed for determination of lecithin/sphingo-myelin ratio to assess the maturity of fetal lungs so that decision regarding induction of labor or continuation of intrauterine transfusions can be made rationally. It is important to remember that babies who have had received a number of intrauterine transfusions with O Rh-negative blood would be born with Rh-negative blood type and their direct Coomb's test would also be negative. They, however, should be immediately exchanged at birth with ORh-negative packed red blood cells to remove the circulating anti-D antibodies and to correct the anemia.

Intravenous Immunoglobulins (IVIG)

In both Rh and ABO hemolytic disease of the newborn, the hemolysis of neonatal red blood cells coated with transplacentally acquired antibodies is mediated by Fc (fragment crystallizable) receptor bearing cells within the reticuloendothelial system. Recent studies have recommended that high dose of IVIG is effective in modifying the hyperbilirubinemia in most cases of Coomb's positive hemolytic anemia. It has been proposed that immunoglobulins block Fc receptors thereby inhibiting hemolysis and reducing formation of bilirubin. It is also believed that IVIG may accelerate the catabolism of endogenous IgG antibodies, thus reducing the levels of circulating pathogenic or immune autoantibodies. In seriously affected Rh-isoimmunized babies, IVIG is given in a dose of 0.5–1.0 g/kg as a slow infusion over 2 hours. When exchange blood transfusion (EBT) is required at birth, IVIG should be given after the EBT. When a subsequent EBT is required due to rising serum bilirubin level, repeat IVIG may be given after the second exchange blood transfusion. IVIG therapy has been shown to reduce the number of EBTs and duration of phototherapy. The therapy has documented benefits and is free from side effects. In view of the relatively milder nature of ABO hemolytic disease of the newborn, IVIG should be used selectively because of its high cost.

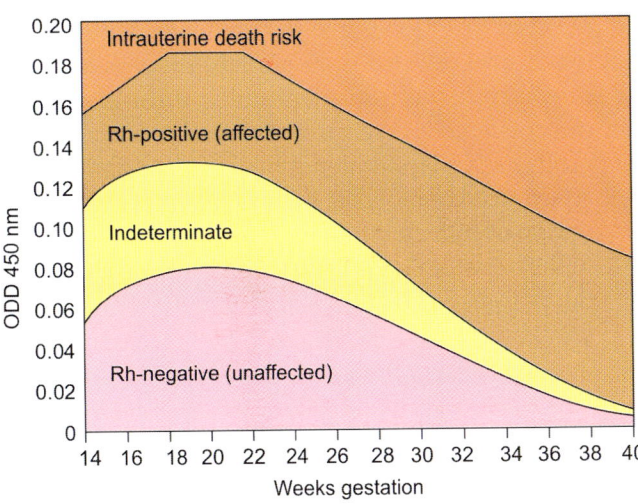

Figure 18.5 Modified Liley's chart for antenatal prediction of severity of fetal disease in rhesus isoimmunization. The optical density difference (ODD) of amniotic fluid is plotted against the gestational age (*Adapted from* Davies PA; Robinson RJ; Scopes JW; Tizard JPM; and Wigglesworth JS. (Eds); Medical Care of Newborn Babies, 1971, *Spastics International Medical Publications, London*).

Jaundice

18

ABO Hemolytic Disease of the Newborn (ABO-HDN)

In view of relatively low incidence of Rh-negative blood group in India, ABO-HDN assumes relatively greater importance. The disease is milder and its severity cannot be predicted antenatally but may be suspected, if there is a past history of ABO-HDN in a previous sibling or if the titer of IgG anti-A or anti-B hemolysins in the mother is more than 1:64. The commonest materno-fetal combinations are O group mother and A or B group fetus. The severity of hemolysis is more in OA incompatibility compared to OB incompatibility. Fetomaternal ABO incompatibility exists in about 25% of pregnancies but hemolytic disease develops in only one in ten such offsprings. Most anti-A and anti-B isohemagglutinins are IgM type and hence not transferred through the placenta. The predilection of having immune IgG antibodies against A or B antigen may run in families. The antibodies may also be produced as an immune response to A and B antigens contained in food, bacteria and vaccines. Low antigenicity of AB factors and their wide distribution in placenta and other body tissues apart from red blood cells, account for the relatively low incidence and milder nature of ABO-HDN. Unlike Rh-HDN, the history of increasing severity of disease in subsequent pregnancies is generally not present in ABO-HDN. Interestingly, the subsequent babies may be more affected or less affected or even spared. The disease is relatively more common in female babies. The ABO antigen sites in the red blood cells of preterm babies are less, explaining the occurrence of relatively milder disease.

The diagnosis is suspected by early onset of jaundice in an A or B group baby of O group mother and mild splenomegaly. Anemia is usually absent. At birth, the disease can be suspected by examining cord blood for elevation of serum bilirubin, presence of maternal IgG anti-A or anti-B antibodies in an antibody-dependent cell-mediated cytotoxicity (ADCC) assay and detection of antigen density of A or B antigens on the red blood cells. Reticulocytosis, spherocytosis and increased fragility of RBCs may be present. Direct Coomb's test is generally negative or weakly positive. The antibodies can be eluted from baby's blood by washing the RBCs twice in saline followed by heating to 56°C to dissociate the antibodies from the antigenic sites. The eluted serum is tested against adult RBCs of known blood group to demonstrate agglutination to confirm the presence of antibodies. High titers of anti-A and anti-B IgG hemolysins can be demonstrated in the maternal serum. The jaundice may reach critical levels to require phototherapy and exchange blood transfusion. Administration of substances rich in AB antigens to mop up circulating antibodies needs to be evaluated.

Nonimmune Hemolytic Anemia

The uncommon causes of hemolytic anemia in the newborn include enyzme defects (G6PD deficiency, pyruvate kinase deficiency), red cell membrane disorders (hereditary spherocytosis and elliptocytosis) and hemoglobinopathies (alpha thalassemia). They are characterized by anemia, hyperbilirubinemia, reticulocytosis and a negative direct antiglobulin test (DAT) or Coomb's test. The diagnosis is confirmed by specific morphology of RBCs on peripheral smear, screening for enzymopathy and hemoglobin electrophoresis.

1. **Glucose-6-phosphate dehydrogenase deficiency**
The deficiency of G6PD in the red blood cells is common amongst people from Mediterranean, Asian and African stock. It is the most common genetic disorder in India. Its incidence in India varies from 5 to 20% among different ethnic groups. In general, G6PD deficiency gene is more frequent in tribes than in non-tribes and relatively high incidence of 16% is found among Parsi, Lambani, south Indian tribal population and north Indian population. The deficiency is inherited as X-linked recessive. Hemolysis may occur spontaneously or following exposure to certain oxidant drugs and infections. The infant may receive the offending drug transplacentally, through breastmilk or directly. Wearing of clothes protected with moth balls (naphthalene) may initiate hemolysis. Apart from hemolysis, there is reduced glucuronidation of bilirubin due to defective G6PD activity in the hepatocytes. Methemoglobin reduction and flourescence are useful screening tests while G6PD tetrazolium cytochemical method is diagnostic to quantify the defect. Sudden, dramatic and unexplained elevation of serum bilirubin in a newborn baby is a characteristic manifestation of G6PD deficiency. Jaundice may occur any time during the neonatal period or subsequently and may be severe enough to require exchange blood transfusion. It is important to remember that following an episode of acute hemolysis, G6PD screening may be unreliable because newly formed RBCs may not be deficient in the enzyme. The screening test should be repeated at 3 months of age.

2. **Hereditary spherocytosis** It is characterized by anemia, hyperbilirubinemia and mild spleno-megaly any time during neonatal period. Laboratory data shows spherocytosis and increased fragility of erythrocytes. Other causes of microspherocytosis and splenomegaly in the newborn, such as ABO incompatibility and infections should be ruled out. *In vitro* abnormal autohemolysis of red blood cells can be corrected by addition of glucose. The abnormality is transmitted as autosomal dominant trait and can be demonstrated in 80% of parents. Splenectomy is curative but should be delayed as long as possible due to increased risk of recurrent pneumococcal infections during infancy. Other uncommon red cell membrane disorders include hereditary elliptocytosis and pyropoikilocytosis.

3. **Homozygous alpha thalassemia** This condition, by and large, is limited to Orientals wherein alpha chain production is deficient while excess gamma chains combine to form Bart's hemoglobin. It is an important cause of non-immunologic hydrops fetalis in South East Asia. The infant is born with severe anemia, gross hepatosplenomegaly and anasarca without any evidences of Rh isoimmuni-zation. The diagnosis is suspected by negative direct Coomb's test and confirmed by identification of Bart and Portland hemoglobin on electrophore-sis. The outcome is generally fatal. The condition is rare in India.

Drugs and Neonatal Jaundice

A large number of drugs may aggravate neonatal jaundice or predispose to occurrence of bilirubin brain damage at lower serum bilirubin levels. The drugs may aggravate neonatal jaundice by causing hemolysis (vitamin K in large doses and drugs causing hemolysis in G6PD deficient infants), blocking Y-acceptor protein (vitamin K and kanamycin) and competing with glucuronyl transferase for hepatic conjugation (novobiocin, moxalactam, gentamicin, kanamycin and chloramphenicol). Drugs may pre-dispose the baby to develop bilirubin brain damage at lower serum bilirubin levels by blocking bilirubin binding sites in the albumin (salicylates, long-acting sulfonamides including sulfasoxazole, sodium benzoate, caffein, lobeline, furosemide, indomethacin, fusidic acid, cedalinid?, kanamycin? and radiographic contrast media). There is sufficient evidence to suggest that infants delivered following oxytocin induction or augmentation of labor develop jaundice earlier and tend to attain higher bilirubin levels. Oxytocin induces hyponatremia and hypo-osmolality in the mother by virtue of its antidiuretic and saluretic effects. These biochemical changes are aggravated by the infusion of electrolyte-free dextrose solution used as a vehicle for administration of oxytocin. Transplacentally trans-mitted hypo-osmolality in the fetal blood leads to enhanced osmotic fragility of red blood cells. The swollen and hyperfragile erythrocytes are easily trapped by the spleen resulting in net higher bilirubin production. Infants born following spinal block with bupivacaine have also increased risk of jaundice. Caution must be exercised while prescribing these medications to pregnant women or jaundiced neonates.

Infections

Intrauterine infections of TORCH complex and Au antigen may cause giant cell hepatitis and jaundice any time during neonatal period. Intrauterine growth retardation, hepatosplenomegaly, petechiae and meningoencephalitis with micro- or hydrocephaly may dominate the clinical picture. Jaundice is an important manifestation of bacterial septicemia and urinary tract infection and should be seriously consi-dered when it first appears after the age of three days and is persistent beyond two weeks of life. The clinical picture is dominated by other systemic features of septicemia. The direct reacting or conjugated bilirubin is more than 15% of the total bilirubin and usually exceeds 2 mg/dL in infants with sepsis or hepatitis. Urine is high colored because direct reacting bilirubin is water-soluble and excreted in the urine. Jaundice is a recognized feature of congenital and neonatal malaria.

Occult or Overt Internal Bleeding

Cephalhematoma, bruising, swallowed maternal blood or internal hemorrhages, such as gastrointestinal bleeding, subcapsular hematoma in the liver and intraventricular hemorrhage or other intracranial bleeds, may cause aggravation of pre-existent jaundice. It must be remembered that about one gram of extravasated hemoglobin contributes to the produc-tion of 35 mg of bilirubin. Whenever serum bilirubin is approaching critical levels, if feasible, the hematoma should be aspirated.

Breast Milk Jaundice

The condition may manifest as persistence of physiological jaundice or it may appear for the first time at the end of first week. It is maximum in intensity between 10 and 14 days but hyperbilirubinemia is never severe enough to need exchange blood transfusion. Multiple factors operate to aggravate jaundice in breastfed babies. Due to inadequate lactation during first few days, there is delay in effective feeding with relative dehydration and hemoconcentration in exclusively breastfed babies. Breastfed babies have greater incidence and severity of physiological jaundice and serum bilirubin may approach 18 mg/dL. There is excessive weight loss of the baby because of inadequate feeding. Colonization of gut is delayed in breastfed infants resulting in greater deconjugation of bilirubin and enhanced enterohepatic circulation. Hepatic conjugation of bilirubin is compromised due to presence of 3-alpha, 20 beta pregnanediol in about 1 to 2% women. High concentrations of unsaturated fatty acids in the human milk due to over activity of lipase may also inhibit hepatic glucuronyl transferase enzyme and Y-acceptor protein. The inhibitory substance in the breast milk is excreted for a period of 2 to 8 weeks and breastfeeding should be continued unless critical levels of bilirubin are achieved.

Almost one-third of breastfed babies are detected to have mild jaundice during 3rd week of life. Babies with breast milk jaundice pass colorless urine and golden yellow stools. Cessation of breastfeeding for about 48 to 72 hours results in prompt fall (2–6 mg/dL) in serum bilirubin and breastfeeding can be re-established without any risk of recurrence of jaundice. However, in view of transient and benign nature of breast milk jaundice, there is no justification to stop breastfeeding. Stoppage of breastfeeding may give a wrong message to the mother causing anxiety and suppression of lactation. Breast milk jaundice should not be considered as a disadvantage of breastfeeding. Instead, it may actually be viewed as an advantage by virtue of additional antioxidant capabilities provided by elevated serum bilirubin levels. It has been shown that aggressive and frequent breastfeeding without any supplementation with plain water or glucose-water is associated with faster resolution of breast milk jaundice.

Cretinism

Prolongation of physiologic jaundice may be the sole manifestation of hypothyroidism in the newborn. The condition should be considered in the differential diagnosis of breast milk jaundice. Inactivity, hypotonia, hoarse cry, poor feeding, constipation and maternal or neonatal goiter should be looked for. All the conditions listed in Table 18.2 should be reviewed and skiagram of knees, T_3, T_4 and TSH levels assayed because early diagnosis of cretinism is mandatory for improved mental prognosis of these children.

Crigler-Najjar Syndrome

It is an autosomal recessive disorder characterized by non-hemolytic unconjugated hyperbilirubinemia due to congenital deficiency of glucuronyl transferase or uridine diphosphate glucuronosyltransferase (UGT1A1 gene). Type I defect is characterized by onset of jaundice at birth, marked severity of jaundice which may lead to kernicterus, secretion of colorless bile lacking in bilirubin glucuronide and lack of response to phenobarbitone. Type II is a milder variant with onset of jaundice between birth and 10 years of age and amelioration of jaundice following phenobarbitone (5 mg/kg/d) therapy. Type I is inherited as autosomal recessive while Type II is autosomal dominant.

Lucey-Driscoll Syndrome

Severe unconjugated hyperbilirubinemia may occur rarely during the first four days of life due to transplacental passage of a glucuronyl transferase inhibiting substance from the mother to the fetus. It is an autosomal recessive disorder due to defective UDP-glucuronosyltransferase 1-1 (UGT1A1 gene). The condition is transient but may sometimes require exchange transfusion to prevent kernicterus.

Gilbert's Syndrome

It is a rare hereditary harmless disorder due to mutation of UGT1A1 gene. It is characterized by episodes of mild jaundice which are triggered by physical stress, exposure to cold, starvation, dehydration and intake of niacin and rifampicin.

Birth Asphyxia, Acidosis, Hypothermia and Hypoglycemia

These metabolic disorders and perinatal distress factors are common among high-risk newborn babies. They may not *per se* aggravate jaundice but often predispose the baby to develop bilirubin encephalopathy at lower serum bilirubin levels (*vide infra*). Hypoxia and hypoglycemia may enhance bilirubin production by stimulating heme catabolism and inhibiting Y-acceptor protein and glucuronyl transferase enzyme. These disorders may damage the integrity of blood–brain barrier.

DANGERS OF HYPERBILIRUBINEMIA

Jaundice in the newborn is a medical emergency because unconjugated hyperbilirubinemia may cause acute bilirubin encephalopathy or bilirubin-induced neurological damage (BIND). The neonatal features of acute bilirubin encephalopathy include lethargy, hypotonia followed by hypertonia, refusal of feeds, shrill cry, "setting sun" sign, fever, convulsions, drowsiness or coma and backward arching of the neck (retrocollis) and trunk (opisthotonos). Moro's response is sluggish or abnormal where sudden extension of arms is not followed by flexion component but is often accompanied with downward rolling of eyeballs, lid lag and peculiar grin (Figure 18.6).

The clinical grading of acute bilirubin encephalopathy is shown in Table 18.4. The manifestations are nonspecific in preterm babies who may die due to apneic attacks and without any seizures. During infancy, the sequelae may manifest as athetoid cerebral palsy, choreoathetosis, brownish staining of teeth, dental–enamel dysplasia, deafness, paralysis of upward gaze and various grades of intellectual retardation and learning disabilities.

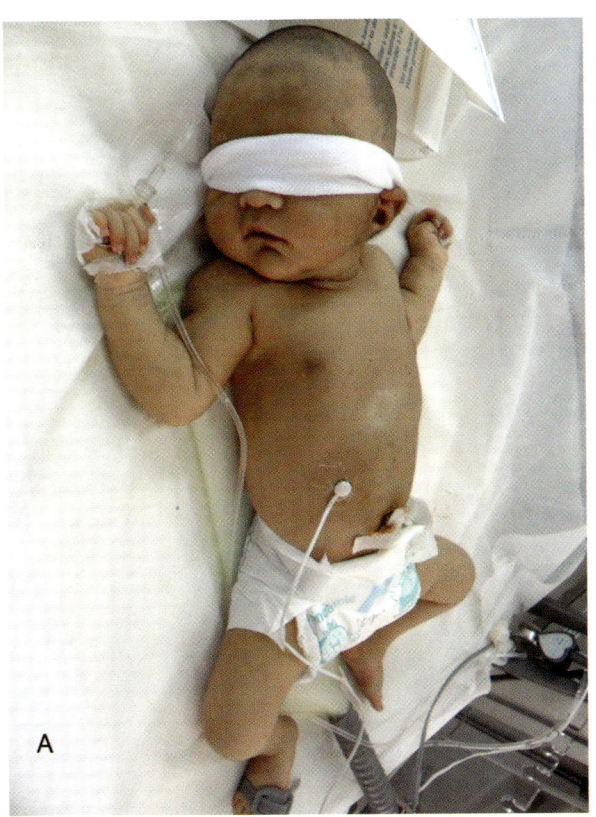 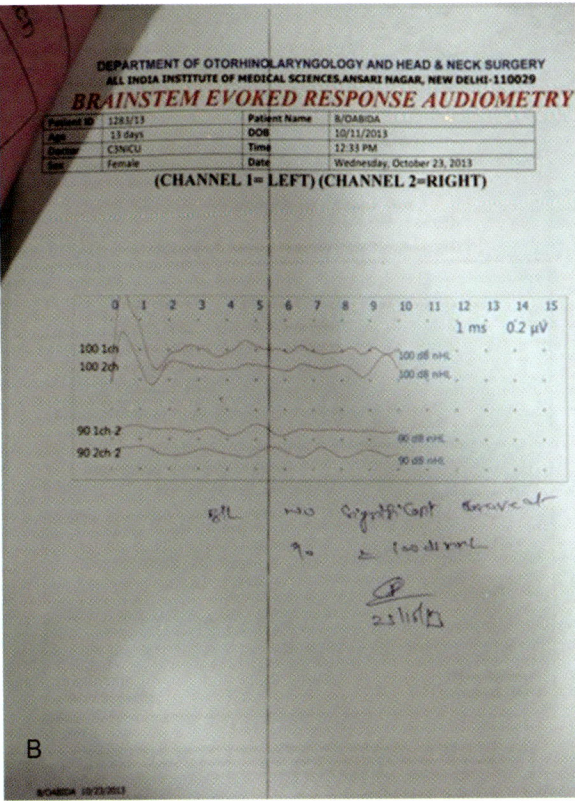

Figure 18.6 (A) Term infant with Rh-hemolytic disease of the newborn with total serum bilirubin level of 20 mg/dL at 48 hours. Infant developed evidences of acute bilirubin encephalopathy on day 4. (B) Portable BERA showed significant suppression of all the waves on both sides.

TABLE 18.4 Clinical scoring of bilirubin-induced neurologic dysfunction (BIND)

Features	Mild (score 1)	Moderate (score 2)	Severe (score 3)
▪ Mental status	Sleepy but arousable and poor feeding	Lethargic and/or irritable with refusal of feeds	Semicoma or coma, apnea, and/or seizures
▪ Muscle tone	Mild hypotonia	Hypo- or hypertonia with mild nuchal or truncal arching	Marked opisthotonos, scissoring or crossing of arms and/or legs
▪ Cry	High pitched	Shrill or shrieky	Inconsolable crying, weak or absent cry
▪ Oculomotor or eye movement	—	—	Sun-set sign with paralysis of upward gaze

Jaundice

18

Pathogenesis of Bilirubin-Induced Brain Damage

The exact pathogenesis of acute bilirubin encephalopathy (ABE) is controversial and complex but is related to the interplay between level of unconjugated bilirubin which is lipid-soluble, gestational maturity of infant and integrity of blood–brain barrier. The major complications of hyperbilirubinemia is bilirubin-induced neurologic dysfunction (BIND) which occurs when circulating bilirubin crosses the blood–brain barrier and binds to brain tissue. Acute bilirubin encephalopathy (ABE) is the acute but reversible form of BIND while kernicterus is the chronic and permanent neurologic sequelae of BIND. Point-of-care brainstem evoked audiometry (BERA) and findings of high T1 signal in globus pallidus and subthalamic nuclei on MRI are diagnostic features of BIND. Till recently, it was generally believed that unconjugated serum bilirubin level of 20 mg/dL or more due to any cause may lead to bilirubin-induced damge in the newborn. There is sufficient evidence to support that among preterm infants, kernicterus may occur at relatively lower serum bilirubin levels and at times serum bilirubin concentrations in excess of 30 mg/dL in term babies may not produce any neurological sequelae.

The bilirubin in plasma exists as albumin bound complex, which cannot premeate through the cell wall. One mole of albumin binds equimolar amount of bilirubin, i.e. one gram of albumin can bind 8.5 mg of bilirubin. When bilirubin binding capacity of albumin is exhausted, either due to deficiency of albumin or continued elevation of unconjugated bilirubin, free bilirubin readily diffuses into the interstitial compartment and binds to tissue proteins. When bilirubin binding capacity of tissue proteins is also exhausted, the free bilirubin seeps across the blood–brain barrier and gains access into the neurons located in the basal ganglia, hippocampus and auditory nuclei (Figure 18.7). Once bilirubin comes into contact with neurons, further damage depends upon availability of hydrogen ions. Bilirubin exists as dianion and combines with hydrogen ion to form bilirubin acid (BH_2) which causes neuronal damage. It is believed that BH_2 has surfactant like property and it positions itself between the lipid bilayer of the membranes to produce manifestations of bilirubin encephalopathy. This step is reversible by early therapeutic intervention thus explaining the reversibility of acute bilirubin encephalopathy by timely exchange blood transfusion.

The concentration of available free bilirubin increases whenever there is hyperbilirubinemia or

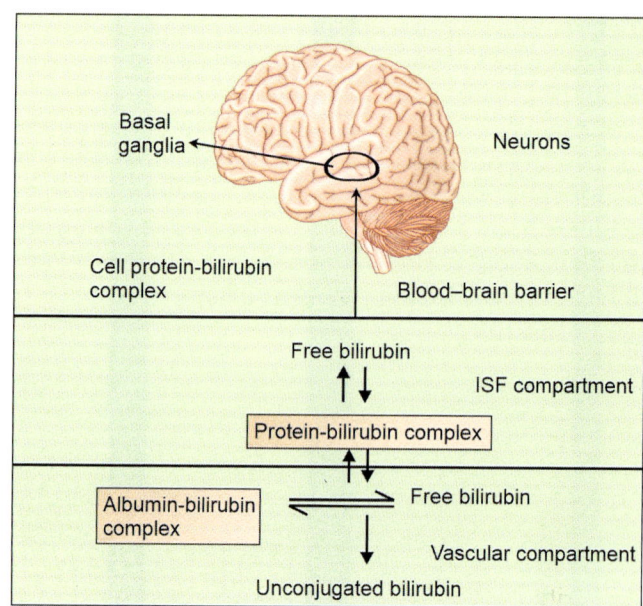

Figure 18.7 Simplified presentation of movements of bilirubin in various fluid compartments in the pathogenesis of kernicterus. ISF, interstitial fluid compartment.

hypoalbuminemia. It has been suggested that serum bilirubin to protein ratio of more than 3.5 may be associated with brain damage. However, it must be remembered that the level of serum albumin may not provide a true estimate of the available bilirubin binding capacity because binding sites in the albumin may also be blocked by H^+ ions and other organic anions, such as salicylates, sulfonamides, free fatty acids, hematin, furosemide, sodium benzoate, indomethacin and certain antibiotics. In the presence of these anions, the bilirubin binding capacity of serum and tissue proteins is compromised and brain damage may develop at lower serum bilirubin levels even in the presence of normal serum protein concentrations. This would explain the greater likelihood of occurrence of bilirubin encephalopathy in seriously ill, acidotic, hypoglycemic and hypoxic preterm babies at relatively lower serum bilirubin concentrations. The residual capacity of the serum albumin to bind dyes, such as BSP (bromosulphthalein) and HBABA (2–4′ hydroxybenzene azobenzoic acid), red cell binding of bilirubin, and salicylate displacement technique, has been employed to predict the occurrence of bilirubin brain damage.

Above hypothesis has been challenged by recent observations that the breakdown of blood–brain barrier may be more critical determinant of kernicterus rather than the level of free bilirubin. This hypothesis is supported by the fact that there is no single level of total or free bilirubin which is completely predictive of bilirubin-induced neurological damage (BIND) in sick premature infants. Among preterm infants dying with or without acute bilirubin encephalopathy, no significant differences have been found between the levels of total or free bilirubin in the two groups. Moreover, analbuminemic humans and mice are known who do not develop kernicterus. It has been shown experimentally that when blood–brain barrier is damaged unilaterally in the rats by infusion of hypertonic solution, subsequent parenteral injection of bilirubin albumin complex, leads to yellow staining or bilirubin encephalopathy on the side in which blood–brain barrier was 'opened' or damaged. These observations suggest that cerebral staining of bilirubin can occur due to entry of even albumin bound bilirubin. It would appear that not only the maturity of the infant or level of unconjugated bilirubin are critical but the integrity of blood–brain barrier is possibly of equal importance in the pathogenesis of bilirubin-induced brain damage. It is difficult to evaluate the integrity of blood–brain barrier but it is well known that it may be damaged or compromised by anoxia, ischemia, inflammation, hyperosmolality, hypercapnia, acidosis and trauma.

Bilirubin staining of brain, as a near terminal event, in the absence of any specific microscopic changes should not be confused with clinicopathological entity of bilirubin encephalopathy. Yellow staining of brain may be seen due to presence of bilirubin in the interstitial tissue rather than neurons. Bilirubin staining and degenerative neuronal changes in acute bilirubin encephalopathy characteristically involve basal ganglia, inferior olivary nucleus, hippocampus, dentate, subthalamic nucleus and nuclei of the floor of 4th ventricle. The classical neurologic signs of acute bilirubin-induced brain damage are not seen among preterm infants because bilirubin staining among them is limited to nuclei of cranial nerves, subthalamus and thalamus.

Biochemical and Biological Determinants of Bilirubin Encephalopathy

Bilirubin Level

During first week of life, total bilirubin is representative of unconjugated bilirubin because conjugated fraction is very small. Clinical assessment of severity of jaundice based on intensity of yellow staining of skin and its cephalopedal progression is reliable with experience. Transcutaneous bilirubinometer, equipped with a photoprobe with reflectometer and computerized spectrophotometer provides digital read out for total bilirubin based upon yellow staining of skin and

subcutaneous tissues. It is non-invasive as probe is applied to the forehead or front of the chest and it is useful screening device for inexperienced residents. The non-invasive TcB measurement is reliable within 2–3 mg/dL of total serum bilirubin (TSB) level obtained by biochemical method. A number of automated sophisticated electronic instruments or bilirubinometers are available which provide a reliable estimate of total serum bilirubin (TSB) on a capillary sample of blood.

The time honored van den Bergh's reaction is widely used for biochemical estimation of total and conjugated bilirubin but it is a sad reality that bilirubin measurements lack accuracy and reliability. Inter-laboratory variability is marked with coefficient of variation of 10 to 12% for total bilirubin and over 20% for conjugated fraction. High performance liquid chromatography (HPLC) is the gold standard method for estimation of TSB but this facility is available in a few centers. There is a need to develop a simple, reliable reproducible method for estimation of total and conjugated bilirubin. The blood sample for bilirubin estimation should be protected against exposure to light. In a term healthy infant, serum bilirubin should not be allowed to cross a level of 25 mg/dL. There is no safe level of bilirubin for preterm infants but efforts should be made to maintain it below 1 mg/dL for every 100 g weight of the infant, viz. for a 1000 g infant, a level up to 10 mg/dL is probably safe.

Bilirubin Protein Ratio

Adequate levels of serum protein are essential for effective binding of bilirubin to prevent its leakage into the interstitial and intracellular compartment. It has been shown that bilirubin protein ratio of 3.5 or more may be associated with development of sequelae of bilirubin encephalopathy. There is a need to check whether serum and tissue proteins are free or blocked by H^+ ions or organic anions and any pharmacologic agent.

Reserve Bilirubin Binding Capacity and Free Bilirubin

HBABA dye binding measures both reserve albumin binding capacity for bilirubin and non-bilirubin binding sites on albumin. HBABA dye binding capacity of less than 50% may be associated with bilirubin brain damage. Salicylate saturation index determines the extent to which albumin is saturated with bilirubin by assessing its displacement on addition of salicylate *in vitro*. In our experience, a salicylate saturation index of 8 or more is associated with bilirubin encephalopathy. Sephadex G-25

Jaundice

18

measures both free and loosely bound bilirubin to albumin. Sephadex column consists of tiny beads of hydrated polymeric material packed into a tube and it actively absorbs both free and loosely albumin-bound bilirubin. The baby is not at risk to develop bilirubin brain damage, if sephadex G-25 column is not yellow stained and level of free and loosely bound bilirubin is less than 0.1 mg/dL. Red blood cell binding of bilirubin has also been utilized to assess the risk of kernicterus. Whenever bilirubin bound to red blood cells exceeds 4 mg/dL, it is considered as unsafe. A front face reflectance fluorometry or semiautomated technique for rapid determination of albumin bound bilirubin, total bilirubin and reserve binding capacity on a drop of blood has been developed. Peroxidase method based on the principle that only free unbound bilirubin can be oxidized by hydrogen as peroxidase in the presence of peroxidase enzyme, has been employed to assess the level of free bilirubin. Bilirubin encephalopathy is unlikely to occur, if the level of free bilirubin remains below 20 nmol/L. *However, it needs to be emphasized that there is no single test till date which can identify the bilirubin or its fraction which is dangerous to the brain.*

Blood–Brain Barrier

Increased permeability of blood–brain barrier or reduced cellular integrity of neurons may predispose to development of acute bilirubin brain damage at lower serum bilirubin levels. Factors determining the integrity of human blood–brain barrier are unknown and there is no way to assess it for clinical purposes. The advent of brainstem evoked response audiometry has made the brainstem and auditory neural pathways accessible to electrophysiological assessment as an early marker of bilirubin encephalopathy and a measure of blood–brain barrier. Somatosensory evoked potentials (which seem to traverse through the basal ganglia) have also been used to assess the neurological integrity in jaundiced infants. Gestational immaturity is associated with greater risk of seepage of bilirubin into the brain by virtue of immaturity of blood–brain barrier. Perinatal distress factors, such as hypoxia, hypothermia, hypoglycemia, acidosis, birth injury and septicemia may damage the integrity of blood–brain barrier and predispose the infant to develop bilirubin-induced brain damage. Some of these metabolic alterations may also adversely operate by virtue of anionic blockage of available bilirubin binding sites in the serum and tissue proteins. Birth asphyxia or CNS damage due to other causes may compromise the activity of bilirubin oxidase system in the brain, which is credited to eliminate bilirubin that seeps into the neurons.

INVESTIGATIONS

Most cases of jaundice in newborn babies are due to physiological causes and do not need any investigations. Investigations are indicated in following high-risk situations which are associated with pathological jaundice.

1. History of severe jaundice or exchange blood transfusion or kernicterus in a previous sibling.
2. Mother O group or Rh-negative.
3. Onset of jaundice within 24 hours or after 72 hours of age.
4. Trunk significantly or distinctly yellow-stained.
5. Sick jaundiced baby.
6. Persistence of jaundice beyond 2 weeks.
7. Jaundiced infant with yellow-colored urine or clay-colored stools.

The nature of investigations depend upon the clinical suspicion of etiology and are mentioned under various clinical situations. Cord blood sample should be collected, if mother's blood type is group O or Rh-negative. Despite all the investigations, no cause of hyperbilirubinemia is found in 25% cases. Most investigations are directed to identify hemolytic, infective and metabolic conditions. *There are no reliable investigations to assess hepatic maturity, quantum of enterohepatic circulation and integrity of blood–brain barrier.*

MANAGEMENT OF HYPERBILIRUBINEMIA

The aim of therapy is to ensure that serum bilirubin is kept at a safe level and brain damage is prevented. Exchange blood transfusion remains the single most effective and reliable method to lower the bilirubin when it approaches critical levels. However, other supportive and therapeutic measures are useful to prevent excessive rise of serum bilirubin and reduce the need for exchange blood transfusion. *It is important to remember that neonatal hyperbilirubinemia is a medical emergency and delay in its management can lead to irreversible brain damage or death.*

Rational management of jaundice in newborn babies is limited by following constraints:

1. There is a lack of reliable laboratory facility for estimation of serum bilirubin level on a micro-sample of blood in most NICUs.
2. There are no uniformly acceptable guidelines for initiating phototherapy or undertaking exchange blood transfusion in neonates of different birth weight and gestation.
3. We do know how to treat hyperbilirubinemia but we do not know when to treat it because there is

yet no single test that can identify the level of bilirubin which is dangerous to the brain.

4. Most NICUs lack the facilities for undertaking bedside evaluation of brainstem evoked responses with a portable machine.

5. The phototherapy units used in most of the neonatal units in our country are unsatisfactory and substandard for providing effective phototherapy because they are not checked for flux or irradiance.

Correlates of Hyperbilirubinemia in Healthy Near-term and Term Babies

In order to reduce hospital costs, most healthy term babies delivered vaginally are discharged from the hospital within 48 hours of delivery. There have been several reports that late-preterm or borderline preterm babies (infants between 35 and 37 weeks gestation) may develop hyperbilirubinemia, which may be overlooked or there may be delay in its recognition, unless the baby is closely monitored. The following guidelines should be followed to reduce the risk of unrecognized hyperbilirubinemia and acute bilirubin encephalopathy in apparently healthy late-preterm and term babies.

1. **Identify risk factors for development of hyperbilirubinemia** History of severe or prolonged jaundice in a previous sibling should alert the pediatrician to be more vigilant. Most cases of Rh-isoimmunization are diagnosed prenatally by estimating titers of anti-D antibodies in the mother by indirect Coomb's test. When mother is O group,

there is a potentiality of ABO incompatibility. In these babies, a cord bilirubin of >2.5 mg/dL can predict development of pathological jaundice (serum bilirubin >15 mg/dL) with a sensitivity of 70% and specificity of 95%. In communities with high incidence of G6PD deficiency (Tribals, Parsis, Punjabis), it is desirable to screen for G6PD deficiency when early discharge is contemplated. Early jaundice (<24 hours), borderline preterm (35–37 weeks), exclusive breastfeeding, bruising and cephalhematoma and history of jaundice in the previous sibling are recognized risk factors for development of hyperbilirubinemia.

2. **Routine screening for serum bilirubin level** Longitudinal studies in near-term healthy babies have shown that serum bilirubin level during first 48 hours is a reliable marker of hyperbilirubinema during first week of life. When serum bilirubin level is estimated at 36–48 hours of life, the risk of subsequent hyperbilirubinemia can be predicted by plotting the bilirubin level on a "hour-specific bilirubin nomogram" (Figure 18.8). When the total serum bilirubin level of the baby falls on the high-risk zone of the nomogram, it is preferable to delay the discharge or monitor serum bilirubin after discharge every 12–24 hours. When serum bilirubin level is 6 mg/dL or more on the first day of life, there is an extremely high risk of development of hyperbilirubinemia and it is preferable to keep the baby under close observation. It is possible to predict serum bilirubin level with a non-invasive transcutaneous bilirubinometer. The

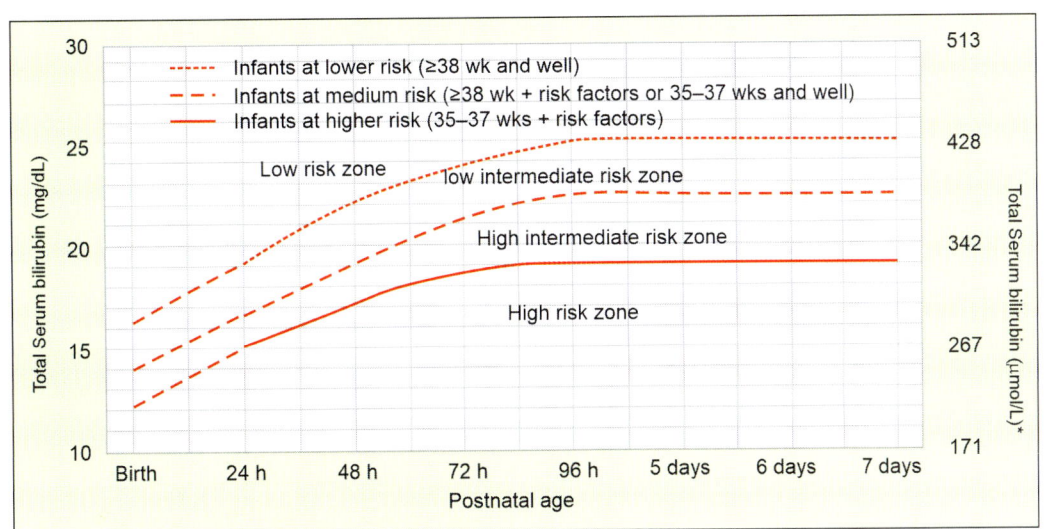

Figure 18.8 Nomogram for assigning risk to near-term well newborn babies based on the hour-specific serum bilirubin values. *Adapted from* AAP Subcommittee on Hyperbilirubinemia, *Pediatrics* 2004; 114:297–316.
*To convert bilirubin values from mg/dL to μmol/L, multiply mg/dL by 17.1.

handheld BiliCheck™ eliminates the interference because of reflectance of skin due to pigmentation and gestational maturity of dermis to provide reliable estimate of serum bilirubin. There is a good linear correlation (r = 0.91) between BiliCheck™ measurement and serum bilirubin estimation by HPLC. However, transcutaneous bilirubin estimation is not reliable when serum bilirubin goes above 15 mg/dL.

3. **End-tidal carbon monoxide estimation** During catabolism of hemoglobin, there is equimolar production of carbon monoxide (CO) and bilirubin. End-tidal CO (EtCO) corrected for room air, is a reliable surrogate of hemolysis and bilirubin production. When this technology is available, an elevated end-tidal CO can identify those infants who are likely to develop hyperbilirubinemia so that their discharge from the hospital can be postponed.

Preventive and Supportive Measures

For prevention of Rh-isoimmunization refer to Chapter 3. Drugs which are known to aggravate jaundice or block the bilirubin binding sites in albumin should be withheld. Vitamin K in large doses should be avoided and naturally occurring vitamin K_1 is preferable for prevention of hemorrhagic disease of the newborn. Perinatal distress factors, such as hypoxia, hypothermia, hypoglycemia and acidosis should be prevented or adequately managed, if unavoidable. It is recommended that the use of phenolic detergents should be avoided in the nursery as far as possible because they may enhance risk of jaundice in the babies.

Adequate feeding Hydration should be maintained and hypoglycemia prevented by early feeding when jaundice is anticipated or already existent. Early feeding augments colonization of gut and reduces enterohepatic circulation. Effective evacuation of meconium is associated with elimination of conjugated bilirubin and stercobilin. Breastfeeding should be given on demand as frequently as baby desires. There is no role of giving extra glucose water to the baby. Breastfeeding may be temporarily withheld for 48 hours, if breast milk jaundice is seriously suspected though most neonatologists do not follow this policy.

Aspiration of cephalhematoma The presence of critical hyperbilirubinemia, i.e. bilirubin of 18 mg/dL or more, in association with a cephalhematoma, is an indication for its aspiration.

Treatment of sepsis and hepatitis When sepsis is suspected, appropriate antibiotics should be administered after collection of blood samples for culture.

There is no role of corticosteroids in the management of giant cell hepatitis. Vitamin K should be used with caution. Avoidance of sucrose would be life saving in infants with hereditary fructosemia.

Phenobarbitone Barbiturates have been shown to induce the maturation of microsomal enzymes, ligandin (Y-acceptor protein) and glucuronyl transferase (UDPGA) thus improving uptake, conjugation and excretion of bilirubin by the liver. Due to lag period of 48 to 72 hours before enzyme activity is induced by phenobarbitone, it is best administered prenatally during 1 to 2 weeks prior to the expected date of delivery or given to the neonate within 24 hours of birth. Its utility is of prophylactic rather than therapeutic nature and is recommended in situations where serious jaundice is anticipated. Prenatal administration of phenobarbitone in a dose of 60–100 mg at night is indicated in an Rh-sensitized mother with a rising titer of indirect Coomb's test. Phenobarbitone in a single dose of 10 mg/kg intramuscular or 5 mg/kg/day in 2 divided doses orally for 3 days is indicated in infants with (i) cord serum bilirubin of >2.5 mg/dL, (ii) early onset of jaundice due to any cause, (iii) difficult or instrumental oxytocin-induced delivery with bruising and cephalhematoma, (iv) G6PD deficiency and (v) Type II Crigler-Najjar syndrome. Its utility is limited in preterm babies. It does not usually produce any sedation or side effects. The enzyme induction properties of phenobarbitone are non-specific and it enhances maturation of several other microsomal enzymes of liver. This may result in enhancement of drug metabolism leading to poor efficacy of chemotherapeutic agents. Phenobarbitone is also known to protect the fetal brain against hypoxic damage and may reduce the incidence of intraventricular hemorrhage.

Clofibrate Clofibrate (Atromid-S) is an organic compound which is used as a lipid-lowering agent. Clofibrate is a more potent inducer of glucuronyl transferase than phenobarbital. In one study, it caused a 100% increase in hepatic bilirubin clearance within one week. Administration of clofibrate (50 mg/kg single oral dose) in healthy term babies with idiopathic hyperbilirubinemia has been shown to reduce serum bilirubin level and need for phototherapy. There are no significant adverse effects. Although clofibrate is more efficacious but it is slow in its action and takes several days to show the beneficial effect. Food and Drug Administration (FDA) has withdrawn clofibrate from the market because of associated long-term morbidity and mortality risk.

MEASURES TO REDUCE SERUM BILIRUBIN

"We do know how to treat hyperbilirubinemia in the newborn but we do not know when to treat it because there is no single test that can identify the level of bilirubin which is dangerous to the brain".

Meharban Singh

Ideally there is a need to have a water-soluble harmless substance or a drug which should bind bilirubin more readily than albumin so that chelated bilirubin can be filtered out in the urine. No such substance as yet is available.

PHOTOTHERAPY

Phototherapy is widely accepted as a relatively safe and effective method for treatment of neonatal hyperbilirubinemia. It has been shown that bilirubin absorbs light maximally at 425–475 nm and light sources whose peak emissions are in this range lower the serum bilirubin levels by several mechanisms. The phototherapy causes photo-oxidation of bilirubin into water-slouble or less lipophilic colorless form of bilirubin. This process is, however, very slow and ineffective. Phototherapy causes configurational photoisomerization wherein E-isomers (4Z 15E, 4E 15E, 4E 15Z) which are more polar water-soluble diazo-negative compounds, are produced. However, configurational isomers are not very stable and they revert back to Z-isomers in the bile duct. Nevertheless, E-isomers are non-toxic and after 8–12 hours of phototherapy, they constitute about 25% of total serum bilirubin. The more efficient mechanism of bilirubin reduction operates through production of stable water-soluble structural-photoisomers of bilirubin, like lumirubin. The photocatabolites of bilirubin are readily excreted in bile, feces and to a lesser extent in urine without any need for conjugation in the liver. Riboflavin appears to catalyze the dermal photo-oxidation of bilirubin but it can induce alterations in intracellular DNA. Phototherapy also enhances hepatic excretion of unconjugated bilirubin into the intestinal lumen.

When to start phototherapy or do an exchange blood transfusion?

In most hospitals in India, phototherapy is over used and misused without any regard for its precise indications and is provided with a phototherapy unit having poor flux or irradiance of doubtful efficacy. Most jaundiced infants are placed under the lights to impress the parents and for pecuniar reasons. It is important to remember that phototherapy is a specialized therapy and specific guidelines and protocol should be followed for its use. Phototherapy is a "drug" and it should be used with due regard for its indications, dose, duration and side effects. There is lack of uniformity or consensus for the level of serum bilirubin at which phototherapy should be started in newborn babies of different birth weights and gestational/postnatal ages. American Academy of Pediatrics recommends that phototherapy should be started, if serum bilirubin approaches the level of 18 mg/dL (15 mg/dL, if baby is having hemolysis or is sick due to sepsis and perinatal distress factors) in a healthy full term newborn baby. The serum bilirubin cut off for exchange blood transfusion in a healthy term baby is taken as 25 mg/dL (Table 18.5). In view of poor quality of phototherapy units in our country, it is

	Total serum bilirubin (mg/dL)			
Age[a] (hours)	Consider phototherapy[b]	Phototherapy[c]	Exchange transfusion if intensive phototherapy fails[d]	Exchange transfusion and intensive phototherapy
≤24[e]	–	–	–	–
25–48	≥12	≥15	≥20	≥25
49–72	≥15	≥18	≥25	≥30
≥72	≥17	≥20	≥25	≥30

TABLE 18.5 Management of idiopathic hyperbilirubinemia in healthy term babies

[a]Jaundice during first 24 hours is always pathological and should be investigated to identify the cause.
[b]Based on individual clinical judgment.
[c]Phototherapy may be discontinued when TSB level falls below 15 mg/dL.
[d]Failure of intensive phototherapy is defined as inability to observe a decline in TSB @ 1–2 mg/dL per 4–6 hours and its inability to keep the TSB levels below the exchange range.
[e]Healthy term infants are unlikely to have jaundice within 24 hours.

Adapted from AAP Clinical Practice Guideline, Subcommittee on Hyperbilirubinemia. Management of hyperbilirubinemia in the healthy term newborn. *Pediatrics* 1994, 94 (4):558–567.

Jaundice

18

recommended that phototherapy may be started early when serum bilirubin approaches 15 mg/dL. There is a strong evidence to suggest that a full term healthy infant with hyperbilirubinemia, in the absence of hemolysis or sepsis, can be managed by phototherapy alone because there is no critical level of jaundice requiring exchange blood transfusion for such an infant.

In near-term or late preterm (35–37 weeks) and term babies, guidelines provided by AAP Subcommittee on Hyperbilirubinemia can be followed for starting phototherapy.

- Use total bilirubin. Do not subtract direct reacting or conjugated bilirubin.
- Risk factors, like isoimmune hemolytic disease, G6PD deficiency, asphyxia, lethargy, temperature instability, sepsis, acidosis or serum albumin <3.0 g/dL should be looked for.
- For well infants between 35 and 37 weeks, use TSB levels for intervention which pertain to the medium risk level. It provides an option to intervene at lower TSB levels for infants closer to 35 weeks and at higher TSB levels for those which are closer to 37 weeks (Figure 18.9).

In preterm babies, depending upon birth weight or gestational age, exchange blood transfusion (EBT) is recommended when serum bilirubin due to any cause approaches 10–20 mg/dL (Table 18.6). Phototherapy is started at a serum bilirubin which is lower by 5 mg/dL from EBT cut off with the hope that effective phototherapy would prevent the need for exchange blood transfusion. After each exchange blood transfusion, the baby should be kept under phototherapy.

TABLE 18.6 Indications for exchange blood transfusion (and phototherapy) in preterm babies

| Birth weight (g) | Total serum bilirubin (mg/dL) | |
	Normal infants	High-risk* infants
Up to 1000	10–12	8–10
1001–1250	12–14	10–12
1251–1500	14–16	12–14
1501–2000	16–18	14–16
2001–2500	18–20	16–18
>2500	20–22	18–20

*High-risk factors include hemolysis, sepsis and perinatal distress factors, like birth asphyxia, hypothermia, hypoglycemia and acidosis. **Start phototherapy at a serum bilirubin level which is lower by 5 mg/dL than EBT level.** Due to increased risk of bilirubin brain damage in high-risk infants, they are managed more aggressively and given an additional allowance of serum bilirubin of 2 mg/dL both for phototherapy and exchange blood transfusion.

Healthy preterm babies rarely require exchange blood transfusion (EBT) except when they have associated adverse factors, like hemolytic disease of the newborn, sepsis, hypoxia and internal hemorrhage. Early phototherapy is recommended in extremely low birth weight babies with perinatal risk factors. There is no role of prophylactic phototherapy in preterm babies. The nursery illumination in general should be improved for better observation of the baby to make an early diagnosis of jaundice. Phototherapy should not be undertaken in centers where round-the-clock facilities for serum bilirubin estimation or exchange blood transfusion are not available.

The Procedure of Phototherapy

The narrow spectral blue light is most effective for phototherapy but it interferes with proper observation of the infant. White daylight fluorescent lamps are quite effective and commonly used in our country. A combination of 4 special blue tubes (Philips TL 52/20 W) and 2 white compact fluorescent 20 watt tubes is useful. Special blue compact fluorescent tubes (CFT) or lamps (Osram 18 W) are more effective. Blue light emitting diodes (LEDs) which emit a narrow spectral band of high intensity light are now available (Figure 18.10). The use of white slings or curtains placed on either side of the infant improves efficacy of phototherapy by reflecting the light on the baby without any wastage. The nude infant is exposed under a portable or fixed light source kept at a distance of about 35 cm from the skin. The distance between the baby and phototherapy unit can be reduced to 15–20 cm to

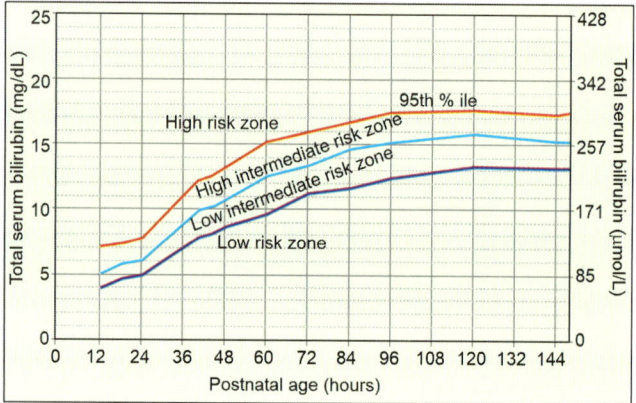

Figure 18.9 Guidelines for providing phototherapy to hospitalized infants of 35 or more weeks' gestation. *Adapted from* AAP Subcommittee on Hyperbilirubinemia. *Pediatrics* 2004; 114(1):297–316.

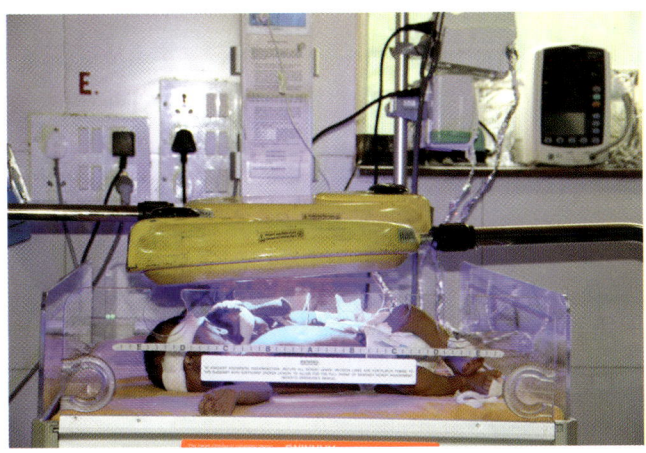

Figure 18.10 Baby under LED phototherapy unit. Note the effective shielding of eyes to protect against retinal damage.

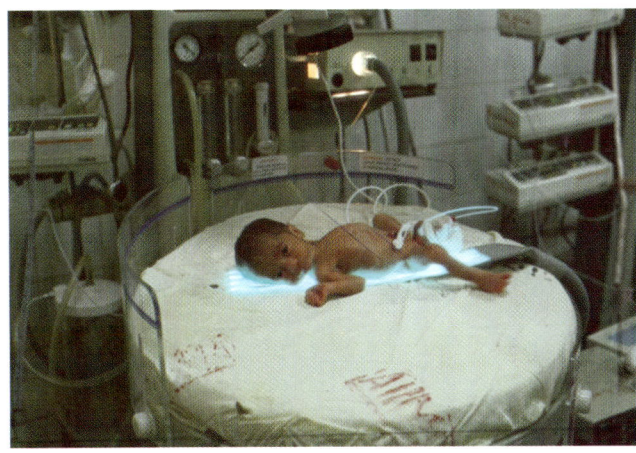

Figure 18.11 Double phototherapy. The baby is lying on a biliblanket and also being provided phototherapy from the top with halogen bulbs.

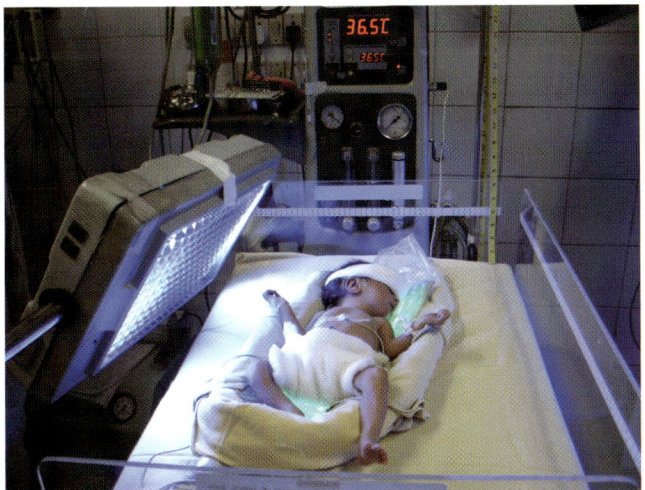

Figure 18.12 Baby under phototherapy with compact fluorescent tubes (CFT).

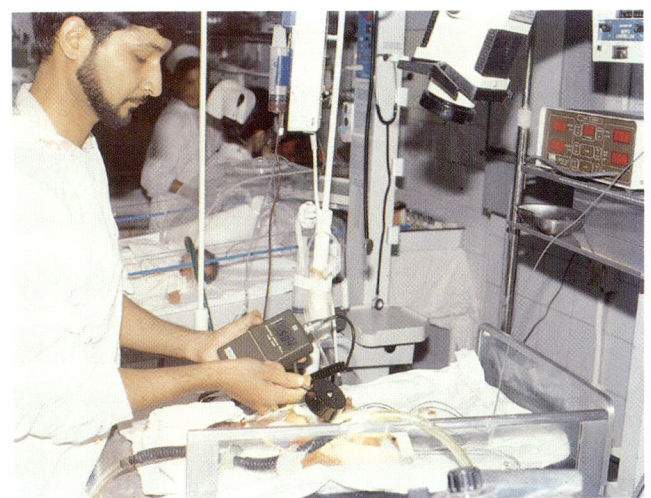

Figure 18.13 The irradiance of phototherapy unit is being checked with a radiometer.

provide more effective or intensive phototherapy. During exposure to light, the eyes must be effectively shielded to prevent retinal damage and a diaper should be kept on to cover the genitals in male infants. Double-light system where total infant is exposed to light both from above and below, is available and is more effective. For effective double surface phototherapy, the infant is placed on a fiberoptic cool biliblanket and provided phototherapy from the top with halogen bulbs (Figure 18.11). The phototherapy units with compact fluorescent tubes are cost-effective and commonly used in India (Figure 18.12).

During phototherapy, infant's position should be changed off and on so that maximal area of skin is exposed to light. For effective phototherapy, it is desirable that minimum spectral irradiance or 'flux' of 15 µW/cm²/nm is available and maintained at the level of infant's skin. The flux or irradiance must be checked once a week with a radiometer and tubes should be replaced when their flux falls below 15 µW/cm²/nm (Figure 18.13). Alternatively, the tubes should be changed after every 3 months or usage of 1000 hours, or when their ends blacken or tubes flicker. Phototherapy for treating hyperbilirubinemia is like giving a "drug" and there is no justification in using substandard light sources for treatment of neonatal jaundice. To filter out ultraviolet rays, the tube lights should be shielded with plastic sheet or plexiglass. Intensive phototherapy should produce a decline in total serum bilirubin of 1–2 mg/dL within 4–6 hours. In a term baby, phototherapy is stopped when TSB levels falls to 13–14 mg/dL. When phototherapy is stopped, there is likely to be a rebound in TSB level by 1–2 mg/dL during next 6–12 hours.

How to ensure effective or intensive phototherapy?

When bilirubin level is rising rapidly due to hemolysis, intensive phototherapy should be provided by delivering irradiance of at least 30 µW/cm²/nm or higher between 400 and 520 nm spectrum. Intensive phototherapy is likely to reduce the level of TSB by 30–40% in 24 hours. The following guidelines can be used to enhance efficacy of phototherapy.

- Reducing distance between phototherapy unit and the baby to 10–15 cm when using CFL/LED lamps.
- Using "special blue" CFL or compact fluorescent tubes (Osram Dulux Blue 18 W).
- Providing "double surface" phototherapy by placing the nude baby on a fiberoptic biliblanket or light-emitting diode (LED) mattress and focusing the phototherapy lights from above. There should be uniform exposure of 60 cm × 30 cm area of skin by the light source ("light footprint").
- Using slings or curtains made of white cloth or aluminum to reflect light on the baby.
- Using high-intensity gallium nitride light-emitting diodes providing narrow spectral band of high intensity light.

Side Effects

Phototherapy is by and large safe but several immediate and late side effects are reported. The common side effects include passage of loose green stools because of transient lactose intolerance and irritant effect of photocatabolites causing increased colonic secretory losses. Hyperthermia, irritability and dehydration due to increased insensible water loss may occur. Body weight and serum osmolality should be monitored. Infants under phototherapy should receive additional (20–40 mL/kg/24 hours) feeds to safeguard against dehydration and hemoconcentration. LED and CFL lights impose less risk of dehydration because they are low heat output devices. Term babies receiving phototherapy should be advised to take breastfeeds every 2 hourly. There is no need to offer extra glucose water in between the feeds. But when weight loss exceeds 10% in first 3–4 days, supplemental formula feeds should be given for 2–3 days.

During exposure to light, infant's skin gets bleached. The clinical evaluation of severity of jaundice becomes unreliable in babies receiving phototherapy and thus serum bilirubin levels should be monitored every 6–8 hourly. Hematocrit or hemoglobin should be checked after every 48 hours because in babies managed with phototherapy there is a greater need for "top-up" blood transfusion since antibodies continue to cause hemolysis. Infants with parenchymal liver disease with biliary obstruction may develop peculiar bronze discoloration of skin due to excessive accumulation of one of the photoisomers designated as lumirubin which is retained and polymerized to bilifuscin imparting brownish discoloration to skin. Phototherapy should be avoided in infants with direct hyperbilirubinemia and congenital porphyria. Some infants may develop flea-bite rash on the trunk or extremities. There is an increased risk of opening up of ductus arteriosus in preterm babies receiving phototherapy.

Recently, phototherapy has been shown to increase mean cerebral blood flow velocity especially in preterm (< 32 weeks) babies. Hypocalcemia may occur during phototherapy due to secretion of melotinin from pineal gland. There is controversial evidence that photo-oxidant damage to red blood cells may cause hemolysis. In some infants, platelet turnover may be increased resulting in lower mean platelet counts but bleeding does not occur. There is theoretical increased risk of developing malignancy of skin later in life. Paradoxically, it has been shown that intermittent phototherapy causes more damage to intracellular DNA as compared to continuous exposure to light. There is experimental evidence to suggest that exposure to light may disturb the circadian rhythm of the sex hormones thus having potential implications regarding onset of puberty and disturbances in future sex behavior.

Exposure to Sunlight

There is no role of exposure of the baby to sunlight for treatment of neonatal jaundice. Sunlight is ineffective for purposes of phototherapy because most of the ultraviolet radiations A and B are absorbed in the atmosphere and only UV radiations with wavelength 315–400 nm reach the earth. Moreover, sunlight is not available round-the-year or round-the-clock and there is a serious risk of producing skin damage due to UV radiations and hyperthermia in summer and hypothermia in winter. The exposure to sunlight is therefore neither safe nor effective for treatment of neonatal hyperbilirubinemia.

Drugs Blocking Enterohepatic Circulation of Bilirubin

Charcoal, agar, polyvinylpyrrolidone and cholestyramine and zinc have been shown to bind unconjugated bilirubin in the gut and prevent its recirculation to the liver.

Agar Agar is a sea-weed extensively used in processing of food. When given orally in a dose of 250 mg every 6 hourly, it binds conjugated bilirubin in the gut and blocks enterohepatic circulation. Its effect is unpredictable and variable.

Cholestyramine Cholestyramine in a dose of 1.5 g/kg/24 hours in four divided doses mixed in milk feeds has been shown to enhance fecal excretion of bilirubin by binding unconjugated bilirubin and bile salts and thus blocking enterohepatic circulation. Duration of phototherapy can be reduced when cholestyramine is administered concomitantly. The infant should be watched for constipation, intestinal obstruction and hyperchloremic acidosis.

Zinc Zinc is credited to inhibit enterohepatic circulation. In a number of randomized controlled trials, zinc gluconate (10 mg/kg/d q 12 hr) has been given to term and near term infants with serum bilirubin >6 mg/dL within first 24 hours of life. Assessment after 5–7 days of intervention did not show any difference in serum bilirubin level and duration of phototherapy in the two groups.

Miscellaneous Drugs

Orotic acid It is metabolic precursor of uridine diphosphate glucuronic acid and thus promotes conjugation of bilirubin. Its utility is limited and cost is prohibitive.

Tin-mesoporphyrin (SnMP) Metalloporphyrins are structural analogues of heme and they inhibit heme oxygenase. It has been shown that tin-porphyrins diminish the production of bile pigments by competitive inhibition of heme oxygenase, a rate-limiting enzyme in heme catabolism. Tin mesoporphyrin (6 μmol/kg single dose IM) has been shown to significantly reduce bilirubin production from a variety of causes. It awaits further therapeutic trials before it can be recommended. Therapy is associated with high incidence of photosensitive skin reactions and potential risk of hepatic and renal toxicity. Phototherapy is contraindicated after administration of tin-mesoporphyrin.

Albumin infusion When administered (1.0 g/kg as 5% salt-free albumin), half to one hour before exchange transfusion, it facilitates more effective removal of bilirubin and also improves the bilirubin binding capacity of the baby. Albumin infusion is followed by elevation of total serum bilirubin because it chelates bilirubin which has seeped into interstitial compartment. The serum bilirubin concentration may not actually rise because of expansion of vascular compartment due to oncotic pressure of infused albumin. Exchange blood transfusion, half to one hour after albumin infusion, is credited to achieve 50% more effective exchange by removal of bilirubin. It is not necessary to give albumin infusion before early exchange transfusion carried out for correction of anemia and its use should be avoided in babies with congestive cardiac failure because of risk of over loading of the circulation. It is rarely used in clinical practice because of exorbitant cost and risk of transmission of viral infections.

EXCHANGE BLOOD TRANSFUSION

It is the most effective and reliable method to reduce bilirubin levels. A number of biological and biochemical parameters should be taken into consideration while deciding to do an exchange blood transfusion for hyperbilirubinemia. *There is as yet no single reliable laboratory parameter that can predict with certainty the risk for development of brain damage due to bilirubin.* Early exchange transfusion with packed red blood cells is done in seriously affected Rh-isoimmunized erythroblastotic babies to correct anemia and remove anti-D antibodies and Rh-positive red blood cells coated with antibodies (Table 18.7). Early exchange blood transfusion is likely to reduce the need for subsequent exchanges and correct anemia and circulatory overload. For subsequent exchange blood transfusion for hyperbilirubinemia due to other causes, there is no "magic" level of bilirubin. Infants complicated by perinatal hypoxia, hypothermia, acidosis, hypoglycemia, sepsis and drugs should be exchanged at a relatively lower serum bilirubin level. Infants with hemolysis should also be exchanged at lower serum bilirubin levels because hematin competes with bilirubin binding sites on the albumin. A lusty term baby with a serum bilirubin level of 20–25 mg/dL at the age of 4 to 5 days should not be hurriedly exchanged because it is anticipated that the improving hepatic maturity would be able to handle the bilirubin load in a day or so.

TABLE 18.7 Early indications for exchange blood transfusion in infants with Rh-hemolytic disease of the newborn

- Cord hemoglobin of <10 g/dL or hematocrit <30%.
- Cord bilirubin of 5 mg/dL or more.
- Unconjugated serum bilirubin of 10 mg/dL within 24 hours or 15 mg/dL within 48 hours or rate of rise of >0.5 mg/dL per hour.

Jaundice

18

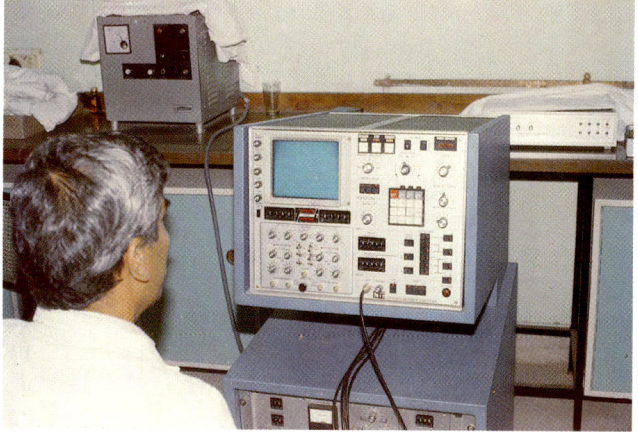

Figure 18.14 Brainstem evoked response audiometry (BERA) being conducted on an infant. It is ideal to have a portable BERA machine for rational management of neonatal hyperbilirubinemia.

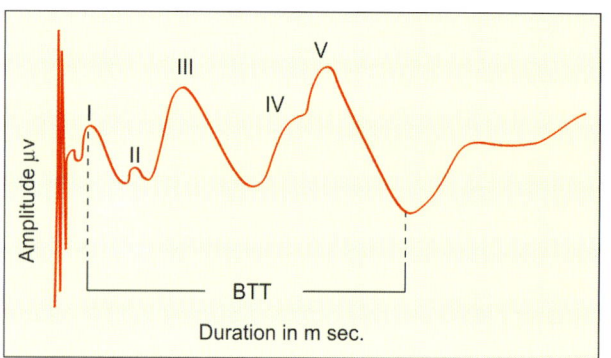

Figure 18.15 The normal BERA waves in a newborn baby. See text for changes due to bilirubin encephalopathy.
BTT; brainstem transmission time

Table 18.4 highlights indications for exchange blood transfusion in preterm babies. When facilities are available, point-of-care brainstem evoked response audiometry can be done to assess the need for exchange blood transfusion (Figure 18.14). Exchange transfusion is indicated, if there is increase in latency and reduced amplitude or absence of waves I, III and IV-V complex (Figure 18.15). Therefore, in an individual infant, the decision for exchange blood transfusion should be based not merely on the level of unconjugated serum bilirubin or availability of bilirubin binding capacity but also on gestational maturity, postnatal age, existence or otherwise of perinatal distress factors, cause of jaundice and findings on brainstem evoked response andiometry. For details regarding procedure of exchange blood transfusion, refer to Chapter 29.

PERSISTENT NEONATAL JAUNDICE

In most infants with physiological jaundice or hyperbilirubinemia due to various causes, jaundice disappears by 2–3 weeks of age. Persistence of jaundice beyond 3 weeks may occur due to unconjugated hyperbilirubinemia or cholestatic disorders.

Persistent Unconjugated Hyperbilirubinemia

When a jaundiced baby is passing colorless urine and yellow or normal-colored stools, the jaundice is likely to be due to elevation of unconjugated bilirubin. The persistent jaundice is more commonly due to non-hemolytic unconjugated hyperbilirubinemia. The commonest cause of persistent unconjugated hyper-bilirubinemia is breast milk jaundice. The condition is benign, serum bilirubin usually ranges between 10 and 15 mg/dL and jaundice may persist up to 6–8 weeks. Other causes of persistent unconjugated jaundice in the newborn include Down syndrome, hypothyroidism, Gilbert syndrome and Crigler-Najjar syndrome. Down syndrome is suspected on the basis of typical phenotype while cretinism may be associated with lethargy, hypotonia, umbilical hernia, temperature instability, dry skin and constipation. Cretinism should be excluded by checking TSH and T_4 levels because it is a treatable cause of mental subnormality. Rarely, ongoing hemolysis due to fetomaternal blood group incompatibility, cephalhematoma, G6PD deficiency, hereditary spherocytosis, malaria, urinary tract infection and pyloric stenosis may cause persistent jaundice.

Persistent Conjugated Hyperbilirubinemia (Cholestatic Disorders)

Conjugated hyperbilirubinemia during early neonatal period is rare. Jaundice is mostly due to elevation of unconjugated bilirubin because of hemolysis, hepatic immaturity and enhanced enterohepatic circulation. For practical purposes, therefore, level of total serum bilirubin (TSB) during first week of life is considered as synonymous with unconjugated bilirubin. Elevation of direct reacting bilirubin by >2.0 mg/dL or >20% of total bilirubin is suggestive of cholestasis disorder. Persistent conjugated hyperbilirubinemia is uncommon during neonatal period and can occur due to a variety of causes (Table 18.8). Most of the conditions listed in Table 18.8 are likely to have first manifestations of the disease after the age of 3 weeks though all have been documented during neonatal period.

Inspissated Bile Syndrome

A proportion of babies seriously affected by Rh-HDN may have prolonged jaundice especially with a high level of direct-reacting bilirubin. During the course of

TABLE 18.8 Causes of prolonged conjugated hyperbilirubinemia in the newborn

- Idiopathic neonatal hepatitis
- Inspissated bile syndrome
- Infections
  - Bacterial sepsis
  - Hepatitis B virus
  - Cytomegalovirus
  - Herpes simplex virus
  - Rubella
  - Coxsackie B virus
  - Echovirus
  - Toxoplasmosis
  - Syphilis
  - Tuberculosis
- Malformations
  - Extrahepatic biliary atresia and hypoplsia, bile duct stenosis, choledochal cyst, intrahepatic biliary atresia and hypoplasia, Alagille syndrome, Bayler's disease, Zellweger's syndrome and congenital hepatic fibrosis
- Metabolic disorders
  - Galactosemia
  - Hereditary fructose intolerance
  - alpha-1 antitrypsin deficiency
  - Tryosinemia
  - Glycogenosis IV
  - Cystic fibrosis
  - Wolman's disease
  - Niemann-Pick's disease
  - Gaucher's disease
  - Dubin-Johnson syndrome
  - Rotor syndrome
  - Hypothyroidism
- Chromosomal disorders
  - Trisomy E
  - Down syndrome
  - Donohue syndrome (leprechaunism)
- Miscellaneous causes
  - Total parenteral nutrition
  - Hypertrophic pyloric stenosis

severe Rh-HDN, conjugated bilirubin may accumulate, because of transient disparity between the maturity of conjugatory and excretory functions of the hepatocytes. The prognosis is generally good and jaundice eventually disappears without any specific therapy but other causes of direct-reacting hyperbilirubinemia especially septicemia should be excluded.

Neonatal Hepatitis

Neonatal hepatitis can occur from a variety of intrauterine viral, parasitic and spirochetal infections. In a large majority of patients with neonatal hepatitis, no cause is identified. In fact, idiopathic neonatal hepatitis account for over 40% of all cases of cholestatic disorders during infancy. Jaundice is usually noted after first week of age and may appear any time up to 3 months of age. Urine and stools are bile-stained. Intermittently, stools may be acholic or clay-colored. Hepatosplenomegaly is seen in almost all patients. Hepatitis B virus may be acquired *in utero*, during delivery or postnatally by maternal contact. Mother is usually asymptomatic hepatitis B carrier and positive for "e" antigen or may have suffered from hepatitis within 2 months before or after delivery. Affected infants are mostly asymptomatic but retain Au antigen positivity for several years. Hepatitis due to intrauterine infections may be associated with growth retardation, meningoencephalitis, ophthalmic manifestations, purpura, anemia and elevation of cord-IgM levels. Infants with herpes simplex, coxsackie-B and echovirus infections manifest with fulminant hepatic necrosis leading to early death.

In most cases of neonatal hepatitis, there is moderate elevation of serum bilirubin with slight preponderance of direct-reacting bilirubin. Transaminases are grossly elevated and there are laboratory evidences of incomplete intrahepatic cholestasis. Etiological diagnosis can be made in a small percentage of patients by demonstration of specific IgM-fluorescent antibodies or by rising titer of hemagglutination inhibition, neutralizing and complement fixing antibodies. Histopathology shows distortion of lobular architecture with massive giant cell transformation and canalicular cholestasis. It would appear that giant cell transformation is a non-specific response on the part of fetal liver from a variety of infective, metabolic and toxic agents. Small number of acute and chronic inflammatory cells may be present in the portal tracts.

Specific therapy is limited to infections caused by Treponema, Toxoplasma and Herpes simplex. Most patients with idiopathic parenchymal liver disease recover spontaneously by one year of age. In about 25% of cases, the chronic liver disease progresses to a stage of micronodular cirrhosis. Corticosteroids do not offer any therapeutic benefit and are not recommended. Infant born to an HBsAg-positive mother should be protected by administration of hepatitis B immune globulin (HBIG) 0.5 mL within 12 hours of birth, and three doses of hepatitis B vaccine given at 0, 1 month and 6 months of age.

Dubin-Johnson Syndrome

It is a rare autosomal recessive, benign disorder with isolated increase in conjugated bilirubin level. Hepatocytes lack the ability to secrete conjugated bilirubin in the bile. The condition occurs due to defect in multiple drug resistance protein 2 gene (ABCC2) located in chromosome 10. The liver is black in color due to polymerized epinephrin metabolites. The diagnosis is based on urinary coproporphyrin I to coproporphyrin III ratio of more than 3:1 and non-visualization of gallbladder on ultrasonography.

Bile Duct Malformations

Bile duct hypoplasia and atresia are rather complex and obscure anomalies posing a therapeutic challenge both to the pediatrician and pediatric surgeon. It is controversial whether all these anomalies are developmental in origin or evolve as a consequence of inflammatory or toxic process in the liver operating after 4 months of gestation. The distinction between developmental and acquired lesion is of therapeutic importance because surgical correction may be life-saving in one, whereas operative interference in a case of progressive inflammatory or metabolic process may be ineffective, unnecessary and often hazardous. Biliary atresia of fetal origin may be associated with splenic malformation (BASM).

Extrahepatic Bile Duct Atresia

It is ten times more common than intrahepatic biliary atresia and may be empirically grouped into operable or correctable type by choledochojejunostomy and previously "inoperable" variant which is currently treated by hepatic portoenterostomy or Kasai's procedure. The condition may be associated with other congenital malformations, like intestinal atresia, dextrocardia, Turner syndrome and polysplenia. Jaundice usually occurs after first week of life. Stools are persistently clay-colored or even cheesy-white. When bilirubin is markedly elevated, "jaundiced" epithelial cells may provide a yellow coating over the surface of stools but stools remain white or acholic in the core. Without surgical correction, all patients develop recurrent cholangitis with progressive biliary cirrhosis and evidences of portal hypertension. Histopathological features are dominated by periportal fibrosis and marked proliferation of interlobular bile ducts. In late stages, histological and biochemical findings in patients with neonatal hepatitis and biliary atresia may be confusingly identical (Table 18.9). Ultrasonography is done to exclude choledochal cyst, identify gallbladder associated vascular malformations and polysplenia or asplenia.

Nuclear scan is best done with 99^m-Technetium trimethylbromo-iminodiacetic acid (Mebrofenin) which is transported to the liver, actively extracted by hepatocytes and then excreted into the biliary system. The infant is primed by giving ursodeoxycholic acid (10–20 mg/kg/d in 2 divided doses) or phenobarbitone (5 mg/kg/d in 2 divided doses) for 5 days. The excretion of radiopharmaceutical into the gut excludes biliary atresia. The specificity of heptobiliary scintigraphy (HBS) is low because absence of biliary excretion of mebrofenin may be seen in some cases of severe neonatal hepatitis, alpha-1 antitrypsin deficiency inspissated bile duct syndrome, and cystic fibrosis.

It is desirable that the diagnosis of biliary atresia should be made by the age of 2 months because success of Kasai's operation is drastically reduced, if it is delayed beyond two months. It seems that hepatic portoenterostomy is effective when there is only hypoplasia of the bile duct which has not yet evolved to an atretic stage.

Intrahepatic Biliary Atresia or Hypoplasia

Alagille Syndrome (ALGS)

It is a rare autosomal disorder with prevalence of 1:100,000 children. Infants with this disorder present with a characteristic clinical picture of cholestasis with other associated anomalies and facial dysmorphism. Anomalies include prominence of forehead, triangular facies, hypertelorism, antimongoloid slant of eyes, flat nasal bridge, malformed low-set ears, pulmonary artery stenosis and defects of anterior vertebral arches (butterfly vertebrae at T3 and T4), and prominent Shwalbe's line in the cornea on slit-lamp examination. Liver biopsy shows prominent inflammatory changes, which progress and produce hypoplasia or ductipenia of bile canaliculi and cholestasis. Jaundice occurs around 4 weeks of age and is associated with marked and rapid elevation of transaminases (GGTP), alkaline phosphatase and lipid fractions. Severe pruritus, xanthomas and steatorrhea provide useful clues for clinical diagnosis.

The diagnosis can be confirmed by finding of JAG1 (Jagged 1) or NOTCH2 (Notch homolog 2) mutations on chromosome 20 p12 by genetic tests. Treatment is primarily medical by improving nutrition and administration of fat-soluble vitamins. Pruritus is treated with ursodeoxycholic acid, rifampin or bile acid binding resins (cholestyramine) and

TABLE 18.9 Differences between neonatal hepatitis and extrahepatic biliary atresia (EHBA)

Features	Neonatal hepatitis	EHBA
• Onset	Anytime during neonatal period	End of first week
• Jaundice	Mild-moderate	Moderate-severe
• Stools	Variable in color	Clay-colored
• Activity and feeding	Normal or slow	Normal
• Hepatosplenomegaly	Early	Late
• Urinary urobilin	+	–
• Stercobilin in stools	+	–
• Serum alkaline phosphatase*	+	++
• SGOT and SGPT*	Severe derangement	Mild to moderate derangement
• Serum alpha-fetoproteins	May be raised	Absent
• Alpha-1 antitrypsin	May be deficient	Generally normal
• Australia antigen	±	–
• Abdominal ultrasonography	Normal	Hypoplastic or ghost gallbladder, choledochal cyst, triangular cord sign, non-visualization of common bile duct, increased diameter of right hepatic artery (>1.5 mm)
• Liver biopsy*	Marked infiltration with inflammatory cells, presence of giant cells and lobular disarray	Hypoplasia, dilatation of bile canaliculi, bile plugs with preservation of basic hepatic lobular architecture.
• Tc 99m-paraisopropyl IDA (iminodiacetic acid) hepatobiliary scintigraphy or HIDA scan	Radioactivity is seen in the intestine	No radioactivity is seen in the intestine even after priming with ursodeoxycholic acid 10–20 mg/d in 2 divided doses for 5 days or phenobarbitone 5 mg/kg/d in 2 divided doses for 5 days
• Peroperative cholangiogram**	Normal	Block may be visualized

*These parameters do not show any distinctive differences after the age of 2 to 3 months.
**It is the gold standard procedure for the diagnosis of EHBA.

antihistaminics. In most children, the progress of the disease slows down by 4–6 years of age. Portoenterostomy (Kasai procedure) is not beneficial and should not be attempted. The end stage liver disease (ESLD) develops in about 20% of affected children and they can be managed by liver transplantation.

MANAGEMENT

Cholestatic Hepatitis

These infants should be managed with low fat, high protein diet supplemented with medium chain triglycerides and 5-times the daily recommended allowances of water-soluble preparations of vitamins A, D, E and K. Breastfed babies would need supplementation with medium chain triglycerides (coconut oil) because they do not require the presence of intraluminal bile acid for their absorption. Vitamin E 25–100 iu/kg should be given daily to safeguard against neurological consequences of vitamin E deficiency during infancy. Vitamin K is given in a dose of 5 mg intramuscularly once a week. Water-soluble vitamins should be given in double the daily recommended allowances. Additional supplements of calcium, phosphate and zinc are advocated. Cholestyramine resin in a dose of 0.25 g/kg per day in 3 to 4 divided doses mixed with fruit juice may relieve pruritus and lower serum bilirubin and cholesterol levels. Alternatively, ursodeoxycholic acid (UDCA) can be given in a dose of 10–15 mg/kg/day in 3 divided doses. Phenobarbitone 5 mg/kg/day alone or in combination with cholestyramine has shown therapeutic benefit and needs further evaluation. Ascites is managed by salt restriction and administration of spironolactone 2–3 mg/kg/day. The disease is slowly progressive but prognosis for survival is good.

Infants with chronic cholestasis and end-stage liver disease can be offered the option of liver transplan-

Jaundice

18

tation. Following the use of newer immunosuppressive agents and cyclosporin A, the survival rates following liver transplantation in children have gone above 75%. The operation is delayed till the infant weighs at least 10 kg. Availability of patient-matched donor liver is the major limiting factor.

Metabolic Disorders

Several inborn errors of metabolism may rarely produce cholestatic jaundice during neonatal period (Table 18.8). Jaundice, vomiting, poor weight gain, hypoglycemia and hepatomegaly are usual clinical findings. There are no specific diagnostic features and these conditions should be considered when there is a strong history of a metabolic disorder in a previous sibling. Hereditary fructose intolerance may produce acute life-threatening features of hepatic necrosis. Urine should be screened for reducing substance and aminoaciduria. Determination of blood glucose, serum protein electrophoresis to identify deficiency of alpha-1 globulin (alpha-1 antitrypsin deficiency) and sweat electrolytes (cystic fibrosis) are necessary to screen these metabolic disorders. The definitive diagnosis of alpha-1 antitrypsin deficiency is based on identification of P_1 phenotype on specialized immunoelectrophoretic typing procedure. Exclusion of lactose and sucrose from diet would prevent further liver damage and is life-saving in patients with galactosemia and hereditary fructosemia, respectively.

Total Parenteral Nutrition (TPN)

Liver dysfunction is the most common complication of TPN. Almost 80% of neonates receiving parenteral alimentation may show elevation of transaminases and clinical jaundice. Cholestasis is more common in very small infants. Infants receiving more than 100 kcal/kg/day may develop hepatomegaly and elevation of transaminases due to lipid deposition. TPN-associated cholestasis may be related to disorder in bile secretion by certain amino acids and deficiency of essential fatty acids. Serious hepatic disease may sometimes develop due to associated sepsis, hepatitis and microabscesses. TPN is contraindicated in infants with pre-existent cholestasis or significant hepatic dysfunction.

Biliary Atresia

Surgical management should be attempted within 2 months of age before the onset of biliary cirrhosis.

Vitamin K 5 mg should be administered intramuscularly to correct prothrombin time. Exploratory laparotomy and direct cholangiography are mandatory to identify the presence and site of obstruction. In few patients with a correctable lesion, it is possible to accomplish direct drainage. Most cases have non-correctable lesions and they are managed by hepatoportoenterostomy as recommended by Kasai. Portahepatis is transected and gut is anastomosed to the proximal surface of the transection site. The success rate of Kasai procedure is almost 90% in "Kasai hands" if performed within 8 weeks of life. When bile flow is not established within next 2–4 weeks, liver transplantation provides the only hope for salvage of these patients. The feasibility of using a "portion of the liver" from adult live donors has circumvented the problem of harvesting age-specific small livers from brain dead children.

ACUTE LIVER FAILURE

Neonatal liver failure (NLF) is rare and carries high mortality if treatment is delayed. The pediatric acute liver failure (PALF) study group defined neonatal ALF as (i) hepatic based coagulopathy (PT ≥20 seconds or INR ≥2) not corrected by vitamin K with or without any evidences of hepatic encephalopathy and (ii) biochemical evidences of acute liver injury. It is suggested that in infants up to the age of 60 days, INR of ≥3 should be used as a cut-off for diagnosis of NLF.

Etiology

The common causes of NLF include gestational alloimmune liver disease (GALD)–neonatal hemachromatosis (NH), inborn errors of metabolism, infections and hematological malignancies. The various causes of NLF are enumerated in Table 18.10.

GALD-NH (gestational alloimmune liver disease (GALD)—neonatal hemachromatosis (NH) is the leading cause of liver failure in the neonatal period. In GALD-NH, liver injury is of fetal onset and usually begins in midgestation. It clinically presents with jaundice, profound coagulopathy (INR 4–10), hypoglycemia, and hydrops fetalis (40–60%). Hepatosplenomegaly is either absent or mild. Apart from evidences of hepatic dysfunction, there is marked elevation of serum ferritin (800–7000 ng/mL), plasma iron and transferrin saturation, whereas transferrin levels are normal or low. The salient clinical features and investigations of neonates with hepatic failure are summarized in Table 18.11.

TABLE 18.10 Common causes of neonatal liver failure

Immune mediated disorder	GALD-NH
Infections	Herpes simplex virus, Hepatitis B virus, Herpesvirus 6, Parvovirus B19, Enteroviruses like Echovirus 11, Coxsackievirus type A and B, Adenovirus, Cytomegalovirus, and septicemia
Metabolic diseases	Galactosemia, tyrosinemia type 1, hereditary fructose intolerance, inborn error of bile acid synthesis, mitochondrial cytopathy, fatty acid oxidation defect, Niemann–Pick disease type C
Hematological	HLH (genetic and acquired due to infections), congenital leukemia, neuroblastoma, Down syndrome associated with myeloproliferative disorders
Vascular disorders and congenital heart diseases	Hepatic vein thrombosis, shock, CHF, hypoplastic left heart, coarctation of aorta, right heart failure, acute myocarditis, severe asphyxia
Drugs	Valproate, acetaminophen (maternal overdose), isoniazid, nitrofurantoin
Idiopathic	'Le foie vide' (hepatic non-regeneration syndrome), giant cell hepatitis

GALD–NH: Gestational alloimmune liver disease–neonatal hemochromatosis, HLH: hemophagocytic lymphohistiocytosis, CHF: Congestive heart failure

TABLE 18.11 Salient clinical features and investigations in neonates with hepatic failure

History	Antenatal history of oligohydramnios, polyhydramnios, birth history, preterm, intrauterine growth restriction, age at presentation, and history of sibling death
Physical examination	Signs of multiorgan dysfunction, jaundice, hepatomegaly, splenomegaly, edema and ascites
Basic investigations	CBC, CRP, blood sugar, blood urea, serum creatinine, albumin and bilirubin, urine routine and reducing substance, culture and antibacterial sensitivity, SGOT/SGPT, GGTP, ALP, APTT, PT, INR, blood pH and lactate level
Specific conditions GALD-NH	Raised ferritin, extrahepatic iron deposition seen by MRI of pancreas or buccal biopsy, TIBC, transferrin saturation
Infections like Herpesvirus, Echovirus, HHV6, Hepatitis B, Adenovirus, and Parvovirus	Viral serology and PCR
Hereditary tyrosinemia	Alfa-fetoprotein, urine succinylacetone,TMS, urine GCMS
Galactosemia	Red cell galactose-1-phosphate uridyl transferase, galactokinase, uridine diphosphate galactose-4-epimerase, serum galactose level
Hereditary fructose intolerance	Aldolase B
Mitochondrial hepatopathy	Lactate-pyruvate molar ratio >20, CSF and blood lactate, mitochondrial DNA, muscle and liver biopsy for quantitative respiratory chain enzyme determination
Fatty acid oxidation defects	Urinary ketones, fasting blood sugar, TMS
Hemophagocytic lymphohistiocytosis and congenital leukemia	Bone marrow examination
Septicemia and shock	Clinical evidences, vital signs and blood culture
Giant cell hepatitis with hemolytic anemia	Coomb's positive hemolytic anemia
Vascular malformations and congenital heart defect	Echocardiography
Maternal medications (paracetamol, isoniazid, valproic acid, nitrofurantoin)	History and drug levels

Abbreviations
GALD–NH: Gestational alloimmune liver disease–neonatal hemochromatosis
CBS: Complete blood count, CRP: C-reactive protein, SGOT: Aspartate aminotransferase, SGPT: Alanine aminotransferase, GGTP: Gamma-glutamyl transpeptidase, ALP: Alkaline phosphatase; APTT: Activated partial thromboplastin time, PT: Prothrombin time, INR: International normalized ratio, TIBC: Total iron binding capacity; TMS: Tandem mass spectrometry; GCMS: Gas chromatography mass spectrometry; PCR: Polymerase chain reaction

Jaundice

18

The general measures include excellent supportive care, minimal handling to minimize changes in intra-cranial pressure, intravenous glucose to maintain blood glucose between 60 and 120 mg/dL, appropriate anti-biotics, antiviral and antifungal agents. Ranitidine is given to prevent gastric bleeding. Liver damage can be reversed in certain metabolic diseases by dietary alterations. When GALD-NH is suspected, it is treated with IVIG along with a cocktail of antioxidants compri-sing of N-acetylcysteine (100 mg/kg/d IV), selenium (3 mg/kg/d IV), vitamin E (25 iu/kg/d oral), prostaglan-din E_1 (0.4 mg/kg/h IV for 2 weeks) and desferioxa-mine 30 mg/kg/d IV until ferritin level is <500 ng/mL). Neonatal orthotopic liver transplantation (OLT) is the only hope in most cases of ALF in neonates.

BIBLIOGRAPHY

Agarwal R, Deorari AK. Unconjugated hyperbilirubinemia in newborns. Current Perspective. Indian Pediatr 2002, 39:30–42.

Alpay F, Sarici SU, Okutan V, et al. High dose intravenous immunoglobulin therapy in neonatal immune hemolytic jaundice. Acta Pediatr 1999, 88 : 216–219.

American Academy of Pediatrics. Subcommittee on Hyperbilirubinemia. Management of hyperbilirubinemia in the newborn infant 35 or more weeks of gestation. Pediatrics 2004, 114:297–316.

Amin SB, Ahlorns C, Orlando MS, et al. Bilirubin and serial auditory brainstem responses in premature infants. Pediatrics 2001, 107 : 664–669.

Bhutani VK, Johnson L, Sivieri EM. Predictive ability of a predischarge hour-specific serum bilirubin for subsequent significant hyperbilirubinemia in healthy term and near-term neonates. Pediatrics 1999, 103:6–14.

Bhutani VK, Gourley GR, Adler S, et al. Non-invasive measurement of total serum bilirubin in a multiracial pre-discharge newborn population to assess the risk of severe hyperbilirubinemia. Pediatrics 2000, 106: e17.

Broderson R. Bilirubin transport in the newborn infant. J Pediatr 1980, 96: 349.

Brouwers HAA, Overbreeke MAM, Ertbruggen IV, et al. What is the best predictor of the severity of ABO-hemolytic disease of the newborn? Lancet 1988, II: 641.

Cashore WJ. Bilirubin and jaundice in the micropremie. Clin Perinatol 2000, 27: 171–179.

Chen HN, Lee ML, Tsao LY. Exchange transfusion using peripheral vessels is safe and effective in newborn infants. Pediatrics 2008, 122: e 905– e 910.

Dennery PA, Seidman DS, Stevenson DK. Neonatal hyperbilirubinemia. N Engl J Med 2001, 344: 581–590.

Deorari AK, Singh M, Ahuja GK, et al. One year outcome of babies with severe neonatal hyperbilirubinemia and reversible abnormality in brainstem evoked responses. Indian Pediatr 1994, 31:915–921.

Dhawan A, Vergani GM. Acute liver failure in neonates. Early Human Development 2005, 81:1005–10.

Diamond I. Kernicterus—Revised concepts of pathogenesis and management. Pediatrics 1966, 38: 539.

Gartner LM, Lee K. Jaundice in breastfed infants. Clin Perinatol 1999, 26: 431–445.

Johnson L, Bhutani VK. The clinical syndrome of bilirubin-induced neurologic dysfunction. Semin Perinatol 2011, 35(3):101–13.

Jokomuljanto S, Qua BS, Surini Y, et al. Efficacy of phototherapy for neonatal jaundice is increased by the use of low cost white reflecting curtains. Arch Dis Child Fetal Neonatal Ed 2006, 91: F 439–F 442.

Levine RL, Fredericks WR, Rapport SI. Entry of bilirubin into the brain due to opening of the blood–brain barrier. Pediatrics 1982, 69: 225.

Liumbruno GM, D'Alessandro A, Rea F, Piccini V, et. al. The role of antenatal immunoprophylaxis in the prevention of maternal-fetal anti-Rh (D) alloimmunization. Blood Transf 2010, 8: 8–16.

Lucey JF. Bilirubin and brain damage—A real mess. Pediatrics 1982, 69: 381.

Maisels MJ, Watchko JF. Treatment of jaundice in low birth weight infants. Arch Dis Child Fetal Neonat Ed 2003, 88–F 459–F 465.

Maisels MJ, Kring EA, Depidder J. Randomized controlled trial of light-emitting diode phototherapy. J Perinatol 2007, 27: 565–567.

Maisels MJ, Mc Donagh AF. Phototherapy for neonatal jaundice. New Engl J Med 2008, 358 (9): 920–928.

Marinez JC, Garcia Ho, otheguy LE, et al. Control of severe hyperbilirubinemia in full term newborn with inhibitor of bilirubin production Sn-mesporphyrin. Pediatrics 1999, 103:1–5.

Mc Donald M. Hidden risks: Early discharge and bilirubin toxicity due to G6PD deficiency. Pediatrics 1995, 96: 734—738.

Moise KJ. The usefulness of middle cerebral artery Doppler assessment in the treatment of fetus at risk for anemia. Am J Obstet and Gynecol 2008, 198: 161–164.

Morriss Bh, Oh W, Tyson JE, et al. Aggressive versus conservative phototherapy for infants with extremely low birth weight. N Engl J Med 2008, 359: 1885–1896.

Newman TB, Maisels MJ. Bilirubin and brain damage: what do we do know? Pediatrics 1989, 83: 1062.

Penn AA, Enzmann DR, Hahn JS, et al. Kernicterus in a full-term infant. Pediatrics 1993, 93: 1003–1006.

Perlman M, Fainmesser P, Sohmer H, Tamari H, Wazy Y, Pevsmer B. Auditory nerve-brainstem evoked responses in hyperbilirubinemic neonates. *Pediatrics* 1983, 72: 658.

Singh M, Patra DP, Vasuki K, Ghai OP. Evaluation of additional criteria for exchange transfusion in the newborn. *Indian Pediatr* 1974, 11: 261.

Singh M, Singhi S. Oxytocin infusion during labor and neonatal jaundice. *Indian Pediatr* 1978, 15: 399.

Singhi S, Singh M. Pathogenesis of oxytocin-induced neonatal hyperbilirubinemia. *Arch Dis Child* 1979, 54: 400.

Sooran-Lunsing I, Woltil HA, Hadders-Algra M. Are moderate degree of hyperbilirubinemia in healthy term neonates really safe for the brain? *Pediatr Res* 2001, 50: 701–705.

Stevenson DK, Verman HJ. Carbon monoxide and bilirubin production in neonates. *Pediatrics* 1997, 100: 252–254.

Stevenson DK, Fanaroff AA, Maisels MJ, *et al*. Prediction of hyperbilirubinemia in near-term and term infants. *Pediatrics* 2001, 108: 31–39.

Subramanian S, Sankar MJ, Deorari AK *et. al*. Evaluation of phototherapy devices used for neonatal hyperbilirubinemia. *Indian Pediatr* 2011, 48: 689–696.

Tan KL. The nature of dose-response relationship of phototherapy for neonatal hyperbilirubinemia. *J Pediatr* 1977, 90: 448.

Taylor S, Whittington P. Neonatal acute liver failure. *Liver Transplant* 2016, 22:677–85.

Thaler MM. Neonatal hyperbilirubinemia. *Seminars Hemat* 1972, 9: 107.

Vreman HJ. Evaluating the efficacy of phototherapy devices. *Indian Pediatr* 2011, 48: 681–682.

Watchko KR, Oski FA. Bilirubin 20 mg/dL—vigintophobia. *Pediatrics* 1983, 71: 660.

Yachha SK. Concensus report on neonatal cholestasis syndrome. Pediatric Gastroenterology Subspeciality Chapter of Indian Academy of Pediatrics. *Indian Pediatr* 2000, 37: 845–851.

Respiratory Disorders

PULMONARY PHYSIOLOGY

During fetal life, lung is a fluid-filled organ receiving 10–15% of cardiac output. It does not subserve any ventilatory function and gas exchange takes place entirely through the placenta. After birth, there are rapid pulmonary and hemodynamic changes and most infants make a smooth transition from intra-uterine to independent extrauterine life. Soon after birth, lung fluid is absorbed and the lungs get filled with air and adequate functional residual capacity (volume of air in the lungs at end-expiration) is quickly attained in term infants. Lung compliance (lung distensibility/lung volume expressed in mL of air per cm of water pressure change per mL of lung volume) and vital capacity increase rapidly and values proportional to the adult are achieved within 8 to 12 hours. Lung compliance (c) = change in lung volume (v)/change in transpulmonary pressure {(Alveolar pressure (Palv)–Pleural pressure (Ppl))}. The blood flow or perfusion of lungs increase by 8- to 10-fold due to fall in high pulmonary vascular resistance resulting in considerable reduction in right-to-left shunting of blood. The pulmonary vasodilation results in part due to increase in arterial oxygen tension, decrease in CO_2 tension, change in pH and partly it is a direct consequence of mechanical effects of inflation. As soon as breathing is established, PaO_2 rises rapidly to between 60 and 80 mm Hg and only about 20% of the cardiac output is shunted from right-to-left.

BLOOD GASES

Arterial blood gases reflect the pulmonary, cardiac and metabolic status of the newborn. Oxygen is carried in the blood in chemical combination with hemoglobin and in solution form. Most of the oxygen is bound to hemoglobin and blood is almost completely saturated

at an arterial oxygen tension of 90 to 100 mm Hg. The relationship between partial pressure of oxygen (oxygen tension) and oxygen saturation as described by the oxygen dissociation curve is depicted in Figure 19.1. The arterial oxygen saturation is the actual oxygen bound to hemoglobin divided by the available capacity of hemoglobin for binding oxygen (one gram of hemoglobin can maximally bind 1.34 mL of oxygen). Due to reduced content of 2, 3-diphosphoglycerate, the oxygen dissociation curve of fetal blood is shifted to the left. At any arterial oxygen tension below 100 mm Hg, fetal arterial blood is more saturated with oxygen. This increased avidity of fetal hemoglobin to readily bind oxygen though advantageous in fetal life poses limitations after birth because at any partial pressure less oxygen is released to the tissues.

The shift of oxygen dissociation curve to the left also makes clinical recognition of hypoxia more difficult. In the newborn, cyanosis is observed at a

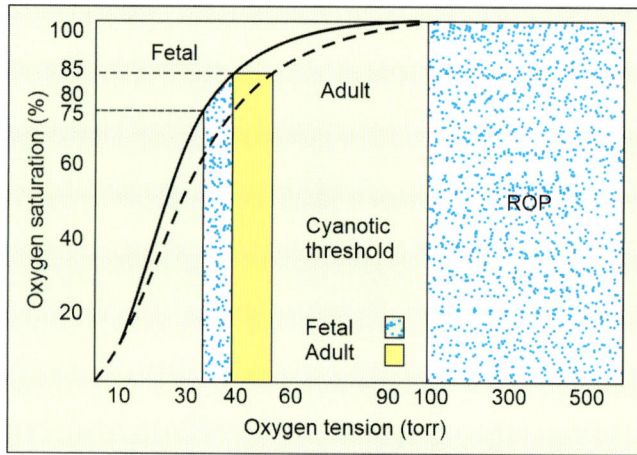

Figure 19.1 Oxygen dissociation curves of fetal and adult hemoglobin.
1 mm Hg is approximately 1 Torr

lower arterial oxygen tension as oxygen saturation of 75–85% (which manifests as cyanosis) is observed at PaO_2 of 32–42 mm Hg. At oxygen tensions above 70–80 mm Hg, arterial oxygen saturation is around 100%. Therefore, hyperoxia cannot be monitored safely by studying arterial oxygen saturation for which oxygen tension values are more informative. Arterial oxygen saturation by pulse oximetry is a useful non-invasive modality to maintain SpO_2 between 85 and 95% in oxygen supplemented preterm babies. In a healthy newborn baby, arterial oxygen and carbon dioxide tensions are maintained between 50 and 80 mm Hg and 35 and 45 mm Hg, respectively.

Acid–Base Parameters

They provide useful information regarding respiratory and metabolic status of the infant. The partial pressure of carbon dioxide ($PaCO_2$) in arterial blood depends upon the functional adequacy of lungs to remove CO_2. The constancy of pH of body fluids is maintained by several compensatory mechanisms and buffer systems. Bicarbonate–carbonic acid system is the most useful buffer and is regulated by Henderson-Hasselbalch equation:

$$pH = 6.1 + \log \frac{HCO_3}{H_2CO_3}$$

or

$$pH = 6.1 + \log \frac{HCO_3}{PaCO_2 \times 0.03}$$

In metabolic acidosis, bicarbonate is reduced either due to its loss in stools or neutralization by accumulation of non-volatile acids. To compensate for fall in bicarbonate, infant hyperventilates to eliminate carbon dioxide to reduce carbonic acid thus lowering arterial PCO_2. In respiratory acidosis due to pulmonary insufficiency (hypoventilation or apnea), there is retention of carbon dioxide with elevation of $PaCO_2$. Elevation of $PaCO_2$ by 1.0 mm Hg lowers pH by 0.08 units. The kidneys attempt compensation by retaining HCO_3 and excreting hydrogen ions. The cause of acidosis and alkalosis, whether metabolic or respiratory, can be determined by measuring blood pH, $PaCO_2$ and HCO_3 (Table 19.1).

Alveolar to Arterial Gas Equation

Alveolar (A) to arterial (a), pO_2 difference (A-aDO_2); and their ratio, i.e. a/ApO_2 are useful estimates of the appropriateness of oxygenation. A simplified working formula to calculate the alveolar pO_2 (ApO_2) is as follows:

$A pO_2$ = inspired pO_2 – arterial pCO_2

The inspired pO_2 = FiO_2 × barometric pressure–water vapor pressure at 37°C. As an example, in an infant who is breathing 40% oxygen ($FiO_2 = 0.4$) and has an arterial pO_2 of 100 mm Hg and pCO_2 of 30 mm Hg, the calculated alveolar pO_2 will be:

$A pO_2$ = 0.4 (760 mm Hg – 47 mm Hg) – 30
= 255 mm Hg

The difference between alveolar pO_2 (ApO_2) and arterial pO_2 (apO_2), expressed as A-aDO_2 in this infant shall be 255–100 = 155 mm Hg. The arterial to alveolar pO_2 ratio, i.e. a/ApO_2 will be 100/255 = 0.39 indicating that 39% of alveolar oxygen is entering into the blood. In normal persons breathing room air, the A-aDO_2 is less than 10 mm Hg (and is up to 200 mm Hg while breathing 100% oxygen). It is preferable to use arterial pO_2 to alveolar pO_2 ratio (a/ApO_2) instead of A-aDO_2 because this ratio does not change with inspired oxygen concentrations. In healthy individuals, a/ApO_2 is more than 0.8, indicating that 80% of alveolar oxygen is entering into the blood. In infants with severe RDS, the ratio may fall to as low as 0.1 to 0.2.

The following additional indicators are useful to assess the adequacy of alveolar ventilation in infants on IPPV:

Ventilation index It is calculated by the equation RR × PIP × $PaCO_2$/1000. The ventilation index of >90 for 4 hours is ominous.

Oxygenation index The oxygenation index (OI) is calculated by the equation MAP × FiO_2(%)/PaO_2. It is a useful index because of ease of calculation. The

TABLE 19.1 Acid–base parameters in clinical situations			
Cause	*pH (7.35–7.45)**	*HCO₃ (24–27 mEq/L)**	*PaCO₂ (35–45 mm Hg)**
1. Metabolic acidosis	↓	↓ ↓	↓
2. Respiratory acidosis	↓	Normal or ↑	↑ ↑
3. Metabolic alkalosis	↑	↑	Normal or ↑
4. Respiratory alkalosis	↑	Normal or ↓	↓

*Normal values in blood. mm Hg is a unit of pressure equivalent to pressure exerted by a mercury column 1.0 mm high at 0°C and standard gravity (1.0 mm Hg = 1.0 torr). In simple or isolated disorders, $PaCO_2$ and HCO_3 levels always change in the same direction.

oxygenation index of more than 15 signify severe respiratory distress while >40 on conventional ventilator on two consecutive blood gases obtained at an interval of 30 minutes is considered as an indication for ECMO.

LUNG SURFACTANT

Surfactant is a complex mixture of phospholipids, proteins and glycoproteins (lecithin and sphingomyelin) that decreases the surface tension of distal airways maintaining adequate functional residual capacity during expiration. The surfactant obtained from mammalian lung lavage consists of 80% phospholipids, 8% neutral lipids and 12% proteins. It increases lung compliance thus preventing collapse of alveoli, so that gas exchange is facilitated throughout the respiratory cycle. The biosynthesis of lecithin (dipalmitoyl phosphatidylcholine) takes place in the microsomal membranes in type II alveolar cells at approximately 20 to 24 weeks of gestation. Phosphatidyl glycerol is synthesized through a series of biochemical steps from its precursor CPD-diglyceride. Myoinositol blocks the synthesis of phosphatidyl glycerol by competing with CPD-diglyceride to form phosphatidyl inositol. As maturity proceeds, cellular and plasma levels of myoinositol decrease, resulting in greater production of phosphatidyl glycerol with enhanced maturity of lungs. The production of phosphatidyl glycerol is compromised, if there is damage to alveolar type II cells by hypoxia, hypothermia, shock, acidosis and antepartum hemorrhage. High levels of fetal insulin in infants of diabetic women are known to interfere with incorporation of choline into lecithin thus producing deficiency of phosphatidyl glycerol in the lungs. Dipalmitoyl phosphatidylcholine (DPPC) is the predominant phospholipid but lesser amounts of unsaturated phosphatidylcholine compounds, phosphatidyl glycerol and phosphatidyl inositol are present in the bovine and porcine lung lavage. In addition, there are four unique surfactant associated apoproteins (SP-A, SP-B, SP-C, SP-D) which facilitate the adsorption of DPPC to the air-liquid interfaces to reduce surface tension.

A variety of conditions are known to enhance and augment the maturity of fetal lungs. The exposure of fetus to chronic stress due to placental dysfunction (toxemia, hypertension, chronic renal disease), maternal narcotic addiction (heroin), prolonged rupture of membranes and sickle-cell disease are associated with enhanced maturity of lungs. Glucocorticoids, whether endogenously released or exogenously administered, thyroxine, catecholamines, prolactin, estrogens, and drugs elevating cyclic AMP are credited to enhance pulmonary maturation. Fetal lung growth is also dependent upon fetal breathing movements and quantity of amniotic fluid. Oligohydramnios due to any cause is associated with hypoplasia of lungs. At identical gestational ages, lung maturity is enhanced in female infants. The fetal lung secretions containing surface-active material travel into hypopharynx and are either swallowed or released into amniotic fluid. Amniotic fluid can be examined for lecithin to sphingomyelin ratio and levels of phosphatidyl glycerol to assess the fetal lung maturity. Depending upon the condition of the mother or wellbeing of the fetus, delivery can be postponed till fetal lungs are mature for extrauterine adaptation.

RESPIRATORY DISTRESS IN NEWBORN BABIES

Respiratory difficulties constitute the commonest cause of morbidity in newborn babies and pulmonary pathology is the most frequent autopsy finding in the neonates. The clinical diagnosis of respiratory distress in the newborn is suspected when the respiratory rate is more than 60 per minute in a quiet resting baby and there are inspiratory costal recessions or expiratory grunt.

Assessment of Severity of RDS

In addition to the severity of above parameters, the presence and intensity of cyanosis and its response to oxygen administration are useful indicators of gravity of the situation. The general alertness and activity, nature of cry, feeding activity and presence or absence of cardiovascular collapse determine the outcome. Apart from taking blood pressure, palpation of peripheral pulsations and color of the baby offers useful information. The severity of RDS can be assessed by Downe's scoring system (Table 19.2). The severity of alterations in acid–base parameters and their relative resistance to specific therapeutic measures suggest poor prognosis. Hypothermia, apneic attacks and disseminated intravascular coagulation are usual terminal events.

Causes

"Diagnosis of a neonatal disorder is based more on the nature of predisposing and associated conditions and antecedent events rather than the clinical manifestations at the time of presentation".

Meharban Singh

Care of the Newborn

19

TABLE 19.2 Downe's scoring system for assessment of severity of respiratory distress

Parameters	Score		
	0	1	2
■ Respiration (rate/min)	<60	60–80	>80
■ Cyanosis (SpO$_2$ <80%)	None in room air	No cyanosis in 40% oxygen	Requiring more than 40% ambient oxygen
■ Retractions	None	Mild	Moderate to severe
■ Grunting	None	Audible with stethoscope	Audible without stethoscope
■ Air entry	Good	Decreased	Barely audible

Downe's score of 7 or more is suggestive of impending respiratory failure

Respiratory distress is a symptom complex secondary to a large number of etiological factors. The list of various disorders causing respiratory distress is summarized in Table 19.3. Newborn baby has a limited capacity to express manifestations of a disease process. Identical and often stereotyped responses are seen from a variety of disorders. Therefore, identification of associated and predisposing conditions is important and often crucial to make an etiologic diagnosis of respiratory distress in the newborn.

RESPIRATORY SYSTEM DISORDERS

The common conditions in this group include aspiration, infections, hyaline membrane disease, massive pulmonary hemorrhage, pneumothorax and congenital malformations. The respiratory distress of pulmonary origin is characterized by tachypnea, marked intercostal retractions and expiratory grunt. Cyanosis is usually mild except in later stages of hyaline membrane disease and certain malformations. The auscultatory findings, though useful for the diagnosis of certain pulmonary malformations, are difficult to elicit or interpret in the newborn due to cross-conduction of sounds and because of the small thoracic cavity. The administration of 100% oxygen is usually followed by elevation of arterial PaO$_2$ to normal level in respiratory system disorders except in terminal stages.

MECONIUM ASPIRATION SYNDROME

Meconium aspiration syndrome (MAS) is one of the most common causes of respiratory distress in term and post-term infants. The overall frequency of meconium stained amniotic fluid (MSAF) varies between 5 and 25% (median 14%). MAS occurs in about 10% of infants born through MSAF. Infants born through MSAF are 100 times more likely to develop respiratory distress compared to their counterparts born through clear amniotic fluid. Passage of meconium *in utero* in vertex presenting babies is suggestive of fetal distress and occurs due to placental dysfunction, post-mature or small-for-dates babies and antepartum hemorrhage. The condition is uncommon in infants below 34 weeks of gestation. Thickly-stained amniotic fluid with particulate matter (pea-soup appearance) and yellow staining of skin, cord and nails are associated with greater risk of development of MAS.

Pathophysiology

The pathophysiology of MAS is extremely complex due to interplay of a number of mechanisms, like airway obstruction, chemical pneumonitis and surfactant dysfunction. Meconium aspiration causes airway obstruction with obstructive emphysema due to ball-valve effect. Due to direct irritation and toxicity of meconium constituents, there is marked alveolar and parenchymal inflammation and edema with leakage of proteins into the airways. There is release of inflammatory mediators, like cytokines (tumor necrosis factor, IL-1B and IL-8). These substances may directly injure the lung parenchyma and lead to vascular leakage, resulting in an injury pattern similar to acute respiratory distress syndrome (ARDS). Meconium adversely affects neutrophil functions by inhibiting oxidative burst and phagocytosis with increased risk of infection. Surfactant dysfunction may occur due to cytotoxic effects of meconium on type II pneumocytes and decreased levels of surfactant proteins A and B (SP-A and SP-B). Proteins, bilirubin, free fatty acids, triglycerides and cholesterol in meconium cause alterations in the phospholipid structure of surfactant which decreases its ability to reduce surface tension.

There is increased airway resistance and reduced compliance of lungs. Pulmonary vasoconstriction occurs due to release of a large number of mediators in the alveoli and bloodstream (leukotrienes,

TABLE 19.3 Causes of respiratory distress in newborn babies

System	Age at onset	Associated or predisposing conditions
Respiratory system		
■ Prenatal and natal aspiration	At birth	Postmaturity, small-for-dates, placental dysfunction, fetal distress, meconium-stained liquor, atelectasis and pneumothorax.
■ Intrauterine pneumonia	1–2 days	Prolonged rupture of membranes, foul smelling liquor, maternal pyrexia during labor and fetal asphyxia.
■ Postnatal aspiration	First week	Preterm, untrained nurse, cleft palate, macroglossia, glossoptosis, retropharyngeal tumor and esophageal atresia.
■ Postnatal pneumonia	1–3 weeks	May follow aspiration and systemic infection.
■ Hyaline membrane disease	1–6 hours	Immaturity, birth asphyxia, Rh-isoimmunization, cesarean section and maternal diabetes mellitus.
■ Massive pulmonary hemorrhage	First week	Small-for-dates, cold injury, disseminated intravascular coagulation, diabetic mother, hyperosmolar sodium bicarbonate injection.
■ Pneumothorax	1–2 days	Aggressive resuscitation, IPPV, meconium aspiration, hyaline membrane disease, hypoplastic lung, and staphylococcal pneumonia.
■ Transient tachypnea	First day	Term baby, cesarean section, maternofetal transfusion.
■ Wilson-Mikity syndrome	1–2 weeks	Very low birth weight babies.
■ Bronchopulmonary dysplasia	2–3 weeks	Prolonged IPPV, oxygen dependence, PDA, overinfusion.
□ Pleural effusion	At birth or later	Hydrops fetalis
□ Congenital malformations of upper respiratory passages	At birth	Choanal atresia, Pierre-Robin syndrome, nasopharyngeal tumor, vascular rings, laryngeal stenosis and web, goiter, etc.
□ Esophageal atresia with tracheoesophageal fistula	First day	Polyhydramnios, single umbilical artery, preterm or small-for-dates babies, congenital cardiac defect, VACTERL association
□ Diaphragmatic hernia	At birth	Hypoplasia of the lung
□ Pulmonary agenesis	At birth	Potter facies, diaphragmatic hernia, and oligohydramnios
□ Lobar emphysema	Variable	May occasionally follow aspiration and tracheomalacia
□ Pulmonary lymphangiectasis	At birth	Lymphedema, chylous ascites and anomalous pulmonary venous drainage
□ Cysts and tumors	Variable	Solitary or multiple cysts and tumors, such as neuroblastoma and teratoma
□ Asphyxiating thoracic dystrophy (Jeune syndrome)	At birth	Hydrocephalus
Cardiovascular system		
Cardiac failure	Variable	Down syndrome, rubella syndrome, large-for-dates, anemia and polycythemia.
Central nervous system		
■ Central nervous system trauma or asphyxia	At birth	Difficult or precipitate delivery
■ Diaphragmatic paralysis	First day	Breech delivery, Erb's palsy
■ Paralysis of intercostal muscles	First week	Myasthenia gravis, Werdnig-Hoffmann disease, congenital poliomyelitis, Guillain-Barré syndrome and myopathies.
Metabolic disorders		
■ Organic acidemias	Variable	Acidosis, hypoglycemia, elevated blood ammonia, seizures, positive family history.

endothelin-1, PGE$_2$) leading to pulmonary persistent hypertension (PPHN) which is associated in one-third of infants with MAS. These pathophysiologic mechanisms lead to atelectasis, air trapping, development of pneumothorax, right-to-left shunting, ventilation-perfusion mismatch (V-Q) and chronic lung disease. The vicious cycle of right-to-left shunting, hypoxemia, hypercapnia, acidosis and pulmonary hypertension, which is frequently associated with MAS, demands high quality of skills, expertise and technology for their management.

MSAF and labor MSAF in preterm gestation may occur due to fetal diarrhea because of listeriosis. In term and post-term infants, MSAF is a reliable correlate of fetal hypoxia. Amnio infusion to dilute meconium is no longer advocated due to increased risk of complications and its futility in preventing MAS. The labor complicated with MSAF should be closely monitored and baby delivered without delay by an emergency cesarean section or assisted vaginal delivery depending upon the status of the cervix and stage of labor.

Delivery room management Thorough oropharyngeal suctioning should be done with a 12 Fr catheter by the obstetrician before delivery of the infant's shoulders. This approach has been recently challenged because despite effective suctioning at birth, some babies may develop MAS due to aspiration of meconium *in utero* during fetal life. Thick-meconium-stained babies, who are depressed at birth, need to be intubated and meconium aspirated by attaching the endotracheal tube directly to a negative pressure source. Positive pressure ventilation should be avoided in the infant until adequate laryngotracheal toilet has been performed to prevent pushing of meconium further into small airways. For further details regarding management of babies born through MSAF at birth, refer to Chapter 6. Aggressive maneuvers, like application of pressure over cricoid region, blockage of epiglottis with fingers and splinting of chest, are condemned due to potential risk of serious complications.

Clinical Features

The aspiration of meconium may occur *in utero*, during process of birth or after birth. *In utero* aspiration of meconium is likely to have more severe clinical course of MAS. Thick pea-soup consistency of MSAF is likely to be associated with MAS compared to thin-consistency MSAF. Most affected infants are term or post-term and may have IUGR and dysmaturity. After resuscitation, initial apnea is followed by progressive respiratory distress with marked suprasternal, intercostal and substernal retractions and grunting. The anteroposterior diameter of chest increases due to progressive obstructive emphysema because of check-valve type of partial obstruction by particulate meconium. The chest may appear emphysematous with variable percussion note, occasional bilateral wet sounds and wheezing. The course is progressive during initial 48–72 hours and may be complicated by PPHN leading to intractable hypoxemia and acidosis. In case of massive meconium aspiration, meconium pigments may be absorbed from lungs and excreted in the urine. Urine may appear dark-brown in color and spectrophotometric examination may show specific absorbance at 450 nm due to presence of meconium pigments. Skiagram of chest is characterized by bilateral hyperaeration due to obstructive emphysema and coarse nodular opacities due to areas of atelectasis and consolidation (Figure 19.2). Hyperaeration as evidenced by hypertransluscence of lungs, horizontal alignment of ribs and depressed domes of diaphragm (at or above 7th intercostal space). The X-ray findings are bilateral, non-uniform and asymmetric. Pulmonary air leaks including pneumothorax commonly complicate the clinical picture.

Management

MAS is the commonest life-threatening respiratory emergency in term babies. Despite intensive management, it is associated with high mortality. Stomach should be washed thoroughly with normal saline to prevent vomiting due to meconium gastritis. Baby

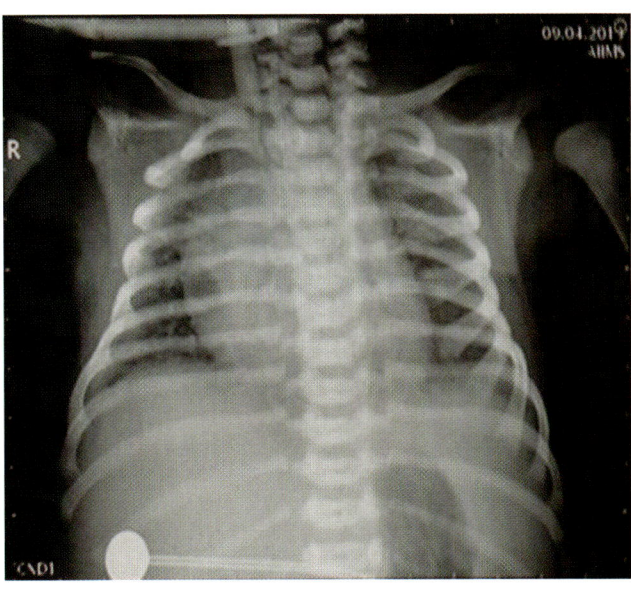

Figure 19.2 Bilateral coarse densities with basal emphysematous changes due to meconium aspiration syndrome.

should be nursed in a thermoneutral environment and given oxygen with a head box. Intravenous fluids should be restricted to two-thirds of the maintenance requirements due to potential risk of SIADH and pulmonary edema. Hypoglycemia, hypocalcemia and hypotension should be looked for and appropriately managed. The role of prophylactic antibiotics is controversial but most neonatologists do administer antibiotics (ampicillin and gentamicin/amikacin) after taking samples for sepsis screen and blood culture. The use of corticosteroids is contraindicated in the management of MAS.

A trial of CPAP may be considered, if FiO_2 requirements exceed 0.4. However, CPAP should be instituted with caution due to increased risk of air trapping and pulmonary air leaks. Assisted ventilation should be provided early when respiratory failure is impending (PaO_2 <50 mm Hg, $PaCO_2$ >60 mm Hg, pH <7.20 despite FiO_2 of 0.6). Infants with MAS are ventilated with high flow rates, increased PIP (30–35 cm H_2O) and short inspiratory time (0.4 sec) to reduce air trapping. Hyperventilation is used to wash out carbon dioxide and produce alkalosis when PPHN sets in. The infant is shifted to high frequency jet or oscillatory ventilation when conventional ventilation is complicated by air leaks. Pneumothorax should be promptly identified and managed by chest drainage. Short term liquid ventilation with perfluorocarbon in experimental animals is associated with reduced lung injury and improved lung mechanics. When PPHN supervenes, therapeutic modalities outlined in Chapter 20 are instituted.

The use of exogenous surfactant is controversial and there are conflicting reports of its therapeutic utility. Early tracheobronchial lavage with diluted surfactant has been shown to reduce the severity of respiratory failure. Surfactant therapy is associated with reduced need for ECMO but there are no differences in other outcome variables. Inhaled nitric oxide (iNO) as a pulmonary vascular relaxing agent is indicated when PPHN complicates the clinical course. It is indicated when mean oxygenation index (Oxygenation index = MAP × FiO_2 (%)/PaO_2) is more than 40. Inhaled nitric oxide causes relaxation of smooth muscles of bronchioles and reduction of pulmonary hypertension. High frequency ventilation, exogenous surfactant and inhaled nitric oxide have reduced the need for ECMO.

Prognosis

Despite advances in the understanding of pathophysiologic mechanisms of MAS and therapeutic advances in the management of respiratory failure and PPHN in newborn babies, outcome of MAS is guarded. The case fatality rates vary between 5% and 35%. There is high risk of cerebral palsy, seizures and mental retardation among survivors depending upon the severity and duration of perinatal hypoxia. These infants are vulnerable to develop recurrent respiratory infections, reactive airway disease and chronic pumonary insufficiency during childhood.

Postnatal Aspiration

This complication, which is readily preventable, is unfortunately common in centers where trained nursing personnel are not available for the care of high-risk babies. Those infants who can suck but have difficulty in swallowing due to immaturity, defective nasopharyngeal mechanisms, such as cleft palate, macroglossia, glossoptosis, pharyngeal membrane, retropharyngeal tumor and esophageal atresia with tracheoesophageal fistula, are likely to get choked and develop aspiration. There may be history of choking or regurgitation during feeds followed by sudden dyspnea and cyanosis. The milk may be sucked from air passages. The localized crepitations and evidences of atelectasis may be detected on clinical and radiological examination. Aspiration of dextrose water produces intense pneumonitis which is worse than aspiration of milk. Aspiration pneumonia most commonly involves right upper lobe area.

INTRAUTERINE AND POSTNATAL PNEUMONIA

In developing countries, pneumonias account for more than 50% cases of respiratory distress in the newborn.

Predisposing Factors

The infection may occur either due to aspiration into lungs or through bloodstream. Premature rupture of membranes, i.e. more than 18 hours interval between the rupture of membranes and birth of the baby, unclean vaginal examinations after the rupture of membranes, foul smelling liquor amnii, febrile maternal illness during peripartal period, fetal hypoxia and prolonged/difficult delivery are important risk factors. The infant may aspirate contaminated liquor amnii *in utero*, if he makes gasping efforts due to fetal hypoxia or aspiration may occur during his passage through birth canal or subsequently. Group-B streptococci (GBS) have been reported to produce a fulminant picture of septicemia and pneumonia which is characterized by early onset of severe respiratory distress, apneic attacks and shock. Perinatal GBS infections are rare in India.

Listeria monocytogenes may also produce intrauterine pneumonia by ascending infection from birth passages. Aspiration of meconium-stained liquor amnii leads to birth asphyxia and severe respiratory distress soon after birth.

Pneumonia may occur during the course of septicemia any time in the neonatal period. Neonates with life-threatening non-infective respiratory and cardiac problems (hyaline membrane disease, CHF) may develop superadded bacterial infection leading to pneumonia. Infants requiring endotracheal intubation and assisted ventilation are also at risk to develop secondary pneumonia. However, among all the predisposing factors, aspiration is most common initiating pathogenetic mechanism. Klebsiella, *E.coli*, Enterobacter, Acinetobacter, *Pseudomonas aeruginosa*, *Staphylococcus aureus* and *albus* are common etiologic agents. Chlamydial infection may produce interstitial pneumonia during 2 to 8 weeks of age. Other unusual organisms include *Ureaplasma urealyticum*, CMV, respiratory syncytial virus (RSV) and *C. albicans*.

Clinical Manifestations

Primary pneumonias are more common among term or post-term infants because of higher incidence of prenatal aspiration because of fetal hypoxia as a result of placental dysfunction. Preterm babies may develop pneumonia postnatally as a consequence of septicemia, aspiration of feeds and assisted ventilation for respiratory failure due to any cause.

The clinical picture is characterized by tachypnea, respiratory distress with subcostal retractions, expiratory grunt and cyanosis. The condition may be heralded by apneic attacks rather than respiratory distress. Cough is rare in a newborn baby. The infant with congenital pneumonia is born following predisposing factors (enumerated *vide supra*) and is often asphyxiated and sick at birth. Respiratory distress is noticed soon after birth or during first 24 hours of life. Auscultatory findings are non-specific and localized or generalized crackles may be audible. The newborn baby may die from pneumonia without manifesting any respiratory distress.

Laboratory Investigations

In all infants with prolonged rupture of membranes or respiratory distress soon after birth, gastric aspirate should be collected in a heparinized tube and examined for cytology. A drop of uncentrifuged stomach aspirate is placed on a clean glass slide and a thick smear is made with the help of another glass slide. After staining with Leishman's stain, total

number of polymorphonuclear leukocytes (lobed nuclei) and epithelial cells are counted in five high-power fields and mean number of cells per one high power field is calculated. The presence of more than 5 polymorphonuclear leukocytes per high power field or when their number exceeds three times the epithelial cell count, it is suggestive of intrauterine or congenital pneumonia. Septic screen may be positive. Bacterial cultures should be sought from liquor amnii, gastric aspirate, throat, external ear, umbilical stump and blood of the baby. In infants with congenital pneumonia, there is a good correlation between the pathogens isolated from throat swab and genital tract.

Skiagram of chest must be taken in all sick infants even when there are no symptoms or signs referrable to the respiratory system. Skiagram of chest may show bilateral opacities or evidences of atelectasis and consolidation. In a case of pneumonia, serial skiagrams would show worsening during next 24 to 48 hours while prompt resolution of bilateral opacities would favor massive meconium aspiration. Pneumonitis in right upper zone is suggestive of postnatal aspiration and tracheoesophageal fistula must be ruled out. Skiagram may show underlying congenital malformations or development of life-threatening complications, like pneumothorax. Point-of-care ultrasonography (POC-USG) by a trained neonatologist is useful for the diagnosis of various conditions causing respiratory distress by taking transthoracic and transabdominal views. Blood gases and acid–base parameters must be monitored to assess the severity of respiratory failure and response to therapy.

Management

Infant should be attached to a vital sign monitor and pulse oximeter for continuous display of vital signs and arterial oxygen saturation. Baby should be nursed in a thermoneutral environment and given oxygen with a head box. Intravenous fluids should be restricted to two-thirds of the maintenance requirements due to potential risk of SIADH. Early and effective intravenous antibiotic therapy is mandatory to improve survival. Refer to Chapter 16 for specific antimicrobial therapy.

Administration of volume expanders like, physiologic saline, plasma and blood is indicated to correct shock. Inotropes may be required to improve cardiac contractions. Metabolic acidosis should be treated by administration of sodium bicarbonate. The goal of therapy is to maintain arterial pH between 7.35 and 7.45, PaO_2 50–80 mm Hg and $PaCO_2$ 35–45 mm Hg. When arterial oxygen tension is <50 mm Hg despite 60% ambient oxygen administered through head box, the baby should be hooked to a CPAP device. When despite effective CPAP, arterial PO_2 remains below 50 mm Hg and pH cannot be corrected to above 7.2 (despite alkali therapy), infant should be intubated and given assisted ventilation. Unlike HMD, compliance of lungs is almost normal in neonates with pneumonia. The initial ventilator settings include PIP 15–25 cm H_2O, PEEP 0–3 cm H_2O, rate 30–40/min and I:E ratio of 1:2. Due to excessive inflammatory exudates, frequent suctioning of endotracheal tube and chest physiotherapy is advised.

Outcome

The prognosis is related to the maturity of the infant and severity or nature of underlying condition and offending organisms. Infants with aspiration of clear fluids do better than those with meconium aspiration syndrome. Early-onset Group B streptococcal infection runs a fulminant course with fatal outcome. Infants with septicemia and systemic manifestations do poorly as compared to those with isolated pneumonia. The mortality varies between 20 and 25%.

Early-onset Group-B Streptococcal Infection

Group-B streptococci (GBS) are the commonest organisms causing infections among newborn babies in several neonatal centers in the West. Early perinatal streptococcal infections lead to respiratory distress syndrome indistinguishable from hyaline membrane disease while late-onset GBS infections generally cause meningitis. Neonatal streptococcal infections have not been commonly documented from India.

The baby is often born following predisposing factors including prolonged rupture of membranes, peripartal febrile maternal illness and prematurity.

Respiratory distress invariably occurs within 3 hours and is complicated by apneic attacks and shock early during the course of illness (Table 19.4). The disease runs a rather fulminant course with poor outcome. X-ray chest appearances are similar to hyaline membrane disease unless additional distinctive features of bilateral coarse lower lobe opacities and increased interstitial markings are present. Pathologically, atypical patchy hyaline membranes are seen infiltrated with inflammatory polymorphs and streptococci. Atelectasis is minimal. Diagnosis is supported by the presence of polymorphs in gastric aspirate and confirmed by demonstration of streptococci in the amniotic fluid, gastric aspirate, blood or lung aspirate.

In addition to general management and ventilatory support, parenteral administration of crystalline penicillin (250,000–450,000 units/kg/d) or ampicillin (200–300 mg/kg/d) may salvage some infants. Transfusion of fresh blood may improve survival by providing opsonic activity against Group-B streptococci. In view of the fact that vaginal colonization rate of streptococci may be as high as 25%, prophylactic use of penicillin is not practical. However, if vaginal GBS colonization is associated with one or more of the following risk factors, intrapartum penicillin (5,000,000 units IV stat followed by 2,500,000 units every 4 hr until delivery) or ampicillin (2 g IV stat followed by 1 g every 4 hr until delivery) is administered for prophylaxis:

1. Previous infant with invasive GBS disease
2. GBS bacteriuria in current pregnancy
3. Labor <37 weeks gestation
4. PROM >12 hours
5. Maternal temperature >38°C.

TABLE 19.4 Differences between RDS due to hyaline membrane disease and early-onset Group-B streptococcal infection		
Criteria	*Hyaline membrane disease*	*Group-B streptococcal infection*
▪ Prolonged rupture of membranes (>18 hours)	Rare	Common (gastric aspirate may show polymorphs and cocci)
▪ Peripartal febrile illness	Rare	Common
▪ Gestational maturity	Invariably preterm	May be preterm
▪ Onset of RDS	During first 6 hours	Always before 3 hours
▪ Apneic attacks	Late	Early
▪ Shock	Late	Early
▪ Course of illness	Variable	Short and fulminant
▪ Peak-inspiratory pressures on a volume-cycled ventilator (cm H_2O)	35–60 (low compliance)	20–35 (high compliance)
▪ X-ray chest	Diffuse granular pattern and air bronchogram	Bilateral course lower lobe opacities and increased interstitial lung markings
▪ Pathological features	Marked atelectasis with typical hyaline membrane formation	Minimal atelectasis with atypical patchy hyaline membranes containing polymorphs and streptococci

HYALINE MEMBRANE DISEASE (HMD)

Idiopathic respiratory distress syndrome or HMD is the commonest cause of neonatal mortality in preterm babies. In our experience, the average overall incidence of HMD is about 10–15 per 1,000 live born affecting 10–15% of preterm babies. The incidence of HMD is inversely proportional to the gestational age. In the West, the highest incidence of around 60% is seen in infants with a gestational age of 26 to 32 weeks. The exact reason for relatively low incidence of HMD in India is unknown but it may partly be due to greater maturity of the low birth weight babies because of high incidence of intrauterine growth retardation, chronic placental dysfunction, infrequent use of general anesthesia for normal deliveries, low neonatal autopsy rate, and lack of awareness.

Pathogenesis

The lack of surfactant due to immaturity of lungs appears to be the basic abnormality. The presence of adequate amount of surface-active material (saturated lecithins and phosphatidyl glycerol) in the air spaces is one of the prerequisites for adequate postnatal pulmonary adaptation. The surface-active material reduces the surface tension to maintain alveolar stability at low pressures so that at the end of expiration alveolar collapse does not occur. Apart from pulmonary immaturity, the production of surface-active material may be compromised by damage to type II alveolar cells due to birth asphyxia, acidosis, hypothermia, Rh-isoimmunization, antepartum hemorrhage and shock. Maternal diabetes mellitus delays maturation of fetal lungs. Infants delivered by emergency cesarean section are also predisposed to develop HMD due to greater chances of perinatal hypoxia. Infants born by elective cesarean section are also at an increased risk of HMD because of lack of adrenergic and steroid hormones which are released during labor. Deficiency of surfactant due to immaturity of lungs or its poor regeneration by damaged type II alveolar cells leads to atelectasis or alveolar collapse. The development of hyaline membranes and characteristic pathological findings of HMD appear to be due to hypoperfusion of the lungs leading to epithelial necrosis and transudation of plasma. The aspiration of amniotic fluid is no longer believed to play any significant role in the formation of hyaline membranes. The combination of end-expiratory alveolar collapse, reduced pulmonary compliance, pulmonary under-perfusion and increased capillary exudation leads to accumulation of CO_2 and reduction in PaO_2 and pH. These metabolic changes lead to constriction of pulmonary arterioles and opening up of right-to-left shunts with perpetuation of hypoxia. Cardiac dysfunction secondary to hypoxia and acidosis may further aggravate the clinical picture.

The Lecithin/Sphingomyelin (L/S) Ratio

The fetal lung secretes fluid containing surface-active material which travels into the posterior pharynx. Most of this is swallowed but a small fraction enters the amniotic fluid. The ratio of lecithin to sphingomyelin in the amniotic fluid can be easily determined by thin-layer chromatography. A sample of amniotic fluid collected by amniocentesis is centrifuged at 1000 rpm for 3–5 minutes and thin layer chromatography (TLC) is performed on the supernatant to estimate the content of lecithin and sphinogmycelin. An L/S ratio of 2 or more is suggestive of adequate lung maturity while a ratio of less than 1.5 is often associated with hyaline membrane disease. Amniotic fluid shake test or density, as assessed by spectrophotometry, is a simple bedside test for assessment of lung maturity. Estimation of phosphatidyl glycerol, however, is most specific indicator of lung maturity and irrespective of L/S ratio, its absence is invariably associated with development of hyaline membrane disease. In women with diabetes mellitus, L/S ratio is unreliable and estimation of amniotic fluid phosphatidyl glycerol levels are mandatory to assess pulmonary maturity.

Gastric aspirate stable microbubble test and click test are useful cot-side screening tests to assess the risk of development of hyaline membrane disease in a high-risk infant. To 0.5 mL of normal saline and 1.0 mL of 95% ethyl alcohol taken in a clean 10 mm × 110 mm test tube, 0.5 mL of gastric aspirate collected within 15 minutes of birth is added. It is vigorously shaken for 15 seconds and allowed to stand for 15 minutes. The surface is inspected for quantum of froth or bubbles. When bubbles cover one-third or less of the liquid surface, the test is negative and indicative of high risk of developing hyaline membrane disease. If froth or bubbles occupy two-thirds or more of the liquid surface, it suggests full pulmonary maturity. The test is unreliable, if gastric aspirate is contaminated with meconium or blood. Rapid test for lung maturity based on mid-infrared spectroscopy of gastric aspirate is highly reliable for prediction of RDS with high sensitivity. In click test, instead of gastric aspirate, 0.2 mL of tracheal aspirate is assessed for production of stable microbubbles with ethyl alcohol.

Respiratory Disorders

19

Diagnosis

The diagnosis of HMD is suspected when there is a clinical triad of tachypnea, expiratory grunt and inspiratory retractions in a prematurely born asphyxiated infant. The babies born to untreated diabetic mothers, severe Rh-isoimmunization and those born by emergency cesarean section are prone to develop HMD. The symptoms may begin at birth or within 6 hours and there is gradual worsening of retractions, grunting and cyanosis during next 24 to 48 hours. The grunting is produced when infant expirates against a closed glottis. It is a compensatory mechanism on the part of the infant to raise end-expiratory alveolar pressure during expiration. The skiagram of chest during early stage shows symmetrical reticulogranular pattern due to scattered atelectasis. The transluscent air-filled bronchi against the airless, solid, atelectic lungs produce characteristic air bronchogram which may extend up to the cardiac border. As the disease progresses, reticulogranular shadows become increasingly confluent leading to formation of ground-glass opacity because of marked underaeration. In the terminal stages, there is complete white out of the lungs which become indistinguishable from the cardiac or mediastinal shadows due to global atelectasis (Figure 19.3). The finding of negative gastric aspirate 'shake test' or "click test" would strongly support the diagnosis of HMD. Serial gastric aspirate shake tests can be done to assess the status of pulmonary maturity during the course of hyaline membrane disease.

The course of HMD is relentlessly progressive and may be complicated by intraventricular hemorrhage manifested by apneic attacks. During recovery when pulmonary venous resistance drops dramatically, left-to-right shunt through PDA may lead to CHF. Disseminated intravascular coagulation may lead to hemorrhagic infarction in the brain or massive pulmonary hemorrhage. Prolonged ventilation may be complicated by air leaks and bronchopulmonary dysplasia. Retinopathy of prematurity may occur because of prolonged hyperoxia. The definitive diagnosis is possible only at autopsy. Grossly, the lungs are acutely congested, totally airless and of liver-like consistency on section. They do not float in water. Acidophilic hyaline material uniformly covers the respiratory bronchioles. Terminal air sacs are completely collapsed and membrane-lined bronchioles or acini are significantly dilated and appear to be separated by thick, intensely congested cellular septa.

Prevention

The premature labor should be suppressed to gain gestational maturity. The induction of labor should preferably be delayed till pulmonary maturity is assured by the results of amniotic fluid L/S ratio or level of phosphatidyl glycerol. When induction of premature labor is unavoidable, whether in the interest of mother or fetus, betamethasone (12 mg IM every 24 hr for 2 doses) or dexamethasone (6 mg IM every 12 hours for 4 doses) should be administered to the mother. Betamethasone has been shown to be more effective than dexamethasone and is associated with reduced risk of side effects. Antenatal steroids can also be given to a diabetic woman at risk of delivering an immature infant. Her insulin requirements may have to be temporarily stepped up for effective control of diabetes mellitus. Pharmacological maturity of lungs can only be achieved, if delivery can be safely postponed for at least 24 hours. There is experimental evidence to suggest that glucocorticoids enter specific receptor cells in the peumocytes to trigger messenger RNA to elaborate surface-active material. Its use is contraindicated, if delivery cannot be safely delayed, viz. eclampsia, febrile chorioamnionitis, severe antepartum hemorrhage and fetal distress as confirmed by positive oxytocin challenge test. There is no prophylactic utility of postnatal administration of corticosteroids. In VLBW babies (gestation <32 weeks) with high-risk factors for RDS, prophylactic surfactant therapy is credited to reduce the severity and complications of RDS. But because of its high cost and restricted availability, it is preferable to administer surfactant as a rescue therapy as soon as the baby is diagnosed to have RDS.

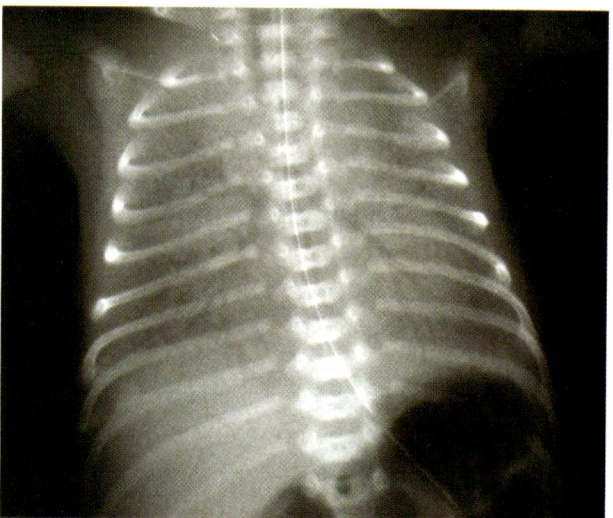

Figure 19.3 Global white out with air bronchogram in an infant with HMD.

Management

Idiopathic respiratory distress syndrome or HMD is the most common life-threatening emergency in newborn babies. The major considerations involved in therapy are to improve ventilation in order to enhance oxygenation, correct acidosis, provide thermoneutral environment and maintain adequate supply of substrate for energy. The goal of therapy is to maintain arterial pH between 7.35 and 7.45, PaO_2 50–80 mm Hg and $PaCO_2$ 35–45 mm Hg. Optimal facilities for supportive care, cardiorespiratory monitoring, oxygen therapy, gasometry and ventilation are required to improve the outcome. The infant should be attached to a vital sign monitor and pulse oximeter for continuous display of vital signs and arterial oxygen saturation. The following clinical observations should be recorded to monitor the progress of the child:

- Rectal or skin temperature hourly until stable and then 4 hourly
- Respiratory rate hourly or continuously
- Severity of retractions and grunting (Silverman and Andersen score)
- Status of peripheral pulses, capillary refill time and blood pressure
- Color
- Apneic episodes
- Activity, responsiveness and cry
- Air entry in the lungs
- Urine output

Intravenous Infusion

It is advisable to start intravenous infusion, preferably through a peripheral vein in all babies with RDS because oral feeding may not be taken by the baby and it is often complicated by risk of aspiration. In infants requiring prolonged ventilation, nasogastric feeding or total parenteral nutrition is needed to prevent tissue catabolism. The volume of maintenance fluids required is guided by the weight, use of phototherapy, radiant warmers and occurrence of SIADH. Sodium bicarbonate, 7.5% solution half diluted with distilled water or two parts of 5% glucose solution should be administrated in a dose of 3 to 8 mEq/kg in 24 hours or the dose of sodium bicarbonate should be calculated on the basis of base deficit to maintain arterial pH above 7.20. Dose of sodium bicarbonate in mEq = base deficit × body weight (kg) × 0.3.

In seriously ill infants, umbilical arterial catheter should be inserted to obtain samples for acid–base parameters and blood gases. The arterial blood samples may also be obtained from temporal, brachial or radial arteries. Transcutaneous continuous monitoring of oxygen or pulse oximetry is a reliable, non-invasive technique which is being increasingly used in many centers. Close surveillance of biochemical variables, such as hypoglycemia, hypocalcemia, hyperkalemia and hyperbilirubinemia is essential to guide the supportive therapy. Administration of volume expanders, like physiologic saline, plasma and blood, is indicated to correct shock. Dopamine may be required to improve cardiac contractions.

Oxygen

The baby's head should be enclosed in a plastic box and oxygen administered to relieve the cyanosis or to achieve the arterial PaO_2 between 50 and 80 mm Hg or arterial oxygen saturation between 90 and 95%. The concentration of ambient oxygen should be checked with an oxygen analyzer whenever baby's condition is assessed. The ambient oxygen concentration should be kept at 5 to 10% higher than the cyanotic threshold of the sick infant. During recovery, ambient oxygen concentration should be reduced by 10% every hour till infant is receiving less than 40% oxygen.

Warmth and Humidity

The skin temperature should be maintained around 36.5°C either by manually altering the temperature of the over head radiant warmer of open care system or by employing servo control system. The infant should be nursed in a thermoneutral environment. Humidity should be maintained above 60%. The chest should not be clothed in order to facilitate the observations but the baby should be enclosed in a perspex heat shield to prevent heat and insensible water loss.

Antibiotics

We routinely administer ampicillin and gentamicin intravenously because of the difficulty of ruling out with certainty the possibility of underlying pulmonary infection. The antibiotics can be taken off after 72 hours, if clinical course and investigations rule out underlying infection. Ampicillin is the drug of choice, if listeriosis is seriously considered. Benzyl penicillin is life saving for treatment of streptococcal pneumonia. During the course of therapy, the antibiotics may have to be changed to treat the superadded infection. Septic screening and periodic cultures from endotracheal tube and blood are needed to guide the antimicrobial therapy. Urine should be examined for budding yeasts and hyphae to rule out candidemia.

Vitamin E

During therapy of RDS, excessive concentrations of oxygen in the arterial blood and respiratory air passages may lead to development of retinopathy of prematurity (ROP) and bronchopulmonary dysplasia, respectively. To prevent damage due to oxygen therapy, it is desirable that FiO_2 should be maintained between 0.4 and 0.6 and PaO_2 should be monitored and kept between 50 and 80 mm Hg. Vitamin E is a biologic antioxidant that inhibits the peroxidation of membrane lipids by free radicals, such as superoxide. There are conflicting reports regarding prophylactic utility of vitamin E for protection against ROP and bronchopulmonary dysplasia. It is recommended that low birth weight babies receiving oxygen therapy may be administered vitamin E in a dose of 100 iu/kg per day intramuscularly from birth onwards in order to maintain blood vitamin E levels between 2.0 and 3.0 iu/dL. Excessive intake of vitamin E may be associated with intracranial hemorrhage and necrotizing enterocolitis (if hyperosomolar oral preparation is used). High dose vitamin E therapy is controversial and should be avoided.

NSAIDs

In preterm infants with RDS, incidence of patent ductus arteriosus is relatively high and may aggravate hypoxemia by opening up of right-to-left shunts and congestive heart failure. During recovery, sudden fall in pulmonary vascular resistance may lead to left-to-right shunt through PDA resulting in CHF. Apart from decongestive measures, indomethacin which is inhibitor of prostaglandin synthetase has been used for pharmacological closure of ductus arteriosus. Indomethacin is administered in a dose of 0.2 mg/kg orally or preferably intravenously every 12-hourly for a total of three doses. Due to its potential toxicity, its use is contraindicated in infants with severe jaundice, bleeding, necrotizing enterocolitis and renal insufficiency. Alternatively, ibuprofen 10 mg/kg stat followed by 5 mg/kg at 24 hr and 48 hr can be given orally or intravenously. Paracetamol is as effective as indomethacin in closing hs-PDA. It is given in a dose of 15 mg/kg orally every 6 hours for 48–72 hours. Early side effects like oliguria, elevation of creatinine and thrombocytopenia are minimal with paracetamol. Surgical closure of ductus is required when NSAIDs fail and infant has intractable congestive heart failure with progressive cardiomegaly and deteriorating pulmonary compliance.

Surfactant

Surfactant therapy is the most important clinical advance in neonatal intensive care in the past 3–4 decades and has been shown by several clinical trials to be useful both for prevention as well as treatment of RDS. The efficacy of surfactant replacement therapy (SRT) in reducing mortality in preterm infants with RDS is proven beyond doubt. It improves oxygenation by resolving atelectases and improving lung compliance. It reduces the duration of ventilatory support, decreases incidence of air leaks and improves survival. Surfactant of human, bovine (Survanta, Surfacten, Infasurf, Calfactant, Alveofact, Neosurf or BLES™) or porcine (Curosurf, Poractant-α) origin and synthetic (Exosurf, DPPC/PG, ALEC, Surfaxin, Venticute) preparations are available. Natural surfactant is slightly more effective than synthetic. The use of surfactant is restricted in developing countries due to its exhorbitant cost and limited availability. Surfactant is now available in Indian market and has been found to be cost-effective by reducing hospital stay and risk of complications. But it must be used with discretion (preferably in babies >1000 g or >28 weeks gestation) and its use should be restricted to NICUs having optimal infrastructure and specially trained nurses. The indications for surfactant therapy and respiratory support in preterm infants with RDS is shown in Figure 19.4. It is possible to use minimally invasive surfactant therapy (MIST) without intubation. An orogastric tube 5 Fr is inserted through the vocal cords with the help of a laryngoscope (Miller 00 blades). The appropriate dose of prewarmed surfactant is administered through OG tube slowly in 30–45s. nCPAP is continued throughout the procedure. The MIST technique has comparable efficacy and outcome compared to more invasive InSurE prcocedure.

Adequate oxygenation, ventilation, perfusion and monitoring should be established before starting "rescue" treatment of RDS with surfactant. It is indicated in premature infants ≥28 weeks gestational age with RDS needing CPAP with ≥50% oxygen or assisted ventilation. Early administration of rescue surfactant therapy is associated with improved outcome. It is administered intratracheally by instillation through a 5 Fr end-hole catheter inserted into the endotracheal tube with the tip of catheter protruding just beyond the end of the endotracheal tube. The dose of Survanta is 100 mg/kg (4 mL/kg available in 4 mL and 8 mL vials) while Curosurf is given in a dose of 100–200 mg/kg (1.25–1.5 mL/kg) and is available as

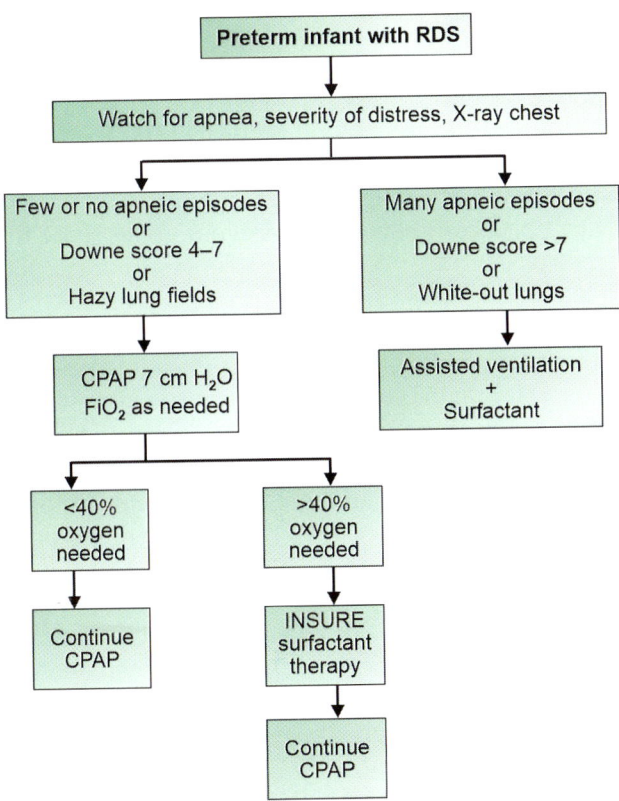

INSURE: In (intubate), Sur (surfactant), E (extubate)
CPAP: Continous positive airway pressure
FiO$_2$: Fractional concentration of oxygen in the inspired air.

Figure 19.4 Flowchart for management of an infant with RDS.

1.5 mL and 2.5 mL vials. It is adminstered through the side port of ET in the ventilator circuit adjacent to the endotracheal tube adapter or through dual lumen ET tube without the need of removing the infant from the ventilator. Recent studies have shown that there is no need to use different positions for administration of surfactant and it should be administered slowly over a 15-minute period in a single dose or two aliquots either through the catheter inserted into the endotracheal tube or a side-port adapter. Infant is kept in a supine position and head is maintained in midline. The previous practice of giving aliquots of surfactant in different positions of the infant is no longer recommended. After bolus administration of surfactant, the infant should be bagged with 40% oxygen or it is allowed to uniformly spread throughout the lungs with the help of assisted ventilation. At the time of administration, the surfactant should not be shaken vigorously and it should be gently swirled to bring it to room temperature. The left over surfactant should be stored in the refrigerator and must be used within 24 hours. Depending upon the severity of disease process, repeat doses may have to be administered after 6–12 hours. However, there is no clear benefit of giving more than 2 doses of Exosurf or 4 doses of Survanta. Natural or animal-derived surfactants are preferred in view of their higher efficacy but they are more expensive.

Surfactant therapy is followed by improved oxygenation requiring reduction of mean airway pressure and FiO$_2$ to prevent development of air leaks and damage to retina and lungs due to hyperoxia. The risk of PDA with left-to-right shunt is higher among treated infants due to sudden fall in pulmonary vascular resistance, following correction of hypoxia and acidosis. The common adverse reactions to surfactant therapy include apnea, hypotension, pulmonary hemorrhage, endotracheal tube blockage and bradycardia. These immediate complications can be reduced by slow administration of surfactant and by decreasing FiO$_2$ and mean airway pressure following administration. Surfactant therapy has not been shown to consistently reduce the incidence of intraventricular hemorrhage, necrotizing enterocolitis, retinopathy of prematurity and chronic lung disease.

Continuous Positive Airway Pressure (CPAP)

Nasal CPAP (nCPAP) coupled with surfactant replacement is the modality of choice for management of preterm infants with RDS in low and middle income countries. Infants with HMD are handicapped by reduced lung compliance and alveolar collapse during expiration. Administration of oxygen under positive pressure ("bubble" CPAP) prevents alveolar collapse and ensures gas exchange throughout the respiratory cycle. Bubble CPAP is indicated and useful in preterm infants with RDS and decreased lung compliance.

It is indicated if arterial oxygen tension remains below 50 mm Hg even when more than 60% oxygen is being administered through a head box. It can also be tried as an initial measure in seriously sick infants with HMD and apneic attacks before attaching them to a ventilator. CPAP can be effectively given through short silastic nasal tubes or short binasal prongs which eliminates the need for endotracheal intubation. INSURE technique (*IN*tubation → *SUR*factant therapy → *E*xtubation) can be followed for administration of surfactant to infants on CPAP inorder to minimize the need for assisted ventilation and attendant complications.

Humidified and warm air–oxygen mixture (maximum flow rate of 5 liters per minute) is passed through T-tube or elbow which is attached to an endotracheal tube or nasal prongs. The screw clamp

Respiratory Disorders

19

on the reservoir bag is used to control the flow of gas and maintain a constant positive pressure within the system. The side arm which is attached with pressure manometer terminates in a water column with a maximum blow off pressure of 15 cm H_2O. Transcutaneous oxygen concentration is monitored. Initially 4 cm H_2O of continuous airway pressure is used. If there is no improvement in clinical condition and arterial blood gases within 15 minutes, airway pressure is gradually increased by increments of 1 cm H_2O up to a maximum of about 8 cm H_2O. The positive pressure at the airways is not completely transmitted to the pleural sac because of severely reduced lung compliance. Therefore, venous return and cardiac output are not compromised. Excessive CO_2 accumulation may occur due to diminished expiration and should be corrected by reducing the airway pressure. An orogastric tube is always placed to decompress swallowed air from stomach.

Weaning from CPAP should be a slow process and it may take several days to disconnect it. Once condition of the infant is stabilized and arterial oxygen tension maintained between 50 and 80 mm Hg, ambient oxygen concentration is gradually reduced by decrements of 5% until it is brought down to 40%. At this stage, CPAP pressure is slowly reduced by 1.0 cm H_2O at a time. During weaning, arterial blood gases should be closely monitored so that ambient oxygen concentration and CPAP pressures are maintained at a level which provides satisfactory oxygenation. When CPAP is 3 to 4 cm and ambient oxygen concentration <40%, the device is removed and infant is placed in an oxygen hood.

Assisted Ventilation

Assisted ventilation can improve survival of infants with severe HMD and respiratory failure from any cause. It is highly specialized and expensive modality of management which cannot be established merely by purchasing a sophisticated ventilator. The essential prerequisites for establishing ventilator facilities are availability of excellent supportive care with experieced medical and nursing personnel, vital sign monitors and round-the-clock facilities for monitoring of blood gases, acid–base parameters and imaging studies. Transcutaneous monitoring of blood gases and pulse oximetry have reduced the need for frequent blood sampling but it has escalated costs and introduced problems of interpretation of changes in blood gases.

Assisted ventilation is needed, if despite 8 cm H_2O CPAP and 60% FiO_2, arterial PO_2 remains below

50 mm Hg, or PCO_2 is greater than 50 mm Hg and pH cannot be maintained above 7.2 (despite alkali therapy). Babies with frequent and prolonged apneic attacks, unresponsive to CPAP or manual IPPV, also require assisted ventilation. In babies with HMD, ventilation with positive end-expiratory pressure (PEEP) is recommended to prevent collapse of the alveoli and bronchioles at the end of respiratory cycle thus allowing gaseous exchange even during expiratory phase. In babies with HMD, initial ventilatory settings include PIP 20–25 cm H_2O, PEEP 4–6 cm H_2O, rate 25–30 breaths/min, inspiratory time 0.3–0.4 sec and FiO_2 between 0.5 and 1.0.

Apart from continuous transcutaneous monitoring, arterial blood gases and pH should be monitored every 4 to 6 hourly. The goal of therapy should be to maintain PaO_2 between 50 and 80 mm Hg, $PaCO_2$ between 35 and 45 mm Hg and pH between 7.3 and 7.4. The baby on ventilator needs to be closely observed all the time for movements of chest, manometer needle and clicking sound of ventilator. During recovery, infant is gradually weaned to patient triggered ventilation (IMV) followed by CPAP before he is completely weaned off. During ventilation, physiotherapy and oropharyngeal and tracheal toilet should receive special attention. For details of newer modalities of assisted ventilation, refer to Chapter 27.

Exchange Blood Transfusion

The role of exchange blood transfusion in the management of HMD is controversial. Improvement in pulmonary ventilation or perfusion or both have been reported following exchange transfusion. Because adult hemoglobin binds oxygen less tightly as compared to fetal hemoglobin, there is a potential risk of retinal damage by oxygen even in the absence of environmental hyperoxia. Moreover, exchange transfusion is a potentially hazardous procedure in a sick infant.

Complications

When there is sudden and unexpected deterioration in the condition of a baby with respiratory distress syndrome, following conditions should be looked for and appropriately managed:
- Intraventricular hemorrhage
- Pnumothorax or air leaks
- Pulmonary infection
- Massive pulmonary hemorrhage
- Hypoglycemia
- Disseminated intravascular coagulation

- Cardiac failure (PDA and infusion overload)
- Severe metabolic alterations

Prognosis

It depends upon the gestational maturity and birth weight of the infant, severity of RDS, associated complications and quality of neonatal care. Outcome is extremely poor in HMD with a case fatality rate of 50% when exogenous surfactant therapy and adequate ventilatory facilities are not available. There is an increased risk of bronchial reactivity, recurrent wheezing and evidences of pulmonary dysfunction on follow-up among survivors of infants with HMD and bronchopulmonary dysplasia. There appears to be an increased risk of a long-lasting damage to any organ when noxious insult operates during the crucial phase of anatomical and functional development. It needs to be emphasized that neonatal disorders not merely carry an exceedingly high mortality but survivors are at an increased risk to develop a life long physical or neuromotor disability due to permanent structural and functional damage to the evolving organs.

MASSIVE PULMONARY HEMORRHAGE

About 5 to 10% of neonatal autopsies show evidences of massive pulmonary hemorrhage. When confluent hemorrhage involves at least two lobes of the lungs it is termed massive pulmonary hemorrhage. The pathogenesis of this disorder is poorly understood, the clinical diagnosis is difficult and outcome is generally fatal. Babies with intrauterine growth retardation, severe hemolytic disease of the newborn, twin gestation, congenital heart disease, PDA, sepsis, cold injury, perinatal distress factors, HMD and those born to a diabetic mother are prone to develop massive pulmonary hemorrhage though this may occur even in a relatively healthy term and preterm babies. Massive pulmonary hemorrhage may be a manifestation of disseminated intravascular coagulation, hemorrhagic pulmonary edema due to acute left heart failure and capillary damage because of bolus injection of hyperosmolar sodium bicarbonate solution. Exogenous surfactant given as a preventive strategy may be associated with increased risk of pulmonary hemorrhage. The incidence of the condition falls as the quality of perinatal services improve. The hemorrhages may be alveolar, interstitial or mixed. It is characterized by sudden apneic attacks or dyspnea associated with frothy blood welling through the nose and the oral cavity. There may or may not be excessive bleeding from the venipuncture sites. Skiagram of chest may show diffuse opacification of one or both lungs and the appearance of air bronchogram.

Maintaining a clear airway, administration of fresh blood transfusion, fresh frozen plasma and furosemide are recommended. The bleeding diathesis should be managed by administration of vitamin K, cryoprecipitate and platlets. Mechanical ventilation with 6 to 8 cm H_2O positive end-expiratory pressure (PEEP) helps to decrease the leakage of hemorrhagic fluid into the alveoli. High-frequency oscillatory or jet ventilation using high mean airway pressure may be more effective and should be tried when facilities are available. Adequate tissue perfusion should be maintained by use of inotropic drugs. The hemodynamically significant PDA (hs-PDA) should be closed by using NSAID, if there are no systemic bleeding manifestations.

PNEUMOTHORAX

Spontaneous pneumothorax occurs in 1 to 2% of newborn babies. It may follow aggressive resuscitation of asphyxiated infant and during CPAP and PEEP ventilation. Additional predisposing factors include meconium aspiration, pulmonary hypoplasia, assisted ventilation and staphylococcal pneumonia. Sudden deterioration of an infant with respiratory distress and cyanosis should alert to the possibility of pneumothorax. Diminished movements of chest and reduced breath sounds with displacement of mediastinum are diagnostic. Prompt bedside diagnosis can be made by transillumination using fiberoptic probe (Figure 19.5). Skiagram of chest AP and cross-table view should be taken to confirm the diagnosis (Figure 19.6). For other details and management, refer to Chapter 29. The practice of administration of 100% oxygen as a therapeutic measure is not recommended due to risk of hyperoxia.

TRANSIENT TACHYPNEA OF THE NEWBORN (TTNB)

The condition is common among term babies born by cesarean section or precipitate delivery. The other risk factors include delayed cord clamping or cord milking, macrosomia, male sex, excessive maternal sedation, prolonged labor with administration of large amount of intravenous fluids to the mother. It is also called as "wet lung syndrome" or type II RDS.

It is characterized by onset of tachypnea in a cesarean-born baby after a few hours of birth. The

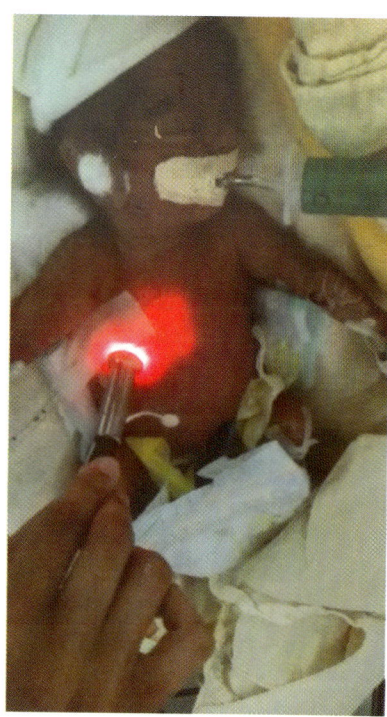

Figure 19.5 Cold light transillumination showing pneumothorax on the right side.

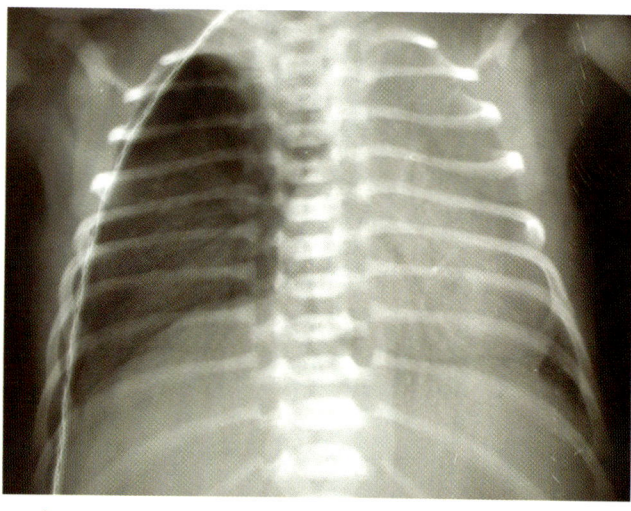

Figure 19.6 Pneumothorax right side following CPAP.

respiratory rate may vary from 80 to 100 per minute, intercostal recessions are absent or minimal, the child remains alert and maintains good color. Some infants may require 40% oxygen to maintain adequate oxygenation. The baby improves within 2 to 3 days without any specific therapy. The condition may represent a mild equivalent of HMD or it may be due to failure of drainage of alveolar fluid through lymphatics which are engorged, thus reducing lung compliance or may simply be due to placental transfusion. It is more common in babies delivered by

cesarean section because lung fluid is normally squeezed out during vaginal delivery. The skiagram of the chest shows hyperinflated lungs, linear streaking at hila due to dilated lymphatics, interlobar fluid and mild cardiomegaly. The diagnosis is made by exclusion of other conditions and benign course of disease. Oxygen should be administered with a head box to maintain SaO$_2$ between 90 and 95%. The role of furosemide is controversial. Oral feeds can be started when respiratory rate is less than 60/min.

Wilson-Mikity Syndrome (Pulmonary Dysmaturity)

This rare condition is limited to babies with a birth weight of less than 1500 g who develop symptoms of mild respiratory distress at the age of 2 to 3 weeks. Skiagram of chest shows diffuse, bilateral, coarse lace-like pattern of infiltrates with areas of hyperaeration due to cystic interstitial emphysema. Symptoms become increasingly severe reaching maximum intensity at about 4–8 weeks after onset. At present, this condition is considered as a part of the spectrum of bronchopulmonary dysplasia. Fatality rate varies between 25 and 50%. Among survivors, symptoms gradually disappear over a period of several weeks and skiagram of chest returns back to normal by 6 months to 2 years of age. Etiology is unknown and pathological changes are nonspecific and dominated by pulmonary fibrosis and uneven pattern of aeration with areas of over-expansion suggestive of obstructive emphysema.

BRONCHOPULMONARY DYSPLASIA (BPD)

Bronchopulmonary dysplasia (BPD) is a chronic lung disorder mostly affecting preterm babies (even term babies may be effected) recovering from respiratory distress syndrome (RDS). The condition has been appropriately renamed as chronic lung disease (CLD). In tertiary care centers, it is recognized to affect almost 15% of preterm babies, the incidence being higher among extremely LBW babies. The incidence of BPD is likely to increase in developing countries following establishment of more effective ventilatory facilities.

Etiology

The etiology of BPD is multifactorial and condition occurs due to interaction between inherent under-development of lungs and use of certain therapeutic modalities, like oxygen administration and assisted ventilation. The most consistent etiologic denominator is barotrauma due to prolonged assisted ventilation irrespective of gestational maturity of the infant. Air leaks producing pulmonary interstitial emphysema (PIE) is a common harbinger of BPD. Infants managed with negative pressure ventilation and oxygen therapy have not been shown to develop this complication. Fluid overload due to overinfusion and increased pulmonary perfusion due to PDA are important predisposing factors. Early development of lung inflammatory changes, increased airway resistance and disordered fibrosis are commonly associated.

Pathophysiology

The pathological changes include mucosal metaplasia, lung inflammation, disruption in the integrity of respiratory epithelium, interstitial fibrosis and smooth muscle hyperplasia. There is interstitial edema and reactive airway disease. There is increased work of breathing demanding more oxygen and calories for maintenance of physical growth and promotion of lung healing. Because of hyperplasia of peri-bronchiolar smooth muscles, pulmonary hypertension supervenes leading to development of chronic cor pulmonale and worsening of clinical condition.

Diagnosis

The earliest evidence of BPD is the delay or difficulty in weaning a preterm baby with RDS from a ventilator. After weaning, the infant continues to have tachypnea, subcostal retractions, wheezing and varying degrees of hypoxemia and hypercapnia. The infant remains oxygen-dependent for several days or months (beyond 28 days of life or 36 weeks of post-conceptional maturity) and does not gain weight. Hypertension may occur due to prolonged use of xanthine derivatives and corticosteroids. The calories are being consumed and wasted to support the work of breathing and promote reparative changes in the lungs rather than for maintenance of physical growth.

The characteristic changes on a plain skiagram of chest evolve over several days and weeks. In the earliest stage, BPD is indistinguishable from severe HMD with difficult and protracted weaning (stage I). In most cases of HMD, lungs return to normal by the end of first week. But in an infant who is destined to develop BPD, streaky densities due to atelectatic patches and air bronchogram persist during second week of life (stage II). Stage III is characterized by areas of translucent cysts (localized emphysema) with streaky densities and hyperaeration of lungs. In due course of time, cystic areas become more widespread and surrounded by dense fibrotic bands with increasing hyperaeration of lungs (stage IV) (Figure 19.7).

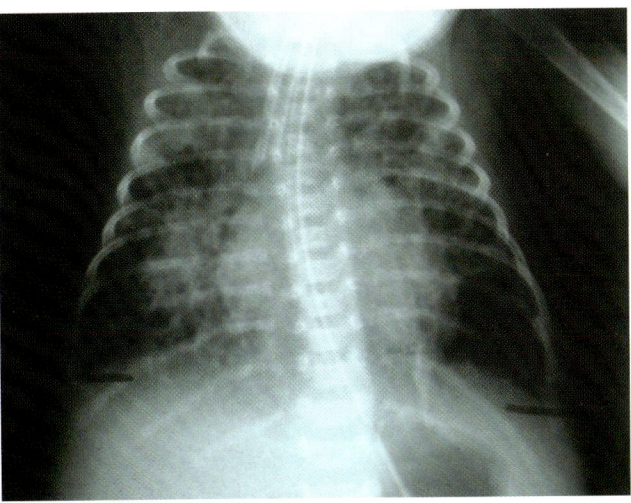

Figure 19.7 Chest X-ray of a preterm baby with postnatal age of 6 weeks showing classical changes of stage 4 broncho-pulmonary dysplasia. There are areas of fibrosis along with emphysematous changes. The costochondral junctions are enlarged due to osteopenia of prematurity.

Arterial blood gases may show low PaO_2, raised $PaCO_2$ and combined respiratory cum metabolic acidosis. EKG may show evidences of right ventricular hypertrophy due to impending cor pulmonale. When indicated, point-of-care echocardiography may be required to exclude existence of PDA. Pulmonary function tests are likely to show evidences of increased airway resistance and decreased lung compliance.

Prevention

The incidence of BPD can be reduced, if etiological factors are carefully controlled during the management of preterm infants with RDS. Improvement in the skills and technology for assisted ventilation of babies with respiratory failure is crucial for reducing pulmonary morbidity and sequelae among NICU survivals. Antenatal administration of dexamethasone when labor starts before 34 weeks of gestation and early administration of surfactant when indicated are known to reduce the incidence and severity of HMD and subsequent development of BPD. Efforts should be made to treat infants with RDS with minimal effective airway pressure and FiO_2 for the shortest duration of time. High frequency jet or oscillatory ventilation is associated with reduced risk of CLD. Intravenous infusion rates should be kept low to prevent pumonary edema and opening up of ductus arteriosus. Pharmacologic closure of ductus should be attempted as soon as PDA is identified. Prophylactic utility of vitamin E and other antioxidants is controversial. There is evidence to suggest that vitamin A

5000 iu IM 3 times weekly for 4 weeks may reduce the incidence of CLD in ELBW babies by 10%.

Treatment

The baby should be nursed in a thermoneutral environment and fluid therapy should be judiciously monitored to prevent over hydration. To meet additional caloric demands of work of breathing, caloric intake should be enhanced to provide 150–200 kcal/kg/d orally or 115 kcal/kg/d through TPN to sustain growth. Intercurrent pulmonary infections should be adequately treated and unusual organisms, like chlamydiae and *Pneumocystis jirovecii*, (previously *P. carinii*) looked for. The arterial oxygen saturation should be maintained between 90 and 95% by administration of humidified oxygen through a head box. Oxygen therapy also helps to sustain physical growth, reduce the risk and delay the development of pulmonary hypertension and cor pulmonale.

Diuretics are useful but care should be taken to maintain electrolyte homeostasis. Furosemide (1 mg/kg daily or every alternate day single dose IM or IV) is the diuretic of choice. Apart from reducing pulmonary edema, furosemide causes vasodilatation, decreases right ventricular end-diastolic volume and pulmonary capillary pressure. There is evidence to suggest that furosemide therapy is associated with improvement in both lung compliance and lung resistance. The side effects of prolonged furosemide therapy include electrolyte imbalance (hyponatremia, metabolic alkalosis due to chloride depletion), hypercalciuria, nephrocalcinosis, osteopenia and ototoxicity. In view of its potent efficacy, furosemide therapy is started when weaning from ventilation is contemplated. As soon as the infant is tolerating enteral feeds and is stable, it is preferable to change over to administration of chlorthiazide (10–20 mg/kg/d q 12 hr oral) and spironolactone (1–3 mg/kg/d q 12 hr oral) because of reduced risk of side effects. Diuretics are continued until the infant no longer requires oxygen therapy. Bronchospasm should be managed by nebulization of salbutamol (0.10–0.15 mL/kg/dose of 5 mg/mL solution q 8 hr). It is effective and relatively free from side effects. Theophylline (6 mg/kg loading dose IV followed by 1–2 mg/kg/d q 8–12 hr for maintenance) is used in infants with severe and recurrent bronchospasm.

A trial of corticosteroids is indicated after 2-weeks of assisted ventilation in an infant with HMD, when it is becoming impossible to wean off a stable patient from a ventilator. A short course of dexamethasone 0.25 mg/kg/dose IV every 12 hourly may be given

for 3 days. If significant improvement is observed in ventilator settings, it should be continued in a gradually decreasing doses over the next 2–6 weeks depending upon the severity of disease process. In view of serious short-term (hypertension, hyperglycemia, GI bleeding, infection) and long-term (poor brain growth, cerebral palsy) side effects of postnatal corticosteroids, the lowest dose should be used for the shortest duration. Hydrocortisone is preferred because of lower risk of adverse effects on central nervous system. The presence of pulmonary infection and PDA contraindicate the use of corticosteroids. Inhaled steroids are effective to facilitate extubation but they have not been shown to reduce the incidence and severity of CLD.

Despite good management, about one-third of infants with BPD succumb to the disease. Survivors have significant long-term mobidity due to pulmonary dysfunction, recurrent respiratory infections, reactive airway disease and neurodevelopmental handicaps.

Pleural Effusion

This may be associated with generalized hydrops fetalis or occur as isolated chylothorax. The baby develops respiratory distress soon after birth and may need urgent thoracocentesis during resuscitation in the labor room. Chylothorax is more common on the right side. It may occur due to traumatic rupture of thoracic duct because of congenital fistula between the thoracic duct and pleural space or due to hypoplasia of lymphatic system. The chemical analysis of pleural aspirate shows presence of fat, cholesterol and protein. Spontaneous recovery usually occurs but at times feeding with medium chain triglycerides is necessary to reduce production of chyle.

Congenital Malformations

Refer to Chapter 25 for surgical causes of respiratory distress.

Pulmonary Agenesis or Hypoplasia

The baby with bilateral pulmonary agenesis may be born dead or dies soon after birth. Diagnosis may be suspected by associated oligohydramnios and Potter facies due to renal agenesis which is characterized by depressed bridge of the nose, anti-mongoloid slant of the eyes, retrognathia and soft flabby low set ears. Hypoplasia of the lungs may occur as an isolated disorder or more often it is associated with diaphragmatic hernia and other space consuming lesions in the thorax. The diagnosis is suspected when difficulty is encountered in inflating the lungs with usual inspiratory pressure while ventilating through endo-tracheal tube. The aggressive efforts for ventilation are often followed by development of pneumothorax. The affected side looks opaque with heart and mediastinum pulled towards the same side because of loss of volume unless there is associated diaphragmatic hernia or pneumothorax. Pulmonary hypertension often complicates the clinical picture.

Pulmonary Lymphangiectasis

This is characterized by respiratory distress and cyanosis dating from birth with progressive fatal course. The diagnosis is aided by detection of either lymphangioma, lymphedema or chylous ascites. The cardiac anomalies, such as anomalous pulmonary venous drainage, has been detected in 50% of the autopsied cases. The skiagram of the chest may reveal lacy reticular pattern, often denser than that seen in HMD and areas of hyperaeration in both the lungs.

Cardiac Failure

It may be impossible at times to differentiate between the respiratory distress of pulmonary origin and due to cardiac failure. The enlarging liver, cyanosis out of proportion to the degree of respiratory distress and its worsening on crying, significant cardiac murmurs and cardiomegaly favor the diagnosis of congestive cardiac failure. The intercostal retractions are either absent or minimal as opposed to the respiratory distress of pulmonary origin. Puffiness or sudden weight gain may also be noticed. The exposure of the baby to an ambient oxygen concentration of 100% fails to raise his arterial PaO_2 above 90 mm Hg in infants with cyanotic congenital heart disease.

Central Nervous System Disorders

CNS Trauma and Birth Asphyxia

It is more often characterized by apneic attacks rather than respiratory distress and clinical picture is dominated by evidences of depression or irritability of central nervous system. In respiratory distress of central origin, breathing is rapid and shallow. Many a times, respiratory distress in such babies is due to associated pulmonary disorders, such as aspiration, hemorrhage and pneumothorax.

Diaphragmatic Paralysis

Following a difficult breech delivery or extraction, the baby may manifest dyspnea soon after birth or it may remain asymptomatic. The diminished respiratory excursions of the diaphragm on the affected side may not be evident clinically. The condition is common in large babies delivered by breech extraction leading to avulsion of nerves of brachial plexus. The diagnosis is often suspected by the associated presence of Erb's paralysis which is seen in about 75% cases of diaphragmatic paralysis. The majority of the cases are on the right side. Roentgenogram of chest may be normal in the neonatal period or may reveal mild elevation of affected dome of diaphragm. As the affected dome of the diaphragm rises higher, the heart may be displaced towards the opposite side. Fluoroscopy shows characteristic paradoxical movements of the paralyzed leaf of the diaphragm with each respiration. Eventration of diaphragm due to protrusion of abdominal contents or aplasia or atrophy is more common on the left side. It is not associated with Erb's palsy and paradoxical movements on breathing are less commonly seen.

Paralysis of Intercostal Muscles

It is characterized by rapid shallow breathing in association with severe hypotonia and paralysis.

Metabolic Disorders

Acidotic breathing may be encountered in babies with diarrhea and dehydration, uremia and organic acidemias especially ketotic hyperglycinemia. Seizures dominate the clinical picture in infants with organic acidemias. Mild tachypnea may occur among preterm infants having late-onset metabolic acidosis. The response to alkali administration is dramatic.

Differential Diagnosis of RDS

The respiratory rate of high-risk infants should be closely monitored during first day of life because most conditions causing respiratory distress manifest during first 24 hours. A careful clinical evaluation should be made to identify the organ system producing respiratory distress (Table 19.5). The age at onset of respiratory distress and presence of associated or predisposing conditions offer useful diagnostic clues (Table 19.3). Gastric aspirate cytology and shake test are useful and simple cot-side tests to screen for intrauterine pneumonia and hyaline membrane disease, respectively. Septic screening and appropriate cultures should be taken to rule out infection. The auscultatory evaluation of chest is often unrewarding in newborn babies. Therefore, reliance should be placed on radiological examination of chest to exclude life-threatening malformations. Serial roentgenograms of chest are useful to assess the progress of disease.

Respiratory Disorders

19

TABLE 19.5 Clinical differences between respiratory distress syndrome on the basis of the system affected

Symptoms and signs	Pulmonary disorders	Cardiac failure	CNS disorders	Metabolic acidosis
■ Tachypnea	Moderate-marked	Moderate-marked	Mild-moderate. Apneic attacks or irregular breathing	Mild-moderate
■ Intercostal recessions	Marked	Absent or minimal	Absent or diaphragmatic	Absent
■ Expiratory grunt	Present	Absent	Absent	Absent
■ Cyanosis	Mild	Severe	Mild	Absent
■ Hepatomegaly	Absent or pushed down	Present	Absent	Absent
■ Mediastinal displacement	May be present	Absent	Rare	Absent
■ Auscultatory findings	Pulmonic findings may or may not be present	Cardiac murmur and abnormalities of heart sounds	Absent	Absent
■ Associated or predisposing features	Immaturity, polyhydramnios, meconium-stained liquor, prolonged rupture of membranes and characteristic facies	Down syndrome, rubella, hydrops fetalis, large-for-dates	Breech delivery, Erb's palsy, hypotonia	Preterm, high protein intake, inborn error of metabolism
■ Stridor	May occur	Rare	Absent or rare	Absent
■ Seizures	Rare	Absent	May occur	Common in association with inborn errors of metabolism.
■ Blood gases	$PaO_2\downarrow$, $PaCO_2\uparrow$	$PaO_2\downarrow$, $PaCO_2$N	PaO_2N, $PaCO_2$N	PaO_2N, $PaCO_2\downarrow$
■ Effect of 100% oxygen on PaO_2	Raised	No effect	Raised	Not needed

Availability of facilities to monitor the status of arterial gases and acid–base parameters is essential to assess the severity and prognosis of the disease process. Respiratory distress syndrome of the newborn cannot be managed adequately, if facilities for gasometry and assessment of acid–base status are either periodic or unavailable.

RECURRENT APNEA

Intermittent cyanosis associated with repeated protracted apneic episodes is generally known as 'recurrent neonatal apnea' or apneic spells. Apnea is defined as cessation of respiration for >20 seconds or cessation of respiration of any duration accompanied by bradycardia (<100 bpm) and/or cyanosis. This is an important cause of mortality and brain damage in immature babies especially those with a gestation of less than 32 weeks. It is characterized by sudden cessation of breathing followed by cyanosis and limpness. Apneic spells of 20 seconds or more in duration are associated with fall in arterial oxygen saturation and bradycardia. Cyanosis appears, if apnea is prolonged up to 30 seconds. After about 20 seconds of apnea, the baby develops bradycardia and may become unresponsive to stimulation. The infant has deceptively good color during the intervals in-between the attacks. Apneic attacks are common in extremely premature babies. Around 20 to 25% of babies weighing less than 1500 g may manifest apneic attacks. The condition demands prompt physical stimulation or artificial ventilation and carries grave prognosis. In term and near term infants, apneic spells are usually associated with serious underlying conditions, like birth asphyxia, sepsis, intracranial hemorrhage, seizures or metabolic disorder. Apnea of prematurity should be differentiated from the following conditions.

Periodic breathing About 30 to 45% of preterm infants breath irregularly, switching easily from predominantly periodic to more regular respirations. It is characterized by following features:

i. Rapid respiratory movements (V) are interrupted by intervals of apnea (A) of more than 3 seconds. Apnea usually lasts 5 to 10 seconds and period of rapid breathing varies from 15 to 20 seconds.

ii. Ratio of duration of breathing to duration of apnea (V/A) should not be more than four or less than one.

iii. The duration of apnea and breathing (A + V) is usually 30 seconds or less.

iv. The periodic breathing occurs for about 2 minutes in a total period of 10 minutes.

The periodic breathing occurs mainly during wakeful state (REM sleep) and baby may abruptly change from one breathing pattern to the other. The period of rapid breathing being more than the duration of apnea, the net ventilation is actually more with resultant respiratory alkalosis and rise in pH. The cyanosis and bradycardia do not occur but administration of oxygen may abolish periodic breathing. The regular breathing pattern is established at a post-conceptional age of 40 weeks. About 50% of full term babies at a height of more than 5,000 feet above sea level may manifest periodic breathing. The absence of crescendo pattern of breathing and presence of definite periodicity distinguish this condition from Cheyne-Stokes breathing.

Cyanotic spell It is defined as sudden attack of cyanosis with slow, shallow and irregular respirations without significant bradycardia. Cyanosis precedes breathing irregularity and apnea never occurs. The cyanotic spells are generally seen in association with pulmonary and cardiac disorders.

Subtle convulsions Sudden tonic convulsions may be followed by cessation of breathing and sometimes cyanosis. At times an apneic attack may lead to a tonic fit due to cerebral anoxia. The sequence of events, however, are different and distinctive. The sudden alteration of tone, twitching, staring look and uprolling of eyes may suggest the possibility of a convulsion. It is usually associated with tachycardia at the onset. The constant monitoring of the baby under aEEG is diagnostic.

Pathophysiology

The exact pathogenesis of recurrent apnea is uncertain. Immaturity of medullary respiratory center with lack of effective respiratory drive appears to be the basic abnormality because the condition is limited to preterm infants. Hypoxemia due to any cause predisposes to apneic attacks. Efferent discharge from medullary respiratory center is highly dependent upon the character and intensity of a variety of afferent impulses to the center. Sudden rise in ambient environmental temperature, vigorous uninterrupted nasopharyngeal suction, neck flexion and lung inflation (Head pardoxical reflex) are known to cause reflex apnea. The apneic attacks are more common during REM sleep which appears to be inhibitory to the medullary centers. There is some evidence to suggest that deficiency of central neurotransmitters (catecholamines) among preterm infants is associated with apneic attacks. The apnea may be central, obstructive or mixed. In central apnea, both the inspiratory effort and airflow cease simultaneously and there are no movements of chest wall. Obstructive apnea is characterized by absence of airflow despite having inspiratory efforts and movements of chest. Obstructive apnea may occur due to sudden collapse of the soft tissue of hypopharynx or due to anomalies in the upper respiratory passages and pulmonary infections.

In most babies, the apneic attacks occur without any premonitory changes in respiration, heart rate and blood pressure. The continuous monitoring of vital functions has shown that apnea is followed by bradycardia and increase in pulse pressure. The bradycardia is either due to direct effect of hypoxia on the heart or as a result of hypoxic stimulation of carotid body chemoreceptors. The rise in pulse pressure during bradycardia appears to be a compensatory phenomenon to increase the stroke volume and maintain the cardiac output. It is only in the very ill preterm baby that this mechanism fails and cardiac output and pulse pressure fall with fatal termination.

Causes and Predisposing Factors

Frequent handling for toilet and feeding may precipitate apneic spells. Raised environmental ambient temperature, vigorous suction and sudden flexion of neck are common triggering factors.

1. **Immaturity** Around 25% of babies with a gestation of less than 32 weeks and/or birth weight of less than 1,500 g are likely to develop apnea of prematurity (AOP). Most cases of AOP present after 1–2 days of life but within first 7 days. Apneic attacks appearing on the first day or after the first week of life are unlikely to be due to AOP.

2. **Pulmonary conditions** Congenital malformations of upper airways, respiratory distress syndrome, pneumonia, pulmonary hemorrhage and aspiration are associated with apneic spells.

3. **Cardiac malformations** Pulmonary atresia, Fallot's tetralogy, transposition of great vessels, total anomalous pulmonary venous return and truncus arteriosus may be associated with apneic attacks. In transient right-to-left shunts, the cyanotic spells may occur.

4. **Neurological disorders** Immaturity, birth trauma with or without intracranial bleeding, congenital central hypoventilation syndrome (Ondine's curse),

congenital myopathy, Werdnig-Hoffmann disease, spinal cord lesions, myasthenia gravis, maternal sedation with pethidine or morphine and accidental intoxication of fetus with a local anesthetic during labor (pudendal block) may be associated with apneic attacks. Seizures should not be mistaken with an apneic spell.

5. **Congenital anomalies** Tracheoesophageal fistula, diaphragmatic hernia, choanal atresia and Pierre-Robin syndrome may be associated with apneic attacks.

6. **Metabolic causes** Hyperbilirubinemia, hypoglycemia, hypocalcemia, acidosis and dehydration should be looked for in infants with apneic attacks.

7. **Infections** Septicemia and meningitis should be seriously considered, if the apneic attacks start after 3 to 4 days of age.

8. **Anemia** is an important cause of apneic attacks in preterm babies.

9. **Methemoglobinemia** Infant may be depressed and hypoxic due to exposure to toxic agents before or after birth, e.g. prilocain (a local anesthetic), aniline dyes, etc.

Assessment of the Infant

The details about the sequence of events, duration of apnea and its frequency, presence or absence of cyanosis and bradycardia should be recorded. Incubator temperature during the apneic episode should be checked. The baby should be clinically screened for any pulmonary and cardiac anomalies. The signs of raised intracranial pressure or other neurological abnormalities, e.g. high-pitched cry, depressed automatic reflexes, diminished general activity and poor feeding should be looked for. A tube should be passed through the nostrils to exclude choanal atresia and down into the stomach to rule out esophageal atresia.

Investigations

Biochemistry Blood should be collected for estimation of glucose, calcium, bilirubin, culture and sensitivity, blood gases and acid–base parameters. In stable babies, capillary blood gas (CBG) values can be assessed to monitor pH and PCO_2 along with pulse oximetry.

Methemoglobin spot test A drop of baby's (patient) blood is placed on a filter paper next to the one from a normal baby (control) and allowed to dry. In methemoglobinemia, the blood spot will appear brown rather than the red of the normal control.

Chest skiagram Pulmonary conditions, like respiratory distress syndrome, aspiration pneumonia, cardiac anomalies and diaphragmatic hernia can be diagnosed on roentgen findings.

EKG should be taken, if cardiac condition is suspected.

Ultrasonography of brain should be done to exclude intraventricular hemorrhage.

aEEG may be required to diagnose subtle seizures.

Management

The severity of the condition and probable cause should be determined. It is essential to diagnose or exclude conditions requiring urgent specialized investigations or operation, e.g. diaphragmatic hernia, tracheoesophageal fistula, subdural hemorrhage, and congenital heart disease.

Monitoring

Due to relatively high incidence of apneic attacks in very low birth weight babies, it is recommended that all infants weighing less than 1800 g should be routinely and continuously monitored during the first two weeks of life. Apnea monitors based on impedance technique which measure changes in electrical resistance across the chest wall during breathing or chest movements recorded by the pressure transducer in an air-filled mattress (ripple type mattress) are satisfactory. Apnea monitors based on chest wall movements are likely to miss obstructive apnea which account for 10% cases of apneic attacks. Infant is continuously monitored and alarm is set for an apneic episode lasting for more than 20 seconds. Since severe episode of an apnea is often followed by bradycardia, a heart rate monitor with an alarm setting for a heart rate of less than 100/minute, serves the dual purpose of heart and respiration monitor and is quite useful in clinical practice. There are combined heart rate and respiration monitors with oscilloscopic display facility. They are more reliable but their cost is prohibitive. Pulse oximeter can be used for dual monitoring of arterial oxygen saturation and heart rate.

General Measures

Handling should be reduced to the bare minimum and infant should be nursed without a pillow. It has been shown that handling and sudden flexion of neck can lower oxygen tension by more than 10 mm Hg. Infant should preferably be nursed in a prone position or kept in a supine position with slight extension of neck.

Stimulation As soon as the baby stops breathing, painful cutaneous stimulation in the form of pinching of skin or tapping on the feet would initiate breathing. Nursing the baby on a rocking water mattress or providing skin-to-skin contact has been shown to reduce the episodes of apneic attacks.

Warmth The baby should be nursed in an incubator with its temperature maintained at the lower end of neutral thermal environment range and without any sudden changes.

Oxygen If facilities for blood gas analysis are not available, oxygen should be given at the lowest concentration necessary to relieve cyanosis. Oxygen should be administered with continuous positive airway pressure (CPAP) through nasal prongs, if apneic attacks are frequent. The oxygen may be continued, if frequency of apneic attacks is reduced. The oxygen administration should be stopped after 6 hours of apnea-free period.

Feeding To avoid aspiration, it is preferable to give intravenous infusion of 10% glucose solution till the apneic attacks are controlled.

Special Measures

Specific therapy is given to treat the underlying condition causing apneic attacks.

Correction of metabolic disorders Hypoglycemia, hypocalcemia and acidosis should be looked for and treated appropriately through intravenous route. For details of therapy, refer to Chapter 24.

Anemia If hematocrit is below 25%, packed red blood cells transfusion is advised.

Antibiotics Apneic attacks starting after 3 days of age are indicative of infection. Septic screening, blood culture and skiagram of chest should be taken in all infants with apneic attacks.

Respiratory stimulants Respiratory stimulants have been used with good results in the management of recurrent apneic attacks of prematurity. The exact mode of their action is uncertain. It has been suggested that xanthine derivatives elevate cyclic-AMP levels by inhibiting cyclic nucleotide phosphodiesterase. Cyclic-AMP is well known to augment the action of a variety of neurotransmitters. Theophylline administration is recommended in a dose of 5 mg/kg intravenously as a loading dose, followed by 2 mg/kg every 8 hours orally or intravenously for maintenance. Therapy is continued till infant is at least 34 weeks mature. Theophylline is methylated to caffeine by preterm infants. Tachycardia and diuresis are common side effects. In resistant cases, theophylline therapy may be supplemented by administration of doxapram in a dose of 0.5 mg/kg per hour as a constant intravenous infusion which is gradually increased to a maximum of 2.5 mg/kg/hr during 48 hours. Doxapram should preferably be avoided due to potential risk of causing jitteriness, seizures, hyperglycemia, abdominal distension and hypertension leading to intraventricular hemorrhage. Respiratory stimulants may aggravate the condition of the baby, if apnea is the manifestation of a seizure.

Caffeine which is a potent centrally acting respiratogenic agent with minimal peripheral side effects unlike theophylline, is equally effective. Caffeine citrate 20 mg/kg intravenously over 30 minutes (equivalent to 10 mg of caffeine base/kg) is followed after 24 hours with maintenance therapy using dosage schedule of 5–10 mg/kg oral in 1 to 2 divided doses daily. Cafirate is available as oral and intravenous solution (20 mg/mL in 3 mL vial). The serum caffeine level should be maintained between 5 and 25 µg/mL. Caffeine benzoate should not be used because it can displace bilirubin from albumin binding sites and predispose the infant to develop kernicterus at lower serum bilirubin levels. Caffein is discontinued after 34–36 weeks of gestational maturity, if no apneic spells occur for 5–7 days. The prophylactic utility of coffee for prevention of apnea of prematurity needs to be evaluated.

Kinesthetic stimulation There is no evidence to suggest that oscillating bed mattress or water bed has any role either in the prevention or treatment of apneic attacks due to prematurity. Kangaroo-mother-care has been shown to control apneic attacks which are resistant to other conventional modes of management.

Artificial ventilation If apneic attacks are occurring despite elevation of ambient FiO_2, nasal CPAP at 4–6 cm H_2O pressure has been found to be effective in obstructive or mixed type of apnea. CPAP may be delivered by short binasal prongs or nasopharyngeal tube. Infants with prolonged or frequent apneic attacks despite CPAP should be intubated and attached to a mechanical ventilator. If lungs are normal, the infant should be ventilated with minimum pressure (PIP 13–14 cm H_2O and PEEP 4–5 cm H_2O), slow rate (20–25/min), small Ti (0.35–0.40 sec) and low FiO_2 (0.4–0.5). The arterial oxygen tension should be maintained between 50 and 80 mm Hg to prevent the risk of retinopathy of prematurity (ROP) and anoxic brain damage.

STRIDOR

Stridor refers to audible noisy breathing due to incomplete obstruction of larynx or the trachea. It can be easily differentiated from pharyngeal moist snore, nasal sounds and wheezing. The baby may be born with stridor or develop it subsequently. It may be constant or intermittent and with or without respiratory difficulty. Feeding difficulty and choking may be associated with stridor due to any cause.

Causes

The obstruction to upper respiratory passages may be intrinsic or extrinsic.

Intrinsic Obstruction

Simple congenital laryngeal stridor The stridor is caused by flaccidity (laryngomalacia) or easy collapsibility of aryepiglottic folds or epiglottis in general. The condition usually manifests by the end of first week or during the second week after birth. The stridor is inspiratory, low pitched vibratory or fluttering in character akin to undulating flutter of curtains when exposed to a blast of wind. It is characteristically intermittent and aggravated by excitement, crying, feeding or sleeping and modified by the posture of the baby. The cry is generally unaffected.

The child is not much inconvenienced by the condition though the loud inspiratory sounds may be frightening to the parents. The respiratory rate may be slightly increased during the height of stridor and respiratory distress with inspiratory chest retractions may be seen. The feeding, general activity and weight gain are satisfactory in uncomplicated cases. The presence of micrognathia and cleft palate may pose additional difficulties in breathing and feeding. The condition disappears spontaneously by six months to one year of age. These infants are, however, prone to develop aspiration of feeds and frequent lung infections.

Tracheomalacia It is a relatively rare condition and is characterized by high-pitched rattling breathing with expiratory stridor. The condition can be easily differentiated from congenital laryngomalacia (Table 19.6).

Congenital laryngeal or tracheal stenosis, atresia and webs Atretic lesions in the upper air passages are incompatible with life and generally remain undetected clinically. Congenital laryngeal stenosis or web is characterized by weak or hoarse cry, labored breathing with markedly diminished air entry in the lungs. In subglottic and tracheal stenosis or hypoplasia, the cry is unaffected and stridor is both inspiratory and expiratory in character.

TABLE 19.6 Salient differences between laryngomalacia and tracheomalacia		
Features	Laryngomalacia	Tracheomalacia
Pathophysiology	Collapse of epiglottis and/or arytenoid cartilages during inspiration	Cartilaginous rings supporting the trachea are soft and tend to collapse during expiration
Clinical features	Most common cause of congenital stridor with onset between 2 and 4 weeks. Coarse low-pitched inspiratory stridor that is worse during agitation, feeding or change of posture. Male to female preponderance of 2:1	High-pitched rattling breathing with expiratory stridor during 4–8 weeks of age. There may be respiratory distress or excercise intolerance
Associated conditions	Uncommon and include diastrophic dysplasia, DiGeorge syndrome, alopecia, XY gonadal dysgenesis, Costello syndrome	Heart defects, gastroesopharngeal reflux disease, developmental delay
Diagnosis	The clinical features are characteristic, laryngoscopy is confirmatory if there is any doubt	Bronchoscopy is confirmatory. The anterior and posterior tracheal walls approximate during expiration
Management	Conservative	CPAP and tracheostomy, if hypoxia is marked
Outcome	Spontaneous resolution by 2 years of age	Majority ameliorate or resolve by 6–12 months of age

Laryngeal cysts or neoplasms Angioma, papilloma, lymphangioma and retention cysts in larynx are characterized by hoarseness, aphonia, stridor and characteristic findings on laryngoscopy.

Laryngeal edema and obstruction due to mucus or meconium Laryngeal edema may occur following traumatic or prolonged endotracheal intubation. The presence of mucus, meconium or blood at the glottis may produce partial obstruction and stridor. Aspiration under direct vision must be carried out in all infants with stridor at birth.

Neurogenic stridor Vocal cord paralysis may be bilateral due to injury to brainstem and in association with Arnold-Chiari malformation or unilateral due to involvement of peripheral nerve. The laryngeal paralysis is most common on the right side because right recurrent laryngeal nerve is longer and hooks around the aorta from front to back. Hoarseness, aphonia and lack of mobility of vocal cords clinches the diagnosis. Hypocalcemia does not manifest with laryngospasm during the neonatal period.

Extrinsic Obstruction

Vascular rings The clinical picture is determined whether it is the compression of trachea or the esophagus that predominates. The stridor is intermittent and both that inspiratory and expiratory in character and is often worsened by flexion of the neck. The infant prefers to keep the head in hyperextension. Cry is normal while brassy or bitonal cough may be intractable. These infants are prone to develop choking and aspiration during feeds and recurrent respiratory infections. Double aortic arch is the commonest anomaly and manifests with severe symptoms early in life. Anomalous innominate and left common carotid artery is characterized by predominant respiratory difficulty while anomalous subclavian artery is either asymptomatic or produces predominant symptoms of esophageal compression. Right aortic arch with left ligamentum arteriosum is often asymptomatic during early childhood.

Tumors of neck and mediastinum The neck should be examined for goiter and lymphangioma while mediastinal mass may produce symptoms of vascular compression.

Diagnosis

Stridor manifesting at birth would suggest the possibilities of laryngeal edema (if intubation had been done), obstruction of glottis with mucus, meconium or blood. The stridor generally disappears following aspiration under direct vision or within 24 hours, if it was due to laryngeal edema. Infants with laryngeal or tracheal atresia and webs are born with severe respiratory difficulty and may die at birth. The persistent or worsening stridor suggests the possibilities of anatomical obstruction or vocal cord paralysis. The cry or voice is affected with laryngeal disorders except in cases of laryngomalacia. Fluttering or undulating character of stridor, best demonstrated by auscultating in front of the nose or mouth is characteristic of laryngomalacia. Tracheal obstruction is characterized by stridor both during inspiration and expiration and brassy hacking cough. The site of obstruction may be localized by auscultating the front of neck in the midline, though relatively short neck of the neonate makes this examination rather difficult. The flexion of neck worsens the respiratory difficulty due to vascular rings and baby prefers to keep his neck hyperextended. Dysphagic symptoms may predominate in infants with vascular rings. The palpation of carotid vessels may show inequality of pulsations on the two sides. The baby should be examined for any micrognathia, glossoptosis, choanal atresia, tumors in the neck and mediastinum. The severity of obstruction is assessed by observing respiratory rate, chest retractions, adequacy of air entry in the lungs and presence of cyanosis.

Laryngoscopic examination gives immediate diagnosis of most of the laryngeal and subglottic disorders. Skiagrams of chest posteroanterior and lateral views are useful to detect any narrowing of trachea and soft tissue swelling. A barium swallow, preferably with a cine-radiography, is helpful for the diagnosis of vascular rings by demonstration of esophageal indentation. Tracheoscopy with or without careful contrast study of trachea is helpful for the diagnosis of tracheal obstruction.

Treatment

Suction of the glottic area under direct vision should be attempted in every baby with stridor at birth. When respiratory difficulty is marked, endotracheal intubation would break open any laryngeal web and relieve obstruction due to stenosis. Infants with laryngeal and tracheal atresia generally die at birth. Intrinsic and extrinsic tumors and cysts require surgical excision. In case of severe laryngeal obstruction, tracheostomy is life saving. Corticosteroids may hasten the recovery in suspected cases of laryngeal edema. Simple congenital laryngeal stridor due to laryngomalacia is a self-limiting condition and does not need any active therapy. Feeding should be supervised in all infants with stridor to avoid aspiration. Gavage feeding is indicated, if respiratory difficulty is marked. Goiter may rapidly regress following administration of triiodothyronine and Lugol's iodine. Subtotal thyroidectomy rather than tracheostomy would be life saving when respiratory distress is marked.

BIBLIOGRAPHY

AAP Committee on Fetus and Newborn. Postnatal corticosteroids to treat or prevent chronic lung disease in preterm infants. *Pediatrics* 2002, 109:330–338.

Ablow RC, Driscoll SG, Effmann EL, et al. A comparison of early-onset Group-B streptococcal neonatal infection and respiratory distress of the newborn. *N Engl J Med* 1976; 294:65.

Aranada JV, Gorman W, Bergsteinsson H, Gun T. Efficiency of caffein in treatment of apnea in the low birth weight infant. *J Pediatr* 1977; 90: 467.

Askie L, Henderson-Smart D, Irwig L, et al. Oxygen saturation targets and outcomes in extremely preterm infants. *N Engl J Med* 2003, 349: 959–967.

Bancalari E, Claure M. Definitions and diagnostic criteria for bronchopulmonary dysplasia. *Semin Perinatol* 2006, 30: 164–170.

Bhartia J. Current options in the management of apnea of prematurity. *Clin Pediatr* 2000, 39: 327–336.

Briniwala MA, Ehrenkranz RA. The role of nutrition in the prevention and management of bronchopulmonary dysplasia. *Semin Perinatol* 2006, 30: 200–208.

Chan KN, Elliman A, Bryan E, Silverman M. Respiratory symptoms in children of low birth weight. *Arch Dis Child* 1989, 64: 1294.

Clearly GM, Wiswell TE. Meconium-stained amniotic fluid and the meconium aspiration syndrome: An update. *Pediatr Clin N Amer* 1998, 45: 511–529.

Dakshinamurti S. Pathophysiologic mechanisms of persistent pulmonary hypertension of the newborn. *Pediatr Pulmonol* 2005, 39: 492–503.

Dargaville PA, South M, MC Dougall PN. Surfactant and surfactant inhibitors in meconium aspiration syndrome. *J Pediatr* 2001, 138: 113–115.

Durand M, Sardesai S, EcEvoy C. Effects of early dexamethasone therapy on pulmonary mechanics and chronic lung disease in very low birth weight infants: A randomized controlled trial. *Pediatrics* 1995, 95: 584–590.

Engle WA. American Academy of Pediatrics Committee on Fetus and Newborn. Surfactant replacement therapy for respiratory distress in the preterm and term neonate. *Pediatrics* 2008, 12: 419–432.

Evans JJ. Prediction of respiratory distress syndrome by shake test on newborn gastric aspirate. *N Engl J Med* 1975, 292: 1113.

Findlay RD, Taeusch HW, Walther FJ. Surfactant replacement therapy for meconium aspiration syndrome. *Pediatrics* 1996, 97: 48–52.

Fraser WD, Hofmeyr J, Lede R. The Amniotransfusion Trial Group. Amnio infusion for the prevention of meconium aspiration syndrome. *N Engl J Med* 2005, 353: 909–917.

Fujiwara T, Maeta H, Chida S, et al. Artificial surfactant therapy in hyaline membrane disease. *Lancet* 1980, 1: 55.

Gerdes JS, Abbasi S, Bhutani VK. Branchopulmonary dysplasia. In: FD Burg, Ellen R Wald, JR Ingelfinger, RA Polin (Eds.) Gellis and Kagan's Current Pediatric Therapy. *WB Saunders Co, Phila* 15th ed. 1998, pp 769–771.

Gluck L, Kulovich MV, Borer RC, Brenner PH, Anderson GC, Spellacy WN. Diagnosis of the respiratory distress syndrome by amniocentesis. *Amer J Obstet Gynec* 1971, 109: 440.

Greenough A, Dimitriou G, Prendergast M, Milner AD. Synchronized mechanical ventilation for respiratory support in newborn infants. *Cochrane Database Syst Rev* 2008, 3: CD000456.

Grier DG, Halliday HL. Management of BPD: guidelines for corticosteroid use. *Drugs* 2005, 65(1): 15–29.

Halliday HL. Recent clinical trials of surfactant treatment for neonate. *Biol Neonate* 2006, 89(4): 323–329.

Jain L, Dudell G. Respiratory transition in infants delivered by cesarean section. *Semin Perinatol* 2006, 30: 296–304.

Jain L, Eaton DC. Physiology of fetal lung fluid clearance and the effect of labor. *Semin Perinatol* 2006, 30:34–43.

Kattwinkel J. Neonatal apnea : Pathogenesis and therapy. *J Pediatr* 1977, 90: 342.

Kinsella JP, Greenough A, Abman SH. Bronchopulmonary dysplasia. *Lancet* 2006, 29: 1421–1431.

Konduri GG. New approaches for persistent pulmonary hypertension of newborn. *Clin Perinatol* 2004, 31: 591–611.

Martin RJ, Miller MJ, Carlo WA. Pathogenesis of apnea in preterm infants. *J Pediatr* 1986, 109: 733.

McCallion N, Davis PG, Morley CJ. Volume-targeted versus pressure-limited ventilation in the neonate. *Cochrane Database Syst Rev* 2005, 3: CD003666.

Murki S, Deorari AK, Vidyasagar D. Use of CPAP and surfactant therapy in newborns with respiratory distress syndrome. *Indian J Pediatr* 2014, 81(5): 481–488.

Murphy BP, Inder TE, Huppi PS, et al. Impaired cerebral gray matter growth after treatment with dexamethasone for neonatal chronic lung disease. *Pediatrics* 2001, 107: 217–221.

Narang A, Nair PM, Bhakoo ON, et al. Management of meconium-stained amniotic fluid: A team approach. *Indian Pediatr* 1993, 30: 9.

Narayan S, Deorari AK. Steroids in perinatology. *Indian Pediatr* 2002, 39: 347–361.

Ostrea EM, Villanueva-Uy ET, Natarajan G, *et al.* Persistent pulmonary hypertension of the newborn. *Pediatr Drugs* 2006, 8: 179–188.

Pfister RH, Soll RF. Initial respiratory support of preterm infants. The role of CPAP, INSURE method and non-invasive ventilation. *Clin Perinatol* 2012, 39: 459–481.

Purandare CN. Fetal lung maturity. *J Obstet Gynecol India.* 2005, 55 (3):215–17.

Rachuri H, Oleti TP, Murki S, Subramanian S. Nethagani J. Diagnostic performance of point of care ultrasonography in identifying the etiology of respiratory distress in neonates. *Indian J Pediatr* 2017, 84 (4):267–70.

Ramanathan R. Surfactant therapy in preterm infants with respiratory distress syndrome and in near-term or term newborns with acute RDS. *J Perinatol* 2006, 26 (Suppl 1): 551–556.

Ramanathan R, Sekar KC, Rasmussen M, Bhatia J, Soll RF. Nasal intermittent positive pressure ventilation after surfactant treatment for respiratory distress syndrome in preterm infants <30 weeks gestation: A randomised controlled trial. *J Perinatol* 2012, 32: 336–343.

Roberts JD, Fineman JR, Morin FC, *et al.* Inhaled nitric oxide and persistent pulmonary hypertension of the newborn. *N Engl J Med* 1997, 336: 605.

Sankar MJ, Deorari AK. Postnatal corticosteroids for chronic lung disease (CLD). *Indian Pediatr* 2007, 44: 531–539.

Schmidt B, Roberts RS, Davis P, *et al.* Caffeine therapy for apnea of prematurity. *N Engl J Med* 2006, 354: 2112–2121.

Shankar V, Paul VK, Deorari AK, Singh M. Do neonates with meconium aspiration syndrome require antibiotics? *Indian J Pediatr* 1995, 62: 327–331.

Shepard FM. Current questions in hyaline membrane disease. *Pediatrics* 1976, 5: 265.

Singh M, Deorari AK, Agarwal R, Paul VK. Assisted ventilation for hyaline membrane disease. *Indian Pediatr* 1995, 32: 1267–1274.

Singh M, Deorari AK. Pneumonias in newborn babies. *Indian J Pediatr* 1995, 62: 293–306.

Suresh GK, Soll RF. Current surfactant use in premature infants. *Clin Perinatol* 2001, 28(3): 671–694.

Sweet DG, Carnielli V, Greisein G, *et al.* European Consensus Guidelines on the Management of Neonatal Respiratory. Distress syndrome in Preterm Infants 2010 update. *Neonatology* 2010, 97: 402–417.

The Neonatal Inhaled Nitric oxide Study Group: Inhaled nitric oxide in full-term infants with hypoxic respiratory failure. *N Engl J Med* 1997, 336: 597.

Thomas S, Verma IC, Singh M, Menon PSN. Spectrum of respiratory distress syndrome in the newborn in North India: A prospective study. *Indian J Pediatr* 1981, 48: 61.

Tomar RS. Ghubiani R, Yadav D. Effect of surfactant therapy using orogastric tube for tracheal catheterization in preterm newborns. *Indian J Pediatr* 2017, 84 (4): 257–61.

Transwell AK, Sherwin E, Smith BT. Single-step gastric aspirate shake test: bedside predictor of neonatal pulmonary morbidity. *Arch Dis Child* 1977, 52: 541.

Velaphi S, Vidyasagar D. Intrapartum and post-delivery management of infants born to mothers with meconium-stained amniotic fluid. Evidence-based recommendations. *Clin Perinatol* 2006, 33: 29–42.

Verder H, Heiring C, Sorensen L. Rapid test for lung maturity based on spectroscopy of gastric aspirate, predicted respiratory distress syndrome with high sensitivity. *Acta Paediatr* 2017, 106 (3): 430–7.

Wiswell TE, Cleary GM. Meconium-stained amniotic fluid and the meconium aspiration syndrome. *Pediatr Clin North Am* 1998, 45: 511–529.

Wiswell TE. Expanded use of surfactant therapy. *Clin Perinatol* 2001, 28: 695–711.

Yu V. Surfactant replacement therapy. *Indian Pediatr* 1998, 35: 1081–1096.

Respiratory Disorders

19

Cardiovascular Disorders

FETAL AND NEONATAL CIRCULATION

The heart assumes its normal four-chambered shape by the end of six weeks of intrauterine life. The oxygenated blood from placenta is returned through the umbilical veins which join the portal vein. Most of the umbilical venous blood is bypassed through ductus venosus to the inferior vena cava and enters the right atrium. In the right atrium, bloodstream is divided into two portions by the inferior margin of septum secundum. Most of the oxygenated blood enters the left atrium through foramen ovale. There it mixes with the small amount of blood returning from the lungs via pulmonary veins and is pumped into left ventricle for distribution to the coronaries, head and upper extremities.

The deoxygenated superior vena caval blood directly traverses through tricuspid valve to enter the right ventricle. A small amount of blood entering the pulmonary trunk flows through the pulmonary circulation while the rest passes through the ductus arteriosus into the descending aorta for distribution into lower extremities. The elevated pulmonary vascular resistance is responsible for this physiological right-to-left shunt through the ductus. During fetal life, no more than 10% of combined right and left ventricular output perfuses through the lungs while placenta receives more than 50% of cardiac output (Figure 20.1).

After birth, with first breath, pulmonary vascular resistance rapidly falls, resulting in increase in pulmonary blood flow. The loss of low resistance placental circulation due to clamping of cord, leads to sudden increase in systemic vascular resistance. As the pressure in the left atrium rises and the pressure on the right side falls, two septa are pressed against each other leading to functional closure of foramen

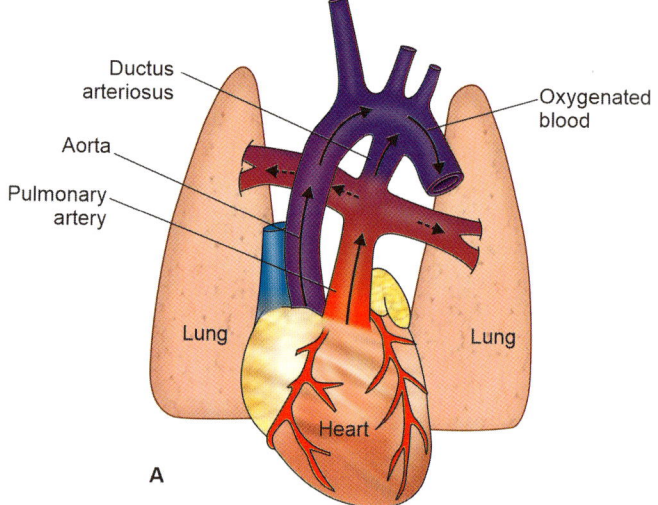

A

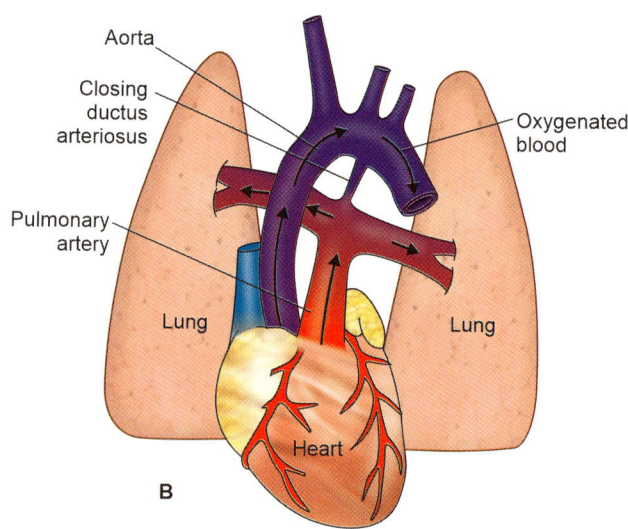

B

Figure 20.1 (A) Normal fetal circulation, (B) Change in pulmonary circulation due to closure of foramen ovale and ductus arteriosus after birth.

ovale. The pressure relations between the aorta and pulmonary trunk are reversed so that a small left-to-right shunt is established through the ductus arteriosus. However, ductus rapidly constricts on exposure to oxygen and by the end of 72 hours it is functionally closed in term babies. The pulmonary vascular resistance continues to fall over several weeks and lowest pulmonary pressure is reached around 8–12 weeks of age.

The main differences between the fetal and post-natal circulation include (i) presence of placental circulation which provides gas exchange to the fetus, (ii) absence of gas exchange in the collapsed lungs with very little flow of blood to the lungs with hardly any pulmonary venous return to left atrium, (iii) presence of ductus venosus which joins the portal vein with inferior vena cava, providing a low resistance bypass for umbilical venous blood to pass through inferior vena cava, (iv) widely open foramen ovale to enable oxygenated blood (through umbilical veins) to reach the left atrium and left ventricle for distribution to the coronaries and the brain, and lastly (v) widely open ductus arteriosus to allow right ventricular blood to reach the descending aorta by bypassing the lungs.

PERSISTENT PULMONARY HYPERTENSION

Most early problems of newborn infants are related to difficulties of adjustments to extrauterine life and are, therefore, unique to this age. Persistence of fetal circulation occurs due to suprasystemic resistance in the pulmonary vascular bed leading to perpetuation of right-to-left shunt through foramen ovale and ductus arteriosus. The condition is now preferably called as persistent pulmonary hypertension of the newborn (PPHN) because it underlines the basic mechanism which leads to persistent fetal circulation (PFC). The condition presents within first 18 hours after birth with marked cyanosis which is out of proportion to the underlying lung disease. It must be distinguished from congenital cyanotic heart disease. The incidence of PPHN varies between 1 and 5 per 1000 live births. The disorder is more common in full term and post-term infants. In preterm infants, RDS and bronchopulmonary dysplasia may be complicated by PPHN.

Etiology

A variety of disorders are known to increase pulmonary vascular resistance. Neonatal pulmonary vessels are hyperreactive to a large number of noxious stimuli. The common predisposing conditions are meconium aspiration syndrome, hypoxia, acidosis, hypoglycemia, fluminant pneumonia, diaphragmatic hernia and hypoplasia of lung. Polycythemia, hyperviscosity and microthrombi can also elevate pulmonary vascular resistance. Excessive muscularization of pulmonary vessels due to chronic intrauterine stress and hypoxia may lead to intractable primary PPHN. The classification and mechanism of production of PPHN is shown in Table 20.1.

TABLE 20.1 Classification of PPHN	
Type	*Mechanism*
Primary PPHN	Excessive muscularization and remodeling of the pulmonary arterial system due to fetal hypoxia and alveolar capillary dysplasia with malalignment of capillaries with the alveoli.
Secondary PPHN	
▪ *Intrapartum asphyxia*	Hypoxia and acidosis cause potent vasoconstriction of pulmonary arteries and lead to perpetuation of fetal circulation. The right-to-left shunt is aggravated and perpetuated by systemic hypotension due to postasphyxial myocardial damage.
▪ *Aspiration and infection*	There is release of vasoactive substances, like endothelin 1, thromboxane A2, leukotrienes, pulmonary microthrombi and suppression of nitric oxide (NO) production.
▪ *Pulmonary hypoplasia*	In infants, pulmonary hypoplasia may occur due to diaphragmatic hernia, congenital lobar emphysema and oligohydramnios (Potter syndrome).
▪ *Maternal drug therapy*	Aspirin and other NSAIDs inhibit synthesis of prostaglandins and may cause premature closure of ductus arteriosus. Maternal smoking and intake of selective serotonin reuptake inhibitors have also been implicated to cause PPHN.
▪ *Maternal diseases*	Case control studies have shown an association between PPHN and maternal diabetes mellitus and urinary tract infection.
▪ *Congenital heart disease*	Obstruction to venous outflow from lungs causes pulmonary hypertension.
▪ *Iatrogenic*	Overzealous ventilation during resuscitation may trigger the development of PHN.

Cardiovascular Disorders

20

Diagnosis

The condition is more common in term and post-term infants. There is a history of fetal distress and meconium-stained liquor. Evidences of perinatal hypoxia and delivery by emergency cesarean section are common antecedents. The infant is severely distressed with deep cyanosis. The severity of respiratory distress and degree of hypoxemia are out of proportion to changes seen on the skiagram of chest. The anteroposterior diameter of chest is increased, if there is aspiration of meconium. Cardiovascular system examination may reveal right ventricular heave, closely split or a single loud second heart sound, gallop rhythm and a systolic murmur at the left sternal border due to tricuspid regurgitation. The existence of predisposing conditions support the diagnosis of PPHN.

Congenital cyanotic heart disease should be ruled out by detailed cardiac evaluation and investigations. Infant is hyperventilated with 100% oxygen (hyperoxia hyperventilation test) to achieve a 'critical' $PaCO_2$ of <25 mm Hg. Following hyperventilation elevation of arterial oxygen tension to >100 mm Hg is suggestive of pulmonary disease and PPHN rather than structural cyanotic heart disease. Preductal (right arm) and postductal (lower extremity), paO_2 difference of >15 mm Hg or arterial oxygen saturation (SaO_2) of >10–20% on simultaneously drawn samples of blood is suggestive of right-to-left shunt at ductal level. The negative test does not exclude the diagnosis of PPHN because shunt could be intrapulmonary or at the level of foramen ovale. Hyperoxia test (obtaining an arterial gas after 15 min of exposure to 100% oxygen) and/or hyperoxia hyperventilation to induce pulmonary vasodilation and improve PaO_2 is no longer practiced because of known adverse effects of hyperoxia and alkalosis in neonates.

EKG may show right ventricular strain or hypertrophy pattern and P-pulmonale. Echocardiographic evidences of PPHN include dilatation of right ventricle and right atrium, leftward deviation of the intraventricular septum, tricuspid regurgitation and right-to-left shunting at the levels of the patent foramen ovale and patent ductus arteriosus. Prolongation of right ventricle systolic time is highly suggestive of PPHN. Right ventricular pre-ejection period to right ventricular ejection time ratio (RVPEP/RVET) usually exceeds 0.5. The cardiac output may be reduced to <150 mL/kg/min. Echocardiographic evaluation should rule out structural cardiac defect although partial anomalous pulmonary venous return cannot be ruled out with certainty. Color Doppler examination is useful to assess the presence of intracardiac or ductal shunting. Polycythemia, hyperviscosity and thrombocytopenia may aggravate the clinical picture and reduce efficacy of vasodilators.

Management

Excellent supportive management, nursing care and ventilatory assistance may salvage some infants with PPHN which has a case fatality rate of 30–60% even in good centers. The correctable underlying problems, like diaphragmatic hernia, polycythemia, hypoglycemia and pneumonia, should be managed. Polycythemia and hyperviscosity should be treated with partial exchange transfusion with normal saline to maintain hematocrit between 50 and 55%. Intravascular volume support with normal saline or packed red blood cells is indicated in infants with volume depletion. External stimuli and unnecessary handling should be minimized because these children are over reactive. Muscle relaxants should be used to reduce hyperreactivity. Sedation with fentanyl (2–5 μg/kg/hour) is often useful. Infant should be ventilated with 100% FiO_2 to correct profound hypoxia to maintain postductal oxygen saturation above 95%. Intermittent hand bagging is useful to improve oxygenation. Acidosis should be corrected by hyperventilation ($PaCO_2$ 20–25 mm Hg) and administration of sodium bicarbonate and attempt should be made to maintain pH between 7.35 and 7.45 to reverse pulmonary vasoconstriction. The use of dopamine to increase systemic vascular resistance and improve contractibility of the heart is recommended. The associated biochemical abnormalities, like hypoglycemia and hypocalcemia, should be treated to provide adequate substrates to the myocardium.

A large number of vasodilators have been tried with variable results because they reduce both pulmonary and systemic pressures. Tolazoline is not a selective pulmonary vasodilator and its use is associated with serious side effects, like hypotension, thrombocytopenia, bleeding and renal dysfunction. It is given as intravenous bolus in a dose of 1–2 mg/kg followed by continuous infusion of 1–2 mg/kg/hour. Infusion of calcium is essential because of fall in the level of ionized calcium due to stress (catabolic release of phosphates) and maintenance of relatively higher pH. Magnesium sulfate by virtue of its potent vasodilatory effects, sedation and muscle relaxation has been used with success in developing countries where nitric oxide is not readily available. A loading dose of 200 mg/kg is given IV over 20 minutes followed by a continuous infusion of 20–150 mg/kg/hr is given to maintain serum magnesium levels between 3.5 and 5.5 mmol/L.

Magnesium antagonises the entry of calcium into smooth muscle cells and is also a potent vasodilatory agent. Adenosine, a purine nucleoside is an effective pulmonary vasodilator by virtue of release of endogenous nitric oxide. It is effective in the treatment of PPHN in preterm babies when administered as a constant infusion at a rate of 30–60 µg/kg/min. Adenosine triphosphate infusion can be tried, if other well-recognized conventional therapies do not succeed.

Nitric oxide (NO) is a potent selective pulmonary vasodilator and has been used with success in developed countries as inhalation therapy. NO is a highly reactive short-lived molecule which is endogenously produced from its precursor arginine by the enzyme NO synthetase. NO is mostly produced in the pulmonary endothelial cells. The molecule enters the adjacent vascular smooth muscle where it binds to the heme component of soluble guanyl cyclase. This leads to production of cGMP-dependent protein kinases resulting in efflux of calcium from cells leading to relaxation of smooth muscles and vasodilatation. Inhaled nitric oxide (iNO) in a low dose (5–20 ppm) is now a standard therapy and modality of choice for the management of PPHN. L-arginine and dipyridamole are useful drugs to facilitate weaning from nitric oxide ventilation which is gradually reduced at the rate of 1.0 PPM. The common side effects of iNO include methemoglobinemia, damage to lungs due to oxygen free radicals and neurotoxicity. In India, medical grade nitric oxide is not readily available and iNO should be introduced in selected tertiary care centers.

Recent experimental studies have documented that intravenous administration of sildenafil, a phosphodiesterase inhibitor, is associated with selective pulmonary vasodilatation which is comparable to iNO therapy. It increases myocardial performance without raising myocardial oxygen consumption by elevation of intracellular levels of cyclic adenosine monophosphate (cAMP). Sildenafil can be given orally in a dose of 3 mg/kg every 6 hours. Recently milrinone, another phosphodiesterase inhibitor, has been used with success. It is given intravenously in a loading dose of 50 µg/kg over 60 minutes followed by a maintenance infusion at a rate of 0.33–0.99 µg/kg/min for 24–72 hours. When underlying predisposing condition is associated with surfactant deficiency (like meconium aspiration syndrome), surfactant replacement therapy is indicated to improve the outcome (Table 20.2).

If there is no significant improvement despite aggressive intensive care, management with high frequency jet ventilation, and extracorporeal membrane oxygenation (ECMO) therapy may salvage some infants in highly specialized centers. The definitive laboratory criteria for institution of ECMO include oxygenation index of >40 in 3 ABGs out of 5 taken 30 minutes apart and A-aDO$_2$ of >600 for 8 hours.

TABLE 20.2 Pharmacological agents for treatment of PPHN			
Agent	Mode of action	Dose	Comments
Inhaled nitric oxide (iNO)	Potent pulmonary vasodilator	20 ppm inhaled for 8d	Expensive, may cause rebound PH, mortality not affected
Sildenafil	Blocks phosphodiesterase 5 (PDE5), potent vasodilator	0.3 mg/kg/dose every 12 hr orally	Improved survival when used with iNO, no rebound PH
Prostanoids (eicosanoids)	They act as "local hormones" by suppressing thromboxane A$_2$ (TXA$_2$) and endogenous production of PGE$_1$ Selective pulmonary vasodilator on inhalation	50–100 ng/kg/min inhaled	Effective in premature babies with PH, can be given SC
Milrinone	It inhibits the action of phosphodiesterase leading to increased intracellular cyclic adenosine monophosphate (cAMP) and calcium. Improves myocardial contractility, decreases pH, acts synergistically with inhaled prostanoids	50 µg/kg/over 60 min followed by maintenance infusion @ 0.33–0.99 µg/kg/min for 24–72 hr	Combination therapy with iNO gives better results
Bosentan	Endothelin receptor antagonist, potent pulmonary vasodilator	2.0–5.5 mg/kg/d orally	Useful in refractory PH

PH, pulmonary hypertension, PPHN; persistent pulmonary hypertension, SC, subcutaneous.

Prognosis

Availability of advanced ventilation facility and iNO therapy has reduced the mortality due to PPHN to less than 25%. The risk of neurodevelopmental sequelae among survivors varies between 15 and 20%. Hyperventilation is known to reduce cerebral perfusion and cause sensorineural hearing loss. Prolonged ventilation may be associated with development of chronic lung disease. The outcome is adversely affected by the following parameters.

1. Labile PaO_2 and inability to reduce $PaCO_2$ despite using PIP of >40 cm H_2O and ventilation rate of over 130/min
2. PaO_2/FiO_2 ratio of <200
3. A-aDO_2 (Alveolar-arterial oxygen difference) >600 (AaDO_2 = P_{atm} – PH_2O × FiO_2 – PaO_2 – $PaCO_2$/RQ)
4. Oxygenation index (OI = MAP × FiO_2 × 100/PaO_2) is increased (mild ≤15, moderate 15–25, severe 25–40 and very severe >40)
5. Low platelet count
6. Low left ventricular output and stroke volume.

PATENT DUCTUS ARTERIOSUS

The patency of ductus arteriosus in fetal life is maintained by prostaglandins E_2 and I_2 (PGE_2 and PGI_2). They are potent vasoactive substances present in every tissue and attain relatively high levels in the fetal blood because they by-pass the lungs by virtue of right-to-left shunts. During fetal life, only 10% of the cardiac output passes through the lungs. The remaining 90% is shunted via the ductus arteriosus to the aorta and systemic circulation. After birth, sudden elevation in oxygen tension and fall in prostaglandin levels triggers the closure of ductus. In a term baby, functional closure of ductus arteriosus occurs within 72 hours while anatomical closure may take several weeks but is generally complete by 3 months of age.

Patent ductus arteriosus (PDA) may occur in 1 in 2000 full term infants as an isolated structural congenital heart lesion which manifests during infancy. A patent ductus may be part of complex cardiac abnormality where survival is dependent on the patency of ductus. The incidence of patent ductus arteriosus is relatively high among preterm infants and is related to gestational immaturity because of increased sensitivity of ductus to prostaglandins. It is estimated that almost one-third of infants with gestational age of 34 weeks or less manifest clinical evidences of patent ductus arteriosus some time during neonatal period. The incidence is much higher among preterm infants with hyaline membrane disease. During recovery from RDS, especially after surfactant therapy, when oxygenation and acidosis improve, there is sudden fall in pulmonary vascular resistance leading to a large left-to-right shunt through the ductus. Spontaneous closure of PDA has been reported in up to 40–67% of very low birth weight (VLBW) infants by 7 days of age.

Prevention

Betamethasone given to women in preterm labor to reduce the severity of RDS has been shown to reduce the incidence of PDA as well. Repeated infusions of normal saline or plasma expanders for hypotension are associated with increased risk of PDA and should be used with caution. During ventilation of preterm babies with RDS, fluid intake should be restricted to 100 mL/kg. Prophylactic use of indomethacin for prevention of PDA is controversial and is not recommended due to potential risk of serious side effects. During phototherapy of extremely preterm babies, some workers recommend shielding of chest wall overlying ductal area to reduce the risk of opening up of ductus.

Clinical Features

PDA should be suspected when a preterm infant being ventilated for RDS does not show the anticipated improvement after 3–4 days or after initial improvement there is sudden deterioration. The possibility of PDA should also be seriousy considered in preterm infants suffering from necrotizing enterocolitis and recurrent apneic attacks. The clinical features generally appear during 4 to 14 days of age. A long harsh ejection systolic murmur at base is the most consistent clinical finding. The murmur is rarely continuous or classical. There may be no murmur when pulmonary vascular resistance is high. The pulmonic component of second heart sound may be accentuated. The peripheral pulses are easily palpable and bounding in character with wide pulse pressure (>25 mm Hg). The precordium may be hyperdynamic. Congestive heart failure may supervene. The differential diagnosis includes arteriovenous fistula, aorticopulmonary window and ruptured sinus of Valsalva. A large PDA (>1.5 mm diameter) with left-to-right shunt in very low birth weight infants can cause pulmonary edema, cardiac failure, pulmonary hemorrhage and increased risk for bronchopulmonary dysplasia.

Diagnosis

Skiagram of chest may show pulmonary plethora and cardiac enlargement. Electrocardiogram is usually

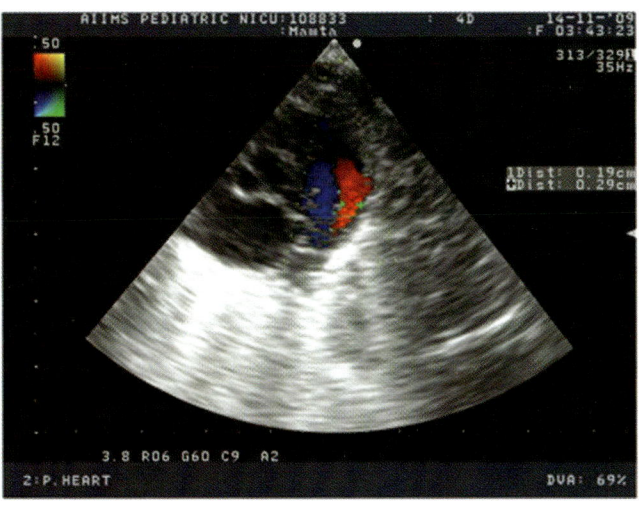

Figure 20.2 Echocardiogram in a preterm baby showing patent ductus arteriosus. The color Doppler shows flow of blood through the ductus (red color).

normal in the newborn period but may show left atrial enlargement and left ventricular hypertrophy in infancy. Significant ventricular hypertrophy or abnormal QRS axis in the newborn period is suggestive of associated congenital heart disease. M-mode echocardiography shows enlargement of left atrial and/or left ventricular end diastolic dimensions. Left atrial to aortic root diameter ratio often exceeds 1.5 and left atrial volume index is increased in infants with hemodynamically significant PDA (hs-PDA). The presence of diastolic pulmonary valve flutter or turbulence (back flow) is also suggestive of patent ductus arteriosus. Direct imaging of PDA using 2-D and pulsed Doppler with color flow imaging is the most sensitive and specific method to confirm the presence of PDA and quantify the amount of shunt (Figure 20.2). The machine is expensive and it has to be wheeled to the NICU.

Biomarkers

A number of biomarkers have been identified in patients with myocardial injury and cardiac dysfunction. Natriuretic peptides are produced either by atria (atrial natriuretic peptide or ANP) or by ventricles (brain natriuretic peptide or BNP). They result in natriuresis, diuresis, arterial vasodilatation and suppression of renin-angiotensin-aldosterone system. BNP and n-terminal pro-BNP have emerged as useful diagnostic markers of hemodynamically significant PDA (hs-PDA) with good sensitivity and specificity. The biomarkers are still at an experimental stage and are not routinely used in clinical practice.

Treatment

Most cases of ductus arteriosus in preterm babies can now be managed successfully by medical therapy. Fluids should be restricted to 80–100 mL/kg/day to reduce volume load to the ventricles. Role of digoxin is controversial and its use is limited to those infants who show frank evidences of congestive heart failure or when indomethacin therapy is contraindicated. Furosemide in a dose of 1–2 mg/kg intravenously every 12 to 24 hours is useful and is routinely recommended. Some workers recommend oral administration of hydrochlorthiazide 1–2 mg/kg/dose twice daily because there is some evidence to suggest that furosemide may promote patency of ductus by stimulating renal prostaglandin E_2 production. In almost two-thirds of cases, uncomplicated with hyaline membrane disease, ductus may close spontaneously within 48 hours of fluid restriction and diuretic therapy.

Prostaglandin-synthetase inhibitors or non-selective cyclo-oxygenase (COX) inhibitors are indicated to promote pharmacological closure of ductus, if conservative measures fail or infant weighs <1000 g. Indomethacin 0.2 mg/kg orally or preferably intravenously as a slow infusion over 30 min is administered every 12-hourly for a total of 3 doses and is effective in 80 to 90% of cases. It is potentially toxic and is contraindicated in infants with thrombocytopenia, bleeding, necrotizing enterocolitis and renal insufficiency. Platelet counts and renal parameters should be checked prior to starting therapy with indomethacin and repeated after 24 hours. Intravenous administration of indomethacin is associated with increase in blood pressure and reduction in cerebral blood flow velocity. It has recently been demonstrated that simultaneous administration of furosemide along with indomethacin effectively counteracts harmful renal side effects of latter. After initial closure of ductus, recurrence may occur in 25% cases which usually responds to a repeat course of indomethacin. Recently, studies have shown that oral ibuprofen 10 mg/kg followed by 5 mg/kg at 24 hours and 48 hours is equally effective and is safer. Paracetamol is equally effective in closing hs-PDA. It is given in a dose of 15 mg/kg orally every 6 hours for 48–72 hours. Early side effects like oliguria, elevation of creatinine and thrombocytopenia are minimal with paracetamol. There is recent evidence to suggest that pharmacological closure of ductus should be attempted only in infants with hypotension and congestive heart failure because treatment is not associated with proven long-term benefits and spontaneous closure of PDA occurs in nearly 50% of affected infants.

Cardiovascular Disorders

20

Surgical ligation of ductus is recommended in infants with intractable congestive heart failure with progressive cardiac enlargement and deteriorating pulmonary compliance and who relapse despite a second course of NSAID. Surgical closure is also indicated, if there are strong contraindications to the use of indomethacin or its administration is associated with serious side effects. The surgical procedure has been successfully performed in the neonatal intensive care unit thus obviating the need for transporting the critically sick ventilator-dependent tiny infant to the operation theater. Surgical ligation may be carried out by thoracotomy or video-assisted thoracoscopy.

CONGENITAL COMPLETE HEART BLOCK

Congenital complete heart block (CCHB) is the most common cardiac cause of fetal and neonatal brady-cardia. It is a disorder of conduction due to abnormality in the AV node with total dissociation between atrial and ventricular contractions. About 60% cases of CCHB are associated with complex cardiac mal-formations, like left atrial isomerism, atrioventricular septal defect, anomalies of great vessels and valvular stenosis or atresia. In 40% cases, there is isolated CCHB in association with maternal systemic lupus erythematosus. The immune-mediated damage to the AV node occurs due to transplacental passage of maternal anti-Ro antibodies (mostly anti-SS-A and occasionally anti-SS-B antibodies). There is an increased association with HLA-DR3 phenotype. CCHB may be picked up in fetal life as early as 16 weeks of gestation. The average ventricular rate is around 60 bpm and varies between 50 and 100 bpm. The atrial rate does not have any fixed time relationship to the ventricular contractions and varies between 140 and 160. M-mode echocardiogram should be done to confirm the diagnosis and exclude structural heart defects. Congestive heart failure may lead to development of hydrops fetalis. In the absence of congestive heart failure, no specific management is required during antenatal period. In the presence of CCHB, the management of labor becomes difficult because cardiotocography becomes unreliable.

When CCHB in fetal life is associated with evidences of congestive heart failure, corticosteroids, azathioprine and plasmapheresis have been tried in mothers with SLE with variable results. There is an on going multicentric trial which is examining the effect of administration of dexamethasone 4 mg daily to the mother who is carrying a baby with CCHB. Isoproterenol administration by cordocentesis has been successfully tried to increase ventricular rate.

Transventricular cardiac pacing during fetal life has been attempted when CCHB is associated with hydrops fetalis and there are no underlying stuctural defects in the heart. The baby should be delivered by cesarean section, if fetal heart rate is <50 bpm or there are evidences of hydrops fetalis.

The neonate with CCHB needs to be closely monitored for heart failure. The heart rate is usually around 50–60 bpm with prominent left ventricular impluse and marked variations in the intensity of first heart sound. EKG shows complete dissociation between auricular and ventricular contractions, wide QRS complexes (>0.10 sec) and prolonged QT interval (>0.44 sec) (Figure 20.3). Echocardiography is indicated to exclude structural cardiac defects, if there are no evidences of SLE in the mother. Asymptomatic infants with a rate of >50 bpm do not need any treatment . Digitalization and diuretics are recommended when there is frank congestive heart failure. Intra-ventricular pacing is indicated when ventricular rate is <50/bpm during waking hours (with QRS >0.10 sec, junctional recovery time >4 sec, pauses in EKG >3 sec) or there is frank congestive heart failure (Figure 20.4). When arrangements are being made for pacing, isoproterenol or atropine may be tried to increase heart rate. The prognosis is good in neonates with isolated CCHB without any structural cardiac defect.

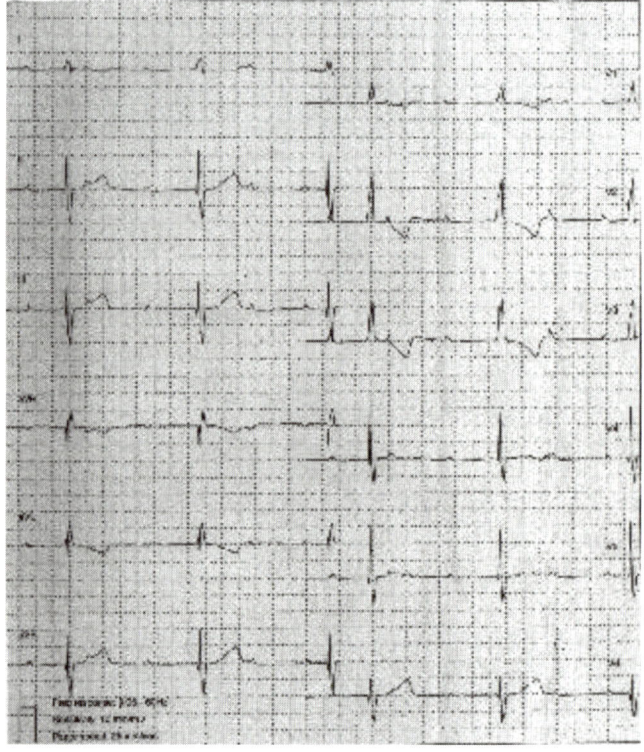

Figure 20.3 EKG showing evidences of complete heart block.

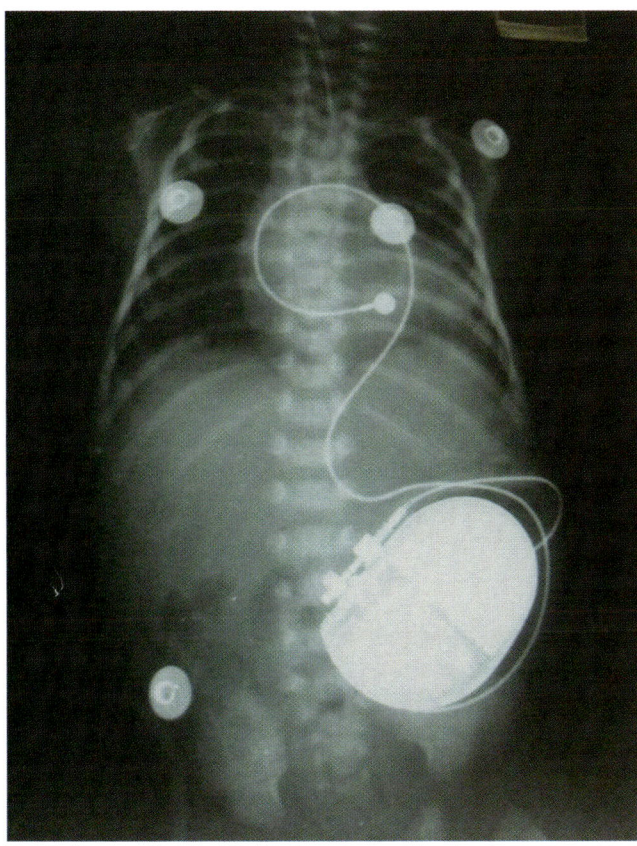

Figure 20.4 Permanent pacemaker in a baby with congenital complete heart block.

SUPRAVENTRICULAR TACHYCARDIA (SVT)

It is the commonest symptomatic arrhythmia in newborn babies. The heart rate is greater than 200 bpm, it is "fixed" without any beat-to-beat variation, P-wave may be hardly discernible but ventricular complexes are normal on EKG. Both onset as well as termination of arrhythmia is rapid and abrupt. Most affected infants do not have any underlying cardiac abnormality but 50% cases may be associated with Wolff-Parkinson-White (WPW) syndrome which is characterized by initial slurred (delta wave) and wide QRS deflection and short PR interval on EKG during recovery from SVT. In a small number of cases, hypertrophic subortic stenosis and Ebstein's anomaly may be associated with WPW syndrome especially among affected female infants.

SVT may occur *in utero* and is diagnosed on the basis of extreme tachycardia. If untreated, it may lead to congestive heart failure and hydrops fetalis. M-mode fetal echocardiography should be done to exclude underlying structural malformations of the heart. The attack can be aborted by administration of digoxin, propranolol, procainamide, quinidine or

verapamil to the mother. If fetal SVT is uncontrolled and there are evidences of fetal hydrops fetalis, the baby should be delivered by emergency cesarean section.

Paroxysmal atrial tachycardia or SVT in the neonate is characterized by tachycardia (>200 bpm), irritability and refusal to feed. Evidences of congestive heart failure may be seen, if SVT is persistent for more than 24 hours. The presence of structural heart disease should be excluded by clinical examination and echocardiography. Adenosine (100 μg/kg IV bolus up to a maximum of 300 μg/kg) is the drug of first choice but its safety in the neonatal period has not been proven. It must be given as rapid IV push because its half-life is only 10 seconds. Intravenous digitalization is recommended in infants without W-P-W syndrome. During digitalis therapy, vagal maneuver, like application of ice pack over the face may be tried in stable infants. Digoxin converts SVT to sinus rhythm in infants without hydrops fetalis. When digoxin is able to achieve sinus rhythm, maintenance therapy is continued for 6 to 12 months. Esmolol 500 μg/kg over 1 minute IV followed by 50 μg/kg/min as constant infusion is the drug of choice in infants with associated WPW syndrome because unlike digoxin it does not cause any antegrade conduction through the accessory pathway. During therapy with beta blockers, infant should be watched for apnea and hypoglycemia. In neonates, verapamil should not be used because of potential risk of sudden death. If the patient is unresponsive to adenosine, cardioversion may be performed followed by maintenance digoxin therapy.

CONGENITAL CARDIAC MALFORMATIONS

Developmental cardiac defects are present in about 10 per 1,000 live newborn babies and about two-thirds of these manifest in the neonatal period. The congenital cardiac malformations which manifest in the newborn period are often severe defects and one-third of these babies die in the neonatal period especially during the first week of life. Cardiac malformation may occur as an isolated anomaly or exist in combination with other complex anomalies, e.g. VATER syndrome (vertebral anomalies, anal atresia, tracheoesophageal fistula, cardiac defects, radial dysplasia) and trisomies 13, 18 and 21. A careful search for other anomalies is essential, because congenital heart disease is associated with at least one non-cardiac malformation in 25% of cases. Table 20.3 depicts various syndromes which are associated with congenital cardiac malformations. Infants of diabetic mothers are predisposed to develop cardiac

TABLE 20.3 Syndromes associated with congenital cardiac malformations		
Syndrome	*Extracardiac features*	*Cardiac anomalies*
Chromosomal anomalies		
Trisomy-13 (Patau syndrome)	Dysmorphism (mid-facial hypoplasia, cleft lip and palate, microophthalmia, coloboma, micrognathia, low-set ears), microcephaly, holoprosencephaly, aplasia of scalp, simian crease, polydactyly, capillary hemangiomas and flexion deformity of fingers.	Over 80% have cardiac defects, VSD is the commonest, PDA may occur.
Trisomy-18 (Edward syndrome)	Hypoplastic baby with facial dysmorphism (dolichocephaly, prominent occiput, short palpebral fissure, low-set ears, micrognathia), short sternum, rocker-bottom feet, overlapping fingers with "clenched fists" and simian crease.	Over 95% have cardiac defects, VSD is most common, valvular regurgitation may occur at multiple sites, PDA may be associated.
Trisomy-21 (Down syndrome)	Facial dysmorphism (brachycephaly, flat occiput, mongoloid slant of eyes, epicanthal folds, Brushfield spots in iris) simian crease, clinodactyly with short fifth finger, marked hypotonia.	40–50% have cardiac defect, common AV canal and VSD are most common. TOF, ASD, PDA and rarely complex cardiac anomalies are associated.
Turner syndrome (monosomy X)	Lymphedema of hands and feet, short webbed neck, facial dysmorphism (triangular face with antimongoloid slant of palpebral fissures, low-set ears) shield-like chest, cubitum valgum and short stature.	25–45% have cardiac defects, coarctation of aorta, bicuspid aortic valve are common.
Syndromes of single-gene defects		
Noonan syndrome (mutations in PTPN 11 gene, SOS 1 gene, and RAF 1, RIT 1 genes)	Hypoplastic baby with facial dysmorphism (hypertelorism, antimongoloid slant of eyes, ptosis, micrognathia, low-set ears), short webbed neck with low hair line, shield-like chest, pectus carinatum or excavatum, cubitum valgum, cryptorchidism and risk of developing leukemia.	Over 50% have cardiac defects namely valvular pulmonic stenosis, ASD, hypertrophic cardiomyopathy.
Holt-Oram syndrome (mutation in TBX 5 gene)	Finger-like triphalangeal or absent thumb, absent or hypoplastic radius, syndactyly and polydactyly.	Over 50% have cardiac defects, ASD, VSD are most common.
Ellis-van Creveld syndrome (mutations EVC and EVC 2 genes on chromosome 4)	Short distal extremities, short stature, polydactyly, respiratory distress, hypoplastic nails, dental anomalies, multiple frenula of upper lip, cleft lip and palate and epispadias.	About 50% have cardiac defects, ASD or common atrium.

(contd.)

TABLE 20.3 Syndromes associated with congenital cardiac malformations (*contd.*)

Syndrome	Extracardiac features	Cardiac anomalies
Gene deletion syndromes		
Williams syndrome (deletion 7q 11)	Facial dysmorphism ("elfin" facies, short palpebral fissure, puffiness, flat nasal bridge, stellate iris, long philtrum, prominent lips), mental subnormality (verbal performance better than motor), and hypercalcemia.	50–70% have cardiac defect, supravalvular aortic stenosis, stenosis of vessels at different sites, i.e. peripheral pulmonary arteries, aorta, renal arteries and coronary arteries.
Sotos syndrome (cerebral gigantism) (NSD 1 mutation and deletion)	Facial dysmorphism (long narrow face, dolichocephaly, bossing of forehead, hypertelorism and thinning of hair over frontotemporal region), over growth of all physical parameters, advanced bone age, neuromotor retardation, seizures, hypotonia and laxity of joints. Behavior disorder, autism, learning disability and phobias are common. Ventricular dilatation, hypoplasia or agenesis of corpus callosum, cerebral and cerebellar atrophy and EEG abnormalities are common.	About 20% of subjects show cardiac anomalies, like PDA, ASD and VSD.
DiGeorge syndrome (Deletion 22 q 11)	Facial dysmorphism (fish mouth deformity, hypertelorism, antimongoloid slant of eyes), hypoplasia or aplasia of thymus and parathyroids, cleft palate or velopharyngeal incompetence, tetany, cell-mediated immune deficiency.	Conotruncal malformations, like interrupted aortic arch, truncus arteriosus and TOF may be associated.
Miscellaneous syndromes		
Alagille syndrome (Jagged 1 gene, NOTCH signalling)	Dysmorphism (micrognathia, broad forehead, deep-set eyes), cholestasis, vertebral and ophthalmological anomalies.	Peripheral pulmonic stenosis is most common.
TAR syndrome (RBM 8A gene mutation and chromosome 1 deletions)	Thrombocytopenia, absent or hypoplastic radii.	About one-third have cardiac defects, TOF, VSD are most common.
VACTERL association (multiple gene defects)	Vertebral defects, anal atresia, cardiac defects, esophageal atresia with tracheoesophageal fistula, radial and renal anomalies, and limb defects.	Around 50% have cardiac defects, VSD is most common.
CHARGE association (mutation of CHD 7 gene)	Facial dysmorphism (broad forehead, square face, facial asymmetry, long nasal tip, ptosis, arched eyebrows, laterally protruding ears), coloboma, heart defects, atresia choanae, retarded growth and development, genital hypoplasia, ear anomalies and deafness, cranial nerve palsies and hypocalcemia.	75–80% have cardiac defects especially conotruncal anomalies, i.e. TOF, double outlet right ventricle, truncus arteriosus, and interrupted aortic arch

anomalies. In neonatal autopsy series, more than 10% of neonatal deaths are associated with serious cardiac anomalies.

In a newborn baby, the diagnosis of the existence of congenital heart disease may be very difficult and differentiation between congestive heart failure and respiratory distress syndrome (RDS) of pulmonary origin may be impossible at times. The early recognition of cardiac anomaly as a cause of respiratory distress, however, has practical implications because surgical intervention is life-saving. The five most frequently encountered cardiac anomalies during first week of life include transposition of the great arteries, hypoplasia of the left heart, tetralogy of Fallot, coarctation of aorta and ventricular septal defect. The classification of congenital heart diseases is shown in Table 20.4.

EVALUATION OF THE NEONATE WITH SUSPECTED CONGENITAL HEART DISEASE

The presence of heart disease should be strongly suspected when at least two of the following features are present in a neonate.

Cardiac Murmur

About 2 to 8% of newborn babies may have a cardiac murmur during the first 2 days of life. Its incidence depends upon the experience, vigilance and enthusiasm of the observer, the quietness of the baby's environment and the age of the baby at the time of examination. The functional murmurs are not associated with any other evidence of cardiac disease and majority of them disappear on follow-up by the age of 3 months. The significant cardiac murmur is often loud, grade III or more and may be associated with an ejection click and abnormalities of the second heart sound. There may be additional evidences of cardiac disease besides the murmur. The presence of murmur is not essential for the diagnosis of heart disease since 20% of infants dying of heart disease in the neonatal period do not have a murmur. In fact, in a severely symptomatic newborn baby, the presence of a soft and insignificant murmur or absence of murmur usually signifies a serious underlying heart disease. Many babies with a left-to-right shunt may not manifest any murmur during the neonatal period. The murmur may appear only after 2 to 4 weeks when the pulmonary vascular resistance and pressure decreases to adult levels. *Therefore, a murmur in the neonatal period does not necessarily indicate the presence of cardiac malformation while absence of a murmur does not rule out congenital heart disease.*

TABLE 20.4 Classification of congenital heart diseases

ACYANOTIC

i. **With shunt**
   - Atrial septal defect
   - Ventricular septal defect
   - Patent ductus arteriosus
   - Aortopulmonary window
   - Aorta-to-right heart, shunt, viz. sinus of Valsalva, aneurysm with fistulae, coronary arterial venous fistula, anomalous pulmonary origin of the left coronary artery
   - Endocardial cushion defect

ii. **With obstruction***
   *Left-sided****:
   - Aortic stenosis
   - Coarctation of aorta
   - Interrupted aortic arch
   - Hypoplastic left heart
   Right-sided:
   - Pulmonary stenosis
   - Ebstein anomaly

CYANOTIC

i. **Decreased pulmonary blood flow**
   - Tetralogy of Fallot
   - Tricuspid atresia
   - Critical pulmonary stenosis or atresia
   - Double outlet right ventricle with PS
   - Single ventricle with PS

ii. **Parallel circulation with poor mixing**
   - d-TGA with intact septum
   - d-TGA with VSD
   - Double outlet right ventricle with subpulmonic VSD

iii. **Complete mixing**
   - Total anomalous pulmonary venous connection
   - Truncus arteriosus
   - Single ventricle without PS

*These anomalies are duct-dependent and they become symptomatic when duct closes after a few days. Administration of oxygen may cause early closure of ductus. The infant should be kept on PGE_1 to maintain the patency of ductus arteriosus till surgical intervention or correction is done.

**These anomalies present with hypotension, poor tissue perfusion and cardiogenic shock.

PS; pulmonary stenosis; VSD, ventricular septal defect, d-TGA; dextro-transposition of the great arteries.

Abnormalities of Pulse

The abnormalities in cardiac rate, rhythm and peripheral pulses are rare as compared to the finding of a cardiac murmur. The rate and rhythm should be evaluated by cardiac auscultation rather than palpation of peripheral pulses which are often difficult to feel in neonates without sufficient experience. A persistent heart rate of more than 200 per minute in a quiet baby is suggestive of paroxysmal atrial tachycardia while a heart rate consistently below 80 per minute suggests complete heart block. *Bradycardia occurs commonly in association with asphyxia, hypothermia, hypothyroidism, raised intracranial tension, hypertension and hyperkalemia.* A rapid and irregular heart rate may rarely occur due to atrial fibrillation, atrial flutter or incomplete AV block. The peripheral pulses would be feeble in aortic stenosis, aortic atresia, severe congestive heart failure and shock. Feeble and delayed pulsations in the femorals suggest coarctation of aorta. The arterial pulsations would be full and bounding in infants with patent ductus arteriosus, AV aneurysm and severe anemia.

Cyanosis

Marked cyanosis in the absence of any respiratory distress is highly suggestive of cyanotic heart disease (exclude methemoglobinemia and polycythemia). The presence of severe RDS with marked retractions of chest and mild cyanosis is more common due to pulmonary rather than cardiac disorders. The important cardiac causes of cyanosis in the newborn include transposition of the great arteries, critical pulmonary stenosis or atresia, tetralogy of Fallot, tricuspid atresia, anomalous pulmonary veins (Table 20.4). The cyanosis due to right-to-left shunt becomes worse when the baby cries. Administration of 100% oxygen in these babies would neither relieve cyanosis nor significantly raise arterial PO_2. When 100% oxygen fails to raise PaO_2 above 50 mm Hg, it is highly suggestive of cyanotic congenital heart disease. The neonate who "fails" a hyperoxia test is likely to have congenital heart disease involving duct-dependent systemic or pulmonary blood flow and should receive prostaglandin E_1 (PGE_1) until definitive diagnosis is made by 2D echocardiography. Differential cyanosis is rare and is difficult to identify clinically. When present it is suggestive of complete transposition of great arteries with pulmonary hypertension and reversed flow through the ductus arteriosus. Pulse oximetry provides a non-invasive method to assess oxygen saturation. Measurement of SaO_2 in the right hand (preductal) should be compared with the foot (postductal) to look for differential cyanosis. Tissue hypoxia due to right-to-left shunt may result in metabolic acidosis and hypothermia. Clubbing of nails generally appears after three to six weeks. Refer to Chapter 26 for detailed evaluation of a cyanotic neonate.

Blood Pressure Abnormalities

Feeble pulses with low blood pressure, poor tissue perfusion or shock are suggestive of obstructive left-sided cardiac lesions. Blood pressure should be recorded in both the arms and legs with an automated Doppler amplification system. Normally blood pressure is higher in the lower extremities compared to the upper. When blood pressure is >10 mm Hg higher in the upper limbs compared to the legs, it is suggestive of conotruncal abnormalities, like coarctation of aorta, arch hypoplasia or interrupted aortic arch. The presence of reversed blood pressure gradient between upper and lower limb extremities is diagnostic of aortic arch abnormalities but its absence does not rule it out.

Cardiac Failure

The recognition of heart failure (HF) may at times be difficult due to similarities between the clinical features of cardiac failure and RDS of pulmonary origin as well as difficulties in the evaluation of cardiac size and jugular venous pressure in a newborn. The useful clinical signs of cardiac failure in the newborn are listed below.

Tachypnea Difficult or slow feeding, rapid and shallow breathing with minimal or no chest retractions and absence of grunting are characteristic. The presence of intense cyanosis rather early during the course of disease favors cardiac failure.

Tachycardia This should be evaluated when the baby is quiet and resting and not after a spell of crying or feeding. Combination of tachypnea and tachycardia is a strong pointer for the presence of cardiac failure. When heart rate is more than 220 bpm it is suggestive of tachyarrhythmia.

Hepatomegaly Progressive enlargement of liver is the most reliable sign of congestive heart failure in a newborn baby. Splenomegaly may also appear.

Edema Puffiness or generalized edema and rapid weight gain of more than 100 g per day are suggestive of cardiac failure. However, facial and pedal edema is a rather late manifestation of cardiac failure in neonates. In heart failure of gradual onset and prolonged duration, inadequate weight gain is more likely because of poor feeding, utilization of energy for breathing effort and tissue hypoxia.

Cardiac enlargement It may not be apparent during the first few days after the onset of cardiac failure. It is difficult to evaluate clinically as well as radiologically.

Cardiovascular Disorders

20

Progressive cardiomegaly, however, is always indicative of congestive cardiac failure.

Auscultatory findings Abnormalities in the cardiac sounds, such as third heart sound, gallop rhythm, a soft first sound or single S_2 and significant cardiac murmur after the age of 12 hours, favor the possibility of underlying developmental defect of the heart. The absence of these findings, however, does not rule out the possibility of cardiac failure.

Miscellaneous features The presence of unexplained vomiting, poor feeding, irritability, sweating (left-to-right shunt) and poor weight gain are additional features suggestive of cardiac failure. It is important to remember that raised jugular venous pressure (due to short neck), peripheral edema (due to recumbent posture), crackles in the chest and pleural effusion are not seen in neonates with cardiac failure.

Abnormalities on X-ray Chest

The presence of thymus shadow and portable nature of study without due regard to the distance between the source of X-rays and the baby, interfere with the evaluation of heart size. The cardiac enlargement may not occur during the first 48 hours after the onset of cardiac failure. The cardiothoracic ratio of more than 60% is taken as an evidence of cardiac enlargement in a newborn baby. Skiagram of chest also provides useful information regarding pulmonary blood flow, location of aortic arch (right or left), specific chamber enlargement, dextrocardia or situs inversus. Infants with situs inversus or situs ambiguous or heterotaxy syndrome (midline stomach bubble) with a left-sided heart are likely to have severe congenital heart defect. The right-sided aortic arch is associated with congenital heart disease in over 90% of patients.

Abnormal Electrocardiogram

The characteristic EKG findings in normal newborn babies are as follows:

Rate Mean 120–130/minute and a range of 90–200/minute.

P-waves Taller than those of older children but their duration is shorter, i.e. 0.02–0.10 seconds.

PR interval 0.06–0.14 seconds. It is maximum on the first day. Heart rate has less significant effect on PR interval in a newborn baby.

Ventricular preponderance In preterm babies up to 32 weeks of gestation, left ventricular preponderance is seen while term babies show right ventricular preponderance. It is characterized by right axis deviation and R/S ratio of more than 1.0 in V1.

T-waves T-waves are upright in right precordial leads and inverted in the left precordial leads during the first 72 hours of life. Subsequently, they are normally inverted in V1 or V3 and upright in V5 and V6.

Q-Tc 0.37–0.48 seconds.

In view of physiological right ventricular preponderance in term babies during the neonatal period, it is important to define the exact criteria of ventricular hypertrophy during this age period.

Right Ventricular Hypertrophy

It is seen in hypoplastic left heart syndrome, pulmonary stenosis, tetralogy of Fallot, total anomalous pulmonary venous drainage and transposition of great arteries. The EKG criteria for the diagnosis of ventricular hypertrophy are listed in Table 20.5. At least two or more of these criteria should be present to permit a definitive diagnosis.

Left Ventricular Hypertrophy

It is seen in grossly preterm babies, hypoplastic right heart syndrome, aortic stenosis, transposition of great vessels, Ebstein's anomaly, endocardial fibroelastosis, truncus arteriosus, and gross immaturity.

Functional Echocardiography

Availability of Doppler and 2D color flow echocardiography has revolutionised the diagnosis and management of congenital heart defects. It is not possible to have round-the-clock services of pediatric

---

TABLE 20.5 Criteria for the diagnosis of ventricular hypertrophy in newborn babies

Right ventricular hypertrophy
- R/S ratio of more than 5 in V1
- R wave in V1 of more than 25 mm, S wave in V5 of more than 15 mm during 1–7 days and 10 mm during 8–30 days
- q wave in V3R and V1
- Upright T wave in V1 after 72 hours of age
- Intrinsicoid deflection of more than 0.03 seconds in V1

Left ventricular hypertrophy
- Absence of normal right axis deviation
- R/S ratio of less than 1 in V1
- S wave in V1 of more than 25 mm and R wave in V5 of more than 15 mm during 1–7 days and 25 mm during 8–30 days
- Inverted T wave in V5 after 72 hours of age
- Intrinsicoid deflection of more than 0.04 second in V5

cardiologists. Most neonates with cardiac problems are too sick to be transported to the cardiac diagnostic facility. A screening cot-side or point-of-care functional or targeted neonatal echocardiography (TNE) should be available in the NICU. It provides sequential or continuous monitoring of the cardiac hemodynamic parameters in critically sick neonates. It is primarily used to assess vascular pressures and flows, myocardial functions and structural heart defects in hemodynamically unstable and sick neonates. The instrument required include two-dimensional (2D) pulsed wave Doppler (PWD) and continuous wave Doppler (CWD) with M-mode facility. In term and preterm infants, a probe frequency range of 7.5–10 MHz provides excellent resolution with adequate tissue penetrations. Infants with severe cyanosis and possibility of complex heart defect should be referred to a pediatric cardiologist for a detailed evaluation and management.

Indications

Functional echocardiography is used for hemodynamic assessment, definitive diagnosis and management of following cardiovascular disorders.

- Perinatal asphyxia with multiorgan dysfunction
- Evaluation of RV and inferior LV systolic and diastolic functions, superior and inferior vena caval blood flow
- Assessment of atrial level shunt (foramen ovale) and hemodynamically significant patent ductus arteriosus (hsPDA)
- Persistent pulmonary hypertension (PPHN)
- Congenital heart disease
- Congenital diaphragmatic hernia
- Shock
- Ultrasound-guided drainage of pericardial effusion, location of umbilical catheters, placement of central line and cannulation for ECMO.

Functional echocardiography provides physiological information in real-time and is increasingly being used in making clinical decisions in the NICU. The role of neonatologist performed cot-side echocardiography is rapidly evolving and is now being considered as an extension of clinical examination to assess hemodynamic status of critically ill neonates. There is an urgent need to develop a structured training program and accreditation process for the neonatologists to develop echocardiographic skills. Standardised and structured training, robust clinical governance and a close collaboration with the pediatric cardiologist are the key elements to ensure patient's safety and professional competence.

CARDIAC FAILURE

Cardiac failure (CF) is defined as inadequate oxygen delivery by the heart or circulatory system to meet the demands of the body. The ratio of non-contractile mass (nuclei, mitochondria and membranes) to the contractile mass is 70% in the fetal heart as compared to 40% in the adult heart. The neonatal heart is thus equipped with poor reserve capacity and is normally working at the upper limit of Frank-Starling curve. A large number of cardiac and non-cardiac conditions are recognized to cause cardiac failure during neonatal period (Table 20.6).

Cardiac malformations The clinical features of congenital cardiac malformations producing cardiac failure during the first month of life are listed in Table 20.7. The definitive diagnosis is often impossible without the aid of M-mode and two-dimensional echocardiography with color Doppler, selective angiocardiography and cardiac catheterization. Availability of point-of-care functional echocardiography (PCFecho) is desirable in the NICU for real-time evaluation of cardiac functions and systemic hemodynamics to make an early diagnosis of life-threatening cardiac malformations.

TABLE 20.6 Common causes of heart failure on the basis of age at onset

Fetal causes
Anemia. Erythroblastosis (Rh-isoimmunization), feto-maternal transfusion, parvovirus B19 infection, alpha thalassemia (hydrops fetalis) and hypoplastic anemia
Arrhythmias. Supraventricular tachycardia, ventricular tachycardia, complete heart block.

First 48 hours
Premature infants. Fluid overload, patent ductus arteriosus, bronchopulmonary dysplasia, hypertension.
Full-term infants. Asphyxial cardiomyopathy, systemic AV fistula, viral myocarditis, polycythemia, sepsis, hypoglycemia, hypocalcemia, complete heart block, congenital thyrotoxicosis and fluid overload.

First week of life
Critical aortic/pulmonary stenosis, hypoplastic left heart syndrome, transposition of great vessels with intact ventricular septum, obstructed total anomalous pulmonary venous connection, coarctation of aorta, Ebstein anomaly

Second week of life
Large ventriculoseptal defect, atrioventricular septal defect, large PDA, unobstructed total anomalous pulmonary venous drainage and truncus arteriosus

1–2 months of life
Large L–R shunts, transposition and malposition complexes, anomalous left coronary artery from pulmonary artery and aorta-pulmonary window.

Cardiovascular Disorders

20

TABLE 20.7 Diagnostic features of various cardiac anomalies in symptomatic neonates

Condition	Age of onset of CHF	Cyanosis	Murmurs and heart sounds	Other clinical features	EKG	X-ray chest	Special investigations	Surgical palliation or correction
■ Hypoplastic left heart syndrome (aortic and mitral atresia)	Within first week. Intractable and rapid course	Mild	Absent or variable, late stenotic murmur and single S_2	Feeble pulses and shock	Severe RVH	Early cardiac enlargement with increased vascularity	Retrograde aortography and echo-cardiography	Norwood procedure during newborn period followed by Fontan operation in childhood. Cardiac transplant is curative
■ Transposition of great vessels with intact ventricular septum	1–2 weeks	Early and deep	None character-istic	Large-for-dates	RVH and later biventri-cular hyper-trophy	Oval or egg-shaped heart with narrow base	Angiocardio-graphy and cardiac catheterization	Balloon atrial septostomy, arterial switch operation
■ Coarctation of aorta (preductal with VSD or PDA)	1–4 weeks	Nil	None character-istic except stenotic murmur across the back	Femoral pulses absent and upper limb blood pressure higher by more than 10 mm Hg than the lower limbs	RVH and later biventri-cular hyper-trophy	Cardiac enlargement with normal to increased vascularity.	Retrograde aortography	Surgical correction
■ Hypoplastic right heart syndrome (pulmonic and tricuspid atresia)	Uncommon except when trans-position of great vessels is associated	Signi-ficant	None character-istic	Abnormal coronary arteries with right ventricular sinusoidal anasta-moses	LVH with left axis deviation in tricuspid atresia and right axis deviation in pulmo-nary atresia	Pulmonary vascularity is reduced	Selective angicardio-graphy	Balloon atrial septostomy and pulmonary valvotomy with Blalock-Taussig shunt
■ Tetralogy of Fallot	Uncommon	Delayed onset except in severe cases	Ejection systolic murmur with single S_2	Anoxic spells	RVH with reduced vascularity	Boot-shaped heart	Cardiac catheteriza-tion	Aorto-pulmonary anastomosis
■ Total anomalous pulmonary venous connection (TAPVC)	1–2 weeks of age	Pulmo-nary ejection systolic murmur, widely split and fixed S_2	Trans-position of great arteries, pulmonary stenosis and coar-ctation of aorta	Right axis deviation with right ventricular hyper-trophy	Cardio-megaly, plethoric lung fields, figure of 8 or snow-man sign after the age of 2 years	Echocardio-graphy	Obstructive TAPVC needs early surgical correction. Postoperatively pulmonary hypertensive crisis may occur	

(contd.)

TABLE 20.7 Diagnostic features of various cardiac anomalies in symptomatic neonates (*contd.*)

Condition	Age of onset of CHF	Cyanosis	Murmurs and heart sounds	Other clinical features	EKG	X-ray chest	Special investigations	Surgical palliation or correction
▪ Large left-to-right shunts (including truncus arteriosus)	2–6 weeks	Nil	Pansystolic murmur with diastolic flow murmur, split S$_2$	Look for signs and symptoms of rubella syndrome and full bounding pulses in PDA and truncus arteriosus	LVH or biventricular hypertrophy	Cardiomegaly with increased pulmonary vascularity	Echocardiography	Ligation of PDA in a term baby or when intractable CHF is present
▪ Persistent pulmonary hypertension	Within 2 hours after birth	Significant	Non-specific systolic murmur may be audible	HMD, meconium aspiration syndrome, hypoglycemia	Normal or RVH	Cardiac enlargement, hyperinflated lungs, flattening of diaphragm and increased pulmonary markings	Echocardiography to exclude congenital heart disease	Not required
▪ Double-outlet right ventricle with VSD	Any time	Uncommon	Loud pansystolic murmur, S$_2$ closely split with loud pulmonic sound.	Trisomy-18, absent thumbs, club feet, malformed jaw, cleft palate, gastrointestinal and genito-urinary anomalies.	Right axis deviation with biventricular hypertrophy	Cardiac enlargement with plethoric lung fields	Angiocardiography	Banding of pulmonary artery needs evaluation
▪ Ebstein's anomaly	Uncommon	Significant	None characteristic, 3rd and 4th heart sounds may be present	None	Tall P waves, prolonged P-R interval, low voltage QRS complexes with right bundle branch block	Box-shaped heart with marked enlargement of right atrium and oligemic lung fields	Cardiac catheterization	None

Note: The conditions have been listed in order of their frequency as a cause of symptomatic heart disease in the newborn period. The characteristics of the murmur are of least diagnostic utility during this age period.

Cardiovascular Disorders

20

Paroxysmal atrial tachycardia The condition has been diagnosed *in utero* by virtue of exceedingly high fetal heart rate. These infants may be born with hydrops fetalis. It is more common in males and is not associated with any cardiac malformation. It is characterized by sudden onset of respiratory distress, vomiting, pallor and refusal to take feeds. The heart rate is over 200 beats per minute and is difficult to count. Electrocardiogram shows heart rate of more than 200 beats per minute without any discernible P waves. The prognosis is good following digoxin and/or propranolol therapy which should be continued for at least one year to safeguard against recurrences. Infant should be carefully evaluated for the presence of Wolff-Parkinson-White syndrome which is characterized by short P-R interval and "slurred" QRS complexes due to accelerated excitation of ventricles.

Complete heart block Complete heart block may be diagnosed *in utero* or after birth by persistent heart rate of less than 100/minute. It is usually asymptomatic but extreme bradycardia (<50/min) may lead to congestive heart failure. In 50% cases, it may be associated with structural heart defects, like corrected transposition of great arteries, atrioventricular septal defect and heterotaxy syndromes (situs ambiguous). It is a useful marker of systemic lupus erythematosus in the mother.

Myocarditis It presents as an unexplained congestive heart failure with a gallop rhythm and muffled first heart sound but without any significant murmur. EKG may show low voltage complexes with depression of ST segment and inversion of T waves. The mother may give history of flu-like illness and pleurodynia due to Coxsackie-B infection before delivery. The prognosis is generally poor.

Severe anemia Hydrops fetalis due to cardiac failure may occur as a result of severe anemia because of any cause.

Arteriovenous fistula Cerebral arteriovenous fistula or hepatic angiomatous malformation may produce intractable cardiac failure. It is important to auscultate the head and liver area in all infants with cardiac failure to identify arteriovenous shunt or vascular malformation. Cardiac flow murmurs are often present. EKG may show presence of biventricular hypertrophy.

Congenital thyrotoxicosis The clinical picture is characterized by maternal history of thyrotoxicosis, evidences of intractable cardiac failure in the baby, tachycardia, diffuse enlargement of goiter, prominent eyes, jitteriness, excessive crying, diarrhea and unsatisfactory weight gain despite good appetite.

Over-loading of circulation Materno-fetal transfusion, polycythemia, excessive hydration by intravenous therapy, acute renal failure and over-loading during exchange transfusion may lead to cardiac failure.

Hypertension Hypertension due to coarctation of aorta, congenital adrenal hyperplasia, renovascular disease, and renal vein thrombosis may result in cardiac decompensation.

Glycogen storage disease The presence of muscular hypotonia and macroglossia should alert the physician to this possibility. Pompe disease (Type 2 GSD) is associated with cardiac involvement. EKG shows left axis deviation, short PR interval and high voltage QRS complexes.

Perinatal distress factors Hypoxia, hypocalcemia, hypoglycemia and acidosis may be associated with cardiac decompensation in newborn babies.

Acute cor pulmonale Cardiac failure may rarely follow persistent pulmonary infection or chronic airway obstruction and bronchopulmonary dysplasia.

Endocardial fibroelastosis It may occasionally manifest in the neonatal period with cardiac failure of insidious onset. There may be history of mumps during pregnancy or a positive family history of similar illness in an earlier sibling. EKG shows left ventricular dominance with inversion of T waves in the left precordial leads.

Management

The neonate who is seriously ill with a suspected cardiac anomaly should be regarded both as a medical and a potential surgical emergency. The baby should preferably be transferred immediately to a center where adequate facilities are available for complete investigations and surgery. With the exception of hypoplastic left heart syndrome, surgical palliation or correction is possible in most of the cardiac anomalies during neonatal period. An effort should be made to stabilize the condition of the baby by medical management of cardiac failure before undertaking special investigations for definitive diagnosis of cardiac malformation.

Position and oxygen therapy The infant should be kept propped up and oxygen administered by raising its concentration to 40% in a plastic box enclosing the baby's head. The handling should be reduced to bare minimum. The supplemental oxygen should be used with caution in infants with left-to-right shunt (due to risk of increasing systemic pressure and reducing pulmonary pressure) and in patients with anatomic outflow obstruction, like hypoplastic left heart syndrome because it may cause early closure of ductus.

Prostaglandins The neonate who "fails" an hyperoxia and hyperventilation test or presents with circulatory collapse or shock is likely to have congenital heart disease involving duct-dependent systemic or pulmonary blood flow and should receive PGE_1 infusion until diagnosis can be confirmed. PGE_1 constant infusion is life saving to maintain the patency of ductus arteriosus in infants with duct-dependent complex congenital cardiac malformations. The palliative management is useful to sustain life till baby is stable to undergo corrective surgery. It is indicated in a large number of congenital cardiac malformations in whom duct-dependent systemic blood flow (hypoplastic left heart syndrome, aortic atresia or stenosis, coarctation of aorta or atresia of aortic arch) and duct-dependent pulmonary blood flow (hypoplastic right heart syndrome, pulmonary stenosis, tricuspid atresia, tetralogy of Fallot and Ebstein anomaly) are crucial for their survival. PGE_1 infusion is indicated in any sick neonate with hypoxemia and cyanosis, even if the cardiac diagnosis is not clear and echocardiographic examination is pending. Its use is contraindicated in infants with total anomalous pulmonary venous return with obstruction, mitral atresia, hypoplastic left heart syndrome (HLHS), and transposition of great arteries with intact ventricular and atrial septum.

One ampoule of PGE_1 (500 µg/mL) is dissolved in 100 mL of dextrose-containing solution to obtain a concentration of 5 µg/mL. The usual starting dose is 0.05–0.40 µg/kg/min. After achieving the desired therapeutic effect, the dose is reduced to as low as 0.005–0.01 µg/kg/min for maintenance. The response to PGE_1 is dramatic, if patency of duct is important for the hemodynamic state of the infant. Failure to respond to infusion of PGE_1 may mean that the initial diagnosis was incorrect, the ductus is either absent or unresponsive to PGE_1. Adverse reactions to PGE_1 include apnea, hypotension, fever, flushing and seizures. PGE_1 infusion makes the ductus friable which should be handled gently during surgery. The infant should preferably be intubated before starting PGE_1 infusion and blood pressure should be closely monitored.

Decongestive Measures

Three types of drugs are used for the management of cardiac failure, viz. preload reducing agents, inotropes and postload reducing agents.

Agents to reduce preload Diuretics decrease the preload by promoting natriuresis. Furosemide 1–2 mg/kg per dose IM or IV every 8 to 12 hours is most suitable. In neonates less than 32 weeks gestation, a single dose should be given in 24 hours. The baby should be weighed before therapy and after every 12 hours and his urine output should be recorded. Spironolactone may be coadministered as a safeguard against development of hypokalemia when prolonged furosemide therapy is needed to protect against hypokalemia. Besides the fluid and electrolyte disturbances, hearing loss is a recognized side effect of furosemide therapy.

Inotropes Digitalis is the most commonly used time honored inotrope. The inotropic action of digitalis is mediated through inhibition of the enzyme Na^+-K^+-ATPase in the myocardial membrane leading to influx of calcium ions into the myocardial muscle fibers. The therapeutic utility of digoxin is limited because the neonatal heart is already working at its peak and has very little reserve. Digoxin has no role in treatment of cardiac failure due to non-cardiac causes.

The total oral digitalizing dose is 0.02–0.04 mg/kg (parenteral dose is 75% of oral dose), the smaller dose is given to preterm infants, seriously affected rhesus isoimmunized babies and infants with myocarditis. Intravenous therapy is generally preferred because of uncertainty of oral and intramuscular absorption. The parenteral dose of digoxin should not exceed three-fourths of the oral dose. One-half of the total digitalizing dose is given as the first dose, one-quarter as the second and third dose after 8 hours and 12 hours, respectively. An electrocardiogram should be obtained before the start of therapy and again before giving the third dose. The next dose of digoxin should be withheld, if heart rate has dropped to less than 100/minute or if PR interval is more than 0.14 seconds. The maintenance dose of digoxin is one-third to one-quarter of total digitalizing dose and should be administered in two divided doses daily. Digitalis is contraindicated in infants with cyanotic spells, idiopathic hypertrophic subaortic stenosis, ventricular tachycardia and obstructive cardiomyopathy in infants of diabetic mothers.

Catecholamines, like dopamine and dobutamine, release endogenous norepinephrine by stimulating B_1 and B_2 receptors, respectively. Dopamine is administered as a constant intravenous infusion @ 5–20 µg/kg/min. The minimum effective dose in preterm babies is 10 µg/kg/min. Dobutamine (5–20 µg/kg/min) is considered as the drug of choice in neonates with cardiac failure due to asphyxia. It is tolerated better because of reduced risk of causing tachycardia or reduction of renal perfusion. It has a lower risk of causing arrhythmia and it reduces after load because of its vasodilatory effect. A combination of low-dose dopamine (up to 5 µg/kg/min) and dobutamine is recommended to minimize the risk of peripheral vasoconstriction induced by high dose of dopamine while maximizing its dopaminergic effects on renal perfusion. Adverse reactions to catecholamines include tachycardia, ventricular arrhythmia and increased after load due to peripheral vasoconstriction especially with dopamine. Amrinone, a selective type III phosphodiesterase inhibitor, is recommended for treatment of cardiac failure following surgical correction of cardiac malformations. It is a useful second line inotropic agent with significant reduction of after load due to vasodilatation and improved relaxation of myocardium during diastole.

Agents to reduce afterload Vasodilators are useful to counteract compensatory systemic vasoconstriction. They decrease the afterload and thus increase the stroke volume. There are three types of vasodilators that can be used for the treatment of cardiac failure, viz. venodilators, arteriolar dilators and combined dilators. ACE-1 inhibitors are useful because they not only suppress the renin-angiotensin-aldosterone axis thereby reducing vasoconstriction, sodium and water retention but also exert a modulator effect on the myocardium. Captopril (0.15–0.20 mg/kg/d q 8–12 hr oral) and enalapril are the commonly used ACE-inhibitors when diuretics and inotropes fail to provide significant relief. In infants with left-to-right shunt, enalapril (0.1–0.4 mg/kg/day orally q 24 hr) provides both hemodynamic as well as clinical improvement. They are contraindicated in infants with bilateral renal artery stenosis, renal dysfunction and the left-sided obstructive lesions, like severe aortic stenosis. They have been shown to adversely affect nephrogenesis in a rat model.

Transport After initial stabilization, the neonate with life-threatening congenital heart disease often needs to be transferred to an institution that provides advanced care in pediatric cardiology and cardiac surgery. Reliable vascular lines should be established, one for administration of PGE_1 and another for delivery of inotropes and other drugs. Umbilical lines placed for resuscitation and stabilization should be left in place during transport because they may be required for cardiac catheterization at the referral center. Infants receiving PGE_1 infusion should be intubated before transport for effective handling of apnea or cardiac arrest during the journey. All intubated neonates should have gastric decompression with a nasogastric or orogastric tube.

Feeding During acute stage, two intravenous lines should be established, one for administration of 10% dextrose (60 mL/kg/day) with supplements of potassium and the other for providing constant infusion of prostaglandins. Subsequently, tube feeding is preferred till respiratory distress is relieved when cup and spoon or bottle feeding with concentrated milk formula should be tried to provide more calories for less effort. The use of low sodium milk is unnecessary when a diuretic is being administered.

Antibiotics Most infants would need antibiotics because pneumonia cannot be excluded with certainty and it is a common comorbidity.

Sedation Phenobarbitone, chloral hydrate or morphine (50 µg/kg SC) is useful in most cases to relieve restlessness and irritability.

Correction of acidosis This would reduce pulmonary vascular resistance and improve myocardial function. Sodium overload should be kept in mind while using sodium bicarbonate.

Environmental temperature Babies with a large left-to-right shunt tend to sweat and have high metabolic rate. They should be nursed in an environmental temperature at the lower end of the neutral range as compared to infants with cyanotic heart disease who may develop hypothermia.

Rotating tourniquet Acute left heart failure with pulmonary edema may benefit by reducing ventricular preload by application of tourniquets to three limbs. They are rotated every 10 to 15 minutes and one limb is left free all the time. Its therapeutic utility is doubtful.

Treatment of the Underlying Cause

Paroxysmal Atrial Tachycardia

Infant may respond to vagal stimulation by doing rectal examination or application of ice bag on the face. Digoxin alone or along with propranolol are useful to prevent recurrence but it is no longer recommended for treatment of an acute attack. Adenosine is the drug of first choice but its safety in the neonatal period has not been proven. Verapamil should not be used in neonates. The direct counter-shock (cardioversion) with 1 watt-sec per kg (maximum of 10 watt-sec) may be required in resistant or hemodynamically unstable cases.

Complete Heart Block

Most neonates with complete congenital heart block do not require any therapy. If signs of heart failure are present or heart rate is very slow (<50/min) treatment with isoproterenol (0.1–0.5 μg/kg/min) may be instituted. Symptomatic infants would invariably need a permanent pacemaker. Intraventricular pacing is indicated when ventricular rate is <50 beats/min during waking hours (with QRS >0.10 sec, junctional recovery time >4 sec and pauses on EKG of more than 3 sec) or when there is gross cardiac failure. In newborn babies, usually transthoracic epicardial pacemaker devices are used.

Myocarditis

These patients tolerate digoxin rather poorly and a lower digitalizing dose should be used. The role of corticosteroids is controversial.

Anemia

Partial exchange transfusion with packed red blood cells (10–20 mL/kg) is recommended, if hematocrit is less than 40%.

Polycythemia

In babies with polycythemia or increased blood volume due to isoimmunization, feto-fetal or maternofetal transfusion and overhydration, the use of furosemide alone is often enough though at times removal of 20 to 40 mL of blood or partial exchange transfusion with normal saline or blood may be life saving.

Hypoglycemia

This should be looked for in all neonates with cardiac failure and treated appropriately.

Thyrotoxicosis

In addition to the use of antithyroid agents, digitalization is essential. In case tachycardia is uncontrolled with digoxin, propranolol has been found useful.

Patent Ductus Arteriosus

Pharmacological closure of patent ductus arteriosus, in preterm babies with RDS, is recommended with indomethacin (0.2 mg/kg IV or oral every 12 hours for 3 doses) or oral ibuprofen 10 mg/kg followed by 5 mg/kg at 24 hours and 48 hours or paracetamol 15 mg/kg oral every 6 hours for 48–72 hours.

AV Aneurysmal Malformation

Vein of Galen malformation and other AV malformations in the brain and liver are rare causes of intractable high output cardiac failure in the newborn period. The infant should be stabilized with a combination of β-adrenergic agonist and vasodilator. The inotrope of choice is dopamine (up to a dose of 10 μg/kg/min) with either sodium nitroprusside (1–5 μg/kg/min) or glyceryl trinitrate (1–5 μg/kg/min). In critically sick babies, phosphodiesterase inhibitors, such as milrinone (0.4–0.75 μg/kg/min), may be life saving. The definitive therapy includes transvenous coil embolization using a femoral or ultrasound-guided transtorcular approach to thrombose the malformed site.

Cardiac Surgery and Percutaneous Transcatheter Cardiac Interventions

One-third of infants with congenital cardiac defects are likely to die during neonatal period because of critical myocardial dysfunction unless urgent surgical intervention is offered to them. Advances in the pediatric cardiac surgery during the past two decades have made surgical correction or palliation possible during infancy and neonatal period for all forms of congenital heart defects. The specific diagnosis of the underlying cardiac defect can now be reliably made by the use of non-invasive high resolution cross-sectional echocardiography and color Doppler imaging especially in critically ill neonates in whom cardiac catheterization and angiocardiography or retrograde aortography is associated with considerable risk. The newer pharmacological agents, like prostaglandin E$_1$ have improved the survival of neonates with critical duct-dependent lesions so that definitive surgery can be undertaken after stabilization of the infant.

A number of cardiac malformations can be managed by cardiac catheterization and by performing palliative procedures. The duct-dependent lesions should be maintained on infusion of PGE$_1$. The baby should be provided excellent supportive care after establishing umbilical venous and arterial lines for resuscitation. The infant should be started on broad spectrum prophylactic antibiotics to cover both Gram-positive and negative organisms. During catheterization, effective measures should be taken to prevent hypothermia. Heparin in a dose of 100 units/kg is given to prevent thrombus formation and reduce the risk of embolization. Table 20.8 summarizes various palliative and corrective interventions and their

TABLE 20.8 Non-invasive cardiac procedures to provide palliation and relief during newborn period

Procedure	Indications
■ Balloon atrial septostomy*	Transposition of great vessels (with intact ventricular and atrial septa), mitral atresia, tricuspid atresia, total anomalous pulmonary venous connection, double outlet right ventricle with restrictive VSD, pulmonary atresia with intact ventricular septum.
■ Balloon valvuloplasty or dilatation of stenotic valves	Critical pulmonic and aortic stenosis
■ Balloon angioplasty	Coarctation of aorta.
■ Stenting	Ductus arteriosus is stented to maintain its patency in duct-dependent cardiac anomalies, peripheral pulmonary stenosis, total anomalous pulmonary venous obstruction, pulmonary artery or right ventricular to pulmonary conduits and coarctation of aorta (awaiting corrective surgery or cardiac transplantation)
■ Coil embolization	Closure of ductus arteriosus, arteriovenous aneurysms and dilated vein of Galen.

*The procedure can be performed up to 3 months of age but best results are seen during first month of life.

indications during the newborn period. Rapid advances in interventional cardiology has made it possible to undertake percutaneous pulmonary and aortic valve replacement and provide a transcatheter closure of the holes in the atrial and ventricular septa.

The current emphasis in pediatric cardiac surgery is to undertake corrective surgery as early as possible. The role of palliative surgery is now limited to babies with hypoplastic pulmonary arteries and those with single ventricle requiring a Fontan type repair by providing direct atriopulmonary anastomosis to bypass the right ventricle. The hitherto inoperable cardiac defects (like hypoplastic left heart syndrome) have been successfully managed by performing two stage Norwood operation and cardiac transplantation in the neonates. Advances in biotechnology have made cardiopulmonary bypass fairly safe even in preterm babies by introduction of newer modality of extracorporeal membrane oxygenation (ECMO). It is obvious that success of neonatal cardiac surgery demands the availability of excellent backup facilities and tertiary level neonatal care facilities with a close coordination between the pediatric cardiac surgeon and the neonatologist.

Cardiac Transplantation

The common indications for cardiac transplantation include end-stage cardiomyopathy, hypoplastic left heart syndrome, single ventricle and palliated heart disease following palliative surgical procedure in an infant with complex congenital heart disease. Cardiac transplantation facilities are available in select centers and procedure is limited by non-availability of cadaveric donors.

SHOCK

Shock is characterized by inability of circulatory system to maintain adequate tissue perfusion leading to hypoxic tissue damage and accumulation of metabolic waste products. It is associated with reduced cardiac output and poor peripheral circulation. Due to lack of routine blood pressure monitoring in newborn babies, the condition is often overlooked. Early recognition and management of shock is desirable to prevent irreversible damage to vital organs and its progression to several life-threatening disorders in the newborn, viz. acute renal failure, disseminated intravascular coagulation, necrotizing enterocolitis, and intraventricular hemorrhage.

Pathophysiology

The basic denominator of shock due to any cause is fall in arterial blood pressure. Arterial pressure is dependent upon cardiac output and vascular resistance (Pressure = flow × resistance). Cardiac output depends upon adequacy of venous return and myocardial contractility. Severe hypoxia, bacterial toxins, anaerobic metabolism and hyperkalemia can adversely affect myocardium. In preterm infants, myocardial contractility is compromised due to higher water content of myocardium. The peripheral vascular resistance is dependent upon tone of blood vessels, volume and viscosity of blood. The tone of pericapillary arterioles depends on the levels of catecholamines and angiotensin. To safeguard vital organs, decrease in perfusion pressure is compensated by shunting of blood to brain and myocardium while blood flow to gut, kidneys and skin is further decreased by vasoconstriction. Tissue hypoxia leads to anaerobic metabolism at the cellular level with accumulation of pyruvic acid and lactic acid. The cellular damage is associated with release of lysosomal enzymes which leak into circulation. Lysosomal enzymes potentiate the production of reticuloendothelial and myocardial inhibitors. Due to decreased availability of energy from anaerobic metabolism, energy-dependent sodium pump starts malfunctioning with influx of sodium and water into cells and efflux of potassium into extracellular fluid. The accumulation of abnormal metabolites, potassium and toxins initiates a vicious cycle which causes further damage to myocardium and blood vessels.

Stages of Shock

The shock can be classified into three stages. The *compensated phase* is characterized by activation of neurohumoral factors that mediate redistribution of blood to vital organs and increase in the heart rate and myocardial contractility. The blood pressure is unstable but is maintained within normal range. When compensatory mechanisms are overwhelmed, the *uncompensated phase* sets in which is characterized by hypotension, poor tissue perfusion (CRT >2s) and worsening of lactic acidosis due to anaerobic metabolism. When effective treatment is delayed, shock may progress to the *irreversible phase* culminating in multiorgan failure and death.

Causes

Depending upon its etiology, shock in the newborn may be classified into three major groups.

Hypovolemic shock It may occur due to acute blood loss or dehydration. Infant may manifest hypovolemic shock at birth due to antepartum hemorrhage, (placenta previa, vasa previa, cord accidents) feto-maternal or twin-to-twin transfusion and ruptured liver or spleen and adrenal hemorrhage. Tight nuchal cord or cord prolapse may be associated with hypovolemia because compression obliterates flow through umbilical vein while flow of blood through umbilical arteries exsanguinates the baby. Bleeding may occur subsequently due to primary or secondary hemorrhagic disease of the newborn. Shock generally appears when at least 20% of blood volume has been lost. Systemic arterial pressure and hematocrit may remain normal immediately following blood loss. Infants with salt-losing variety of congenital adrenal hyperplasia manifest with diarrhea, vomiting and hypotension during early neonatal period. There is potential risk of adrenal insufficiency among infants born to mothers who received prolonged corticosteroid therapy during pregnancy.

Cardiogenic shock The cardiogenic shock due to myocardial dysfunction may occur due to perinatal hypoxia (hypoxic–ischemic cardiomyopathy), acidosis, congenital cardiac defects with inflow or outflow obstruction, cardiomyopathy, myocarditis, cardiac tamponade, and arrhythmias. Tachypnea, tachycardia, cardiomegaly and elevation of right or left atrial pressures with low cardiac output are often associated. Central venous pressure is elevated but frank clinical evidences of congestive heart failure are often absent due to its sudden onset and rapid fulminant course. Point-of-care echocardiography is useful to assess the myocardial functions for selection of appropriate therapy.

Septic shock It is the most common type of shock and is generally associated with Gram-negative septicemia. Various exotoxins and endotoxins are released in the circulation causing damage to the myocardium and peripheral blood vessels. There is abnormal peripheral vasoregulation due to increased or altered endothelial nitric oxide (NO) production and immaturity of neurovascular pathways. The systemic inflammatory response (SIRS) to infection may cause damage to multiple organs. The clinical picture is often complicated by patent ductus arteriosus (PDA) and persistent pulmonary hypertension (PPHN). There is some experimental evidence to suggest that plasma of septic animals contains certain factors which make adrenal cortex unresponsive to endogenous ACTH.

Clinical Features

History and antecedent conditions should be reviewed to identify various predisposing conditions known to cause shock. Infant looks pale (despite satisfactory hematocrit), lethargic and hypotonic. Tachycardia, tachypnea, circumoral grayish discoloration may be present. Extremities are cold while trunk is relatively warm. The heater output display of the incubator or open care system is elevated in an attempt to keep the baby warm. A disparity of more than 1.5°C between core temperature and peripheral skin temperature is suggestive of circulatory failure. Capillary refilling time as checked by blanching of the upper chest is increased to more than 2 seconds due to sluggish peripheral circulation (to assess CRT, count one, two, pink). There may be gross disparity between arterial oxygen tension and arterial oxygen saturation. Decreased activity, cold extremities and delayed capillary refill time are present several hours before the actual fall in blood pressure. Arterial pulsations are feeble or absent and blood pressure is low (normal blood pressure in a term infant is 60/40 mm Hg). In preterm babies, shock is suspected, if systemic mean arterial pressure (MAP) is less than gestational age in weeks. Sclerema may develop in terminal stages. Central venous pressure is elevated in cardiogenic and septic shock whereas it is low in infants with hypovolemia. Due to reduced renal perfusion, oliguria (urine output <0.5 mL/kg/hr) and anuria supervene.

If unrecognized and untreated, the clinical picture of shock may be dominated by manifestations of ischemic damage to capillaries and internal organs. Disseminated intravascular coagulation, acute renal failure, necrotizing enterocolitis, pulmonary hemorrhage and periventricular–intraventricular hemorrhage may dominate the clinical picture. Shock is an important predisposing factor in the pathogenesis of these conditions but may be overlooked, if all high-risk infants are not routinely monitored for their blood pressure.

Laboratory Investigations

The infant should be attached to a multichannel vital sign monitor including non-invasive BP monitor and pulse oximeter. Urine bag should be attached or urinary catheter inserted for accurate estimate of urine output. Blood should be examined for complete blood counts, hematocrit, sepsis screen, C-reactive protein, procalcitonin and presepsin. Blood glucose, serum electrolytes (Na, K, Ca), renal and liver function tests and blood coagulation profile should be assessed at baseline and during the course of therapy. Arterial blood gases, acid–base parameters, serum lactate and pyruvate levels, should be checked. Blood and/or CSF examination and culture and antibiotic sensitivity pattern of the isolates is mandatory. Skiagram of chest for pneumonia or aspiration and abdomen for paralytic ileus and NEC should be taken. When congenital heart disease is suspected, EKG and two-dimensional color Doppler echocardiography are advocated for precise diagnosis of cardiac defect. Ultrasonography of head and abdomen is indicated for diagnosis of periventricular–intraventricular hemorrhage, leukomalacia, adrenal hemorrhage and rupture of liver or spleen. Additional investigations may be required depending upon associated conditions and complications.

Management

Early recognition of shock and its management is essential to prevent anoxic damage to vital organs. Monitoring of blood pressure in critically sick neonates should become a routine in the NICU. The specific management is related to the underlying pathophysiologic mechanism and etiological factors contributing to shock. Central venous pressure (CVP) and arterial blood pressure should be monitored to guide therapy. Monitoring of CVP in term and late preterms is useful for rational management of shock but it is technically difficult in preterm babies. The catheter can be placed in the right atrium or in the intrathoracic part of superior or inferior vena cava through the umbilical vein or percutaneously through the external jugular vein. CVP should be maintained between 5 and 8 cm H_2O.

Infant should be nursed in a thermoneutral environment to minimize the oxygen and glucose requirements. Intravenous line should be established with a medicath and volume expanders (physiological saline, Ringer's lactate, fresh frozen plasma and blood) should be administered rapidly in a dose of 10–20 mL/kg to maintain CVP above 5 cm H_2O. Hypoxia, acidosis, hypoglycemia and electrolyte abnormalities should be looked for and corrected by appropriate therapy. Bolus injection of undiluted 7.5% solution of sodium bicarbonate should be avoided to prevent occurrence of intracranial and pulmonary hemorrhage. Calcium gluconate (1 mL/kg of 10% solution IV slowly) administration is useful by virtue of its positive inotropic effects on the heart. Blood transfusion should be given to raise blood volume and correct anemia, if hematocrit is below 40%. Disseminated intravascular conagulation should be managed by administration of vitamin K, fresh frozen plasma and exchange transfusion with fresh heparinized blood. Appropriate antibiotics must be administered parenterally depending upon the bacterial ecology of the NICU.

Myocardial contractility can be improved by inotropic effects of sympathomimetic amines and digoxin. Dopamine has both alpha and beta adenergic effects and should be used in amounts up to 10 μg/kg/minute with the aid of a constant infusion pump. Higher doses of dopamine may aggravate pulmonary vasoconstriction which usually exists in neonates with hypoxia and septic shock. Dobutamine, a drug synthesized from isoproterenol, is a strong inotrope with mild vascular effects. Dobutamine is suitable in neonates with low cardiac output but with normal or increased peripheral vascular resistance. Dobutamine is administered as a constant infusion at a rate of 5–20 μg/kg/minute. Epinephrine increases myocardial contractility and peripheral vascular resistance and can be used in infants who do not respond to dopamine. Epinephrine is useful in neonates with sepsis when low perfusion is because of peripheral vasodilatation. The starting dose is 0.05–0.1 μg/kg/minute and can be increased rapidly as needed while dopamine infusion rates are reduced. Epinephrine is an effective adjunct therapy to dopamine because cardiac norepinephrine stores are readily depleted with prolonged dopamine infusion. Isoproterenol is a pure beta-adrenergic stimulator with marked inotropic and chronotropic properties, which may produce cardiac arrhythmias. In infants with cardiogenic shock, administration of isoproterenol (0.1–0.5 μg/kg/min) and digoxin is beneficial. Milrinone and amrinone (3 mg/kg IV bolus followed by 5–20 mg/kg/min constant infusion) are phosphodiesterase III inhibitors and have potent inotropic effect and also reduce after load by virtue of their vasodilator effect (Figure 20.5).

Administration of hydrocortisone in pharmacological doses for treatment of septic shock in newborn babies has not been evaluated but there is some evidence that it may improve cardiac index and microcirculation. Hydrocortisone 1 mg/kg IV every 8 hours may be tried for 2–3 days. Hydrocortisone is preferred over dexamethasone because of its mineralocorticoid effect but there is potential risk of adverse long-term neurologic effects. The therapeutic utility of naloxone to antagonize the effect of endorphins released in response to stress of fulminant sepsis has not been studied in newborn babies. Pentoxyphylline, a xanthine derivative, has been shown to improve capillary blood flow by reducing blood viscosity and increasing deformability of RBCs. Methylene blue (1 mg/kg slow infusion over one hour), a soluble guanylate cyclate inhibitor, has been shown to improve the outcome of septic shock by inhibiting synthesis of nitric oxide (NO).

Pericardiocentesis may be life-saving for treatment of cardiac tamponade due to pneumopericardium. Procedure is accomplished through subxiphoid approach by directing the needle towards the left shoulder at an angle of 30° to 45° from the skin. The position of the needle can be electrocardiographically monitored by connecting it to a chest lead with an alligator clamp, when ST elevation or ectopic beat would indicate that it has established contact with epicardium. In infants with cardiogenic shock due to tachyarrhythmias, direct current cardioversion may be life-saving.

Monitoring

The following parameters should be monitored during the course of treatment:

- Vital signs and arterial oxygen tension (PaO_2)
- Central venous pressure (CVP) should be maintained between 5 and 8 cm H_2O.
- Capillary refill time
- Mean arterial blood pressure on NIBP monitor or intra-arterial line

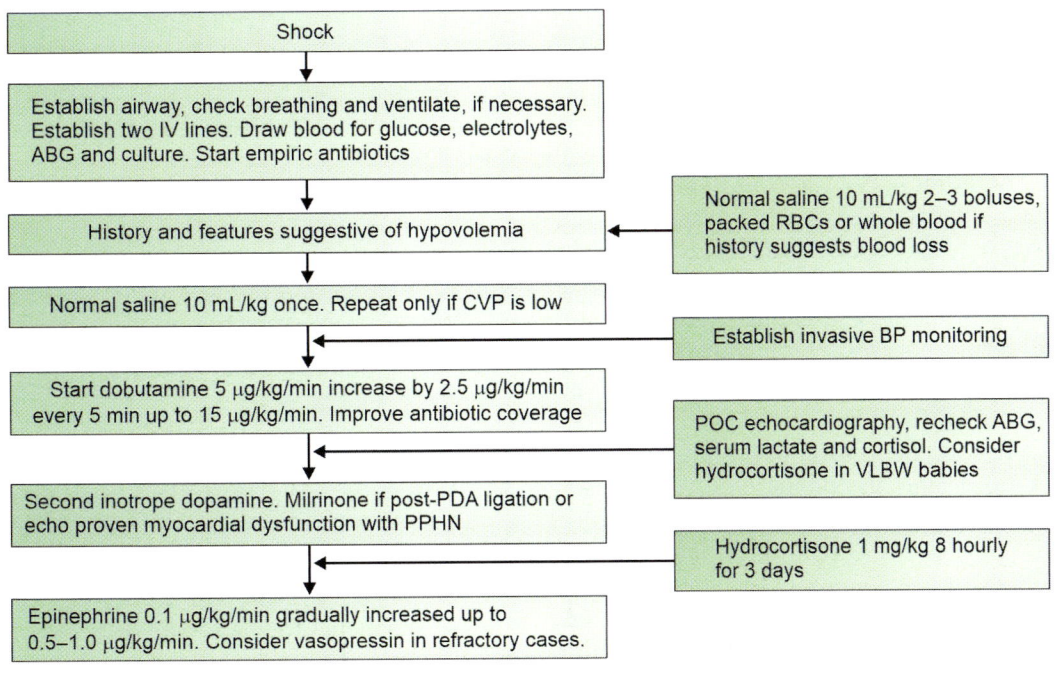

Abbreviations:
CVP: Central venous pressure, ABG: Arterial blood gases, POC: Point-of-care
VLBW: Very low birth weight, PPHN: Persistent pulmonary hypertension

Figure 20.5 Algorithm for management of neonatal shock.

Cardiovascular Disorders

20

- Urine output
- Base deficit, blood pH, cortisol and lactate level
- Point-of-care echocardiography by neonatologist. Superior vena cava (SVC) flow should be maintained above 40 mL/kg/min to ensure adequate cerebral blood flow.

Biochemical improvement in the aforementioned parameters is suggestive of gradual recovery and favorable outcome.

HYPERTENSION

Though uncommon it is often missed because of lack of routine monitoring of blood pressure in newborn babies. With the availability of non-invasive ultrasonic Doppler system, it is reported that hypertension may be seen in 2.5% of admissions in the intensive care nursery. In the newborn babies, hypertension has been defined as systemic blood pressure greater than 90/60 mm Hg in term infants and greater than 80/50 mm Hg in preterm infants. In almost two-thirds of infants, hypertension is due to renal artery thrombosis which may be caused by umbilical artery catheterization, sepsis, and disseminated intravascular coagulation. The increased use of indewelling umbilical artery catheters has led to increased incidence of renal artery thrombosis and hypertension. Additional causes include renal artery stenosis, renal vein thrombosis, congenital renal anomalies, neuroblastoma, congenital adrenal hyperplasia, thyrotoxicosis, Cushing's disease and coarctation of aorta. Raised intracrainal tension, fluid overload, polycythemia, hypernatremia, hypercalcemia, closure of abdominal wall defects, bronchopulmonary dysplasia and administration of phenylepherine, theophylline, doxapram and corticosteroids may cause transient elevation of blood pressure. It has been observed that crying alone can increase both systolic and diastolic blood pressure values in full term infants by as much as 20 mm Hg.

The diagnosis is made on recording the blood pressure because there are no diagnostic clinical symptoms and signs. The presence of predisposing and etiologic conditions should alert the neonatologist to closely monitor the blood pressure. There may be clinical evidences of congestive heart failure, patent ductus arteriosus, intracranial bleed, abnormal pulses and enlargement of kidneys. Urinalysis may show proteinuria and hematuria. There may be biochemical evidences of renal dysfunction. Elevated palsma renin activity is of doubtful utility. CT scan and radionuclide scintigraphy may show evidences of structural abnormalities and disturbances of renal plasma flow.

Renovascular disease is characterized by decreased effective renal plasma flow, decreased urine flow rate and an increased concentration of iodohippurate. Percutaneous femoral angiography is reserved for severely hypertensive neonates in whom renal scan is non-diagnostic.

Mild hypertension would respond to sodium restriction and diuretics. The safe antihypertensives during newborn period include hydralazine (1–8 mg/kg/d q 6–8 hr IV, PO), propranolol (0.5–5.0 mg/kg/day q 6–8 hr PO) and methyldopa (5–50 mg/kg/d q 8 hr PO). Extreme elevation of blood pressure is best treated with intravenous administration of diazoxide (2–5 mg/kg/dose q 20 to 30 min) or nitroprusside (0.5–5.0 µg/kg/min IV constant infusion). Recently, captopril has been successfully used in intractable cases of neonatal hypertension associated with elevated levels of plasma renin. It acts primarily by inhibiting the enzymes that convert angiotensin I to angiotension II and is administered in a dose of 0.1–0.4 mg/kg per dose orally every 8–12 hours. The medications are usually tapered, if blood pressure remains normal for 4 to 8 weeks. Nephrectomy is indicated, if intractable hypertension is caused by unilateral renal disease.

BIBLIOGRAPHY

Adelman RD. Neonatal hypertension. *Ann Nestle* 1984, 42/1: 32–42.

Arando JV, Thomas R. Systemic review: Intravenous ibuprofen in preterm newborns. *Semin Perinatol* 2006, 30(3): 114–120.

Archer N. Patent ductus arteriosus in the newborn. *Arch Dis Child* 1993, 69: 529–532.

Bhat BV, Palakkal N. Management of shock in neonates. *Indian J Pediatr* 2015, 82(10):923–9.

Bhat R, Das UG. Management of patent ductus arteriosus in premature infants. *Indian J Pediatr* 2015, 82(1):53–60.

Bhat R, Fisher E, Raju TNK, Vidyasagar D. Patent ductus arteriosus. Recent advances in diagnosis and management. *Pediatr Clin N Amer* 1982, 29: 1117.

Blake KD, Davenport SLH, Hall BD, et al. CHARGE association: An update and review for the primary pediatrician. *Clin Pediatr* 1998, 37: 159–174.

Bucciarellia RL, Egan EA, Gessner IH, Etizman DV. Persistence of fetal cardiopulmonary circulation. *Pediatrics* 1976, 58: 192.

Castenada AR, Mayer JE, Jones RA, et al. The neonate with critical congenital heart disease: Repair—A surgical challenge. *J Thorac Cardiovasc Surg* 1989, 98: 896.

Dakshinamurti S. Pathophysiologic mechanisms of persistent pulmonary hypertension of the newborn. *Pediatr Pulmonol* 2005, 39: 492–503.

Ferguson EC, Krishnamurthy R, Oldham SAA. Classic imaging signs of congenital cardiovascular abnormalities. *Radio Graphics* 2007, 27:1323–34.

Filippi L, Poggi C, Serafini L, Fiorim P. Terlipressin as rescue treatment of refractory shock in a neonate. *Acta Paediatr* 2008, 97(4): 500–502.

Friedman WF, Heyman MA. Commentary—New thoughts on an old problem: Patent ductus arteriosus in the premature infant. *J Pediatr* 1977, 90: 338.

Gupta SK. Clinical approach to a neonate with cyanosis. *Indian J Pediatr* 2015, 82(11):1050–60.

Hammerman C, Yousefzadeh D, Choi JH, Bui KC. Persistent pulmonary hypertension of the newborn. Managing the unmanageable? *Clin Perinatol* 1989, 16: 137.

Hastreite AR, Abella JB. The eectrocardiogram in the newborn period. *J Pediatr* 1971, 78: 146.

Kinsella JP, Abman SH. Inhaled nitric oxide: Current and future uses in neonates. *Semin Perinatol* 2000, 24(6): 387–395.

Konduri GG. New approaches for persistent pulmonary hypertension of newborn. *Clin Perinatol* 2004, 31: 591–611.

Lambert E, Canent R, Hohn A. Congenital cardiac defects in the newborn. A review of the conditions causing death or severe distress in the first month of life. *Pediatrics* 1966, 37:343.

Lee C, Mason LJ. Pediatric cardiac emergencies. *Anesth Clin N Am* 2001, 19: 286–309.

Liske MR, Greeley CS, Law DJ, *et al.* Report of the Tennessee Task Force on screening newborn infants for critical congenital heart disease. *Pediatrics* 2006, 118(4): e1250–e1256.

Marino BS, Bird GL, Wernovsky G. Diagnosis and management of the newborn with suspected congenital heart disease. *Clin Perinatol* 2001, 28: 91–136.

Mistry K, Gupta C. Neonatal hypertension. *NeoReviews* 2017, 18:357–71.

Ostrea EM, Villanueva-Uy ET, Natarajan G, *et al.* Persistent pulmonary hypertension of the newborn. *Pediatr Drugs* 2006, 8: 179–188.

Rein AJ, Omokhodion SI, Nir A, *et al.* Significance of a cardiac murmur as the sole clinical sign in the newborn. *Clin Pediatr* 2000, 39 (9): 511–520.

Rosenberg AA. Outcome in term infants treated with inhaled nitric oxide. *J Pediatr* 2002, 140 (3): 284–287.

Sasi A, Deorari AK. Patent ductus arteriosus in preterm infants. *Indian Pediatr* 2011, 48: 301–308.

Saxena A. Drug therapy of cardiac disease in children. Working Group on Management of Congenital Heart Diseases in India. *Indian Pediatr* 2009, 46: 310–338.

Saxena A. Working Group on Management of Congenital Heart Diseases in India. Concensus on timing of intervention for common congenital heart diseases. *Indian Pediatr* 2008, 45: 117–126.

Seri I, Noori S. Diagnosis and treatment of hypotension outside the transition period. *Early Hum Develop* 2005, 81: 405–411.

Shah SS, Ohlsson A. Ibuprofen for prevention of PDA in preterm and/or low birth weight infants. *Cochrane Database Syst Rev* 2006, (1): CD 004213.

Sharma V, Berkelhamer S, Lakshminrusimha S. Persistent pulmonary hypertension of the newborn. *Maternal Hlth Neonatal Perinatol* 2015, 1:14–69.

Shekerdemian LS, Ravn HB, Penny DJ. Intravenous sildenafil lowers pulmonary vascular resistance in a model of neonatal pulmonary hypertension. *Am J Resp Crit Care Med* 2002, 15: 165 (8): 1098–1102.

Siassi B, Blanco C, Cabal LA, Coran AG. Incidence and clinical features of patent ductus arteriosus in low birth weight infants. A prospective analysis of 150 consecutive born infants. *Pediatrics* 1976, 57: 347.

Singh HP, Hurley RM, Myers TF. Neonatal hypertension: Incidence and risk factors. *Amer J Heart* 1992, 5: 51–55.

Singh Y, Katheria A, Tissot C. Functional echocardiography in the neonatal intensive care unit. *Indian Pediatr* 2018, 55:417–24.

Singh Y, Gupta S, Grover AM, Gandhi A, Thomson J, Qureshi S, *et al.* Neonatologist performed echocardiography (NoPE): Training and accreditation in UK. *Eur J Pediatr* 2016, 175:281–7.

Southall DP, Vullimay DG, Davies MJ, Anderson RH, Shinebourne, EA, Honhson AN. A new look at the neonatal electrocardiogram. *Brit Med J* 1976, 2: 615.

Vanhaesebrouk S, Zonneberg I, Vandervoot P, *et al.* Conservative treatment for patent ductus arteriosus in the preterm. *Arch Dis Child Fetal Neonatal Ed* 2007, 92: F 244–F 247.

Walsh-Sukys Mc, Tyson JE, Wright LL, *et al.* Persistent pulmonary hypertension of the newborn : Practice variation and outcome. *Pediatrics* 2000, 105: 14–18.

Wolfson B. Radiologic interpretation of congenital heart disease. *Clin Perinatol* 2001, 28 (1): 71–78.

Wynn JL, Wong HR. Pathophysiology and treatment of septic shock in neonates. *Clin Perinatol* 2010, 37(2): 439–479.

Cardiovascular Disorders

20

Renal Disorders

PHYSIOLOGICAL CONSIDERATIONS

During intrauterine life, homeostasis of the fetus is dependent upon integrity of placenta which admirably looks after fetal nutrition, respiration, metabolism and excretion of waste products. Therefore, there are no fluid, electrolyte or biochemical disturbances at birth in infants born with bilateral renal agenesis. Serum creatinine level may be high at birth reflecting maternal levels and it declines within 1–2 weeks to 0.5 mg/dL. Urine is produced from about 10th–12th gestational weeks and it contributes towards formation and adequacy of amniotic fluid. Renal blood flow accounts for only 2–3% of cardiac output in fetal life compared to 15–18% in the newborn and 20–25% in the adult. Bilateral renal agenesis or hypoplasia is associated with oligohydramnios. Fetal oliguria is an important cause of pulmonary hypoplasia, postural abnormalities (squashed fetus) and contractures of joints.

At birth, combined weight of kidneys is about 25 g and fetal lobulations are present. Medulla is much thicker than cortex and there is relative predominance of glomerular over the tubular tissue. At birth, renal blood flow rapidly increases to 15 to 18% of cardiac output by increase in systemic blood pressure, decrease in renal vascular resistance and increase in the ratio of inner to outer cortical blood flow. The uncorrected rate of glomerular filtration in the newborn is around 4 mL/minute (approximately 1 mL/min/kg body weight) and glomerular filteration efficiency is about one-fourth of an adult. After birth, the GFR rises quickly, doubling by 2 weeks of age and reaching the adult level by one year of age. The newborn baby is ill-equipped to dispose off excess water and solute load effectively and efficiently.

Fractional excretion of sodium (FENa) which is a measure of kidney's ability to reabsorb sodium is usually less than 2% in a term newborn baby. Due to high degree of anabolism and because of rapid growth, the solute load or excretory burden to the kidneys is minimal. Functionally, juxtamedullary nephron is more mature as compared to glomeruli. Nevertheless urinary concentration ability of neonatal kidneys is limited to approximately 700 mOsm/L (500 mOsm/L in preterm infants and 800 mOsm/L in term infants) as compared to 1400 mOsm/L in older children. Apart from reduced tubular reabsorption capacity, the principal reason for low maximal urinary osmolality is reduced availability or filteration of urea in the newborn. In a healthy newborn, there is almost complete anabolism of protein and relatively small quantity of urea is available for excretion. The rapid growth and anabolism during early life has been referred to as "third kidney" because it reduces solute load and excretory demands on the kidneys. In contrast, both preterm and term infants can dilute their urine with a minimal urine osmolality of 50 mOsm/L.

Newborn baby is prone to develop acidosis because of renal tubular immaturity. There is inappropriate loss of amino acids, phosphates, and bicarbonates filtered through the glomeruli due to defective tubular reabsorption. The maximal rate of tubular reabsorption is also low. The renal threshold for bicarbonate is low and, therefore, it cannot be conserved. There is increased production of organic acids and inability to produce H^+ ions and excrete strongly acidic urine. During first few days of life, the renal excretion of ammonia is directly proportional to gestational age. The capacity of kidneys to produce ammonia and titrable acid is limited. Lactic acidosis secondary to tissue hypoxia and hypercarbia secondary to respiratory failure further worsens the systemic acidosis.

Functional inadequacy of glomeruli and tubules is more marked in preterm babies. Nephrogenesis is not completed until about 34 weeks of gestation and blood flow to renal cortex is low. GFR of VLBW babies is less than 25% of a term infant when adjusted for surface area. They are thus more handicapped to handle fluid or solute load and are unable to effectively reabsorb or conserve bicarbonate and amino acids. Preterm infants are prone to develop metabolic acidosis when exposed to additional protein load. Their excretory capacity to eliminate solute and drugs is limited. In a sick preterm infant, sepsis, hypoxia, hypotension, patent ductus arteriosus, acidosis and catabolism impose additional burden to immature kidneys. Indomethacin and high-dose dopamine may further reduce GFR. It is not uncommon for a sick VLBW infant to show elevation in serum urea and creatinine concentration despite adequate hydration. In preterm babies, urinary sodium losses are high because of increased FENa of 3–6%. They are prone to develop hyponatremia which is further aggravated because of excessive intake of fluids. They should be provided with high sodium intake of up to 10 mEq/kg/day. Renal calcium excretion is greater in VLBW babies with increased risk of osteopenia of prematurity and nephrocalcinosis. Postnatal functional maturation of kidneys is rapid and by about 3 months of age they achieve complete maturity.

The time of passage of first urine after birth is variable and depends upon when urine was last passed *in utero* and adequacy of feeding after birth. Most newborn babies pass urine within 12 hours after birth and almost all do so by 48 hours. Urine output is low during first 2 to 3 days in exclusively breastfed babies due to inadequacy of lactation. Subsequently, urine output varies between 1 and 5 mL/kg/hour and frequency of voiding is marked due to small capacity of urinary bladder and poor concentration ability of the kidneys. Infants may void 15–20 times in 24 hours. *Some infants may cry before passing urine due to unpleasant sensation of full bladder, become quiet or dazed while passing urine and resume crying after evacuation due to discomfort of wet diaper.* This is a normal pattern and should not be mistaken with bladder neck obstruction. Stream of micturition is also characteristic in the newborn. Unlike an adult, there is no hesitancy and voiding terminates abruptly without any dribbling or straining efforts to expel residual urine.

LABORATORY EVALUATION

Urinalysis

Examination of freshly voided specimen of urine or a sample obtained through suprapubic puncture provides useful information. Urine can also be readily collected by applying gentle pressure over the suprapubic area to evacuate the bladder. Urinary osmolality ranges from 60–600 mOsm/L with a pH of 6.0 to 7.0. Specific gravity ranges between 1.021 and 1.025 in term infants. Excessive excretion of urates in the newborn may stain the diaper pink and give false-positive result for proteinuria, if tested with trichloracetic acid. Proteinuria in excess of 30 mg/dL in a random sample is abnormal and calls for further studies. Transitory glycosuria in the first week of life may be seen in 20% of preterm infants. Microscopic examination may normally show few epithelial cells but no leukocytes or red blood cells. Timed collection of urine with a bag or test tube is essential to assess the adequacy of urinary output (Figure 21.1).

Serum Chemistry

The concentration of blood urea is markedly affected by the protein intake and rate of anabolism. Serum blood urea nitrogen (BUN) values vary between 5 and 20 mg/dL. (BUN is approximately one-half of blood urea values.) In sick infants with hypoxia and sepsis, BUN may rise by virtue of enhanced tissue catabolism even when protein intake is restricted. Renal insufficiency is suspected, if BUN is greater than 20 mg/dL or rises at a rate of 5 mg/dL/day or higher. During first two weeks of life or so, serum creatinine values in the newborn approach normal adult values of 0.5–1.0 mg/dL as a reflection of maternal creatinine level. Subsequently serum creatinine levels are low and vary between 0.1 and 0.2 mg/dL among healthy infants. Relatively low serum creatinine levels in newborn babies pose technical difficulties for their accurate laboratory analysis. Nevertheless, endogenous creatinine clearance provides a useful measure of GFR under usual clinical circumstances. Electrolytes should

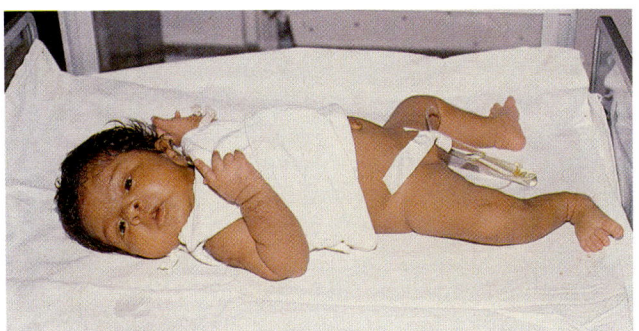

Figure 21.1 Urine collection in a test tube in a male infant. The urine can be withdrawn with the help of a catheter and syringe after each evacuation. In a female infant, bag is used for urine collection.

Renal Disorders

21

be monitored while keeping in mind physiological hyperkalemia during first week of life. Birth asphyxia, RDS, pulmonary air leaks, positive pressure ventilation, hyperglycemia, hypothyroidism, cerebral edema and intracranial infection and hemorrhage may be associated with syndrome of inappropriate secretion of ADH (SIADH). It is characterized by features of water-intoxication as evidenced by hypo-osmolality and low levels of serum electrolytes and calcium.

Glomerular and Tubular Functions

Estimation of glomerular filtration rate (GFR) in an infant is important when either an intrinsic renal abnormality is suspected or drug therapy with a potentially nephrotoxic agent needs to be monitored. Estimation of endogenous creatinine clearance, inulin clearance and ^{51}Cr-EDTA clearance is technically difficult in neonates. Plasma creatinine levels can be used to calculate GFR as follows: GFR (mL per min per 1.73 m^2) = KL/Pcr, where L represents body length in cm, Pcr is plasma concentration of creatinine in mg/dL and K is a constant, representing urinary creatinine excretion per unit body weight. The values of K for preterm (<34 weeks) and term babies are 0.34 and 0.44, respectively.

The fractional excretion of sodium (FENa) represents the percent of filtered sodium that is excreted in the urine and serves as a good index of glomerulotubular balance. It is calculated by the formula:

$$FENa\ (\%) = \frac{Urine\ sodium \times Serum\ creatinine}{Serum\ sodium \times Urine\ creatinine} \times 100$$

In term infants, FENa is usually less than 2% but the values are higher in preterm infants (5–10% in infants <34 weeks) who have poor tubular reabsorption of sodium and hence require higher daily maintenance allowances of sodium (4–6 mEq/kg/day).

Morphologic Evaluation

Oligohydramnios, obstructive uropathy or anuria, renal mass, hematuria, facial dysmorphism or ear anomalies are useful indicators for assessment of functional anatomy of kidneys and urinary tract. Ultrasonography of the kidneys is non-invasive and most useful in identifying congenital renal malformations. Nephrosonography can identify kidney size, differentiate between solid versus cystic mass and localize obstruction. Radionuclide evaluation with ^{131}I - Hippuran renal scan and renogram are equally safe to assess renal perfusion, parenchymatous functions and excretory abnormalities. Technetium 99m-diethylene triamine penta-acetic acid (DTPA) and mercaptoacetyltriglycine (MAG3) istopes are handled by glomerular filteration

and can be used to assess renal blood flow and renal function. They can be used to differentiate obstructive from non-obstructive hydronephrosis after intravenous administration of furosemide. Isotopes that bind to the renal tubules, such as technitium 99 m-dimercaptosuccinic acid (DMSA), produce static images and are used to assess anatomical changes in the renal cortex.

Intravenous pyelography is potentially hazardous in the newborn and may be followed by complications of cortical ischemia, medullary necrosis, and pulmonary edema due to osmolar load of contrast. No preparation or dehydration prior to the procedure is necessary. Air provides a good contrast which can be enhanced by injection of air into stomach or giving a carbonated drink. Hypaque 50% (diatrizoate sodium or amidotrizoate) in a dose of 3 mL/kg is injected intravenously through a peripheral vein cannulated via medicath. In view of the profound osmolarity of 1600 mOsm/L of 50% hypaque, it is desirable to inject the contrast slowly over 90 seconds period. The films should be taken every 15 to 30 minutes over next 4 hours in view of slow excretion of the dye in newborn babies. Procedure is contraindicated in the presence of dehydration, congestive heart failure and renal insufficiency. Plain skiagram of abdomen may not show kidney outlines due to lack of perinephric fat. Excretory urography would delineate site, size and functions of kidneys and define status of calyces, pelves, ureters and bladder. Voiding cystourethrography, in continuation of intravenous pyelography or by instillation of 15% solution of contrast through urethra, is essential for evaluation of obstructive uropathy (Figure 21.2). For confirmation of diagnosis of renal vein thrombosis, inferior vena cavogram is mandatory.

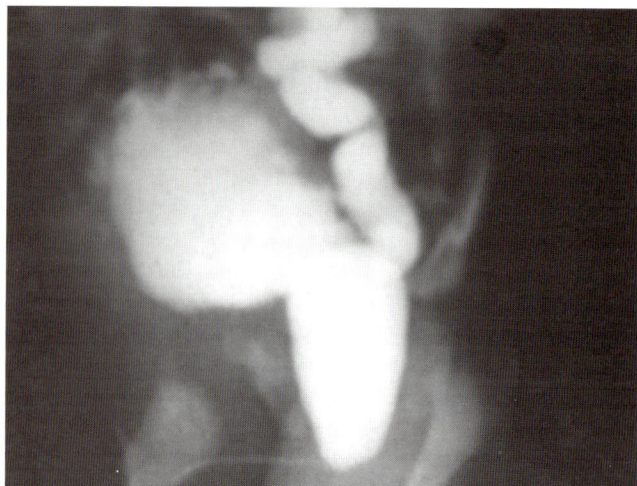

Figure 21.2 Micturating cystourethrogram showing enlarged bladder with diverticulum and mega ureter due to posterior urethral valve.

Prenatal Ultrasound

Antenatal ultrasonography can detect fetal genito-urinary abnormalities in 0.3 to 0.5% of pregnancies. Hydronephrosis is the commonest abnormality, unilateral being more common than the bilateral disease due to pelvicalyceal junction abnormalities or bladder neck obstruction. Antenatal management of fetal hydronephrosis is controversial. Ultrasound examination can also reliably diagnose multicystic dysplastic kidney (MCDK), especially when there is unilateral involvement. All neonates with abnormal ultrasound study of the fetal urinary tract should be re-evaluated at 72 hours after birth. Early re-evaluation is not recommended to avoid a false-negative result because of physiologic decreased urine output during this period. If the sonographic findings are negative at 72 hours, a repeat study is done at the age of one month because milder grades of hydronephrosis may be missed because of physiologic dehydration during early life. Infants showing hydronephrosis should undergo voiding cystourethrography (contrast or radionuclide) to diagnose obstruction or vesicoureteric reflux. A renal isotope scan by using Tc-99m-labeled diethylene triamine penta-acetic acid (DTPA) with furosemide is recommended to study the differential functions of each kidney. Until a definitive diagnosis is made, chemoprophylaxis with cephalexin (50 mg/kg/d) or amoxycillin (15 mg/kg/d) single daily dose may be instituted, though it is controversial at present because of risk of emergence of resistant strains of bacteria. Postnatal management of antenatally detected hydronephrosis is summarized in Figure 21.3.

COMMON RENAL DISORDERS

Developmental defects, infections, circulatory disorders including vascular occlusion causing renal insufficiency comprise large majority of renal disorders in the newborn. Apart from life-threatening malformations, other developmental genitourinary defects are often silent in the newborn and manifest later in life. Symptoms of urinary tract infection are often vague and non-specific because of difficulties in identification of dysuria or frequency of voiding. Renal insufficiency is common and of critical impor-

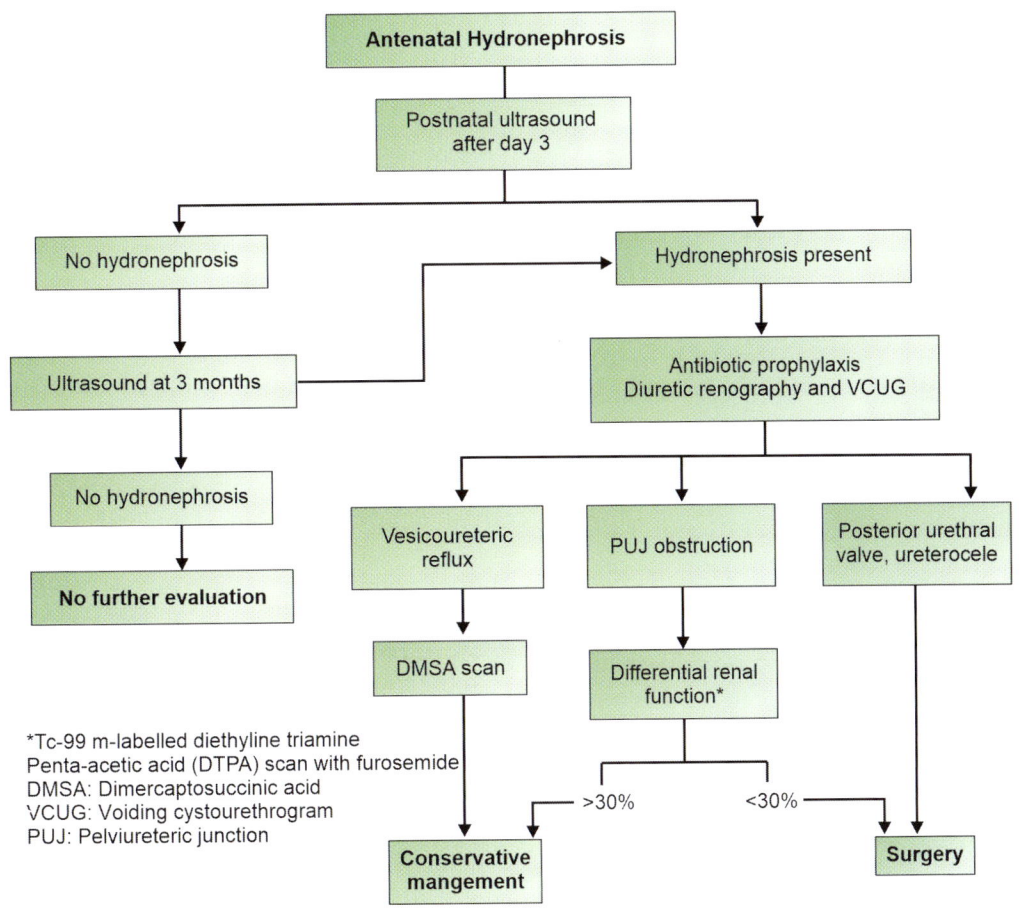

Figure 21.3 Algorithm for management of antenatally detected hydronephrosis.

tance because of frequent use of aminoglycosides which are nephrotoxic. It is often unrecognized due to low index of suspicion and difficulties in collection of satisfactory samples of urine and lack of reliable and simple laboratory tests to assess renal functions in the newborn.

Hematuria

Hematuria is defined as 5 red blood cells per high power field and is uncommon in newborn babies. Passage of red-colored urine is frightening for parents and is indicative of hematuria although presence of urates, bile pigments and porphyrins in urine may also produce similar discoloration. Microscopic hematuria in a female infant is most commonly due to contamination with physiological vaginal bleeding. Blood may enter the urine at any point in the urinary system from the kidneys to the urethra. The common causes of hematuria include hypoxic–ischemic damage resulting in cortical and/or medullary necrosis, acute tubular necrosis, hemorrhagic disease of the newborn, renal vein or artery thrombosis, infection, obstructive uropathy, congenital syphilis, nephrocalcinosis, neoplasia, severe thrombocytopenia and disseminated intravascular coagulopathy. Hematuria may occur following suprapubic bladder aspiration or catheterization and intravenous pyelography or angiocardiography. Examination of freshly voided urine specimen to detect the presence of red blood cells or other type of casts is helpful to differentiate between the hematuria from upper and lower urinary tract. The presence of casts, which are produced in tubules, is pathognomonic of parenchymal renal disease. It would also differentiate between hematuria and hemoglobinuria but if urine is not examined immediately after collection, red blood cells may hemolyze on standing.

Renal Vein Thrombosis

The condition is more common among male infants and occlusion may be unilateral or bilateral. The main causes include dehydration, polycythemia, anoxia, reduced renal blood flow due to shock and hyperosmolality. Babies born to diabetic mothers are particularly susceptible because of polycythemia, dehydration due to osmotic diuresis, platelet hyperfunction and increased synthesis of prostaglandin endoperoxides. The thrombotic process may start *in utero*. The presence of hematuria, enlarged kidneys, hypertension, thrombocytopenia and evidences of intravascular coagulation suggest the diagnosis. Polycythemia, hyperosmolality, microangiopathic hemolytic anemia, thrombocytopenia and low fibrin

levels should be looked for. Nephrosonography with Doppler ultrasound followed by inferior vena cavogram would clinch the diagnosis.

The underlying predisposing factors, such as dehydration, polycythemia and shock, should be corrected. Role of anticoagulation is controversial especially in unilateral cases. In bilateral cases with evidences of DIC, anticoagulation can be achieved by administration of heparin 100 units/kg stat followed by continuous intravenous infusion of 25 to 50 units/kg/hour to maintain PTT of 1.5 times of normal. Oliguric infants should be treated on the lines of acute renal failure.

Renal Artery Thrombosis

The condition is limited to use of indwelling umbilical artery catheterization. It is characterized by hematuria, hypertension and renal insufficiency. Diagnosis can be suspected by an ultrasound examination and confirmed by angiography. Medical management is preferred over surgical thrombectomy. Indwelling catheter should be removed followed by use of thrombolytic agent and antihypertensive drugs. Most unilateral cases have satisfactory renal function and normal blood pressure by 2 years of age.

ACUTE RENAL FAILURE (ARF)

Renal insufficiency due to acute kidney injury (AKI) is common in high-risk newborn babies and its incidence varies depending upon the criteria used for diagnosis. It is suspected either by azotemia (serum creatinine level >1.5 mg/dL or rising by 0.3 mg/dL/d) or GFR <35 mL/min/1.73 m^2 or oliguria, which is defined as urine output of less than 1.0 mL/kg/hour. In non-oliguric renal failure (35% cases), which can occur following birth asphyxia, urine output is normal. The incidence of oliguric renal failure varies between 6 and 8% of NICU admissions and it accounts for 5% of all deaths in the NICU. In 2004, the Acute Dialysis Quality Initiative (ADQI) proposed an AKI classification system called "**R**isk, **I**njury, **F**ailure, **L**oss, **E**nd-stage kidney disease (RIFLE)" to promote a consistent definition of AKI. The Kidney Disease Improving Global Outcomes (KDIGO) classification of neonatal AKI is summarized in Table 21.1.

Etiology

The cause of ARF may be prerenal (reduced renal perfusion due to hypovolemia and shock), renal (intrinsic renal disease) or postrenal (obstructive uropathy). Hypoxia and shock are major contributory factors in

TABLE 21.1 Kidney Disease Improving Global Outcomes (KDIGO) classification for neonatal acute kidney injury		
Stage	*Serum creatinine*	*Urine output*
0	No change or rise <0.3 mg/dL	≥1 mL/kg/h
1	Rise by ≥0.3 mg/dL within 48 h or rise ≥1.5–1.9 of the reference value within 7d	0.5–1.0 mL/kg/h
2	Rise by ≥2.0–2.9 mg/dL of the reference value	0.3–0.5 mL/kg/h
3	Rise by ≥3.0 mg/dL of the reference value or >2.5 mg/dL rise with renal replacement therapy	≤0.3 mL/kg/h

the development of prerenal ARF. Hypovolemia due to loss of blood, fluids, and electrolytes when severe and prolonged may lead to acute cortical or tubular necrosis. Renal arterial or venous thrombosis as a consequence of disseminated coagulopathy and toxic or drug-induced nephropathy are additional causes of damage to renal parenchyma. Renal tubular necrosis may also result from tubular luminal obstruction because of uric acid nephropathy, hemoglobinuria and myoglobinuria. Congenital renal malformations, such as bilateral renal agenesis, hypoplasia, dysplasia, and polycystic disease should be excluded. Post-renal ARF may be caused by obstructive uropathy (Table 21.2).

Diagnosis

Oliguria or anuria and progressive azotemia confirm the diagnosis. BUN of greater than 20 mg/dL and serum creatinine of more than 1.0 mg/dL are useful indicators of ARF or AKI. Catabolic states, such as sepsis, starvation, tissue necrosis, dehydration and sequestered bleeding, may result in elevated urea levels despite normal renal function. The level of BUN should also be correlated with daily intake of protein by the infant. Electrolytes should be monitored. There is rise in serum potassium, magnesium and phosphorus and fall in calcium levels. During first 7 to 10 days of life, potassium may be normally as high as 7 mEq/L due to leakage from the cells. Prerenal failure and renal tubular necrosis should be differentiated clinically and by urinary/plasma ratios of solutes. A urinary/plasma osmolality ratio (UOsm/POsm) of less than 1.0 is suggestive of intrinsic renal failure (Table 21.3). Urinalysis may show granular or hyaline casts, RBCs, tubular cells and proteinuria in neonates with intrinsic renal disease. A number of early non-invasive biomarkers of AKI, such as serum cystatin C (CysC), urinary interleukin-18 (IL-18), serum and urinary

TABLE 21.2 Major causes of acute kidney injury in the newborn

Prerenal (75–80%)
Reduced renal perfusion
Shock
Asphyxia neonatorum or hypoxia due to any cause
Sepsis
Dehydration
Blood loss
Fetomaternal or twin-to-twin hemorrhage
Surgery
Drugs
Maternal intake of captopril, indomethacin or NSAIDs
Poycythemia
Congestive heart failure

Intrinsic renal (10–15%)
Congenital renal anomalies
Agenesis
Dysplasia
Hypoplasia
Polycystic kidneys
Acute tubular necrosis
Reduced renal perfusion due to prerenal causes
Nephrotoxic drugs (indomethacin, aminoglycosides, tolazoline, amphotericin B, vancomycin, captopril, furosemide, diethylene glycol)
Hyperosmotic contrast dyes
Uric acid nephropathy
Vascular
Disseminated intravascular coagulation
Venous thrombosis
Arterial thrombosis
Cortical necrosis
Inflammatory
Syphilis
Toxoplasmosis
Pyelonephritis

Postrenal (5%)
Obstructive uropathy
Posterior urethral valves
Urethral stricture
Urethral diverticulum
Imperforate prepuce
Ureterocele
Ureteropelvic or ureterovesical obstruction
Extrinsic tumors

Neurogenic bladder

TABLE 21.3 Laboratory and clinical differences between prerenal and intrinsic renal failure in neonates

Parameters	Prerenal failure	Intrinsic renal failure
Urine specific gravity	>1.014	<1.014
UOsm (mOsm/L)	>500	<300
UNa (mEq/L)	<20	>40
FENa (%)*	<1.0	>3.0
Renal failure index**	<1	>4 (term) or >8 (preterm)
UOsm/POsm	>1.5	<1.0
Serum BUN/Cr	>20	<20
Urine Cr/Plasma Cr	>25	<10
Response to volume infusion with or without diuretic	Increased urine output	No effect

$$*\text{FENa (\%)} = \frac{\text{Urine sodium} \times \text{Serum creatinine}}{\text{Serum sodium} \times \text{Urine creatinine}} \times 100$$

$$**\text{Renal failure index} = \frac{\text{Urine Na} \times \text{Serum creatinine}}{\text{Urine creatinine}} \times 100$$

neutrophil gelatinase-associated lipocalin (N-GAL), kidney molecule-1 (KIM-1), osteopontin (OPN), and beta-2 microglobulin (β_2MG), have been identified but they need validation in neonates. Ultrasonography of abdomen is done to exclude polycystic or dysplastic kidneys and obstructive uropathy due to posterior urethral valves. Renal Doppler studies are useful for the diagnosis of vascular thrombosis.

Management

The principles of management of ARF in the neonates are the same as in the older children. When hypovolemia or prerenal failure is suspected, administer isotonic saline 20 mL/kg intravenously in one hour. If urine flow is not established, furosemide 1–2 mg/kg is administered intravenously after correction of dehydration to force diuresis. If no response is seen, some workers recommend second dose of furosemide 3 to 5 mg/kg intravenously before diagnosing intrinsic ARF. Dopamine or dobutamine in a "renal dose" (2–4 μg/kg/min infusion) is used at times to provide inotropic support to the heart and improve renal perfusion. Postrenal failure is managed by urgent drainage of urinary bladder to relieve back pressure followed by definitive surgery. For an obstructive lesion to produce ARF, it must be assumed that lesion is either bilateral or patient has only a single kidney.

ARF due to established intrinsic renal disease is managed by maintenance of water, electrolytes, hydrogen ions and provision of adequate nutrition. Fluid intake should be restricted to insensible water loss (25–40 mL/kg/24 hours) plus urinary output.

Depending upon gestation, postnatal age, use of radiant warmer and phototherapy, insensible water loss in preterm babies may vary between 40 and 100 mL/kg/day. Potassium and phosphates should be withheld while calcium should be administered. Hyperkalemia (>6 mEq/L) should be treated by administration of calcium, sodium bicarbonate, glucose with insulin (2.5 units/100 mL of 10% dextrose) and salbutamol nebulization (2.5 mg in 2 doses 2 hours apart). Sodium is administered to replace its loss in urine and to correct any hyponatremia. When hyponatremia is severe (Na <120 mEq/L) or associated with seizures, it should be corrected by administration of 3% hypertonic saline in a dose of 5 mL/kg over 4 hours. Acidosis should be corrected by administration of sodium bicarbonate or THAM and pH maintained between 7.25 and 7.35. It must be remembered that acidemia should be corrected only after correcting hypocalcemia to prevent tetany. The dose of calcium gluconate is 50–100 mg/kg (0.5–0.1 mL/kg of 10% calcium gluconate) 3 to 4 times per day intravenously. Hypertension should be looked for and appropriately managed. There is some evidence to suggest that prophylactic administration of theophylline, an adenosine antagonist, in term infants with birth asphyxia reduces the risk of renal dysfunction. When given in a single low dose (5–8 mg/kg) it has been found to be protective against post asphyxial AKI. The management of various complications of AKI are summarized in Table 21.4.

Protein intake should be restricted to 0.5 g/kg per day and minimal caloric intake of at least 40 kcal/kg/day should be ensured by administration of

TABLE 21.4 Management of various complications of AKI

Complication	Treatment	Remarks
Fluid overload	**Fluid restriction** Insensible water losses (400 mL/m²/d); add urine output and other losses; 5–10% dextrose for insensible losses; N/5 saline for urine output	Monitor other losses and replace as appropriate, consider dialysis
Pulmonary edema	Oxygen; furosemide 2–4 mg/kg iv	Monitor CVP; consider dialysis
Hypertension	**Symptomatic** Sodium nitroprusside 0.5–8 mg/kg/min infusion; furosemide 2–4 mg/kg iv; nifedipine 0.3–0.5 mg/kg oral/sublingual	In emergency, reduce blood pressure by 1/3rd of the desired reduction during first 6–8 hr, 1/3rd over next 12–24 hr and the final 1/3rd slowly over 2–3 days
	Asymptomatic Nifedipine SR, amlodipine, prazosin or atenolol	
Metabolic acidosis	Sodium bicarbonate (IV or oral) if bicarbonate level is <15 mEq/L or pH <7.2	Watch for fluid overload, hypernatremia, hypocalcemia; and consider dialysis
Hyperkalemia	**Emergency** Calcium gluconate (10%) 0.5–1 mL/kg over 5–10 minutes iv	Stabilizes cell membranes; prevents arrhythmias
	Salbutamol 5–10 mg nebulized	Shifts potassium into cells
	Less critical Sodium bicarbonate (7.5%) 1–2 mL/kg over 15 minutes	Shifts potassium into cells
	Dextrose (10%) 0.5–1 g/kg and insulin 0.1–0.2 U/kg	Requires monitoring of blood glucose
	Calcium or sodium resonium (kayexalate) 1 g/kg per day	Given orally or rectally, can be repeated every 4 hours
Hyponatremia	Fluid restriction; if there is sensorial alteration or seizures 3% saline 6–12 mL/kg over 30–90 minutes	Hyponatremia is usually dilutional; 12 mL/kg of 3% saline raises sodium by 10 mEq/L
Severe anemia	Packed red blood cells 3–5 mL/kg; consider exchange transfusion	Monitor blood pressure, fluid overload
Hyperphosphatemia	Phosphate binders (calcium carbonate, acetate; aluminium milk products, phosphate)	Avoid high phosphate foods like milk products and high protein diet

glucose polymers (polycose) and corn oil. Urinary output should be closely monitored. Infant should be weighed every 12-hours and daily weight loss of 0.5–1.0% of weight is expected and desirable when management is satisfactory. Electrolytes should be frequently monitored and serum calcium x phosphate product should not be allowed to exceed 70. Nephrotoxic drugs should be stopped or their dosage reduced to safe levels. Tolazoline, aminoglycosides and indomethacin are contraindicated when there are evidences of renal failure.

Peritoneal dialysis is indicated when despite adequate medical management there is critical hyperkalemia, azotemia and pulmonary edema although unlike older children no absolute criteria for peritoneal dialysis are available in the newborn. Neonates with AKI are often hypoxic and cannot metabolize lactate contained in conventional dialysis solution. It is desirable to prepare a dialysis solution where lactate is replaced by bicarbonate. Since calcium may get precipitated in the solution containing bicarbonate, it should not be incorporated in such a dialysate and

administered separately intravenously. When prolonged peritoneal dialysis is anticipated, a Tenckhoff catheter should be used. For details of peritoneal dialysis refer to Chapter 29. In end-stage renal disease, renal replacement therapy is being increasingly used with success.

Prognosis

The outcome depends upon the underlying cause/s and associated congenital anomalies. Acute renal failure *per se* is seldom the cause of death when fluid homeostasis and electrolyte balance is maintained. Non-oliguric AKI has a better prognosis in neonates. The outcome is poor in infants with septicemia, NEC, disseminated intravascular coagulation and multiorgan failure. The long-term abnormalities in GFR and tubular functions can persist in 25% of the neonates and may progress to chronic kidney disease (CKD). After recovery, the infant should be kept under follow-up for several years because abnormalities in renal function may reappear anytime later in life.

Renal Disorders

21

RENAL MALFORMATIONS

Most congenital anomalies of kidneys and urinary tract (CAKUT) are asymptomatic during neonatal period and are picked up on follow-up. Serious malformations with obvious manifestations during early life are often incompatible with life. Renal malformations are associated with a large number of hereditary disorders, associations and chromosomal abnormalities. Affected infants are either born dead or die soon after due to progressive renal failure, sepsis or because of associated anomalies in other vital organs. Unusual delay or difficulty in passing urine, oliguria or anuria, palpable renal mass and facial dysmorphism due to oligohydramnios often alert the neonatologist to the possibility of underlying renal anomalies. Potter facies is characterized by large low-set ears with folded helices, squashed face with small receding chin and compressed nose, and epicanthal folds with anti-mongoloid slant of eyes. A prominent skin fold arising from inner canthus and passing obliquely under both eyes, give a wizened old man-look to the infant (Figure 21.4). Pectus excavatum and widely spaced or supernumerary nipples may be associated with some renal abnormalities. Infants with unilateral multicystic dysplastic kidney (MCDK) are usually asymptomatic although the affected kidney has no

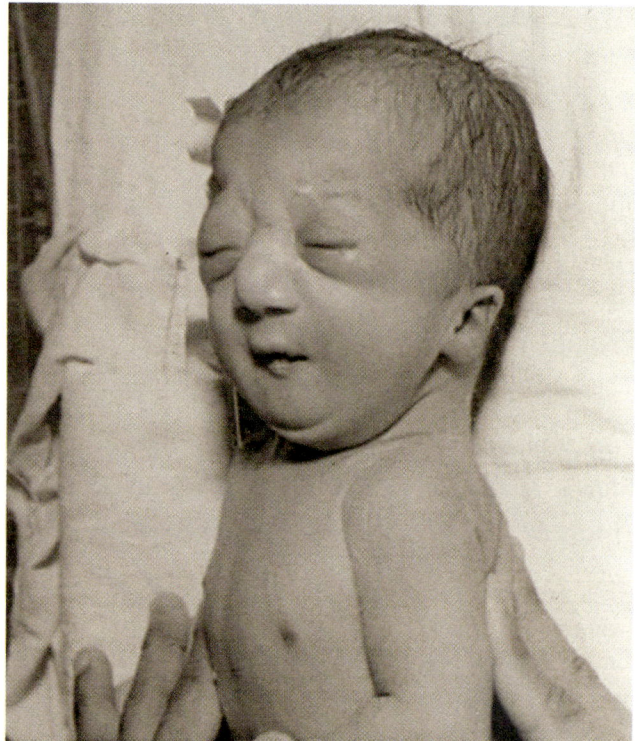

Figure 21.4 Potter facies showing receding chin, flat nose, low-set ears and prominent skin folds below the eyes.

renal function as demonstrated by DMSA renal scan. There is general agreement that surgical removal of symptomatic unilateral MCDK is indicated, if it is associated with hypertension or infection and when a large kidney is causing respiratory difficulty.

Bilateral Renal Agenesis and Dysplasia

Most affected infants are males either prematurely born or growth retarded. Oligohydramnios, single umbilical artery, amnion nodosum, Potter facies, club feet and bowed legs are often associated. Its incidence is reported as one in 4,000 deliveries. Almost half the subjects are stillborn. Those born alive, develop severe respiratory distress because of associated pulmonary hypoplasia. Pneumothorax is common following attempts for resuscitation at birth. Other associated internal malformations include esophageal, duodenal and anal atresia, colonic agenesis and Meckel's diverticulum. Infants surviving from respiratory difficulties succumb to progressive renal failure within a few days. Bilateral renal aplasia or multicystic-dysplasia present identical clinical picture and can only be differentiated at autopsy. Meckel's syndrome is described wherein polycystic kidneys are associated with occipital encephalocele, eye abnormalities, cleft lip or palate, congenital heart defects, genetic anomalies, hepatic fibrosis, and polydactyly.

Enlarged Kidneys

Kidneys in newborn babies are at a lower position, right being lower than the left. Lower pole of both the kidneys may be palpable by bimanual examination due to laxity of abdominal wall. The vast majority of all palpable abdominal masses in the newborn are renal in origin. Horseshoe-shaped or fused kidney, which is commonest anomaly, may sometimes be suspected on clinical examination. Bilateral enlargement of kidneys is most commonly seen due to renal malformations, such as hydronephrosis because of obstructive uropathy, polycystic disease and renal vein thrombosis. A smooth renal mass is most likley to be the result of hydronephrosis or renal vein thrombosis whereas an irregular surface suggests cystic malformation or tumor. A unilateral irregular lumbar mass should be considered as malignant unless proved otherwise. Hemihypertrophy should be looked for and is known to be associated with Wilms' tumor, adrenal and hepatic tumors and visceral hemangiomas. Kidney masses due to developmental defects are often associated with oligohydramnios, single umbilical artery and Potter facies which must be enquired into and looked for.

Obstructive Uropathy

Developmental obstruction of the urinary tract produces dilatation above the site of lesion and a retrograde rise in hydrostatic pressure causing structural and functional damage to the kidneys. Severe cases of lower urinary tract obstruction manifest during the newborn period while milder ones are detected during later infancy and childhood. There is marked abdominal distension with enlarged hydronephrotic kidneys and distended urinary bladder. Ascites due to leakage of urine through ruptured pelvis, calix or ureter is common. Ascitic fluid would contain urea and other urinous elements. Urethral obstruction may be associated with congenital absence of abdominal musculature or so-called prune-belly syndrome (Eagle-Barret syndrome) in which flabby abdominal wall gives an appearance of dried prune (Figure 21.5). Apart from gross evidences of dilatation of whole urinary tract and kidneys, it is associated with undescended testes and large flaccid phallus because of grossly dilated urethra. Other congenital malformations, such as pulmonary hypoplasia, malrotation of gut and imperforate anus, may be associated. Like most other renal malformations, obstructive uropathy is also more common among male infants. The cause of obstruction may be posterior urethral valve, urethral atresia and urethral diverticulum.

The obstructive uropathy should be considered as an emergency and urgent action should be taken to identify the cause and relieve the obstruction. Catheter evacuation of bladder should be attempted with due aseptic precautions. If the procedure fails, emergency suprapubic cystostomy and nephrostomy is indicated after correction of any fluid and electrolyte disturbances. Associated urinary tract infection should be identified and managed with appropriate antibiotics. Early recognition and management of obstructive urinary tract anomalies offer the best hope for

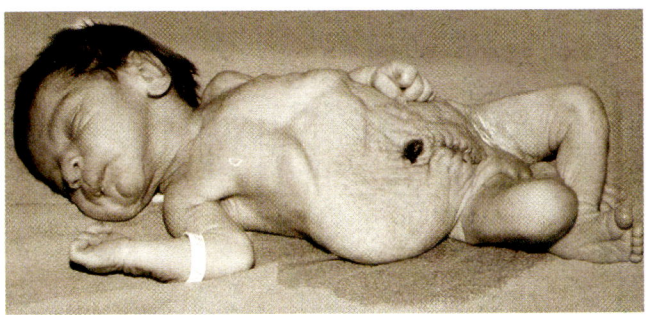

Figure 21.5 Prune-belly syndrome. Note prune-like abdomen and large flaccid phallus.

prevention of further renal damage and intact survival of the afflicted infants.

CONGENITAL NEPHROTIC SYNDROME

Finnish type of familial congenital nephrotic syndrome of unknown etiology is a rare condition in the newborn. It is an autosomal recessive disorder. The disease starts in intrauterine life as evidenced by elevated protein content of amniotic fluid and large placenta. Amniotic fluid and maternal serum alpha-fetoproteins are elevated and serve as useful markers for antenatal diagnosis in subsequent siblings. Most infants are prematurely born with intrauterine growth retardation and polycythemia. Proteinuria is present from first day of life but edema may occur anytime during 4 to 8 weeks of age. Serum IgG levels are low. Histopathology may show characteristic microcystic changes in proximal convoluted tubules and other non-specific sclerotic and proliferative changes in the glomeruli. The condition should be differentiated from renal parenchymatous involvement due to intrauterine infections by syphilis, toxoplasmosis, CMV, and renal vein thrombosis. Serum immunoglobulins of both IgG and IgM class would be elevated in infants with intrauterine infections. Treatment of congenital nephrotic syndrome is supportive to provide additional proteins, prevention and early management of infections. Diuretics and restriction of sodium intake may be helpful to reduce the edema. Steroids and immunosuppressive drugs are not effective. Most infants succumb to sepsis during first 6 months of life. Kidney transplant is the only hope for prolonged survival.

URINARY TRACT INFECTION

Most cases of urinary tract infection in the newborn occur as a consequence of systemic infection. Kidneys are affected as a result of bacteremia or septicemia. Unlike ascending urinary tract infections in older children, which are more common in girls, pyelonephritis in the newborn afflicts boys more often. This is in consonance with higher incidence of sepsis and renal developmental defects among male neonates. The offending organisms causing urinary tract infection are similar to those causing septicemia and include mostly Gram-negative bacteria, *E.coli*, Klebsiella, Entrobacter species, Acinetobacter, Proteus, enterococci, and *Pseudomonas aeruginosa*.

There are no specific clinical features and urinary tract infection should be ruled out in all infants suspected to have septicemia. Clinical picture is dominated by features of septicemia. Isolated urinary tract infection produces milder symptoms in the form of poor weight gain, lethargy, diarrhea, vomiting and elevation of blood urea. Jaundice, hepatomegaly and hemolytic anemia occurs, if there is underlying septicemia. Infected and inflamed kidneys may become enlarged and palpable.

Satisfactory urine specimen for routine and microscopic studies can be collected in a sterile plastic bag or with a test tube in a male infant. To avoid contamination, external genitals should be thoroughly washed with soap and water. After application of bag, baby should be checked every 10 to 15 minutes to avoid unnecessary stagnation of urine in the bag. If infant moves his bowels or bag has been in place for more than an hour, the procedure should be repeated and a new bag affixed. Urine collection with a bag is not satisfactory for culture studies due to risk of contamination. Suprapubic aspiration of bladder is easy, safe and acceptable method to obtain clean specimen of urine. Catheterization of bladder for collection of urine specimen is not recommended in the newborn period. The presence of more than 5 leukocytes per HPF in a clean catch uncentrifuged specimen of urine is significant. Isolation of bacteria in excess of 10^4 per mL, on two occasions, is considered as confirmatory evidence for true bacteriuria. Lower colony counts, mixed cultures and isolation of different organisms on repeat study are indicative of contamination. The quantitation or colony count is not necessary, if urine sample is obtained by suprapubic aspiration when any bacterial growth would be considered as significant. The incidence of asymptomatic bacteriuria varies between 0.5% of term infants and 1 to 3% of preterm infants.

The details and principles of specific antibacterial therapy are the same as outlined for the management of septicemia. Ampicillin and an aminoglycoside through parenteral route is recommended for 10–14 days. The dosage should be adjusted depending upon the functional status of kidneys. Urologic investigations are unwarranted unless there are obvious evidences of obstructive uropathy. However, if infection recurs or is difficult to eradicate, appropriate urological investigations should be conducted during follow-up.

NEPHROCALCINOSIS

Nephrocalcinosis is usually associated with hypercalciuric state. Furosemide, methylxanthines, glucocorticoids and vitamin D administration are associated with increased urinary excretion of calcium and nephrocalcinosis. Secondary hyperoxaluria in association with parenteral nutrition and hyperphosphaturia facilitate the deposition of calcium crystals in the kidneys. Primary oxalosis, renal tubular acidosis and urinary tract infection are uncommon causes of nephrocalcinosis and renal stones. There are increasing reports of nephrocalcinosis in very LBW babies. The diagnosis is made on ultrasound examination of the kidneys. There is no specific treatment but drugs that cause hypercalciuria should be stopped. In infants with bronchopulmonary dysplasia when prolonged diuretic therapy is required, it is preferable to give thiazide diuretic and provide supplements of magnesium. There is no significant renal dysfunction and most cases resolve spontaneously by the end of first year. However, significant tubular dysfunction may persist during childhood.

ABDOMINAL MASSES

Abdominal masses are uncommon during newborn period but when present they often pose a diagnostic dilemma. Abdominal lump may be noticed at birth or appear anytime later. Infants with bilateral dysplastic or multicystic kidneys and severe obstructive uropathy may be stillborn. Abdominal palpation in a quiet and relaxed newborn, about one hour after feed, can be accomplished with ease to identify pathological enlargement of any viscera. Liver edge and lower poles of kidneys (especially right kidney which is lower) can be felt in most newborns. Urinary bladder is an abdominal organ during neonatal period and is often palpable as a suprapubic mass. Renal masses are far more common and any lump in the flanks should be considered as renal in origin unless proved otherwise. Common causes of abdominal masses are listed in Table 21.5.

Discrete, freely mobile almost wandering masses are most commonly due to duplication of gut, mesenteric cyst or ovarian cyst. Transillumination must be done as a routine to differentiate between a cystic and solid lump because tense cystic mass may feel rather firm on palpation. *Solid lumps in the newborn should be considered as potentially malignant unless proved otherwise by biopsy.* For proper evaluation of pelvic mass by palpation and rectal examination (use smallest finger), it is essential that urinary bladder must be emptied by gentle suprapubic pressure. Laboratory investigations are done to identify any evidences of blood loss or bleeding diathesis and to assess functional status of kidneys. Fall in hematocrit may suggest subcapsular hematoma or adrenal hematoma and thrombocytopenia may be associated with hepatic hemangioma and renal vein thrombosis.

TABLE 21.5 Abdominal masses in the newborn

Hepatic masses
  Subcapsular hematoma
  Hemangioma and hamartoma
  Lymphangioma
  Choledochal cyst
  Hepatoblastoma

Renal masses
  Cystic
  Hydronephrosis
  Multicystic dysplastic kidneys
  Polycystic kidneys
  Adrenal hematoma
  Solid
  Renal vein thrombosis
  Wilms' tumor
  Mesoblastic nephroma
  Hamartoma
  Neuroblastoma

Intraperitoneal masses
  Meconium ileus
  Meconium peritonitis with pseudocyst
  Mesenteric cyst
  Duplication of gut
  Ovarian cyst

Pelvic masses
  Hydrocolpos or hematocolpos
  Teratoma
  Neuroblastoma
  Ectopic kidney
  Anterior meningocele

Plain skiagrams of chest and abdomen may provide useful information. Bony calcification or dental vestiges may be seen in retroperitoneal teratoma. Meconium ileus and meconium peritonitis with or without meconium pseudocyst is associated with signs of intestinal obstruction. Diffuse blotchy calcification is suggestive of meconium peritonitis while a rim of calcification around a mass is diagnostic of adrenal hematoma. Ultrasound scanning is a safe and accurate tool to delineate the origin and nature of an intra-abdominal lump and must be undertaken in all cases as an investigation of first choice. Radionuclide scans of liver and kidneys provide useful information when lumps are associated with these organs. Excretory pyelography is advised in a case of unilateral solid mass to differentiate between Wilms' tumor and neuroblastoma. Cystogram obtained by instillation of 15% hypaque through a urethral catheter is indicated when obstructive uropathy is suspected. Prophylactic administration of amoxicillin 20 mg/kg/

day oral, one day before and 2 days after the procedure of micturiting cystourethrography is recommended. Venacavogram through femoral vein is mandatory for confirmation of diagnosis of renal vein thrombosis. Barium enema studies with water-soluble barium or diluted hypaque are indicated when intraperitoneal mass in relation to gastrointestinal tract is suspected.

Hepatic Masses

Diffuse enlargement of liver in the newborn occurs most commonly due to congestive heart failure, hepatitis, cholangitis and microabscesses.

Subcapsular hematoma Rapid onset of anemia, shock and enlarged liver at or soon after birth in an infant born following breech extraction is suggestive of subcapsular hematoma. The hematoma may continue to enlarge after birth and may rupture into peritoneal cavity producing hemorrhagic ascites and progressive anemia and jaundice. Administration of vitamin K and urgent correction of shock with blood transfusion is mandatory. Surgical intervention is necessary in those cases where hematoma has ruptured.

Hemangioma In infants with unexplained enlargement of liver or congestive heart failure, liver area should be auscultated to identify any bruit due to hemangioma and arteriovenous fistula. Cutaneous hemangiomas should be looked for and are often associated. Platelets may be trapped in the hemangiomatous web resulting in thrombocytopenia. Aortography is confirmatory to outline vascular tumor of liver while biopsy is contraindicated and may prove fatal. Corticosteroids in large doses are beneficial. Subtotal hepatectomy or ligation of hepatic artery is indicated when steroid therapy fails. In general, irradiation therapy is avoided in the newborn period due to its carcinogenic potential and adverse effects on growth.

Lymphangioma Lobular hepatic mass which is compressible and associated with visible or intraperitoneal lymphangioma, is suggestive of lymphangioma of liver. Surgical excision or partial hepatectomy is necessary depending upon the size of the tumor.

Choledochal cyst There is cystic dilatation/s from any part of the biliary tract. The anomaly is extremely rare and usually present in infancy. Girls are 4 times more affected than boys. The clinical features are vague and include nausea, vomiting, cholestatic jaundice, pain in right hypochondrium and fever due to cholangitis. Cyst is rarely palpable. Liver function tests, ultrasonography and CT scans are useful screening tests. Magnetic resonance cholangiopancreatography (MRCP) and Technitium-99m (^{99m}Tc) hepatoiminodiacetic acid

(HIDA) scintigraphy are useful non-invasive tests to confirm the diagnosis. The cyst is excised followed by reconstruction of the biliary tree with hepatico-jejunostomy in a Roux-en-y fashion.

Hepatoblastoma Hepatoblastoma is exceedingly rare in newborn period. Elevation of alpha-fetoprotein may not be diagnostic of hepatoblastoma because hepatic injury or dysfunction due to any cause is associated with nonspecific elevation of alpha-fetoproteins during the newborn period.

RENAL MASSES

Renal masses are by far the most frequent cause of abdominal lump in the newborn. Oligohydramnios, single umbilical artery and Potter facies are often associated with a variety of malformations of kidneys and its drainage system. Developmental kidney diseases with severe oligohydramnios include autosomal recessive polycystic kidney disease, bilateral renal agenesis, bilateral multicystic dysplastic kidneys, and complete ureteral obstruction. Urinous ascites is diagnostic of obstructive uropathy. Presence of hypertension would also favor the possibility of renal lump.

Hydronephrosis Obstructive uropathy at birth is typically characterized by presence of three abdominal masses, two kidneys and the bladder. Infants with severe obstruction may have ascites due to leakage of urine into peritoneal cavity as a result of hydrostatic rupture of the pelvis or ureter. Decompression of kidneys should be achieved by urgent drainage of bladder and pelves. Site of obstruction is identified by contrast cystography and corrective surgery performed subsequently after stabilization of the infant.

Multicystic dysplastic kidneys (MCDK) Bilateral renal dysplasia is not compatible with life because they are associated with pulmonary hypoplasia and affected children are either stillborn or die soon after birth. Therefore, most cases of multicystic kidneys present as unilateral, nodular but transilluminant cystic mass in the flank. They can be reliably diagnosed by current imaging techniques with an accuracy of more than 90%. The infant should be evaluated for associated anomalies (cardiac, esophageal, anorectal, pelvi-ureteric obstruction on the opposite side). Nephrectomy is indicated, if affected kidney is non-functional and associated with hypertension and pyelonephritis or renal mass is causing respiratory difficulty.

Polycystic kidneys They present as bilateral diffuse and massive enlargement of both kidneys in the absence of any evidences of obstructive uropathy. The condition is familial and transmitted as autosomal recessive. There is progressive renal insufficiency and death. Renal transplantation is the only hope for these patients. Autosomal recessive polycystic kidney disease (ARPKD) is usually associated with hepatic fibrosis and/or dilated bile ducts. Hepatic involvement may progress to liver failure requiring transplantation in adolescence.

Adrenal hematoma It is an extremely rare cause of abdominal mass and often detected at autopsy. The usual predisposing conditions include birth trauma, asphyxia and DIC. The right gland is more commonly involved and in 8 to 10% cases adrenal hemorrhage may be bilateral. Rim of calcification at the margin of swelling on X-ray examination is diagnostic.

Renal vein thrombosis (*see* page 416 for details)

Wilms' tumor Solid tumors of the kidney are mostly unilateral. Excretory pyelography shows that function of kidneys is preserved while renal collecting system is grossly distorted and splayed. Wilms' tumor may be associated with hemihypertrophy and aniridia which should be looked for in any infant having abdominal lump. The principles of management are the same as in older children but radiation therapy is often avoided during newborn period.

Mesoblastic nephroma It is the most common intrarenal tumor seen in the newborn. Among tumors, it is second only to sacrococcygeal teratoma in frequency in the newborn. It is generally a benign tumor but has all the clinical features resembling Wilms' tumor. In mesoblastic nephroma, there is no clear cut interface between the tumor and adjacent normal renal tissue. Ultrasound reveals a solid mass within the kidney with low-level ring pattern of echoes. Surgical excision of tumor or nephrectomy is curative.

Neuroblastoma Abdominal neuroblastoma in the newborn mostly arises from adrenal medulla thus displacing the adjacent kidney downwards and outwards. It is the most common malignancy in neonates accounting for at least 50% of all neonatal malignant tumors. The tumor is more likely to be malignant in the newborn period. Skiagram of abdomen may show typical punctate calcification. Examination of bone marrow, urinary catecholamines and skeletal survey may provide diagnostic clues. Intravenous pyelography would confirm that the tumor is extrarenal causing classical displacement of the kidney upon which the tumor rests. Prognosis of infantile neuroblastoma is better compared to those arising later in life.

Hamartoma It is a benign tumor of the kidneys which is made up of an abnormal mixture of healthy cells and tissues. Simple surgical excision is curative.

INTRAPERITONEAL MASSES

Most intraperitoneal masses are usually discrete, well defined and freely mobile in all the abdominal quadrants.

Meconium ileus In mucoviscidosis, ileum is obstructed by thick putty-like meconium and associated with abdominal distension and vomiting. Vague, ill-defined boggy masses of thick meconium are felt in mid-abdomen. Skiagram of abdomen shows evidences of intestinal obstruction with typical ground-glass appearance of inspissated meconium. Sweat chloride content is characteristically high in these infants. The test is unreliable, if less than 100 mg sweat is collected. It should be repeated when infant is 3–4 weeks old. Stool should be examined for tryptic activity. Take 1:5 or 1:10 dilution of meconium in normal saline and place it on the gelatin side of undeveloped X-ray film. The film should be incubated at 37°C for one hour. If trypsin activity is present, the gelatin is dissolved. Absence of trypsin is suggestive of cystic fibrosis and complete intestinal obstruction due to any cause.

Meconium peritonitis with pseudocysts In some infants with small gut atresia, perforation of proximal bowel wall may occur in intrauterine life. Extravasated intestinal contents are walled off by the surrounding intestinal loops and a psudocyst filled with thin green fluid develops within the abdominal cavity. Examination shows an ill-defined immobile inflammatory mass of varying consistency in association with signs of intestinal obstruction and calcification on X-rays. The pseudocyst can be evacuated and removed and intestinal continuity established by excision of atretic gut.

Mesenteric cyst Lymphatic cyst in the mesentery is characterized by its oblique location in conformity with peritoneal attachment and is freely mobile in horizontal plane from one quadrant to the other.

Duplication of gut Cystic duplication of small bowel may develop in association with duodenum, jejunum or terminal ileum. They produce symptoms of subacute intestinal obstruction with acute episodes of volvulus. The duplication mass is cystic and remarkably mobile except when arising from duodenum. Barium meal examination may show distorsion of affected segment of gut.

Ovarian cyst It is characterized by a large, easily palpable and amazingly mobile mass on one or both sides. Due to long pedicle, torsion is a potential complication.

PELVIC MASSES

Hydrocolpos or hematocolpos It produces a large midline suprapubic mass secondary to either imperforate hymen, distal vaginal atresia or absence of vagina. The mass persists even after evacuation of urinary bladder. Examination of perineum shows bluish-colored bulge in the vestibule in case of imperforate hymen. Intestinal obstruction and hydronephrosis may occur due to pressure. Because of compression of blood vessels, edema and cyanosis of legs may be observed. Incision of hymen with drainage of retained blood and secretions from uterus and vagina is curative. Infants with vaginal atresia require an abdominoperineal operation with vaginoplasty. The condition should not be confused with labial adhesions when the inner lips (labia minora) of the vulva stick together. The condition can be treated by gentle attempts to manually break the adhesions over a period of few days.

Teratoma, neuroblastoma, ectopic kidney and anterior meningocele account for other pelvic masses during neonatal period. Sacrococcygeal teratomas present no difficulty in clinical diagnosis (Figure 21.6). Skiagrams of spine, excretory pyelography and barium enema are recommended to delineate these masses. Abdominal neuroblastoma, Wilms' tumor and teratoma account for more than one-half of the total malignancies encountered during newborn period.

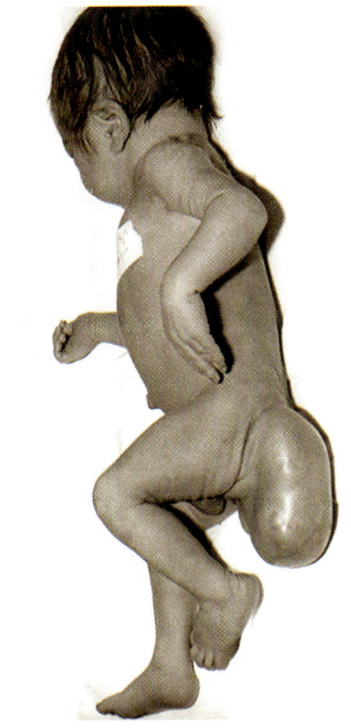

Figure 21.6 Typical appearances of sacrococcygeal teratoma.

Renal Disorders

21

Sarcoma botryoides It is a grape-like tumor that arises from the edge of vulva or vagina. When small it can be confused with a normal posterior vaginal tag. Intravenous pyelography is useful to exclude obstructing ureterocele and biopsy is diagnostic.

BIBLIOGRAPHY

Agras PI, Tarcan A, Baskin E, Cengiz N, Gurakan B, Saatci U. Acute renal failure in the neonatal period. *Renal Failure* 2004, 26: 305–309.

Al-Wassia H, Alshaikh B, Sauve R. Prophylactic theophylline for the prevention of severe renal dysfunction in term and post-term neonates with perinatal asphyxia: a systematic review and meta-analysis of randomized controlled trials. *J Perinatol* 2013, 33: 271.

Anand SK, Northway JD, Crussi FG. Acute renal failure in newborn infants. *J Pediatr* 1978, 92: 985.

Annabelle NC, Minnie MS. Acute renal failure management in the neonate. *Neo Reviews* 2005, 6: e369–e376.

Askenazi D, Abitbol C, Boohaker L, *et al.* Optimizing the AKI definition during first postnatal week using Assessment of Worldwide Acute Kidney Injury Epidemiology in Neonates (AWAKEN) Cohort. *Pediatr Res* 2019, 85:329.

Bakr A, Eid R, Allam NA, Saleh H. Neonatal acute kidney injury: Diagnostic and therapeutic challenges. *J Nephrol Res* 2018, 4(1):130–4.

Bakr AF. Prophylactic theophylline to prevent renal dysfunction in newborns exposed to perinatal asphyxia: a study in a developing country. *Pediatr Nephrol.* 2005, 20: 1249–52.

Bartone FF, Mazer MJ, Anderson JE, *et al.* Diagnosis and treatment of fluid filled renal structures in children with ultrasonography and percutaneous puncture. *Urology* 1980, 16: 432.

Bhatt GC, Gogia P, Bitzan M, Das RR. Theophylline and aminophylline for prevention of acute kidney injury in neonates and children: a systematic review. *Arch Dis Child* 2019, 0:1–10. doi: 10.1136 archdischild. 2018–315805.

Chandler JC, Gauderer MWL. The neonate with an abdominal mass. *Pediatr Clin N Am* 2004, 51: 979–997.

Cohen MD. Intravenous urography in neonates and infants. *Br J Radiol* 1979, 52: 942.

Coulthard MG, Vernon B. Managing acute renal failure in very low birth weight infants. *Arch Dis Child* 1995, 73: F187–F192.

Eslami Z, Shajari A, Kheirandish M, Heidary A. Theophylline for prevention of kidney dysfunction in neonates with severe asphyxia. *Iranian J Kidney Dis* 2009, 3:222–6.

Garrette R and Franken E. Neonatal ascites: Perirenal urinary extravasation with bladder outlet obstruction. *J Urol* 1969, 102: 627.

Gouyon JB, Guinard JP. Management of acute renal failure in newborns. *Pediatr Nephrol* 2000, 14: 1037–1044.

Hartman GE, Shochat SJ. Abdominal mass lesions in the newborn: diagnosis and treatment. *Clin Perinatol* 1989, 16: 123.

Henderson KD, Torch EM. Differential diagnosis of abdominal masses in the neonate. *Pediatr Clin N Amer* 1977, 24: 605.

Kidney Disease Improving Global Outcomes (KDIGO). Acute Kidney Injury Working Group. KDIGO Clinical Practice Guidelines for Acute Kidney Injury. *Kidney International Suppl 1*, 2012, 2: 1–138.

Kohli HS, Bhalla D, Sud K, *et al.* Acute peritoneal dialysis in neonates: comparison of two types of peritoneal access. *Pediatr Nephrol* 1999, 13: 241–244.

Koralkar R, Ambalavanan N, Levitan EB, *et al.* Acute kidney injury reduces survival in very low birth weight infants. *Pediatr Res* 2011, 69: 354.

Maherzi M, Guignard JP, Torrado A. Urinary tract infection in high-risk newborn infants. *Pediatrics* 1979, 62: 521.

Marsha ML, Annbelle NC, Peter DY. Neonatal peritoneal dialysis. *Neo Reviews* 2005, 6: e369–e376.

Moghal NE, Embleton ND. Management of acute renal failure in the newborn. *Semin Fetal Neonatal Med* 2006, 11: 207–213.

Norman ME, Asadi FK. A prospective study of acute renal failure in the newborn infant. *Pediatrics* 1979, 63: 475.

Ravindra LM, John AK, Sudhir VS, *et al.* Acute Kidney Injury Network: report of an initiative to improve outcomes in acute kidney injury. *Critical Care* 2007, 11: R 31.

Ricciz Z, Cruz DN, Ronco C. Classification and staging of acute kidney injury: beyond the RIFLE and AKIN criteria. *Nature Rev Nephrol* 2011, 7: 201–208.

Ross B, Cowett RM, Oh W. Renal functions in low birth weight infants during the first two months of life. *Pediatr Res* 1977, 11: 1162.

Selewski DT, Jordan BK, Askenazi DJ, *et al.* Acute kidney injury in asphyxiated newborn treated with therapeutic hypothermia. *J Pediatr* 2013, 162: 725.

Shaffer FE, Norman ME. Renal function and renal failure in the newborn. *Clin Perinatol* 1989, 16: 199.

Sheldon CA, Gonzalez R, Mauer SM, *et al.* Obstructive uropathy, renal failure and sepsis in the neonate: A surgical emergency. *Urology* 1980, 16: 457.

Tank ES, Carey TC, Seifert AL. Management of neonatal urinary ascites. *Urology* 1970, 16: 270.

Neurological Disorders

Brain is the first organ that differentiates during embryonic life. Its size at birth is relatively large as compared to other organs and its weight at birth is one-half of the weight of adult brain (other organs being 1/20th of adult size). At birth body weight is 5% of an adult while the brain size is about 60% of an adult. Its size is not significantly affected by intra-uterine malnutrition. The most susceptible areas of brain to perinatal damage include basal ganglia, rhinencephalon, dentate and auditory nuclei and vestibular system. Brain in a newborn baby functions mostly at a subcortical level because babies born without cerebral hemispheres are indistinguishable in behavior from normal newborn infants and cerebral motor defects do not generally manifest in the neonatal period. Neurological examination has a limited localizing value for cerebral lesions in the newborn period. The presence of some degree of visual fixation and ability to turn head towards diffuse light, occurrence of neonatal seizures of cerebral origin and elicitation of evoked cortical responses on electroencephalogram suggest that cerebral cortex does function to some extent even in a newborn baby.

NEUROLOGICAL EXAMINATION

The lack of cooperation and proper 'state'* of the baby poses practical difficulties. Therefore, emphasis is laid on thorough observation which is likely to be most informative and least disturbing to the infant. The neurological examination is best performed about two hours after the last feed when baby is in 'state' 3 or 4 but normal babies remain in these 'states' only for 10–15%

of the time. The examination should never be attempted immediately after the feed because some babies may vomit, if they are handled or disturbed. Most babies fall asleep after a feed. The infant should be completely undressed in a warm, well illuminated and quiet room. The physician's hands should be warm and clean.

Purpose of Neurological Examination

Routine neurologic examination in a healthy term baby is unnecessary. The information regarding activity, behavior and feeding pattern of the baby as reported by the mother or nurse, absence of any abnormalities of skull and spine and symmetry of spontaneous movements of limbs on the two sides are enough to rule out any significant neurological abnormalities. There is no need to 'inflict' Moro reflex on these apparently normal babies. In general, a detailed neonatal neurological examination is usually done for the following purposes:

1. Diagnosis of acute neurological illness.
2. Prognosis for future neurological development following perinatal hazards and neurological illness.
3. Assessment of gestational age.

The Approach for Examination

Inspection of the newborn baby is most informative and should be accorded the maximum time.

General Observations

The 'containers' of the central nervous system (skull and spine) should be carefully examined to exclude any traumatic or developmental defects. 'State' of the

---

*'States' of wakefulness in a neonate. State 1. Deep sleep with regular respirations. State 2. Light sleep with eyes closed, occasional movements of eyelids, lips, fingers, etc. and irregular respirations (REM sleep). State 3. Eyes open with no gross body movements (quiet wakefulness). State 4. Eyes open with gross body movements. State 5. Eyes open or closed and crying.

baby and cry should be recorded. High-pitched shrill cry may signify the presence of cerebral irritability.

Skull

The occipitofrontal circumference (OFC) should be measured after 24 hours of birth when caput succedaneum, molding and over-riding of sutures would have disappeared. The head circumference may be greater by more 3.0 cm as compared to the chest circumference at the level of nipples in preterm, small-for-dates, and hydrocephalic infants. Abnormalities of shape, symmetry and swellings (cephalhematoma and encephalocele) should be looked for. Transient 'setting sun' sign may be normally seen in some neonates. If persistent and exaggerated, it suggests hydrocephalus and acute bilirubin encephalopathy. It is suggestive of raised intracranial tension because of compression of orbital plate or brainstem irritation.

During the first 48 hours, skull bones overlap each other due to molding. A wide range of normal variations in the size of anterior fontanel and sutural separation makes their interpretation difficult. Hydrocephalus should be suspected only when head circumference is increased. Sagittal suture may be separated up to 0.50 to 0.75 cm during the first fortnight due to the rapid growth of the brain outstripping the bony growth of the calvarium. Generally squamoparietal sutures are not separated except in hydrocephalus but may be open in preterm and small-for-dates babies without hydrocephalus. A ridge at metopic suture (midline on forehead) is normal while sutural ridges at other places suggest craniosynostosis. Auscultation of skull may reveal a bruit in infants with arteriovenous fistula or angiomatous malformation.

Transillumination should be done as a routine in all cases. The torch should be fitted with a circular tightly fitting rubber foam ring over its front end to ensure close contact of the torch to the baby's scalp. A fiberoptic cold light source can be used for transillumination. Normally, the halo of light around the rim of the illuminator extends up to one centimeter in the occipital region and about two centimeters in the frontal region in term babies. Excessive transillumination is seen whenever the abnormal collection of fluid at any intracranial site is within one centimeter of the inner table of skull. In large collections of fluids and in infants with hydranencephaly or porencephaly, the whole skull may glow with light.

Spine

Exclude spina bifida and associated anomalies, tuft of hair, dermal sinus and fracture of the spine.

Cranial Nerves

Examination of cranial nerves has limited usefulness. For examination of second and eighth cranial nerve, refer to the section on special senses. For examination of third, fourth and sixth cranial nerves, the baby should be held in the arms in a diffuse light when he may open eyes spontaneously. Ptosis and inability to close the eye should be looked for. Doll's eye movements should be tested to detect any ocular palsy. Nystagmoid movements may be seen normally. For assessment of fifth and seventh nerves, when you tap the nasion, the eyes close. This evaluates movements of the upper face (Figure 22.1). Rooting reflex gives information about the lower half of the face (Figure 22.2). Asymmetry of the face on crying is a useful sign of facial palsy. In partial facial palsy, mandible alone may deviate to one side as the baby cries. Corneal reflex is absent when trigeminal nerve is affected. Look for nasal regurgitation during feeds and elicit the gag reflex for evaluation of ninth and tenth cranial nerves. Asymmetry of tongue is seen due to involvement of the twelfth nerve.

Fundus

The examination of fundus is of limited value in a newborn baby. Satisfactory pupillary dilatation can be achieved with instillation of a mixture of 2.5% phenylephrine and 0.5% tropicamide eye drops every 10 minutes up to 3 times. The disc is normally pale and devoid of foveal reflex during the first three months of life. Papilledema as a sign of raised intracranial tension is rare because rising tension is easily buffered by sutural diastasis. Retinal hemorrhages are commonly encountered but are of no clinical

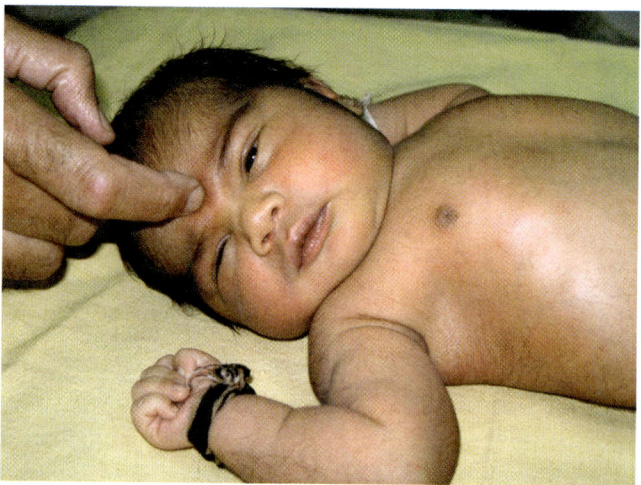

Figure 22.1 Glabellar tap. Gentle tap on the nasion results in a brisk closure of the eyelids. The response may be asymmetric when upper face is paralysed.

less than 29–31 weeks of gestation, during raised intracranial tension and posterior fossa compression. In a newborn baby, the dilated pupils give poor prediction regarding the side or site of intracranial hemorrhage.

2. The baby responds to bright light by blinking.
3. Head turns towards diffuse light after 32 weeks of gestation.
4. The baby shows attention or follows a moving red ball after 34 weeks of gestation.
5. Opticokinetic nystagmus is present.

Hearing Clinical examination for hearing in the newborn is not reliable. The baby is watched for the following responses, after giving a sound stimulus of 500 to 1000 cycles per second (temple bell, whistle, beating of *thali* with a spoon). The method of producing sound should not produce a whiff of air.

Startle response, blinking of eyes, sudden change in the activity with greater alertness and change in the heart rate.

The positive responses both for visual attention and hearing signify lack of generalized neurological disturbances. Negative response, however, is of little significance because many variables may affect this.

Motor Functions

Spontaneous movements The range and symmetry of spontaneous movements should be observed. Watch and record in detail any tremors (jitteriness) and convulsions.

Muscle tone The normal term neonate is rather hypertonic while preterm babies are hypotonic. Increase or decrease in tone must be significant before it is regarded as abnormal. Differences in muscle tone between the two sides of the body have greater localizing value. The baby's head must be kept in the midline, while assessing the muscle tone, otherwise asymmetric tonic neck reflex (ATNR) may influence muscle tone unequally on the two sides.

Tendon jerks The deep tendon jerks are rather variable in neonates and are generally brisk. Knee jerk in the newborn is normally followed by contraction of adductors of both hips (crossed adductor spread). Ankle clonus may elicit up to eight jerks in normal babies but if 10 to 12 uninterrupted jerks are obtained, it is abnormal. The tendon jerks are of poor diagnostic utility except in infants with peripheral nerve and spinal cord injuries.

Primitive Reflexes

The newborn babies have a large number of primitive reflexes which are brainstem-mediated automatic

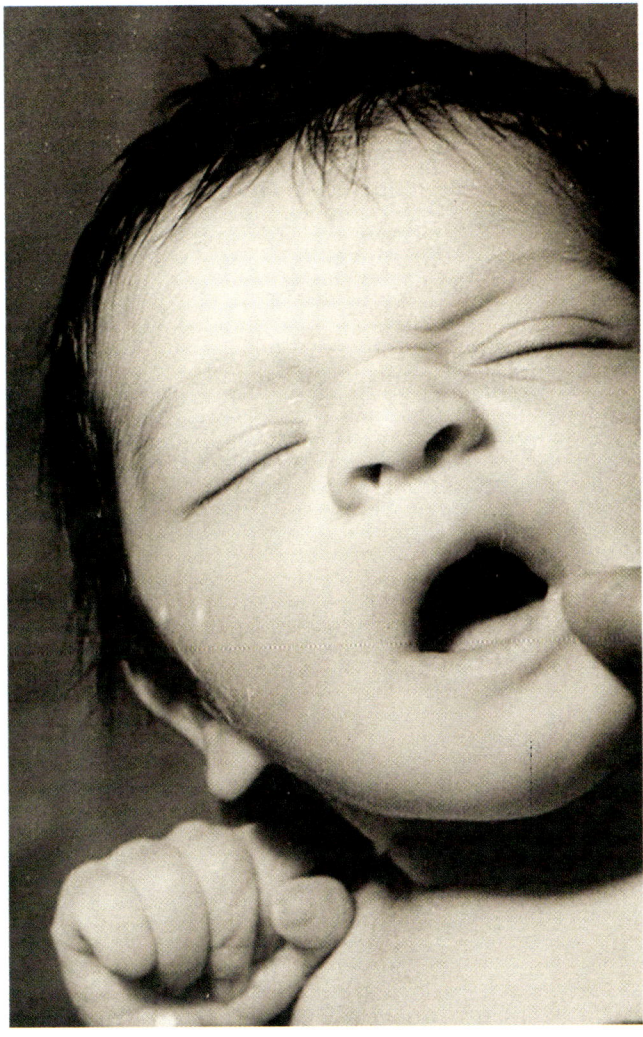

Figure 22.2 Rooting reflex. The baby opens his mouth, turns towards the side of stimulus when angle of the mouth is touched. It enables the infant to instinctively 'root' for the nipple during breastfeeding.

significance. Large subhyaloid hemorrhages are seen in intracranial bleeding in the subarachnoid and subdural spaces. Choroidoretinopathy is suggestive of certain intrauterine infections. Refer to Chapter 26 for screening of retinopathy of prematurity (ROP).

Special Senses

They can be tested only during 'states' 3 to 4 otherwise the interpretation is unreliable.

Vision The visual fixation and attention must be assessed with due patience and care because these are the only functions at birth which indicate the integrity of cerebral hemispheres. The visual acuity in a term newborn baby is around 20/150.

1. The size of pupils and their reaction to light should be recorded. Pupils do not react to light in babies

responses. It is time consuming and tiring both for the baby and physician to try to elicit all automatic reflexes. The following reflexes are useful for clinical purposes and one should observe whether the response is sluggish, normal or exaggerated and symmetric or asymmetric.

Moro reflex The Moro reflex or startle response is the most useful. The baby should be held supine over the right hand and arm. The flexed head is suddenly allowed to drop by about 30°. A positive response consists of rapid abduction and extension of upper limbs and opening of hands followed by slower adduction and flexion or embrace equivalent (Figure 22.3). The infant may cry. The response can also be elicited by pulling a supine infant by holding at both hands

(as in traction response). When angulation occurs between the head and trunk, the hands are sharply released to cause sudden extension of neck.

The response may be depressed or absent in infants with cerebral depression. Exaggerated or jumpy response may be obtained in cases of cerebral irritability due to hypoxic-ischemic encephalopahty, brainstem damage and infants with blindness. The Moro reflex may be incomplete in babies with a gestation of less than 35 weeks. Asymmetric Moro response may suggest brachial palsy and fracture of clavicle or humerus. In babies with acute bilirubin encephalopathy, the Moro response is often characteristic. The sudden extension of arms is not followed by flexion component but often accompanied with downward rolling of eyeballs ('setting sun' sign), lid lag and a peculiar grin.

Glabellar tap Tapping of nasion is followed by closure of eyes in infants above 30 weeks gestation.

Rooting and sucking responses Stimulation of angle of mouth or lips would initiate rooting and sucking in infants above 34 weeks gestation. The mother or nurse's report regarding feeding behavior of the baby is more informative.

Asymmetrical tonic neck reflex (ATNR) When the baby's head is turned to one side, the ipsilateral arm and leg gets extended while contralateral limbs are flexed. If a baby constantly or persistently maintains the tonic neck posture, it is abnormal and may signify future development of cerebral plasy (Figure 22.4).

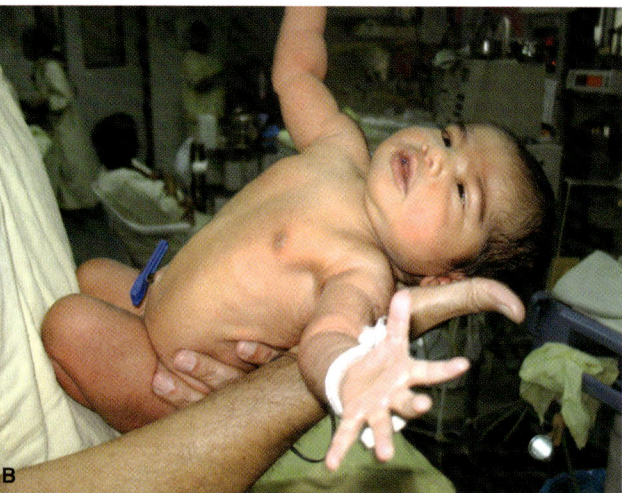

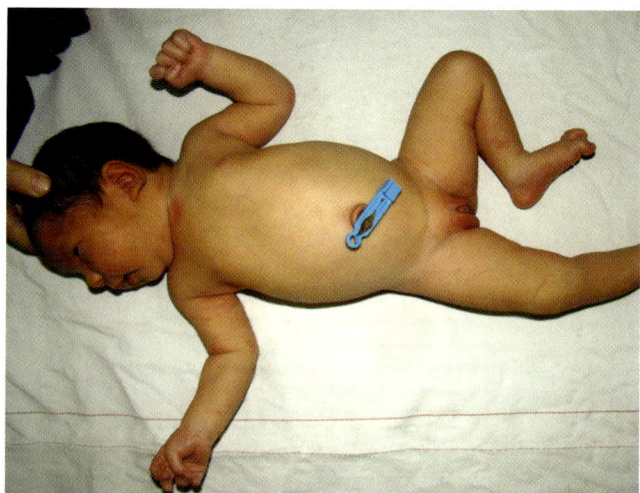

Figure 22.3 Moro reflex. (A) The infant is held supine over the arm and head is supported over the palm. (B) Sudden extension of the flexed head by letting it drop by 30° results in abduction and extension of upper limbs followed by adduction and flexion or embrace equivalent.

Figure 22.4 Tonic neck reflex. In a supine infant when head is turned to one side, the extremities facing the head are extended while limbs on the opposite side are flexed. Persistent neck tonic posture in an infant is suggestive of cerebral palsy.

Traction reflex The supine baby when pulled up by holding at the wrists, his ability to flex the arms and neck should be observed.

Palmar and plantar grasp The finger is placed on the palmar surface of fingers or plantar surface of toes of the baby to elicit grasp or flexion of toes (Figure 22.5). Stroke dorsum of the hand to persuade the baby to open the hand.

Most primitive reflexes disappear between 3 and 4 months of age and their persistence is considered as an early sign of cerebral palsy.

Sensory Functions

Sensory testing is of limited value in the newborn. The response to painful stimuli should be assessed, if injury or disease of peripheral nerves or spinal cord is suspected (Figure 22.6). The anal reflex must be elicited in infants with neural tube defects.

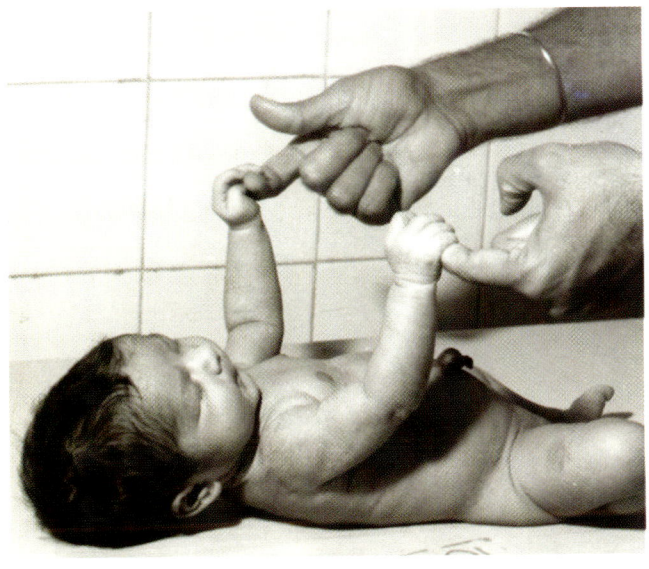

Figure 22.5 Grasp reflex. Healthy term infant can be lifted off the cot by virtue of his strong palmar grasp.

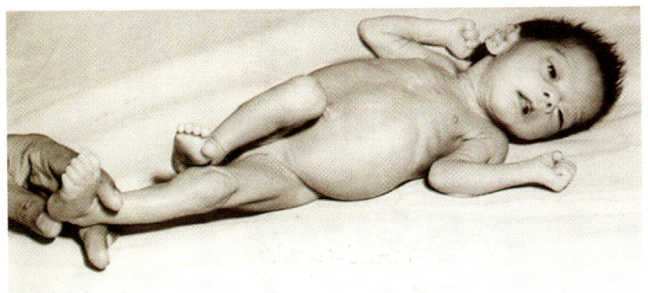

Figure 22.6 Crossed extension reflex. The left foot is being given a painful stimulus. The unstimulated right leg is flexed followed by abduction and extension as if to ward off the painful stimulus. The reflex operates through spinal arc.

The newborn baby has a limited capacity to respond to a wide variety of disorders in the central nervous system. This explains poor correlation between clinical manifestations and underlying pathological process. There is lack of clarity or overlap in pathological expression of various disorders with the exception of kernicterus and intracranial hemorrhage. The baby whose brain functions have been disturbed due to perinatal hazards such as birth trauma, hypoxia, biochemical disorders (especially hypoglycemia and hyperbilirubinemia) and pre- or post-natal infections may show the following features.

Cerebral Depression

It is characterized by lethargy, refusal of feeds, reduction in muscle tone and lack of spontaneous movements. The primitive reflexes and deep tendon jerks may be diminished or absent. It may be associated with lack of visual attention and fixation. Respiratory failure may manifest with apneic attacks and cyanosis.

Cerebral Irritability or Hyperexcitability

During this phase, the spontaneous movements and muscle tone may be increased. The baby shows excessive jitteriness or tremulous movements spontaneously or following various stimuli. The cry is shrill and high pitched. It is often difficult to quieten or console the child. The primitive reflexes may be variable or exaggerated. Cerebral irritability may be followed by cerebral depression and *vice versa.*

Lateralized Abnormality or Hemi-syndrome

There may be definite and consistent asymmetry of spontaneous movements, muscle tone, tendon jerks and primitive reflexes. Injuries to the peripheral nerves rather than cerebral disorders are generally responsible for involvement of a limb. Neonatal stroke due to blockage of anterior cerebral artery may manifest as focal seizures and hemiplegia.

Seizures

They are indicative of a serious underlying hypoxia, cerebral disorder or biochemical abnormality.

Floppiness

Severe floppiness of cerebral origin is associated with features of cerebral depression as opposed to hypotonia of peripheral origin. Respiratory distress may dominate the clinical picture, when paralysis of diaphragm or intercostal muscles is associated.

Neurological Disorders

22

INTRACRANIAL HEMORRHAGE

The clinical localization of site of intracranial hemorrhage is often difficult because of lack of specific neurological features. The presence or absence of associated or predisposing factors and time of onset of symptoms may offer useful clues (Table 22.1). Moreover, clinically it may be impossible to differentiate between neurologic manifestations of perinatal hypoxia and intracranial hemorrhage. Hypoxia may predispose to the development of intracranial bleeding and *vice versa*.

TABLE 22.1 Types of intracranial hemorrhage and their clinical features

Site	Source of bleeding	Predisposing factors	Age at onset and specific clinical features	Prognosis
Intraventricular	Rupture of subependymal vessels with germinal layer hemorrhage	Immaturity, hypoxia, hypercapnia, precipitate delivery, RDS and rapid injection of hyperosmolar sodium bicarbnonate	Onset at any time. Bulging anterior fontanel, apneic attacks, hypotonia and subtle seizures. Ventricular tap would show blood-stained CSF	Variable with hydrocephalus in survivors
Subarachnoid	Bridging veins or small vascular channels derived from involuting anastomoses between leptomeningeal arteries	Any class of baby with or without history of birth trauma and asphyxia	Seizures, bulging anterior fontanel and blood-stained CSF	Good but there is risk of hydrocephalus
Intracerebral a. *Superficial*	Superficial vessels	Immaturity, hypothermia, acidosis, shock and rhesus incompatibility	Usually during first 48 hours, may be later	Related to primary disease
b. *Hemorrhagic infarction*	Embolic arterial occlusion, venous or arterial thrombosis	Gram-negative infections, DIC and polycythemia	Features of septicemia and secondary hemorrhagic disease of the newborn	Often fatal
c. *Deep cerebral*	Extension from intraventricular hemorrhage or rupture of major vessels	Immaturity, perinatal distress factors and trauma	First 48 hours, catastrophic manifestations	Usually fatal
Intracerebellar	Primary intracerebellar hemorrhagic infarction, extension from intraventricular or subarachnoid hemorrhage, traumatic laceration or rupture of major veins or occipital sinus	Preterm babies, perinatal hypoxia and birth trauma	Early on day one or delayed up to 2–3 weeks, signs of brainstem compression like apneic attacks, skew deviation of eyes, facial paresis, flaccid quadriparesis and evidences of raised intracranial tension	Uniformly fatal outcome in preterm babies
Subdural	Rupture of great cerebral vein or cerebral vein in the region of superior sagittal sinus, laceration of tentorium and falx	Large baby with traumatic delivery, difficult forceps, breech or brow presentation	After 48 hours. Lateralized findings may be present. Subdural tap may help but should be attempted only when suspicion is strong	Often fatal

Note: Unexplained jaundice and anemia in a newborn baby should arouse the suspicion of internal hemorrhage.

Care of the Newborn

22

Apart from lumbar puncture and occasionally ventricular tap, other specialized neurologic investigations especially cranial ultrasonography and CT scan are of great diagnostic utility in the newborn. Ultrasonic imaging of structures adjacent to the bone, i.e. the subdural space, is often inadequate and best evaluated by CT or MRI scan. Examination of CSF is essential to exclude meningitis and subarachnoid bleeding. When blood-stained CSF is obtained, traumatic tap should be excluded.

Treatment

The treatment is mostly symptomatic and supportive. Vitamin K 1 to 2 mg should be given intramuscularly to correct any associated coagulation defect. Administration of coagulation factors have not been demonstrated to be of any prophylactic or therapeutic utility. Chloral hydrate or phenobarbitone are useful for control of cerebral irritability. The seizures should be managed symptomatically.

Brain edema and raised intracranial tension may be associated with perinatal hypoxia and intracranial bleeding. The definitive diagnosis of raised intracranial tension is difficult during the neonatal period but should be strongly suspected in the presence of marked features of cerebral depression and bulging anterior fontanel. The use of dexamethasone (1.0 mg 12 hourly for 3–4 days) and mannitol (1.0 g/kg as 20% solution IV over 20 min for 3–4 doses in term babies with raised ICP) is controversial and should preferably be avoided. Sudden reduction in cerebral volume following mannitol administration may lead to rupture of cerebral veins and aggravation of bleeding. Tapping of cerebrospinal fluid through lumbar or ventricular site relieves intracranial tension.

Supportive measures Handling of the baby should be reduced to the barest minimum. Vital signs should be monitored and any apneic attacks should be managed by physical stimulation and artificial ventilation, if the attacks are prolonged. Temperature regulation should receive due attention because these infants are liable to develop hypothermia, if hypothalamus is damaged. Fluids should be restricted to two-thirds of the maintenance requirements due to increased risk of inappropriate secretion of antidiuretic hormone. Anemia and jaundice should be looked for and appropriately managed.

Primary Subarachnoid Hemorrhage

Subarachnoid hemorrhage may be primary or secondary due to extension from subdural, or intraventricular hemorrhage. Primary subarachnoid hemorrhage is relatively common and second only in frequency to intraventricular hemorrhage. The predisposing factors and pathogenesis of primary subarachnoid hemorrhage are not known. The bleeding usually occurs from bridging veins or small vascular channels derived from involuting anastomoses between leptomeningeal arteries. No specific predisposing factors are known but there is higher association with birth trauma and asphyxia. Most cases are asymptomatic and diagnosed on autopsy as an associated pathology. The occurrence of seizures on the second or third day of life in a well baby is suggestive of subarachnoid hemorrhage. Prognosis is excellent though hydrocephalus may develop during follow-up. Rarely, massive subarachnoid hemorrhage may prove fatal. Ultrasonography is relatively insensitive to detect subarachnoid hemorrhage because of normal increase in echogenicity around the periphery of the brain. Cerebrospinal fluid examination may show presence of crenated red blood cells, elevation of protein and xanthochromia. The treatment is symptomatic and supportive. Prognosis is good.

INTRAVENTRICULAR HEMORRHAGE

Germinal matrix or periventricular-intraventricular hemorrhage is the most common cause of intracranial bleeding and neurological damage in very LBW babies. It occurs in approximately 15 to 20% of all infants weighing less than 1500 g or having gestational maturity of less than 32 weeks. The availability of real-time ultrasound scanning with portable instruments has provided definitive means for early diagnosis and follow up of high-risk LBW infants who are susceptible to develop intraventricular hemorrhage and its sequelae.

Pathogenesis

The pathogenesis of periventricular–intraventricular hemorrhage is still imperfectly understood. It is dependent upon the interplay of anatomical and physiological immaturity of developing cerebral vasculature of preterm babies exposed to hazards of perinatal hypoxia and its consequences. The periventricular capillaries in germinal matrix of preterm babies are structurally deficient in smooth muscle, collagen or elastin. These delicate immature capillaries lie unsupported in the soft gelatinous matrix of germinal layer. They are thus vulnerable to direct hypoxic or hydrostatic insult from a variety of life-threatening complications. The vulnerability of periventricular region to hemorrhage is further enhanced because this area is preferentially overperfused and provided with excessive amount of fibrinolytic activity. The cerebral blood flow in preterm infants is pressure-passive and any rise in arterial pressure is directly transmitted to the capillaries. Elevation in the arterial pressure may occur due to hypoxia and hypercapnia in the perinatal period. Rough handling, tracheal suctioning, administration of xanthine derivatives may cause sudden elevation of arterial blood pressure with rupture of capillaries in the germinal matrix. Diving reflex, which is rather immature and over-reactive in preterm babies may lead to preferential shunting of blood to the brain. Rapid infusion of volume expanders and hyperosmolar solutions of glucose or sodium bicarbonate further aggravates these physiological responses.

Apart from direct transmission of arterial pressure through pressure-passive cerebral vasculature, passive venous congestion may also elevate pressure in the periventricular capillaries. Birth asphyxia and postnatal hypoxia due to apneic attacks or RDS may elevate venous pressure by virtue of hypoxic cardiac failure. Positive pressure ventilation with PEEP and pneumothorax are also associated with elevation of venous pressure leading to congestion in the intracerebral capillaries (Figure 22.7). The bleeding occurs into periventricular germinal layer matrix. It may remain small and localized or rupture through ependyma into the ventricular system or extend into cerebral parenchyma causing leukomalacia and porencephalic cyst. Progressive hydrocephalus is a common sequelae.

Clinical Features

The clinical features of periventricular–intraventricular hemorrhage may be absent, subtle or life-threatening. The onset of hemorrhage is usually during the first two days of life (especially during first 12 hours). In critically sick preterm babies having RDS, apneic attacks, patent ductus arteriosus, assisted ventilation, CPAP and pneumothorax, intraventricular hemorrhage may have onset anytime during neonatal period. There are no diagnostic clinical features of intraventricular hemorrhage. Unexplained fall in hematocrit and changes in muscle tone may be the only manifesta-

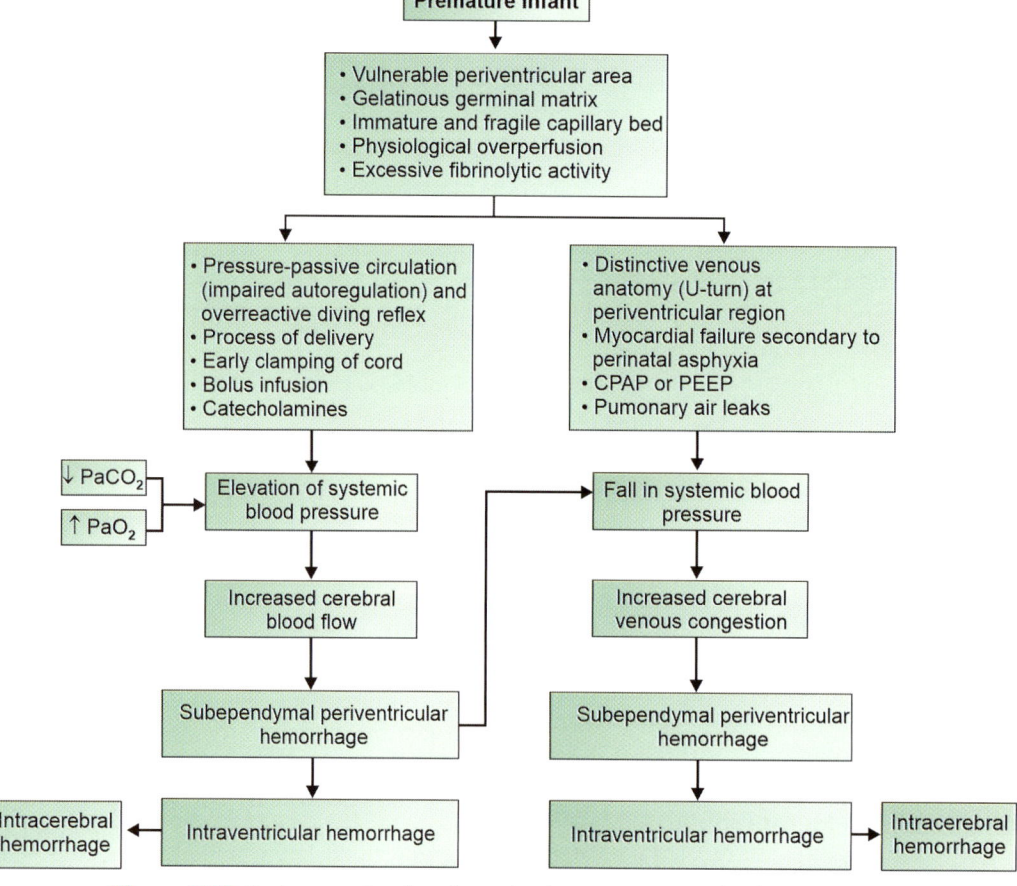

Figure 22.7 Pathogenesis of periventricular–intraventricular hemorrhage.

tions. Infants with moderate hemorrhage may manifest apathy, lethargy, hypotonia, increase in popliteal angle, skew deviation or downward rolling of eyeballs. Anemia and hyperbilirubinemia without apparent cause should alert to the possibility of internal bleeding. In infants with massive hemorrhage with rupture into ventricles or extension into cerebral hemispheres, clinical picture is characterized by catastrophic neurological deterioration. Infant is unresponsive with generalized hypotonia, non-reactive pupils, apneic attacks and vasomotor instability. Apart from neurological signs, shock, pallor, jaundice, bradycardia, temperature instability and metabolic acidosis may dominate the clinical picture. Acute hydrocephalus may be evidenced by bulging anterior fontanel. Intracranial pressure should be monitored with a non-invasive pressure monitor.

Diagnosis

The clinical picture is not characteristic and in about 50% of patients, there are no clinical manifestations. Sudden unexplained fall in hematocrit or rise in serum bilirubin should arouse the clinical suspicion of massive periventricular–intraventricular hemorrhage. Lumbar puncture is a useful screening procedure and cerebrospinal fluid may show elevated number of red blood cells, raised proteins and xanthochromia. Diagnosis can be confirmed by point-of-care or neonatologist based ultrasound scanning with a portable high resolution sector scan using anterior fontanel as an acoustic window. *Infants with a birth weight of <1500 g or gestational age of less than 32 weeks should be routinely screened by ultrasound examination of head at the ages of 2 days, 7 days, 21 days and before discharge.* When IVH is diagnosed, weekly ultrasonic evaluation is recommended till ventricular size is stabilized. Early diagnosis does not offer any theraputic advantage at this stage. The hemorrhage in the germinal matrix is identified as an echogenic focus over the head of caudate nucleus and/or caudo-thalamic notch. The subependymal hemorrhage is generally bilateral. The hemorrhage may increase in size and rupture through the ependyma into the lateral ventricle to produce an echogenic hematoma. Progressive posthemorrhagic hydrocephalus may follow due to obstructive arachnoiditis in the posterior fossa. Massive hemorrhage may extend laterally into the cerebrum which is associated with catastrophic acute manifestations and extremely high incidence of neuromotor sequelae among the survivors.

During recovery and following resorption of extravasated blood, subependymal and porencephalic cysts may be seen on ultrasound examination. On the basis of severity, size and extension of periventricular–intraventricular hemorrhage, it is classified into four grades. In Grade I, hemorrhage is limited to subependymal germinal matrix with no or minimal intraventricular hemorrhage (<10% of ventricular area). It carries excellent prognosis and immediate and late outcome is identical with preterm infants without any hemorrhage. In Grade II, intraventricular hematoma occupies up to 50% of ventricular area while in Grade III, hemorrhage distends lateral ventricles and occupies more than 50% of ventricular area on parasagittal view. The rupture or extension of hemorrhages laterally into the cerebral tissue is designated as Grade IV and carries ominous immediate and late outcome (Figure 22.8). There is evidence to suggest that cerebral hemorrhage may actually be periventricular hemorrhagic infarction rather than extension of IVH because ependymal lining of the lateral ventricle is usually intact. During follow-up, weekly or fortnightly ultrasound examination is necessary to follow the trend of hydrocephalus and development of subependymal and porencephalic cysts. For evaluation of intracranial hemorrhage, CT scan does not offer any additional diagnostic advantages. The procedure is also handicapped by the need for transporting a critically sick and unstable baby to the CT-room and dangers of ionizing radiation during multiple follow-up studies.

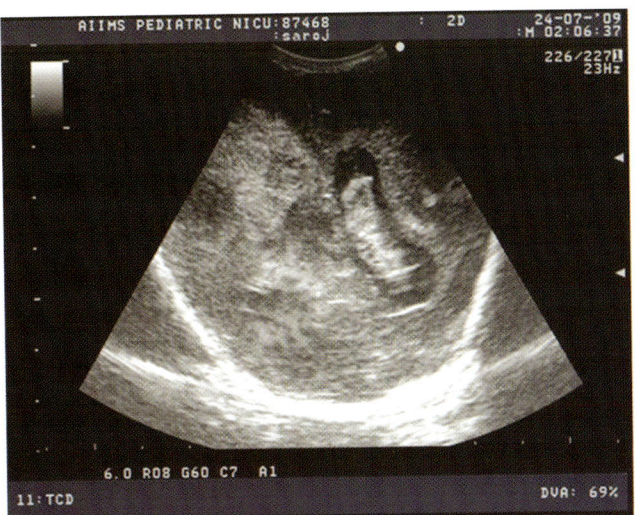

Figure 22.8 Cranial ultrasonogram in a premature baby showing grade 4 intraventricular hemorrhage. There is periventricular hemorrhagic infarction on the right side along with dilatation of the left ventricle which is filled with blood.

Neurological Disorders

22

In view of relatively high incidence and poor outcome of intraventricular hemorrhage, premature birth should be postponed by administration of tocolytic agents. Antenatal administration of corticosteroids, when labor sets in before 34 weeks of gestation, is associated with reduction of incidence and severity of both RDS and IVH. Delivery of high-risk preterm infant should preferably take place in a specialized center where adequate facilities are available for peripartal fetal monitoring to ensure early identification of fetal hypoxia and effective management of birth asphyxia. Delayed clamping of cord (≥1.0 min) is associated with reduced risk of IVH. Monitoring of blood pressure to prevent undue fluctuations, avoidance of excessive handling and bolus administration of colloids and sodium bicarbonate are crucial to prevent intraventricular hemorrhage. There is some controversial evidence to suggest that use of pancuronium bromide during assisted ventilation of babies with RDS may reduce the incidence and severity of IVH. The prophylactic administration of antenatal and postnatal phenobarbitone for prevention of IVH is no longer recommended. There is no concensus or universal acceptance of prophylactic administration of indomethacin for prevention of IVH and PDA due to its potential side effects of thrombocytopenia, reducing tissue perfusion and causing ischemic changes in vital organs. The prophylactic utility of ethamsylate, a capillary-stabilizing agent is controversial.

There is no specific or satisfactory therapy. Affected infants should be closely monitored to maintain optimal blood pressure, oxygenation and acid–base status. Suctioning and handling should be gentle and kept to the barest minimum. Severe anemia and bleeding manifestations should be corrected by administration of packed red blood cells and blood components. Following intraventricular hemorrhage, cerebral perfusion may be reduced due to rise in CSF pressure.

Hydrocephalus may develop in 25% of infants with IVH. It is characterized by rapidly increasing head size, bulging anterior fontanel, brainstem signs including "sunset eyes" and progressive ventricular dilatation. When intracranial pressure is elevated, removal of 10 to 12 mL of CSF at frequent intervals is therapeutically useful. Serial lumbar punctures are useful when the ventricles remain in communication with the lumbar subarachnoid space, or in grade I and II IVH. Glycerol in a starting dose of 1 g/kg is administered orally every six hours when progressive ventricular dilatation is noticed on follow-up ultrasound

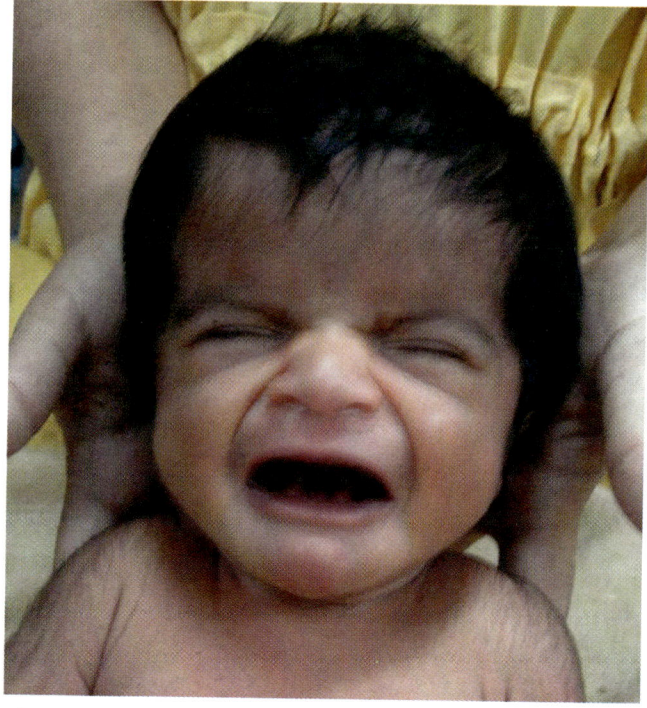

Figure 22.9 Hydrocephalus following IVH in a preterm baby.

scanning. After one week, the dose of glycerol is increased to 2 g/kg per dose. Alternatively acetazolamide, a carbonic anhydrase inhibitor, in a dose of 50–100 mg/kg/day q 6 hr combined with furosemide (1 mg/kg/dose q 12 hr) can be used. The prolonged administration of diuretics is associated with the risk of development of hypercalciuria (urinary calcium to creatinine ratio of >0.21), nephrocalcinosis and deafness. Hydrocephalus in association with increased intracranial pressure is managed with external ventricular drainage or ventriculoperitoneal shunt (Figure 22.9). The protocol for management of hydrocephalus following IVH is summarized in (Figure 22.10).

The outcome is related to the severity and extension of intraventricular hemorrhage, immaturity of the infant and nature of the underlying predisposing conditions. Hydrocephalus and neurological sequelae may occur in about 50% of survivors.

NEUROLOGICAL SEQUELAE OF HYPOXIC–ISCHEMIC ENCEPHALOPATHY

Acute life-threatening syndrome of hypoxic-ischemic encephalopathy (HIE) is discussed in detail in Chapter 6. The major concern of perinatal hypoxia is the development of cerebral palsy (CP) and neuromotor disability during childhood. Cerebral palsy which is defined as non-progressive, non-familial motor disorder

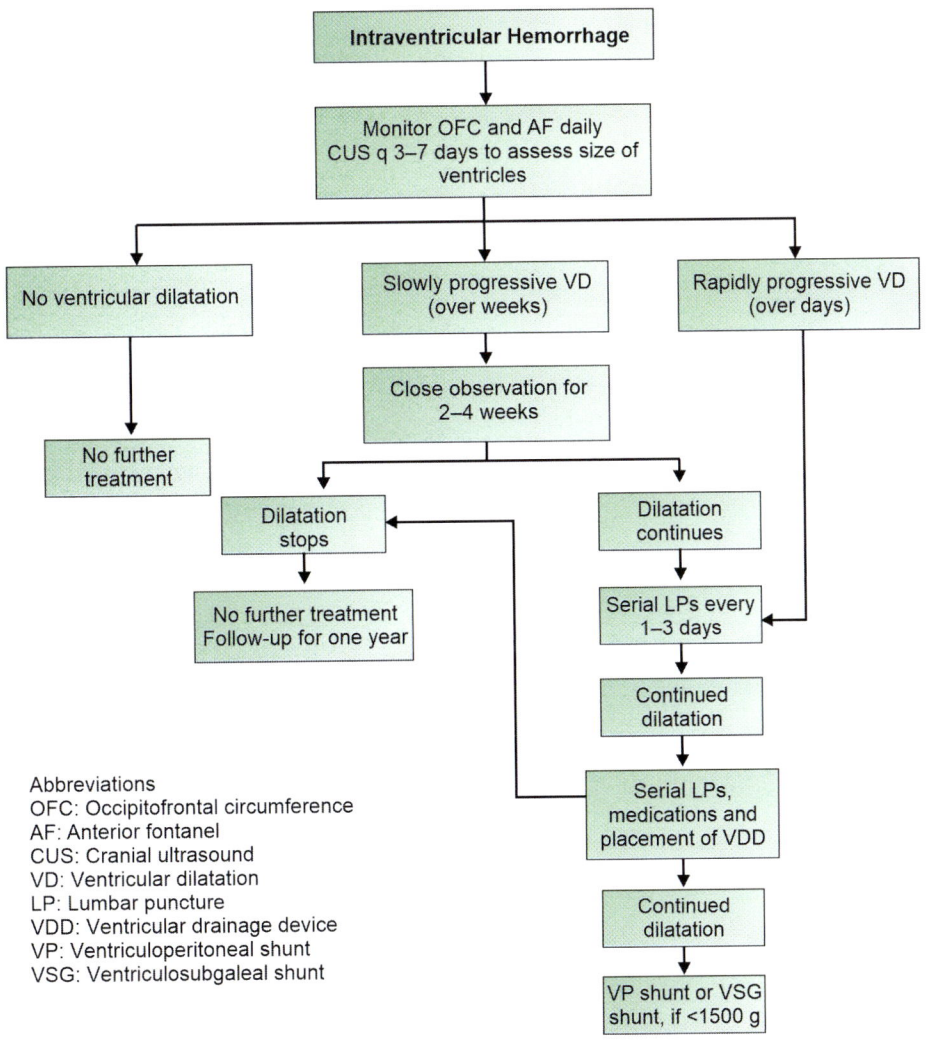

Figure 22.10 Algorithm for management of ventricular dilatation following intraventricular hemorrhage.

of cerebral origin affects approximately 2 to 3 per 1000 infants. The origin of brain injury resulting in CP may date back to the antepartum, peripartum and postnatal (during first year of life) period. There is increasing evidence that most cases of brain injury associated with CP are not related to perinatal events. There is overwhelming evidence to suggest that 70 to 80% cases of CP are antepartum in origin. It is well known that many infants with asphyxia may have normal neuromotor development and many children with CP do not have any adverse perinatal events. Almost one-half of children with CP have normal intelligence and one-fourth are severely retarded. When CP is associated with severe mental retardation, it is more likely to be due to adverse peripartum events. Isolated severe mental retardation without CP is more likely to be due to genetic, viral, metabolic or developmental origin rather than HIE. The neuropathologic syndromes of hypoxic-ischemic cerebral injury with their neuro-

motor outcomes during infancy and childhood are described below.

1. **Parasagittal cerebral injury** This injury classically occurs in term babies with severe birth asphyxia. There is bilateral necrosis of cortical and adjacent subcortical white matter involving the superior medial and posterior aspects of the parieto-occipital cerebral hemispheres. The necrosis occurs within the border zones which are referred to as watershed areas between the end branches of the major cerebral vessels. These regions are extremely vulnerable to decrease in the cerebral perfusion pressure. Parasagittal cerebral injury is best demonstrated by technetium brain scan and MRI rather than CT scan. The most common long-term sequelae of this injury is spastic quadriplegia wherein upper extremities are more severely affected than the lower extremities.

2. **Periventricular leukomalacia (PVL)** This is the leading ischemic lesion affecting 15–30% of preterm infants below 32 weeks (<1500 g) of gestation. There is bilateral necrosis of white matter adjacent to the external angles of the lateral ventricles involving the centrum semiovale, optic and auditory radiations. This region of cerebral white matter is traversed by descending fibers from motor cortex subserving functions of lower extremities. The long-term manifestations include spastic diplegia (lower limbs are more severely affected than upper limbs), visual and cognitive deficits. Electrophysiological and behavioral tests of higher visual and auditory functions are usually abnormal.

The exact pathogenesis is uncertain but perinatal hypoxia, premature separation of placenta and chorioamnionitis are recognized predisposing factors. Postnatal hypoxia (RDS, assisted ventilation, pulmonary air leak syndrome, etc.), sepsis and shock may also cause PVL. The two key features for pathogenesis of leukomalacia include (i) hypoxia-ischemia affecting watershed regions of the white matter and (ii) vulnerability of the periventricular white matter of the premature infants. There are both focal necrosis (which becomes cystic) and diffuse white matter lesions.

There are no clinical markers of PVL during neonatal period. In severe PVL, spasticity of lower limbs may be detected at 40 weeks of postconceptional maturity. Serial ultrasound scans should be performed in preterm babies to make an early diagnosis of PVL (Figures 22.11 and 22.12). Based on cranial ultrasound scans, PVL is graded as shown in Table 22.2.

There is no specific therapy for PVL which is the leading cause of spastic diplegia in preterm babies. Other neuromotor sequelae include visual and auditory abnormalities, strabismus, nystagmus, visual field defects, perceptual or behavior problems and learning difficulties. Efforts should be made to prevent PVL by providing gentle, humanized, optimal and developmentally supportive care to preterm VLBW infants. Physiotherapy (active and passive movements) and early stimulation is advised.

3. **Focal or multifocal ischemic brain necrosis** It is characterized by injury to all the cellular elements caused by an infarction in the region of vascular distribution. The middle cerebral artery is the most common vascular territory affected, with the left side twice as commonly involved as the right side. Neuropathologic sequelae include porencephaly,

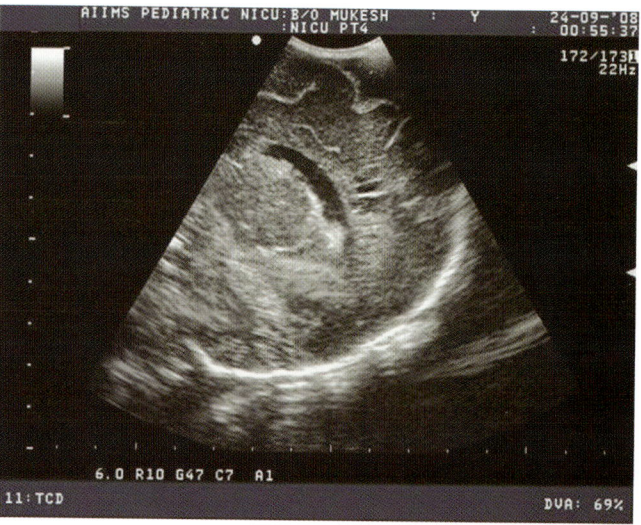

A

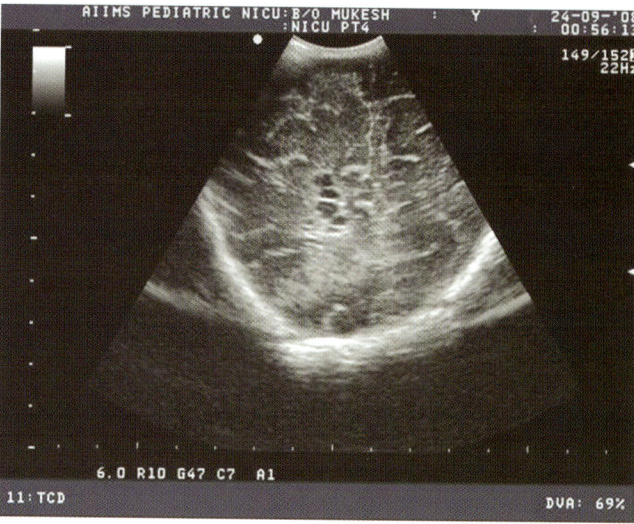

B

Figure 22.11 Cranial ultrasonogram of a 3 weeks old preterm baby. (A) Coronal section, (B) Sagittal section showing cystic lesions suggestive of periventricular leukomalacia.

multicystic encephalomalacia, and hydranencephaly. The long-term neurologic sequelae usually include spastic hemiplegia, quadriplegia and/or seizures.

4. **Status marmoratus** This is the least common form of CNS lesion due to perinatal hypoxia-ischemia complex and is characterized by selective neuronal injury within the region of basal ganglia, i.e. thalamus, caudate nucleus, globus pallidus, and putamen. The abnormal myelin pattern provides a marbled appearance to the basal ganglia. It is generally associated with other neuropathologic manifestations described *vide-supra*. In an isolated form, the long-term neurologic manifestations of this lesion are choreoathetosis (dystonic cerebral palsy).

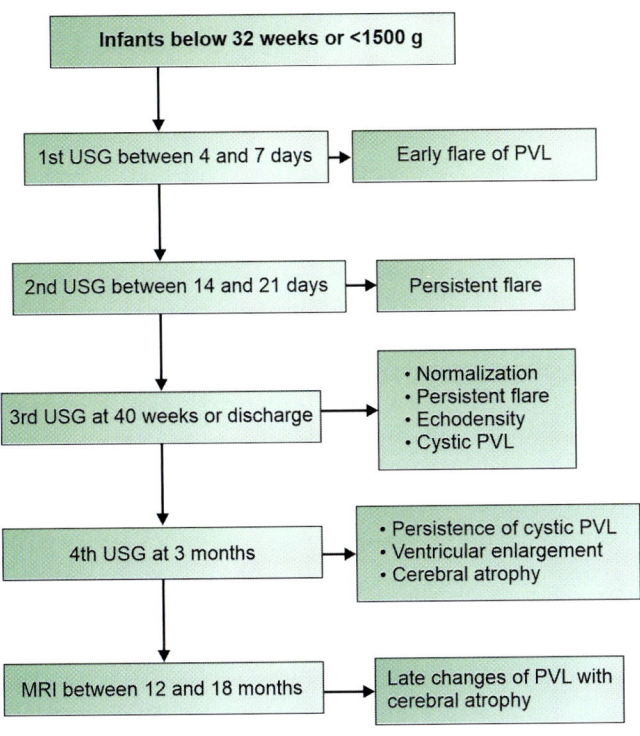

Figure 22.12 Algorithm for diagnosis of PVL.

TABLE 22.2 Grading of PVL (de Vries)	
■ Grade I	Persistence of echodensities or flare for >7 days
■ Grade II	Flare leads to formation of small localized frontoparietal cysts
■ Grade III	Extensive cystic fronto-parieto-occipital leukomalacia
■ Grade IV	Extensive subcortical cysts

Adapted from de Vries LS, *et al.* Ultrasound abnormalities preceding cerebral palsy in high-risk preterm infants. *J Pediatr* 2004, 144(6):815-20.

5. **Selective neuronal necrosis (SNN)** The patchy neuropathologic lesions of SNN are invariably associated with other neuropathologic manifestations described above. The hypoxic or excitotoxic damage due to amino acids selectively involves hippocampus, lateral geniculate body, thalamus, caudate nucleus, putamen, globus pallidus, motor nuclei of the fifth and seventh cranial nerves and dorsal vagal nuclei. The long-term sequelae include mental retardation, tone abnormalities and seizures.

BIRTH TRAUMA TO CENTRAL NERVOUS SYSTEM

Intracranial Injury

The improved obstetrical management and early resort to cesarean section has reduced the incidence of birth trauma. Precipitate delivery or difficult forceps and vacuum extraction in a large baby, extraction of breech and other abnormal presentations may be associated with intracranial hemorrhage. The baby is generally asphyxiated at birth and spontaneous respirations may not be established even after resuscitation. The abnormal neurological behavior (cerebral depression or irritability) often manifests within the first 48 hours of life. The differentiation between the isolated perinatal hypoxia and intracranial birth injury is difficult and is guided by the nature of events during delivery rather than by any specific syndrome of neurological manifestations.

Spinal Cord Transection

This relatively rare form of birth injury follows difficult breech extraction when fracture of cervical spine or avulsion of cervical cord may occur. Sometimes, a click or crack may be heard during delivery. It is characterized by flaccid paraplegia, with retention of urine and overflow incontinence. Respiratory failure due to diaphragmatic paralysis may dominate the clinical picture. Sensations may be dulled or absent below the site of lesion. Prognosis is grave.

Peripheral Nerve Palsies

Facial Palsy

It may occur with or without forceps application. Facial asymmetry, inability to close the eye and absent rooting reflex on the affected side suggest the diagnosis (Figure 22.13). The recovery is excellent and complete. By and large, most peripheral nerve injuries in the newborn carry a good prognosis because of greater regenerative power and short length of nerves. Bilateral facial palsy or its association with 6th nerve paralysis suggests a central lesion such as agenesis of seventh nerve nucleus (Möebius syndrome). The infant is unable to smile, close the eyes or move them from side-to-side. The condition may be associated with anomalies of hands, feet and chest wall (Poland syndrome).

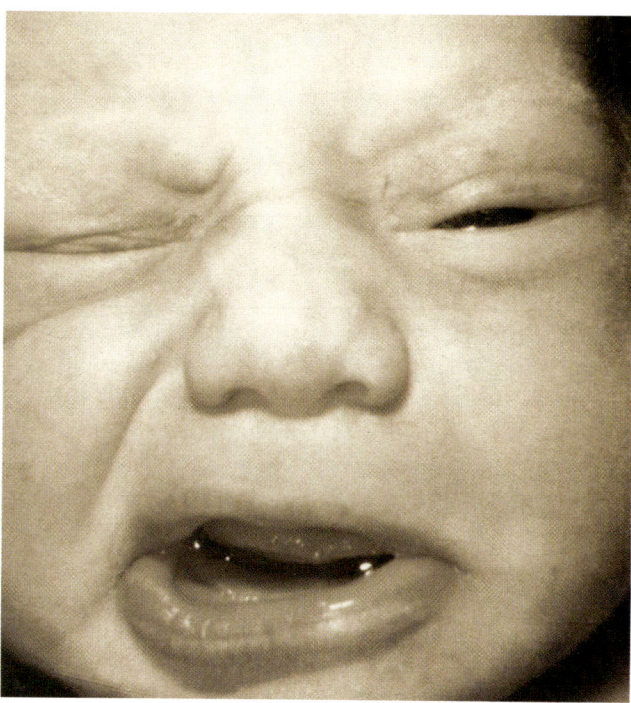

Figure 22.13 Facial palsy on the left side.

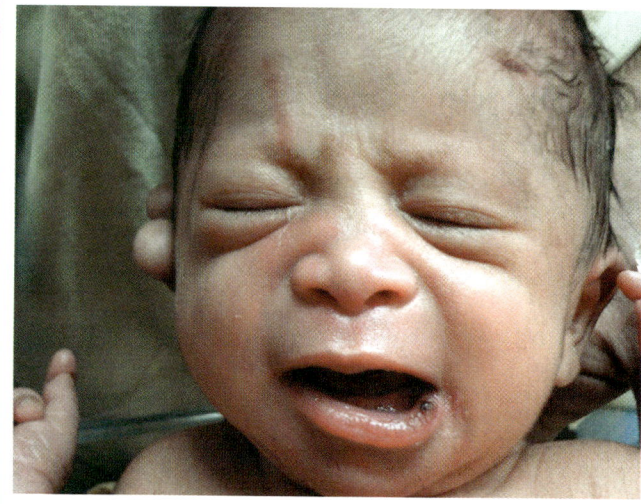

Figure 22.14 Congenital absence of depressor anguli oris muscle on the right side.

Partial facial palsy or *congenital absence* or *hypoplasia* of *depressor anguli oris* muscle is a relatively frequent condition. Facial asymmetry on crying is limited to the corner of the mouth and mandible which gets pulled downwards on the normal side (Figure 22.14). Eye closure is unaffected but depth of nasolabial fold is flattened on the normal side. There is high incidence of cardiovascular, genitourinary and skeletal anomalies associated with congenital absence or hypoplasia of depressor anguli oris muscle.

Brachial Plexus Palsy

Avulsion of brachial nerve roots may occur during difficult breech extraction or shoulder impaction especially in a large baby.

Erb's palsy When upper cervical roots (C5, C6) are affected, the arm hangs limply, adducted and internally rotated with elbow extended and pronated (Figure 22.15). Arm recoil is lost. Respiratory distress may occur, if diaphragmatic paralysis is associated. The lack of spontaneous movements and asymmetric Moro response would favour the diagnosis of Erb's palsy. It may be associated with fracture of clavicle or involvement of lower cervical roots. Skiagram of the shoulder should be taken to rule out associated bony injuries.

Klumpke's palsy The involvement of lower cervical nerve roots (C7, C8, T1) manifests as wrist drop and flaccid paralysis of hand with absent grasp response. The presence of miosis, ptosis and anhidrosis (Horner's syndrome) though uncommon would suggest associated damage to the cervical sympathetic chain of the first thoracic root.

The arm should be kept in the position of abduction and external rotation at the shoulder and flexion of elbow in infants with Erb's palsy. In Klumpke's palsy, cotton or rubber ball should be placed in the baby's hand to avoid contractures. Massage and passive movements of muscles would aid recovery which is generally complete but may take a few weeks or months. In severe cases especially when associated with laceration of nerves, the affected limb may remain permanently short and stunted. Electromyography and nerve-conduction studies can distinguish between avulsion of nerves and stretch injury. The lesions of the upper brachial plexus have a better prognosis than those of lower or total plexus. If paralysis persists for more than 3 months, neuroplasty is indicated.

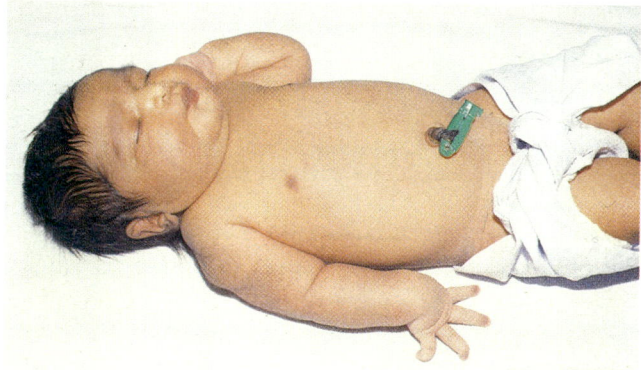

Figure 22.15 Erb's palsy on the right side in a large-for-dates baby of a mother with diabetes mellitus.

Phrenic Nerve Palsy

Phrenic nerve injury, though rare, is often associated with upper brachial palsy. Diaphragmatic paralysis results in irregular labored thoracic breathing without any visible abdominal movements. The diaphragm is elevated on the affected side and breath sounds are diminished. The characteristic see-saw movements of two sides of diaphgram during respiration is obvious on fluoroscopic examination. The paradoxical movements of diaphragm (upward with each inspiration) on fluoroscopy or ultrasonography is diagnostic. There is no specific therapy but baby should be placed on the affected side. Administration of oxygen, CPAP and gavage feeding, depending upon the severity of respiratory difficulty, are often indicated. The recovery is usually complete but the course may be complicated by respiratory infections. At times when recovery is incomplete, the weak, flabby and elevated leaf of diaphragm may manifest as eventration during infancy. In symptomatic cases, diaphragmatic plication may be needed.

CNS MALFORMATIONS

Brain is a relatively common site for malformations. The abnormalities in size, shape and symmetry of the head and face often suggest underlying congenital malformations. The presence of any ectodermal dysplasia and spinal deformities should alert to the possibility of associated abnormalities in the central nervous system.

Neural Tube Defects

Neural tube defects (NTDs) are the most common congenital malformations affecting the brain and spinal cord. The incidence of NTDs varies between 0.5 and 10/1000 live births in different regions of India. The neural tube is formed during 3rd week of embryonic life when midline ectoderm becomes the neural plate under the inductive influence of the overlying mesoderm. The neural plate rapidly evolves through neural groove followed by formation of a neural tube which closes or is covered by 4th week of embryogenesis. The failure of closure of neural tube leads to development of various NTDs namely anencephaly, encephalocele, and spina bifida with meningocele or meningomyelocele.

The incidence of NTDs show wide variations and is influenced by race, ethnicity, nutritional status, geographic location and socioeconomic status. The well recognized etiological factors associated with NTDs include folic acid deficiency, prenatal exposure to antiepileptic drugs (especially valproate and carbamazepine), folic acid antagonists (aminopterin), maternal fever, diabetes mellitus and irradiation. There is controversial association between NTDs and deficiency of zinc and choline during pregnancy. Neural tube defects may be associated with trisomies 13 and 18, triploidy and Meckel syndrome. The risk of recurrence of NTD after one affected pregnancy is 2–3% and may approach 10% if two previous pregnancies are affected. Intake of periconceptional (before conception and up to 8 weeks of gestation) folate 0.4 mg daily is a well-recognized strategy to prevent occurrence of NTDs. In a high-risk pregnancy (previous NTD-affected pregnancy), folic acid is given in a dose of 4 mg per day. In India, because most pregnancies are not planned, the timely administration of supplements of folic acid, presents a formidable challenge to health care professionals. Fortification of staple foods with folic acid is a reliable strategy in regions of the world with high incidence of NTD.

Types of Neural Tube Defects

Primary neural tube defects They are due to primary failure of closure of the neural tube or its disruption during 18–25 days of gestation. They account for 95% of NTDs and include myelomeningocele, encephalocele (mostly occipital) and anencephaly. They are usually associated with Arnold-Chiari malformation which is characterized by malformation of pons and medulla, downward displacement of cerebellum, medulla and fourth ventricle into the upper cervical cord with resultant aqueductal block leading to development of hydrocephalus. Myelomeningocele is discussed in detail in Chapter 25.

Secondary neural tube defects In about 5% of NTDs, there is abnormal development of lower sacral or coccygeal segments during secondary neurulation. These lesions are covered with skin and are rarely associated with hydrocephaly or neurological deficits. They include meningocele, lipomeningocele and spina bifida occulta or closed NTD which may be associated with split cord malformation or diastematomyelia with tethering of spinal cord and sacral agenesis (Figures 22.16 and 22.17). The cutaneous markers for spina bifida occulta include hairy patch, sacral dimple or sinus, capillary hemangioma, caudal appendage or lipoma. These infants should undergo detailed neurological examination of lower limbs and MRI scan of the spine.

Neurological Disorders

22

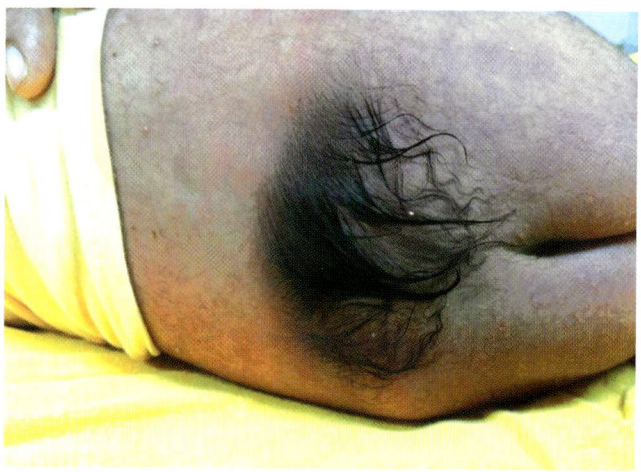

Figure 22.16 Tuft of hair over the sacrum. Infant had spina bifida occulta and diastematomyelia.

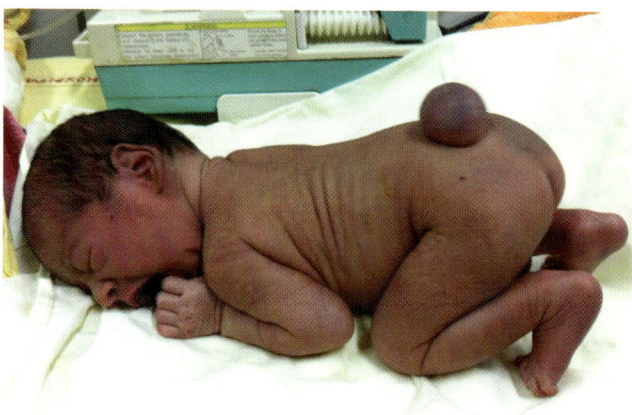

Figure 22.17 Meningocele covered with skin. There were no neurological deficits.

Anencephaly

It is a lethal congenital malformation in which both cerebral hemispheres and several other areas of brain are absent. Its average incidence in India varies between 0.5 and 3.0/1000 deliveries and is comparable with prevalence of meningomyelocele. A variety of agents including folic acid antagonists, valproic acid and clomiphene have been implicated. The condition can be diagnosed antenatally by detection of elevated levels of alpha-fetoproteins in the maternal serum and amniotic fluid around 14 to 16 weeks of gestation. If a woman has given birth to one affected child, the chances of recurrence are 5%. Among affected infants there is a slight preponderance of females. Most infants are stillborn but those born alive die within few hours or days. The frontal bones and vault are deficient and deformed brain is exposed to view. Eyes are bulging like those of a frog due to defective orbits

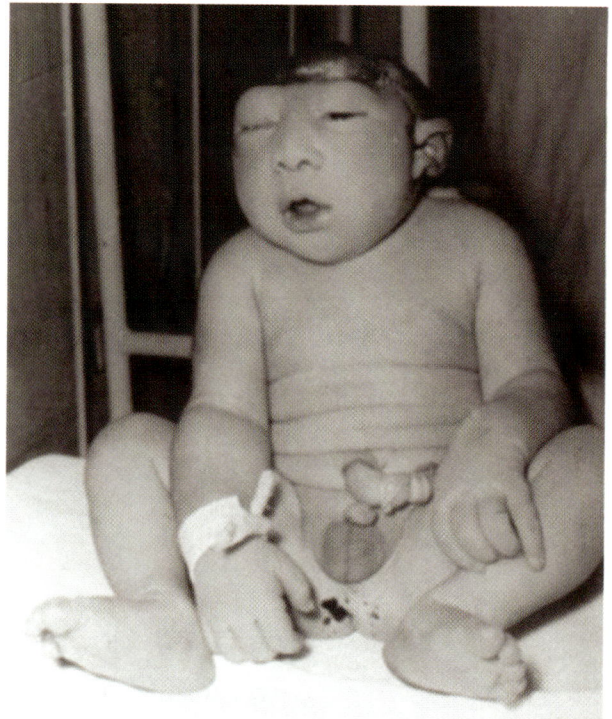

Figure 22.18 Live born infant with anencephaly. Upper extremities are rather well developed in these infants.

(Figure 22.18). The condition is often associated with polyhydramnios, large thymus and extremely small adrenals with almost total lack of fetal cortex and hypoplastic lungs. The brainstem and cerebellum may be partially developed and pituitary gland is often absent. Hyperreflexia is common but there is no decerebrate rigidity. A detailed neurological and behavioral assessment with particular reference to evaluation of visual fixation should be undertaken in live born infants with anencephaly as it may offer useful clues to the normal neurological and endocrine functions at this age. It is unethical to harvest organs from anencephalic infants for transplantation before they are brain dead although they are all destined to die.

Holoprosencephaly

It is a rare developmental disorder of the brain due to defective cleavage of the forebrain or prosencephalon with failure of the forebrain to divide into hemispheres or lobes. The risk factors include maternal diabetes mellitus and various chromosomal abnormalities (Trisomy 13 and 18) and deletions. In severe cases, prenatal diagnosis can be made by ultrasonography after 10th week of gestation. Facial dysmorphism is common and include cyclopia, cebocephaly (monkey-head with close set eyes), premaxillary agenesis and single central incisor tooth. Depending upon the degree of cleavage abnormality, MRI shows single ventricle, absent falx cerebri and fused basal ganglia. The morbidity and mortality is extremely high.

Lissencephaly

It literally means smooth brain and occurs because of defective neuronal migration during the 12th–24th weeks of gestation resulting in lack of development of brain grooves (sulci) and folds (gyri). The affected infants display microcephaly, severe psychomotor retardation, failure to thrive, seizures, and spasticity or hypotonia. The cause is unknown and condition may occur due to fetal viral infection or genetic mutation. The diagnosis is usually made by cranial ultrasonography, computed tomography (CT) or magnetic resonance imaging (Figure 22.19). Cerebral atrophy is associated with dilatation of ventricles. Treatment is supportive and symptomatic and outcome is usually dismal.

Agenesis of Corpus Callosum

Corpus callosum is a large C-shaped bundle of nerve fibers that connects two cerebral hemispheres. Agenesis of corpus callosum (ACC) occurs in 1:1000–4000 live births. It is inherited as an autosomal recessive or an X-linked dominant trait. It is a heterogeneous disorder without any characteristic clinical features. The usual abnormalities include difficulty in feeding and/or swallowing, hypertelorism, hypotonia, seizures, hearing and visual problems. Some patients may have severe behavioral and

cognitive disabilities. They exhibit atypical facial scanning with reduced attention to the eyes of others during conversation. ACC may be associated with a number of chromosomal deletion syndromes including Dandy-Walker syndrome. The condition is suspected on sonography of the brain and diagnosis can be readily confirmed by CT scan and MRI.

Hydrocephalus

Hydrocephalus occurs due to imbalance between the production of CSF and its drainage and resorption. The diagnosis is based on head circumference of more than 97th percentile for the gestational age, bulging anterior fontanel and 'setting sun' sign. The separation of sutures in the absence of above signs should not be taken as an evidence of hydrocephalus.

The commonest cause of hydrocephalus is Arnold-Chiari malformation in association with myelomeningocele. The cerebellar tonsils and part of the meninges and cord protrude through the foramen magnum and incompletely close the spinal canal. The obstructive hydrocephalus may also occur due to congenital aqueductal stenosis and obstruction at the outlet of foramina of fourth ventricle. Hydrocephalus may also be acquired due to intraventricular or subarachnoid hemorrhage, intrauterine infections especially toxoplasmosis and neonatal meningitis. The rate of head growth should be checked weekly and therapeutic response (except in infants with Arnold-Chiari malformation) to acetazolamide 50–100 mg/kg per day q 6 hr orally for 2–4 weeks should be assessed. During first 3 months of life, normal head growth velocity is 2 cm per month. In cases of rapidly progressive hydrocephalus, ventriculoatrial shunt should not be delayed.

Hydranencephaly

It is a rare birth defect with absence of cerebral hemispheres due to infection, vascular insult, exposure to environmental toxin or trauma after first trimester of pregnancy. The cerebral hemispheres are reduced to paper thickness in this condition and intracranial contents appear like a bag of cerebrospinal fluid. The diagnosis is clinched by demonstrating uniform glow of whole cranium on transillumination. The prognosis for neurological and mental development is grave in this condition in spite of the shunt operation. Like infants with anencephaly, the neurological behavior of these babies should also be studied in detail, as they provide a useful experimental model for understanding the role of cerebral hemispheres in the newborn.

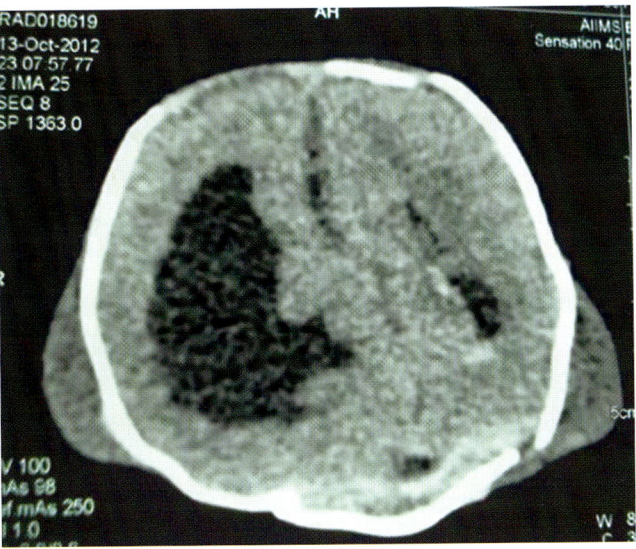

Figure 22.19 MRI showing lissencephaly in a one month old infant with intractable seizures.

Microcephaly

The head size of less than 3rd percentile for weight or period of gestation may result either due to craniosynostosis or arrested and altered brain growth. The baby should be investigated for the possibility of various intrauterine infections including zika virus. Skiagram of skull should be taken to look for intracranial calcification and craniosynostosis.

Midline Spinal Abnormalities

The midline congenital dermal sinus above the level of second sacral vertebra invariably communicates with theca and predisposes to the development of ascending meningitis which may be recurrent. Unlike pilonidal dimples, communicating dermal sinuses must be excised as early as possible. The presence of midline hairy patch or nevus demands complete neurological examination of lower limbs and evaluation of bladder and bowel functions. X-ray spine must be taken to exclude any underlying spinal abnormality such as diastematomyelia.

JITTERINESS

Many normal infants or those with cerebral excitability often show coarse tremors or jitteriness. In tremors, the rate of movements is identical in either direction, whereas clonic tonic seizures show a rapid alteration of fast and slow phase of movements. Jitteriness is not accompanied by abnormalities of gaze and is aggravated by touching the baby. It is abolished by passive flexion of the limb. Jitteriness is often exaggerated by physical and photic stimulation and when marked in intensity or frequency, it is indicative of the same implications as neonatal seizures. Jitteriness is considered to be clinically significant, if it occurs when the infant is quiet and alert. There are no associated eye or facial movements, autonomic changes or aEEG abnormalities.

Causes

Normal infants Many healthy term infants manifest transient jitteriness during the first 48 hours or so. The tremors are of short amplitude and brief duration. Jitteriness is more common in a crying infant and is associated with visual inattentiveness. Physiological jitteriness is reduced while infant is sucking. Elevated serum norephinephrine levels have been documented in healthy term infants with jitteriness.

Cerebral hyperexcitability Perinatal hypoxia, cerebral edema and raised intracranial tension due to any cause may manifest as jitteriness in addition to other features suggestive of cerebral irritability.

Hypoglycemia Jitteriness is a common symptom of hypoglycemia.

Hypocalcemia Jitteriness is a recognized manifestation of hypocalcemia.

Hypomagnesemia Low serum magnesium levels have been documented in jittery infants.

Congenital thyrotoxicosis Infants are hyperalert, restless and jittery.

Infants of diabetic mothers Excessive tremulousness may be seen even in the absence of hypoglycemia or hypocalcemia. Polycythemia may predispose to jitteriness.

Narcotic withdrawal syndrome Prolonged gestational intake of pethidine, morphine, heroin, alcohol, diazepam and barbiturates, may lead to withdrawal symptoms in the form of excessive jitteriness or seizures in the newborn baby.

Drug toxicity Administration of large doses of phenothiazines to the mother may manifest with toxic symptoms in the baby which may persist for a few days or weeks. Atropine derivatives given orally for abdominal colic or local instillation of ephedrine nose drops should be used with caution due to their potential risk of toxicity particularly in low birth weight babies.

Treatment

An effort should be made to identify the cause in infants with significant or marked jitteriness. The specific biochemical abnormality should be managed as described under the management of neonatal seizures. In a large majority of jittery infants, no cause is identified. The tremulousness disappears spontaneously or following administration of phenobarbitone or chloral hydrate.

NEONATAL SEIZURES

In the newborn infant, seizures may occur due to an underlying cerebral or biochemical abnormality. Seizures are more common in newborn period than in any other phase of human life. Their incidence varies from 0.5 to 0.8% in term babies and 6–12% in babies weighing less than 1500 g. Newborn babies do not manifest febrile convulsions. Jitteriness which is characterized by stimulus-sensitive rhythmic tremors peculiar to newborn babies should not be confused with seizures.

Types of Seizures

Generalized tonic and clonic convulsions, as in grandmal epilepsy, are not seen in the neonates. Due to incomplete development of axons, dendritic processes, arborization and poor myelination, the manifestations are more subtle and pleomorphic. The severity of convulsive movements is related to the size of the baby. Larger the baby, more powerful are the twitchings. Manifest seizures are uncommon among preterm infants. The clinical morphology of the seizures generally offers little clue to the etiology or prognosis.

Subtle seizures or motor automatisms They account for over 50% of all seizures and are more common in preterm babies. They can be easily missed. Jerking of eyes (with or without conjugate deviation), blinking or fluttering of eyelids, staring look, sucking, chewing, or smacking orobuccal movements and apneic attacks are included among subtle seizures. Oral, facial and lingual phenomena are common due to advanced maturation of the limbic system. There is tachycardia at the onset followed by bradycardia after the apnea and hypoxemia. EEG may be normal because seizures have onset from the brainstem or deep cortical structures. In sick neonates, aEEG monitoring is recommended to detect "electrographic-only" seizures.

Multifocal clonic seizures without Jacksonian pattern Tonic convulsive movements migrate haphazardly from one limb to another. The twitchings may be predominantly limited to one side of the body. They may occur due to hypoxic-ischemic encephalopathy and birth trauma.

Focal clonic seizures They are well localized and often associated with loss of consciousness. Even focal seizures in a newborn baby are a manifestation of bilateral cerebral disturbance. They are common due to metabolic disorder, birth trauma and cerebral infarction. Right-sided clonic seizures are most commonly due to blockage of left middle cerebral artery.

Tonic seizures There is generalized stiffening, akin to decerebrate (tonic extension of all limbs) or decorticate (flexion of upper limbs and extension of lower limbs) posturing and may be associated with stertorous breathing and eye signs or occasional clonic jerks. They may be associated with intraventricular hemorrhage and acute bilirubin encephalopathy. In general, the prognosis of tonic seizures is poor.

Myoclonic seizures Sudden jerky movements produced by episodic contractions of a group of muscles are uncommon in the newborn. These may occur in babies with developmental defects including anencephaly. Typical triad of hypsarrhythmia on electroencephalogram, massive myoclonic spasms and mental retardation may develop during infancy (infantile or salaam spasms). The onset is characteristically around 4 months of age and the condition is also called as West syndrome.

Apnea as a manifestation of seizures Apneic attacks with bradycardia are common in extremely preterm babies as a manifestation of immaturity of respiratory center. Subtle seizures in term babies may manifest with apneic attacks. During convulsive apnea, the heart rate either remains normal or there may be tachycardia. It is often associated with subtle seizures like eye opening, staring gaze and conjugate deviation of eyes. EEG may show abnormalities. The inadvertent use of respiratory stimulants in these babies may worsen the seizure activity.

Causes

Unlike older children, neonatal seizures are rarely idiopathic. Biochemical abnormalities are a common correlate of seizures in newborn babies. The salient causes of convulsions in the newborn, in the decreasing order of their frequency, are given below.

Perinatal complications Birth asphyxia and intracranial injuries together account for about half of the neonatal seizures. In babies with 5-minute Apgar score of less than 3, the convulsions may occur on the first day of life due to hypoxic-ischemic encephalopathy. The convulsive manifestations of intracranial bleed appear between 2 and 7 days of age. Cephalhematoma or fracture of skull and bulging anterior fontanel due to raised intracranial tension may be associated. The cerebrospinal fluid is often blood stained or xanthochromic. In subarachnoid hemorrhage, seizures commonly occur on second or third day and during the interictal period infant is alert and normal. There may be associated metabolic complications like hypocalcemia, hypoglycemia and CNS infection.

Hypocalcemia Hypocalcemia (serum calcium <7 mg/dL) is the commonest biochemical abnormality causing neonatal seizures. Convulsions occur on the first day or at the end of the first week. In the absence of perinatal complications, the prognosis in this group is excellent.

Hypoglycemia In neonates, hypoglycemia is diagnosed when blood glucose level is <40 mg/dL, irrespective of period of gestation. The diagnosis is suspected, if any of the situations known to predispose to hypoglycemia such as immaturity, severe IUGR, large-for-dates

TABLE 22.3 Common causes of neonatal seizures with their frequency and clinical correlates

Cause	Frequency	Clinical correlates
Hypoxic-ischemic encephalopathy	30–50%	Perinatal hypoxia, Apgar score ≤3 at 5 min later
Metabolic disorders Hypoglycemia, hypocalcemia, hypomagnesemia, hypo/hypernatremia	5–20%	Preterm, infant of diabetic mother, IUGR infant, acute kidney damage, pre-eclampsia
Intracranial hemorrhage	5–15%	Sudden pallor, lethargy, coma, confirmed on USG
CNS malformation	6–15%	Well baby, dysmorphism, microcephaly
Meningitis (fetal and neonatal)	2–15%	Inconsolable crying, fever, bulging anterior fontanel, IUGR
Cerebral infarction	4–12%	Hemiplegia or monoplegia, disseminated coagulopathy, dehydration
Inborn errors of metabolism	3–5%	Refractory seizures, history of sibling deaths and consanguinity
Acute bilirubin encephalopathy	1–2%	Hyperbilirubinemia due to Rh and ABO incompatiblity, leaky blood–brain barrier
Maternal drug withdrawal	1%	History of maternal drug intake
Benign idiopathic neonatal seizures	1%	5th day seizures
Neonatal epilepsy syndromes	<1%	Benign sleep myoclonus, exaggerated startle response
Idiopathic	4–5%	Family history of seizures

babies, Rhesus isoimmunization, and infants of diabetic mothers coexist.

Infections Intrauterine infections or neonatal septicemia may be associated with meningitis. About one-third of patients with neonatal menigitis, present with convulsions. The clinical diagnosis of meningitis in the newborn is often difficult. Therefore, lumbar puncture is mandatory in all babies with seizures to exclude this potentially treatable condition. Tetanus neonatorum is an important cause of spasms which should not be confused with convulsions.

Inborn errors of metabolism If convulsions are intractable to therapy and when there is a history of consanguinity or a similar disorder in the previous sibling, metabolic causes should be excluded. Symptoms appear after introduction of milk feeding. Apart from seizures, look for evidences of vomiting, severe jaundice, hepatosplenomegaly, virilization and malodorous urine.

Developmental defects Presence of facial or caput asymmetry should arouse the suspicion of underlying developmental defect of brain such as microcephaly, hydrocephalus, dysgenesis (heterotopias, neuronal disorganization or migration), microgyria, porencephaly, lissencephaly, hydranencephaly and agenesis of corpus callosum.

Acute systemic illness The babies with severe respiratory distress and septicemia may develop fits as a result of hemorrhagic infarction because of disseminated intravascular coagulation and hypoxia.

The frequency and correlates of common causes of seizures in neonates are given in Table 22.3.

Miscellaneous Conditions

Neonatal narcotic withdrawal or abstinence syndrome The babies born to the mother addicted to heroin, or diamorphine hydrochloride, morphine, methadone or alcohol, may manifest with characteristic withdrawal symptoms like irritability, high-pitched cry, tremors, hypertonicity, vomiting, diarrhea and tachycardia after 48 hours of birth. The withdrawal symptoms are mediated through release of epinephrine when baby is no longer exposed to maternal opioids after birth.

Hereditary hyperekplexia (Stiff baby syndrome) It is a rare familial disorder with hyperactive startle, generalized myoclonus, severe hypertonia, apnea and bradycardia. It is caused by defects in glycinergic neurotransmission. There is a good response to benzodiazepines especially clonazepam.

Drug toxicity The use of large doses of phenothiazines for the management of eclampsia may lead to phenothiazine toxicity in the neonate as evidenced by excessive jitteriness, rigidity and opisthotonos. Theophylline, doxapram, propylene glycol (diluent in IV nutritional formulation) can cause seizures in newborn babies.

Local anesthetics During paracervical block, inadvertent injection of local anesthetic into the fetal scalp may result in intractable convulsions. Pupils are usually dilated and non-reactive to light and doll's eye phenomenon is lost due to complete external ophthalmoplegia. Careful examination of the scalp may show the needle mark.

Hypomagnesemia The suspicion is aroused when in a baby with hypocalcemia, biochemical or therapeutic improvement does not occur with calcium therapy alone.

Pyridoxine dependency It is a rare autosomal recessive disorder of an enzyme involved in production of inhibitory neurotransmitter GABA and presents with early-onset intractable seizures. Prolonged maternal administration of vitamin B$_6$ during pregnancy may predispose to this condition. The levels of pyridoxal-5-phosphate in the cerebrospinal fluid of affected infants are low. Seizures may be focal or generalized having onset during first 12 hours and are resistant to conventional therapy. There are no characteristic features but condition should be suspected in any infant having intractable cryptogenic focal seizures with developmental retardation having onset during first 18 months of life. Irritability, restlessness, crying and vomiting may precede the seizures. There may be a history of severe or fatal cryptogenic convulsive disorder in a sibling. There may be consanguinity among the parents. EEG may show generalized bursts of bilaterally synchronous high voltage 1–4 Hz activity with interspersed spikes. Seizures are controlled with intravenous administration of 50–100 mg pyridoxine and they reappear within 3 weeks of withdrawal of pyridoxine.

Dyselectrolytemia Hypo- and hypernatremic states may be associated with convulsions.

Benign Seizures in Neonates

Benign neonatal sleep myoclonus. It has onset during first week of life and occurs as synchronous myoclonic jerks during REM sleep in preterm babies. There are no seizures when baby is awake, EEG is normal and seizures spontaneously disappear by 2 months of age.

Benign familial neonatal convulsions occur as self-limiting isolated clonic seizures on second or third day of life. The condition is autosomal dominant with spontaneous recovery within 1–6 months of age.

Benign idiopathic "fifth day" seizures. The multifocal clonic seizures classicaly occur on day 5 and usually disappear on day 15. The cause is unknown though low CSF zinc level has been reported in a few cases.

Diagnosis

The time of onset of seizures (Table 22.4), positive family history of convulsions in the previous sibling(s) (Table 22.5) and presence of associated conditions provide useful clues to the clinical diagnosis. The readily treatable conditions like metabolic disorders (hypocalcemia, hypoglycemia) and bacterial meningitis must be identified promptly. The following investigations are often necessary for precise etiological diagnosis and for assessment of prognosis.

First-line investigations Check hematocrit, blood glucose, calcium, phosphorus, magnesium, sodium, venous pH and base excess. Hypocalcemia can be rapidly suspected by looking for prolonged QTc interval (>0.2 sec) on EKG. CSF examination and blood culture should be taken in all cases to exclude pyogenic meningitis. Cot-side cranial ultrasound and EEG should be done once metabolic disorders are excluded.

TABLE 22.4 Age of onset of convulsions

First day

Hypoxic-ischemic encephalopathy, cerebral contusion, 'first day' hypocalcemia, pyridoxine dependency, accidental injection of local anesthetic into fetal scalp.

Between 1 and 3 day

Intracranial hemorrhage, hypoglycemia, narcotic withdrawal and inborn error of metabolism.

4th to 7th day

Tetany, meningitis, TORCH infections, developmental malformations, acute bilirubin encephalopathy, and benign neonatal seizures.

1–4 weeks

Late-onset hypocalcemia, sepsis, progressive hydrocephalus, herpes encephalitis, inborn error of metabolism, cerebral dysgenesis and epileptic syndromes.

TABLE 22.5 Seizures with recurrence in sibship

- Inborn errors of metabolism.
  Maple syrup urine disease, hyperglycinemias, organic acidemias, proline aminoaciduria, galactosemia, glycogen storage disease and fructose intolerance.
- Developmental defects of central nervous system.
- Narcotic abstinence (withdrawal) syndrome.
- Pyridoxine dependency.
- Hyperbilirubinemia due to rhesus isoimmunization.
- Benign familial seizures.

Neurological Disorders

22

Second-line investigations When convulsions persist and first-line investigations are unable to identify the cause, non-contrast CT scan and MRI of brain is advised to exclude structural or developmental defects like cerebral dysgenesis, lissencephaly and neuronal migration disorders. Appropriate tests including serology for TORCH infections should be undertaken to exclude intrauterine infections. Screening tests for exclusion of inborn error of metabolism include ABG, anion gap, blood ammonia, lactate/pyruvate level, plasma and urinary amino acid profile (high performance liquid chromatography or tandem mass spectrometry). If facilities exist, mother's urine and baby's meconium should be screened for maternal drug abuse. Therapeutic trial with pyridoxine is usually reserved as a last resort.

Electroencephalography

Polygraphic EEG recording and video monitoring have greatly facilitated classification and management of neonatal seizures. A conventional 10–20 channel continuous EEG for at least one hour with due modifications for neonates and concurrent video recording is the gold standard for monitoring seizures in the newborns. In the NICU, a 2-channel bed side EEG in combination with amplitude integrated EEG (aEEG) is reliable for screening purposes (Figure 22.20). Automated EEG has a low accuracy for seizure detection compared to conventional EEG and may miss brief episodes of low voltage focal seizures. Neonatal seizures may be associated with EEG abnormalities and at times EEG abnormalities are seen without any clinical seizures ("EEG-only" seizures). EEG should be recorded by a skilled technician and interpreted by a specially trained physician. Apart from electro-encephalographic abnormalities, it is important to assess background activity and maturation pattern of EEG. The 5–7 Hz "comb-like" rhythm on EEG is suggestive of maple syrup urine disease. Patients with pyridoxine-dependency may have generalized 1–4 Hz sharp and slow wave activity. Herpes encephalitis is characterized by multifocal periodic pattern on EEG. Unifocal diphasic spike or sharp wave pattern carries good prognosis. Multiple foci with periods of virtual electrical silence interrupted by bursts of irregular, polymorphic and asynchronous activity or flat EEG denote poor outcome. In neonatal EEG, interpretation of background activity and identification of maturation changes are more important than the epileptiform abnormalities.

Management

After taking relevant blood samples and collection of cerebrospinal fluid, intravenous line should be established in a peripheral vein. This facilitates injection of medicines and avoids risk of aspiration of feeds. Infant should be nursed in a thermoneutral environment and special attention should be paid to his perfusion (by checking capillary refill time and blood pressure) and ventilation. Biochemical abnormalities should be looked for and treated appropriately.

EKG shows QoTc >0.2 sec or serum calcium <7 mg/dL Calcium gluconate 200 mg/kg of 10% solution (2 mL/kg) diluted with equal volume of water is injected slowly in 5–10 minutes under cardiac monitoring. For maintenance, repeat the same dose through constant infusion every 6–8 hr. Give 0.2 mL/kg 50% solution of magnesium sulfate 1M two doses 12 hours apart, if there is no or poor response to calcium therapy.

Dextrostix shows hypoglycemia (<40 mg/dL) Glucose 5–10 mL/kg of 10% solution as a bolus followed by 10% dextrose at a rate of 8 mg/kg/minute. The blood glucose should be maintained between 70 and 120 mg/dL. For details refer to management protocol for hypoglycemia in Chapter 24.

When seizures persist even after correction of hypocalcemia, and hypoglycemia, anticonvulsants should be given.

Anticonvulsant Therapy

Phenobarbital has been the gold standard for management of neonatal seizures for over 90 years. In case

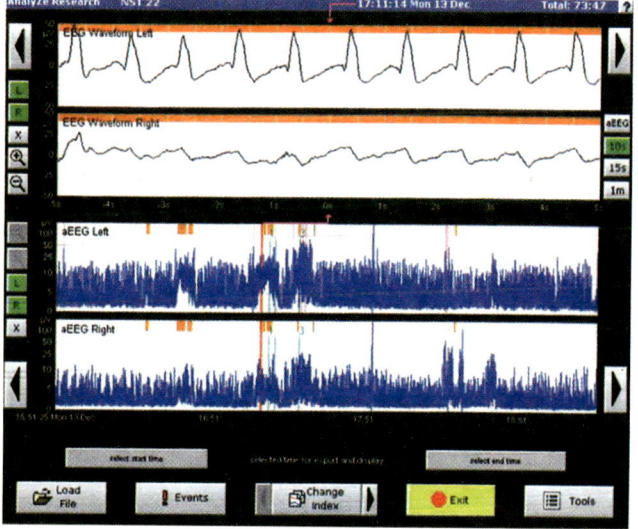

Figure 22.20 Screenshot of aEEG trace demonstrating seizures.

there is no improvement and/or no biochemical abnormality has been detected, parenteral loading dose of phenobarbitone 20 mg/kg is administered slowly intravenously over 20 minutes. If there is no response in 15 minutes, additional doses of phenobarbitone 10 mg/kg every 15 minutes are administered intravenously till the seizures are controlled or a total dose of 40 mg/kg has been given. If convulsions are still uncontrolled despite maximal dose of phenobarbitone, phenytoin is administered intravenously in a loading dose of 20 mg/kg. It is diluted in normal saline and administered slowly at a rate of 1 mg/kg/min. Fosphenytoin, a pro-drug of phenytoin, is preferred because of its solubility in standard intravenous solutions, neutral pH, feasibility to administer at a faster rate and lack of necrosis of subcutaneous tissues on extravasation. It is given in a loading dose of 15–20 mg/kg IV. Fosphenytoin 1.5 mg is equivalent to 1.0 mg phenytoin and is expressed as phenytoin equivalents (PE). The maintenance therapy with phenobarbitone and phenytoin is started after 12 hours of loading dose and given in a dose of 5 mg/kg/day in two divided doses.

If convulsions are intractable and baby is in a status convulsicus, give lorazepam 50 μg/kg IV slowly over 2–5 min. Diazepam should be avoided as it has a short duration of action, carries the risk of inducing apneic attacks and may predispose the baby to develop kernicterus by displacement of bilirubin from the binding sites in the protein because it contains sodium benzoate as a preservative. Alternatively, clonazepam 100–200 μg/kg can be given IV over 30 sec. Benzodiazepines can be repeated as and when needed. Midazolam 0.05–0.15 mg/kg/dose is effective when given through intramuscular route because it is highly soluble in water. Paraldehyde can also be given in a dose of 200–400 mg/kg deep IM as 5% solution in 5% dextrose or diluted with double volume of olive oil or coconut oil and given per rectum. Lidocaine 2 mg/kg IV bolus followed by 6 mg/kg/hr as a constant infusion has been used with success to abort intractable seizures. However, it should never be co-administered with phenytoin due to potential risk of myocardial damage and arrhythmia. Levetiracetam is given in a loading dose of 50 mg/kg IV followed by maintenance dose of 5 mg/kg every 8–12 hours. Topiramate is safe in newborn period but no parenteral formulation is available. Sodium valproate 20 mg/kg oral or IV as a loading dose followed by 10 mg/kg every 12 hr has been used in newborn babies. It is associated with a serious risk of hepatotoxicity. Vigabatrin in a dose of 50 mg/kg/day has been used in neonates with refractory infantile spasms. Newer antiepileptic agents, levetiracetam and topiramate are being used as add-on agents because of their efficacy, better tolerability and safety profile. Refer to Figure 22.21 for stepwise management of neonatal seizures.

Specific Situations

Perinatal complications The associated metabolic disorders like hypoglycemia, hypocalcemia and hyponatremia due to inappropriate secretion of ADH should be recognized and promptly treated. The use of hypertonic mannitol and furosemide may be considered for relief of cerebral edema in term babies with severe hypoxic-ischemic encephalopathy. There is no role of dexamethasone for relief of cerebral edema. Selective cooling of brain or total body moderate hypothermia (core temperature <34°C) is being increasingly used in the management of neonates with hypoxic-ischemic encephalopathy. It raises the threshold for seizures by reducing release of excitatory neurotransmitters. A recent study has shown that there is no effect of hypothermia on pharmacokinetics of phenobarital but time taken to normalization of EEG background is reduced suggesting neuroprotective effect of hypothermia.

Diuretic therapy and gastric lavage are effective to enhance excretion of inadvertently injected local anesthetic into infant's scalp during pudendal block.

Infections Appropriate and early antibiotic therapy for bacterial meningitis is likely to improve survival and reduce the risk of sequelae.

Pyridoxine-dependent Seizures

Give pyridoxine 100 mg IV under EEG control and close clinical observation. Repeat 100 mg pyridoxine IV every 10 min till seizures are controlled or a cumulative dose of 500 mg is given. In the absence of suitable intravenous formulation of pyridoxine in India, it is given intramuscularly (1.0 mL neurobion provides 50 mg pyridoxine) and 1.0 mL each may be administered intramuscularly in the anterolateral aspect of each thigh. Watch for prolonged depression of cerebral activity or vital functions during next 12 hours. The maintenance dose of pyridoxine is 5 mg/kg (or 50 mg/d) single oral dose daily. If pyridoxine is stopped, seizures would reappear within 3 weeks. There is no need to administer any other anticonvulsant agent in infants with pyridoxine-dependent seizures.

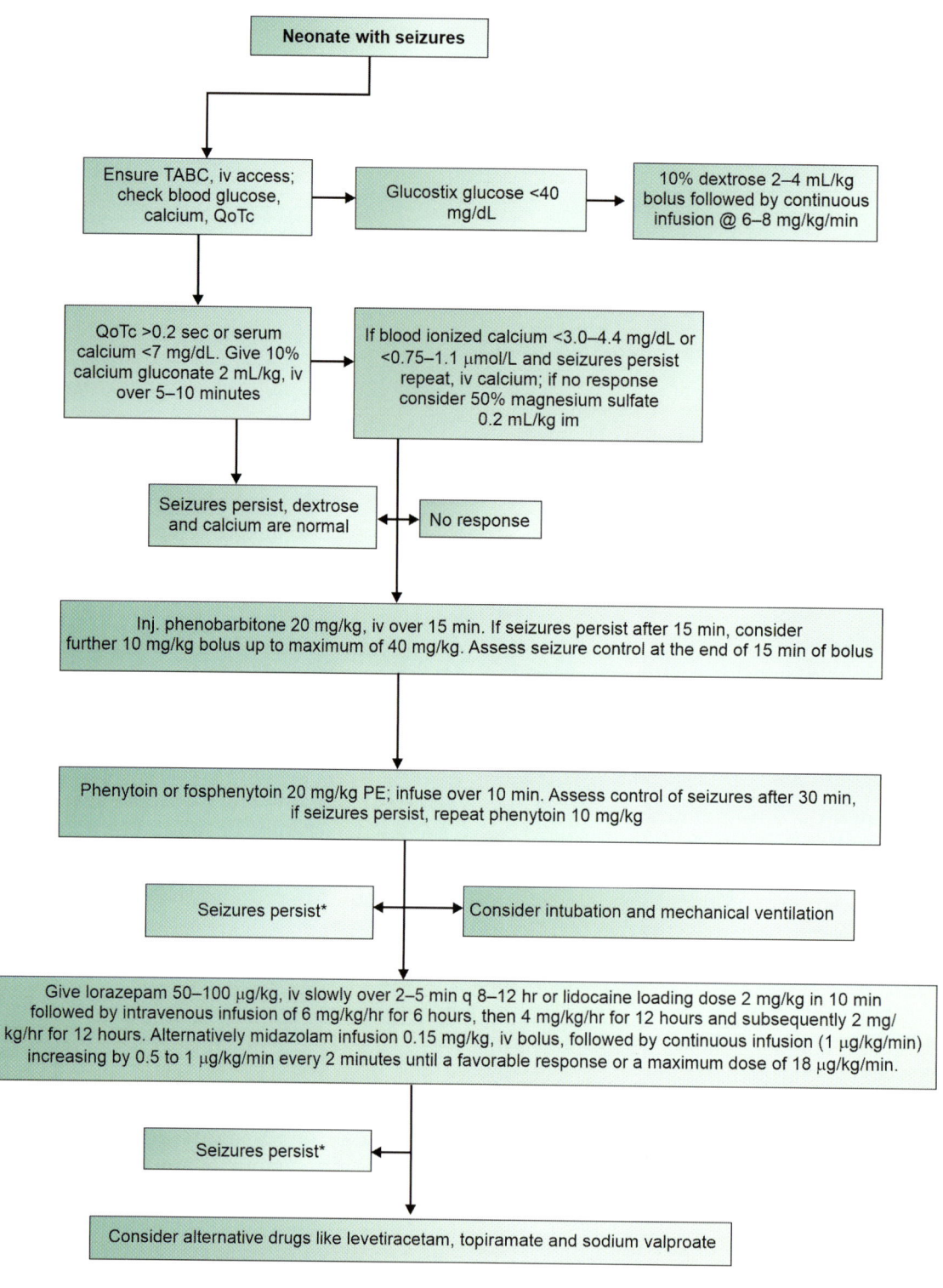

Figure 22.21 Flowchart for management of neonatal seizures

Exchange blood transfusion is indicated in the following situations:

- Life-threatening metabolic disorder.
- Accidental injection of local anesthetic to the fetus.
- Transplacental transfer of maternal chlorpropamide to the fetus.
- Acute bilirubin encephalopathy.

Inborn errors of metabolism Prompt cessation of milk feeding while trying to identify the underlying metabolic defect, may be life saving.

Narcotic withdrawal syndrome Administration of phenobarbitone (5–8 mg/kg/d in 2 div doses) or diluted Tr. opium or paregoric 2 drops/kg every 4–6 hr and attention to hydration would be life saving. Diazepam, clonidine and chlorpromazine are less effective. The sedatives should be tapered off slowly and cautiously.

Duration of Anticonvulsant Therapy

The duration of anticonvulsant therapy is guided by the neurological status of the infant at discharge, cause of the seizures and EEG findings. All anticonvulsants are stopped except phenobarbitone when seizures are controlled. At discharge, if CNS examination is normal, phenobarbitone may be stopped. Phenobarbitone is continued, if there are any CNS abnormalities at the time of discharge and infant is re-assessed at one month. If there is no recurrence of seizures, CNS examination, EEG and CT scan or MRI are normal, phenobarbitone is tapered over next 2 weeks. When phenobarbitone is continued, child is evaluated at the age of 3 months.

The infant is treated like a case of epilepsy, if seizures are recurrent or there are any evidences of neuromotor disability and/or EEG abnormalities at 4 months. Additional and alternative anticonvulsants may have to be administered when prolonged anti-convulsant therapy is required.

Prognosis

About one-fourth of neonates with convulsions die and amongst survivors prognosis regarding recurrence of seizures and neuromotor sequelae is determined by the underlying disease process and EEG findings. The onset of seizures within 24 hours of age, presence of myoclonic seizures or stiffening attacks and their persistence for more than 48 hours suggest poor outcome. Prematurity, perinatal hypoxia, birth injury leading to intraventricular or subdural hemorrhage, developmental abnormalities, metabolic seizures, hypoglycemia and meningitis are associated with high rate of sequelae. Uncomplicated hypocalcemia, narcotic withdrawal and subarachnoid hemorrhage carry good prognosis. A normal interictal EEG is associated with a good outcome. Flat or periodic and polyphasic EEG signifies poor prognosis. The overall risk of epilepsy and brain damage among survivors of neonatal seizures is 30 to 40%.

FLOPPY NEONATE

A normal term infant is 'hypertonic' by adult standards and it is difficult to completely extend his limbs. Preterm infants are normally hypotonic and muscle tone increases as the gestational maturity proceeds.

Assessment of Tone

For assessment of active and passive tone, refer to Chapter 7 for evaluation of gestational age. Paralysis of respiratory muscles may be characterized by rapid shallow breathing which may dominate the clinical picture.

Causes and Diagnosis

The diagnosis of the precise cause of hypotonia may be very difficult without detailed investigations including muscle biopsy which is most useful.

Cerebral Disorders

Birth asphyxia, intracranial hemorrhage, sedative drugs, severe generalized illness such as septicemia and respiratory distress may be associated with hypotonia. The diagnosis is suggested by lethargy, poor feeding, lack of alertness, poor Moro response, seizures and normal or increased deep tendon reflexes. When a child with atonic diplegia is suspended upright by holding under the arms, flexion of hips may occur (Foerster sign). It must be borne in mind that alterness of the baby is a distinctive feature of hypotonia due to non-cerebral causes. No specific investigations are generally needed except cranial ultrasonography and MRI but if organic acidemia is suspected as a cause of floppiness, plasma and urinary amino acid chromatography should be asked for.

Spinal Cord Injury

Spinal cord transection is rarely seen in modern obstetric practice. Severe trauma to cervical cord during difficult breech extraction manifests with bilateral brachial palsy, flaccid paralysis of all the limbs and retention of urine with overflow incontinence. The child would be alert unless there is associated intra-cranial injury. The sense of pain may be blunted though it is difficult to evaluate. Deep tendon reflexes may be normal or increased. Skiagrams of the cervical spine should be taken to exclude any fracture of the vertebral body or transverse process. Electromyography (EMG) and muscle biopsy are generally non-contributory.

Anterior Horn Cell Disorders

Werdnig-Hoffmann disease (spinal muscular atrophy) It is characterized by sluggish fetal movements and fasciculations of tongue. Most of the normal newborn babies have 'restless' tongues thus making the evaluation for fasciculations difficult. The baby is fully alert but the feeding and cry may be poor because of marked weakness of neck muscles. Tachypnea may be marked due to paralysis of intercostal muscles. The deep tendon reflexes are absent. EMG shows a neurogenic disorder and muscle biopsy may reveal neurogenic group atrophy. Family history of affected sibling may be obtained as it is inherited as an autosomal recessive disorder.

Benign congenital hypotonia It is a benign condition with neonatal hypotonia which markedly improves or disappears with age. The diagnosis is made by exclusion. There is no evidence of central or peripheral nervous system involvement and muscle biopsy does not show any histochemical or ultra-structural abnormalities.

Congenital Guillain-Barré disease It is a rare disorder and may be suspected by finding albuminocytologic dissociation in the cerebrospinal fluid which is difficult to interpret in a newborn baby.

Neuromuscular Junction Disorders

Myasthenia gravis neonatorum It may manifest in about 12% of babies born to mothers with the disease. It is characterized by floppiness, normal alertness, pooling of oral secretions, poor feeding, feeble cry and generalized muscular weakness appearing 2 to 3 days after birth. The facial weakness manifests by mask-like face, open mouth and staring look but unlike adult myasthenic patients, external ophthalmoplegia and ptosis are rare. Deep tendon jerks are usually normal. EMG may show non-specific changes. Therapeutic trial with intramuscular injection of edrophonium chloride (tensilon) 1.0 mg or neostigmine methyl sulfate 0.1 mg clinches the diagnosis. After confirmation of the diagnosis, treatment should be continued with injection neostigmine methyl sulfate 0.1–0.5 mg about 10 minutes before each feed for 1 to 2 days followed by oral neostigmine bromide

1.0–4.0 mg half an hour before each feed. The condition is transient and therapy may be tapered off in 3 to 4 weeks.

Muscle Disorders

Congenital myopathies These are characterized by sluggish fetal movements, decreased muscle mass or wasting and sluggish deep tendon jerks. The babies are alert and they cry and feed normally. EMG and muscle biopsy demonstrate myopathic pattern. Creatine phosphokinase estimation is generally unnecessary because Duchenne pseudohypertrophic muscular dystrophy does not manifest in the neonatal period. History of an affected sibling may be obtained.

Glycogen storage disease The diagnosis may be supported by macroglossia, cardiomegaly and generalized hypotonia.

Hereditary Connective Tissue Disorders

Marfan syndrome Phenotype is characterized by thin and long body frame, thin and long spider-like fingers, muscular hypoplasia and marked hypermobility of joints with genu recurvatum. Bilateral subluxation of lenses and dilatation of aortic root with aortic regurgitation are commonly associated.

Ehlers-Danlos syndrome It is characterized by loose, hyperextensible and stretchable skin, hypermobile joints, easy bruisability and generalized fragility of various connective tissues. The facial features may include hypertelorism, epicanthic folds, high-arched palate and hypermobile tongue which can be stretched to touch the tip of the nose.

Miscellaneous Conditions

Down syndrome Hypotonia is a constant feature and its presence should alert the physician to look for other evidences of Down syndrome.

Cretinism Hypotonia, inactivity, poor cry, constipation and persistence of physiological jaundice are usual clinical features during neonatal period.

Prader-Willi syndrome The diagnosis is often retrospective when these babies manifest mental retardation, obesity and diabetes mellitus later in life. The hypotonia improves with time and mental retardation becomes apparant as child grows. The presence of undescended testes and micropenis are the only clues in the neonatal period in the affected male children. Exact cause is unknown but it appears to be due to CNS disorder affecting hypothalamus.

Zellweger syndrome Cerebrohepatorenal syndrome due to peroxisomal defect is characterized by facial dysmorphism (dolicho-turricephaly, prominent forehead, epicanthal folds, wide anterior fontanel, high-arched palate), eye abnormalities (cataract, glaucoma, corneal clouding, brushfield spots, pigmentary degeneration of retina) profound hypotonia, hepatomegaly, cortical cysts in the kidneys, cholestasis and seizures due to neuronal heterotropia in cerebral white matter. Skeletal muscle fibers may show degeneration and cytoplasmic vacuoles. All of the peroxisomal disorders can be diagnosed prenatally.

Primary carnitine deficiency It is a rare inborn error of metabolism which is characterized by inability to use certain fats for energy particularly during fasting. The clinical features include muscle weakness, hypotonia, encephalopathy, cardiomyopathy and hypoglycemia. The diagnosis is based on low carnitine levels and identification of mutations in the SLC22A5 gene. The condition can be ameliorated by giving supplements of L-carnitine.

Joubert syndrome It is an autosomal recessive disorder with underdevelopment or absence of cerebellar vermis and malformed brainstem. Features of facial dysmorphism include broad forehead, arched eyebrows, ptosis, hypertelorism, low-set ears and a triangle-shaped mouth. Hypotonia and ataxia occur early. Other features include episodes of slow or rapid breathing, abnormal eye movements (ocular motor apraxia), and delayed neuromotor development. MRI shows characteristic molar tooth sign at appendix of cerebellum.

BIBLIOGRAPHY

Ahmann PA, Lazzara A, Dykes FD, *et al*. Intraventricular hemorrhage in the high-risk preterm infant: incidence and outcome. *Ann Neurol* 1980; 7: 118.

Alistair GSP. Neonatal meningitis in the new millennium. *Neo Reviews* 2003; 4: 73.

American Academy of Pediatrics, Committee on Genetics. Folic acid for the prevention of neural tube defects. *Pediatrics* 1999; 104: 325–327.

Ancel PY, Livine F. Laroque B, *et al*. Cerebral palsy among very preterm children in relation to gestational age and neonatal ultrasound abnormalities. The EPIPAGE cohort study. *Pediatrics* 2006; 117: 828–835.

Andreolli A, Turco EC, Pedrazzi G, Beghi E, Pisani F. Incidence of epilepsy after neonatal seizures: A population-based study. *Neuroepidemiology* 2019, 52:144–51.

Banker B, Larroche J. Periventricular leukomalacia of infancy. *Arch Neurol* 1962; 7: 386–410.

Bassan H, Feldman HA, Limperopoulos, *et al*. Periventricular hemorrhagic infarction: Risk factors and neonatal outcome. *Pediatr Neurol* 2006; 35: 85–92.

Bol KA, Collins JS, Kirby RS. The National Birth Defect Prevention Network. Survival of infants with neural tube defects in the presence of folic acid fortification. *Pediatrics* 2006; 117: 803.

Carin MAR, Linda S deVries. Pharmacology review: lidocaine for neonatal seizure management. *Neo Reviews* 2008; 9: e 585–e 589.

Co JPT, Elia M, Engel J, *et al*. Proposal of an algorithm for diagnosis and treatment of neonatal seizures in developing countries. Epilepsia 2007; 48(6): 1158–64.

Decourten GM, Rabinowicz T. Intraventricular hemorrhage in premature infants : Reappraisal and new hypothesis. *Dev Med Child Neurol* 1981; 23: 389.

Dubowitz V (Ed.). The Floppy Infant. *Clinics in Developmental Medicine,* 1969; No. 31.

Evans D, Levene M. Neonatal seizures. *Arch Dis Child Fetal Neonat Ed* 1998; 78: F70–F75.

Glass HC, Wirrell E. Controversies in neonatal seizures management. *J Child Neurol* 2009; 24(5): 591–599.

Goh YI, Bollano E, Eierson TR, *et al*. Prenatal multivitamin supplementation and rates of congenital anomalies: A meta-analysis. *J Obstet Gynaecol Canada* 2006; 28: 680.

Gospe SM. Current perspectives on pyridoxine-dependent seizures. *J Pediatr* 1998; 132: 919–923.

Grant EG. Sonography of the premature brain : Intracranial hemorrhage and periventricular leucomalacia. *Neuroradiology* 1986; 28: 476.

Jensen FE. Neonatal seizures: an update on mechanisms and management. *Clin Perinatol* 2009, 36(4):881–900.

Jhonson K, Gerada C, Greenough A. Treatment of neonatal abstinence syndrome. *Arch Dis Child Fetal Neonatal Ed* 2003; 88: F2–F5.

Maria A, Gupta A, Agarwal R, Sreenivas V, Paul VK, Deorari AK. Incidence of periventricular leukomalacia among a cohort of very low birth weight neonates (<1500). *Indian Pediatr* 2006, 43:210–16.

Massingdale TW, Buttross S. Survey of treatment practices for neonatal seizures. *J Perinatol* 1993; 13: 107–110.

Olson DM. Neonatal seizures. *Neo Rev* 2012; 13: e 213–e 223.

Paine RS and Oppe TF. In: Neurological Examination of Children. Clinics in Developmental Medicine 20/21. *Spastics Society Medical Education and Information Unit,* 1966.

Paine RS, Brazelton TB, Donovan DE, Drorbaugh JE, Hubbell JP and Sears EM. Evaluation of postural reflexes in normal infants and in the presence of chronic brain syndrome. *Neurology* 1964; 14: 1036.

Paine RS. Neurological examination of infants and children. *Pediatr Clin N Am* 1960; 7: 471.

Painter MJ, Scher MS, Stein MD, *et al.* Phenobarbitone compared with phenytoin for treatment of neonatal seizures. *N Engl J Med* 1999; 341: 485–489.

Parker S, Zuckerman B, Bauchner H, *et al.* Jitteriness in fullterm neonates: Prevalence and correlates. *Pediatrics* 1990; 85: 17.

Patra K, Wilson-Costello D, Taylor HG, *et al.* Grades I-II intraventricular hemorrhage in extremely low birth weight infants: Effects on neurodevelopment. *J Pediatr* 2006; 149: 169–173.

Perlman JM. Intrapartum hypoxic-ischemic cerebral injury and subsequent cerebral palsy: Medicolegal issues. *Pediatrics* 1997; 99: 851–859.

Prechtl HFR. The neurological examination of the full term newborn infant. *Clinics in Developmental Medicine, No. 63,* 1977.

Pressler RM, Mangum B. Newly emerging therapies for neonatal seizures. *Semin Fetal Neonatal Med* 2013; 18: 216–223.

Riviello JJ. Drug therapy for neonatal seizures. *Pharmacol Rev* 2004; 5: e215–e220.

Robinson R. Cerebral function in the newborn. *Develop Med Child Neurol* 1988; 8: 561.

Ronen GM, Buckley D, Penney S, Streiner DL Long-term prognosis in children with neonatal seizures: a population-based study. *Neurology* 2007; 69: 1816–1822.

Rose AL and Lombroso CT. Neonatal seizure state—A study of clinical, pathological and electroencephalographic features in 137 full-term babies with a long-term follow up. *Pediatrics* 1970; 45: 404.

Shellhaas RA, Shoita AI, Clancy RR. Sensitivity of amplitude integrated electroencephalography for neonatal seizure detection. *Pediatrics* 2007; 120: 770–777.

Shoemaker MT, Rotenberg JS. Levetiracetam for the treatment of neonatal seizures. *J Child Neurol* 2007; 22: 95–98.

Soul JS, Eichenwald E, Walter G, *et al.* CSF removal in infantile post hemorrhagic hydrocephalus results in significant improvement in cerebral hemodynamics. *Pediatr Res* 2004; 55: 872–876.

Tekgul H, Gauvreau K, Soul J, *et al.* The current etiologic profile and neurodevelopmental outcome of seizures in term newborn infants. *Pediatrics* 2006; 117: 1270–1280.

Vesoulis ZA, Mathur AM. Advances in management of neonatal seizures. *Indian J Pediatr* 2014; 81(6): 592–598.

Volpe JJ (ed). Neonatal seizures. In: Neurology of the Newborn. 5th ed. *Philadelphia: WB Saunders and Co* 2008; pp 203–244.

Volpe JJ. Neonatal intraventricular hemorrhage. *N Engl J Med* 1981; 304: 886–891.

Woodward LJ, Anderson PJ, Austin NC, *et al.* Neonatal MRI to predict neurodevelopmental outcomes in preterm infants. *N Engl J Med* 2006; 355: 685–694.

Yamamoto H, Aihara M, Nijima S, *et al.* Treatment with midazolam and lidocaine for status epilepticus in neonates. *Brain Develop* 2007; 29: 559–564.

Zupanc ML. Neonatal seizures. *Pediatr Clin North Am* 2004; 51(4): 961–978.

Hematologic Problems

BLEEDING DISORDERS

Severe hemorrhage in the newborn is uncommon but it is a life-threatening emergency which demands urgent and preferably fresh blood transfusion. Most of the coagulation factors with the exception of Factors I, V, VII and platelets are reduced in the normal newborn babies. The preterm baby has added hazards of increased vascular permeability and inability to-effectively utilize vitamin K for synthesis of coagulation factors.

Causes

The bleeding may occur *in utero* or after birth.

Fetal Hemorrhage

This may be associated with twin-to-twin transfusion, fetomaternal hemorrhage, antepartum hemorrhage from fetal aspect of placenta (placenta previa, abruptio placentae), administration of coumarin anticoagulants to mother and accidental incision of placenta during cesarean section. The baby is severely pale and in shock and should be differentiated from asphyxia pallida (*see* Chapter 6).

Neonatal Hemorrhage

Bleeding may occur due to defective coagulation, thrombocytopenia or combined coagulation and platelet defects.

DEFECTIVE COAGULATION

Hemorrhagic Disease of the Newborn

Newborn babies are predisposed to develop vitamin K deficiency and hemorrhagic manifestations or vitamin K-dependent bleeding. Vitamin K is required for the synthesis of coagulation Factors II (prothrombin),

VII, IX and X by a process of carboxylation of glutamic acid in vitamin K-dependent proteins. Transplacental passage of vitamin K is minimal and hepatic storage of vitamin K in the newborn is limited (25% of adult stores). The maternal to cord plasma ratio of vitamin K is 1:30 and only 10% of vitamin K administered to the mother reaches the fetus. In healthy mothers, plasma vitamin K concentration is 1–2 mg/L while in cord blood it is usually less than 0.05 mg/L. The endogenous production of vitamin K in the neonates is limited because of relative sterility of gut. Vitamin K-responsive hemorrhagic disease of the newborn occurs in 1 in 200–400 infants not given vitamin K at birth. The incidence of bleeding due to vitamin K deficiency is 15–20-fold higher in exclusively breast-fed infants as compared to formula-fed infants. The plasma half life of vitamin K is less than 72 hours but it may be stored in the healthy liver for up to one month.

a. **Early-HDN** Severe life-threatening hemorrhagic manifestations are seen *in utero* or within 24 hours of life. The site of bleeding is usually concealed inside the body cavities, like cranium, thorax, and abdomen. Subcutaneous hemorrhages, large ecchymoses and even external bleeding may be seen. Vitamin K deficiency occurs *in utero* due to maternal intake of warfarin, anticonvulsants (especially phenytoin and phenobarbitone), INH, rifampicin, salicylates, and broad-spectrum antibiotics.

b. **Classical-HDN** The classical variety of hemorrhagic disease of the newborn is most common and occurs due to physiological vitamin K deficiency in the newborn period which is further aggravated by inadequate intake of vitamin K due to breast-feeding. The reported incidence of the disease is 0.25–0.5%. The vitamin K content of human milk (1–9 µg/L) is one-fourth of cow's milk. Relatively low concentration of vitamin K in breast milk is due to low maternal intake of vitamin K_1 and poor transfer of vitamin K to breast milk. A single dose of vitamin K 5 mg IM to lactating women increases the concentration of vitamin K in breast-milk to 8 ±3.7 µg/dL. The quantity of milk ingested during first few days is rather small and may be inadequate to meet the daily requirements of vitamin K (12 µg/day). The colonization of gut is delayed by flora known to synthesize vitamin K endogenously. In exclusively breastfed babies, gut is colonized by bifidobacteria which do not synthesize vitamin K. The classical-HDN usually manifests during 2nd and 3rd (up to 1–7 days) day of life and is characterized by bleeding from umbilical stump, nose, GI tract and following a surgical procedure such as circumcision. The manifestations are not very severe and disease can be readily managed by administration of vitamin K.

c. **Late-HDN** The bleeding manifestations occur after first week (usually 2–16 weeks) of life. The condition is rare in formula fed infants and in infants who had received injectable vitamin K at birth. The infant may be apparently healthy but more often there are predisposing conditions which are known to produce vitamin K deficiency, viz. chronic diarrhea, malabsorption, hepatic cholestasis, prolonged administration of broad-spectrum antibiotics, and mucoviscidosis. The bleeding may occur from any site but more commonly from intracranial vessels, mucous membranes, skin and GI tract. It is a life-threatening condition with a mortality risk of 2%.

Diagnosis

The association of predisposing factors and age at onset of bleeding offer useful clues. The infants with hemorrhagic disease of the newborn do not appear ill or toxic which easily differentiates them from disseminated intravascular coagulation. The laboratory parameters pertaining to vitamin K-dependent coagulation factors are deranged. The clotting time, prothrombin time, partial thromboplastin time and thrombotest are all prolonged. Serum vitamin K levels are difficult to measure but levels of "Proteins induced in vitamin K absence" (PIVKA-II) are specific and provide a sensitive index of vitamin K deficiency. In the absence of vitamin K, synthesized prothrombin circulates in its non-carboxylated form which is measured as PIVKA. PIVKA-II levels are elevated in infants with vitamin K deficiency due to any cause and can be estimated by HPLC, ELISA or crossed immunoelectrophoresis.

VITAMIN K PROPHYLAXIS

American Academy of Pediatrics recommends that all newborn babies should receive 0.5–1.0 mg (0.5 mg in infants <1500 g) vitamin K_1 intramuscularly at birth to prevent HDN. However, these recommendations are not uniformly accepted and adopted in all countries. There is evidence to suggest that incidence of classical-HDN is higher among exclusively breastfed babies as compared to formula fed infants. However, there are numerous biological advantages of human milk and despite the available scientific evidence pertaining to HDN, it is difficult to comprehend that healthy term babies fed on breast milk are predisposed to develop classical-HDN. It is against the basic tenets of nature and commonsense that a ready-made food produced by nature is deficient in an important nutrient and is unable to serve the nutritional needs of a healthy baby. The incidence of classical HDN is merely 0.1% in most neonatal units in the developing countries. It is well known that colostrum has higher content of vitamin K and it is possible that vitamin K in the human milk has enhanced bioavailability and absorption. Due to the common practice of giving prelacteal and prolacteal feeds, despite specific instructions against their use, it is possible that there may be early colonization of gut even in breastfed babies resulting in reduced incidence of classical HDN.

In India, it is difficult to follow the policy of administration of vitamin K to babies born at home or community health care facilities. Oral preparation of vitamin K is not available and one would have to give 1000 injections of vitamin K to prevent one case of classical HDN which can be easily diagnosed and promptly managed by therapeutic administration of vitamin K. There are logistic difficulties, inherent risks of intramuscular injections and above all danger of inadvertent administration of high dose of vitamin K_3 (menadione sodium bisulphite which is available as 10 mg/mL formulation) which can lead to severe hemolysis, jaundice and even kernicterus. Because of relatively high incidence of G6PD deficiency in India, administration of synthetic vitamin K to all newborn babies do have a potential risk of causing hemolytic jaundice. However, in hospital born babies, most pediatricians administer prophylactic vitamin K. In view of the fact that plasma half life of vitamin K is only 72 hours and its storage in a healthy liver is limited up to one month, it is difficult to comprehend that parenteral administration of a single dose of vitamin K can prevent late onset HDN which may occur as late as 16 weeks (even up to one year by some workers!). Till a safe and suitable preparation of oral vitamin K is available, it is preferable to follow a selective vitamin K prophylaxis policy (Table 23.1).

Treatment

Classical-HDN can be prevented by administration of vitamin K 0.5–1.0 mg intramuscular (or 1–2 mg oral) to all newborn babies at birth. Initial concerns regarding the risk of development of lymphoreticular malignancy following administration of injectable vitamin K at birth have been found to be untrue. The non-availability of oral preparation of vitamin K in India is posing logistic difficulties to pursue this policy. Naturally occurring lipid-soluble vitamin K_1 (phylloquinone or phytonadione) and K_2 (menaquinone) are rapid in action and are non-toxic even in high doses. Vitamin K_1 is present in green leafy vegetables while vitamin K_2 is synthesized in the gut by bacterial flora. The water-soluble synthetic preparation of vitamin K_3 (menadione sodium bisulfite) is potentially toxic and can cause hemolysis and severe jaundice by blocking glutathione metabolism in the red blood cells. The water soluble preparation, however, is readily absorbed from the gut without any bile salts. There is a need to have a suitable licensed preparation of oral

---

TABLE 23.1 Indications for prophylactic administration of vitamin K during neonatal period

- **At birth**
  - Maternal intake of drugs, like anticonvulsants (phenytoin, phenobarbitone), warfarin, salicylates and antitubercular agents (rifampicin, INH).

- **Infants admitted to the NICU**
  - Birth weight <2000 g, or gestation <36 weeks
  - Traumatic and difficult deliveries
  - Birth asphyxia
  - Grossly SFD or LFD babies
  - Congenital malformations requiring surgical intervention

- **Subsequently**
  - Administration of broad-spectrum antibiotics*
  - Total parenteral nutrition*
  - Cholestatic hepatitis
  - Chronic diarrhea or malabsorption
  - Prior to surgery

*Administer weekly 1.0 mg vitamin K IV

---

vitamin K_1 (one drop to provide 1.0 mg vitamin K) for convenience and safety for administration to all newborn babies at birth in developing countries. The oral dose of vitamin K is double of the parenteral dose.

The therapeutic dose of vitamin K for treatment of classical-HDN is 1 to 2 mg intravenously or subcutaneously which is followed by dramatic response with correction of coagulation abnormalities within 24 hours. It should not be given intramuscularly due to risk of development of hematoma. Infants predisposed to develop early-HDN (as evidenced by maternal intake of drugs known to deplete coagulation factors) should receive vitamin K_1 2 mg intravenously at birth. They may be delivered by cesarean section to to reduce the risk of trauma due to vaginal delivery. High-risk infants, predisposed to develop late-HDN due to chronic diarrhea, cholestasis, and sterilization of gut should receive daily supplements of 50–100 µg of vitamin K or monthly intramuscular injection of 1.0 mg of vitamin K till underlying disorder is controlled. For life-threatening hemorrhage, administration of vitamin K should be followed with 10 to 20 mL/kg of fresh frozen plasma. In any hemorrhagic disorder, if more than 20% blood has been lost or if there are evidences of shock, immediate blood transfusion would be life saving.

Hepatic Insufficiency

Liver damage due to hepatitis, anoxia, immaturity, metabolic disorders such as galactosemia, fructosemia and severe rhesus isoimmunization may lead to deficiency of coagulation factors which are manufactured in the liver. Jaundice and other evidences of hepatic dysfunction would be associated. There is no thrombocytopenia.

Inherited Deficiency of Coagulation Factors

Classical hemophilia (AHG or Factor VIII deficiency), Christmas disease (PTC or Factor IX deficiency), von Willebrand's disease and afibrinogenemia may manifest in the neonatal period, if deficiency is marked. Neither Factor VIII nor Factor IX crosses the placenta. Nearly one-third to one-half of patients with hemophilia develop bleeding during the neonatal period. Bleeding may follow circumcision, heel-stick punctures and umbilical stump. Intracranial bleeding may occur following traumatic delivery. The PTT is prolonged but PT and platelet count are always normal.

Maternal Medications

The deficiency of vitamin K-dependent coagulation factors may be induced in the fetus, if mother has received prolonged therapy with coumarin derivatives, salicylates, barbiturates, phenytoin, mysoline, primidone, INH and rifampicin during pregnancy. Mother should be given 10 mg vitamin K intramuscularly 24 hours before delivery. The bleeding can be prevented or controlled readily by administration of vitamin K to the baby.

THROMBOCYTOPENIA OR QUALITATIVE DEFECTS OF PLATELETS

Megakaryocytes are seen in the yolk sac by 5 weeks of gestation and in the liver and spleen by 10 weeks. The fetal platelet count is around $1,50,000/mm^3$ at the end of first trimester. Platelet count increases linearly as pregnancy advances attaining a mean count of $2,70,000/mm^3$ at 40 weeks.

Functional disorders of platelets may be congenital (Glanzmann's thrombasthenia) or acquired as a consequence of drugs administered to the mother or the infant (aspirin, indomethacin, phenothiazines, furosemide, tricyclic antidepressants, theophylline, and sodium valproate). Thrombocytopenia is diagnosed, if platelet count is less than $100,000/mm^3$. In a peripheral smear finding of 3 to 10 platelets per oil immersion field is considered as normal (multiply this number by 15,000–20,000 to get rough platelet count).

Immune Disorders

Passively transferred from the mother Idiopathic thrombocytopenic purpura and systemic lupus erythematosus may be associated with thrombocytopenia in the baby. Infact, thrombocytopenia in the neonate may be the presenting sign of ITP or SLE in an asymptomatic mother. There may be maternal history of ITP, maternal thrombocytopenia and antiplatelet IgG antibodies in the mother. When disease is active, mother should receive corticosteroid therapy for 10 to 14 days prior to delivery. Certain drugs such as sulfonamides, sedormid, quinine and quinidine, when taken by the pregnant woman, get tagged to the platelets to confer them antigenic properties. The platelet antibodies are transferred to the fetus through the placenta and cause damage and destruction of fetal platelets. In all these situations, maternal thromboyctopenia is also associated.

Platelet isoimmunization Platelet group incompatibility between the mother and fetus may result in platelet isoimmunization or alloimmunization on the analogy of rhesus incompatibility. The incidence of clinically manifest neonatal alloimmune thrombocytopenia (NAIT) is 1 in 1500 pregnancies and HPA-1

or HPA-4 antigen system is most commonly implicated. The mother will not have any thrombocytopenia but would show high titers of complement fixing antibodies (anti-HPA-1 or 4) against baby's platelets. There may be family history of neonatal thrombocytopenia in successive pregnancies. Almost one-half of the patients may manifest with fetal intracranial hemorrhage. After birth, platelet count may continue to fall for a week or so and then it gradually rises during 1–12 weeks of age.

Depression of Megakaryocytes in the Bone Marrow

Septicemia, intrauterine infections especially rubella, cytomegalovirus, toxoplasmosis and syphilis may be associated with thrombocytopenia and hepatic damage. Maternal medications with thiazides, tolbutamide, vancomycin and hydralazine during pregnancy may cause reduction in white blood cells and megakaryocytes in the bone marrow. Heparin administration to the mother may be associated with thrombocytopenia by formation of an antibody that crossreacts with platelets and endothelium. Congenital leukemia may be associated with thrombocytopenia. Neutropenia and thrombocytopenia have been documented in association with severe Rh-HDN due to marked erythropoiesis in the bone marrow.

Hereditary Disorders

Wiskott-Aldrich syndrome (WAS), a sex-linked recessive disorder, is characterized by triad of infantile eczema, recurrent viral and bacterial infections and thrombocytopenia. Children with recurrent infections or abnormal immunoglobulin levels should receive timely IVIG infusions. All patients should receive *Pneumocystis jerovecii* prophylaxis with administration trimethoprim-sulfamethoxazole or an equivalent agent. Deformity and shortening of forearm due to absent radii in association with amegakaryocytic bone marrow has been documented. Congenital pancytopenia (Fanconi's anemia) with or without associated anomalies is a rare cause of thrombocytopenia during neonatal period. The rare genetic syndromes of thrombocytopenia include familial macrothrombocytopenias (Bernard-Soulier syndrome, May-Hegglin anomaly), chromosomal disorders (Trisomy 13,18, 21,Turner syndrome), Noonan syndrome, Alport syndrome and inherited metabolic disorders.

Sequestration of Platelets

Thrombocytopenia may occur in association with giant hemangioma (Kasabach-Merritt syndrome), indwelling catheters, renal vein thrombosis, polycythemia, necrotizing enterocolitis, intracardiac thrombosis, placental vascular thrombi (pre-eclampsia, eclampsia) and cyanotic congenital heart disease. Babies born to mothers with PIH, especially those born preterm and growth retarded, are likely to have both thrombocytopenia and neutropenia. The mechanism of neutropenia appears to be decreased production because of an unidentified inhibitor while the cause of thrombocytopenia is not clear. PIH-related thrombocytopenia presents at birth, reaches its nadir on day 2 or 3 and usually resolves within 7–10 days.

Idiopathic Thrombocytopenia

In about 60% cases of neonatal thrombocytopenia, no cause is found even on detailed investigations. The platelet count usually varies between 50,000 and 100,000/mm^3 and invariably resolves by day 10.

COMBINED COAGULATION AND PLATELET DEFECTS

Disseminated Intravascular Coagulation (DIC)

It is an important cause of bleeding in sick preterm babies and occurs in about 10% of sick infants admitted to the NICU. The various predisposing factors include immaturity, septicemia, asphyxia, hypothermia, acidosis, hyaline membrane disease, shock and severe rhesus isoimmunization. Tissue or endothelial damage due to necrotizing enterocolitis and abruptio placentae results in release of thromboplastin material. The stagnation of red blood cells due to poor peripheral circulation as a result of hypothermia and shock leads to anoxic tissue damage which initiates intravascular coagulation. The release of thromboplastic material from disintegrating red blood cells and their precursors in patients with severe rhesus isoimmunization may further activate coagulation. The accumulation of fibrin thrombi in various organs may be cleared by reticuloendothelial system or by activation of fibrinolytic system. The resultant accumulation of fibrin degradation products (FDP) by latter mechanism further aggravates bleeding manifestations as they are known to interfere with conversion of fibrinogen to fibrin and cause platelet dysfunction. The widespread intravascular coagulation leads to consumption of platelets and other coagulation factors.

Clinical Features

The clinical picture is dominated by the predisposing factors or underlying disease process that initiated the widespread intravascular coagulation. The infant is critically ill and is often hypothermic, acidotic, hypovolemic, and anemic. Tissue hypoxia due to extensive areas of thrombosis may produce localizing symptoms in the form of purpura fulminans, necrotizing enterocolitis and cerebral infarction. The generalized bleeding tendency is manifest by oozing from venipuncture sites, intracranial and pulmonary hemorrhage.

Diagnosis

The laboratory evidences for the diagnosis of disseminated intravascular coagulation include thrombocytopenia, fragmented erythrocytes due to microangiopathy, prolonged PT and PTT, plasma fibrinogen of less than 100 mg/dL; abnormal reports of screening tests for Factors V and VIII (thrombotest of 10% or less and thromboplastin generation test of greater than 20 seconds), presence of circulating fibrin degradation products (>100 μg/dL) and demonstration of intravascular fibrin in the tissues of those babies who succumb to hemorrhagic diathesis. Elevated levels of d-dimers (>0.5 mg/mL) in blood are diagnostic of DIC, deep vein thrombosis and pulmonary embolism. d-Dimers are formed by action of plasmin on the fibrin clot.

Vascular Defects

In preterm babies, the presence of increased vascular permeability may aggravate bleeding. Germinal layer hemorrhage with resultant periventricular-intraventricular bleeding is believed to be caused by anoxic and hypercapnic capillary damage in preterm babies. Acute peptic ulceration and hematemesis may occur following asphyxia and intracranial birth trauma. Bleeding may occur from hemangioma and vascular malformations of the skin or gastrointestinal tract.

Local or Traumatic Causes

These may or may not be associated with any coagulation disorder or vascular defect.

  i. Umbilical cord bleeding due to slipped ligatures or laceration of cord during delivery.
 ii. Bruising and petechiae on the presenting part due to increased cephalic venous pressure.
iii. Traumatic bleeding because of stiff catheters, tubes, rectal thermometer, etc.
 iv. Cephalhematoma and subgaleal hemorrhage.
  v. Capsular tears in the liver or spleen. The bleeding from these sites commonly follows difficult breech extraction.

Hematologic Problems

23

vi. Gastrointestinal bleeding. Swallowed maternal blood, acute peptic ulceration, perforation of gut, volvulus and necrotizing enterocolitis should be considered in the differential diagnosis. In neonates with gastrointestinal bleeding, X-ray abdomen must be taken as a routine to exclude perforation.

vii. Subconjunctival hemorrhage. These occur possibly due to increased cerebral venous pressure during passage through the birth canal. Large babies of multiparous mothers and those of Negro or Asiatic origin are more susceptible to develop subconjunctival hemorrhages.

viii. Retinal hemorrhage. These are common in normal babies and are of no pathological significance but may be associated with polycythemia and increased viscosity of blood. They may at times be large and subhyaloid but vision is invariably spared.

Clinical Features due to Bleeding

The site and severity of blood loss would determine the clinical manifestations. Bleeding from gastro-intestinal tract, umbilical cord and subaponeurotic scalp hemorrhage are common in association with classical hemorrhagic disease of the newborn while intracranial and pulmonary hemorrhages are usually seen in association with disseminated intravascular coagulation. The excessive bleeding from injection sites may occur in both the conditions. The presence of clinical signs of acute blood loss such as pallor, rapid breathing, rising heart rate and falling blood pressure indicate that baby has lost at least 10% of his blood volume. An accurate estimation of previous and concurrent blood loss should be maintained to guide therapy. The level of hemoglobin and hematocit immediately following acute blood loss is of limited value and they should be repeated 12 hours later when full hemodilution would have taken place. The presence of internal hemorrhage and collection of blood in tissues contribute to excessive bilirubin production due to disintegration of red blood cells and may manifest as hyperbilirubinemia.

Diagnosis

When vomiting of blood and melena is the sole manifestation during the first 48 hours, the possibility of swallowed maternal blood should be excluded by doing the **Apt and Downey test** as follows:

One part of vomitus or stool is mixed with 5 parts of distilled water and centrifuged. The supernatant should be pink before proceeding further. Add 1 mL of 1% sodium hydroxide solution to the supernatant and wait for 1 to 2 minutes. If the solution changes to yellow-brown color, it favors the possibility of swallowed maternal blood (adult hemoglobin gets denatured by the alkali) while in case of fetal blood the solution remains pink and unaltered. Two controls should be run alongside by taking two drops of blood each from a baby and an adult and by repeating the procedure.

A detailed history should be taken regarding various drugs taken by the mother during pregnancy and her health status with particular reference to any bleeding diathesis. Mother's VDRL, rhesus blood group and any possibility of infective illness during pregnancy should be checked. The type, site and age at onset of bleeding offer useful diagnostic clues. The feeding schedule and status of vitamin K prophylaxis should be enquired. On the basis of clinical examination, the bleeding neonate should be classified into "sick" and "well" neonate which offers useful diagnostic clues as shown in Table 23.2. The flowcharts outline the clinical approach for further investigations and diagnosis of bleeding disorder (Figures 23.1 and 23.2). The blood sample must be collected for coagulation studies and other investigations before giving transfusion otherwise retrospective diagnosis of the cause would remain uncertain.

Management

In all cases of bleeding in a newborn baby, vitamin K* 2 mg intravenous or subcutaneous should be given as soon as blood has been collected for investigations. If the baby has any clinical signs of blood loss or if estimated blood loss exceeds 20% of his blood volume, a blood transfusion should be given immediately. The amount to be transfused depends upon the estimate of blood loss failing which 30 mL/kg may be given for the first transfusion. The initial 20–40 mL of blood should be given rapidly for which umbilical vein catheterization may be preferred. In cases of severe anemia due to prolonged slow bleeding, partial exchange blood transfusion is recommended to avoid over loading the circulation. The vital signs, concurrent estimate of blood loss, hemoglobin and hematocrit should be monitored to determine the need for subsequent transfusions. In gastrointestinal bleeding, X-ray abdomen

---

*Naturally occurring vitamins K_1 (phylloquinone) and K_2 (menaquinone) are preferred because of rapidity of response and lack of any risk of producing hyperbilirubinemia.

TABLE 23.2 Simple diagnostic approach in a bleeding neonate

Platelets	PT	PTT	Diagnostic possibilities
"Sick" neonate			
Decreased	Increased	Increased	Disseminated intravascular coagulation
Decreased	Normal	Normal	Platelet-consumption (infection, necrotizing enterocolitis, vascular thromboses, giant hemangioma, polycythemia)
Normal	Increased	Increased	Liver disease, heparinization
Normal	Normal	Normal	Altered vascular integrity (e.g. extreme prematurity, severe hypoxia and acidosis, hyperosmolality).
"Well" neonate			
Decreased	Normal	Normal	Immune thrombocytopenia, thrombosis, hypoplasia of bone marrow
Normal	Increased	Increased	Hemorrhagic disease of the newborn
Normal	Normal	Increased	Hereditary clotting factor deficiencies
Normal	Normal	Normal	Bleeding due to local factors (trauma, anatomic abnormalities), qualitative platelet abnormalities (rare), disrupted vessel from anatomical lesion (e.g. ulcer, hemangioma), swallowed maternal blood.

Adapted from Pramanik AK. The bleeding neonate. In: Medical Emergencies in Children. Singh M (*Ed.*) CBS Publishers and Distributors Pvt Ltd, New Delhi Revised 5th ed. 2016, 306–336.

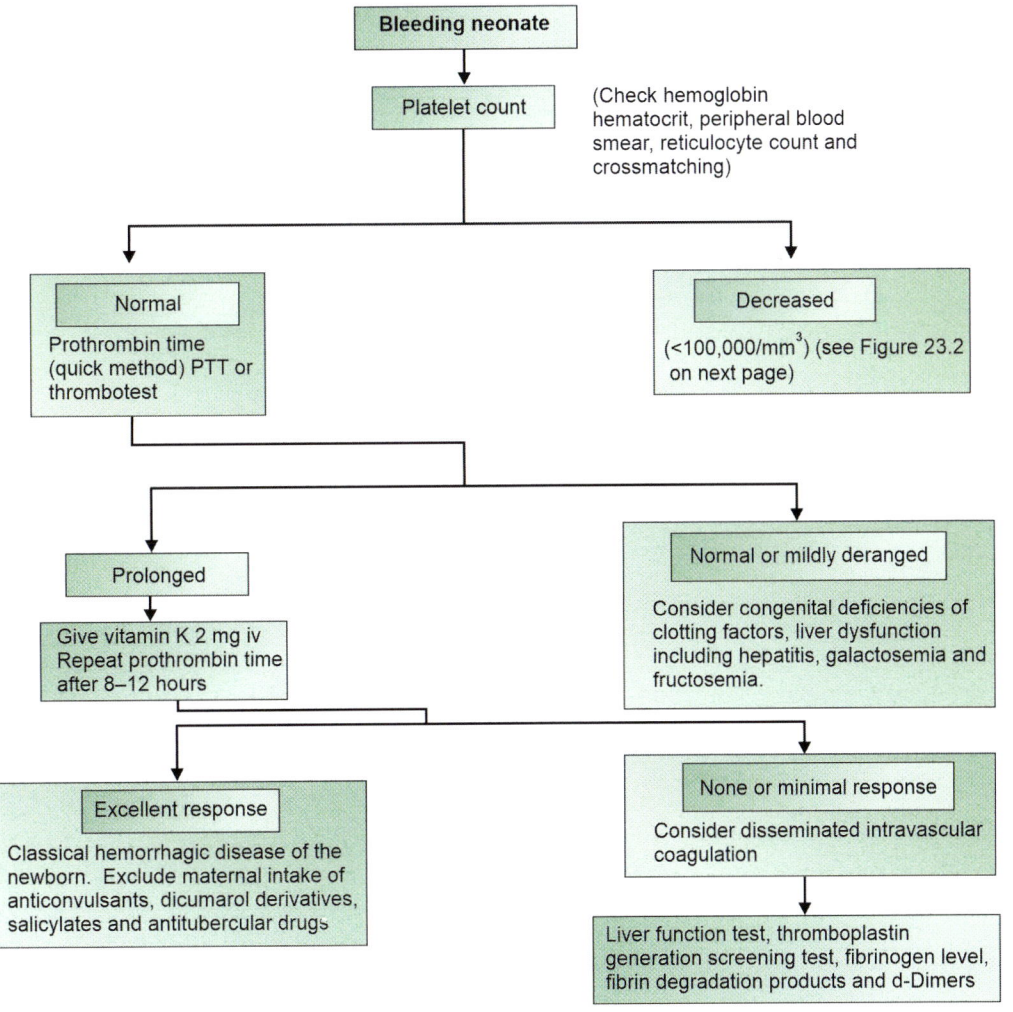

Figure 23.1 Algorithm for an approach to a bleeding neonate.

Hematologic Problems

23

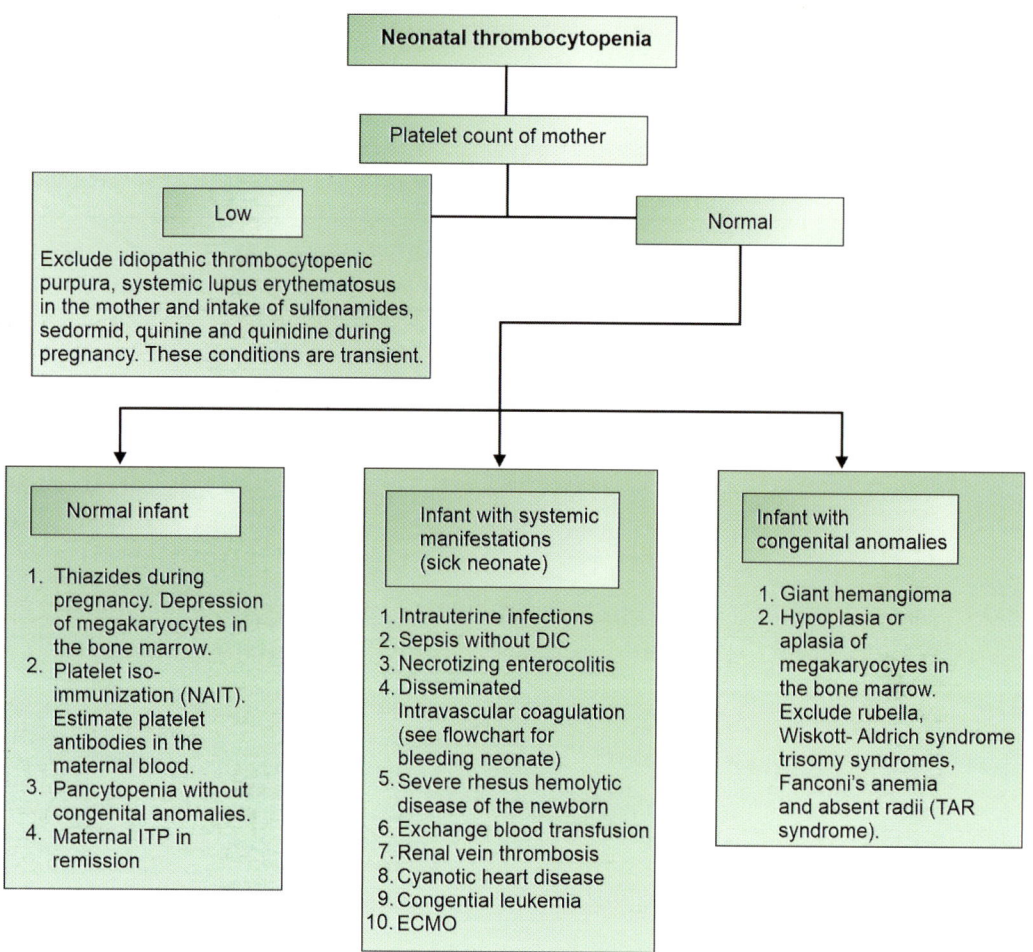

Figure 23.2 Algorithm for diagnostic approach to thrombocytopenia in a neonate.
NAIT: Neonatal alloimmune thrombocytopenia, ECMO: Extracorporeal membrane oxygenation, ITP: Idiopathic thrombocytopenic purpura, TAR: Thrombocytopenia and absent radii.

must be taken to exclude perforation and other surgical conditions.

If thrombocytopenia or deficiency of clotting factors is present, it is best to use fresh blood for transfusion. When facilities are available, fresh platelet infusions are ideal for the treatment of thrombocytopenia from any cause and fresh frozen plasma transfusion is more useful when deficiency of clotting factors do not respond to administration of vitamin K. In patients with disseminated intravascular coagulation, treatment should be initiated with fresh frozen plasma 10–15 mL/kg and one unit of fresh platelet concentrate every 12 to 24 hours. When fresh frozen plasma and platelet concentrate are not available, frequent administration of fresh blood (10–15 mL/kg every 12–24 hours) may prove life saving. If bleeding is intractable, exchange transfusion with fresh heparinized or CPD blood may be tried though its role is controversial. It removes circulating fibrin degradation products and provides clotting factors and platelets. The tissue oxygenation

is also improved by exchange transfusion because adult hemoglobin has lower affinity for oxygen which is readily released to the tissues. The use of heparin is controversial. It is indicated in infants with wide spread thrombosis with gangrenous necrosis of skin (purpura fulminans). Heparin is given as a bolus of 25–35 units/kg followed by 10–15 units/kg/hr as a continuous infusion to maintain activated partial thromboplastin time (aPTT) and international normalized ratio (INR) at 1.5 to 2 times of normal. Administration of appropriate antibiotics and supportive therapy to correct shock, hypoxia, acidosis and hypothermia must receive due attention. The outcome is generally poor in these patients because of involvement of vital organs by the hemorrhagic manifestations.

Infants with symptomatic thrombocytopenia, due to maternal lupus erythematosus, may need short term corticosteroid therapy. The mother with active ITP should receive a course of corticosteroid therapy for 10 to 14 days prior to delivery. The use of IVIG to the mother is controversial. The infant should preferably be delivered by cesarean section and given short course of prednisolone 2 mg/kg/day. Recently, some workers have successfully used high doses of intravenous gamma globulins (0.4 g/kg/day IV for 2 to 5 days or 1 g/kg/day for 2 days) in these infants. Pancytopenia on rare occasions may respond to cortisone and/or testosterone.

Alloimmune fetal thrombocytopenia is rare and occurs when mother is human platelet antigen (PIA-1) negative while father or fetus is PIA-1 positive. There may be history of recurrent fetal hemorrhages including a similar history among mother's sister/s. Intravenous immunoglobulins (IVIG) and prenatal steroids to the mother and platelet transfusion to the fetus through cordocentesis are useful. Infant should preferably be delivered by cesarean section. Mother's platelets should be collected 24 hours before delivery. They should be washed and suspended in plasma to get rid of PIA-1 or PIA-4 antibodies present in the maternal serum. Platelet transfusion is given to the baby, if there is active bleeding or platelet count is <20,000/mm³. Random donor platelets are used, if there is serious bleeding and PIA-1 negative platelets are not available. The giant hemangioma with Kasabach-Merritt syndrome is treated with platelet transfusion, clotting factors, prednisolone and alpha-interferon. Spontaneous involution occurs by 1 to 2 years and surgical excision should be limited to intractable cases.

Irradiated CMV-negative platelet concentrate, preferably ABO compatible, should be used to treat thrombocytopenia. Platelet transfusion is given, if platelet count is less than 100,000/mm³ in a baby having active bleeding or less than 30,000/mm³ (<50,000/mm³ in babies <1500 g) in an asymptomatic baby. One unit of platelet prepared from whole blood or by platelet pharesis is usually sufficient to increase the platelet count by approximately 100,000/mm³ in a 3 kg infant. The normal half-life of transfused platelets is 4–5 days. After transfusion, platelet count should be checked after 6 hours. When there is a good increment in platelet count, it is indicative of platelet under production and good prognosis. However, a poor platelet increment suggests platelet consumption disorder and relatively poor outcome. There is a growing evidence that inadequate megakaryocytopoiesis is a major cause of neonatal thrombocytopenia. In the near future, rhTPO (recombinant human thrombopoietin) and interleukin-11, which is a hematopoietic growth factor, are likely to be used to enhance megakaryocytopoiesis.

ANEMIA

Fetal Erythropoiesis

During fetal life, erythropoiesis begins by about 6th gestational week. Fetal erythropoiesis is endogenously controlled by erythropoietin produced by the fetus because maternal erythropoietin does not cross the placenta. The increased affinity of fetal hemoglobin for uptake of oxygen is related to low levels of 2, 3-diphosphoglycerate (2, 3-DPG). During fetal life, RBC production is rapid because of high levels of erythropoietin which is mostly produced in fetal liver. The switch over from fetal to adult hemoglobin synthesis follows a sigmoid curve and by 30 to 32 weeks of gestation, hemoglobin A is being produced in significant amounts. The red blood cells containing adult hemoglobin have higher levels of 2, 3-DPG with gradual rightward shift of hemoglobin-oxygen dissociation curve facilitating release of oxygen to the tissues.

The level of hemoglobin at birth is unrelated to the nutritional status of the mother but infants born to iron deficient mothers are likely to have poor stores of iron and greater incidence and severity of late-onset physiological anemia. At term, cord hemoglobin is 14–18 g/dL with hematocrit of 50 to 55%. The hemoglobin and hematocrit values in the capillary blood sample are about 5% higher than the simultaneous venous sample, due to stasis in the capillaries with transudation of plasma. During the first 6 hours, hemoglobin and hematocrit rises due to the effect of placental transfusion and delay in feeding. Subsequently, a gradual fall in hemoglobin continues up to 8 to 12 weeks of age when it reaches a level of 11 g/dL. At term, cord blood contains 5 to 10 nucleated red blood cells per 100 white blood cells. The evidences of hyperactive red cell proliferation at birth disappear by the end of first week indicating that hypoxic stimulation to red cell production *in utero* is lost following a rise in arterial oxygen tension to 95% after birth (fetal aortic saturation is around 45%). The gradual fall in hemoglobin during early life occurs because of following factors:

a. The newer red blood cells are smaller in size and have lower hemoglobin content.

b. The production of red blood cells and hemoglobin does not keep pace with body growth and increase in blood volume.

c. The fetal hyperactivity of bone marrow is replaced by relative hypoactivity due to low levels of erythropoietin during the phase of change over from fetal to adult hemoglobin production.

The infant may be born anemic or develop anemia after a few days or weeks.

Hemorrhagic Anemia

About 5 to 10% cases of neonatal anemia are due to blood loss.

Fetal Hemorrhage

The fetal bleeding may occur from placenta, umbilical cord or inside the fetal tissues. The bleeding from umbilical cord and placenta may manifest with antepartum hemorrhage which can be tested for the presence of fetal blood.

Placental Bleeding

Bleeding may occur due to placenta previa, abruptio placentae with or without retroplacental hemorrhage or clots and accidental bleeding, rupture of marginal sinus and accidental incision of placenta during cesarean section.

Twin-to-twin transfusion It occurs in about 15% of monochorionic twins having arteriovenous shunts in the placenta. The recipient twin would be large and plethoric while the donor twin is small, anemic and malnourished but both have an identical risk of morbidity. Hemoglobin difference of greater than 5 g per 100 mL between the two twins is suggestive of twin-to-twin transfusion.

Fetomaternal transfusion Fetomaternal hemorrhage of mild nature occurs in almost 50% of pregnancies but may be severe enough to cause anemia in about 1%. It may be chronic and manifest as iron deficiency anemia at birth with or without cardiac failure or more commonly acute fetomaternal hemorrhage during delivery manifests with severe anemia and shock. Chronic fetal-to-maternal hemorrhage is characterized by anemia, reticulocytosis (>10%) and presence of fetal RBCs in maternal circulation (Kleihauer-Betke count). External podalic version, amniocentesis, cesarean section (baby is held above the level of mother) and manual removal of placenta often predispose and aggravate fetomaternal hemorrhage. Tight nuchal cord may lead to fetoplacental bleeding.

Bleeding from Umbilical Cord

Rupture of normal cord The rupture or laceration of normal umbilical cord is rare but may occur, if it is short and following precipitate unattended delivery.

Rupture of diseased cord Aneurysm or focal weakness of umbilical cord due to intrauterine infections such as syphilis may predispose to rupture.

Anomalous vessels of cord Velamentous insertion of cord, when the umbilical cord inserts in the membranes a variable distance proximal to the placental surface, predisposes to the occurrence of bleeding from umbilical vessels unsupported by Wharton's jelly. Bleeding may occur in a case of vasa previa where the umbilical vessels are lying over the cervical os.

Internal Hemorrhage in the Fetus

Fetal hemorrhage may occur due to deficiency of vitamin K dependent factors following maternal intake of coumarin derivatives, salicylates, anticonvulsants, INH and rifampicin. In alloimmune thrombocytopenia, fetal hemorrhage may occur but it is rare in cases of autoimmune thrombocytopenia. Capsular tears in the liver and spleen can occur following difficult breech extraction and would manifest with severe anemia and shock at birth.

Neonatal Hemorrhage

Hemorrhage in the newborn may be associated with a variety of disorders. The common causes of neonatal bleeding include cephalhematoma or subgaleal blood loss, bleeding from umbilical stump, GI bleeding (vitamin K deficiency, stress ulcer, NEC, nasogastric catheter), intraventricular hemorrhage and disseminated intravascular coagulation. Iatrogenic blood loss following frequent blood sampling for various investigations is a relatively frequent cause of anemia in a sick neonate. It should be remembered that removal of about 10 mL of blood from a neonate, weighing 1500 g constitutes a loss of about 8% of his blood volume (equivalent to about 400 mL of blood in an adult).

Hemolytic Anemia

Hemolysis is the most frequent cause of anemia in the newborn though the clinical picture is often dominated by jaundice and hepatosplenomegaly rather than anemia.

Isoimmunization due to fetomaternal blood group incompatibility In addition to early anemia in severely affected infants, anemia of sufficient severity may manifest after 2 to 4 weeks due to continuing hemolysis.

Congenital hemolytic anemia Glucose-6-phosphate dehydrogenase deficiency, pyruvate-kinase deficiency, hereditary spherocytosis and elliptocytosis may occasionally manifest in the newborn. Homozygous alpha thalassemia often manifests with life-threatening anemia and hydrops at birth. Maternal autoimmune hemolytic disease, lupus erythematosus and drug-induced Heinz body formation may rarely cause fetal hemolytic anemia.

Infections Hemolysis, bone narrow depression, disseminated intravascular coagulation, and blood loss may all contribute to the development of anemia in various fetal and neonatal infections.

Anemia of Prematurity

Preterm babies often become significantly anemic after 4 to 8 weeks. Physiological anemia is early and more severe in preterm babies due to rapid growth velocity and reduced materno-fetal transfer of vitamin E, folic acid, vitamin B_{12} and iron. RBC survival is reduced in preterm babies compared to the term. Early administration of iron (2–4 mg/kg/d) does not modify the course of early physiological anemia of prematurity but would prevent the occurrence of late-onset physiological anemia around 6 to 8 months of age. In babies weighing less than 1800 g, folic acid deficiency may exist but its role in the development of early-onset anemia of prematurity is doubtful. Vitamin E dependent hemolytic anemia has been reported in very low birth weight babies (<1500 g). There is excessive iatrogenic loss of blood due to frequent sampling. The nadir of hemoglobin of 9 g/dL is seen around 6–8 weeks in infants below 1500 g or <32 weeks gestation.

Miscellaneous Conditions

Anemia following exchange blood transfusion Exchange transfusion in the newborn baby is often followed by anemia because of low hemoglobin content of CPD-blood used for exchange. Folic acid deficiency may also occur because folic acid content of stored adult red blood cells is lower compared to fetal red cells.

Pancytopenia or erythroid hypoplasia (Diamond-Blackfan syndrome) Congenital red cell aplasia (erythrogenesis imperfecta) may manifest in the newborn period with anemia, reticulocytopenia, triphalangeal thumbs and Turner syndrome.

Leukemia It is rare. It is often associated with Down syndrome and the peripheral blood picture is suggestive of acute myeloblastic type. The clinical picture is characterized by anemia, hepatosplenomegaly, bleeding manifestations and discrete firm purple subcutaneous nodules. The outlook is generally poor and death occurs within 3 months of age.

Osteopetrosis Severe anemia, thrombocytopenia, hepatosplenomegaly, optic atrophy and hydrops fetalis may be present at birth. There is generalized increase in bone density.

TORCH infections Intrauterine infections especially rubella and parvovirus infection may be associated with anemia and thrombocytopenia.

Diagnosis

Infants born with acute blood loss during or before delivery are often limp, pale and in shock. They must be differentiated from severely asphyxiated babies with circulatory collapse because of life-saving therapeutic implications (refer to Chapter 6). The presence of antepartum hemorrhage and evidence of blood loss from placenta and/or umbilical cord should alert to the possibility of fetal hemorrhage. The vaginal blood can be tested for the presence of fetal hemoglobin. Initial hematocrit (which must be done on venous blood) may be normal but repeat hematocrit after 4–8 hours may reveal low hematocrit following hemodilution.

The hematological evidences of iron deficiency anemia at birth would suggest the possibility of chronic feto-fetal or feto-maternal hemorrhage. The presence of jaundice with or without hepatosplenomegaly is suggestive of hemolytic anemia and perinatal infections which can be confirmed by appropriate laboratory tests. The presence of reticulocytosis in cord blood is characteristic of hemolytic states but may also be seen in preterm babies, intrauterine growth retardation, perinatal hypoxia, chronic feto-maternal transfusion and cyanotic heart disease. Reticulocyte count is low in infections and bone marrow hypoplasia.

The diagnosis and severity of fetomaternal hemorrhage can be confirmed by testing maternal blood by **Kleihauer-Betke technique**.

Principle

At acidic pH, adult hemoglobin can be eluted from intact red blood cells while fetal hemoglobin is resistant to acid elution. The fetal red blood cells remain darkly stained while adult red blood cells would appear like ghost cells following acid elution.

Reagents

- Ethanol 80%
- Citric acid 0.1 M (stock solution A)

- Disodium hydrogen phosphate 0.2 M (stock solution B). For working buffer (pH 3.3) 73.4 parts of stock solution A are mixed with 26.6 parts of stock solution B
- Acid hematoxylin
- Eosin B 0.1%.

Procedure

1. Fill staining dish with buffer solution and incubate at 37 °C for 15 minutes.
2. Make a thin smear of maternal blood (may be diluted with normal saline) on a glass slide. Oxalated or finger prick blood may be taken. Make control smears from a newborn baby and normal adult.
3. Fix the slides by covering with 80% ethanol for 5 minutes. Rinse in tap water and dry.
4. Immerse the slides in buffer solution for 5 minutes. Agitate at 1 and 3 minutes.
5. Rinse in tap water and dry.
6. Stain with acid hematoxylin for 3 minutes and rinse with tap water. Stain with eosin for 4 minutes and rinse with tap water and let dry.
7. Count total RBCs/HPF in 5 fields and calculate the mean RBC count/HPF. Count the fetal (deeply staining) RBCs in 30 high power fields and calculate their percentage. Fetal cell count of 1% is equivalent to about 50 mL of fetal blood loss.

Kleihauer technique is more sensitive as compared to estimation of fetal hemoglobin in maternal blood. The fetal hemoglobin would rise by only 1% following 50 mL of fetomaternal hemorrhage. Moreover, all fetal red blood cells may not contain 100% fetal hemoglobin but for Kleihauer count, fetal hemoglobin content of up to 20% is good enough to pick up fetal red blood cells. The presence of maternal thalassemia minor, sickle cell anemia and hereditary persistence of fetal hemoglobin may give false positive indication of fetomaternal hemorrahge by acid elution technique of Kleihauer. On the other hand, the presence of fetomaternal ABO incompatibility may give false negative result because fetal cells may be eliminated by maternal antibodies.

Management

The presence of acute blood loss with tachycardia and circulatory collapse at birth should be treated with immediate blood transfusion. Estimation of hemoglobin or hematocrit at birth may not show any evidence of blood loss unless it is repeated 4 to 8 hours later when anemia may be manifest. The amount of blood to be transfused depends upon the estimate of blood loss which can be assessed by Kleihauer-Betke technique and from blood volume or arterial pressure of the infant. Initially 20–30 mL/kg should be given rapidly to correct shock and in a life-threatening situation, O Rh negative blood may be given without crossmatching. Infants with severe erythroblastosis with cord hemoglobin of 10 g or less per 100 mL should receive partial exchange transfusion with packed red blood cells. Administration of furosemide and monitoring of venous pressure during the procedure would safeguard against cardiac failure. For management of blood loss following neonatal bleeding, refer to p 460.

Babies with early anemia of prematurity rarely need blood transfusion and it should be avoided, if reticulocyte response is good. The fall of hemoglobin to less than 8 g/dL (hematocrit <25%) due to any cause or presence of symptoms, such as feeding difficulty, breathlessness, apneic attacks, tachycardia and poor weight gain, is best treated by giving blood transfusion to raise hemoglobin level up to 12 g per 100 mL. During transfusion, care should be taken to avoid precipitating cardiac failure and baby should be watched closely for tachypnea and tachycardia. For detailed indications and risk of blood transfusion in newborn babies, refer to p 470. The use of recombinant human erythropoietin (rh-EPO) is limited due to its exhorbitant cost and controversial benefits. Its use may reduce the frequency and volume of RBC transfusions in VLBW babies. It may be given to clinically stable infants with a birth weight of <1500 g or gestation of <32 weeks, infants with bronchopulmonary dysplasia and cyanotic congenital heart disease. It is given in a dose of 600–750 iu/kg once a week subcutaneously for 2–6 weeks or up to the post conceptional maturity of 36 weeks. Iron supplementation should be provided orally in a dose of 4–6 mg/kg/d in two divided doses. Adequate intake of protein is also essential for optimal response to rh-EPO therapy.

In view of low iron stores in infants born to anemic mothers and relatively high incidence of maternal anemia in developing countries, all term babies should receive prophylactic iron (2 mg/kg/day) after 12 weeks of age. Iron supplementation (2–4 mg/kg/d) is started in preterm babies as soon as full enteral feeds are established. Iron prophylaxis does not modify the course of early anemia of prematurity but incidence of late physiological anemia around 6 months of age is reduced. Folic acid supplementation is recommended to all low birth weight babies and those who undergo exchange blood transfusion. Infants with a birth weight of less than 1500 g shall benefit by receiving vitamin E (15 iu/day) till they reach a conceptional age of about 36 weeks. Effective use of ultramicro-techniques for blood sampling is essential to prevent the occurrence of iatrogenic anemia.

POLYCYTHEMIA AND HYPERVISCOSITY

Polycythemia or 'thick' blood syndrome is a relatively common disorder and occurs in about 2 to 4% of all newborns. The incidence varies depending upon the obstetrical practice of early or delayed clamping of cord and the time of sampling. It is uncommon in preterm babies because hematocrit progressively increases as gestation advances. Hyperviscosity is associated with reduced blood flow or perfusion to various organs resulting in a variety of symptoms and signs of organ dysfunction. The major determinants of blood viscosity are number of erythrocytes, erythrocyte deformability, plasma proteins especially level of fibrinogen and lipids. *The diagnosis of polycythemia is made when venous or central hematocrit is greater than 65%.* Capillary blood hematocrit is usually higher than venous due to stasis and extravasation of fluid through capillaries. However, capillary blood obtained after warming the heel is quite satisfactory for routine screening of all newborn babies after the age of 4 hours. Infants with a capillary hematocrit level of 70% or more should be further investigated. When facilities exist, viscosity of venous blood should be measured with a microviscometer and shear rates greater than two standard deviations from the mean are suggestive of hyperviscosity. The relationship between hematocrit and viscosity is linear up to hematocrit of 60% but viscosity increases exponentially when hematocrit rises beyond 70%. Almost one-half of infants with polycythemia exhibit hyperviscosity.

Etiology

Delayed clamping or milking of cord is an important cause of polycythemia and hypervolemia. When clamping of cord is delayed more than three minutes after birth, a 30% increase in blood volume is noted. Materno-fetal transfusion occurs when baby is held too low following vaginal delivery. Twin-to-twin transfusion syndrome is an important cause of polycythemia in the recepient twin. Hematocrit and hemoglobin must be routinely checked in all cases of monochorionic twins. Infants of diabetic and sometimes thyrotoxic mothers have higher incidence of polycythemia. Hyperinsulinemia in the fetus is associated with increased levels of erythropoietin. Elevated blood glucose levels and osmotic diuresis in infants of diabetic women may lead to hyperviscosity

and its consequences out of proportion to levels of hematocrit. Polycythemia is common in infants with intrauterine growth retardation due to chronic placental insufficiency or postmaturity, high altitude habitat and maternal smoking. Other relatively uncommon causes of polycythemia include congenital adrenal hyperplasia, Beckwith-Wiedemann syndrome, cretinism, cyanotic congenital heart disease, and trisomy 13, 18 and 21 syndromes. Hemoconcentration due to dehydration may cause transient elevation of hematocrit and hyperviscosity.

Clinical Features

A variety of symptoms and signs may be produced because of sluggish circulation and hypoperfusion of various organs. Clinical manifestations referable to every system of the body have been documented. Cardiopulmonary features are characterized by tachypnea, tachycardia, cyanosis and cardiomegaly. Some of these infants present with a symptom complex of persistent fetal circulation and mimic congenital cyanotic heart disease. Central nervous system manifestations are characterized by apathy, lethargy, hypotonia and poor feeding. These features of CNS depression are often followed by irritability, tremulousness and seizures over next few hours. Transient renal failure or insufficiency may occur due to reduced perfusion of kidneys. Polycythemia and increased fragmentation of red blood cells may be associated with hyperbilirubinemia. Thrombocytopenia and sludging is associated with hypercoagulable state which can produce thrombotic complications including renal vein thrombosis. Engorgement of penis may lead to priapism. Hypoglycemia, hypocalcemia and hypomagnesemia are common metabolic complications especially in small-for-dates babies. Hypoglycemia may be intractable unless polycythemia is corrected. These metabolic alterations may account for some of the CNS manifestations. Necrotizing enterocolitis, especially following umbilical catheterization for exchange plasma transfusion is more common among polycythemic infants due to greater chances of mesenteric thrombosis.

Treatment

Unusual delay in clamping the cord should be avoided in high-risk situations for polycythemia. Hydration should be maintained by early feeding and hemoconcentration due to dehydration should be corrected by infusion of fluids. Hematocrit should be routinely checked at the age of 12 to 24 hours in all infants at

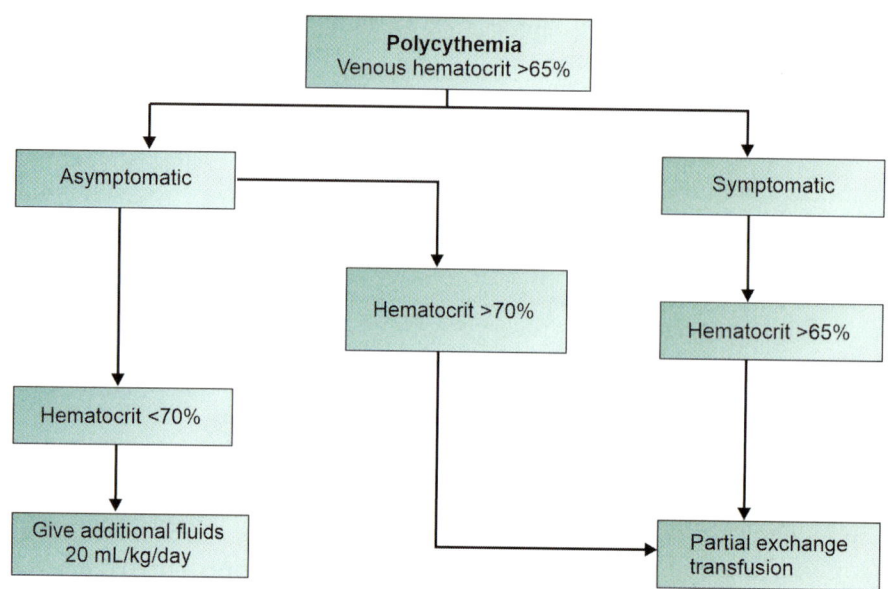

Figure 23.3 Algorithm for management of polycythemia.

increased risk to develop polycythemia (small-for-dates, large-for-dates, IDMs, twins, pre-eclampsia, eclampsia). Serum glucose, calcium and bilirubin should be monitored and appropriately managed. Hydration status should be assessed by recording weight, serum sodium, BUN and urinary specific gravity or osmolality. Phenobarbitone may be given for prophylaxis against hyperbilirubinemia to a large, polycythemic and bruised baby of a diabetic mother. Phlebotomy and/or partial plasma exchange transfusion are satisfactory procedures to reduce viscosity in symptomatic infants. The indications for partial exchange transfusion depend upon the level of venous hematocrit and whether infant is symptomatic or asymptomatic (Figure 23.3).

Partial exchange transfusion through umbilical route with fresh frozen plasma or physiological saline is the preferred mode of therapy. Exchange transfusion with physiological saline is associated with greater reduction in viscosity. The volume for exchange is determined by the following calculation:

$$\frac{\text{Observed venous Hct} - \text{Desired venous Hct}}{\text{Observed venous Hct}} \times \frac{\text{Blood}}{\text{volume}}$$

The desired venous hematocrit is taken as 50% and blood volume is calculated on the basis of 80 mL/kg and 100 mL/kg for term and preterm babies, respectively. Central venous pressure should be monitored during the procedure. Hematocrit and hemoglobin estimation should be repeated at the end of procedure. There are conflicting reports regarding the neurological

outcome of asymptomatic polycythemic infants on follow-up irrespective of treatment. Among symptomatic infants, preliminary follow-up observations suggest that neurologic sequelae are significantly less among infants treated with exchange transfusion.

ARTERIAL AND VENOUS THROMBOSES

Neonates have increased risk of thrombus formation due to decreased levels of protein C, protein S, plasminogen, anti-thrombin III and reduced prostacyclin-regenerating activity. Platelets aggregate and stick together more easily in neonates. The highest incidence of thrombosis in otherwise healthy subjects is seen during neonatal period.

Risk Factors

Preterm babies are more vulnerable to develop thrombosis because of decreased levels of antithrombin III and greater need for insertion of indwelling vascular catheters. Infants with birth asphyxia, polycythemia, congenital heart disease and IDMs are at an increased risk to develop thrombotic complications. Insertion of indwelling vascular catheters for diagnostic and therapeutic purposes is the leading cause of development of thrombosis.

Arterial Thrombosis

The clinical signs depend upon the vessel involved and site of obstruction. Thrombosis of peripheral artery is characterized by evidences of decreased perfusion, pallor, reduced pulsations and ischemic skin changes. Aortic thrombosis is characterized by reduced pulsations and perfusion of lower extremities, increased differential in blood pressure between upper and lower extremities, hypertension, hematuria, oliguria and congestive heart failure. Ultrasound with Doppler color flow imaging provides non-invasive technology for diagnosis. Radiographic contrast study may be required for confirmatory evidence, if ultrasound examination is inconclusive.

Treatment

Unnecessary arterial catheterization should be avoided. Heparinised saline (0.5–1.0 unit/mL) should be infused at a rate of 1–2 mL/hr with the help of an infusion pump to prevent the development of arterial thrombosis. When arterial thrombosis is diagnosed, the indwelling catheter should be removed and heparin therapy started. Heparin should be given through a dedicated IV line in a loading dose of 75 units/kg over 10 minutes followed by continuous infusion of 25 units/kg/hr. The partial thromboplastin time should be maintained at 2 to 3 times (60–85 seconds) of control. Check PT/PTT 4 hours after the loading dose and every 12–24 hours subsequently. Low molecular weight (LMW) heparin (2 mg/kg/dose) can be given subcutaneously every 12 hour and is safer with less stringent need for laboratory monitoring. If heparin therapy fails, urokinase may be given locally through the indwelling catheter or systemically to dissolve the thrombus. If there is no improvement and fibrinogen level remains high, consider infusion of 10 mL/kg of fresh frozen plasma. Tissue plasminogen activator (tPA) is available as an alternative to urokinase therapy. tPA is currently thrombolytic agent of choice due to reduced risk of allergic reactions and short half-life. If there is life-threatening bleeding due to thrombolytic therapy, cryoprecipitate (1 unit/5 kg) and amino caproic acid (100 mg/kg IV every 6 hr) may be life saving. Surgical thrombectomy should be avoided due to high risk of mortality.

Venous Thrombosis

The commonest cause of venous thrombosis is insertion of a central venous line (CVL). Spontaneous thrombosis of renal veins can occur in infants of diabetic mothers and polycythemic babies. The signs of venous obstruction include swelling and distension of veins proximal to the site of obstruction. Renal vein thrombosis presents with a triad of enlarged kidney, hematuria and thrombocytopenia. Ultrasound examination is a useful non-invasive method for the diagnosis of thrombosis of a major vein. Radiographic contrast study through central venous line would confirm the diagnosis, if ultrasound examination is equivocal. Venography through peripheral vessels in the upper extremities may provide diagnostic information in some cases.

Treatment

The CVL should be kept patent by constant infusion of heparinised saline (0.5–1.0 unit/mL) at a rate of 1–2 mL/hr to prevent development of venous thrombosis. Medical therapy is preferred over surgical thrombectomy. Urokinase infusion at a rate of 150 units/kg/hr through CVL may dissolve the thrombus. If the CVL is completely blocked, the catheter should be removed and heparin therapy started *vide-supra*. Heparin and thrombolytic therapy should not be given concurrently. During anticoagulation or thrombolytic therapy, intramuscular injections and arterial punctures should be avoided. Administration of fresh frozen plasma (10 mL/kg) often complements anticoagulation therapy.

TRANSFUSION OF BLOOD AND BLOOD COMPONENTS

Blood transfusion is a hazardous procedure in newborn babies with a potential risk of transmission of several diseases especially CMV in preterm infants. There is a risk of development of graft-versus-host disease (GVHD) which can be prevented by irradiation of blood especially in infants with combined immunodeficiency disorder. In neonates, component therapy is preferred because of lower risk of complications compared to whole blood transfusion. As many as 70–80% of very LBW babies require at least one transfusion. The development of iatrogenic anemia should be prevented by using microbiochemical techniques and keeping a close watch and monitoring of blood sampling. It must be kept in mind that removal of 10 mL of blood from a 1500 g neonate constitutes a loss of about 8% of his blood volume which is equivalent to about 400 mL blood in an adult.

Whole Blood and Red Blood Cell Transfusion

In order to reduce the risk of blood-borne diseases and prevent occurrence of host-versus-graft disease, it is preferable to avoid whole blood transfusion except in cases of acute blood loss with hypotension. Leukocyte-depleted red cell pack is preferred to reduce the risk of transmission of CMV, if testing facilities for its screening are not available. Red cell suspension is prepared by removing the plasma and suspending the RBCs in a diluent solution which is specially formulated to increase their shelf life. A unit of packed red blood cells has a volume of about 250 mL with a hematocrit of 70–80% and contains all type of cells including leukocytes and platelets. The packed RBCs can be suspended in fresh-frozen plasma (FFP) to reconstitute whole blood. Ideally FFP should be used from the same donor bag from which the packed RBCs was produced. Alternatively, AB group FFP can be used from a different donor. The final product should be used within 24 hours of reconstitution and it has the same characteristics as whole blood except for reduced plateletes.

Indications

1. Severe anemia (Hb <8 g/dL), congestive heart failure or hydrops fetalis due to chronic *in utero* anemia (Rh-isoimmunization, fetomaternal hemorrhage, twin-to-twin transfusion, fetal hemorrhage). It is preferable to do partial exchange transfusion with packed RBCs to correct anemia while avoiding volume overload.
2. Acute blood loss (>20% blood volume) due to placenta previa, abruptio placentae, rupture of the cord, hemorrhagic disease of the newborn with hypotension or cardiorespiratory signs.
3. Post-exchange top up transfusion.
4. Neonatal anemia
5. Major surgery

It is recommended to use restrictive blood transfusion indications especially in preterm infants on the basis of hemoglobin or hematocrit and the clinical status of the neonate.

  i. Hematocrit of <40% in neonates having acute cardiorespiratory insufficiency, requiring ventilator support.
 ii. Hematocrit of <30% in a symptomatic baby (lethargy, poor feeding, tachycardia, and poor weight gain, etc.)
iii. Hematocirt of <20% in an asymptomatic baby.

Donor Blood

The blood should be collected from non-professional voluntary donors and screened for HBV, HCV, HIV, CMV, VDRL and malaria. Avoid use of blood from first or second degree relatives because of increased risk of graft versus host disease (GVHD) especially in preterm babies due to immaturity of immune system. The blood is collected in a sterile, disposable, plastic pack containing CPD (citrate, phosphate, dextrose and often adenine) as an anticoagulant preservative solution. The ratio of blood to anticoagulent is maintained around 7:1. The blood should be depleted of leukocytes to reduce the risk of transmission of viral infections especially CMV. The use of on-line filters during transfusion are recommended to reduce transfusion of leukocytes. A single unit of blood should be apportioned to a quadruple pack system (piggy back) to reduce wastage and avoid exposure to multiple donors. These packs can be fractionated into different components at the time of use. Dedicated small units should be earmarked for multiple transfusions to the same baby to reduce exposure to multiple donors for reducing the risk of transmission of blood-borne diseases and sensitization. Identify infants who are likely to receive multiple transfusions and try to infuse them with blood/blood products fractionated from a single donor unit as far as possible.

Walking donor program is not acceptable by most blood banks in India because screening concept is applied to collected blood and not the walking donor who can get re-infected anytime. If facilities are available, the blood should be irradiated before transfusion to reduce the risk of host-versus-graft disease. Indications for gamma irradiation of blood include (i) intrauterine transfusion of RBCs and platelets, (ii) postnatal transfusion of neonates who received fetal transfusion, (iii) neonates weighing <1500 g or gestation <32 weeks, (iv) donation from first or second degree relatives, and (v) neonates with congenital or acquired immunodeficiency state. Transfusion of adult RBCs provides the added benefit of lowered oxygen affinity, which augments oxygen delivery to the tissues. But it is associated with an increased risk of development of ROP in preterm infants.

Procedure

Fresh blood (5–7 days old) should be used for exchange transfusion while blood with valid shelf life is acceptable for simple or top up transfusion. When exchange transfusion is performed for sepsis and sclerema, use fresh (<6 hours old) non-refrigerated blood. The storage of blood beyond a few days has adverse consequences in newborn babies because of several biochemical and biological alterations (Table 23.3).

TABLE 23.3 Adverse effects of storage on whole blood

- Reduction in the pH due to accumulation of pyruvate and lactate.
- Rise in the plasma potassium concentration.
- Progressive reduction in the red cell content of 2, 3 diphosphoglycerate (2, 3 DPG) which may lead to reduction of oxygen at the tissue level.
- Loss of all platelet functions within 48 hours of storage.
- Reduction in Factor VIII to 10–20% of normal within 48 hours of storage.

The blood should be allowed to get warm slowly at room temperature without using any active warming procedure. The recommended volume of transfusion is 20–40 mL/kg for whole blood and 10–15 mL/kg for packed red blood cells. In anemia due to chronic blood loss, packed RBC volume to be transfused is calculated by the formula:

$$\frac{\text{Blood volume} \times (\text{desired Hct} - \text{actual Hct})}{\text{Hct of packed RBCs being transfused}}$$

The rate of infusion should be restricted to 5 mL/kg/hr to prevent cardiac over load. In infants with active bleeding, transfuse at a rate of 10–20 mL/kg/hr while monitoring vital signs. In infants with impending heart failure, do not exceed transfusion rate of 2 mL/kg/hr. Intravenous furosemide 0.5–1.0 mg/kg may be given during the transfusion to prevent worsening of heart failure. Microaggregate (20–40 microns) blood filters or 3rd generation adsorption filters should be used to sieve off leukocytes during transfusion. Microaggregate filtration is effective in prevention of transfusion associated complications like respiratory insufficiency, graft-versus-host disease, transfusion of viruses, thrombocytopenia and immuno-modulation in newborn babies (Table 23.4).

Exchange Blood Transfusion

Indications

1. Treatment of ABO and Rh-isoimmunization (to reduce serum bilirubin, remove antibodies and antibody coated RBCs, and correct anemia).

TABLE 23.4 Complications of blood transfusion in newborn babies*

- Volume overload with cardiac failure.
- Transfusion or allergic reactions, immune-related hemolysis due to mismatch.
- Electrolyte (hyperkalemia, hypocalcemia), acid–base disturbances and hypoglycemia.
- Risk of transmission of infections like hepatitis B and C, HIV, cytomegalovirus, syphilis and malaria.
- Graft-versus-host disease.
- Iron overload.
- Oxidant damage to tissues with increased risk of ROP .
- Transfusion-related acute lung injury (TRALI).
- Alloimmunization.
- Hypothermia following transfusion of cold blood.

*The risk of complications is higher in neonates with a birth weight of <1500 g or gestation <32 weeks.

---

2. Severe anemia with cardiac decompensation (partial exchange with packed RBCs).
3. Controversial indications like life-threatening septicemia, sclerema, inborn error of metabolism and disseminated intravascular coagulation.

Choice of Blood

1. *Rh incompatibility*
   i. Blood arranged before birth: ORh negative crossmatched against mother.
   ii. Blood arranged after birth: Rh negative blood of baby's ABO group crossmatched against infant and mother.
2. *ABO incompatibility* Rh matched O group blood crossmatched with mother.
3. *Other indications* Blood group of infant cross-matched against infant and mother.

Blood Volume to be Exchanged

Exchange is done with double the blood volume of the baby (160–200 mL/kg, the larger volume refers to preterm babies). The double volume exchange removes about 90% of red blood cells and 50% of circulating bilirubin. Refer to Chapter 29 for detailed guidelines for the procedure of exchange blood transfusion.

Platelet Transfusion

Indications

The indications for platelet transfusion are summarized in Table 23.5.

Collection and Storage

Free flow blood should be collected from fresh venepuncture site without using plastic cannula. Platelets can be obtained from multiple random donors (RDP) or from a single donor. Single donor platelets (SDP) are obtained by a process called plateletpheresis wherein RBCs and platelet-poor plasma is returned back to the donor. The procedure is repeated 4–6 times to yield 4–6 units of platelets from one donor. The concentration of platelets is higher in SDP (3×10^{11}/unit) compared to RDP (0.5×10^{10}/unit). SDP units are associated with relatively lower risk of allo-immunization and transmission of viral diseases compared to platelet units obtained from pooled donor blood. Nevertheless, in clinical practice, RDP units are adequate to treat thrombocytopenia. In neonates with severe and prolonged thrombocytopenia, it is preferable to use single donor platelets for administration of multiple platelet transfusions. Platelet packs are more likely to be contaminated with bacteria because

| Platelet count mm³ | Bleeding | | Immune status | |
	Present	Absent	AITP*	NAIT**
< 30,000	Transfuse	Consider transfusion	Transfuse, if infant is bleeding or IVIG is not available	Transfuse, if bleeding
30–49,000	Transfuse	Transfuse, if postnatal age <1 week, weight <1.0 kg, sick baby with sepsis or DIC, IVH grade 3–4 or surgery*** is required	Transfuse, if unstable or bleeding	Transfuse, if bleeding
50–99,000	Transfuse	Avoid	Avoid	Transfuse, if bleeding
>100,000	There is no need to transfuse platelets			

TABLE 23.5 Indications for platelet transfusion

*AITP: Autoimmune thrombocytopenia

**NAIT: Neonatal alloimmune thrombocytopenia

***During surgery, platelet count should be maintained above 100,000/mm³

they are stored at room temperature (24°C). The platelet bag should be placed on an agitator. The shelf life of platelets is maximum of 5 days when stored in special bags. One unit of platelets is contained in a volume of 50 mL (platelets 5×10^{10}) which can be concentrated to a volume of 10–20 mL prior to infusion. Platelet packs contain leukocytes, plasma and some red blood cells. Ideally group-specific platelets should be used. Blood filter should not be used during transfusion of platelets as it will considerably reduce the number of platelets. In Rh-negative girl infants, platelets obtained from Rh negative donor should be used to prevent Rh sensitization.

Procedure

It is ideal to have blood group-specific platelet concentrate but in practice it is acceptable to transfuse platelets without crossmatching. In case of neonatal isoimmune thrombocytopenia, maternal platelets are concentrated and resuspended in appropriate serum to reduce infusion of maternal plasma which is laden with platelet antibodies. Check the quality of stored platelets by holding the bag against light and turning it upside down to look for "swirling movements". Platelets should never be transfused through umbilical or central vein or arterial line due to risk of thrombosis. The platelet concentrate should be transfused through a peripheral line slowly during 4 hours in a dose of 0.1 unit/kg which is expected to raise the platelet count by 40,000/mm³. Platelet count should be checked after one hour of completion of transfusion and then every 24 hours to maintain platelet count above 100,000/mm³.

Granulocyte Transfusion

It is not feasible to provide transfusion of granulocytes in developing countries because of non-availability of cell separators and prohibitive cost of collection and irradiation. There is potential risk of transmission of CMV during granulocyte transfusion. It is important that granulocytes should be transfused as soon as possible after collection but no later than 24 hours.

Indications

i. Sepsis with lack of clinical improvement after 48 hours of appropriate antibiotic therapy.
ii. Neutrophil count of <3000/mm³ during first week of life and <1000/mm³ after the age of one week.
iii. Bone marrow having <10% nucleated neutrophils or peripheral blood having >70% immature polymorphonuclear leukocytes.

Procedure

Administer $1–2 \times 10^9$ granulocytes/kg in a volume of 10–15 mL/kg every 12–24 hours. The aim of therapy is to raise the granulocyte count above 3000/mm³ in infants <1 week of age and >1000/mm³ in older neonates. The granulocyte count must be sustained and maintained for at least 48 hours for desired therapeutic benefit.

Fresh Frozen Plasma (FFP)

Plasma is prepared by centrifugation or by the process of plasmapheresis within 8 hours of collection of blood. Freshly obtained plasma is kept frozen at –20°C or lower to preserve the labile coagulation factors

(Factors II, VII, X and XI). It contains albumin, antibodies and coagulation factors. Fresh frozen plasma can be stored at –20°C up to one year. FFP is useful for infusion of albumin, clotting factors and immunoglobulins.

Indications

i. Sick neonates with unspecified coagulation disorder due to sepsis, DIC, NEC and hepatitis, etc.

ii. Hemorrhagic disease of the newborn with massive blood loss.

iii. Reconstitution of packed RBCs for exchange transfusion.

iv. Before undertaking invasive procedure in an infant having PT/PTTK (partial thromboplastin time with kaolin) 1.5–2 times of normal value.

v. Severe anticoagulant protein deficiency.

FFP should not be used for prevention of intraventricular hemorrhage, or supportive treatment of sepsis.

Procedure

Use type-specific product or AB-negative FFP without crossmatching. Transfuse through a microaggregate filter. The pack should be thawed in a water bath maintained between 30°C and 37°C. For volume expansion give 10–20 mL/kg over 30 minutes. To replace clotting factors, administer 15–20 mL/kg every 8 to 12 hours. After thawing, it should be administered immediately because there is a rapid fall in the concentration of coagulation factors.

Cryoprecipitate

It is rarely required but may be used in infants with Factors VIII and XIII deficiency, afibrinogenemia or hypofibrinogenemia, von Willebrand disease and control of bleeding during anticoagulation and thrombolytic therapy. It is prepared from fresh frozen plasma by collecting the precipitate formed during controlled thawing. The precipitate is then refrozen within one hour in 10–15 mL of donor plasma and kept stored below –18°C for a period up to one year. It provides 80–100 iu of Factor VIII, 100–250 mg of fibrinogen, 40–60 mg fibronectin, 40–70% von Willebrand factor and 30% of Factor XIII of the donor plasma. It is useful for replacement of various coagulation Factors. Cryoprecipitate can be used without compatibility testing and is transfused @ 2 units/kg body weight of the recepient.

Albumin Transfusion

The available standard albumin solutions are in 5% and 20% concentration with 96% albumin and 4% globulin. They are available in large volume packs which need to be divided into smaller aliquotes under laminar flow to reduce wastage. It is used for volume expansion for treatment of shock, for raising serum albumin concentration before exchange blood transfusion and for treatment of hypoproteinemia. Albumin 0.5–1.0 g/kg (10–20 mL/kg of 5% solution) is infused intravenously over 2 to 4 hours. There is no need for compatibility testing or use of filter during its administration. The maximum daily dose is 6 g/kg. It should be used with caution in infants with anemia and impending congestive heart failure. Avoid administration of 25% solution due to risk of development of intraventricular hemorrhage. It is expensive and there is a potential risk of transmission of viral infections because it is prepared from a large pool of donated human plasma.

BIBLIOGRAPHY

AAP Committee on Fetus and Newborn. Controversies concerning vitamin K and the newborn. *Pediatrics* 2003, 112: 191–192.

Antret-Leca E, Jonville-Bera AP. Vitamin K in neonates: How to administer, when and to whom. *Pediatr Drugs* 2001, 3: 1–8.

Bakshi S, Deorari AK, Roy S, Paul VK, Singh M. Prevention of subclinical vitamin K deficiency based on PIVKA II levels: Oral versus intramuscular route. *Indian Pediatr* 1996, 33: 1040.

Bell EF, Strauss RG, Widness JA. Randomized trial of liberal versus restrictive guidelines for red blood transfusion in preterm infants. *Pediatrics* 2005, 115: 1685.

Boulton F. Transfusion guidelines for neonates and older children. *Brit J Haemat* 2004, 124: 433–453.

Buchanan GR. Coagulation disorders in the neonate. *Pediatr Clin N Amer* 1986, 33: 203.

Burrows RF. Perinatal thrombocytopenia. *Clin Perinatol* 1995, 22: 779

Chalmers EA. Epidemiology of venous thromboembolism in neonates and children. *Thromb Res* 2006, 118: 3–12.

Chessell JM and Wigglesworth JS. Secondary hemorrhagic disease of the newborn. *Arch Dis Child* 1970, 45: 539.

Chines DB, McKenzie SE, Siegel DL, *et al*. Immune thrombocytopenic purpura. *N Engl J Med* 2002, 13: 995.

Deorari AK, Paul VK, Shreshtha L, Singh M. Symptomatic neonatal polycythemia: Comparison of partial exchange transfusion with saline versus plasma. *Indian Pediatr* 1995, 32: 1167–1171.

Hematologic Problems

23

474 Dzik WH. Leucoreduction of blood components. *Curr Opin Hematol* 2002, 9(6): 521–526.

Galel SA, Fontaine MJ. Hazards of neonatal blood transfusion. *Neo Reviews* 2006, 7: e69–e75.

Goldberg K, Wirth FH and Hathaway EE, *et al.* Neonatal hyperviscosity. Effects of partial plasma exchange. *Pediatrics* 1982, 69; 419.

Kaplan C. Immune thrombocytopenia in the fetus and newborn: diagnosis and therapy. *Trans Clin Biol* 2001, 8: 311–314.

Kelton JG. Management of the pregnant patient with idiopathic thrombocytopenic purpura. *Ann Int Med* 1983, 99: 796.

Kiefel V, Bassier D, Kroll H, *et al.* Antigen-positive platelet transfusion in neonatal alloimmune thrombocytopenia (NAIT). *Blood* 2006, 107: 3761–3763.

Kothari SS, Verma S, Wasir HS. Thrombolytic therapy in infants and children. *Amer Heart J* 1994, 127: 651.

Michaels LA, Gurian M, Hegyi T, *et al.* Low molecular weight heparin in the treatment of venous and arterial thromboses in the premature infant. *Pediatrics* 2004, 114: 703–707.

Mihatsch WA, Braegger C, Bronsky J, *et al.* Prevention of vitamin K deficiency bleeding in newborn infants: A position paper by the ESPGHAN Commitee on Nutrition. *JPGN* 2016, 63:123–29.

Monagle P, Chan A, Massicotte P, *et al.* Antithrombotic therapy in children. *Chest* 2004, 126: S645–S687.

Murray NA, Howarth LJ, McCloy MP, *et al.* Platelet transfusion in the management of severe thrombocytopenia in neonatal intensive care unit patients. *Transfus Med* 2002, 12: 35–41.

Ng E, Loewy AD. Position statement: Guidelines for vitamin K prophylaxis in newborns: A joint statement of the Canadian Paediatric Society and the College of Family Physicians of Canada. *Canada Fam Physician* 2018,65:736–9.

Ohls RK. Trnsfusions in the preterm infant. *Neo Reviews* 2007, 8(9): e377–e386.

Rennie JM, Kesall AWR. Vitamin K prophylaxis in the newborn-again. *Arch Dis Child* 1994, 70: 248–251.

Rothenberg T. Partial plasma exchange transfusion in polycythemic neonates. *Arch Dis Child* 2002, 86(1): 60–62.

Sillers L, Slambrouk CV, Lapping-Carr G. Neonatal thrombocytopenia: Etiology and diagnosis. *Pediatr Ann* 2015, 44(7):e175–e180.

Singh M. Vitamin K during infancy: current status and recommendations. *Indian Pediatr* 1997, 34: 708–712.

Sola MC, Vecchio AD, Rimsza LM. Evaluation and treatment of thrombocytopenia in the neonatal intensive care unit. *Clin Perinatol* 2000, 27(3), 655.

Stockman JA. Anemia of prematurity: current concepts in the issues of when to transfuse. *Pediatr Clin North Am* 1986, 33: 11.

Strauss RG. Controversies in the management of the anemia of prematurity using single-donor red blood cell transfusion and/or recombinant human erythropoietin. *Trans Med Rev* 2006, 20: 34–44.

Strauss RG. Erythropoietin and neonatal anemia. *N Engl J Med* 1994, 330:1227.

Venkatesh V, Khan R, Curley A, *et al.* The safety and efficacy of red cell transfusions in neonates: A systematic review of randomized controlled trials. *Brit J Haematol* 2012, 158: 370.

Venkatesh V, Khan R, Curley A, *et al.* How we decide when a neonate needs transfusion. *Brit J Haematol* 2013, 160: 421.

Watchko JF. Common hematologic problems in the newborn. *Pediatr Clin* 2015, 62(2): 509–24.

Wexner EJ. Neonatal polycythemia and hyperviscosity. *Clin Perinatol* 1995, 22: 693.

Whitehall JS, Patole SK, Campbell P. Recombinant human erythropoietin in anemia of prematurity. *Indian Pediatr* 1999, 36: 17–27.

Whyte RK, Jefferies AL. Red blood cell transfusion in newborn infants. *Paediatr Child Health* 2014, 19(4): 213–217.

Whyte RK, Kriplani H. Low versus high hemoglobin concentration threshold for blood transfusion for preventing morbidity and mortality in very low birth weight infants *Cochraine Database Syst Rev* 2011: CD000512.

Williams JA. Christ WM. Erythropoietin—Not yet a standard treatment for anemia of prematurity. *Pediatrics* 1995, 95: 9–10.

Metabolic Disorders

Metabolic disorders are relatively common during newborn period as compared to any other age group. Most life-threatening inborn errors of metabolism (IEM) manifest during newborn period and account for significant proportion of unexplained deaths. High incidence of metabolic derangements in newborn babies, especially among preterm infants, is due to physiological and biochemical immaturity. Symptomatic metabolic disorders are associated with increased risk of neuromotor disability on follow-up among the survivors. It is, therefore, essential that high-risk infants should be routinely screened for common metabolic disturbances, such as hypoglycemia and hypocalcemia. Their incidence and severity can be reduced by adopting appropriate feeding regimen and timely institution of supplements. The symptomatic metabolic disorders carry relatively high mortality but timely intervention and therapy is associated with dramatic response and improved quality of life.

HYPOGLYCEMIA

Blood glucose concentrations in the newborn baby, irrespective of its birth weight and gestational age, are generally lower than those found in older children and adults. The infant is born with a blood glucose concentration of 60–70% of the maternal level and it falls during first 24 hours, the lowest value is seen at the age of three hours. This is followed by a transient rise in blood glucose level during next 24 hours and again dangerously low levels may be encountered at the age of 3 to 4 days before stability is achieved.

There is a controversy and confusion regarding the universally accepted definition of hypoglycemia in the newborn baby. The operational threshold for hypoglycemia is defined as "that concentration of plasma or whole blood glucose at which the clinician should consider intervention, based on the currently available evidence in the literature". Most workers agree that a true blood glucose level of less than 40 mg/dL (irrespective of period of gestation), if associated with symptoms of hypoglycemia or if confirmed on repeat analysis in asymptomatic babies, is indicative of hypoglycemia (1.0 mmol/L of glucose is equivalent to 18.02 mg/dL).

Predisposing Conditions

Intrauterine Growth Retardation

In malnourished babies and smaller of the discordant twins, the liver weight is much reduced whereas the brain weight remains within normal limits so that the ratio of brain weight to liver weight is greater than five. This discrepancy in the size of the utilizer (brain) and provider (liver glycogen) of glucose leads to hypoglycemia. The other predisposing factors in these babies include higher incidence of fetal and neonatal asphyxia, raised basal metabolic rate and higher oxygen uptake, excessive responsiveness to insulin, inability to increase adrenaline output in response to hypoglycemia and possibly disturbed hypothalamic mechanism in the brain. Hypoglycemia occurs in about 15% of small-for-dates babies and is often symptomatic especially in male babies. It generally manifests between 24 and 72 hours and is preventable by early feeding. Some infants with IUGR and perinatal asphyxia may have protracted hypoglycemia for several months and may need treatment with diazoxide.

Maternal Diabetes Mellitus

The fetus by virtue of being exposed to high concentrations of glucose *in utero* responds by hyperplasia of islet cells of pancreas. The high insulin concentrations may lead to hypoglycemia in about 50% of such babies which is observed mostly during first 12 hours after birth and is asymptomatic in majority of infants. About one-fifth of babies born to mothers with gestational diabetes mellitus may show hypoglycemia. The administration of chlorpropamide during the latter part of pregnancy may lead to intractable hypoglycemia in the baby which may need exchange blood transfusion.

Immaturity

There is a direct correlation between blood glucose levels and gestational maturity and birth weight of the baby. The low hepatic glycogen stores and relatively high incidence of hypoxia, hypothermia and respiratory distress syndrome in these babies contribute to hypoglycemia. Maternal tocolytic therapy with beta-sympathomimetic agents (ritodrine, isoxsuprine, salbutamol, terbutaline) can predispose to hypoglycemia. These agents decrease peripheral utilization of glucose leading to hyperglycemia in the mother and hyperinsulinemia in the fetus. The incidence of hypoglycemia in preterm babies varies between 5 and 10% and is higher in babies with a birth weight of less than 50th percentile for their gestational age. About three-fourths of hypoglycemic low birth weight babies are symptomatic.

Erythroblastosis Fetalis due to Rhesus Incompatibility

The hyperplasia of islet-cells of pancreas may lead to asymptomatic hypoglycemia during the first 24 hours of life in about 5% of babies with erythroblastosis. The incidence of hypoglycemia is directly related to the severity of rhesus hemolytic disease. There is some evidence to suggest that breakdown products of hemolyzed red blood cells (glutathion) inactivates circulating insulin leading to hyperplasia of islet cells to maintain adequate insulin levels. Exchange transfusion with heparinized blood is associated with hypoglycemia while following exchange transfusion with CPD-blood, rebound hypoglycemia may occur.

Miscellaneous Disorders

Hypoglycemia is common following severe birth asphyxia, hypothermia, septicemia and polycythemia. Rarely, recurrent and often intractable hypoglycemia may occur due to a number of metabolic and developmental disorders. They include glycogen storage disease, galactosemia, fructosemia, maple syrup urine disease, organic acidemias, adrenal insufficiency, leucine sensitivity, and insulinoma. Large-for-dates infants due to any cause (maternal diabetes, erythroblastosis fetalis, Wiedemann-Beckwith syndrome, transposition of great vessels) are associated with islet cell hyperplasia and are predisposed to develop hypoglycemia. Their overgrowth appears to be due to consumption of large quantities of glucose *in utero*. Therefore, their organs are replete with glycogen. The hypoglycemia would be provoked by milk feeding in leucine sensitivity, galactosemia, fructosemia (sucrose added to the milk) and in some cases of islet cell hyperplasia and tumor. Maternal therapy with beta blockers especially propranolol and oral hypoglycemic agents is also associated with neonatal hypoglycemia. Neonatal hypoglycemia can be classified on the basis of underlying pathophysiological mechanism (Table 24.1).

TABLE 24.1 Classification of neonatal hypoglycemia on the basis of underlying physiologic mechanisms

Fetal/neonatal hyperinsulinism
- Maternal diabetes mellitus
- Erythroblastosis fetalis
- Wiedemann-Beckwith syndrome
- Transposition of great vessels
- Maternal therapy with beta-sympathomimetic tocolytic agents (ritodrine, isoxsuprine, salbutamol, terbutaline) and propranolol.
- Insulin producing tumors (nesidioblastosis, islet cell adenoma, islet cell dysmaturity).
- Leucine-sensitivity

Decreased glycogen stores and/or increased utilization of glucose
- Intrauterine growth retardation
- Prematurity
- Birth asphyxia
- Hypothermia
- Polycythemia
- Septicemia
- Starvation

Miscellaneous conditions
- Inborn errors of metabolism (glycogen storage disease, galactosemia, fructose intolerance, fatty acid oxidation disorders, defective ketone synthesis, glutaric aciduria type 2, maple syrup urine disease, congenital adrenal hyperplasia, cretinism).
- Maternal therapy with chlorpropamide and beta-blockers (propranolol and labetalol?).
- Exchange transfusion with heparinized or ACD/CPD blood.
- Congenital hypopituitarism.

Indications for Routine Monitoring of Blood Glucose

In order to prevent brain damage, blood glucose should be routinely estimated in the following high-risk situations.

- Small-for-dates babies and smaller of the discordant twins.
- Infants of diabetic mothers or those with a birth weight of above 90th percentile for their period of gestation.
- Preterm infants <35 weeks gestation.
- Rhesus hemolytic disease of the newborn.
- Babies with prolonged hypoxia, hypothermia, polycythemia, septicemia, cardiac failure, midline syndromic defects and suspected metabolic disorders.
- Infants born to mothers receiving therapy with intravenous glucose, terbutaline, propranolol and oral hypoglycemic agent.
- Infants on IV fluids or total parenteral nutrition.
- Babies with symptoms suggestive of hypoglycemia.

The routine monitoring of blood glucose in above high-risk situations is recommended at 2 hours after birth and thereafter 4–6 hourly for the first 48 hours. The blood sample should be collected just before administration of the feed. In babies born to diabetic mothers, glucose screening is done during first 12 hours. Following exchange transfusion with CPD blood, glucose level should be checked 2 hours after the procedure to detect rebound hypoglycemia. In a symptomatic infant with hypoglycemia on a feed trial, blood glucose should be checked after one hour of feed.

Methods for Estimation of Blood Glucose

It is imperative to measure the level of true glucose rather than the reducing ability of the blood either by glucose oxidase, glucose electrode and Nelson and Somogyi methods. The blood glucose level is the sum total of glucose in the plasma and red blood cells, although the latter is unavailable to the brain. The rapid glycolysis of red cell glucose demands that whenever there is delay in doing the estimation, sample should be stored in the refrigerator or should be immediately precipitated with sodium fluoride to inhibit glycolysis otherwise falsely low values of glucose may be obtained. If these precautions are not taken, the glucose level of sample may drop at a rate of 15–20 mg/100 mL/hour. Glucose strips (dextrostix) are very useful and essential for screening glucose on

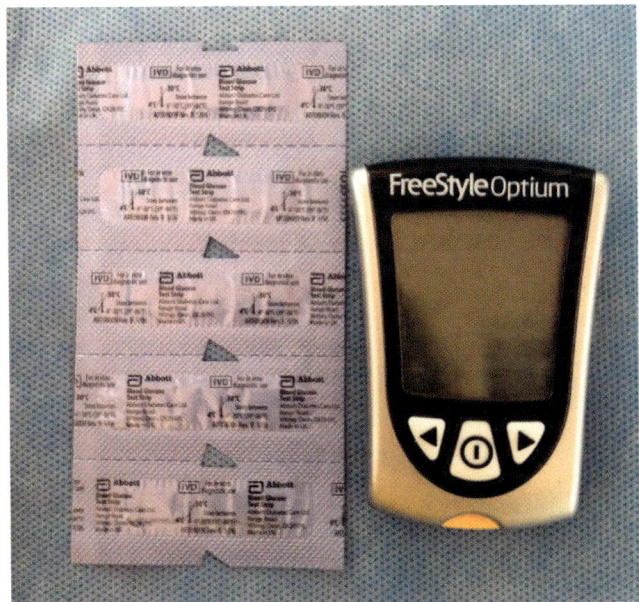

Figure 24.1 Glucometer for screening blood glucose with the help of dextrostix.

capillary samples with the help of a dextrometer (Figure 24.1). They are not accurate for monitoring low glucose levels. Reagent strips measure whole blood glucose which is 15% lower than plasma level. If dextrostix reveals blood glucose concentration of less than 40 mg/dL, treatment should not be delayed while one is awaiting confirmation of hypoglycemia by laboratory study.

Clinical Manifestations

There are no pathognomonic symptoms of hypoglycemia in the newborn and there is poor correlation between the level of blood glucose and symptomatology. The various factors which result in poor correlation between blood glucose concentration and development of symptoms include probable utilization of lactate and glycerol as an alternative substrate by the brain, reduced peripheral utilization of glucose rather than the total or red cell glucose content and susceptibility or threshold of brain to hypoglycemic insult which may be altered by anoxia, hypothermia, and intracranial injury.

Irritability of the central nervous system is manifested by jitteriness, coarse tremors, twitchings and convulsions. Jitteriness alone is not a reliable sign of hypoglycemia. The babies may manifest with refusal of feeds, apathy, limpness and coma. Episodes of apnea with cyanosis and tachypnea with irregular breathing may occur due to hypoglycemia in preterm babies. There may be episodes of sudden pallor, limpness and hypothermia. Tachycardia and sweating may occur because of excessive catecholamine secretion. Cardiomegaly and occasionally cardiac failure may occur in hypoglycemic babies. Septicemic babies may also have associated hypoglycemia.

In view of the fact that there are no diagnostic symptoms or signs of hypoglycemia and above clinical manifestations can occur from a variety of causes, the proof of hypoglycemic etiology of symptoms rests solely upon their prompt disappearance on administration of intravenous glucose.

Diagnosis

Asymptomatic hypoglycemia The true blood glucose level is below 40 mg/dL (plasma glucose <45 mg/dL) on two occasions in a baby without any clinical symptoms of hypoglycemia.

Symptomatic hypoglycemia The diagnosis is made on the basis of Whipple's triad: (i) Presence of symptoms attributable to hypoglycemia, (ii) low true blood glucose documented by an accurate and sensitive laboratory method and (iii) disappearance of clinical symptoms when blood glucose level is normalized. If the clinical symptoms or signs attributed to hypoglycemia are not resolved on administration of glucose, other diagnostic possibilities should be considered.

Prevention

Infants at increased risk to develop hypoglycemia (SFDs, LFDs, IGDMs, IDMs, smaller of the twin) should receive sugar-fortified feeds. The infant should be nursed in a thermoneutral environment so that glucose is not wasted for metabolic thermogenesis. First feed should be given within first hour of birth. Breastfeeding should be continued and formula feeds fortified with 5 g sucrose/dL should be offered every 2-hourly during first 3 days of life. Instead of adding sucrose, formula feeds can be prepared in 5% dextrose water. The mother should not be asked to buy the feeding bottle or the formula which should be provided from the nursery. The supplementary feeds should be given with a cup and spoon. Blood glucose should be checked after one hour of complementary feed. After 3 days of age, the infant should receive exclusive breastfeeding. If hypoglycemia develops despite administration of fortified feeds, the protocol for management of hypoglycemia should be followed.

Treatment

Symptomatic cases In symptomatic cases, therapy should be administered immediately after withdrawing

a blood sample for glucose estimation. The baby should be kept warm by nursing in a thermoneutral environment. In a symptomatic infant with seizures, give 5–10 mL/kg of 10% dextrose intravenously as a bolus. In the absence of seizures, symptomatic infant is given a mini-bolus of 2 mL/kg of 10% dextrose. This is followed by continuous infusion of 10% dextrose at a rate of 6 mg/kg/minute preferably with the help of an infusion pump. Calculate separately glucose intake (mg/kg/min) and water requirements everyday. For example, if fluid requirement is 80 mL/kg/d, it works out to be 0.055 mL/kg/min. In this case, 10% dextrose (100 mg dextrose/mL) would provide the glucose infusion rate of 5.5 mg/kg/min while 15% dextrose (150 mg/mL) solution would provide 8.25 mg glucose/kg/min. Depending upon the daily fluid requirements, the concentration of dextrose solution to be infused can be worked out to provide the desired amount of constant delivery of glucose. The maximal glucose concentration is usually limited to 15% to safeguard against the risk of thrombophlebitis. To prepare 14.5% solution of dextrose, add 30 mL of 25% dextrose (7.5 g dextrose) to 70 mL of 10% dextrose (7.0 g dextrose). The calculator shown in Figure 24.2 is useful for estimation

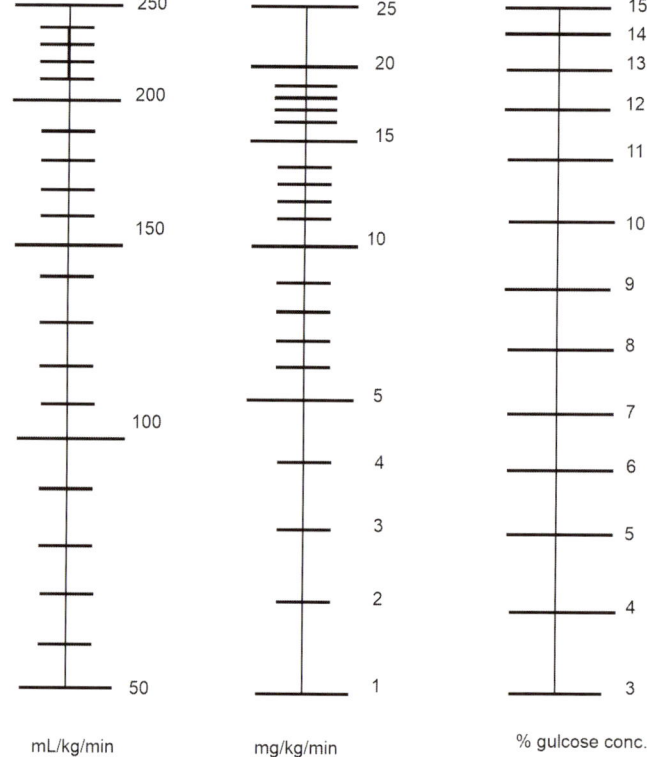

mL/kg/min   mg/kg/min   % gulcose conc.

Figure 24.2 Glucose drip calculator. Use a plastic ruler to calculate interconversion of glucose concentration parameters to calculate the infusion rate of glucose.

of rate and concentration of glucose solution needed for ensuring desired infusion of glucose.

Blood glucose is monitored every 2 hours. The glucose infusion rate is gradually increased by 2 mg/kg/minute every hourly till a maximum infusion rate of 12 mg/kg/minute is reached or the blood glucose has crossed the level of 40 mg/dL. The glucose level should be checked after 30 min of each change in infusion rate. When blood glucose level crosses 60 mg/dL, glucose infusion rate is gradually tapered with decrements of 2 mg/kg/minute every 6 hourly till glucose infusion rate comes down to 4 mg/kg/minute with satisfactory blood glucose values (>50 mg/dL). The blood glucose level should be maintained between 60 and 100 mg/dL. Hyperglycemia should be avoided as it is also known to cause brain damage. Oral feeds are introduced gradually when glucose infusion is being tapered. The infant is completely weaned off intravenous infusion when his blood glucose values are stable at an infusion rate of 4 mg/kg/minute. Refer to algorithm for step-wise management of hypoglycemia (Figure 24.3).

Resistant or Persistent Hypoglycemia

The most common cause of recurrent and persistent hypoglycemia in the newborn period is congenital hyperinsulinism (CHI). In an intractable case, if despite maintaining the maximal glucose infusion rate of 12 mg/kg/minute, hypoglycemia is uncorrected, hydrocortisone hemisuccinate 5 mg/kg should be given intravenously every 12 hr. In babies with hypoglycemia due to maternal diabetes mellitus or erythroblastosis, glucagon (100–300 µg/kg/dose up to 3 doses IM) and/or epinephrine may be given because these infants are replete with glycogen. Glucagon acts by mobilizing hepatic glycogen stores, enhancing gluconeogenesis and promoting ketogenesis. These agents are not recommended for malnourished and preterm babies. In infants with persistent and recurrent hypoglycemia beyond first week of life, nesidioblastosis, islet cell adenoma and inborn errors of metabolism should be excluded. Diazoxide (10–25 mg/kg/day in 3 to 4 divided doses slowly intravenously or orally) is useful to control the glucose-induced release of insulin. Diazoxide acts by keeping K_{ATP} channels of the beta-cells of the pancreas open, thereby reducing the secretion of insulin. In intractable cases, octreotide, a synthetic somatostatin,

is administered subcutaneously in a dose of 5–20 µg/kg/d q 8–12 hours. These infants should be managed in a tertiary care center. When glucose requirements are very high (>12 mg/kg/min) or hypoglycemia persists for more than 7 days, endocrine evaluation is mandatory. Infants with congenital hyperinsulinism should be assessed for hyperammonemia (leucine sensitive hypoglycemia) and positron emission tomography scan using fluorine-18L-3, 4-dihydroxyphenylalanine isotope (18F-DOPA-PET) to identify whether it is focal or diffuse involvement of the pancreas. Infants with focal involvement of pancreas are managed with laparoscopic focal lesionectomy while diffuse forms of CHI that do not respond to medical therapy are managed by near total pancreatectomy with lifelong supplements of insulin and pancreatic enzymes.

Asymptomatic cases The management is identical as in symptomatic cases but diagnosis should be confirmed by repeating blood glucose estimation. Bolus administration of glucose is not recommended in asymptomatic babies. Asymptomatic infant of a diabetic mother may be managed with sugar-fortified feeds expectantly for the first 4 hours or so. Oral glucose or feeding alone are not enough once hypoglycemia has occurred because oral glucose is more likely to stimulate insulin release as compared to intravenous glucose infusion.

Dextrose Infusion Rate

Glucose infusion rate (GIR) depends upon the concentration of dextrose in the infusate and rate of infusion. It is calculated as follows:

$$1.\ GIR^* = \frac{\%\ dextrose\ infused \times Rate\ of\ infusion\ (mL/kg/hr)}{Weight\ (kg) \times 6}$$

$$2.\ GIR^* = \frac{\%\ dextrose\ infused \times Rate\ of\ infusion\ (mL/kg/d)}{144}$$

3. $GIR^* = \%$ dextrose infused $\times$ Rate of infusion (mL/kg/d) $\times 0.007$

*GIR: Glucose infusion rate mg/kg/min.

The glucose infusion rates can be directly read from the Table 24.2 or checked from the dextrose infusion calculator (Figure 24.2). Many NICUs have computerized provider order entry systems that automatically calculate the GIR.

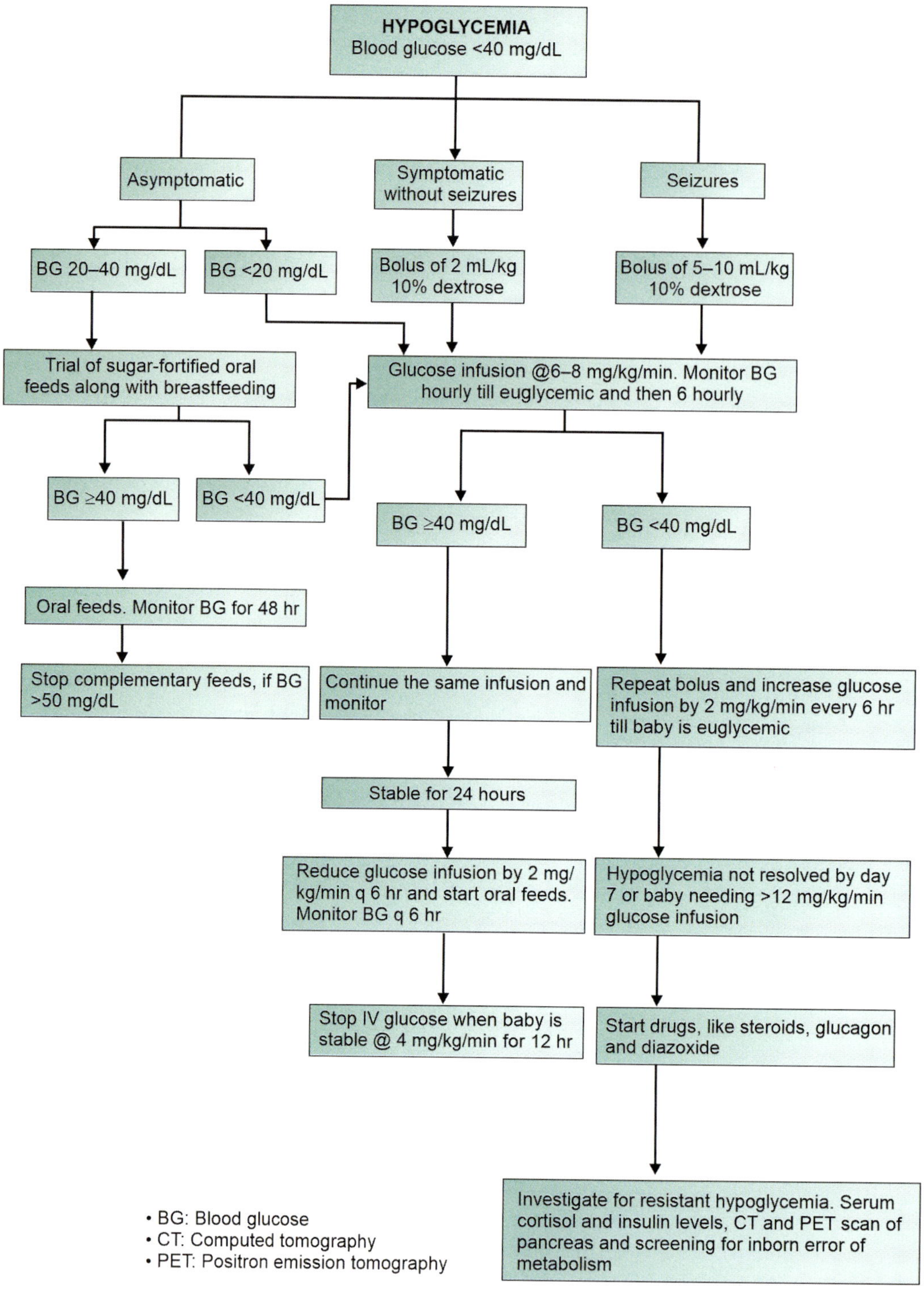

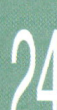
24

HYPOGLYCEMIA
Blood glucose <40 mg/dL

Asymptomatic

Symptomatic without seizures

Seizures

BG 20–40 mg/dL

BG <20 mg/dL

Bolus of 2 mL/kg 10% dextrose

Bolus of 5–10 mL/kg 10% dextrose

Trial of sugar-fortified oral feeds along with breastfeeding

Glucose infusion @6–8 mg/kg/min. Monitor BG hourly till euglycemic and then 6 hourly

BG ≥40 mg/dL

BG <40 mg/dL

BG ≥40 mg/dL

BG <40 mg/dL

Oral feeds. Monitor BG for 48 hr

Stop complementary feeds, if BG >50 mg/dL

Continue the same infusion and monitor

Repeat bolus and increase glucose infusion by 2 mg/kg/min every 6 hr till baby is euglycemic

Stable for 24 hours

Reduce glucose infusion by 2 mg/kg/min q 6 hr and start oral feeds. Monitor BG q 6 hr

Hypoglycemia not resolved by day 7 or baby needing >12 mg/kg/min glucose infusion

Stop IV glucose when baby is stable @ 4 mg/kg/min for 12 hr

Start drugs, like steroids, glucagon and diazoxide

Investigate for resistant hypoglycemia. Serum cortisol and insulin levels, CT and PET scan of pancreas and screening for inborn error of metabolism

- BG: Blood glucose
- CT: Computed tomography
- PET: Positron emission tomography

Key points:
- Check blood glucose after 30 min of every change in infusion rate.
- Reduce glucose infusion rate, if last 2 blood glucose values are >50 mg/dL.
- In case of resistant hypoglycemia, exclude polycythemia.
- Oral feeding helps in better glycemic control and should be initiated/continued along with intravenous therapy.
- There is no role of drugs in infants with IUGR.
- Stop hydrocortisone in 3–5 days.

Figure 24.3 Algorithm for management of hypoglycemia.

TABLE 24.2 Glucose infusion rates (mg/kg/min) at various infusion rates and percentage of dextrose solution

Intake of fluids mL/kg/hr (mL/kg/d)	5% dextrose	10% dextrose	15% dextrose
3 (72)	2.5	5.0	7.5
4 (96)	3.2	6.5	9.6
5 (120)	4.1	8.3	12.3
6 (144)	5.0	10.0	15.0
7 (168)	5.8	11.6	17.4

Prognosis

Untreated symptomatic hypoglycemia may terminate fatally. Histopathology shows fragmentation of neuronal nuclei and loss of Nissl bodies with increased granularity of cytoplasm. Similar changes may also be seen in neonates dying of severe hypoxia. Among survivors of symptomatic hypoglycemia, 50% may be mentally retarded or manifest cerebral palsy with myoclonic or generalized seizures. The associated factors, such as immaturity and perinatal asphyxia *per se* may be responsible for neonatal sequelae rather than hypoglycemia. It has also been postulated that subsequent mental handicap may be as a result of underlying brain defect which may have also contributed to the development of hypoglycemia. The prognosis of hypoglycemia is generally poor in babies with congenital hyperinsulinism, inborn errors of metabolism and Wiedemann-Beckwith syndrome. In asymptomatic hypoglycemic babies of diabetic mothers, the outcome is excellent.

HYPERGLYCEMIA

This is relatively rare in the neonate and is diagnosed when whole-blood glucose level exceeds 125 mg/dL or plasma glucose value is more than 145 mg/dL. Glucose infusion rate of more than 6.0 mg/kg/min in newborn babies may be associated with hyperglycemia. The condition may occur following intravenous glucose infusion, exchange transfusion with citrate phosphate dextrose (CPD) blood and in anencephalic baby due to poor utilization of glucose. Cerebral utilization of glucose may also be reduced in meningitis, meningoencephalitis and intracranial hemorrhage leading to elevation of blood glucose levels. Extremely low birth weight babies may not utilize 10% dextrose leading to hyperglycemia. Transient hyperglycemia may occur during the stress of hypoxia in a large baby when hepatic and cardiac glycogen is broken down to provide glucose to the brain. Administration of caffeine and aminophylline to preterm infants for the management of apneic attacks may lead to hyperglycemia due to activation of hepatic glycogenolysis and inhibition of glycogen synthesis. Neonatal infections may rarely cause hyperglycemia by imposing added stress to an already impaired carbohydrate metabolism. Premature infants requiring mechanical ventilation or other painful procedures may develop hyperglycemia due to endogenous release of catecholamines and other "stress" hormones.

Neonatal diabetes mellitus is a rare condition diagnosed by onset of hyperglycemia before first month of life that lasts for at least 2 weeks and requires insulin therapy. The etiology is unknown but most cases occur among small-for-gestational age infants. Family history of diabetes mellitus may be obatained in one-third of cases. Almost 50% cases are permanent while the rest are transient (lasting for 17 days to 5 years) with or without recurrence in later life. The onset of diabetes mellitus after the age of one month and its association with HLA-DR3 and DR4 increases the likelihood of permanent diabetes mellitus. Wolcott-Rallison syndrome (WRS) is a rare autosomal recessive disorder characterized by diabetes mellitus having onset between 1 and 3 months of age and is associated with multiple epiphyseal dysplasias, osteopenia, renal and hepatic impairment and poor long-term mental prognosis. Hyperglycemia leads to hyperosmolarity as each 18 mg/dL rise in blood glucose concentration leads to increase in serum osmolarity by 1 mOsm/L. The infant may present with sudden weight loss due to dehydration as a result of osmotic diuresis accompanied by fever and failure to thrive in the absence of diarrhea or vomiting. Blood glucose levels may approach 2,000 mg/per/dL but ketonuria is mild or absent due to effective tubular reabsorption of ketoacids in the newborn babies. Hyperosmolar state may lead to contraction of intracellular volume of brain with potential risk of intracranial hemorrhage. The condition should be managed by intravenous rehydration and administration of insulin in a dose of 0.5–3.0 units/kg/day q 6 hr subcutaneously which may need to be continued for a period of few weeks. The mental prognosis is guarded in infants with protracted hyperglycemia.

HYPOCALCEMIA

Calcium Homeostasis

Body calcium exists in two major compartments, skeleton (99%) and extracellular fluid (1%). Calcium in the extracellular fluid is present in three forms, (i) bound to albumin (40%), (ii) bound to anions, like

Metabolic Disorders

24

phosphorus, citrate, sulfate and lactate (10%) and (iii) free ionized form (50%). Ionized calcium is essential for several biochemical processes including blood coagulation, neuromuscular excitability, integrity of cell membranes and production of certain enzymes.

Both calcium and maternal parathyroid hormone cross the placenta. There is an active transport of calcium and phosphorus to the fetus from maternal sources and fetal concentrations of calcium are about 1.0 mg/dL higher than the maternal. Most of placental transport of calcium takes place during last trimester of pregnancy so that prematurely born infants have deficient stores of calcium. Small-for-dates infants usually have normal serum calcium levels and stores of calcium in the body. The mean serum calcium in the cord blood varies between 9 and 12 mg/dL. Parathormone and 1, 25-dihydroxyvitamin D are the main calcium-regulating hormones. Parathormone mobilizes calcium from bones, increases calcium reabsorption in renal tubules and stimulates renal production of 1,25 $(OH)_2$ D_3. The biologically active 1,25 $(OH)_2$ D_3 increases intestinal calcium and phosphate absorption and mobilizes calcium and phosphate from bones.

Serum calcium level falls after birth especially in preterm babies and a state of physiological hypocalcemia is achieved during 24 to 36 hours of age. Parathyroid gland of the newborn is sluggish to respond due to its suppression by maternal parathormone in fetal life. Due to reduced GFR and defective tubular reabsorption in the newborn, kidney is unable to excrete phosphorus. Thus during first few days after birth, serum calcium falls and phosphorus level rises. A number of situations can accentuate this physiological fall in serum calcium leading to severe or symptomatic hypocalcemia. The neuromuscular irritability is related to the amount of ionized calcium rather than the protein bound or total serum calcium.

Ionized calcium is the only biologically available form of calcium but for routine clinical purposes, measurement of serum total calcium level is adequate. *Serum calcium of less than 8.0 mg/dL (<2 mmol/L) in term infants and <7.0 mg/dL (or ionized calcium <4 mg/dL or <1.0 mmol/L) in preterm infants during the first four weeks of life is designated as neonatal hypocalcemia* (calcium 1.0 mg/dL is equivalent to 0.25 mmol/L or 0.5 mEq/L). Serum phosphorus is generally raised to more than 6 mg 100 mL except in cases associated with hypomagnesemia. Hypoglycemia may be associated with hypocalcemia in some babies particularly following glucagon therapy.

Causes

Early-onset Hypocalcemia (First 3 Days)

Immaturity There is a direct correlation between birth weight and serum calcium. About 50% of infants weighing less than 2,500 g and 75% of those weighing less than 1,500 g may show transient self-limited hypocalcemia during first 24 hours of life. Various factors which predispose low birth weight babies to develop hypocalcemia include low calcium stores due to early birth, delayed feeding, renal immaturity and reduced glomerular filtration rate leading to retention of phosphates, hypoproteinemia, frequent administration of sodium bicarbonate solution and respiratory distress syndrome. During acidosis, calcium is mobilized from the bones and excreted. Following correction of acidosis with sodium bicarbonate, calcium goes back into the bones leading to hypocalcemia. There is a fall in ionized calcium level when acidosis is overcorrected. The incidence of hypocalcemia in low birth weight babies is unrelated to the nature and mode of delivery.

Maternal diabetes mellitus About 25 to 50% of babies born to diabetic mothers may develop hypocalcemia which is believed to be due to immaturity and hypercorticism though the evidence for latter is controversial. Hypercalcitonemia, hypoparathyroidism, abnormal vitamin D metabolism and hyperphosphatemia have been implicated by different workers. The macrosomia associated with IDM may increase demand for calcium.

Complications during delivery Perinatal hypoxia, difficult and prolonged delivery, emergency cesarean section especially following a trial of labor, toxemia and antepartum hemorrhage are associated with high incidence (10–30%) of hypocalcemia. The contributory factors appear to be tissue catabolism with release of phosphorus and increased cortisone release because of stress of complicated delivery. Serum phosphorus is generally raised in these situations. It is also associated with release of calcitonin and hypoxic renal insufficiency. In high-risk babies, serum calcium should be checked at 24 and 48 hours of age.

Late-onset Hypocalcemia (Classical Neonatal Tetany)

It is characterized by onset of tetany at the age of 5 to 10 days in healthy term babies receiving animal milk or formula feeding. The ingestion of cow's milk with high phosphate content or low calcium/phosphorus ratio (Ca : P ratios of cow's and human milk are 1.3:1 and 2.2:1, respectively) leads to hyperphosphatemia and hypocalcemia in the neonate. There is transient deficiency of parathyroid hormone or lack of end organ responsiveness to produce phosphate diuresis. This hypothesis fails to explain the rarity of this type of tetany in preterm babies.

Uncommon Conditions

Maternal hyperparathyroidism Maternal hypercalcemia and raised parathyroid hormone levels are reflected in fetal circulation, thus leading to suppression of fetal parathyroid glands. It is important to estimate maternal serum calcium, phosphorus and alkaline phosphatase levels and obtain skiagrams of hands in all cases of tetany of late onset.

Idiopathic hypoparathyroidism This rare condition may be suspected by the findings of low serum calcium, raised serum phosphorus of permanent or recurrent nature in the absence of renal insufficiency, steatorrhea and rickets.

Vitamin D deficiency It is uncommon and may occur due to maternal anticonvulsant therapy or deficiency of vitamin D. Neonatal causes include exclusive breastfeeding, renal insufficiency, nephrosis, hepatobiliary disease and malabsorption.

Hypomagnesemia It decreases synthesis and secretion of parathyroid hormone leading to hypocalcemia. Hypocalcemia cannot be corrected by calcium therapy alone unless magnesium is given.

DiGeorge sequence or CATCH 22 syndrome It is characterized by hypocalcemia due to thymic aplasia with lymphopenia and recurrent infections in association with absent parathyroid glands. Dysmorphic features with hypoplasia or absence of third and fourth branchial pouch structures, defective ears, short philtrum, cleft palate or velopharyngeal incompetence with congenital defects of the aortic arch and heart may be associated. There is deletion on chromosome 22 (22 q 11 deletion).

Hypoproteinemia Total serum calcium may be low but tetany generally does not manifest due to satisfactory levels of ionized calcium. In general, plasma calcium concentration falls by 0.8 mg/dL (0.2 mmol/L) for every 1.0 g/dL fall in serum albumin level.

Congenital rickets Maternal osteomalacia may rarely lead to congenital rickets manifesting before the age of 3 months. Because of relative deficiency of vitamin D in breast milk, exclusively breastfed infants are at an increased risk to develop rickets.

Exchange transfusion Exchange transfusion with citrated blood may result in lowered levels of serum ionized calcium though the total serum calcium is unaltered. However, symptoms of hypocalcemia are rare.

Electrolyte disturbances Acidosis, especially following correction by administration of sodium bicarbonate, may lead to tetany. Excessive sodium intake may reduce serum calcium levels by increasing urinary calcium losses.

Renal disorders Both glomerular as well as renal tubular defects may lead to hypocalcemia. Acute renal failure is often associated with hyperphosphatemia and hypocalcemia. Renal dysfunction may impair the production of 1, 25-dihydroxyvitamin D_3.

Phototherapy There is some evidence that phototherapy may reduce the pineal secretion of melatonin which is known to block the effect of cortisol on uptake of calcium by the bone. Reduced levels of melatonin are likely to cause hypocalcemia due to unchecked effect of cortisol.

Furosemide therapy It is known to cause hypercalciuria leading to hypocalcemia especially in preterm babies who have deficient stores of calcium.

Intravenous lipid infusion Elevated levels of free fatty acids may mop up calcium by forming insoluble soaps. *In vitro*, a rise of 5 mmol/L of free fatty acids has been shown to decrease serum ionized calcium by 0.6 mg/dL.

Clinical Features

There are no dignostic features of hypocalcemia and many cases are asymptomatic and transient. Early symptoms in preterm babies include shallow rapid breathing with transient episodes of apneic attacks and cyanosis. Exaggerated neuromuscular activity may be manifest by excessive jitteriness, especially in response to various external stimuli, such as touch, sound and light. Hypocalcemia is the commonest biochemical abnormality seen in association with neonatal convulsions. Some babies may show sustained ankle clonus and positive peroneal sign though Chvostek's sign can be elicited in normal babies in the absence of hypocalcemia. The affected babies remain characteristically alert and their behavior and activity is unaffected even in the presence of muscle spasms as opposed to infants with hypoglycemia. The periods of muscular excitability may alternate with phases of immobility and hypotonia. Some babies may have high-pitched squeaky cry and episodes of laryngospasm.

Diagnosis

High index of suspicion and routine monitoring of high-risk babies vulnerable to develop hypocalcemia, is mandatory to make an early diagnosis. Low serum calcium (<8.0 mg/dL) is diagnostic but it is time consuming and demands relatively a large volume of blood sample. Electrocardiogram is useful and reliable to suspect hypocalcemia and monitor response to therapy. EKG may show 2:1 atrioventricular block with low voltage and prolonged QoT due to prolongation of ST interval. QoTc is more reliable and is calculated as follows:

$$QoTc = \frac{QoT\ (sec)}{\sqrt{R - R\ interval\ (sec)}}$$

Wherein QoT interval is calculated from the origin of Q wave to the beginning of T wave. *QoTc of more than 0.2 seconds is highly suggestive of hypocalcemia.* Before administration of calcium, blood sample should be collected for serum calcium, phosphorus and alkaline phosphatase. Hyperparathyroidism in the mother should be excluded by estimating serum paratharmone, calcium, phosphorus, alkaline phosphatase and evaluating skiagram of hands. The unusual causes of late-onset neonatal hypocalcemia should be looked for and excluded by appropriate investigations including 1,25 $(OH)_2$ D_3, and parathormone (PTH) level. Elevated serum phosphate suggest excessive phosphate intake, renal insufficiency or hypoparathyroidism. Absence of thymic shadow on skiagram of chest is suggestive of DiGeorge syndrome. Echocardiography may be required to exclude underlying cardiac anomaly in infants with DiGeorge and CATCH 22 syndrome. Ophthalmic examination for cataracts and CT scan of brain is advised for exclusion of pseudohypoparathyroidism.

Management

Asymptomatic Babies

Give 2 mL/kg/dose of 10% calcium gluconate intravenously after dilution with equal volume of 5% dextrose every 6 hourly and continue for 48 hours once EKG had returned back to normal. If infant is orally fed, calcium gluconate 10% solution (2 mL/kg every 6 hourly) can be given through oral route for treatment of asymptomatic hypocalcemia.

Symptomatic Babies

Parenteral therapy is indicated in the presence of extreme irritability, convulsions and apneic attacks. Calcium gluconate 10% solution (2 mL/kg or 20 mg elemental calcium/kg) diluted with equal volume of 5% dextrose should be injected slowly at a rate of less than 1.0 mL per minute through an established intravenous line with continuous monitoring of heart rate. It should never be infused through the umbilical vein

due to risk of development of hepatic necrosis, if the catheter is lodged in a branch of the portal vein. The maximal dose recommended is 10 mL for full term and 5 mL for preterm babies. It is followed by 8 mL kg/day of 10% calcium gluconate solution (75 mg/kg/day of elemental calcium) as a constant infusion for at least 48 hours after EKG had returned back to normal. *The injection should never be given intramuscularly because of risk of tissue necrosis and it should not be added to infusion solutions containing sodium bicarbonate because of risk of producing precipitate of calcium carbonate.* It should be used with caution in babies receiving digitalis and in hypokalemic states. If hypocalcemia is unresponsive to calcium therapy, magnesium sulfate (0.2 mL/kg of 50% solution intramuscular in 2 doses 12 hours apart) should be administered. This should be followed by maintenance oral dose of 0.2 mL/kg of 50% magnesium sulfate once daily for 3 days. Extravasation of calcium containing solution into subcutaneous tissue is dangerous and may lead to tissue necrosis. Indentify extravasation early and inject hyaluronidase SC at the site of extravasation (15–30 units in one mL of normal saline). There is no role of vitamin D in the management of neonatal hypocalcemia.

Resistant Hypocalcemia

Infants with prolonged and/or resistant hypocalcemia should be investigated for hypomagnesemia and other unusual causes. Elevated phosphate levels in the absence of exogenous phosphate load (cow's milk) and presence of normal renal functions are suggestive of hypoparathyroidism. These neonates need supplementation with calcium (50 mg/kg/d q 8 hr) and 1, 25 $(OH)_2$ D_3 or calcitriol (0.5–1.0 µg/day). Therapy may be stopped after 6 weeks in infants born to mothers with hyperparathyroidism.

Prophylaxis

Infants at increased risk to develop hypocalcemia (preterm <1500 g, birth asphyxia, IDMs) should receive elemental calcium 35–45 mg/kg/day. Calcium gluconate 10% solution (elemental calcium 9 mg in each 1.0 mL) 1 mL/kg/dose diluted with equal volume of distilled water should be given intravenously every 6-hourly for 48–72 hours or till oral feeds with supplements of calcium are started.

Calcium and Phosphorus Supplements

In view of low stores of calcium and phosphorus and rapid growth velocity of preterm babies, they must receive adequate supplements of calcium and phosphorus to prevent osteopenia of prematurity. The calcium/phosphorus ratio of the milk formula should be at least 2:1 to avoid excessive phosphorus load as a safeguard against late onset tetany of the newborn. Infants weighing less than 1500 g and receiving EBM should be given daily supplements of elemental calcium of 160 mg/kg and phosphorus 80 mg/kg with a suitable oral preparation containing two parts of calcium and one part of phosphorus. There is no need for supplements when human milk fortifier is used to supplement EBM. The supplements should be continued till the postconceptional maturity of 38 weeks or weight of 2000 g.

Vitamin D

Exclusively breastfed infants should receive daily supplements of 400–600 iu of vitamin D because breast milk is deficient in vitamin D. There is no role of administration of vitamin D for treatment of early and late-onset hypocalcemia in newborn babies. Pharmacological doses of vitamin D (5000 iu/d) are indicated for treatment of osteopenia of prematurity. Vitamin D analogues (dihydrotachysterol and calcitriol) are used for treatment of hypocalcemia due to chronic renal dysfunction and DiGeorge syndrome.

Prognosis

In hypocalcemic fits, the prognosis regarding mental development is excellent. If hypocalcemia is due to natal complications, the prognosis is determined by the nature and severity of associated conditions.

OSTEOPENIA OF PREMATURITY

Preterm babies especially those below 1500 g are born with poor stores of calcium and phosphorus because 80% of skeletal uptake of these minerals occurs during the last trimester of pregnancy. They have poor intestinal absorption of calcium and impaired conversion of vitamin D into its active metabolites. Feeding with human breast milk provides approximately 40–50 mg/kg/day of calcium and 30–40 mg/kg/day phosphorus which is inadequate to meet the daily needs of 210–250 mg/kg/day and 100–125 mg/kg/day of calcium and phosphorus respectively. Consequently, osteopenia of prematurity or metabolic bone disease (MBD) is a significant hazard and even rickets may occasionally develop in preterm babies. The incidence is inversely related to the gestational age. If adequate supplements of calcium and phosphorus are not provided, it affects 20–30% of VLBW babies (<1500 g) and 60–75% of ELBW babies (<1000 g).

Etiology

The principal cause of osteopenia or metabolic bone disease of prematurity is reduced stores of calcium and phosphorus because of preterm birth. There are several risk factors which predispose to osteopenia of prematurity. Feeding with unfortified human milk or parenteral nutrition without adequate supplements of calcium and phosphorus may lead to development of osteopenia or even frank rickets. Administration of certain drugs especially loop diuretics (furosemide), corticosteroids and methylxanthines may lead to increased urinary losses of calcium. Acquired or congenital tubular defects may be associated with phosphaturia. Vitamin D deficiency is not an important cause of osteopenia but may contribute some role in infants with cholestatic hepatitis. Infants with bronchopulmonary dysplasia and prolonged administration of furosemide therapy are specially vulnerable to develop osteopenia of prematurity. Congenital rickets may be seen in infants born to mothers with osteomalacia, hypoparathyroidism and prolonged therapy with magnesium sulfate. Salient risk factors for metabolic bone disease of prematurity are listed in Table 24.3.

TABLE 24.3 Risk factors for metabolic bone disease of prematurity	
Antenatal	*Postnatal*
■ Pre-eclampsia	■ Prolonged TPN >4 weeks
■ Placental insufficiency	■ Sepsis
■ Chorioamnionitis	■ Necrotizing anterocolitis
■ Nuromuscular disorders	■ Bronchopulmonary dysplasia
■ Genetic polymorphisms (vitamin D receptor, estrogen, collagen alpha 1 genes)	■ Cholestasis
■ Male gender	■ Renal dysfunction
	■ Medications (loop diuretics, methylxanthines, gluco-corticoids)

Metabolic Disorders

24

Clinical Features

The clinical manifestations are subtle and may be easily overlooked. Clinical and biochemical manifestations may be seen around 2 to 4 months of postnatal age. There is hypotonia and decreased linear growth. The softening of chest bones may lead to respiratory difficulties and delay in weaning from ventilator. There may be prominence of forehead, dolichocephaly, wide anterior fontanel, widened cranial sutures and craniotabes (softening and flattening of occiput). There may be widening of wrists, knees and ankles with rachitic rosary due to swelling of the costochondral junctions (Figure 24.4). The ribs may be pulled posteriorly at the insertion of diaphragm producing Harrison's groove. Pathologic fractures may occur spontaneously or on excessive handling. Chest physiotherapy must be done gently and with due care in these infants to safeguard against development of fracture of ribs.

Diagnosis

Serum calcium is usually within normal range while there is significant hypophosphatemia (<4 mg/dL) and marked elevation of alkaline phosphatase (>1000 iu/L). Alkaline phosphatase is also elevated in infants with cholestatic hepatitis. There is hypercalciuria with elevated urinary calcium to creatinine ratio. The serum levels of $25(OH)D_3$ are usually low or borderline. Skiagram of chest taken for evaluation of RDS may provide useful clues for osteopenia or decreased mineralization by showing widening of costochondral junctions (Figure 24.5). Koo has proposed following grading on skiagrams of wrists: Grade I. There is loss of dense white line at metaphysis and increase in

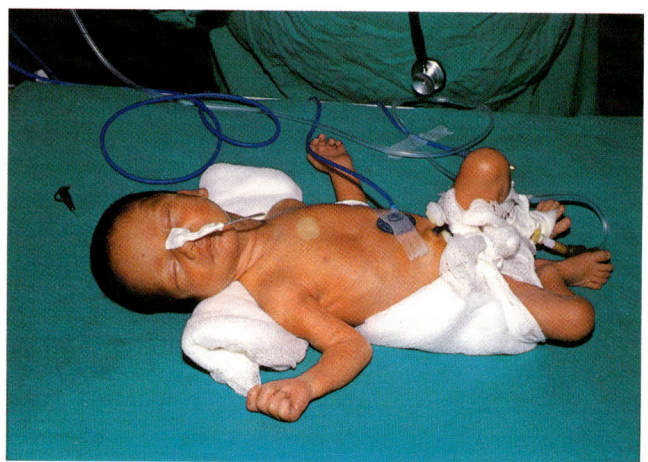

Figure 24.4 Prominent forehead with widening of costochondral junctions and wrists due to osteopenia of prematurity.

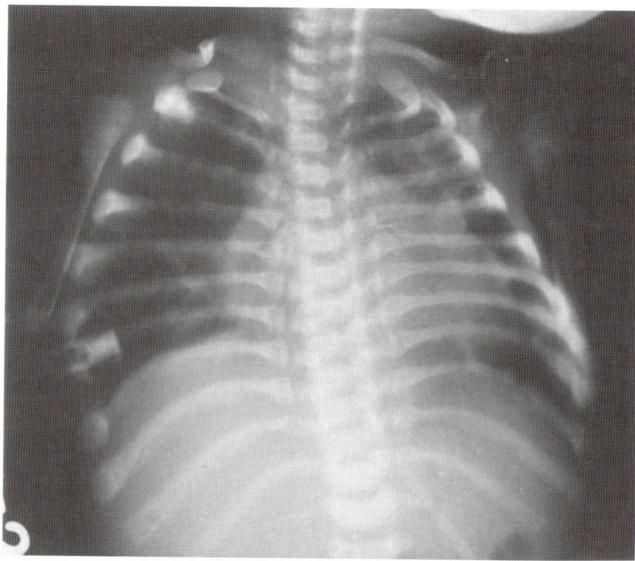

Figure 24.5 Widening of costochondral junctions on X-ray chest taken to exclude bronchopulmonary dysplasia.

submetaphyseal lucency with thinning of cortex (osteopenia). Grade II. Flaying and irregularity of metaphysis with splaying and cupping (rickets). Grade III. The aforementioned changes are associated with fractures. Quantitative ultrasound (QUS) is a useful screening modality while dual energy X-ray absorptiometry (DEXA) is the gold standard technique to assess bone mineral density (BMD). Photon densitometry is an excellent tool for measurement of bone mineral content but is reserved for research purposes.

Management

Prevention EBM-fed infants with a birth weight of <1500 g should receive daily oral supplements of calcium 160 mg/kg, phosphorus 80 mg/kg and vitamin D 400–600 iu till they achieve a postconceptional maturity of 38 weeks. In clinical practice, it is achieved by administration of ostocalcium syrup (7.5–10.0 mL/kg/d) or tablet (1.0–1.5 tablet/kg/d) given in divided doses mixed with EBM three times a day. Infants receiving intravenous therapy or parenteral nutrition should receive these supplements parenterally. The calcium and phosphate concentration in the TPN solution should be 30 mg/dL and 20 mg/dL, respectively. Potassium phosphate should be added first in the TPN solution followed by calcium salt to avoid precipitation.

Treatment Osteopenia of prematurity is treated with supplements of calcium, phosphorus and vitamin D 400–800 iu daily. Therapy is usually continued for a period of 3 months. At times high doses (5,000–10,000 iu/day) of vitamin D are required to correct biochemical and skeletal abnormalities. Infants with defective vitamin D metabolism respond better to dihydrotachysterol or calcitriol therapy. Gentle massage and passive movements of limbs are associated with enhanced mineralization and growth of bones.

HYPERCALCEMIA

Neonatal hypercalcemia (serum calcium level >11.0 mg/dL or serum ionized calcium level >5.0 mg/dL) is uncommon. It is usually asymptomatic and discovered incidentally on routine screening. The common causes include primary hyperparathyroidism, congenital transitory hyperparathyroidism in association with maternal hypoparathyroidism, congenital hypophosphatasia, subcutaneous fat necrosis, hypervitaminosis A and D and use of thiazide diuretics. Low phosphate intake in preterm infants fed with unsupplemented human milk or total parenteral nutrition may develop hypercalcemia due to excessive production of 1, 25 dihydroxyvitamin D. Williams syndrome is characterized by intrauterine growth retardation, idiopathic hypercalcemia, "elfin" facies, supravalvular aortic stenosis or peripheral pulmonic stenosis and psychomotor retardation. Blue diaper syndrome is a rare cause of unexplained hypercalcemia. There is a metabolic defect in intestinal transport of tryptophan with excretion of blue-colored tryptophan metabolites (indicanuria) which stain the diaper blue.

The clinical features of hypercalcemia are nonspecific and include craniotabes, poor feeding, hypotonia, vomiting, polyuria, constipation, fractures (hyperparathyroidism), hypertension and nephrocalcinosis. In hyperparathyroidism, serum calcium and alkaline phosphatase are elevated while phosphorus is low. PTH level is raised with demineralization and subperiosteal resorption of bones of hands and wrists. Alkaline phosphatase level is low in infants with hypophosphatasia. Excessive intake of vitamin D may be associated with elevated levels of 25 $(OH)_2$ D.

Life-threatening hypercalcemia is treated by volume expansion with normal saline and furosemide (1 mg/kg IV q 8 hr). Oral or parenteral phosphates (3.0–5.0 mg/dL) should be given to preterm infants with hypophosphatemia. Cortisone (10 mg/kg/d) or methylprednisolone (2 mg/kg/d) is effective to correct hypercalcemia due to hypervitaminosis A and D and subcutaneous fat necrosis. Low-calcium and low-vitamin D diet is recommended in infants with hypervitaminosis A or D, subcutaneous fat necrosis

and Williams syndrome. Calcitonin is a potent inhibitor of bone resorption but its effect is not sustained. Parathyroidectomy with autologous re-implantation may be indicated in intractable cases with severe persistent neonatal hyperparathyroidism.

HYPOMAGNESEMIA

This rare metabolic defect may occur in association with hypocalcemia, intrauterine growth retardation, severe diarrhea and following massive resection of gut. Decreased serum magnesium levels have been reported in infants of toxemic or diabetic mothers and following exchange blood transfusion with citrated blood. The average serum magnesium level during first week of life is 1.5 ±0.12 mEq/L. Hypomagnesemia should be suspected, if hypocalcemia is unresponsive to calcium therapy. The phosphate level is generally normal and babies may be slightly edematous. The condition can be treated by administration of 0.2 mL/kg of 50% magnesium sulfate solution (1 mL of 50% magnesium sulfate solution provides 4 mEq of magnesium) intramuscularly one or two injections followed by oral supplementation of magnesium in a dose of 30 mg per day for 3 to 4 days.

LATE METABOLIC ACIDOSIS

Most pediatricians are quite conversant with occurrence of metabolic acidosis amongst seriously ill newborn babies with severe birth apshyxia, respiratory failure and respiratory distress syndrome during first two days of life. However, relatively frequent development of metabolic acidosis among healthy preterm formula-fed infants having onset during late first week or early second week of life is not generally recognized.

Pathogenesis

Renal immaturity and relatively high net dietary acid (protein) load are considered to be two main risk factors determining the occurrence and severity of late-onset metabolic acidosis. The condition is rare among infants fed with human or humanized milk. Intestinal shunting of base resulting in increased excretion of bicarbonate in the urine and stools, and liberation of H^+ ions from bone during mineralization are additional contributory factors. Preterm infants are unable to handle an excessive endogenous acid load of dietary protein intake due to immaturity of renal and intestinal acid–base regulatory mechanisms. The acid excretion rate of preterm infants is only 0.4 mmol/100 mg of excreted nitrogen in term infants. Excessive proliferation of E. coli flora of gut on artificial feeds is

Metabolic Disorders

24

held responsible for occurrence of semiloose or loose stools by a mechanism similar to that seen in blind-loop syndrome.

Clinical Features

The condition is limited to preterm babies and its incidence is directly related to the degree of immaturity. Disturbances in early neonatal weight gain pattern are invariable. Excessive initial weight loss (>10%), failure to regain birth weight by two weeks and poor weight gain velocity of less than 1.0% of body weight, or sudden unexplained drop in weight, should be looked for. Lethargy, slow feeding and circumoral grayish unhealthy hue should alert to the possibility of late metabolic acidosis. Occurrence of mild diarrhea should not be mistaken for bacterial infection. Tachypnea occurs due to respiratory attempts at compensation of acidosis. Hypothermia may also occur. Reflex activity, however, is well maintained unlike septicemia. The diagnosis is confirmed by demonstration of pH <7.35 and base deficit of more than 5 mmol/L with CO_2 TOT of <21 mM after the third day of life.

Treatment

The protein intake among preterm infants should be restricted to 4 g/kg/day because higher intakes are associated with frequent development of metabolic acidosis. This can be achieved by administration of humanized milk (whey-predominant) or expressed breast milk. The occurrence of late-onset metabolic acidosis should be identified by its characteristic clinical profile and differentiated from septicemia. Therapy with oral 7.5% sodium bicarbonate (dose calculated as 0.6 × body weight × base deficit) is followed by prompt recovery. Sodium bicarbonate therapy should be continued for a period of 2 weeks or till gestational maturity of 36 weeks is achieved. It is associated with rapid gain in weight and improvement in the general appearance, wellbeing and activity of the infant. Prophylactic alkalinization of milk, by administration of 0.5–1.0 mL of 7.5% sodium bicarbonate with each feed, can be given to formula fed infants with a gestational age of 32 weeks or less.

INBORN ERRORS OF METABOLISM (IEM)

Genetically determined deficiency of a specific enzyme may manifest as a life-threatening metabolic disorder in the newborn period. The excessive accumulation of metabolites, before the enzyme block or deficiency of end product may prove harmful to the rapidly growing tissues of the infant. The incomplete defects and those dependent upon exposure to certain environmental factors may not produce any recognizable illness in the newborn period. Early diagnosis and institution of effective treatment may salvage some of the infants with serious metabolic defects and prevent brain damage in others. The overall incidence of IEMs is around 3–4 per 1000 live births. Over 300 genetic defects related to synthesis, metabolism, transport and storage of biochemical compounds have been identified. Around 30% of inborn errors of metabolism are associated with involvement of central nervous system. It is estimated that almost 20% of acute life-threatening illnesses in newborn babies are attributed to an inherited metabolic disorder. The signs and symptoms of a hereditary metabolic disease can mimic almost any pediatric disease. The presence of an inborn error of metabolism should be suspected in the following situations.

1. Previous history of unexplained neonatal deaths, unexplained seizures and mental retardation or of a known metabolic disorder. Infants with such a history must be thoroughly screened for a possible metabolic defect even in the absence of any problems in the neonatal period. Routine screening for relatively common conditions, such as phenylketonuria though practiced in certain countries, is currently not feasible for developing countries in view of different needs and priorities.
2. The development of evidences of unexplained (after exclusion of sepsis, hypoxic–ischemic encephalopathy and hypoglycemia) cerebral depression with refusal of feeds, unresponsiveness, profound hypotonia, respiratory distress or apneic attacks and seizures are useful markers of inborn error of metabolism.
3. The abnormal smell either from the baby or his urine and presence of ketonuria should also arouse the suspicion of a congenital metabolic disorder (Table 24.4). The clinical picture may be indistinguishable from fulminant septicemia and at times both may coexist.
4. Unexplained vomiting and/or diarrhea, dehydration, hepatosplenomegaly, jaundice and bleeding manifestations should be investigated for a possible metabolic defect.
5. Failure to thrive despite adequate feeding and in the absence of any infection.
6. Cardiomyopathy, arrhythmia and hypotonia may occur in infants with long-chain fatty acid oxidation defects, mitochondrial respiratory-chain defects and neonatal form of Pompe disease.

7. Facial dysmorphism and phenotypic abnormalities may be seen in a number of inborn errors of metabolism (Table 24.5).

8. Unexplained severe metabolic acidosis.

9. Acute fatty liver or HELPP (**h**emolysis, **e**levated **l**iver enzymes and **l**ow **p**latelet counts) during **p**regnancy in women carrying fetuses with long-chain-3 hydroxyacyl-coenzyme dehydrogenase deficiency (LCHADD).

10. Consanguinity among parents.

TABLE 24.4 Abnormal urinary and body odor*

Disease	Nature of odor
▪ Cystinuria and homocystinuria	Sulphurous
▪ Hawkinsinuria	Chlorine-like or swimming pool
▪ Isovaleric acidemia and glutaric acidemia type II	Sweaty feet or ripe cheese
▪ Maple syrup urine disease	Maple syrup or burnt sugar
▪ Methionine malabsorption	Boiled cabbage
▪ Multiple carboxylase deficiency	Cat urine
▪ Phenylketonuria	Mousy or musty odor
▪ Tyrosinemia, hypermethio-nemia, trimethylaminuria	Rotten fish
▪ Tyrosinemia type I	Rancid butter

*Unusual odor is more readily smelt in a sample of frozen urine because organic compounds with different freezing points concentrate on the top. A filter paper soaked with urine can be smelled. (Akin to perfume selection in a cosmetic outlet!)

TABLE 24.5 Inborn errors of metabolism with dysmorphic features

Disorder	Dysmorphic features
Peroxisomal disorders (Zellweger syndrome)	Prominent forehead, large fontanel, flat nasal bridge, epicanthal folds, hypoplastic supraorbital ridges.
Pyruvate dehydrogenase deficiency	Epicanthal folds, flat nasal bridge, small nose with anteverted flared nostrils and long philtrum.
Glutaric aciduria type II	Macrocephaly, high forehead, flat nasal bridge, short anteverted nose, ear anomalies, hypospadias and rocker-bottom feet.
Cholesterol biosynthetic defects (Smith-Lemli-Opitz syndrome)	Epicanthal folds, flat nasal bridge, cataracts, syndactyly of toes and genital abnormalities.
Congenital disorders of glycosylation	Inverted nipples, lipodystrophy
Lysosomal storage disorders	Hurler-like phenotype

In a multicentric study conducted by Indian Council of Medical Research, it was found that inborn errors of metabolism account for 5% cases of mental retardation. The studies conducted at the Genetics Division of AIIMS, New Delhi revealed that hereditary metabolic disorders accounted for 10% cases of mental retardation. The common neurometabolic disorders include organic acidurias, amino acidopathies, urea cycle disorders, mucopolysaccharidosis, congenital lactic acidosis, peroxisomal disorders and fatty acid oxidation disorders. It is estimated that maple syrup urine disease, organic acidurias, urea cycle defects and non-ketotic hyperglycinemias account for over 65% cases of inborn errors of metabolism.

Diagnosis

There is a need to develop sophisticated biochemical diagnostic facilities in selected advanced or regional genetic centers in the country. The currently available facilities for a definitive diagnosis of inborn errors of metabolism are rather unsatisfactory. The nature and sequence of investigations depends upon the clinical suspicion of the underlying metabolic disorder. Availability of facilities for monitoring blood ammonia and acid–base parameters is crucial for pursuing an algorithmic approach for the diagnosis of common neurometabolic disorders. The most common neurometabolic disorders in order of their frequency include aminoacidopathies, organic acidurias, urea cycle disorders, congenital lactic acidosis and peroxisomal disorders (Table 24.6). In a baby with life-threatening CNS manifestations, presence of abnormalities on CT scan or MRI study usually rules out a metabolic disorder. However, abnormalities on brain scan may be seen in infants with lactic acidosis syndromes (Leigh disease) and lysosomal or peroxisomal metabolism disorder. Agenesis of corpus callosum is commonly associated in infants with non-ketotic hyperglycinemia.

Complete blood counts Bone marrrow suppression with neutropenia and thrombocytopenia is an important feature of a number of organic acidemias, like isovaleric, methylmalonic and propionic acidemia.

Urinalysis Reducing substance in urine is seen in patients with galactosemia, diabetes mellitus, hereditary fructose intolerance, pentosuria, Fanconi syndrome and renal glycosuria. The Clinitest detects presence of galactose and glucose but not fructose. A positive reaction with Clinitest should be investigated further with the Clinistix reaction (glucose oxidase) which is specific for glucose. Urine should be

TABLE 24.6 Inborn errors of metabolism having onset in the newborn period

- **Aminoacidopathies**
  Maple syrup urine disease
  Nonketotic hyperglycinemia
  Homocystinuria
  Sulfite oxidase deficiency
  Tyrosinemia type I and III
- **Organic acidurias**
  Methylmalonic aciduria
  Propionic aciduria
  Isovaleric aciduria
  Multiple carboxylase deficiency
  Glutaric aciduria type I
- **Hyperammonemias**
  Ornithine carbamylase deficiency
  Citrullinemia
  Argininosuccinate lyase deficiency
  Phosphate synthetase deficiency
  Triple H syndrome
- **Congenital lactic acidemias**
  Respiratory chain disorders
  Pyruvate dehydrogenase deficiency
  Pyruvate carboxylase deficiency
  Krebs cycle disorders
- **Glycogen storage disorders**
  Glucose-6-phosphate dehydrogenase deficiency
  Fructose disphosphate deficiency
  Glycogen storage diseases III and IV
- **Fatty acid oxidation disorders**
  Idiopathic systemic carnitine deficiency
  Palmitoyl carnitine transferase deficiency
  Multiple acyl-CoA dehydrogenase deficiency
  Medium and long chain acyl-CoA dehydrogenase deficiency
- **Peroxisomal disorders**
  Zellweger syndrome
  Neonatal adrenoleukodystrophy
  X-linked adrenoleukodystrophy
  Adrenomyeloneuropathy
  Infantile Refsum
  Rhizomelic chondrodysplasia punctata

examined for ketonuria and ketoacidemia by high voltage electrophoresis and gas liquid chromatography. The presence of ketones with normoglycemia is suggestive of propionic acidemia. The absence of ketones in association with hypoglycemia suggests the possibility of defective fatty acid oxidation. It may occur due to increased insulin secretion caused by an insulinoma, or it may represent a defect in mitochondrial fatty acid oxidation or ketogenesis. Ferric chloride test may be positive in patients with phenylketonuria (green), maple syrup urine disease (green-gray), tyrosinemia (fading green), histidinemia (blue-green), alkaptonuria (dark-brown) and ketosis (light-green). Cot-side urine screen for reducing substance, ferric chloride, DNPH (chalky-white precipitate) and nitroprusside (red-purple) test provides useful information (Table 24.7).

Biochemical Screening

Four biochemical tests are particularly useful for screening and broad classification of IEMs, i.e. arterial blood pH, blood lactate, blood ammonia and urinary ketones (Table 24.8).

Blood glucose Hypoglycemia commonly occurs with organic acidurias, galactosemia, glycogen storage disease type I, hereditary fructose intolerance, tyrosinemia type I, systemic carnitine deficiency, glutaric acidemia type II and hyperglycerolemia. Non-ketotic hypoglycemia is the hallmark in infants with defects of fatty acid oxidation. Hypoglycemia may be intermittent or intractable and precipitated by an intercurrent illness (Figure 24.6).

Acid–base parameters and electrolytes Electrolytes are generally normal unless there is severe vomiting or diarrhea. The bicarbonate level may be low in patients with organic and aminoacidurias. Metabolic acidosis with increased anion gap (≥ 16) is seen in patients with organic acidemias, fatty acid oxidation disorder, glycogen storage disease type I, hereditary fructose intolerance, renal tubular acidosis, glutaric

TABLE 24.7 Urine screen for neurometabolic disorders

Disorder	Ferric chloride	DNPH*	Reducing substance	Nitroprusside test
Phenlyketonuria	+	+	−	−
Galactosemia	−	−	+	−
Organic aciduria	+	+	−	−
Aminoaciduria	−	+	−	−
Homocystinuria	−	−	−	+

*DNPH: Dinitrophenyl hydrazine

TABLE 24.8 Biochemical screening for inborn errors of metabolism

Group	Acidosis	Elevated lactate	Elevated ammonia	Ketosis	Diagnosis
I	–	–	–	+	Maple syrup urine disease
II	+	–	–	+	Organic aciduria
III	+	+	–	+	Lactic acidosis
IV	–	–	+	–	Urea cycle disorder
V	–	–	–	–	Non-ketotic hyperglycinemia, peroxisomal disorder, phenylketonuria, galactosemia and sulfite oxidase deficiency

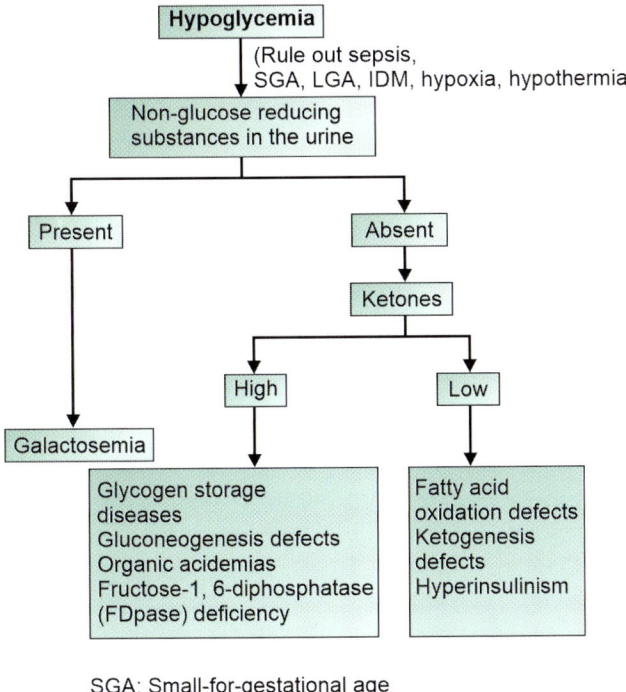

SGA: Small-for-gestational age
LGA: Large-for-gestational age
IDM: Infant of diabetic mother

Figure 24.6 Algorithm for protracted hypoglycemia in a newborn baby.

acidemia type II and mitochondrial disorders (Figure 24.7). Absence of metabolic acidosis, however, does not rule out the possibility of organic acidurias.

Liver enzymes Galactosemia is the most common metabolic cause of liver disease in the neonate. Hepatic dysfunction as evidenced by elevated transaminase levels is common in a number of metabolic disorders including organic acidurias, aminoacidurias, glycogen storage disease, hereditary fructose intolerance, lysosomal storage disease, mitochondrial disorders and peroxisomal disorders. Cholestatic jaundice with failure to thrive may occur due to alpha-1-antitrypsin deficiency.

Lactate and pyruvate levels Altered pyruvate metabolism leads to lactic acidosis in many metabolic conditions including mitochondrial disease, pyruvate metabolism defects, glycogen storage disease, organic aciduria and aminoacidurias (Figure 24.7). Lactic acidosis is commonly seen in critically sick neonates with poor tissue perfusion due to dehydration, seizures, shock, congenital heart disease and intracranial bleeding. Lactate level should be tested on arterial blood which should be collected after 2 hours of fast.

Plasma ammonia level This is one of the most useful screening tool for diagnosis of a metabolic disorder (Figure 24.8). Blood sample for ammonia should be collected after 4–6 hours of fasting and processed without delay. Blood ammonia levels are elevated 10 to 100 times (500–1500 µmol/L) in urea cycle disorders and two to three times in mitochondrial disorders and organic acidemias and aminoacidopathies.

Plasma carnitine This test is usually available in a reference biochemical laboratory. Patients with organic acidurias generally have a low plasma free carnitine level (<20 mmol/L) and an elevated acyl-carnitine/free carnitine ratio (>0.4). The presence of low free carnitine or elevated acylcarnitine/free carnitine ratio should prompt studies for organic acidurias and peroxisomal defects. Carnitine therapy may provide therapeutic utility in these patients.

Plasma amino acids In infants with elevated blood ammonia level or liver enzymes, plasma amino acid profile should be studied. Urinary organic acid pattern is a useful screening method. There may be no characteristic plasma or urinary amino acid abnormalities in two most common disorders of urea degradation, i.e. carbamyl phosphate synthetase deficiency and ornithine transcarbamylase deficiency. These disorders can thus be confused with other hyperammonemic encephalopathies, such as Reye syndrome, organic acidurias associated with hyperammonemia and lysine protein intolerance.

Spinal fluid Amino acid profile of CSF is recommended when a defect of glycine cleavage is suspected.

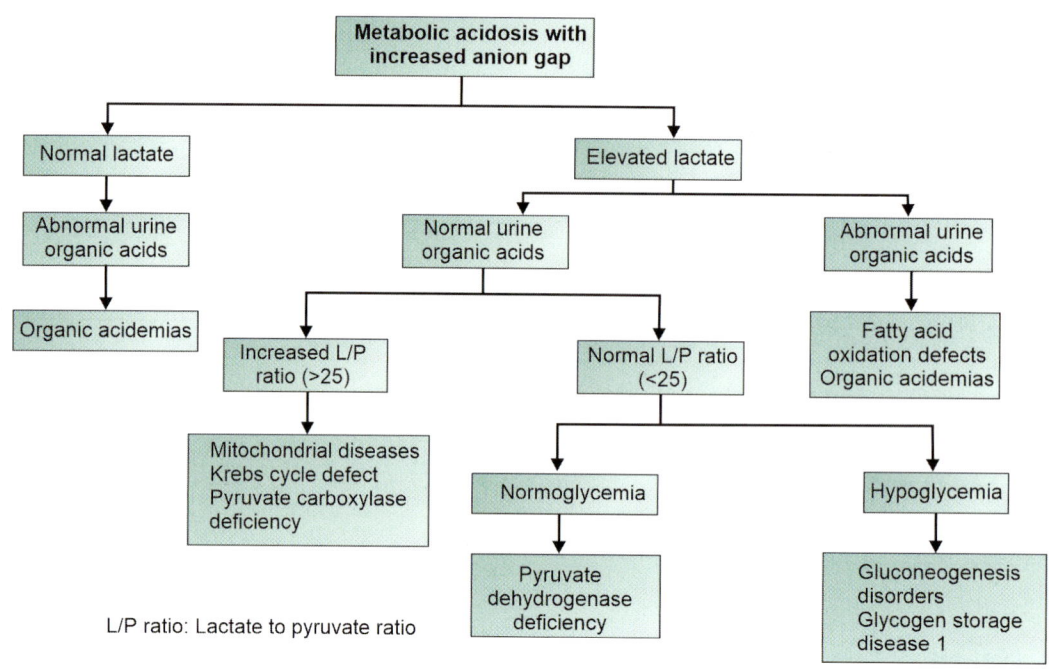

Figure 24.7 Algorithm for metabolic acidosis with increased anion gap in a newborn baby suspected to have IEM.

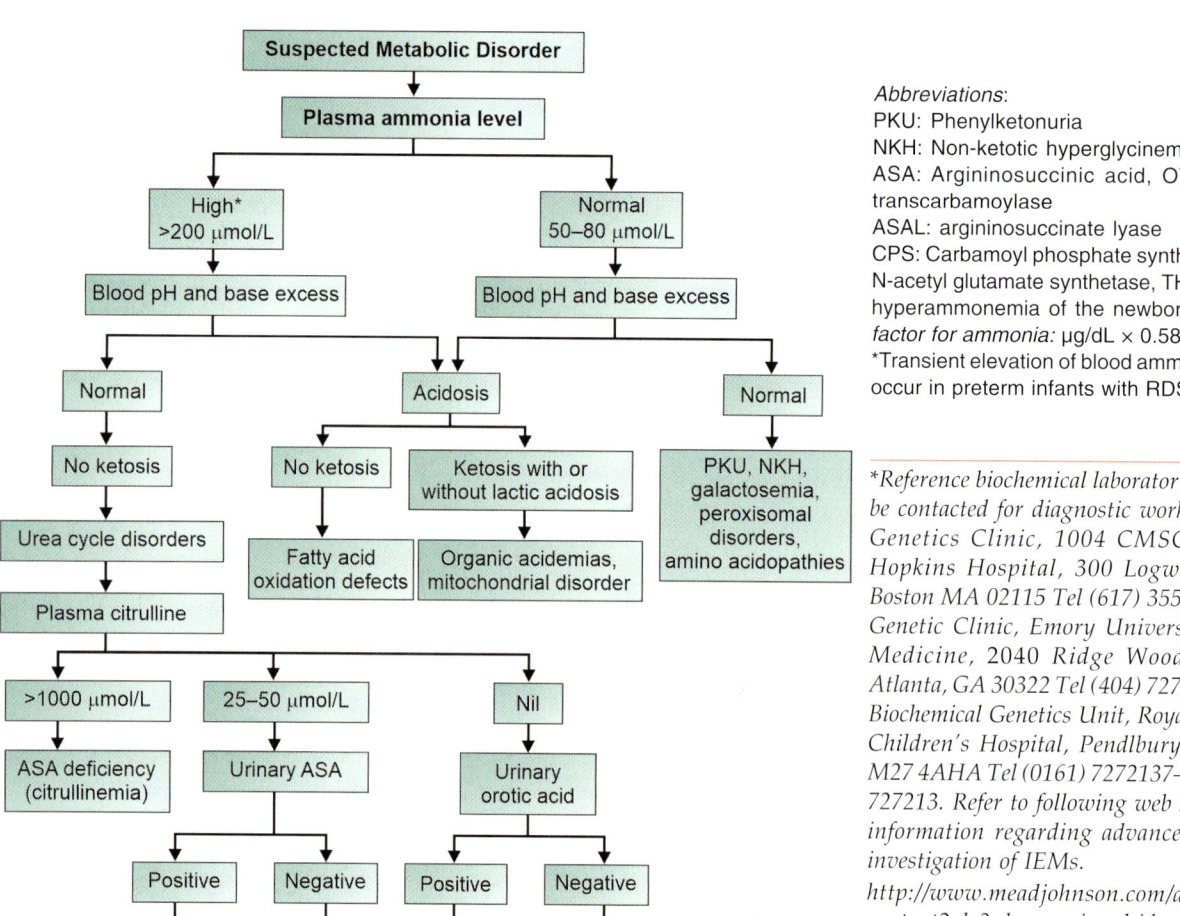

Abbreviations:
PKU: Phenylketonuria
NKH: Non-ketotic hyperglycinemia
ASA: Argininosuccinic acid, OTC: Ornithine transcarbamoylase
ASAL: argininosuccinate lyase
CPS: Carbamoyl phosphate synthetase, NAGS: N-acetyl glutamate synthetase, THAN: Transient hyperammonemia of the newborn. *Conversion factor for ammonia*: µg/dL × 0.5872 = µmol/L.
*Transient elevation of blood ammonia level may occur in preterm infants with RDS

Reference biochemical laboratories which may be contacted for diagnostic workup: Pediatric Genetics Clinic, 1004 CMSC, The Johns Hopkins Hospital, 300 Logwood Avenue, Boston MA 02115 Tel (617) 355 6394, Emory Genetic Clinic, Emory University School of Medicine, 2040 Ridge Wood Drive NE, Atlanta, GA 30322 Tel (404) 7275731, Willink Biochemical Genetics Unit, Royal Manchester Children's Hospital, Pendlbury, Manchester M27 4AHA Tel (0161) 7272137–8, Fax (0161) 727213. Refer to following web sites for more information regarding advanced centers for investigation of IEMs.
http://www.meadjohnson.com/app/iwp/HCP content2.do? dm = mj and id = /HCP_Home Product.Information product. Descriptions http://www.geneclinics.org

Figure 24.8 Diagnostic approach for IEM based on plasma ammonia level.

Care of the Newborn

24

This defect is characterized by encephalopathy, burst suppression pattern on EEG and partial or complete agenesis of corpus callosum.

Specific enzyme studies The aforementioned tests are useful to diagnose organic acidopathies, amino-acidopathies and urea cycle defects. In the absence of elevation of blood ammonia and lack of metabolic acidosis, defects of carbohydrate metabolism and peroxisomal disorder should be considered and ruled out by specific tests. Skin biopsy for fibroblast cultures for enzymatic assays or DNA studies and biopsy of other body tissues, like liver, kidney and muscle is obtained for assay of enzymes and mitochondrial electron transport pathways (Table 24.9). In infants with hypotonia and progressive muscle weakness, muscle carnitine levels should be assayed. Patients with autosomal recessive carnitine muscle membrane transport defect show excellent response to carnitine therapy.

Biochemical Autopsy

When a neonate is terminally ill with an hereditary metabolic disorder, appropriate samples of body fluids and tissues should be collected and stored. In the event of death, tissue samples should be collected as early as possible preferably within 12 hours of death. The frozen or lyophilized specimens can later be sent to a laboratory* specially equipped for detailed biochemical studies. Specimens can also be transported on filter paper strips after seeking guidance from the laboratory.

1. **Blood** Collect 5–10 mL blood with absolute aseptic precautions. Keep 1–2 mL in heparin for chromosomal studies and 4–5 mL in EDTA for DNA studies at room temperature and 4°C, respectively. Keep measured aliquots of whole blood, plasma and leukocytes separately frozen at –20°C. Dispatch the samples by courier, so that they reach the laboratory within 48 hr of collection.
2. **Urine** Measured volume should be lyophilized or stored at –20°C.
3. **Spinal fluid** Lyophilize or store at –20°C.
4. **Skin biopsy** Two samples of 3–5 mm square should be taken from a well-perfused area of trunk. Clean the area with alcohol/spirit followed by normal saline. Keep the biopsy in sterile saline and transport in a special culture medium at 4°C for chromosomal analysis and enzyme assay.
5. Specimens from muscle, liver, kidney, heart and brain should be kept frozen and transported in dry ice or liquid nitrogen for biochemical studies, histochemistry, routine and electron microscopy.
6. Clinical photography for assessment of dysmorphism.
7. Radiographic infantogram to evaluate any skeletal dysplasia.

Management

The high-risk infant in whom inborn error of metabolism is anticipated should be kept nil orally and given 10% dextrose infusion. During acute life-threatening situation in a symptomatic infant, milk feeding is stopped and 10% dextrose infusion with intralipid is started to prevent endogenous tissue protein catabolism. Hypoglycemia should be managed as per standard protocol. Ringer's lactate should not be used for fluid and electrolyte therapy in a child with a known or suspected metabolic disorder. Metabolic acidosis should be corrected with sodium bicarbonate. The infant should be nursed in a thermoneutral environment and should be assisted to have adequate ventilation and tissue perfusion. In a life-threatening situation, exchange blood transfusion may have limited therapeutic utility while hemodialysis effectively eliminates toxic metabolites. When blood ammonia level exceeds 600 μg/dL or there is intractable metabolic acidosis, hemodialysis is life-saving. Most cases would require antibiotics for treatment of septicemia and for sterilization of gut to reduce synthesis of organic acids.

Parenteral administration of cocktail of vitamins and cofactors (100–1000 times of physiological dose) is useful in several cases of vitamin-responsive enzyme deficiencies (Table 24.10). In infants with hyperammonemia, sodium benzoate 250 mg/kg in 10% dextrose should be given at a rate of 20 mg/kg over 1–2 hr, followed by constant infusion of 250–500 mg/kg during 24 hr. Arginine or citrulline is given to infants with urea cycle defects. L-carnitine (50–300 mg/kg/d IV or 200–800 mg/kg/d oral) is recommended for patients with organic aciduria, mitochondrial disorders and conditions characterized by low free carnitine or elevated acylcarnitine to free carnitine ratio. In patients with mitochondrial encephalopathy, steroid therapy has been shown to reduce serum lactate and pyruvate levels.

The infant should be kept NPO till his mental status and vital signs are stable. Oral feeds should be gradually introduced beginning with protein intake of 0.5 g/kg/d which can be gradually increased up to 1.5 g/kg/d. The offending substrate should be eliminated and limiting amino acid or cofactor provided in the diet depending upon the specific

TABLE 24.9 Diagnostic features of acute life-threatening metabolic disorders in neonates

Disorder	Screening features	Definitive diagnosis
Adenosine deminase deficiency	Combined immunodeficiency features	Adenosine deaminase
Adrenogenital syndrome	Virilization, vomiting, dehydration, hyponatremia and hyperkalemia, urinary 17-ketosteroids	Urinary pregnentriol, serum 17-hydroxy-progesterone, dehydroepiandrosterone, 21-hydroxylase
Argininoscuccinic acidemia	Coarse short friable hair, elevated blood ammonia, urinary arginosuccinate	Argininosuccinate lyase assay in various tissues
Citrullinemia	Elevated blood ammonia and citrulline	Argininosuccinate synthetase
Fructose intolerance	Jaundice, hepatosplenomegaly, hypoglycemia and fructosuria	Hepatic fructose-1-phosphate-aldolase
Galactosemia	Feeding difficulties, poor weight gain, jaundice, hepatosplenomegaly, cataracts, hypoglycemia, reducing substance in urine and galactose in blood	Galactose-1-phosphate-uridyltransferase (GALT)
Glycogenosis	Doll-like facies, hypoglycemia, hepatomegaly	Glucose-6-phosphatase
Hyperammonemia (carbamyl phosphate synthetase and ornithine transcarbamylase deficiency)	Elevated blood ammonia, orotic aciduria in OTC deficiency	Ornithine transcarbamylase, carbamyl phosphate synthetase
Hyperglycinemia, non-ketotic	Seizures, hiccups, hypotonia and glycinemia	Glycine-serine conversion
Hyperglycinemia, ketotic	Acidosis, seizures, leukopenia, thrombocytopenia, glycinemia and glycinuria	Propionyl-coenzyme A carboxylase
Hypervalinemia	Valinuria	Hypervalinemia, valine-α-ketoglutarate transaminase
Isovaleric acidemia	Vomitings, acidosis, lethargy, convulsions and coma. "sweaty feet" smell,* isovaleryl glycinuria	Isovaleric acidemia
Lactic acidemia	Acidosis, growth retardation, ataxia, and hypoglycemia	Elevated lactic acid and alanine in blood and urine. Pyruvate decarboxylase
Maple syrup urine disease	Acidosis, hypoglycemia, seizures, maple syrup odor*, branched-chain aminoaciduria	Branched-chain aminoacidemia and branched-chain ketoacid decarboxylase
Methylmalonic acidemia**	Acidosis, hypoglycemia, neutropenia, methylmalonic aciduria	Methylmalonic acid in urine and blood, methyl-malonyl-CoA mutase
Peroxisomal disorders	Dysmorphism, encephalopathy, severe hypotonia, muscle weakness, seizures, deafness, eye abnormalities	Elevated very long chain fatty acid, phytanic acid and low or abnormal peroxisomes
Phenylketonuria	Vomiting, blond hair, blue eyes, eczema, mental retardation, microcephaly, musty odor, Guthrie test positive	Phenylalanine hydroxylase
Propionic acidemia	Acidosis with a large anion gap, ketosis, hypoglycemia, neutropenia, thrombocytopenia, hyperglycinemia	Propionic acidemia, propionyl CoA carboxylase
Pyroglytamic acidemia	Acidosis	Pyroglytamic acid in urine and blood and glutathione synthetase assay in fibroblasts

*Unusual odor is more readily smelt in frozen urine because organic compounds with different freezing points concentrate on the top.
**Severe liver dysfunction and organic acidemias may also be associated with elevated blood ammonia levels.

TABLE 24.10 Cofactor and limiting amino acid therapy in IEM

Disorder	Vitamin/cofactor	Dose (mg/d)	Amino acid supplement
Pheynlketonuria	—	—	Tyrosine
Neonatal tryosinemia	Vitamin C	50–100	—
Classical homocystinuria	Pyridoxine and folic acid	100–500 and 10–20	Cystine
Hartnup disease	Niacin	100–250	—
Mitochondrial disorder	Riboflavin	100–150	—
Maple syrup urine disease	Thiamine	10–20	—
Methylmalonic acidemia	B_{12}	1.0–3.0	Bicarbonate
Multiple carboxylase deficiency	Biotin	5–20	—
Isovaleric acidemia	—	—	Glycine and L-carnitine
Hawkinsinuria	Vitamin C	1000	—
Hyperammonemia	Sodium benzoate	250–500	—
Primary CoQ10 deficiency	Coenzyme Q10	2–15	—

diagnosis. The advice of a referral metabolic center and an experienced dietician is extremely useful in specific metabolic situations. For specific nutritionl requirements and availability of dietary formulations for various inborn errors of metabolism, refer to website: http://www.icmrmetbionetindia.org/nutritiousnews.aspx.

Dietary Restrictions

A galactose-free (lactose-free) diet is likely to quickly reverse the symptoms and prevent cataracts, liver damage and mental retardation in patients with galactosemia. Neonates with PKU should be given a protein substitute which is phenylalanine-free but otherwise nutritionally complete. In patients with glycogen storage disease, hypoglycemia can be prevented by frequent feeds during the day and continuous nasogastric feeding at night. Raw corn starch (2 g/kg every 6 hours) has been shown to be effective to prevent hypoglycemia in older children with glycogen storage disease 1, and fatty acid oxidation disorders. Children with hyperammonemia are given low-protein (1.4 g/kg) diet containing essential amino acids and adequate calories. It is desirable to seek the guidance of an experienced dietition to ensure adequate intake of essential amino acids, fatty acids, minerals and vitamins to children with IEM.

Specific Therapy

Genetic disorders cannot be cured but their symptoms can be ameliorated or handicap can be prevented through several therapeutic approaches.

Replacement therapy Thyroxine replacement prevents mental retardation in children with thyroid dyshormonogenesis, cortisone suppresses the excess of ACTH production and androgen synthesis in congenital adrenal hyperplasia (CAH) and administration of Factor VIII/IX prevents bleeding in cases of hemophilia. Specific enzymes are available for replacement therapy in patients with Gaucher disease, Hurler syndrome, Morquios syndrome, Fabry disease, and Pompe disease but their availability is limited and cost is prohibitive.

Reducing accumulation of toxic metabolite In lactose intolerance and galactosemia, lactose-free milk is given. The infant with phenylketonuria is given a diet low in phenylalanine to prevent brain damage. Certain drugs, like allopurinol, inhibits xanthine oxidase and thus reduces the synthesis of uric acid in patients with gout.

Promoting excretion of toxins The excretion of certain toxic metabolites can be promoted by administration of chelating agents, viz. d-penicillamine promotes excretion of copper in patients with Wilson disease and desferrioxamine is useful to chelate iron in cases of thalassemia and hemochromatosis.

Induction of enzymes Phenobarbitone is useful for inducing the hepatic microsomal enzyme glucuronyl transferase in infants with Crigler-Najjar syndrome.

Avoidance of certain drugs Certain drugs which are known to precipitate adverse symptoms in metabolic disorders, for example, barbiturates in porphyria hepatica and oxidative agents in glucose-6-phosphate dehydrogenase deficiency, should be avoided.

Gene Therapy

Gene therapy with replacement of abnormal gene is curative but is still in experimental stage. Gene therapy has been tried in patients with adenosine deaminase deficiency (ADA), Duchenne muscular dystrophy, familial hypercholesterolemia and certain cancers. The

Metabolic Disorders

24

aim is to replace the defective gene with the normal gene. This is done by using a viral or non-viral vector for introducing the normal functioning gene. The normal gene may be introduced directly into the defective body organ, i.e. *in vivo* or more often the process is achieved *in vitro* followed by its transfer into the patient.

Organ Transplantation

Transplantation of liver or bone marrow is used for treatment of several inborn errors of metabolism and genetic immunologic or hematologic disorders. A successful transplant is essentially curative, though there are significant risks and complications.

Disorders of Amino Acid Metabolism

Hereditary Hyperglycinemias

It represents a group of disorders in amino acid metabolism characterized by life-threatening elevation of glycine in the body fluids. There are at least two forms of hyperglycinemia, each representing a distinct disease. They are inherited as autosomal recessive disorders.

Ketotic hyperglycinemia due to defective conversion of serine to glycerine is characterized by acute episodes of ketoacidosis precipitated by infection or intake of protein. Clinical manifestations include vomiting, neutropenia, thrombocytopenia, coma and early death. Survivors are left with severe mental retardation and osteoporosis. Ketotic hyperglycinemia may coexist with both propionic acidemia and methylmalonic acidemia.

Non-ketotic hyperglycinemia due to failure of conversion of glycine to carbon dioxide and hydroxymethyl tetrahydrofolic acid, also produces life-threatening clinical picture in the newborn baby. After one or two days of milk feeding, the baby becomes lethargic, unresponsive, markedly hypotonic and depressed. Myoclonic jerks or generalized seizures, hiccups and apneic attacks soon appear and terminate fatally. Mental retardation is invariable in survivors. EEG shows the characteristic burst suppression pattern. The diagnosis is suspected by finding elevated levels of glycine in body fluids and an elevated CSF to plasma glycine ratio. Measurement of glycine cleavage system activity in hepatocytes confirms the diagnosis.

Maple Syrup Urine Disease (MSUD)

The defective oxidative decarboxylation of branched-chain keto acids results in elevation of branched-chain amino acids leucine, isoleucine and valine. The symptoms appear after one week and include poor feeding, lethargy, vomiting, hypertonicity, muscular rigidity, opisthotonos and convulsions. The clinical features are due to accumulation of metabolites especially leucine which also leads to hypoglycemia. The characteristic 'burnt sugar' like smell of urine is highly suggestive of maple syrup urine disease and should be looked for in all neonates with acute unexplained systemic disorder. The useful screening tests include ferric chloride (navy blue color), DNPH (yellow precipitate) and Guthrie test. Elevated plasma and urine levels of leucine, isoleucine, valine and their respective keto acids are diagnostic of MSUD. Urine DNPH screening test is positive. Hemodialysis is life-saving to eliminate branched-chain amino acids and their metabolites from the body fluids. The infant should be kept on a low branched-chain amino acid diet throughout life. Liver transplantation is curative.

Disorders of Carbohydrate Metabolism

Galactosemia

It is inherited as an autosomal recessive trait and occurs due to deficiency of galactose-1-phosphate uridyltransferase (GALT) or galactokinase deficiency. The symptoms appear after 1 to 2 weeks of milk feeding and include poor feeding, lethargy, vomiting and unsatisfactory weight gain. Persistence of physiological jaundice, hepatosplenomegaly and bleeding manifestations would suggest associated hepatic damage. Lethargy, irritability and seizures due to hypoglycemia are common. They have increased risk to develop sepsis due to *E. coli*. Cataracts appear after 2 to 6 weeks of age. Cirrhosis and neuromotor retardation are common in untreated cases.

Urinalysis would show the presence of reducing substance which can be identified as galactose by sugar chromatography. Newborn babies receiving lactose-free formula will not show galactose in the urine. Proteinuria and abnormal aminoaciduria are also present. Total reducing substances in the blood would be much higher than the true glucose. The diagnosis is confirmed by demonstration of galactose-1-phosphate uridyltransferase (GALT) deficiency in the red blood cells or fibroblasts. Semiquantitative assay of blood for GALT is used for newborn screening program and is known as Beutler test. Exclusion of lactose (milk) from the diet is followed by prompt improvement and further hepatic and cerebral damage due to galactose can be avoided.

Hereditary Fructose Intolerance

There is deficiency of fructose-1, 6-biphosphate aldolase (aldolase B) in the liver which leads to rise in intracellular concentration of fructose-1-phosphate. The condition is inherited as an autosomal recessive trait. The symptoms appear when the infant is started on artificial feeds containing sucrose or fructose. The clinical picture, by and large, is similar to galactosemia. It is characterized by vomiting, failure to gain weight, hypoglycemia, seizures, jaundice and hepatosplenomegaly. Neuromotor development is usually unaffected. Urinalysis reveals reducing substance (which can be identified as fructose by sugar chromatography) and non-specific proteinuria and aminoaciduria. Estimation of blood sugar would show high levels of total reducing substance and markedly reduced true glucose level. Intravenous fructose tolerance test (3 g per m^2) is followed by profound hypoglycemia and fall in serum inorganic phosphorus. The test should, however, be avoided or but conducted with great care in a newborn baby. The diagnosis is confirmed by assay of fructose aldolase activity in the liver and DNA analysis of point mutations of the aldolase B gene.

Blood fructose levels are variable and not diagnostic in cases of fructose intolerance. Withdrawal of fructose, sucrose and sorbitol from the diet is followed by prompt clinical recovery. Hemorrhagic manifestations would respond to administration of vitamin K.

Glycogen Storage Disease-Type 1

Glucose-6-phosphatase deficiency may manifest in the neonatal period with recurrent acidosis and hypoglycemia. The mode of inheritance is autosomal recessive. The characteristic physical findings include a round doll-like facies and protuberant abdomen due to marked hepatomegaly. There is no splenomegaly or cardiomegaly. Laboratory findings include hypoglycemia, which appear falsely low because of displacement by lipids. Following glycogen stimulation, glucose levels do not rise but lactate levels increase significantly. The treatment is aimed at maintaining euglycemia by oral intake of uncooked corn starch and continuous nasogastric feeds at night. Orthotopic liver transplantation is curative.

Disaccharidase Deficiency

Primary lactose or sucrose isomaltase deficiency is rare in the newborn period and most cases of lactose intolerance are secondary to acute infective diarrhea. Physiological lactase deficiency may be an expression of immaturity in an occasional very low birth weight baby. Diarrhea with frothy sour smelling stools is associated with marked abdominal distension and perianal soreness which are suggestive of disaccharidase deficiency. Stool pH of less than 6, presence of reducing substance in the stools and increased excretion of hydrogen in breath are useful screening tests. Lactose tolerance test, intestinal biopsy and enzyme assay would confirm the diagnosis. Lactose-free diet or provision of lactose-free milk formula is followed by gradual recovery.

Disorders of Steroid Metabolism

Congenital adrenal hyperplasia with salt-losing syndrome may present as a life-threatening condition in the newborn period and demands early recognition. One-third of infants with 21-hydroxylase deficiency and majority of those with 3 beta-hydroxysteroid dehydrogenase deficiency are salt losers. The diagnosis is easy in a female infant with signs of virilization but evidences of isosexual precocity in males do not manifest in the neonatal period. Male infants with 3 beta-hydroxysteroid dehydrogenase deficiency can be identified with hypospadias and cryptorchidism. Vomiting, with or without diarrhea, dehydration and failure to thrive are common features during neonatal period. Hyponatremia, hyperkalemia and hypoglycemia offer useful clues for further investigations. Skeletal maturation may be advanced.

Diagnosis

Serum electrolytes In salt-wasting type of CAH, there is hyponatremia and hyperkalemia.

Random urine sample The ratio of cortisol precursors to cortisol, i.e. cortisone and its metabolites (11-oxygenation index), if greater than 1.0 is suggestive of congenital adrenal hyperplasia.

24-hour urine sample It is often difficult to obtain 24-hour urine sample, particularly when external genitalia are ambiguous or female type.

1. *17-Ketosteroids* The diagnostic levels are greater than 1 mg/24 hours.
2. *Pregnanetriol* Elevated in infants with 21-hydroxylase defect.
3. *Tetrahydro-compound S* Elevated in 11-hydroxylase defect.
4. *Dehydroepiandrosterone* Elevated in 3 beta-hydroxysteroid dehydrogenase defect.

Plasma endocrine profile Elevated serum 17-hydroxyprogesterone (17-OHP), markedly lowered serum cortisol, raised serum levels of dehydroepiandrosterone sulfate (DHEAS) and testosterone are diagnostic of CAH due to 21-hydroxylase and 11-β-hydroxylase deficiency.

Management

During salt-losing crises or when vomiting is present, hydrocortisone acetate in a dose of 5 mg every 8-hours intravenously is given during first 3 days and subsequently reduced to 2.5 mg every 12 hourly. Cortisone acetate can be substituted orally once the clinical condition stabilizes and continued throughout life in a dose of 5 mg in the morning and 10 mg in the evening. Administration of mineralocorticoid, desoxycorticosterone acetate (DOCA) in a dose of 1.0–2.0 mg per day may be necessary to ensure sodium retention. When DOCA is not available, fludrocortisone 0.1–0.2 mg per day in 3 to 4 divided doses is given orally along with 2–4 g of sodium chloride every day in the milk feeds. The maintenance cortisone would be required throughout life and dosage may have to be increased at the onset of any infection. Vaginal reconstruction and clitorectomy may be required and should be undertaken around adolescence.

Disorders of Homeostasis and Red Cell Enzymes

Hereditary disorders of coagulation are briefly described in Chapter 23. Severe jaundice in a newborn baby can occur due to deficiency of glucuronyl transferase (Crigler-Najjar syndrome) or as a result of hereditary hemolytic anemia because of deficiency of glucose-6-phosphate dehydrogenase, pyruvate kinase, hereditary spherocytosis and elliptocytosis.

Prevention of IEMs

In view of unsatisfactory management of most genetic disorders, preventive strategies should be effectively harnessed to prevent the birth of affected children.

Carrier Screening

It is possible to detect the carrier state in a number of autosomal and X-linked disorders. In high-risk families or communities, it is important to assess the carrier state in order to provide genetic counseling to prospective couples before marriage. Estimation of HbA$_2$ level is useful for detection of beta thalassemia carrier state. Female carriers of Duchenne muscular dystrophy may show high serum levels of creatine phosphokinase (CPK) while relatively low level of G-6-PD enzyme in the RBCs is suggestive of carrier state of glucose-6-phosphate dehydrogenase deficiency.

Molecular techniques are now being increasingly used for detection of carrier state.

Prenatal Diagnosis

In a number of genetic disorders, it is possible to make antenatal diagnosis of a genetic disorder and offer selective termination of pregnancy, if fetus is affected with a lethal or untreatable disabling genetic disorder. The prenatal screening and diagnostic facilities are offered when family or mother is high-risk to give birth to a child with chromosomal or genetic disorder.

Non-invasive screening Three-dimensional ultrasonography and fetoscopy are useful for diagnosis of facial dysmorphism and congenital malformations. High levels of alpha-fetoprotein in maternal blood is a sensitive marker for open neural tube defects. Alpha-fetoprotein and estriol is low whereas hCG is high in pregnancies with Down syndrome (Triple test).

Invasive prenatal testing Chorionic villus sampling (around 12 weeks) and amniocentesis (16–18 weeks) are used for karyotyping, DNA-based studies and enzyme assays. Amniotic fluid is the preferred sample for chromosomal studies and chorionic villus biopsy for DNA-based tests.

NEWBORN SCREENING PROGRAM

"Newborn screening is a public health intervention that involves a simple blood test to identify many life-threatening genetic illnesses before any symptoms begin".

Lucille Roybal-Allard

There are a number of metabolic or genetic disorders that do not produce any obvious symptoms or signs in early newborn period but may produce serious disability or life-threatening manifestations when these infants are started on oral feeds. In developed countries, routine screening is done at birth to exclude over 40–50 metabolic disorders. In India, universal metabolic screening is neither required nor feasible because of lack of technology and logistical difficulties because many deliveries are not taking place at health care facilities. When we cannot tackle a number of visible or gross neonatal health problems, it is illogical to create cost-intensive strategies to identify "invisible" or "hidden" inborn errors of metabolism. It is more logical and cost-effective to ensure that every pregnant woman receives good quality antenatal care, delivers at a health care facility and is provided with essential newborn care.

In India, it is recommended that metabolic screening should be limited to conditions which have high incidence, availability of a simple and robust screening test and effective treatment. These conditions include hypothyroidism, G6PD deficiency, congenital adrenal hyperplasia, phenylketonuria, galactosemia, hemoglobinopathies and cystic fibrosis. The second approach is to identify high-risk families with history of inborn error of metabolism in the family members or previous sibling/s and unexplained neonatal deaths or disability. When high-risk parents are planning to have another baby, antenatal diagnosis should be attempted with the help of chorionic villus sampling and if fetus is affected, the mother can be offered an option of medical termination of pregnancy.

According to WHO, the genetic services should be gradually introduced in countries with infant mortality rate (IMR) of less than 50 per 1000 live births. Considering the prevalence of various inborn errors of metabolism and huge financial implications of universal screening for low-middle income countries (LMICs), it is recommended to pursue the following practical approach for newborn screening in India.

Category A (all newborns) Screening for hearing and hypothyroidism should be universal while screening for congenital adrenal hyperplasia (CAH), sickle cell disease and hemaglobinopathies should be introduced in a phased manner especially in high-risk populations. The screening for hearing is discussed in Chapter 28.

Category B (high-risk families) The screening is done when there is high likelihood of a genetic disorder in the family viz. unexplained life-threatening, neonatal disorder (after exclusion of common causes including sepsis), history of consanguinity, unexplained sibling death(s), neuromotor disability, mental retardation or seizure disorder. The conditions which should be seriously considered and ruled out include phenylketonuria, galactosemia, cystic fibrosis, homocystinuria, alkaptonuria, biotinidase deficiency, maple syrup urine disease, medium-chain acyl-CoA dehydrogenase deficiency, tyrosinemia and fatty acid oxidation defects.

Category C (Familes who demand or/and can afford.) The screening facilities for 40–50 inherited metabolic disorders can be offered to well-to-do families in urban health care settings where facilities are available to send appropriate blood samples to a reliable laboratory.

There is a need to gradually introduce newborn screening program in India with a special focus on type and timing of blood sample, financial implications and sound logistics. In general, cord blood is not suitable for newborn screening because of adverse effects of stress of labor (release of catecholamines and TSH) and lack of toxic metabolites and biochemical byproducts which appear after 24–48 hours of age or later when oral feeds are introduced. Screening is done by measuring the metabolites and enzyme activity in the whole blood samples collected on specialized filter paper having "circles" for collecting blood spots. The screening tests usually have high sensitivity but may lack in specificity. It is best to collect a blood sample after 72 hours and within 7 days of life on a special filter paper. Infants screened before 24 hours of life should be rescreened at 2 weeks of age to detect posible missed cases. In case of G6PD screening, blood sample should be collected before blood transfusion. If the baby had been screened after the episode of hemolysis or blood transfusion, the test should be repeated after 4 months of transfusion or hemolysis in order to ensure that baby's mature RBCs (and not the donor's RBCs) are tested.

Screening test results should be confirmed by definitive or high technology analytical tests, like tandem mass spectrometry (TMS), combined gas-liquid chromatography and mass spectrometry (GC/MS), enzyme assays and DNA probes. It is recommended that all sick neonates, especially when diagnosis of sepsis is unlikely or ruled out, should be screened for a metabolic disorder at the age of 7 days or later. The gestational age and birth weight should be intimated to the screening laboratory for proper interpretation of test results. At times administration of antibiotics may interfere with the test results of certain metabolic disorders, like galactosemia and phenylketonuria. Information about panels of diseases being tested in different parts of the world is available on the website of the International Society for Neonatal Screening (ISNS) at http://www.isns.neoscreening. org/.

Neonatal Thyroid Screening

Availability of a sensitive and specific radioimmunoassay (RIA) method for assay of thyroid hormone has simplified the screening program to assess neonatal thyroid status. The cord blood collected on filter paper strips is satisfactory and reliable for screening purposes. Screening is done by mass estimation of T_4 levels but definitive diagnosis of congenital hypothyroidism is based on elevated TSH levels. T_4 screening is more sensitive with high frequency of false positives especially in LBW and preterm babies. TSH screening is more specific but should be done after 48–72 hours. The computed international survey data has suggested a worldwide prevalence of primary congenital hypothyroidism in the range of one per 1000 to 4,000 infants. Recently, it has been shown that infants born to mothers belonging to endemic iodine deficient belt in India have higher risk of neonatal hypothyroidism.

Thyroid screening should be universal and should never be overlooked, if family hails from an iodine deficient area, mother is suspected to have a thyroid disorder or if infant shows any evidences of hypothyroidism, like prolonged physiological jaundice beyond 2 weeks, lethargy, constipation, poor temperature control and delayed osseous development. Examine cord blood or baby's blood after 3–4 postnatal days for TSH and T_4.

TSH level of >50 mIU/L in cord blood is diagnostic of neonatal hypothyroidism. T_4 may be normal or low (<8 µg/dL in cord blood) in these infants. After day 3, TSH level of >20 mIU/L is suggestive of congenital hypothyroidism. After 3 weeks of age, the upper limit of TSH is 10 mIU/L. It is important to remember that low levels of T_4 in association with normal levels of TSH may be seen in preterm infants due to immaturity of hypothalamic-pituitary-thyroid axis or deficiency of thyroxine binding globulin. Repeat T_4 levels after 3–4 weeks are usually normal. Transient hypothyroidism with elevated TSH and low T_4 has been described in infants born to mothers who were given vaginal douches with povidone iodine solution during perinatal period. Early diagnosis of hypothyroid state and its therapy within 2 weeks of age is mandatory for normal physical and mental development. Thyroxine-deficient neonates born to iodine deficient mothers do not receive sufficient thyroxine or iodine from breast milk. They must be treated with therapeutic doses of iodine and thyroxine to ensure that T_4 levels are maintained between 8 and 12 µg/dL. T_4 levels below 8 µg/dL are unsatisfactory to maintain optimal physical and mental growth. During therapy, monitoring of TSH levels is unreliable during early infancy because it may remain relatively high in some babies even when effective replacement therapy is being given.

BIBLIOGRAPHY

Abrams SA, Hawthorne KM, Placencia JL, et al. Micronutrient requirements of high-risk infants. Clin Perinatol 2014, 41:347–61.

American Academy of Pediatrics Committee on Genetics. Issues in newborn screening. Pediatrics 1992, 89:345.

Arya VB, Senniappan S, Guemes M, Hussain K. Neonatal hypoglycemia. Indian J Pediatr 2014, 81(1):58–65.

Augustine AM, Jana AK, Kuruvilla KA, Danda S, Lepcha A, Ebenezer J, et al. Neonatal hearing screening: Experience from a tertiary care hospital in southern India. Indian Pediatr 2014, 51:179–83.

Bear A, Cornblath M, Gentz J, Kellum M, Persson Bengt, Zeterstrom R, Haworth JC. Neonatal hypoglycemia—A discussion. J Pediatr 1971, 79:314.

Bolouyt N, Van Kempe A, Offringa M. Neurodevelopment after neonatal hypoglycemia: A systematic review and design of an optimal future study. Pediatrics 2006, 117: 2231–2243.

Burton BK. Inborn errors of metabolism in infancy. A guide to diagnosis. Pediatrics 1998:102:e69.

Buyukgebiz A. Newborn screening of congenital hypothyroidism. J Pediatr Endocrinol Metab 2006, 19(11): 1291–1298.

Carmencita DP, Bradford LT. Newborn screening in the Asia Pacific region. J Inherit Metab Dis 2007, 30: 490–506.

Chakrapani A. Detection of inborn errors of metabolism in the newborn. Arch Dis Child Neonatal Ed 2001, 84 : 205.

Chaves-Carballo E. Detection of inherited neurometabolic disorders: A pratical clinical approach. Pediatr Clin N Amer 1992, 39:801–819.

Cornblath M, Howdon JM, Williams AF, et al. Controversies regarding definition of neonatal hypoglycemia: Suggested operational thresholds. Pediatrics 2000, 105:1141–1145.

Cornblath M, Ichord R. Hypoglycemia in the neonate. Semin Perinatol 2000, 24:136–149.

Crombez E, Koch R, Cederbaum S. Pitfalls in newborn screening. J Pediatr 2005, 147:119–120.

Danks DM. Management of newborn babies in whom serious metabolic illness is anticipated. Arch Dis Child 1974, 49:576.

Desai MP, Colaco MP, Ajgaonkar AR, et al. Neonatal screening for congenital hypothyroidism in a developing country: Problems and strategies. Indian J Pediatr 1987, 54:571–581.

Desai MP, Sharma R, Riaz I, Sudhanshu S, Parikh R, Bhatia V. Newborn screening guidelines for congenital hypothyroidism in India: Recommendations of the Indian Society for Pediatric and Adolescent Endocrinology (ISPAE)-Part I screening and confirmation of diagnosis. Indian J Pediatr 2018, 85(6):440–7.

Enns GM, Pockman S. Diagnosing inborn errors of metabolism in the newborn: laboratory investigations. Neo Reviews 2001, 2:192.

Faienza MF, D'Amato E, Natale MP, et al. Metabolic bone disease of prematurity: Diagnosis and management. Front Pediatr 2019, 7:143.

Fisher DA. Second International conference on neonatal thyroid screening : Progress report. J Pediatr 1983, 102 : 653.

Fisher DA, Klein AH. Thyroid development and disorders of thyroid function in the newborn. New Engl J Med 1981, 304:702–712.

Gentz J, Persson B, Zetterstorm O. On the diagnosis of symptomatic neonatal hypoglycemia. *Acta Paediatr Scand* 2008, 58: 449–459.

Gupta N, Kabra M. Acute management of sick infants with suspected inborn errors of metabolism. *Indian J Pediatr* 2011, 78:854–859.

Hawthorne KM, Abrams SA. Safety and efficacy of human milk fortification for very low birth weight infants. *Nutr Rev* 2004, 62: 482–485.

Holtzman NA. Expanding newborn screening *JAMA* 2003, 290: 2608–2608.

Hsu HC, Levine MA. Perinatal calcium metabolism: Physiology and pathophysiology. *Semin Neonatol* 2004, 9: 23–36.

Hughes IA. Congenital adrenal hyperplasia: a life long disorder. *Hormone Res* 2007, 68 (suppl 5): 84–89.

ICMR Task Force on Inherited Metabolic Disorders. The journey of newborn screening: Inception to conclusion. *Indian J Pediatr* 2018, 86(11):933–4.

Juneja A, Sultan A, Bhatnagar S. Wilcott-Rallison syndrome. *J Indian Soc Pedod Prev Dent* 2012, 30:250–3.

Kabra M. Dietary management of inborn errors of metabolism. *Indian J Pediatr* 2002. 69:421–26.

Kamath SS, Newborn screening in India. *Indian Pediatr* 2015, 52:373–4.

Kapoor S, Kabra M. Newborn screening in India: current perspectives. *Indian Pediatr* 2010, 47:219–224.

Keen JH. Significance of hypocalcemia in neonatal convulsions. *Arch Dis Child* 1969, 44:356.

Kochupillai N, Godebole MW, Pandav CS, Karmarkar MG, Ahuja MMS. Neonatal thyroid status in iodine deficient environment of the sub-Himalayan region. *Indian J Med Res* 1984, 80:293.

Koh THHG, Eyre JA, Aynsley-Green A. Neonatal hypoglycemia—the controversy regarding definition. *Arch Dis Child* 1988, 63:1386.

Koo WWK, Gupta JM, Nayanar VV, et al. Skeletal changes in preterm infants. *Arch Dis Child* 1982, 57:447–452.

Koo WWK, Tsang RC. Building better bones: calcium, magnesium, phosphorous and vitamin D. In: Nutrition During Infancy : Principles and Practice. Reginald C Tsang, Stanley H Zlotkin, Buford L Nichols, James W Hanseneds. *Digital Educational Publishing, Inc.* 2005.

Kumta NB. Inborn errors of metabolism: An Indian perspective. *Indian J Pediatr* 2005, 72(4):325–332.

Leonard JV, Morris AAM. Inborn errors of metabolism around time of birth. *Lancet* 2000, 356:583.

Levy P, Shapira E. State-of-the-art of biochemical genetics. *Amer J Dis Child* 1993, 147:1153–1158.

Litmanovitz I, Dolfin T, Friedland O, et al. Early physical activity intervention prevents disease of bone strength in very low birth weight infants. *Pediatrics* 2003, 112 (1):15–19.

Lucas A, Morley R. Outcome of neonatal hypoglycemia. *Brit Med J* 1999, 318:194–196.

Merke DP, Bornstein SR. Congenital adrenal hyperplasia. *Lancet* 2005, 365:2125–2136.

Mirzahi A, London RD and Gribets D. Neonatal hypocalcemia. Its causes and treatment. *N Engl J Med* 1968, 278:1163.

Nyhn WL. An approach to the diagnosis of overwhelming metabolic disease in early infancy. In: Current Problems in Pediatrics vol. VII. *Year Book Medical Publishers Inc. Chicago*, 1977.

O'Brien D, Goodman SI. The critically ill child. Acute metabolic disease in infancy and early childhood. *Pediatrics* 1970, 46:620.

Ranlov P, Siggaard Anderson O. Late metabolic acidosis in premature infants: Prevalence and significance. *Acta Paediatr Scand* 1965, 54:531.

Rayannavar A, Calabria AC. Screening for metabolic bone disease of prematurity. *Semin Fetal Neonatal Med* 2020 Feb, 25(1) 101086. doi:10.1016/j.siny.2020101086. Epub 2020 Jan 16.

Saudubray JM, Ogier H, Bonnefont JP, et al. Clinical approach to inherited metabolic diseases in the neonatal period: A 20 year survey. *J Inherit Metab Dis* 1989,12 (suppl 1):25.

Saudubray JM, Gracia-Cazorla A. Inborn errors of metabolism overview: Pathophysiology, manifestations, evaluation and management. *Pediatr Clin North Am* 2018, 65(2):179–208.

Seashore MR, et al. Metabolic disease of the neonate and young infant. *Semin Perinatol* 1993, 17:318.

Sharma S, Kumar P, Agarwal R, Kabra M, Deorari AK, Paul VK. Approach to inborn errors of metabolism presenting in the neonate. *Indian J Pediatr* 2008, 75(3):271–6.

Singhi S, Marwah RK, Singh M. Late metabolic acidosis in the preterm infants: clinical profile and response to oral sodium bicarbonate therapy. *Indian J Med Res* 1979, 69:440.

Sperling MA, Menon RK. Differential diagnosis and management of neonatal hypoglycemia. *Pediatr Clin North Am* 2004, 51:703–723.

Tada K, Kure S, Kume A, Hiraga K. Non-ketotic hyperglycinemia: molecular lesion, diagnosis and pathophysiology. *J Inherit Metabol Dis* 1993,16:691.

Verma IC, Bijarnia-Mahay S, Jhingan G, Verma J. Newborn screening need of the hour. *Indian J Pediatr* 2015, 82(1):61–70.

Wilcken B. Problems in the management of urea cycle disorders. *Mol Genet Metab* 2004, 81 (suppl):S86–S91.

Wybregt SH, Reisner SH, Patel RJ, Nellhaus G, Cornblath M. The incidence of neonatal hypoglycemia in a nursery for premature infants. *J Pediatr* 1964, 64:796.

Surgical Conditions

MEDICAL MANAGEMENT OF SURGICAL NEONATES

The improved survival rates for complex surgical conditions of the newborn babies have been achieved by improvements in the skills of pediatric surgeons, introduction of minimally invasive surgical techniques, increased understanding regarding the problems of homeostasis and physiological needs of sick preterm babies and availability of non-invasive technology for continuous monitoring of vital parameters in neonates. The specific details regarding medical management of various surgical conditions are given along with broad principles governing the perioperative management of newborn babies. A close cooperation and coordination between the pediatric surgeon, neonatologist, anesthetist, neonatal nurses, respiratory therapist and pharmacist is essential to improve the outcome of the surgical neonate. The medical management is directed to ensure adequate ventilation (and oxygenation), satisfactory tissue perfusion (effective circulation), thermoneutral environment, supply of adequate amounts of fluids, electrolytes and calories, maintenance of biochemical homeostasis and prevention of nosocomial infections (Table 25.1).

Preoperative Management

Early diagnosis of a surgical condition in the neonate is important because operative success and outcome is directly related to the time taken to diagnose and prepare the infant for surgery. It needs to be emphasized that one-day-old infant is a good surgical risk and no preoperative management may be required in such cases. Delay in the diagnosis is likely to lead to complications, disturbances of fluids and electrolytes and compromised status of tissue perfusion and oxygenation depending upon the nature of the

developmental defect. The condition of the infant should be stabilized by parenteral administration of fluids and electrolytes to provide maintenance needs, correct any deficits and replenish on-going concurrent losses. The third-space fluid losses are known to occur in a variety of abdominal conditions, such as NEC, peritonitis, gastroschisis, omphalocele and intestinal obstruction. Inadequate replacement of these losses (which are difficult to quantify) can lead to hypovolemia and shock. Infusion of 5% albumin, plasma and whole blood may be required to maintain blood pressure.

Fluid losses due to vomiting and nasogastric aspiration should be replaced as 0.45% saline in dextrose. Persistent and protracted vomiting due to pyloric stensosis can lead to hypochloremic alkalosis with hypokalemia which is corrected by administration of sodium chloride and potassium chloride. Apart from adequate hydration and satisfactory perfusion, status of ventilation (as evidenced by normal arterial blood gases and pH) and biochemical parameters (electrolytes, calcium, glucose and BUN) should be maintained within normal limits before undertaking major surgery. *Vitamin K 0.5–1.0 mg IV or IM must be given to all neonates before surgery.* A suitable antibiotic should be administered to an infected neonate and those requiring major abdominal surgery. Adequate amount of crossmatched blood should be arranged. The infant should be taken to the operation theater in a transport incubator to ensure that his body temperature and ventilation are normal before induction of anesthesia.

Intraoperative Management

The aim of surgical management is not merely to correct the abnormality but also to ensure that minimal metabolic stress is imposed during the procedure. The major concerns during surgery include the risk of cold

TABLE 25.1 Principles of perioperative medical management of newborns

1. Ensure adequate ventilation
- Maintain pH 7.35–7.45, arterial PO_2 50–80 mm Hg, $PaCO_2$ 35–45 mm Hg
- Ensure optimal position, posture, suction, open airways, relieve abdominal distension, provide oxygen with head box, CPAP and ventilation.
- Monitor breathing rate, color, apneic attacks and oxygen saturation.

2. Maintain tissue perfusion
- Ensure adequacy of cardiac contractions and circulating blood volume.
- Check losses due to vomiting, nasogastric aspiration, intestinal obstruction (third space losses), gastroschisis, bleeding, and operative blood loss and ileostomy fluid losses, etc.
- Give vitamin K before surgery.
- Monitor pulse, capillary refill time (<2 sec over upper chest), blood pressure*, pH, central venous pressure.

3. Provide thermoneutral environment
- Nurse and operate under servo-control system.
- Avoid unnecessary exposure, give fluids, blood and blood products after warming to body temperature.

4. Supply fluids, electrolytes and calories
- Establish a reliable intravenous access.
- Check sources of fluid and electrolyte losses and assess status of hydration.
- Provide maintenance needs of fluids, electrolytes and calories, replenish deficits and concurrent on-going losses.
- Monitor weight, hydration status, urine output, plasma and urine osmolality and serum electrolytes.
- Start total parenteral nutrition, if starvation is prolonged beyond 5 days.

5. Maintain biochemical homeostasis
pH, acid–base parameters, electrolytes, calcium, glucose, BUN and bilirubin should be monitored.

6. Prevent nosocomial infections
- Ensure strict asepsis and handwashing
- "Septic screening" for early diagnosis of sepsis
- Prophylactic antibiotics following major surgery or during assisted ventilation.

*It is useful to maintain mean arterial blood pressure just above the gestation of the baby in weeks, i.e. around 32 mm Hg in a baby of 32 weeks gestation.

stress and need for making an accurate assessment of blood loss and third-space losses of fluids to prevent hypovolemia and shock. During major surgery, infant should be attached to an electronic thermometer, ECG oscilloscope, non-invasive blood pressure monitor and pulse oximeter. The baby should be placed on a circulating warm water mattress or enclosed in a fiberoptic hot pipe system to create a warm microenvironment during surgery. The overhead radiant warmer is ineffective because baby is covered with thick drapes and it interferes with OT lights and movements of the anesthetist and surgeon. Fluids, blood and blood products must be warmed to 37°C before infusion. Accurate estimate of blood loss during surgery should be maintained preferably by weighing dry and blood-soaked guaze pads on an accurate electronic weighing scale. It must be remembered that loss of 20 mL of blood in a 1500 g infant amounts to a loss of 15% of his blood volume (equivalent to 750 mL of blood loss in an adult).

During surgery, the maintenance fluid requirement should be provided by infusion of one-fourth saline-dextrose solution at a rate of 4 mL/kg/hour. The infusion rate of glucose should not exceed 4–6 mg/kg/minute to prevent the risk of hyperglycemia. In addition to the maintenance fluid needs and blood loss, the third-space fluid losses due to translocation of tissue fluid by surgical dissection and damage must be replaced. During major abdominal surgery, third-space losses are replenished by administration of a dextrose-free solution like Ringer's lactate at a rate of 10–15 mL/kg/hour. Transfusion of large volumes of blood can lead to hyperkalemia and hypocalcemia which should be specifically looked for on the ECG monitor. During a prolonged surgical procedure, frequent monitoring of hematocrit, pH, glucose and electrolytes is advocated.

Postoperative Management

Infant should be transferred to NICU and attached to a vital sign monitor, electronic thermometer, non-invasive blood pressure monitor and pulse oximeter. Urine bag must be attached and urine output maintained between 1and 3 mL/kg/hr with an osmolality between 150 and 400 mOsm/L or specific gravity 1005–1015. He should be nursed in an intensive care incubator or open care system with a facility for servo-controlling the body temperature. Hematocrit, electrolytes, glucose, calcium, blood gases and osmolality should be checked as soon as possible. *Acidosis in the presence of normal arterial oxygen and carbon dioxide tension is a very sensitive index of unsatisfactory tissue perfusion in a newborn baby.* It should be promptly treated by rapid administration of 20 mL/kg of physiological saline or fresh frozen plasma (FFP) over a period of one hour. Sodium bicarbonate can be administered as a slow infusion over 4 to 6 hours. Postoperatively, many infants demonstrate hyponatremia and fluid retention due to inappropriate secretion of antidiuretic hormone which is released during surgery in response to hypoxia, hemorrhage, hypotension, anesthesia and pain. During first 48 hours postoperatively, maintenance fluids should be restricted to two-thirds of the recommended volume. The gastric aspirate should be replaced by one-half strength physiological saline while ileostomy losses are replenished with physiological saline. Tissue breakdown and catabolic state during surgery may be followed by hyperkalemia which needs to be monitored by keeping a close watch on the ECG tracing. The supplements of potassium should be withheld till adequate urine flow is established.

The infant should be closely watched clinically and by periodic septic screening to identify occurrence of nosocomial infection as early as possible. The role of administration of large doses of immune globulins for prevention of bacterial infections is controversial. Fresh frozen plasma should be administered on every alternate day to provide proteins, complement, lysozyme, and coagulation factors. There is no significant difference in the rates of amino acid oxidation, protein degradation or synthesis and caloric needs during pre- and postoperative period in newborn babies. When enteral feeding cannot be established by fifth postoperative day, it is desirable to start total parenteral nutrition to reverse the catabolic state in order to promote healing and growth. Adequate supplements of vitamins and calcium is essential during postoperative management.

The emotional and physical needs of the surgical neonate should not be overlooked in the maze of catheters and sensors. It is often forgotten that newborn babies also feel pain. Infact they feel more pain because they are more delicate but they are unable to complain and the tiny ones cannot even cry. A number of adverse physiological and biochemical consequences have been demonstrated in neonates exposed to painful stimuli. Pain is associated with rise in blood pressure, increase in heart rate, elevation of intracranial pressure and fall in arterial oxygen saturation. Depending upon the nature of the surgical procedure, pain can be safely controlled by administration of morphine in a loading dose of 50 µg/kg followed by continuous infusion of morphine at a rate of 10–15 µg/kg per hour. Fentanyl in a loading dose of 10 µg/kg followed by constant infusion at a rate of 1–5 µg/kg/hour also provides adequate analgesia and sedation. The toxic side effects of both morphine and fentanyl can be effectively reversed by administration of naloxone.

OPTIMAL TIMING FOR SURGERY

Life-Threatening Surgical Conditions

Early diagnosis and rational medical management of congenital malformations is crucial to enhance survival. Immediate or early surgery is life-saving in following life-threatening surgical conditions. Most of these malformations are present in fetal life and surgical correction is required to save life or prevent complications. However, the condition of the baby should be stabilized before undertaking major surgery.

1. Diaphragmatic hernia
2. Esophageal atresia with/without tracheo-esophageal fistula
3. Tension pneumothorax
4. Lobar emphysema
5. Intestinal obstruction, supralevator anorectal malformation
6. Necrotizing enterocolitis with perforation
7. Gastroschisis
8. Ruptured omphalocele
9. Leaking meningomyelocele
10. Acute abscesses

Various other surgical conditions can be subdivided into following two groups depending upon the need for urgent or elective surgery. In several situations, surgery may not be requried because the condition may get corrected spontaneously, viz. umbilical hernia, hydrocele, sternomastoid tumor, hemangioma and ventriculoseptal defect. At times, extensive surgery is postponed till baby can withstand it or when organs are fully developed for best cosmetic results.

Emergency Surgical Conditions

Infants with inguinal hernia, cystic hygroma, meningomyelocele with thin sac should be operated as soon as diagnosed. Sacrococcygeal teratoma should be operated within two weeks after birth and infants with congenital hypertrophic pyloric stenosis are operated around 4–5 weeks of age. Infants with biliary atresia must be operated within 8–12 weeks of age. Infants with talipes equinovarus and congenital dislocation of hips should receive physiotherapy and special plaster casts within first week after birth. The casts would need removal and refixing every 1–2 weeks depending upon the severity of abnormality.

Elective Surgical Conditions

Surgery can be delayed for optimal cosmetic results till the deformed organs can be handled and resected with ease. A number of conditions are self-limiting

TABLE 25.2 Elective surgical conditions with optimal timing for their surgery

Condition	Timing for surgery	Condition	Timing for surgery
▪ Biliary atresia, congenital	4–6 weeks (preferably within 12 weeks)	▪ Hydrocele ▪ Hypospadias	After 2 years
▪ Cleft lip	Usually at 2–3 months. Ideally it should be operated in the neonatal period for good cosmetic results.	□ Meatotomy □ Chordee correction □ Urethroplasty ▪ Indirect inguinal hernia	Any time after birth Around 6 months 18–24 months In preterm babies at corrected age of 2 months.
▪ Cleft palate	9–18 months		At the time of diagnosis in healthy term babies
▪ Ectopic anus in the vestibular region	2–3 months	▪ Perineal ectopic testis ▪ Phimosis*	At the time of diagnosis
▪ Epispadias		□ Prepucial separation	Around one year of age
□ Chordee correction	Around one year of age	□ Circumcision	After 2–3 years
□ Urethroplasty	6 months to one year after chordee correction	▪ Sternomastoid tumor	Physiotherapy soon after birth and tenotomy around one year of age, if torticollis persists
▪ Exstrophy bladder			
□ Bladder closure	Within 48 hours		
□ Bladder neck repair and anti-reflux surgery	After 2 years	▪ Syndactyly ▪ Tongue-tie	1–2 years Around one year, if parents insist
□ Urethroplasty	After achieving continence		
□ Augmentation cystoplasty	8–10 years	▪ Umbilical hernia	After 4–5 years
▪ Hemangioma	5–6 years	▪ Undescended testes	12–15 months. Surgery may be done earlier, if it is associated with inguinal hernia
▪ Hirschsprung's disease	Between 12 and 15 months (body weight 10 kg) or 6 months after colostomy		

*Application of steroid cream after gentle retraction of prepuce for 3–4 weeks corrects the abnormality by breaking the adhesions in most infants.

and may resolve spontaneously while a delay in surgical correction in others may lead to irrversible organ damage and permanent sequelae. Table 25.2 gives the list of common conditions with optimal timing for their surgical correction.

GASTROINTESTINAL OBSTRUCTION

Obstruction in the gastrointestinal tract may occur at any site from esophagus to anus. These conditions may be divided into three broad groups for practical considerations.

Esophageal Atresia and Tracheoesophageal Fistula

Upper part of esophagus is developed from retropharyngeal segment and the lower part from pregastric segment of the first part of primitive gut. At four weeks of gestation, the laryngotracheal groove is formed. Two longitudinal furrows develop and separate the respiratory primordium from esophagus. Deviation or altered cellular growth of the septum results in formation of fistulae between esophagus and trachea.

Six types of esophageal anomalies are recognized. The classification of Gross is widely used, with designations extending from A to F (Figure 25.1). Type-A esophageal atresia consists of a blind upper

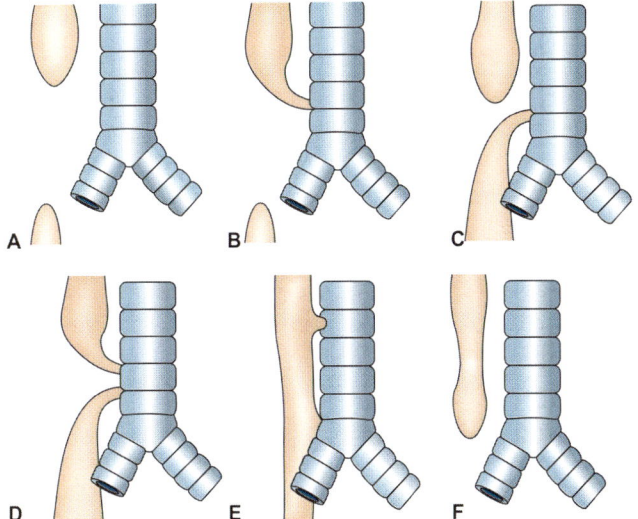

Figure 25.1A to F Different types of esophageal atresia with tracheoesophageal fistula based upon classification by Gross. Type-C accounts for almost 90% of cases.

and a blind lower esophageal segment without any tracheoesophageal fistula. In the B, C and D forms, there is an associated tracheoesophageal fistula either from the upper esophageal segment (Type B), lower esophageal segment (Type C) or from both segments

(Type D). The E variant refers to H-type of tracheo-esophageal fistula without any esophageal atresia. Congenital stenosis or narrowing of esophagus without atresia or fistula is designated as type F. The type-C esophageal atresia is far more common (about 87%) than others while types E and F are rarely diagnosed in the neonatal period.

Clinical Features

The presence of maternal polyhydramnios and single umbilical artery should alert the pediatrician to look for atresia of the upper digestive tract. About 20% of affected infants are either preterm or growth retarded. The affected baby has excessive drooling, saliva is frothy and there is choking and cyanosis with the first feed. Overflow of milk and saliva from esophagus and regurgitation of secretions through the fistulous tract (when present) into the lungs result in aspiration pneumonia. Over one-third of infants with esophageal atresia have other major associated anomalies of heart, gastrointestinal and genitourinary systems. The anomalies of VACTERL association, namely **V**ertebral defects, **A**nal anomalies, **C**ardiac defects, **TE**F with esophageal atresia, **R**enal defects and **L**imb anomalies should be looked for.

Diagnosis

A stiff red rubber catheter cannot be passed into stomach and it may get arrested at a distance of 8 to 10 cm from the mouth. If a polythene catheter is used, it may get coiled up in the upper pouch of esophagus and accumulated secretions may be mistaken for stomach contents. The latter should have acidic pH. X-ray chest may show upper esophageal pouch due to air as a contrast (Figure 25.2). A skiagram may be obtained with a catheter having radiopaque end *in situ*. An air bubble is seen in the stomach, if there is a communication between the lower part of the eso-phagus and trachea (as in the commonest variety). In esophageal atresia without tracheoesophageal fistula, abdomen is scaphoid and there is no air bubble in the stomach. The plain film may also show associated vertebral anomalies. Lungs may show atelectasis or aspiration pneumonia in the right upper zone. Con-trast material is seldom needed to outline the upper esophageal pouch. Water-soluble non-ionic contrast medium (omnipaque) may be used provided it is aspirated immediately after taking the radiographs.

Management

The baby should be nursed supine with head raised to 45° to reduce reflux of gastric contents into the

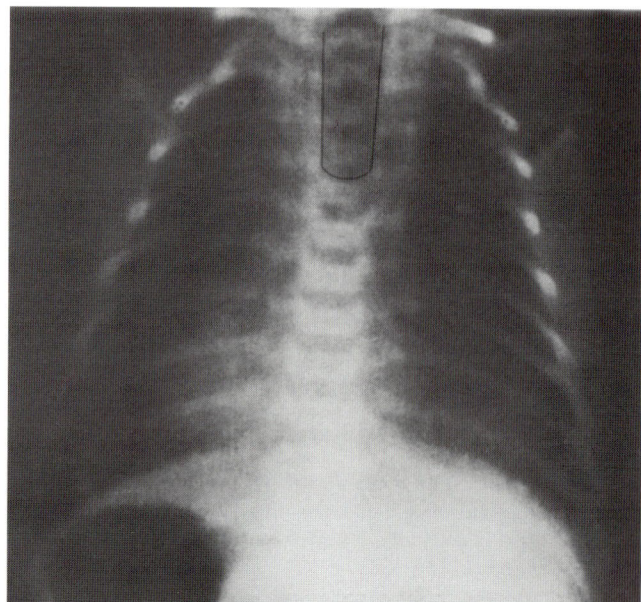

Figure 25.2 Upper esophageal pouch visualized without any contrast.

fistula. The esophageal pouch should be sucked with a multiple end-hole suction catheter every 5 minutes or continuously with gentle negative pressure of about 15–35 cm H_2O. Antibiotics and intravenous fluids should be administered. Ligation of fistula and eso-phageal anastomosis through extrapleural route is pe-formed as early as possible as a single stage opera-tion to prevent aspiration pneumonia. When atretic segment is long, feeding gastrostomy and ligation of fistula is undertaken initially followed by plastic repair of esophagus after 6 to 8 weeks.

Prognosis

The prognosis depends upon how soon the diagnosis is made, whether penumonitis has occurred or not, the size and maturity of the baby, existence of serious anomalies, such as congenital heart disease and urogenital defects, experience of the surgeon and standard of medical and nursing care of the NICU. In most pediatric surgical units, the mortality has been reduced to less than 20%.

Obstruction beyond Esophagus and up to Rectum

Intestinal obstruction in the newborn is almost equally contributed by three groups of anomalies, i.e. intestinal atresia, malrotation and anorectal anomalies. Among intestinal atresias, duodenal atresia is the commonest and accounts for one-half of the cases. Trisomy-21 with duodenal atresia is the commonest association and is seen in one-half of the cases. Approximately 20% of all patients with neonatal intestinal obstruction are associated with cardiac, genitourinary, vertebral and chromosomal anomalies (Trisomy-21 with duodenal atresia and VATER anomalies comprising of **v**ertebral, **a**nal atresia, **t**racheoesophageal fistula, **r**adial and **r**enal dysplasia). Malrotation of the bowel may be associated with other GI abnormalities, like diaphragmatic hernia, annular pancreas, bowel atresias and omphalocele. Hirschsprung's disease, by and large, is limited to term babies, while one-third of infants with intestinal atresia are preterm.

Intestinal obstruction is characterized by vomiting, abdominal distension and failure to pass meconium in various combinations depending upon the site, type and cause of obstruction.

Vomiting

Many neonates vomit on the first day due to gastritis as a result of amniotic fluid ingestion. It responds to stomach wash and is never persistent. Later on, occasional regurgitation following feeds due to improper technique of feeding and aerophagy is common. The persistent and projectile vomiting, especially if it is bile-stained (yellow-green color), suggests upper intestinal obstruction. Bilious vomiting is most commonly due to malrotation of gut unless proved otherwise. The vomiting is more severe and early in onset in high intestinal obstruction and is delayed in distal obstruction. In gastroesophageal reflux, vomiting characteristically occurs as soon as the baby is returned to the cot after the feed. When held upright, the baby does not vomit. In hypertrophic plyoric stenosis, vomiting generally starts after two weeks of age, it is large, non-bilious and projectile. Unlike possetting due to aerophagy, these babies do not gain weight satisfactorily, are constipated and become emaciated.

Abdominal Distension

It is more pathognomonic but may be absent, mild or localized to the epigastrium in cases of high intestinal obstruction. It is marked and generalized in distal obstruction. Abdominal distension may also occur in preterm babies due to hypotonia and small capacity of stomach, functional ileus, respiratory distress syndrome, following artificial ventilation or CPAP, peritonitis, absence of abdominal musculature, ascites and hydronephrosis.

Failure to Pass Meconium

If a newborn baby has not passed meconium by 24 hours of age, he needs to be investigated for intestinal obstruction. Some infants who have passed meconium *in utero*, may not evacuate within 24 hours after birth. The passage of two or three small grayish meconium stools do not exclude small gut atresia or stenosis because colonic meconium may be evacuated. At times the child may pass meconium through abnormal orifices, such as ectopic anus, vagina, urethra, and vitellointestinal duct. When a newborn baby passes satisfactory meconium stools for 3 to 4 days and then suddenly develops features of acute intestinal obstruction, conditons like septicemia and peritonitis with paralytic ileus, midgut volvulus, necrotizing enterocolitis, perforation and rarely instussusception should be seriously considered. When bilious vomiting is associated with bleeding per rectum or occult blood in stools, it is suggestive of malrotation, midgut volvulus and necrotizing enterocolitis (NEC).

Clinical Examination

The baby with septicemia, necrotizing enterocolitis and volvulus may look very sick, lethargic, hypothermic, sclerematous and in shock. Orifices at the bottom should be checked for their site and size. Peristalsis may be visible but even normal preterm babies may also show visible peristaltic waves due to thin abdominal wall. The hallmark of pyloric stenosis is palpable ovoid or "olive" shaped mass due to hypertrophied pylorus. The pylorus should be explored with fingers of left hand by palpating gently but deeply lateral to the edge of right rectus muscle about 2–3 cm above and to the right of umbilicus while infant is being fed on the left breast. Hypertrophic pyloric stenosis is characterized by triad of projectile non-bilious vomiting, visible peristalsis from left to right in upper abdomen and palpable pyloric tumor. A vague ill-defined lump and abnormal meconium may be felt in meconium peritonitis, volvulus, meconium ileus, necrotizing enterocolitis and inspissated milk syndrome. In mucoviscidosis, meconium may be felt as "clay-like" mass in the right lower abdomen. Abdominal wall may show edema and redness in cases of peritonitis and volvulus.

The baby should be examined for evidences of any other associated anomalies which may modify the prognosis. About 30% cases of duodenal atresia are seen in infants with Down syndrome. Hydration and electrolyte status should be assessed. Rectal examination (use little finger) may help to exclude anorectal stenosis. The possibility of Hirschsprung's disease should be suspected, if there is a narrow rectal segment. Withdrawal of finger in such cases results in explosive passage of meconium with significant abdominal deflation. When gastric aspirate exceeds 20 mL or if it is bilious or fecal, it is very suggestive of upper intestinal obstruction.

Radiological Examination

Plain skiagram of abdomen in supine, upright and cross-table lateral views (if a mass is felt), without the use of contrast material, is informative and should be taken before gastric decompression. Air serves as an excellent contrast at this age period. Pyloric stenosis or atresia shows single air bubble or dilated stomach while duodenal atresia is characterized by double bubble sign (Figure 25.3). Distal duodenal atresia or jejunal atresia may show triple bubble sign (Figure 25.4). Small gut atresia shows dilatation of loops of intestine with several air fluid levels (Figure 25.5). The distal gut may be completely airless as air takes about 6 to 8 hours to reach the colon. In distal obstruction due to Hirschsprung's disease, meconium plug syndrome and paralytic ileus, there is increased amount of air throughout the gut but no air fluid levels are visualized. It is difficult to differentiate between the shadows due to large or small gut in the newborn on plain skiagrams. Necrotizing enterocolitis is characterized by increased air shadows, pneumatosis intestinalis, perforation and air along the portal tract. The presence

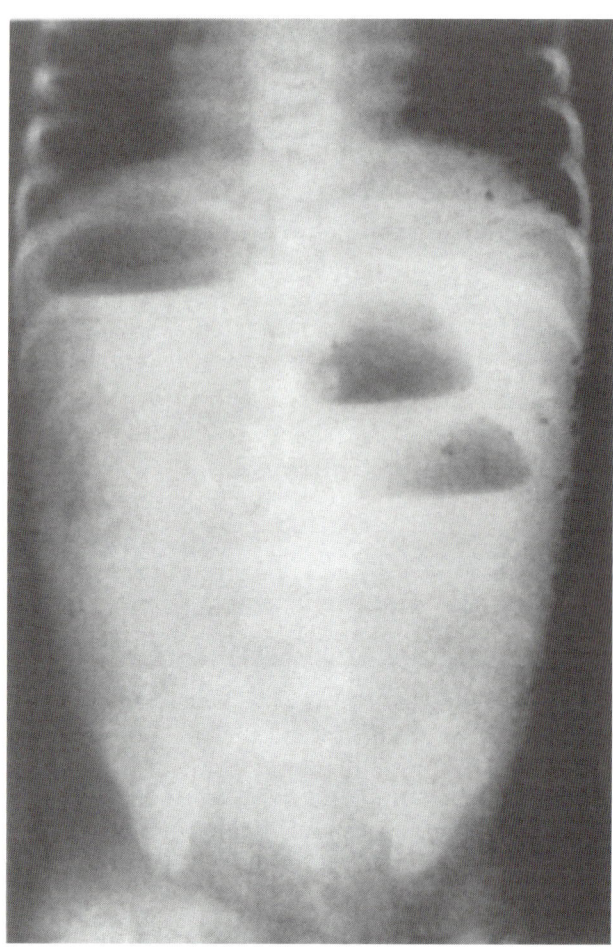

Figure 25.4 Triple bubble sign. The infant had jejunal atresia.

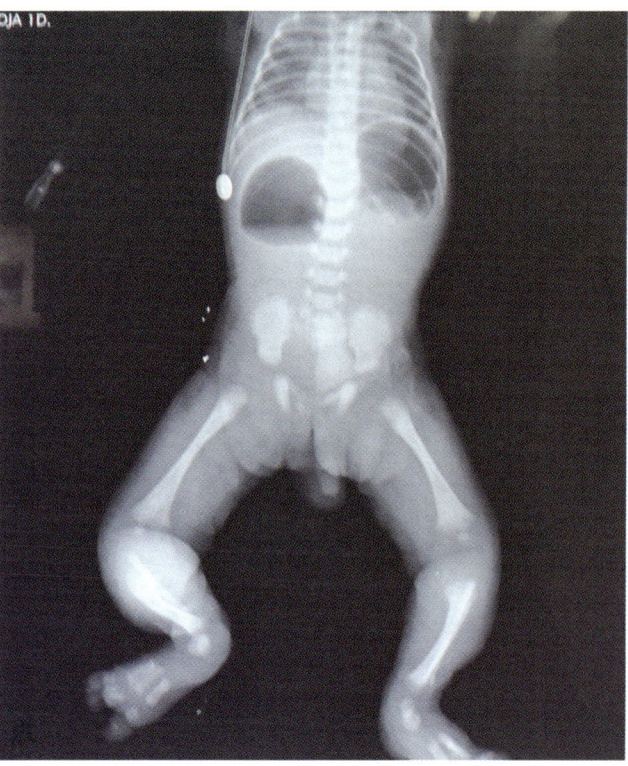

Figure 25.3 Double bubble sign. The infant had duodenal obstruction due to annular pancreas.

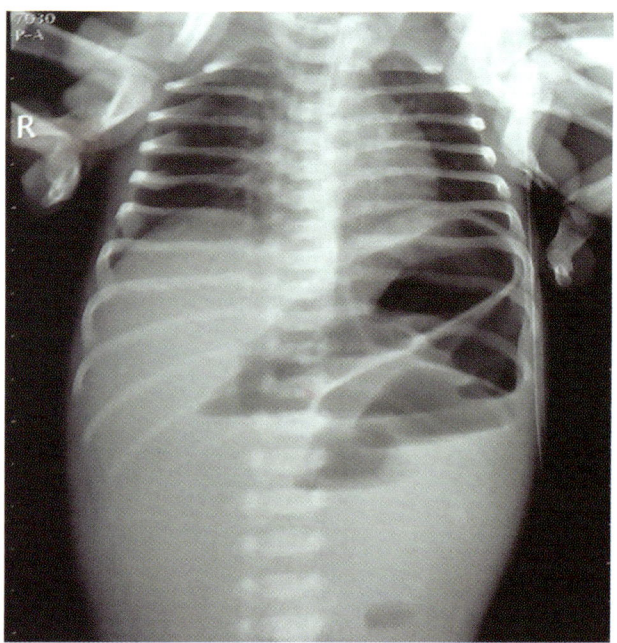

Figure 25.5 Multiple air fluid levels due to small gut atresia.

of calcification suggests fetal meconium peritonitis. In meconium ileus, plain skiagram of abdomen may show "soap bubble appearance" due to mixing of swallowed air with abnormal meconium. The diagnosis of mucoviscidosis or cystic fibrosis as a cause of meconium peritonitis can be confirmed by polymerase chain reaction because estimation of sweat electrolytes and tryptic activity of stools are unreliable in the neonatal period.

In persistent or projectile non-bilious vomiting in a term infant after the age of 2 weeks, ultrasonography of upper abdomen should be done. Pyloric muscle thickness of >4.0 mm and pyloric canal length of >15 mm is diagnostic of hypertrophic pyloric stenosis. The presence of hypoechoic rings of hypertrophied muscle around the hyperechoic pyloric mucosa may produce a "target sign".

Non-flocculable barium, as a contrast medium, is preferred to gastrografin. The latter is a 70% solution with an osmolarity of 1900 mOsm/L and may attract three times its volume of water into the intestinal lumen causing dehydration and even collapse. Barium swallow is indicated for the diagnosis of gastroesophageal reflux, hiatus hernia and pyloric stenosis (string sign). Barium enema is occasionally undertaken to diagnose malrotation of gut which may be associated with duodenal or Ladds bands and volvulus (Figure 25.6). Malrotation may be associated with other GI anomalies, like diaphragmatic hernia, annular pancreas, bowel atresia and omphalocele. Midgut volvulus with strangulation is characterized by gasless abdomen, dilated thick-walled bowel loops mainly on the right side of abdomen and absence of blood flow through superior mesenteric artery on color Doppler ultrasonography. In small gut atresia, barium enema demonstrates microcolon (Figure 25.7). About 90% cases of Hirschsprung's disease can be diagnosed in the neonatal period by finding a narrow rectal segment with funnel-shaped dilatation at the level of transition zone and marked dilatation of the proximal colon (Figure 25.8). Barium enema should be done without any preparation and barium should be diluted with normal saline before instillation. Postevacuation films after 24 hours often show persistence of contrast in the left colon. Rectal manometeric studies may provide useful supportive information. In normal subjects, distension of rectum is followed by relaxation of the internal sphincter and contraction of external sphincter whereas in patients with Hirschsprung's disease there is contraction of the internal sphincter. During surgery, mucosal rectal biopsy can be taken through a transperitoneal approach with frozen-

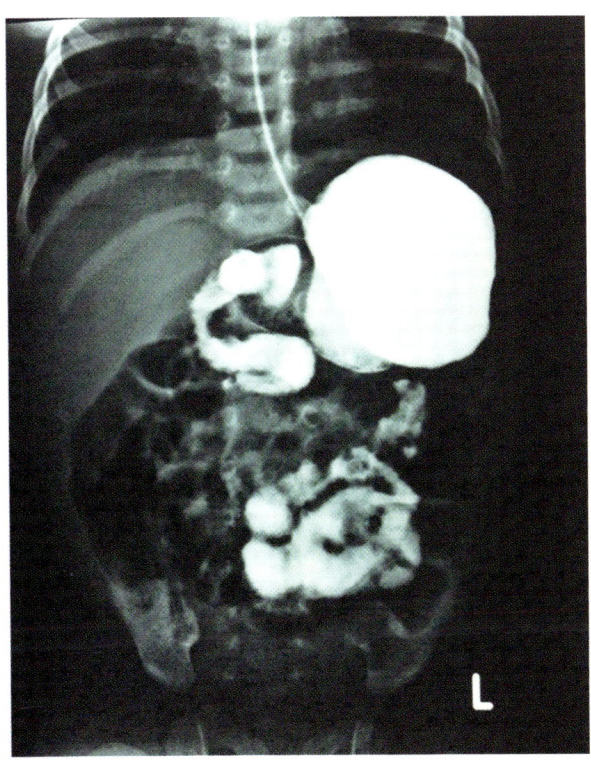

Figure 25.6 Barium meal follow through in a 15 days old neonate with cork screw malrotation of gut. The duodenojejunal junction is located to the right of the midline with entire gut loops displaced towards the right side of the abdomen.

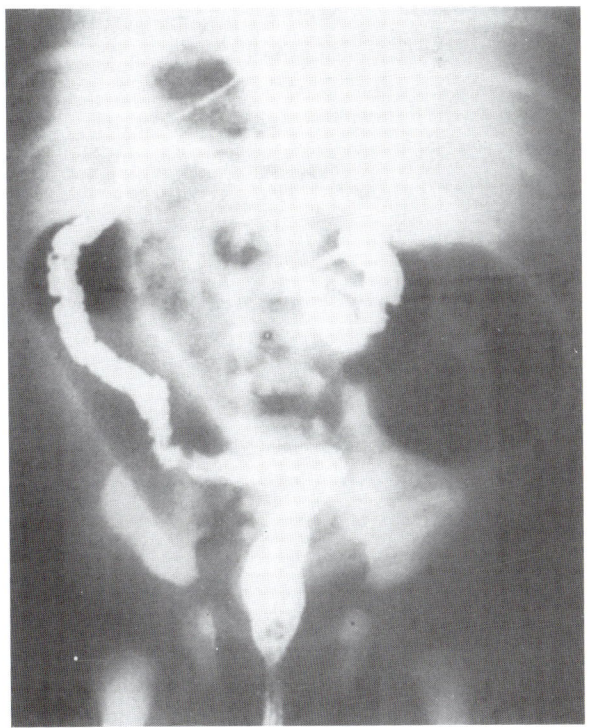

Figure 25.7 Typical appearance of microcolon due to ileal atresia.

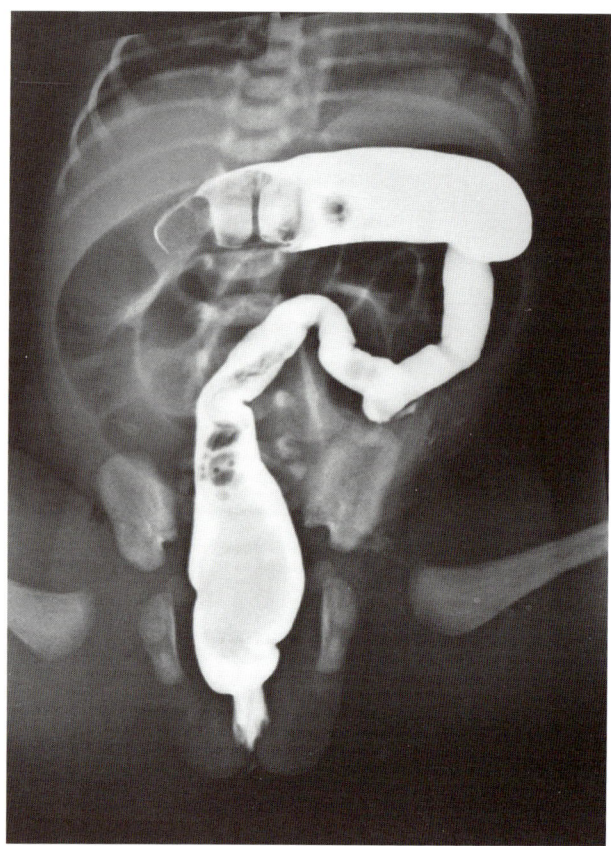

Figure 25.8 Barium enema showing typical appearances of Hirschsprung disease.

section confirmation of aganglionosis. In infants with equivocal radiographic findings, transanal suction rectal biopsy should be taken at different levels, viz. 3 cm, 5 cm, 7 cm from the anal verge before undertaking laparotomy. The biopsy specimen is placed on a small piece of filter paper, quickly frozen and stained with acetylcholinestrase. Absence of ganglion cells and presence of increased number of acetylcholinesterase positive nerve fibers in the lamina propria and muscularis mucosa are suggestive of Hirschsprung's disease.

Management

During the first week of life, fluid requirements for daily maintenance needs are 60–120 mL/kg. These can be given as one-fifth isotonic saline in 10% glucose solution. Additional fluid requirements for correcting the deficit should be assessed by weight loss, severity of dehydration and concurrent losses. Provision should be made for replacing concurrent losses in the vomitus. These should be replaced before the patient is submitted to surgery. Patients with suspected septicemia, peritonitis and necrotizing enterocolitis should be managed with intravenous fluids, gastric aspiration, appropriate antibiotics and maintenance

of normal body temperature. *Vitamin K 0.5–1.0 mg intramuscularly should be routinely administered before any neonatal surgery.* Meconium plug syndrome may be associated in infants of diabetic mothers and cystic fibrosis. Digital examination of the rectum and introduction of 2 to 3 mL of glycerine in normal saline at a distance of about 3 to 5 cm from anal orifice facilitates the passage of meconium plug. These cases should be followed up for Hirschsprung's disease. Meglumine diatrizoate (gastrografin) or sodium diatrizoate (hypaque) 1:4 dilution can be administered as a therapeutic enema in a well-hydrated infant. Acetylcysteine by enema or orally has been tried successfully to relieve obstruction due to meconium ileus. N-acetylcysteine 5 mL of 10% solution is given orally every 6 hours for 5 days. This form of therapy is not generally recommended because some cases of meconium ileus have associated small gut atresia or perforation.

The surgical management consists of bypassing the obstruction with end-to-end anastomosis or ileostomy/colostomy. The entire gut must be diligently examined to identify all the atretic lesions which may be at multiple sites. Postoperatively, maintenance fluid requirements should be limited to two-thirds of the usual physiologic needs. Gastric aspirate should be replaced by half isotonic saline and ileostomy losses by isotonic saline. Intravenous alimentation may have to be prolonged, if large portion of the gut has been excised. Plasma (20 mL/kg) or 5% salt free albumin (1.0 g/kg) should be administered twice a week. Oral feeding can be introduced very gradually when the gastric aspirate is minimal, abdominal distension is absent, bowel sounds are audible and baby is passing meconium again.

Prognosis

The mortality depends upon the age at diagnosis, type of defect, size of the baby, presence of other associated anomalies and adequacy of pre-, para- and postoperative management. In specialized centers with optimal perioperative medical management, the mortality due to neonatal intestinal obstruction has been reduced to less than 5%. Short gut syndrome with poor physical growth and unsatisfactory nutritional status may occur following extensive resection of small gut.

ANORECTAL ANOMALIES

Malformations at the distal most end of gastrointestinal tract are most common and affect one in 4000 live births. They can be easily identified at birth by proper inspection of the perineum to ascertain the site and size of anal orifice. During embryogenesis, cloaca (common genitourinary cum fecal channel) is divided into urogenital sinus ventrally and rectum dorsally by downward growth of urorectal septum. Urogenital sinus subsequently evolves into urethra and lower third of vagina in the female and posterior urethra in the male. The development of perineum is associated with posterior displacement of the lower part of rectum and anal orifice. The classification of anorectal anomalies is based on the arrest of this sequence of development. There may be either failure on the part of urorectal septum to divide the cloaca completely or failure of posterior migration of rectum in the perineum.

Classification

Anorectal anomalies present with a wide spectrum of malformations as shown in Table 25.3. Most male babies have high anomalies (supralevator) while reverse is true in female babies. Female babies usually have a fistula from the terminal end of the bowel opening externally in the vestibule or vagina while in male babies fistulous connection is at a higher level and is not visible on clinical examination. Perineum and vestibule should be examined in lithotomy position with a magnifying glass and shadowless bright light.

TABLE 25.3 Classification of anorectal malformations

Male	Female
High	
Anorectal agenesis with recto-prostatic or rectovesical fistula	Anorectal agenesis with rectovaginal fistula
Without fistula	Without fistula
Rectal atresia*	Rectal atresia*
Intermediate	
Rectobulbar fistula	Rectovaginal fistula
Rectourethral fistula (black eye urethra)	Rectovestibular fistula
Anal agenesis without fistula	Anal agenesis without fistula
Low	
Anocutaneous or perineal fistula	Anovestibular fistula
	Anocutaneous or perineal fistula
Anal stenosis	Anal stenosis
Complex malformations	Cloacal malformations

*Normal anal orifice is present but catheter cannot be passed beyond 2 cm.

In a male infant, there is imperforate anus (rectal atresia) with rectovesical or more commonly recto-urethral fistula. Alternatively, failure of posterior migration of rectum may lead to development of ectopic anus or rectoperineal fistula. Fistulous opening may be located anywhere in the median perineal raphe between scrotum and normal position of anus (Figure 25.9A). Generally, perineal opening is extremely small but at times a bead of meconium may be seen gaping through it. Due to relatively small fistulous opening of rectum, male infant with anorectal malformation often shows evidences of intestinal obstruction.

In girls, imperforate anus (rectal atresia) may be associated with rectovaginal or rectovestibular fistula. In cases of rectovestibular fistula, anal orifice is located in the vestibule between introitus and fourchette. This opening can be easily missed unless carefully looked for with a sterile probe under bright light. In some cases, defective posterior migration of distal end of rectum results in formation of ectopic anus which opens as a rectoperineal fistula anywhere between fourchette and normal location of anus (Figure 25.9B).

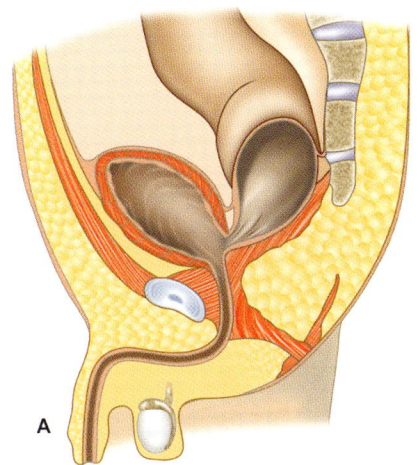

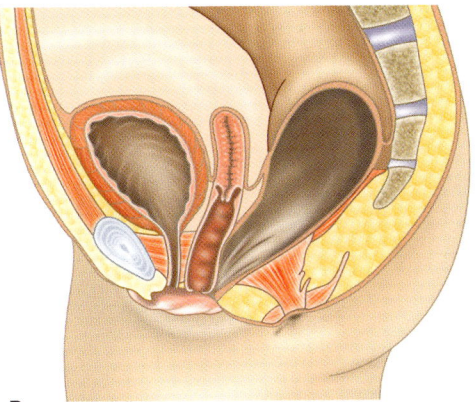

Figure 25.9 (A) Anorectal anomalies in a male child, (B) Anorectal anomalies in a female child.

The ecotopic rectal opening in the female, irrespective of its location in vagina, vestibule or perineum is usually reasonably large and generally there are no symptoms of intestinal obstruction. Rarely, there is only one perineal opening in the female due to persistent cloaca forming a common channel with urethera, vagina and rectum. Such an infant may show signs of intestinal obstruction.

Clinical Features

Unrecognized anorectal malformations in boys may produce symptoms of intestinal obstruction due to relatively small size of rectal opening. Careful inspection of perineum at birth is essential to identify the location and size of the anal opening. Imperforate anus without any visible ectopic opening in the perineum should be investigated to find out whether the defect is above ('high' type) the levator ani or below ('low' type) it. The infant with a flat bottom without any dimple or anal impulse on crying is suggestive of a 'high' anomaly (Figure 25.10).

Lateral invertogram with a lead marker at usual anal site to see the distance between gas in rectal pouch and perineum is often unnecessary. Instead, lateral cross-table skiagram of a prone infant with buttocks elevated (knee-chest position) is quite satisfactory because in this position rectum would be highest and distal most gas bubble can be identified. Skiagram

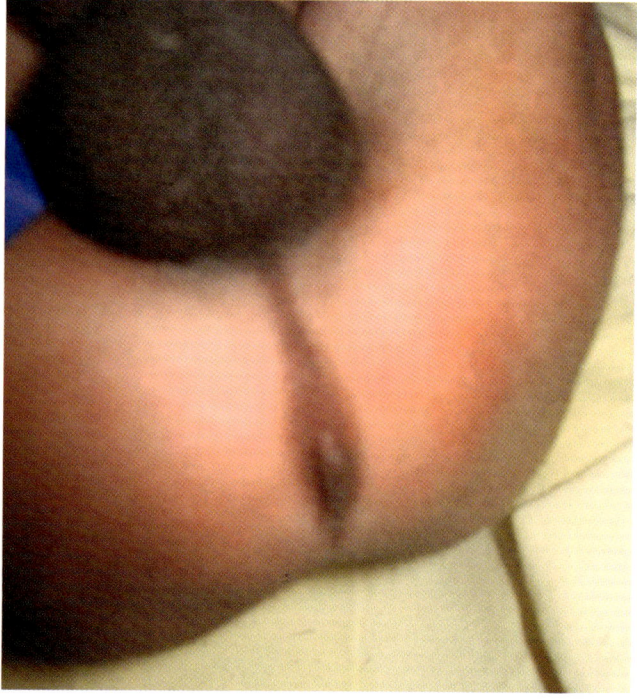

Figure 25.10 Imperforate anus in a male neonate. There was no anal impulse on crying.

should be taken after at least 18 hours of birth, because it takes time for the gas to reach rectum. If the distal colonic gas shadow is above the level of pubococcyx line (which corresponds to puborectalis sling), it is indicative of 'high' defect. Some workers have suggested that M-line (M stands for muscle), an horizontal line passing through upper two-thirds and lower one-third of ischium, is a more reliable indicator of the position of levator ani muscle to classify the anomaly into 'high' and 'low' types. X-ray tube should be centered in a true lateral position over the buttock region for proper delineation of ischium. Passage of meconium through urethra or presence of gas in the urinary bladder should be looked for and are indicative of 'high' anomaly. Skiagrams should be carefully evaluated for presence of vertebral defects and sacral agenesis. Sacral agenesis is associated with 'high' anomaly, neurogenic bladder, lack of perineal sensations or 'puckering' at the anal dimple on pinprick and impotence in later life. Fistulogram after injection of contrast is mandatory to outline the exact tract of fistula and its anatomical connections.

About 20 to 70% of infants with anorectal anomalies have additional major internal malformations which must be screened clinically and identified by appropriate investigations. One-third of infants with anorectal malformations have urinary tract anomalies. Associated anomalies have been given an acronym of VATER complex which stands for **v**ertebral defects, **v**ascular abnormalities (ventricular septal defect, single umbilical artery), **a**nal atresia, **t**racheoesophageal fistula with **e**sophageal atresia, **r**adial and **r**enal dysplasia. Cardiovascular and chromosomal anomalies (trisomy 18 and 21) have also been reported.

Management

Prognosis and surgical staging are guided by the type of anorectal anomaly and the nature of associated malformations. In most cases of low anomalies, modified cut-back operation or perineal anoplasty is all that is required in the neonatal period. In male infants with symptoms of intestinal obstruction due to extremely tiny perineal orifice or a female infant with cloacal abnormality, colostomy is required as an emergency measure. *When in doubt regarding the nature of anomaly, it is always better to do a colostomy rather than explore the perineum which may cause damage to the sphincters.* Pelvic colostomy is preferable over transverse colostomy because of solid consistency of stools and less area of absorption of urine refluxing from the colo-urinary fistula. Diarrheal episodes are handled more safely in case of pelvic colostomy. After 4–6 months of age, when infant weighs around 5 kg, definitive surgery can be undertaken. If the terminal end of bowel extends below second sacral vertebra on a distal cologram, posterior sagittal anorectoplasty can be undertaken.

In high lesions, it is recommended to use a dual approach by combining abdominal and posterior sagittal approaches, tackling either procedure first and then turning the baby over. Exposure through the posterior sagittal approach enables an accurate placement of the bowel through the puborectalis sling to ensure satisfactory continence. After two weeks of definitive surgery, daily dilatation of neorectum is regularly practised to ensure adequate calibre of anal canal. Six to eight weeks after definitive surgery, the diverting colostomy is closed. During follow-up especially in cases of supralevator anorectal mal-formations, toilet training is advised. Specific attention should be paid to the diet to prevent constipation or loose stools, development of gastrocolic reflex, timing and training for defection with the help of sibling and rectal wash out, if needed. All efforts should be made to ensure that the rectum is not allowed to dilate due to constipation.

INTESTINAL PERFORATION

The child may be born with perforation or may develop it postnatally.

Fetal Intestinal Perforation

In small gut atresia, meconium ileus, fetal volvulus, intussusception, the gut may rupture leading to meconium peritonitis. In the west, mucoviscidosis is the leading cause of meconium peritonitis. The extravasated meconium may cause intense chemical and foreign body reaction which may get walled off by the surrounding intestinal loops to produce a pseudocyst. Skiagram of abdomen may show calci-fication and opaque metaphyseal bands parallel to the epiphyseal plate at the ends of long bones, ileum and scapula (Figure 25.11).

Postnatal Intestinal Perforation

Besides perforation due to acute intestinal obstruction, perforation of the stomach may follow nasogastric intubation, intracranial birth injury with acute peptic ulceration, congenital deficiency of gastric musculature especially over the greater curvature and intake of indomethacin. Gastric perforation may occur sponta-neously in a relatively healthy infant. It is characterized by hematemesis, bilious vomiting, abdominal distension

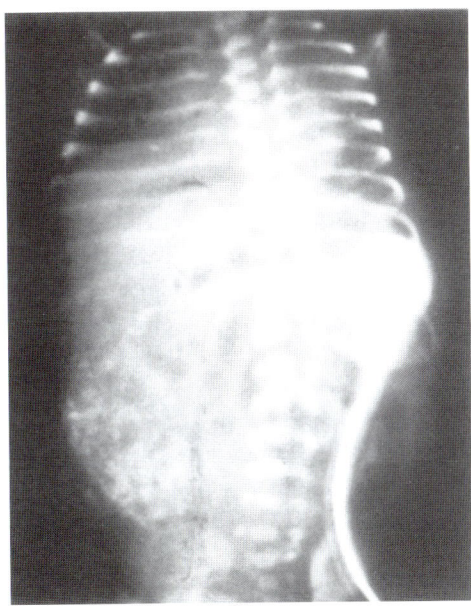

Figure 25.11 Meconium peritonitis due to fetal intestinal perforation with calcification in the right iliac region.

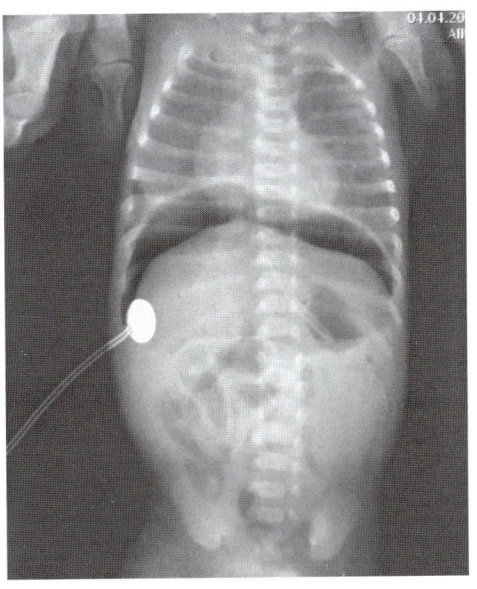

Figure 25.12 Air under the diaphragm due to intestinal perforation because of jejunal atresia.

and obliteration of hepatic dullness. Pneumoperito-neum and trapped air in the stomach wall will be seen on skiagrams of abdomen. *In all infants with gastro-intestinal bleeding, skiagram of abdomen in supine and upright posture must be taken to rule out perforation.* Early surgery is indicated, if there is massive bleeding or in association with perforation. Intestinal obstruction due to small gut atresia or cork screw malrotation may lead to perforation of gut (Figure 25.12). The pneumo-peritoneum needs emergency decompression, if breathing is being interfered with.

NECROTIZING ENTEROCOLITIS

Necrotizing enterocolitis (NEC) in the newborn has been recognized long since but of late there is an upsurge in its incidence in neonatal special care units throughout the world. Its incidence is variable among different centers and even in a given center its occurrence varies from time-to-time depending upon the bacterial ecology of the neonatal intensive care unit (NICU), feeding practices, obstetric resuscitation procedures and other variables. At times, a number of cases appear in a 'cluster' or as outbreaks. The overall incidence varies between 1 and 3/1000 live births or 5 to 10% of admissions to the NICU.

Epidemiology

The disease is mostly limited (90%) to low birth weight preterm babies due to immaturity of the gastro-intestinal tract. Preterm babies are vulnerable to develop NEC because of high incidence of perinatal distress factors, stasis of gut because of autonomic immaturity, poor barrier functions of gut or immune defences, lack of feeding with human milk and higher incidence of nosocomial infections. Among term infants with NEC, almost one-half are small-for-gestational age or dysmature. Various predisposing factors include prematurity (especially <34 weeks), perinatal hypoxia, active resuscitation, RDS/apnea or both, assisted ventilation, acidosis, hypoxia, shock, umbilical artery catherization, use of H_2 blockers or indomethacin and early or large-volume nasogastric formula feedings. The protective or trophic role of human milk and probiotics for prevention of NEC is well accepted.

Pathogenesis

The exact etiology of NEC is unknown and its pathogenesis is multifactorial and complex. It would appear that intestinal mucosal injury due to or as a consequence of ischemia is the core pathogenetic mechanism. Perinatal hypoxia, hypovolemia or shock because of various predisposing factors leads to a situation akin to "diving reflex" resulting in mesenteric vasospasm in order to divert the blood to vital organs to enhance their perfusion. The net reduction in intestinal perfusion with or without mesenteric vasospasm or thrombosis, leads to ischemic mucosal injury (Figure 25.13). Additional or direct mucosal damage due to large volume of intragastric feedings and bacterial toxins (neuraminidase) elaborated by invasion of anaerobic microorganisms aggravate mucosal injury. There is increasing evidence to support the critical role of platelet activating factor (PAF) and other inflammatory mediators, like leukotrienes, interleukins and tumor necrosis factor in the pathogenesis of NEC. The mucosal necrosis leads to intestinal dysfunction with

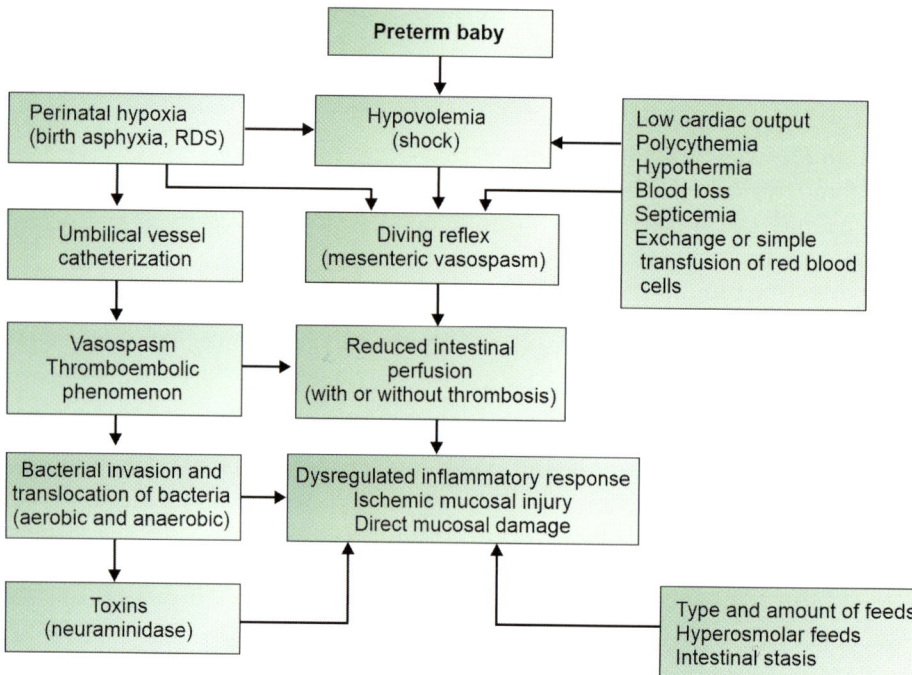

Figure 25.13 Pathogenesis of necrotizing enterocolitis. Perinatal hypoxia and shock appear to initiate intestinal mucosal ischemia in a preterm baby.
Adapted from Touloukian RJ. Neonatal enterocolitis. *Surg Clin North Am* 1976, 56: 281.

functional intestinal obstruction characterized by delayed gastric and small gut emptying, bilious vomiting and abdominal distension. Feeding with large volume of hyperosmolar feeds (formula feeds, 10% dextrose, human milk fortifier, vitamin E, calcium gluconate, etc.) at this stage would aggravate mucosal damage and may be associated with leakage of undigested protein antigens into portal circulation. The hepatic Kupffer cells may be unable to contain or eliminate these antigens, resulting in systemic endotoxemia and shock with further aggravation and perpetuation of ischemic damage to intestinal mucosa. Mucosal necrosis and bleeding manifests as fresh or occult blood in stools. Enteric bacteria cause fermentation of undigested feeds leading to production of hydrogen gas which enters through mucosal breaks to produce blebs of pneumatosis intestinalis and portal venous gas.

Clinical Features

Preterm or sick newborn babies should be closely watched for development of NEC. The symptoms may appear after 96 hours of initiation of oral feeding. Disease may occur anytime during neonatal period but majority of cases occur within first 10 days of life. The onset may be insidious or explosive and at times delayed. Functional intestinal obstruction as evidenced by abdominal distension and retention of milk in the stomach in a sick-looking LBW baby is the earliest marker of the disease. Early signs are indistinguishable from neonatal sepsis. The full blown clinical picture is characterized by triad of abdominal distension, gastrointestinal bleeding and pneumatosis intestinalis (air in the bowel wall) on abdominal radiography.

Further progress of the disease can be arrested, if oral feedings are withheld at this stage. The clinical picture is characterized by progressive abdominal distension and blood-streaked loose stools or occult blood in stools in a sick preterm baby. Gastric emptying is delayed and peristalsis is reduced or absent. Bilious vomiting may provide decompression, if gastric aspiration is delayed. Infant looks sick, pale and lethargic with circumoral grayish discoloration. Thermal instability and hypotension are frequent. Apneic attacks, generalized bleeding (due to DIC) and sclerema herald poor outcome. About one-half of patients develop transmural necrosis and perforation resulting in peritonitis and free air under the right dome of the diaphragm. The presence of ascites, erythema and edema of abdominal wall and localized mass or rigidity over right lower quadrant of abdomen should alert to the possibility of intestinal perforation.

Candidemia produces an identical clinical picture and must be excluded. The modified Bell's staging criteria for NEC along with treatment options are shown in Table 25.4.

Investigations

Leukocytosis, thrombocytopenia, metabolic acidosis and hyponatremia are commonly associated. Serial skiagrams of abdomen, supine, cross-table lateral and oblique views, should be taken every 12-hour during the course of NEC. Depending upon the stage of the disease, gaseous distension, dilated fixed loops of bowel, pneumatosis intestinalis, portal vein gas, and pneumoperitoneum may be seen on X-rays (Figures 25.14 and 25.15). Pneumatosis intestinalis, the pathognomonic feature of NEC, is present in 85% of patients. Sonographic detection of portal air may help in making an early diagnosis. Overt or occult blood in the stools is invariably present. Reducing substance (positive stool clinitest) due to unabsorbed lactose in stools may be positive. Elevated hydrogen gas in the breath is a useful marker of the disease. Following perforation, meconium pigments may be absorbed in the bloodstream and excreted in the urine. The meconium pigment is different than bilirubin and gives a specific absorbance at 405 nm. Spectrophotometric examination of urine may show meconium index of more than 1.0. At times, urine may appear dark-brown or green when large amounts of meconium pigment is excreted. Urine should be examined for budding yeasts and hyphae to rule out systemic candidiasis. Serological test for identification of T-antigen in blood would confirm the co-existence of anaerobic bacterial infection in the gut. Elevated alpha-fetoproteins are indicative of associated hypoxic damage to the liver. Electrolytes, hematocrit, and coagulation status should be monitored during the course of therapy. Serial measurements of C-reactive protein (CRP) are helpful in the diagnosis and assessment of response to therapy. Blood and stool cultures for aerobic and anaerobic organisms are mandatory.

Differential Diagnosis

The insidious onset, characteristic clinical picture and radiological findings of pneumatosis intestinalis are diagnostic. The triad of thrombocytopenia, persistent metabolic acidosis and intractable hyponatremia is usually present. Feeding intolerance in a sick preterm baby may be confused with early stage of NEC. Sepsis and pneumonia may cause ileus without NEC. Acute surgical abdomen due to malrotation with midgut

TABLE 25.4 Modified Bell's staging criteria for NEC

Stage	Systemic signs	Abdominal signs	Radiologic signs	Treatment
IA—Suspected NEC	Temperature instability, apnea, bradycardia and lethargy	Elevated pre-gavage residuals, mild abdominal distension, emesis, guaiac-positive stool	Normal or intestinal dilatation, mild ileus	NPO, antibiotics for 3 days pending culture report
IB—Suspected NEC	Same as above	Bright-red blood per rectum	Same as above	Same as above
IIA—Definite NEC Midly ill	Same as above	Same as above, plus absent bowel sounds	Intestinal dilatation, ileus, pneumatosis intestinalis	NPO, antibiotics for 7–10 days
IIB—Definite NEC Moderately ill	Same as above, plus metabolic acidosis and thrombocytopenia	Same as above, plus absent bowel sounds, definite abdominal tenderness, abdominal cellulitis or right lower quadrant mass	Same as IIA, plus portal vein gas, doubtful ascites	NPO, antibiotics for 14 days, sodium bicarbonate for acidosis
IIIA—Advanced NEC Severely ill, bowel intact	Same as IIB, plus hypotension, bradycardia, severe apnea, combined respiratory and metabolic acidosis, disseminated intravascular coagulation, neutropenia	Same as above, plus signs of generalized peritonitis, marked tenderness and distension of abdomen	Same as IIB, plus definite ascites	Same as above, plus 200 mL/kg fluids, inotropic agents, assisted ventilation, paracentesis
IIIB—Advanced NEC Severely ill, bowel perforated	Same as IIIA	Same as IIIA	Same as IIB, plus pneumoperitoneum	Same as above, plus surgical intervention

NPO; nil per OS or nothing by mouth

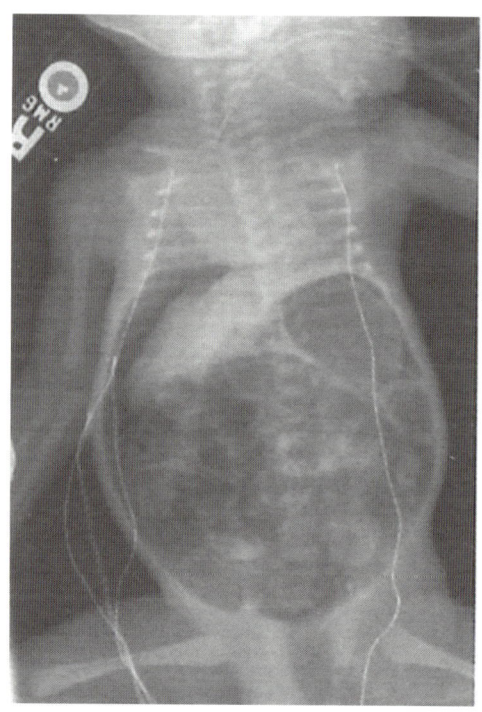

Figure 25.14 Plain X-ray abdomen erect showing gas under the diaphragm in a preterm infant with necrotizing enterocolitis.

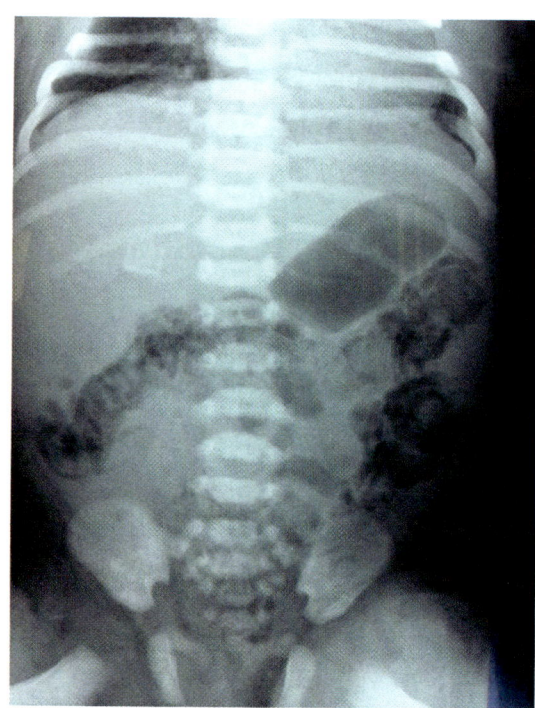

Figure 25.15 Typical appearances of pneumatosis intestinalis in an infant with necrotizing enterocolitis.

volvulus, intussusception, gastric perforation and thrombosis of mesenteric vessels may present rather acutely as a catastrophe. The presence of diarrhea and blood in stool is suggestive of infectious enterocolitis due to *Campylobacter* species rather than NEC. Candidemia may mimic early features of NEC and must be excluded by appropriate culture studies.

Treatment

Early recognition of NEC and vigorous medical management has reduced the need for surgery. Nevertheless, the condition should be managed under close guidance and supervision of a pediatric surgeon so that when indicated surgery is not unnecessarily delayed. If there are any umbilical catheters, they should be promptly removed. Intravenous line should be established to administer fluids, electrolytes and drugs. Pharmacological support with low doses of dopamine (3–5 µg/kg/min) is useful to improve splanchnic and renal blood flow. The fluid requirements are markedly increased due to abdominal fluid sequestration (3rd space losses), peritonitis and septic shock. Oral feedings should be stopped for 7 to 14 days and gastric aspiration preferably by slow continuous suction with a wide-bored catheter (Fr 10 or 12) is advised. Total parenteral nutrition (TPN) is instituted and by and large outcome in cases of NEC is related to the feasibility and availability of TPN.

Systemic antibiotics, depending upon the prevailing spectrum of bacterial pathogens in a particular NICU, are administered intravenously. Piperacillin-tozabactam is a useful broad-spectrum antibiotic and can be used as a single agent. The role of oral colistin (10–15 mg/kg/dL) or gentamicin is controversial. Metronidazol 15 mg/kg IV loading dose followed by 7.5 mg/kg/dose every 12 hours may be administered to treat associated anaerobic infection. Fresh frozen plasma (10 mL/kg/day) is recommended on every alternate day to provide complement, humoral immune factors, coagulation factors and to improve blood volume to correct shock. The blood lost through glastrointestinal bleeding or through sampling should be replaced.

Diluted enteral feedings with EBM are started in small amounts when abdominal distension disappears, gastric aspirate is negligible, intestinal peristalsis is audible and there is no occult blood in the stools. The stomach should be aspirated before each feed and next feed should be omitted or its volume reduced, if aspirate contains bile/milk or exceeds 5 mL. The weaning from intravenous to oral alimentation in cases of NEC should be extremely slow, cautious and

controlled. Most cases of NEC can be managed conservatively but surgery is indicated in following situations:

1. Bowel perforation as evidenced by pneumoperitoneum or portal venous gas on plain abdominal radiograph.
2. Full thickness necrosis of bowel wall with impending perforation as evidenced by dilated loop of intestine that remains unchanged in position and shape for more than 24 hours on serial radiographs.
3. Peritonitis as suggested by ascites, abdominal mass, induration and erythema of abdominal wall and localized abdominal rigidity. Aspiration of brown-colored or meconium-stained ascitic fluid (or ascitic fluid showing bacteria on Gram's stain) is indicative of intestinal gangrene and perforation.

The necrotic portion of the gut is excised and end-to-end anastomosis is established or enterostomy is performed. The abdomen is closed after placing a drain in the peritoneal cavity. The conservative therapy is continued and oral feedings are initiated with extreme caution in operated cases. In ELBW (<1000 g) or unstable babies, peritoneal drainage is established under local anesthesia and exploratory laparotomy is delayed.

Prognosis

Early NEC without perforation is likely to have outcome akin to neonatal sepsis. Depending upon the stage of the disease, quality of supportive care and availability of parenteral nutrition, the case fatality rates vary between 20 and 50%. Infants requiring surgical intervention are likely to have growth retardation, osteopenia, neuromotor delay and parenteral nutrition-related complications. Common gastrointestinal sequelae include strictures, enteric fistulas, short bowel syndrome, malabsorption and chronic diarrhea.

Prevention

Even following aggressive therapeutic efforts, the mortality in cases of established NEC varies between 15 and 30% in the West. Because of greater awareness of predisposing factors and improved understanding of pathogenetic mechanisms underlying NEC, it has been possible to reduce the incidence of the condition. Antenatal administration of corticosteroids, when labor starts prematurely, is credited to reduce the risk of NEC. Perinatal hypoxia, RDS/apnea, hypovolemic shock and other predisposing situations should be prevented and managed promptly to circumvent "diving reflex". Oral feeding should be delayed in sick

LBW babies and whenever poor perfusion of bowel is suspected. The enteral feeding should be small, iso-osmolar (preferably human milk) and its volume should be increased gradually and cautiously. The stomach should be aspirated before each feed and next feed should be omitted or reduced, if aspirate contains bile/milk or if its volume exceeds 50% of the amount administered in the last feed. The double-blind controlled trials have failed to demonstrate any prophylactic utility of administration of oral antibiotics to high-risk LBW babies for prevention of NEC. Recently, it has been shown that oral administration of immuno-globulins (75% IgA and 25% IgG) to high-risk preterm infants may reduce the incidence of NEC. Trials are being conducted to assess the role of platelet aggravating factor (PAF) antagonists to reduce the incidence of NEC. Administration of probiotics to preterm babies are credited to reduce the risk of NEC. Studies are ongoing to determine which organisms are most effective and their safety and side effects.

Iatrogenic Perforation

Perforation of the gut has been known to occur following insertion of rectal thermometer and introduction of tubes from above or below especially when due care is not exercised. The use of soft polyvinyl catheters, gentleness and proper technique of introduction of rectal thermometer (by directing it posteriorly) are recommended for avoiding these mishaps.

RESPIRATORY SURGICAL EMERGENCIES

Respiratory distress is a common life-threatening situation at birth or after few hours and early decision is mandatory to find out whether the problem is medical or needs urgent surgical correction. The common surgical conditions are discussed below.

Choanal Atresia

The normal newborn baby breathes entirely through his nose except when crying. In choanal atresia, the baby has severe respiratory difficulty dating back from birth because the posterior nasal air passage is blocked by a bony or membranous septum. Breathing improves and color returns to normal as soon as the baby starts crying. Infants are obligatory nose breathers until about 4 months of age. Unilateral atresia may be asymptomatic. It comes to light during feeding or when the other nostril is blocked due to upper respiratory tract infection. No breath sounds are audible while listening over the nostrils with a stethoscope. The inability to pass a catheter through

the posterior nasopharynx confirms the diagnosis. Diagnosis can be established by instilling a small amount of water-soluble contrast agent into the posterior nares and obtaining a skiagram of the skull in the lateral position. CT scan of nasal passages is a useful non-invasive method to confirm the diagnosis. Oral airway should be inserted and the baby fed with a tube. The presence of bilateral choanal atresia should alert the pediatrician to look for other components of CHARGE association, such as **C**oloboma, **H**eart defect, **A**tresia choanae, **R**etarded growth and development, **G**enital hypoplasia, **E**ar anomalies with deafness. Surgical correction may be deferred till the age of 2 to 3 months when the nasal passages are bigger.

Pierre Robin Syndrome

The essential features of this syndrome include micrognathia and retrognathia, backward displacement of the tongue (glossoptosis) causing respiratory difficulty and attacks of cyanosis (Figure 25.16). A U-shaped midline cleft palate or high-arched palate are often associated but are not essential features of the syndrome. There may be feeding difficulties due to cleft palate and incoordinated sucking and swallowing.

In its early recognition lies half the management. The baby should be nursed in a prone position with an oral plastic airway. The infant's head in prone position may be lifted off the mattress by a length of tube gauze suspended from a drip stand and attached

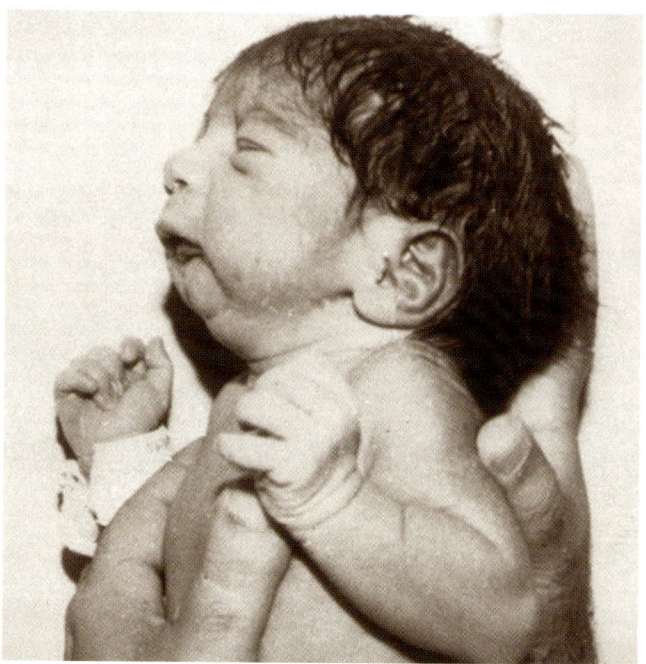

Figure 25.16 Typical appearances of micrognathia and retrognathia in an infant with Pierre Robin syndrome.

to the head with adhesive plaster. In this position, the tongue is held forward by gravity, without any risk of glossoptosis. In some cases, artificial tongue tie may be produced surgically by making the under surface of tongue, floor of the mouth and inside of lower lip raw and suturing these. Alternatively, tongue may be kept pulled out with the help of a suture to prevent glossoptosis. Initially, tube feeding should be carried out. Later on feeding with a spoon or *paladay*, long nipple and a large hole of flanged teat are satisfactory. The mandible grows and by two to three months of age, glossoptosis disappears. The child would need the plastic repair of palate by the age of about one year.

Esophageal Atresia with Tracheoesophageal Fistula

Respiratory distress and choking with cyanosis suggest this condition. Refer to Chapter 19 for details of respiratory emergencies due to developmental defects.

CONGENITAL DIAPHRAGMATIC HERNIA

These are generally false hernias as they do not have a peritoneal sac. Herniation occurs early in fetal life before the peritoneal lining is formed. The persistence of pleuroperitoneal canal results in herniation of abdominal contents into the thorax, commonly on the left side. The incidence of the condition varies between 1 per 2000 and 5000 live births. Polyhydramnios is associated in 75% of cases. Around 50% cases are associated with other anomalies especially neural tube defects, cardiac defects, intestinal malrotation and trisomy syndromes (trisomy 13, 18 and 45 XO). The diaphragmatic hernia is about three to four times more common on the left as compared to the right side. Mediastinum is displaced and there is compression or hypoplasia of ipsilateral lung.

Fetal Diagnosis

Polyhydramnios and ultrasonography after 16 weeks of gestation can pick up diaphragmatic hernia. The severity of lung hypoplasia determines the outcome. Lung-to-head (LHR) ratio of <1.0 is associated with 100% mortality while a ratio of >1.4 is associated with good prognosis. In advanced centers, *ex utero* intrapartum treatment (EXIT) procedure has been successfully conducted to reduce severity of lung hypoplasia and improve the outcome. Prenatal diagnosis of diaphragmatic hernia alerts the attending neonatologist to take prompt management decisions, like elective intubation and avoidance of bag and mask ventilation. Differential diagnoses include diaphragmatic eventration, congenital cystic adenomatoid malformation (CCAM), pulmonary sequestration and bronchogenic cyst.

Clinical Features

These infants usually have difficulty in resuscitation. Spontaneous breathing is established inadequately and baby has deep labored gasping respirations. Diminished air entry and occasional tinkling peristaltic sounds on the left side with the displacement of heart to the right, suggest the diagnosis. The abdomen usually appears flat or scaphoid. The clinical differentiation from pneumothorax may be difficult. Urgent skiagram of the chest, posteroanterior and lateral views, should be taken in all babies with difficult resuscitation. Diagnosis is confirmed by finding bowel loops in the thorax but difficulty may occasionally arise, if bowel is still airless (Figure 25.17). Because of hypoplastic lung, these infants are very prone to develop pneumothorax on the contralateral side due to rupture of normal lung unless great care is taken while ventilating them.

Treatment

Alertness and prompt action at birth is vital for salvaging these babies, who may die in the labor room. Ventilation should be maintained by endotracheal

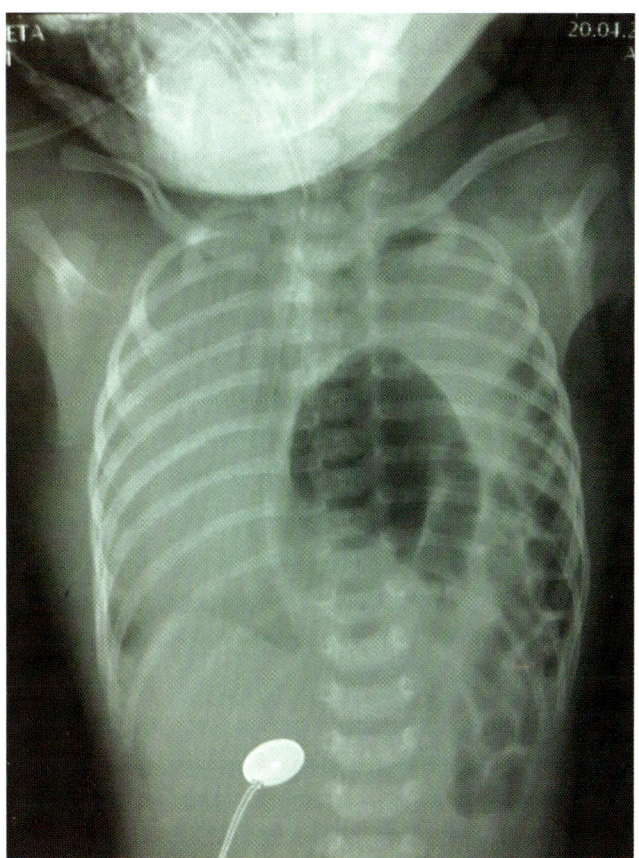

Figure 25.17 Diaphragmatic hernia. The intestinal loops in the left hemithorax have pushed the heart towards right side.

tube and assisted respiration by hand or machine, if spontaneous efforts are weak. *Resuscitation with a bag and mask should never be attempted in these cases as it causes gaseous distension of bowel with worsening of respiratory difficulty.* The head end should be raised and stomach contents including air should be aspirated frequently to reduce distension of the bowel. The infant should preferably be nursed in a lateral decubitus with affected side down to reduce mediastinal displacement.

Surgical reduction of hernia should be undertaken as soon as possible after correction of derangements in blood gases and pH. Peripheral venous and arterial lines should be established as umbilical lines may need to be removed during surgery. These infants are extremely sensitive to fluid overload, maintenance fluid requirements should be restricted to 30 mL/kg/day. The prognosis is related to the degree of pulmonary compression and hypoplasia of lung. Pulmonary hypertension due to hypertrophy of arterial wall of small arteries may cause persistent cyanosis as a result of right-to-left shunt. They should preferably be ventilated with a rapid rate (60–80/minute), low inspiratory pressure (up to 20 cm H_2O) and FiO_2 of 100% from the beginning irrespective of initial PaO_2. The inspiratory pressure should be kept low due to potential risk of damage or rupture of the alveoli of the contralateral lung and permissive hypercapnia is preferred.

High frequency oscillatory ventilation and assist-control mode of ventilation are ideal for these infants. Extracorporeal membrane oxygenation (ECMO) and nitric oxide inhalation therapy are associated with improved survival. These infants are vulnerable to develop persistent pulmonary hypertension which adversely affects their prognosis. The condition carries a high mortality rate of 40% despite advances in the management of critically sick newborn babies. Early onset of symptoms and herniation of the liver into the thorax are associated with poor outcome.

Fetal Surgery

In fetuses with severe CDH where a part of liver has herniated into fetal chest cavity and/or the lung (normal side) to head ratio (LHR) is less than or equal to 1.0, fetoscopic endoluminal tracheal occlusion (FETO) is done between 26 and 28 weeks of gestation to obstruct the normal flow of fetal lung fluid. The build up of tracheal pressure and fluid content promotes the growth of lungs and reduces risk of hypoplasia of the lungs. Fetus is delivered through a keyhole incision in the abdominal wall and uterus of the mother. A tiny detachable balloon or clip is placed in the fetal trachea. Around 34 weeks of gestation, EXIT (*ex utero intrapartum treatment*) procedure is performed. It is a specialised cesarean section, wherein the baby is partially delivered through an abdominal incision. The baby remains attached by its umbilical cord to the placenta and a pediatric otolaryngologist removes the balloon or clip to establish an airway so that the fetus can breathe. After completion of EXIT procedure, the umbilical cord is clamped and then cut to deliver the baby and complete the remainder of the C-section procedure. Fetoscopic endotracheal occlusion (FETENDO) and EXIT procedures are highly skill oriented but have not given the desired dividends regarding improved outcome.

Prognosis

Despite advances in intensive care of neonates, CDH is associated with a relatively high risk of morbidity and mortality. The adverse prognostic factors include early (<20 weeks) herniation of bowel into the chest, herniation of liver, early onset of symptoms, severe abnormalities in PaO_2 and $PaCO_2$ in room air, co-existing cardiac anomalies, pulmonary hypertension and severity of pulmonary hypoplasia. Prenatal USG lung (contralateral)-to-head ratio (LHR) is a useful prognostic marker. The LHR of <1.0 is associated with 100% mortality, 1.0–1.4 with 38% survival and >1.4 with 100% survival.

Laryngeal Web

Infant is severely asphyxiated at birth and is likely to die unless web is perforated by a stiff endotracheal tube or a bronchoscope.

Congenital Lobar Emphysema

The condition may occur as a congenital malformation or an acquired cyst due to partial obstruction with mucus or a meconium plug. Because of air trapping, there is progressive development of emphysema of a lobe with compression of surrounding structures and respiratory distress. Elective intubation of the opposite bronchus or high-frequency ventilation may cause resolution of the lobar emphysema. When conservative measures fail, bronchoscopy should be performed to remove any obstructing material or rupture the bronchogenic cyst. Surgical resection is done as a last resort, if palliative measures are unsuccessful.

Cystic Adenomatoid Malformation

It is characterized by cystic dysplasia or hamartomatous malformation of the lung involving a lobe. Skiagram of chest shows a cystic mass with displacement of mediastinum to the opposite side. The condition may be confused with diaphragmatic hernia. Surgical excision is recommended because there is risk of malignant transformation in untreated cases.

Pneumothorax

Spontaneous pneumothorax is more common in the newborn than at any other age in childhood. The common predisposing factors include meconium aspiration, hypoplastic lung, aggressive attempts at resuscitation, CPAP and intermittent positive pressure ventilation. The baby may develop respiratory distress and cyanosis soon after spontaneous breathing is established. The clinical signs may be difficult to interpret. Mediastinal shift perhaps is the most reliable sign. X-ray chest would show collapsed lung with translucent air shadow without any lung markings. The tension pneumothorax is suggested by the displacement of mediastinum, herniation of lung across the midline, widened intercostal spaces and depressed diaphragm (Figure 25.18).

In tension pneumothorax, immediate drainage of air with needle puncture should be attempted either at second intercostal space one centimeter away from the sternal border or in the fourth intercostal space in the anterior axillary line. This should be followed by constant closed drainage by using continuous suction pressure of about minus 2 cm H_2O (*see* Chapter 19 for details). Administration of 100% oxygen is followed by rapid resorption of pleural air but is no longer advocated due to potential risk of hyperoxia. The child should be administered appropriate antibiotics.

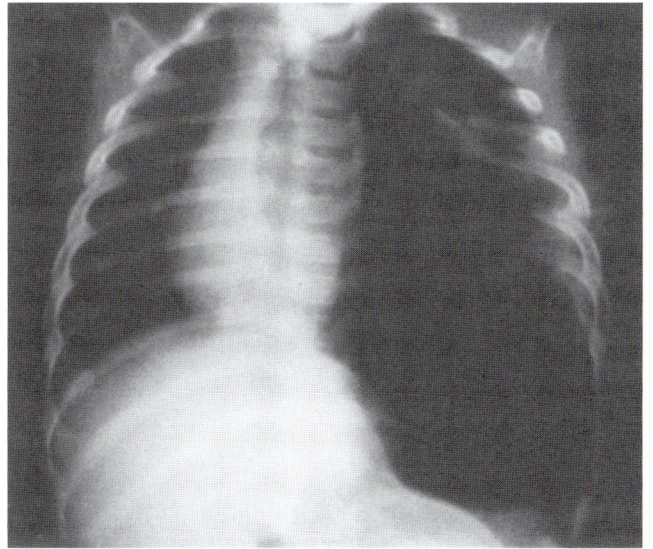

Figure 25.18 Tension pneumothorax on the left side.

UROLOGICAL CONDITIONS

Most newborn babies pass urine within 24 hours of birth and all do so by 48 hours. If the child does not pass urine by 48 hours, check for history of oligohydramnios and look for facial abnormalities, such as large low set ears, flat nose, and recession of chin (Potter facies). These dysmorphic features may be associated with renal agenesis. Abdomen should be examined for ascites, enlarged kidneys and full bladder which would suggest obstructive uropathy. Inability to retract the foreskin is normal at this age and should not be diagnosed as phimosis. The presence of single umbilical artery, absent abdominal wall musculature and anorectal anomalies are commonly associated with genitourinary abnormalities (*see* Chapter 21).

In most cases of alleged non-passage of urine by 48 hours, provision of extra fluids, compression of bladder area during examination and application of urine bag are enough and most babies are likely to void during the next 4 to 6 hours. The opportunity of watching the male baby to void should be utilized to make sure that it conforms to the normal pattern, i.e. stream is adequate and forceful, neither sprays or dribbles nor stops intermittently. Some babies cry before passing urine due to uncomfortable sensation of full bladder and this should not be mistaken as a sign of urinary obstruction. The suspected renal mass in a neonate should be investigated preferably by ultrasonography and radionuclide renal scan or CT scan rather than excretory urography. Any solid intra-abdominal mass in a newborn baby should be considered as malignant unless proved otherwise.

AMBIGUOUS EXTERNAL GENITALIA

Neonates with ambiguous external genitals pose difficulties in assigning the gender at birth. They often pose a diagnostic challenge. The underlying metabolic disorder, such as salt losing type of adrenogenital syndrome, may present as a life-threatening emergency. Early decision to assign the sex is necessary to spare the family serious anxiety and embarrassment and prevent emotional problems in the affected children. The genetic sex is determined at the time of fertilization. Disorder of sexual differentiation can occur due to chromosomal, hormonal and gonadal defects which form the basis for their classification. For example, an XX chromosomal individual with ambiguous external genitals is classified as a female pseudohermaphrodite while an XY individual with atypical external genitalia is designated as male pseudohermaphrodite. Infants having both ovaries and testes, irrespective of their chromosomal sex, are called true hermaphrodites.

Both male (Wolffian) and the female (Müllerian) genital ducts are present in the fetus by the sixth week of gestation. Fetal testes play an important role in sex differentiation during embryogenesis. Fetal testes elaborate testosterone which is converted to dihydrotestosterone with the help of 5-alpha reductase which is responsible for masculinization by channeling the differentiation of Wolffian ducts into epididymis, vas deferens and seminal vesicles. In addition, fetal testes secrete Müllerian regressive factor (MRF) which causes involution of Müllerian system with regression or non-development of fallopian tube, uterus and upper third of vagina. Thus in the absence of functioning fetal testes, all fetuses are destined to differentiate their Müllerian anlage into female external genitals. Testes are formed approximately at 7 weeks of gestation, whereas ovarian development does not occur until the 13th to 16th week of gestation. Phenotypic sex is established at the end of first trimester. If a female fetus is exposed to excessive androgens during the first trimester, her clitoris and labioscrotal folds will virilize and may appear indistinguishable from a normal male phallus and scrotum but the latter would be empty. In the second and third trimesters, male phallic growth and scrotal maturation is dependent on testicular androgens produced under the influence of gonadotropins from the fetal pituitary.

Classification and Diagnostic Work-up

From a practical and clinical standpoint, newborn babies with ambiguous external genitalia are best grouped as follows:

1. *Neonates with ambiguous genitalia but having a uterus*
   a. With ovaries
   b. With testes
2. *Neonates with ambiguous genitalia but without a uterus*
3. *Hypospadias group*

Anatomy of external genitals must be carefully assessed and presence of uterus should be ascertained. Uterus at birth is relatively large and firm due to influence of maternal hormones and can be palpated with ease on rectal examination. When in doubt, ultrasonography is extremely useful to identify the uterus. Conventional radiographic contrast studies, after instillation of dye into the vagina or urogenital

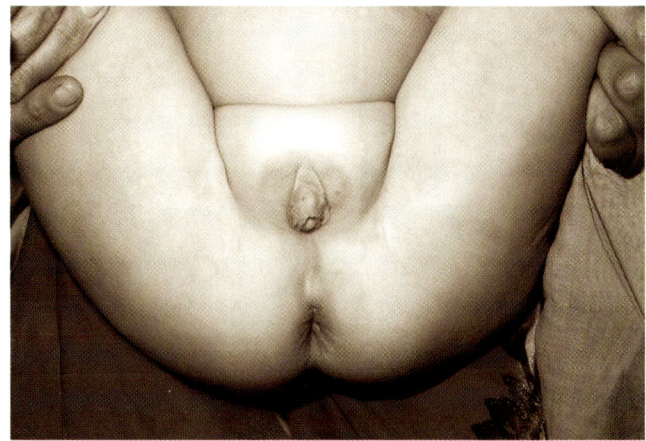

Figure 25.19 Ambiguous external genitalia in an XX infant.

sinus, are indicated to delineate vagina and cervix. The presence of cervix is always associated with a uterus. Examination of external genitalia should include assessment of the size and shape of phallus, location of urethral meatus and vaginal introitus or presence of a common opening of urogenital sinus or cloaca (Figure 25.19). *Penis is identified by one midline frenulum while clitoris has two paramedian frenula on its ventral surface.* Shape and size of scrotum and labia should be checked and gonads looked for. Both ovary and testis may be present within the scrotum, labia or inguinal canal or there may be no identifiable gonads. The presence of increased pigmentation of breast areola and scrotum is suggestive of adrenogenital syndrome due to increased ACTH secretion. A buccal smear for Barr bodies followed by complete karyotyping is essential to find chromosomal sex and any excess or deficiency of sex chromosomes. Rapid karyotyping can be performed by using fluorescent *in situ* hybridization (FISH) technique. In all infants with ambiguous genitalia, adrenogenital syndrome should be ruled out by estimation of serum electrolytes, 17-hydroxyprogesterone (17-OHP) and urinary 17-ketosteroids and pregnanetriol. At times, gonadal biopsy or laparotomy is indicated, if diagnosis cannot be reached by careful physical examination, radiological, sonographic, chromosomal and biochemical studies.

Neonates with Ambiguous Genitalia and Uterus but without Apparent Testes

Female Pseudohermaphroditism

It is the commonest type of intersexuality. Infant is genetically female (46 XX karyotype) with masculinization of external genitals either due to maternal ingestion of androgens during pregnancy, maternal virilizing tumor or endogenous production of androgens by the fetus because of defective biosynthesis of adrenal corticoids. There may be a family history of unexplained deaths in early infancy. Adrenogenital syndrome accounts for approximately 70% of all cases of intersexuality and about one-half of these infants display salt wasting or hypertension. The basic biochemical defect is an enzymic block interfering with the production of cortisol, leading to an excessive accumulation of androgenic steroids. The most common types of enzyme deficiency are 21-hydroxylase (salt loser) and 11-beta-hydroxylase (hypertension). The clinical features are characterized by ambiguous genitalia with hypertrophied clitoris and a separate perineal urethra. Hyperpigmentation of breast areola and labia is often present and uterus is easily recognized by rectal examination or sonography. Infant with salt wasting type of defect presents as life-threatening emergency with vomiting, dehydration, hyponatremia, hyperkalemia, hypoglycemia and shock. Elevated urinary 17-ketosteroids would confirm the diagnosis.

Therapy by administration of isotonic saline with dextrose and glucocorticoids is initiated as an emergency measure while awaiting the reports of hormonal assays. Hydrocortisone in a dose of 5 mg every 8-hour intravenously is given during first 3 days and subsequently reduced to 2.5 mg every 12 hourly. Cortisone acetate can be given orally once clinical condition stabilizes and is continued for life (5 mg in the morning and 10 mg in the evening). Administration of a mineralocorticoid, desoxycorticosterone (DOCA) in a dose of 1.0–2.0 mg/day IM may be necessary to ensure sodium retention. When DOCA is not available, fludrocortisone 0.1–0.2 mg/day in 3–4 divided doses is given orally along with 4–8 g sodium chloride every day in milk feeds. Clitoral hypertrophy may regress following early cortisone therapy but if clitoris is unsightly and fails to regress, clitoral amputation is indicated. With effective replacement hormonal therapy, these children have the best prognosis for sexual performance and can lead normal reproductive life.

Females with Urogenital Sinus Anomalies

These female (46 XX) infants have serious developmental defects of urogenital and anorectal region leading to exstrophy, cloaca and anorectal anomalies. They need detailed radiological and endoscopic examination for outlining the exact anatomy of various structures in the perineum. Infants with vaginal atresia or imperforate hymen with hydrocalpos at birth would

require urgent surgical intervention and drainage. Vaginoplasty and reconstruction surgery is deferred to later childhood.

Neonates with Ambiguous Genitalia, Uterus and Gonads

True Hermaphroditism

True hermaphrodites are uncommon and are characterized by ambiguous genitalia with uterus and palpable external gonads. Genetic sex may be male, female or mosaic. Gonadal tissue may have various combinations of ovary, testis, and ovotestis. Variations in the consistency of gonads may suggest existence of both ovary (which is smaller, higher and feels more firm) and testis. Laparotomy and gonadal biopsy is indicated in these infants to document the diagnosis of true hermaphroditism and to differentiate them from male pseudohermaphroditism with dysgenetic testis or mixed gonadal dysgenesis. The increase in serum testosterone concentration following hCG stimulation indicates the presence of testicular tissue.

Male Pseudohermaphroditism

The deficiency of Müllerian regressive factor (MRF) in a genetically male infant leads to development of ambiguous genitalia, uterus and testes. There are two forms of male pseudohermaphrodites. The presence of Y chromosome and palpable gonad easily differentiates them from female pseudohermaphrodites. Infants with dysgenetic testes often have XO-XY karyotype, whereas male pseudohermaphrodites with mixed gonadal dysgenesis may have either XO-XY or 45 X, 46 XY complement. The incidence of malignancy in dysgenetic testes is higher.

Neonates with Ambiguous Genitalia and without Demonstrable Uterus

These infants have 46 XY karyotype and palpable or undescended testes.

Male Pseudohermaphrodites with Lipoid Hyperplasia

These genetically male infants have ambiguous genitalia and hypoplastic vagina and clitoris. Testes are undescended and skin shows hyperpigmentation. The hormonal block is believed to be a lack of conversion of cholesterol to pregnenolone due to deficiency of desmolase resulting in deficient production of all steroids (including androgens) and accumulation of cholesterol in the adrenal gland. They may die due to vascular collapse and hyponatremia because of urinary loss of salt. Plasma 17-hydroxycorticoids and urinary 17-ketosteroids are both reduced.

Incomplete Testicular Feminization
(Complete Androgen Insensitivity Syndrome, Lubs Syndrome, Gilbert-Dreyfus Syndrome, Reifenstein Syndrome)

There is variable and often minor ambiguity of external genitals including hypospadias. The diagnosis is often delayed till puberty when these children fail to show development of secondary sex characters. There is gynecomastia and delay in appearance of facial and pubic hair. Testosterone and luteinizing hormones (LH) are elevated because the basic defect is endorgan unresponsiveness to androgens.

Hypospadias Group

Infants with urethral opening at scrotal junction or perineum (perineoscrotal hypopadias) and cryptorchidism are associated with sexual disorders in 30% of cases. Hypospadias may be associated with a variety of sexual disorders including male pseudo-hermaphroditism, true hermaphrodite, mixed gonadal dysgenesis and incomplete testicular feminization. Male infants with deficiency of 3 beta-hydroxysteroid dehydrogenase are characterized by hypospadias in association with life-threatening features of salt losing. This enzyme is also required for biosynthesis of testicular hormones and its absence leads to incomplete virilization of males during fetal life.

Micropenis

The normal length of penis of a full-term male infant is at least 2.5 cm measured stretched from the pubis ramus to the tip of the glans. The causes of microphallus with or without cryptorchidism include septo-optic dysplasia or Kallman's syndrome, Prader-Willi syndrome, Robinow syndrome, Klinefelter syndrome, Carpenter syndrome, Meckel-Gruber syndrome, Noonan syndrome, de Lange syndrome, trisomy 21, Fanconi syndrome and fetal hydantoin syndrome. Panhypopituitarism is characterized by microphallus, hypoglycemia and hyperbilirubinemia. The penile length can be increased by administration of testosterone enanthate 25 mg IM every month for 3 months.

Assigning the Gender for Rearing

An early decision should be taken to assign a gender to the infant to avoid future embarrassment to the parents and emotional trauma to the child. Children are believed to establish gender identity by 18 to 24 months of age. The sex of rearing is decided on the basis of genetic or gonadal sex of the infant. Majority of infants with sexual disorders should be raised as females because anatomically and functionally most defects are more compatible with passive female phenotype. There is some evidence to suggest that sexually incompetent females can adjust to life better than sexually incompetent males. The female external genitals can be more easily reconstructed with plastic repair to produce anatomically functional female. It is impossible to surgically construct functionally adequate external genitals in a male. The parents must be taken into confidence and explained about the reasons for assigning a particular sex to the child. They must also be told about the long-term plan of management, need for reconstructive repair, ultimate sexual and reproductive capabilities of the child and questions concerning future marriage.

Nonretractable Prepuce (Phimosis)

The foreskin is not retractable at birth in all newborn babies. Even by one year of age, foreskin is not retractable in up to 50% of boys. This does not cause any problem or difficulty in passing urine. Ballooning of prepuce during micturition is normal in infants. The development of persistent nappy rash due to use of a diaper may lead to scarring of the prepuce. It can be managed by dilatation of prepucial orifice by breaking the adhesions. Gentle retraction of prepuce with local application of steroid cream may break the adhesions thus avoiding the need for surgical intervention.

Circumcision is often done at birth as a religious ritual in certain communities. The procedure is done on medical grounds, if there is a tight prepuce beyond 2 years of age especially when it is associated with recurrent balanitis or urinary tract infection. The procedure should be done by a pediatric surgeon under dorsal penile block or subcutaneous ring block. There is recent evidence to suggest that there is reduced risk of HIV, urinary tract infection, squamous cell carcinoma of penis, sexually transmitted genital ulcer and carcinoma cervix (among spouse) in circumcised males.

Exstrophy of Bladder

It is characterized by anterior abdominal wall defect with exposed urinary bladder, epispadias and several variants of cloaca and widely separated pubic rami. The exposed bladder mucosa should be covered with a plastic wrap to keep it moist. The mucosa should not be touched with latex gloves because of high risk of allergy to latex. The bladder should be reconstructed by turn-in procedure and lengthening of phallus as early as possible followed by reconstruction of bladder neck at 5–7 years of age. The condition is not associated with other abnormalities and carries good prognosis. Cloacal exstrophy is a complex anomaly and demands high level of surgical skills for reconstruction and gender assignment.

Hydrometrocolpos

In this condition, a membrane completely covers the vaginal orifice (imperforate hymen) leading to accumulation of uterine and vaginal secretions. There is progressive dilatation of uterus and vagina with bulging of hymen. There may be swelling and cyanosis of lower extremities and features of compression of bladder and rectum. The condition is managed by incision of hymen and drainage of mucus and secretions. If condition is missed in the neonatal period, spontaneous resolution may occur. When diagnosis is delayed until puberty there is reappearance of hydrometrocalpos following menstruation.

Miscellaneous Conditions

Cleft Lip and Cleft Palate

Bilateral cleft lip is an obvious and disfiguring deformity while isolated cleft palate may be missed, if oral cavity is not inspected. These malformations may occur separately or together (Figure 25.20). In isolated central cleft palate, other anomalies may be associated and it is genetically a distinct entity (Figure 25.21). Orofacial defects and chromosomal anomalies are commonly associated. The baby's profile should be seen to detect micro- or retrognathia in order to exclude Pierre Robin syndrome. Ventricular septal defect may be associated because closure of the ventricular septum occurs at the same time as the fusion of frontonasal processes with the maxillary process. Bilateral cleft of the primary and secondary palates is a consistent feature of trisomy 13–15 (D-trisomy, Patau syndrome).

The parents are often very upset to see the deformed child and need reassurance and alleviation of guilt feelings. Gavage feeding for first few days followed by feeding with a spoon or *paladay* are often satisfactory. The infant should be held with his head raised or upright and feeding given slowly to avoid choking, aspiration and otitis media. Spoon feeding is generally most satisfactory but baby must be offered dummy

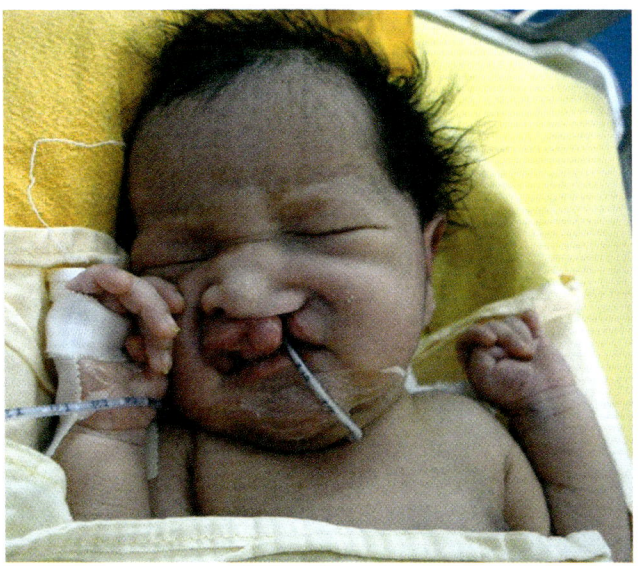

Figure 25.20 Bilateral cleft of the primary and secondary palates.

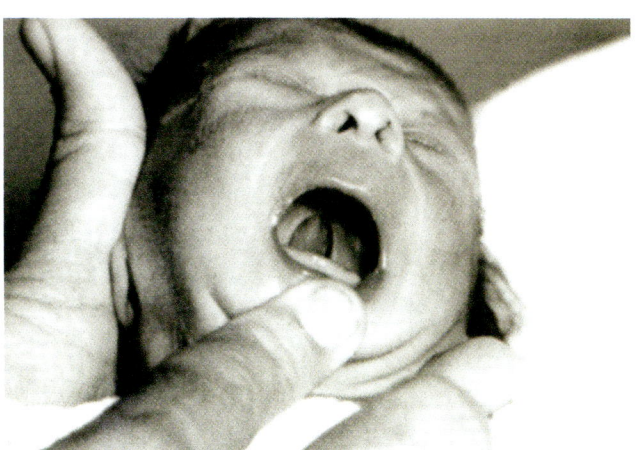

Figure 25.21 Isolated cleft palate. The infant also had ventricular septal defect.

nipple in between the feeds to give him experience of sucking which also improves the muscular control of the tongue and helps the growth of mandible. Palatal plate or obturator may be used to occlude the defect while feeding. Bottle feeding may be done with a long nipple or a flanged teat which can block the defect. Premaxilla, if jutting forward, should be aligned with the alveolar margins by applying graded traction with the help of an elastic belt. It is desirable that cleft lip should be repaired before the baby leaves the hospital as it is of great psychological advantage to the parents. The repair of cleft palate is deferred till the age of about one year. The common complications include recurrent ear infections, lack of clarity of speech and nasal intonation and dental problems, like cleft alveolus leading to displacement, rotation or non-eruption of permanent teeth which may require dental and orthodontic treatment.

EXOMPHALOS (OMPHALOCELE)

The abdominal contents protrude through the umbilicus (Figure 25.22). The opening in the umbilical cord may vary in size from 2 to 15 cm. The gut is covered with peritoneum and amnion and the umbilical cord joins the hernial sac at some point. Occasionally, sac may be ruptured before birth as indicated by dull and thickened covering membranes. Infants with a large omphalocele should be delivered by cesarean section to prevent rupture of the sac. The child should be examined for presence of any other evidences of Beckwith-Wiedemann syndrome, trisomies 13, 18, 21, malrotation of the gut and cardiac, genitourinary and skeletal defects. Large omphaloceles are often associated with respiratory distress due to interference with respiratory mechanics. The baby should be nursed supine and hernial contents lifted off anteriorly with the help of a string to relieve abdominal compression. Stomach should be decompressed by continuous nasogastric suction. All cases should preferably be managed conservatively by application of 1% mercurochrome solution every hour till the exposed area epithelializes. The operation may to be delayed till the age of 2 to 3 months. When sac is ruptured, it should be encased in a bowel bag (Vi-Drape® isolation bag) followed by early surgical repair. Large defects require prosthesis for closure.

GASTROSCHISIS

The abdominal contents herniate out through the abdominal wall lateral to the umbilical cord. The abdominal wall defect is usually less than 5 cm and viscera (usually colon and small intestine) protruding through the defect are not covered by peritoneal sac (Figure 25.23). The intestinal loops appear thickened, opaque and matted and may be associated with atresia or stenosis of the gut in 10% of cases. Unlike exomphalos, these infants do not have any other non-enteric congenital malformations. Nasogastric tube should be inserted for decompression. Cover the exposed intestines with warm saline-soaked gauze and wrap the baby in a dry sterile towel to prevent heat loss. Establish an intravenous line in an upper extremity. Because of absence of sac, the primary closure should be attempted as an emergency procedure within 6 hours of age. These infants require intensive medical management with total parenteral nutrition.

MYELOMENINGOCELE

Prenatal diagnosis can be made by estimation of maternal serum alpha-fetoprotein (AFP) and prenatal ultrasound examination along with determination of amniotic fluid AFP and acetylcholinesterase. There is no difficulty in making the diagnosis at birth and the speculation whether it is myelocele, myelomeningocele

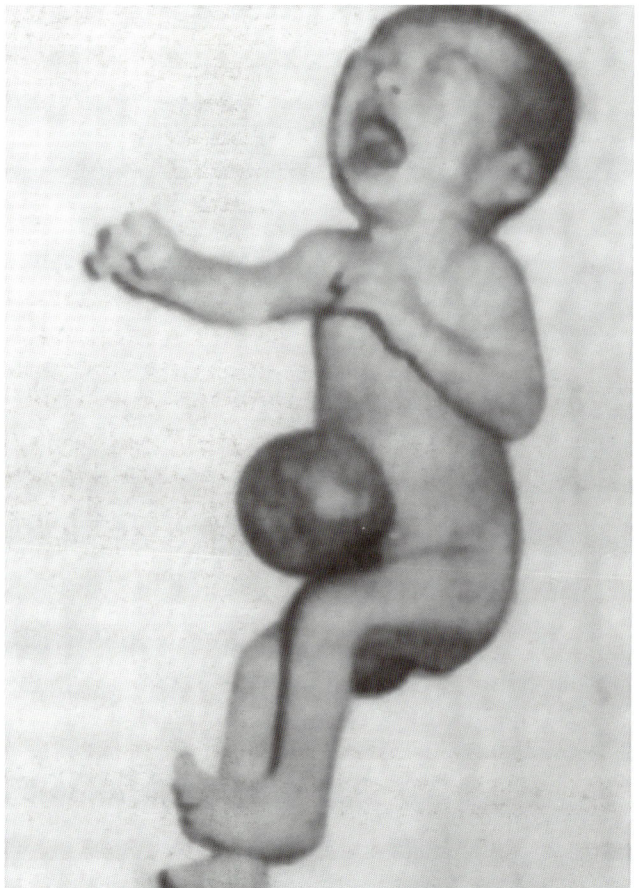

Figure 25.22 Infant with exomphalos. Other evidences of Beckwith-Wiedemann syndrome should be looked for.

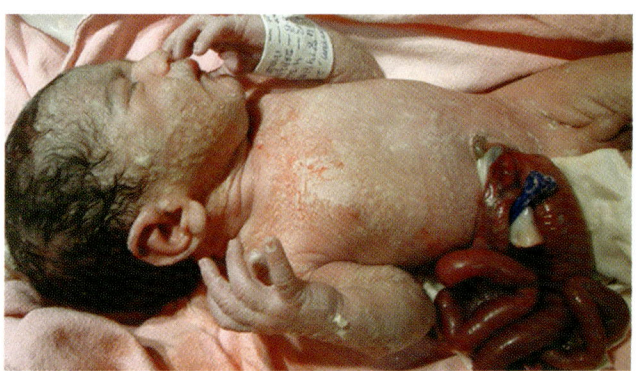

Figure 25.23 Gastroschisis in a newborn baby at birth.

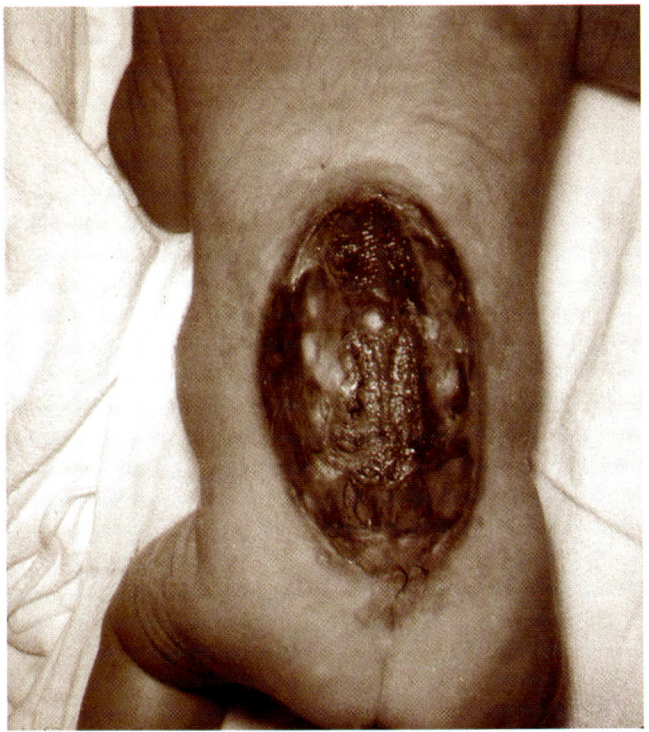

Figure 25.24 Open meningomyelocele.

or meningocele is of doubtful theoretical value (Figure 25.24). Most cases of myelomeningocele show exposed deformed neural tissue surrounded by bluish membranes with oozing of cerebrospinal fluid. It is often associated with Arnold-Chiari malformation and hydrocephalus is either present at birth or appears later. All newborns with neural tube defects should be screened for the presence of congenital heart disease, renal malformations and structural defects of the airways, GI tract, spine, ribs and hips. Lower limbs should be examined for severity of paralysis, deformities of bones and contractures. Spontaneous movements, withdrawal response to painful stimulus, plantar grasp and deep tendon jerks should be elicited. Look for anal reflex, patulous anus and dribbling incontinence, with or without palpable bladder. Neurogenic bladder, vesicoureteral reflux and hydronephrosis may be associated.

The defects which are covered by skin do not need urgent treatment but others should be closed soon after birth because they are likely to get infected. The baby should be nursed prone and the sac should be kept covered with a sterile saline-moistened gauze sponge to prevent infection and fluid loss. Ventriculo-peritoneal shunt procedure for hydrocephalus is required sooner or later (Figure 25.25). Urinary retention should be dealt by periodic compression of bladder and baby followed up for development of any

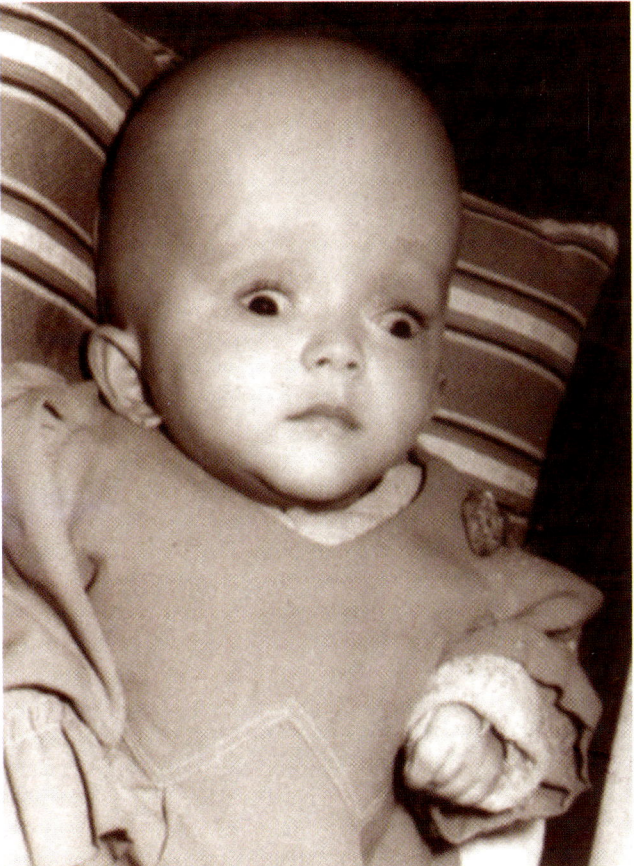

Figure 25.25 Hydrocephalus in an infant who was operated for meningocele during neonatal period.

urinary infection. The treatment demands a close team work between the surgeon, pediatric neurologist, physiotherapist and social worker. The radical treatment is contraindicated, if it is associated with severe paralysis of lower limbs, extensive kyphosis, severe hydrocephalus, and if other major anomalies are present. The exact cause is unknown. The recognized high-risk factors include male gender, primiparous mother, maternal smoking, excessive intake of alcohol and coffee. There is evidence to suggest that *in utero* closure of myelomeningocele may reduce the risk of Arnold-Chiari malformation and improve the neuromotor outcome. The neural tube defects can be prevented by periconceptional supplementation with folic acid.

TALIPS EQUINOVARUS (CLUBFOOT)

This abnormality is probably related to *in-utero* posture because it is more common in first born infants and pregnancies associated with oligohydramnios. The incidence of anomaly varies between 0.5 and 8 per 1000 live births. It is characterized by plantar flexion

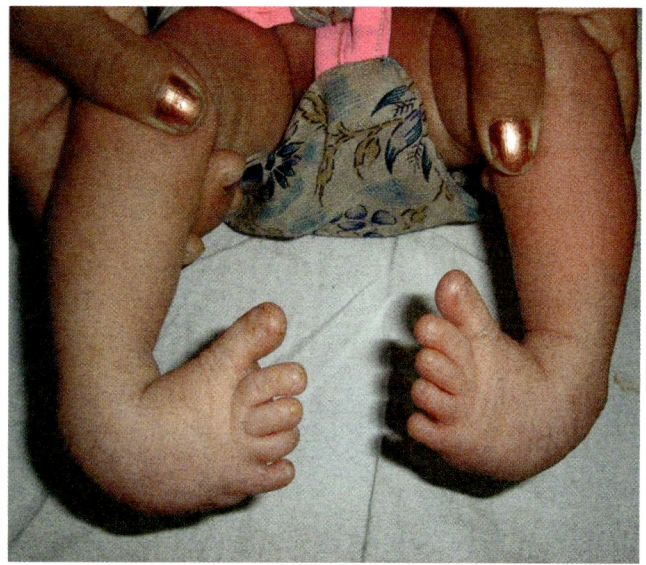

Figure 25.26 Bilateral clubfeet.

(equinus) and inversion (varus) of the ankle and adduction of forefoot (Figure 25.26). The term "clubfoot" refers to the way the foot is positioned at a sharp angle to the ankle, like the head of a golf club. The dorsiflexion of the foot is limited and unlike normal babies the dorsum of the foot cannot be made to touch the front of the shin. Skin may be puckered or grooved on the medial side of the foot. In bilateral cases, spine should be examined for meningocele and any tuft of hair to suggest dermoid or diastematomyelia. All the joints should be examined to exclude arthrogryposis multiplex. In mild cases, manipulations (eversion and dorsiflexion) alone are enough to correct the anomaly. In established or ankylosed cases, immediate advice of orthopedic surgeon should be sought for early manipulations and plaster applications. The corrective casts should be applied as soon after the birth as possible.

Treatment

The parents should be prepared for a long period of treatment and reassured that foot would become entirely normal and the child would be able to walk and dance without any difficulty. The Ponseti method of treatment has become standard of care. The treatment should be started after 5–7 days of age. All the deformities are corrected simultaneously by application of long-leg cast with knee(s) kept flexed at 90°. The plaster of paris or fiberglass cast is changed weekly for a total of 5–6 castings. Associated developmental dysplasia of hips (DDH) should be excluded by clinical examination and sonography and should be simultaneously managed. After completion of casting protocol, braces are used to maintain the correction and prevent the relapse of club feet. After completion of Ponseti protocol and manipulations, the residual equinus is corrected by percutaneous Achilles tenotomy (PAT). After the surgical procedure, the long leg cast is applied and left in place for 3 weeks.

CALCANEOVALGUS DEFORMITY

The deformity of foot is like a mirror image of club foot and occurs due to *in utero* cramped up position. The ankle is dorsiflexed and foot is abducted, everted or pronated. The dorsum of the foot is maintained close to the shin. Most cases can be managed by physiotherapy by passive plantar flexion and inversion of foot. When foot cannot be plantar flexed to neutral position and there is fixed or rigid calcaneovalgus deformity, the condition is managed by graded application of plaster casts over 6–8 weeks as in the case of club feet.

GENU RECURVATUM

It is a benign disorder characterized by hyperextension of the knees due to laxity of ligaments or abnormal *in utero* positioning. The condition is usually bilateral. Skiagram of the knees should be taken to exclude subluxation. In dislocation of knees, the tibia is shifted anteriorly and laterally in relation to the femur. Congenital fibrosis of the quadriceps is frequently associated with the subluxation and dislocation of knees. Genu recurvatum is treated by passive streching exercises and repeated cast changes to provide stability to the knee joints. The subluxated and dislocated knee is best managed by open reduction because stretching exercises and cast changes may result in damage to the epiphyseal plate.

CONGENITAL DISLOCATION OF HIPS (CDH)

The condition is now called "developmental" dysplasia of the hip (DDH) which denotes a spectrum of hip abnormalities (immature hip, mild acetabular dysplasia, dislocatable hip and subluxated hip), which may progress to frank dislocation. The incidence of DDH varies from 10 to 35 per 1,000 live born infants. Most cases of DDH are unilateral with left hip being more commonly affected. The dislocation is bilateral in about 20% of cases. The exact etiology is unknown. The condition is more common among first born, postterm or large infants and female babies delivered following breech presentation. The prolonged gestation is associated with increase in the maternal hormones which may account for the laxity of the hip joint. Other risk factors include oligohydramnios, congenital torticollis, club feet and metatarsus adductus. The increased frequency of hip abnormalities in the family members of the affected children is suggestive of genetic predisposition of CDH. Genetic studies on DDH families have identified key genes (GDF5, IL6, TGF-B1, PAPPA2, ASPN, TBX4) which may play a role in DDH.

The routine examination of hips of all infants by Ortolani-Barlow maneuver is essential for early diagnosis (refer to Chapter 7). The click may not be audible in the newborn baby but the middle finger on the greater trochanter can be guided to feel the entry of the femoral head into the acetabulum. The limitation of abduction is not generally seen during the neonatal period because it occurs due to shortening of adductors in infants with relatively long-standing dislocation. The femoral pulse may not be readily felt on the affected side. At times asymmetry of skin creases over buttocks or labia and shortening of leg may offer clue to the diagnosis. The X-rays should be taken with both hips extended and legs held in 45° abduction and full internal rotation. The femoral head is displaced upwards and laterally on the affected side (Figure 25.27). On the normal side, the upward projection of longitudinal axis of femur crosses the spine at the lumbosacral junction. If the hip is dislocated, a similar projection of the long axis of the femur passes above the bony edge of acetabulum and crosses the lumbar spine at a higher level. The conventional skiagrams of hips may not show any abnormalities. Ultrasound examination of hip joints provides diagnostic information after one month of age. There is high incidence of false-positive reports during newborn period. Dynamic assessment of stability of the hip on real-time multiplanar ultrasonography with a 7 MHz linear transducer is useful for the diagnosis of DDH. After 6 months of age, radiography is useful for diagnosis of DDH.

Treatment

The key to successful treatment is early diagnosis and commencing treatment before 6 weeks of age. A number of devices are available to maintain the legs in abduction and external rotation. Pavlik harness is a dynamic splint that maintains the hip in flexion and abduction (frog position). The success rates with Pavlik harness varies between 80 and 96.7% with avascular necrosis (AVN) risk of 0–28%. Von Rosen splint has virtually replaced Pavlik harness (Figure 22.28). It is associated with a success rate of 99% and risk of AVN merely 0.6%. The recovery is generally complete in a period of about 3–4 months.

In teratologic type of CDH, femoral head does not relocate into acetabulum on flexion and abduction and Ortolani sign is absent. In unilateral cases, there is shortening of leg and asymmetry of the gluteal folds. These infants are best treated by loop traction, adductor tenotomy, open reduction, use of modified Denis Browne bar or splint followed by physiotherapy.

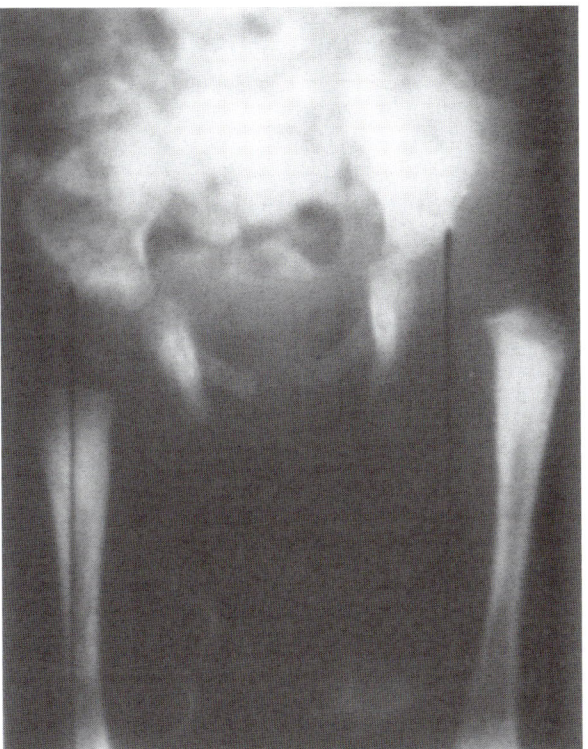

Figure 25.27 Congenital dislocation of hip on left side. The femoral head is displaced upwards and laterally.

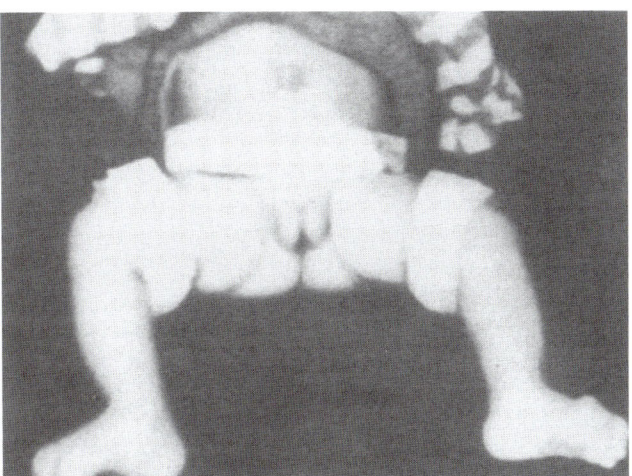

Figure 25.28 Infant restrained with indigenously fabricated von Rosen splint to maintain both hips in abduction and rotation.

Achildi O, Grewal H. Congenital anomalies of the esophagus. *Otolaryngol Clin North Am* 2007, 40: 219–244.

Adzick NS, Nance ML. Medical Progress : Pediatric surgery (second of two parts). *N Engl J Med* 2000, 342: 1726.

Agarwala S, Mitra DK. Timing of surgery for common pediatric surgical conditions. *Indian J Pediatr* 1996, 63: 769–774.

American Academy of Pediatrics. Committee on Genetics : Evaluation of the newborn with developmental anomalies of the external genitalia. *Pediatrics* 2000, 106: 138.

American Academy of Pediatrics. Committee on Bioethics. Fetal therapy: Ethical considerations. *Pediatrics* 1999, 103: 1061.

Barlow TG. Early diagnosis and treatment of congenital dislocation of the hip. *J Bone Joint Surg.* 1962, 44:292–301.

Barry JE, Auldist AW. The VATER association—one end of spectrum of anomalies. *Amer J Dis Child* 1974, 128: 769.

Bhatnagar SN, Sarin YK. Management of congenital diaphragmatic hernia in newborn: Paradigm shift and ethical issues. *Indian J Pediatr* 2017, 84(8):629–35.

Boles ET. Imperforate anus. Symposium on neonatal surgery. *Clin Perinatol* 1979, 6: 149–161.

Cyvin KB. Congenital dislocation of the hip joint. *Acta Paediatr Scand* 1978, Supplement, 263.

Dennison WM. The Pierre Robin syndrome. *Pediatrics* 1965, 36: 366.

Dillon PW, Cilley RE. Newborn surgical emergencies. *Pediatr Cl N Amer* 1993, 40: 1289.

Godbole P, Stringer MD. Bilious vomiting in the newborn: how often is it pathologic? *J Pediatr Surg* 2002, 6: 909–911.

Gupta DK, Sharma S, Azizkhan RG (Eds). Pediatric Surgery: Diagnosis and Management volume I and II *Jaypee Bros Medical Publishers, New Delhi* , 2009.

Hammerman C, Kaplan M. Germ warfare: Probiotics in defence of the premature gut. *Clin Perinatol* 2004, 31: 489–500.

Howat JM, Wilkinson AW. Functional intestinal obstruction in the neonate. *Arch Dis Child* 1970, 45: 800.

Hughes IA, Hauk C, Ahmad SF, *et al.* LWPES Concensus Group: Concensus statement on management of intersex disorders. *Arch Dis Child* 2006, 91: 554–563.

Jani JC, Nikolaides KH. Fetal surgery for severe congenital diaphragmatic hernia. *Ultrasound Obstet Gynecol* 2012, 39:7–9.

Jobe AH. Fetal surgery for myelomeningocele. *N Engl J Med* 2002, 347: 4–6.

Kasivajjula H, Maheshwari A. Pathophysiology and current management of necrotizing enterocolitis. *Indian J Pediatr* 2014, 81(5): 489–497.

Kastenberg ZJ, Sylvester KG. The surgical management of necrotizing enterocolitis. *Clin Perinatol* 2013, 40: 135–148.

Keckler SJ, Peter SD, Valusek PA, *et al.* VACTERL anomalies in patients with esophageal atresia: An updated delineation of the spectrum and review of the literature. *Pediatr Surg Int* 2007, 4: 309–313.

Kliegman RM, Fanaroff AA. Necrotizing enterocolitis. *N Eng J Med* 1984, 310: 1092.

Kosloske AM. Surgery of necrotizing enterocolitis. *World J Surg* 1985, 9: 277.

Kunisaki SM, Barnewolt CE, *et al.* Ex-utero intrapartum treatment with extracorporeal membrane oxygenation for severe congenital diaphragmatic hernia. *J Pediatr Surg* 2007, 42:98–104.

Kureel SN, Malik GK. Anorectal malformations: Practical tips. *J Neonatol* 2007, 21: 233–237.

Lin T, Pimpalwar A. Minimally invasive surgery in neonates and infants. *J Indian Assoc Pediatr Surg* 2010,15(1):2–8.

Liu Y, Zhao D, Zhao L, Li H, Yang X. Congenital club foot: Early recognition and conservative management for preventing late disabilities. *Indian J Pediatr* 2016, 83(11):1266–74.

Lorber J. Spina bifida cystica—Results of treatment of 270 consecutive cases with criteria for selection for the future. *Arch Dis Child* 1972, 47: 854.

Louie JP. Essential diagnosis of abdominal emergencies in the first year of life. *Emerg Med Clin N Am* 2007, 25: 1009–1040.

Moss R, Dimmitt RA, Barnhart DC, *et al.* Laparotomy versus peritoneal drainage for necrotizing enterocolitis and perforation. *N Engl J Med* 2006, 354: 2225–2234.

Narasimharao KL, Prasad GR, Katariya S. Prone cross table lateral view: An alternative to invertogram in imperforate anus. *Am J Roentgenol* 1983, 140: 227–229.

Neu J, Walkar WA. Necrotizing enterocolitis. *N Engl J Med* 2011, 364: 255–264.

Pena A. Surgical correction of high imperforate anus. *World J Surg* 1985, 9: 236.

Richardon WR. Surgical emergencies on the day of birth. *Amer J Dis Child* 1961, 102: 164.

Ross AJ. Intestinal obstruction in the newborn. *Pediatr Rev* 1994, 15: 338.

Shabtai L, Specht SC, Herzenberg JE. Worldwide spread of the Ponseti method for club foot. *World J Orthop* 2014, 5:585–90.

Schnitzer JJ, Donahoe PK. Surgical treatment of congenital adrenal hyperplasia. *Endocrinol Metab Clin North Am* 2001, 30: 137.

Sillen U, Hagherg S, Rubenson A, *et al.* Management of esophageal atresia : Review of 16 year's experience. *J Pediatr Surg* 1988, 23: 805.

Talbert JL, Felman AG, De Busk FL. Gastrointestinal surgical emergencies in the newborn infant. *J Pediatr* 1970, 76: 783.

Tomlinson J, O'Dowd D, Fernandes JA. Managing developmental dysplasia of the hip. *Indian J Pediatr* 2016, 83(11):1275–79.

Touloukian RJ. Neonatal necrotizing enterocolitis. *Surg Clin North Am* 1976, 56: 281.

Ugwu RO, Okoro PE. Pattern, outcome and challenges of neonatal surgical cases in a tertiary teaching hospital. *Afr J Paediatr Surg* 2013, 10(3):226–30.

Walker GM, Neilson A, Young D, Raine PAM. Color of bile vomiting in intestinal obstruction in the newborn: Questionnaire study. *Brit Med J* 2006, 332: 1363–1365.

Walsh MC, Kliegman RM. Necrotizing enterocolitis: Treatment based on staging criteria. *Pediatr Clin N Amer* 1986, 1:179–202.

Wilkinson AW. Congenital anomalies of anus and rectum. *Arch Dis Child* 1972, 47: 960.

Yazheck S, Ndaye M, Kalin AH. Omphalocele: A 25-year experience. *J Pediatr Surg* 1986, 21: 761.

Miscellaneous Conditions

BIRTH INJURIES

Birth injuries include avoidable and unavoidable trauma sustained by the infant during the process of birth. The injury may occur antenatally, intrapartum or during resuscitation. The incidence of birth injuries in a particular country or a center reflects the standard of obstetrical services in that place. The common risk factors for birth injuries include primiparity, osteomalacia or short stature of mother, cephalopelvic disproportion, prolonged or precipitate labor, abnormal malpresentation, versions, torques, tractions, instrumental delivery and vacuum extraction. Low birth weight or preterm babies and large-for-dates or overgrown babies and infants with congenital anomalies are at an increased risk to develop birth injuries. Over the years, obstetrical vigilance and early resort to cesarean section has considerably reduced the incidence of serious mechanical birth injuries though the reduction in perinatal hypoxic brain damage has not been generally impressive.

Superficial Abrasions

These occur over the sites of forceps or vacuum application. Accidental incision of the baby may occur during cesarean section. The gaping incised wound may require stitching and should be protected from infection by local application of 1.0% aqueous solution of mercurochrome.

Petechiae and Bruising

Following prolonged delivery, the presenting part of the baby may show cyanotic bluish tinge, petechiae and bruises (traumatic cyanosis). The infant looks rather mauled and deceptively ill. Spontaneous recovery occurs within 2 to 3 days. Subconjunctival hemorrhages are commonly seen in healthy babies and they disappear spontaneously.

Cephalhematoma

Subperiosteal collection of blood may occur following normal or complicated delivery due to rupture of superficial veins between the skull and periosteum. Predisposing factors for this are uncertain. A cystic or fluctuant swelling limited by suture lines appears after a few hours of birth and at times on the second day. The edges of the swelling may give a false impression of depressed skull fracture due to organized rim of cephalhematoma. The overlying scalp may show discoloration.

The swelling may appear at any site but unilateral parietal cephalhematomas are most common (Figure 26.1). The condition should be differentiated from caput succedaneum which is characterized by diffuse edematous non-fluctuant swelling of soft tissues on the presenting part of the scalp. It is present

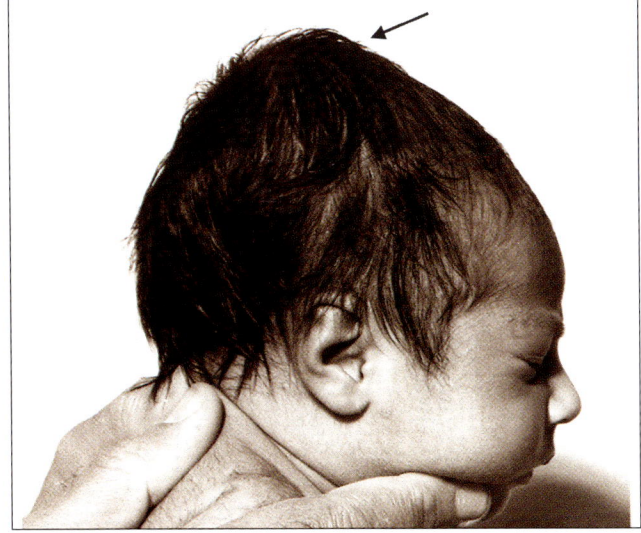

Figure 26.1 Arrow points to cephalhematoma over parietal region in an infant born following spontaneous vaginal delivery.

at birth and often disappears within 24 hours and is not limited by suture lines. Cranial meningocele or encephalocele is located in midline over the occipital region and can be differentiated from cephalhematoma by positive crying impulse and associated bone defect. At times, massive subaponeurotic collection of blood under the scalp may be seen in babies born by vacuum extraction (subgaleal hematoma). In view of its location over the surface of periosteum, it is not limited by suture lines. Hematoma may extend to involve entire calvarium leading to periorbital and auricular edema and ecchymoses. The blood collection may be massive causing hypovolemia or shock and hyperbilirubinemia.

Most cephalhematomas spontaneously disappear after a variable period of few days or weeks depending upon their size. Vitamin K 1–2 mg intramuscularly should be given to correct any coexistent coagulation defect, especially in cases of subaponeurotic collection of blood. In a case of subgaleal hematoma, a pressure dressing of scalp is useful to prevent further bleeding. The incision and drainage is indicated only when cephalhematoma gets infected or if it is contributing to critical hyperbilirubinemia. Phototherapy may be required for treatment of hyperbilirubinemia. Hemoglobin should be checked to assess need for blood transfusion.

Fractures

Skull

Ability of the skull to mold during the delivery protects it from injury during normal uncomplicated labor. Linear skull fractures may be associated in one-fourth of infants with cephalhematoma and are of no therapeutic significance. The depressed fractures may occur due to compression as a result of forceps or against the maternal symphysis pubis and sacral promontory. These also disappear spontaneously but at times surgical elevation may be required, if there are associated neurological manifestations.

Clavicle

Fracture of calvicle is the most common and often follows breech extraction or shoulder impaction. The fracture of clavicle may occur following uncomplicated vaginal delivery. The reported incidence of fractured calvicle varies between 0.2 and 3.5%. The baby cries due to pain when handled. Most newborn infants with fracture of clavicle have no or minimal physical findings. A greenstick fracture may be asymptomatic at birth and picked up by callus formation at 7 to 10 days of age. The movements of affected limb may be limited and Moro reflex may by asymmetric. The crepitus may be elicited at the site of fracture and supraclavicular depression on the affected side is often obliterated. The associated fracture of the humerus and Erb's palsy should be looked for and excluded. The prognosis is excellent and callus may form within one week. Immobilization of the arm on the affected side can be achieved by pinning the infant's sleeve to the shirt or by wrapping the limb. Paracetamol (10–15 mg/kg/dose) is a safe analgesic for use in newborn babies.

Humerus

The forcible manipulations and pulling at baby's arm during delivery may result in fracture of the humerus which is commonest at the junction between upper one-third and the lower two-thirds of humerus. The diagnosis is suspected by pain and limitation of movements of the affected limb, asymmetric Moro response and crepitus at the site of fracture. The strapping of the arm by the side of chest for two weeks is recommended for immobilization. The prognosis is excellent unless the epiphysis is damaged, in which case the limb may be permanently shortened.

Femur

Fracture of femur is rare and caused by forcible manipulation of legs during breech extraction. Spontaneous healing with excess callus formation occurs without any splintage. However, better results are obtained by overhead traction–suspension of both lower extremities, even if the fracture is unilateral and application of a spica cast for 4 weeks. In infants with more than one fracture, osteogenesis imperfecta should be ruled out (Figure 26.2).

Birth Trauma to Central Nervous System

For intracranial birth trauma and perinatal hypoxia, spinal cord transection and injuries to peripheral nerves, refer to Chapter 22.

Visceral Trauma

Capsular laceration of liver and spleen and adrenal hemorrhage may follow difficult breech extraction. The damage may also occur due to over-zealous attempts at external cardiac massage. The hemorrhage may remain concealed as subcapsular hematoma or capsule may rupture with blood flowing into the peritoneal cavity. The baby may manifest severe pallor, tachycardia and evidences of shock. The presence of and flexing the neck towards unaffected side. The majority of these tumors resolve spontaneously by six months to one year of age. If torticollis persists beyond one year, surgical correction may be undertaken.

CYANOSIS

The delivery of oxygen to the tissues depends on the fraction of inspired oxygen concentration (FiO_2), lung ventilation, cardiac output, hemoglobin concentration and dissociation of oxygen from hemoglobin to the tissues. Peripheral cyanosis is seen in majority of normal babies at birth and subsequently whenever they are given a bath or exposed to cold. Traumatic cyanosis and petechiae may appear on the presenting part following difficult delivery and is again benign in nature.

Oxygen Dissociation Curve

Most of the oxygen in blood is bound to hemoglobin (one gram of hemoglobin can maximally bind 1.34 mL of oxygen). The oxygen dissociation curve of the fetal blood is shifted to the left due to lower content of 2, 3-diphosphoglycerate in the fetal hemoglobin. It readily binds oxygen at lower arterial oxygen tensions to achieve higher oxygen saturation. However, at any partial pressure (PaO_2), less oxygen is released to the tissues. Due to the shift of the oxygen dissociation curve, clinical recognition of hypoxia is delayed because cyanosis appears at a relatively lower oxygen tension in newborn infants.

Classification

Based on the severity of hypoxia and nature of the underlying cardiac defect, cyanosis is classified as peripheral cyanosis or acrocyanosis, central cyanosis and differential cyanosis. Acrocyanosis is limited to the extremities and lips and occurs due to local vasoconstriction, and sluggish circulation due to cold stress. There are no abnormalities in arterial oxygen tension (PaO_2) and saturation (SpO_2). It is benign condition but at times it may be an early correlate of serious disorders like sepsis, hypoglycemia or low cardiac output. Central cyanosis is characterized by uniform discoloration of skin and mucosal surfaces. When cyanosis is more pronounced in the lower limb than the upper limb, it is called differential cyanosis. It may not be clinically obvious and is best diagnosed by preductal (right arm) and postductal (any lower extremity) SpO_2 difference >10–20% and PaO_2 difference of >15 mm Hg on simultaneously drawn samples of blood is suggestive of right-to-left shunt

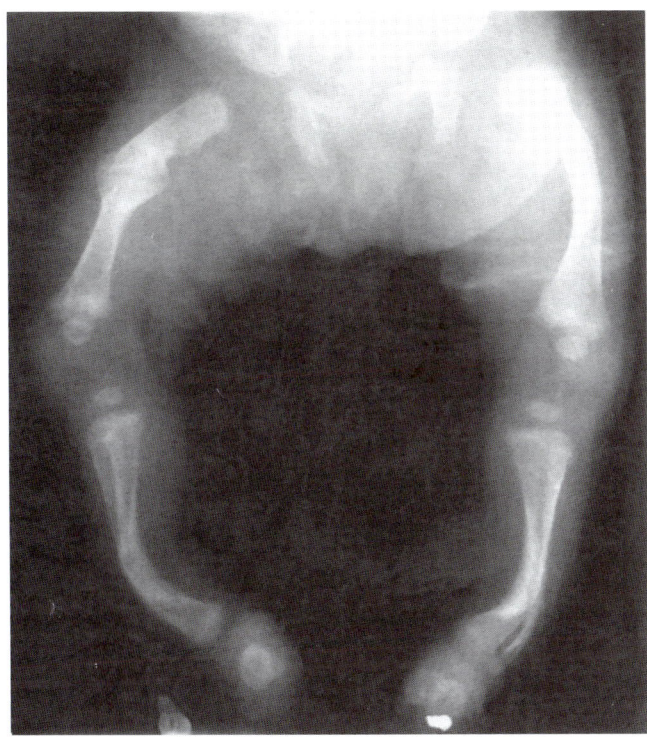

Figure 26.2 Multiple fractures with callus formation in a neonate with osteogenesis imperfecta.

shifting dullness may suggest the existence of blood in the peritoneal cavity which can be aspirated for diagnostic purposes. Enlargement of liver in association with clinical evidence of blood loss should alert the physician to the possibility of subcapsular hematoma. Abdominal ultrasonography is useful to confirm the diagnosis. Hyperbilirubinemia may occur as in other cases of internal hemorrhage in the tissues and body organs. Early recognition and administration of vitamin K and blood transfusion with monitoring of central venous or arterial pressure may salvage some of these babies. Surgical laparotomy is usually required to seal the bleeding site in the liver or spleen. Adrenal hemorrhage is rarely diagnosed in life but when detected at autopsy it is impossible to say whether it was the result of direct trauma, anoxia or endotoxin shock.

Sternomastoid 'Tumor'

During the second week of life, a firm mass 1–2 cm in diameter may be noted in the midportion of the sternomastoid muscle. It is believed to be either a small hematoma from injury to the muscle at birth or due to fibromatous malformation of the muscle. The attention to the condition is often directed by the presence of torticollis on the affected side. The mother should be advised to overextend the affected muscle by turning the infant's head in the opposite direction at ductal level. It occurs because of reversal of blood flow across patent ductus arteriosus (PDA) because of persistent pulmonary hypertension of newborn (PPHN), coarctation of aorta (CoA) or interrupted aortic arch (IAA). In the absence of PPHN, differential cyanosis is virtually diagnostic of cyanotic CHD. When PPHN or CoA are associated with transposition of great arteries (TGA), lower limbs are less cyanosed than the upper limbs (reverse differential cyanosis).

Causes

The causes of cyanosis can be remembered by an acronym ABCDE (Table 26.1). Respiratory and cardiac conditions are leading causes of hypoxia and cyanosis.

Clinical Signs of Hypoxia

Cyanosis The development of cyanosis depends upon concentration and character of hemoglobin, arterial oxygen saturation or tension, and cutaneous perfusion. Cyanosis occurs when more than 3 g/dL of reduced or desaturated hemoglobin is present in the capillaries. It generally manifests as circumoral bluish-gray discoloration and appears when arterial oxygen tension (PaO_2) or partial pressure of oxygen in arterial blood falls below 40 mm Hg or when oxygen saturation of the arterial blood (SpO_2) is less than 85%. Polycythemic babies may manifest cyanosis more readily while onset of cyanosis is delayed in babies with anemia. In very small preterm babies, even with low arterial oxygen tension, their skin may be pink due to direct diffusion of ambient oxygen through the thin skin. At times, clinical differentiation between peripheral and central cyanosis may be difficult. During capillary blood sampling, if in a cyanosed baby, pink blood flows out from a prewarmed heel, it favors the possibility of peripheral cyanosis.

Heart rate A fixed heart rate of 120 per minute or bradycardia is commonly seen in hypoxic babies.

Activity Instead of restlessness which is characteristic of suffocation, the newborn hypoxic baby becomes lethargic and unresponsive.

Hypothermia Lack of oxygen would impair metabolism of brown fat, thus resulting in fall of baby's core temperature. The skin temperature over the sites of brown fat would be the first to drop.

Acidosis Hypoxia leads to anaerobic tissue metabolism resulting in metabolic acidosis. Rapid breathing may be a manifestation of underlying cardiopulmonary disorder causing hypoxia or may occur as a compensatory phenomenon.

Indications for Oxygen Therapy

1. Birth asphyxia
2. Hypoxemia (SpO_2 <85% or PaO_2 <50 mm Hg) in room air
3. Cyanosis (exclude congenital cyanotic heart disease without cardiac failure and methemoglobinemia)
4. Respiratory distress due to hyaline membrane disease, pneumonia, cardiac failure and congenital malformations. Oxygen therapy is indicated, if respiratory distress is worsening or if any of the above clinical features of hypoxia are evident or if arterial oxygen tension is less than 40 mm Hg or arterial oxygen saturation is less than 85%.
5. Hypothermia
6. Recurrent apneic attacks
7. Pneumothorax or pneumomediastinum. Inhalation of 100% oxygen would facilitate earlier resorption of air but drainage of air is life-saving in a case of tension pneumothorax.

TABLE 26.1 Causes of cyanosis in neonates	
A. Airway	Choanal atresia, micrognathia, Pierre Robin sequence, laryngomalacia, vocal cord palsy, tracheal stenosis, vascular ring, cystic hygroma or other neck masses.
B. Breathing	*Parenchymal disorders*: Hyaline membrane disease, aspiration, pneumonia, pulmonary hemorrhage, lymphangiectasia, pulmonary edema.
	Non-parenchymal disorders: Pneumothorax, pleural effusion, congenital diaphragmatic hernia, congenital cystic adenomatoid malformation, congenital lobar emphysema, diaphragmatic palsy.
C. Circulation	Persistent pulmonary hypertension of the newborn, pulmonary arteriovenous fistula, cyanotic congenital heart diseases, low cardiac output states.
D. Defective hemoglobin	Methemoglobinemia, sulfhemoglobinemia, hemoglobin M.
E. Eclectic (etcetera or etc.)	Sepsis, hypoglycemia, polycythemia, CNS depression, apnea of prematurity.

Sources of Oxygen

Oxygen supply systems include compressed gas cylinders (1800–2400 psi), centralized pipe gas supply (around 50 psi) and oxygen concentrators. Compressed gas cylinders provide a high-pressure supply of 100% medical grade oxygen which is allowed to flow through a down regulating valve before being delivered through a flow-meter gauge. Gas cylinders are used in small hospitals and provide back-up facility in case of failure of the central supply. Oxygen concentrator is an electrical device with a molecular "sieve" to extract oxygen from the air by filtering out nitrogen, water vapors and other trace gases. The polymeric membrane concentrators can deliver 50 to 90% oxygen at a flow rate up to 10 L/min. Portable oxygen concentrators can be plugged into a vehicle DC adapter and they can run both on the mains as well as battery power.

Modes of Oxygen Administration

Breathing infant Ambient oxygen concentration should be raised to 40% or more depending upon the need. The aim is either relief of cyanosis or maintenance of arterial PO_2 between 50 and 80 mm Hg. The baby's head should be enclosed in a perspex box (Figure 26.3) and oxygen is allowed to flow inside the box rather than the incubator to reduce wastage and achieve better ambient oxygen concentration around the face. A gas flow of 2–3 L/kg/min is necessary to avoid accumulation of carbon dioxide in the box. In deeply cyanosed babies, 100% oxygen can be administered through a tightly fitting oronasal mask for a period of 10 to 15 minutes. Oxygen can also be

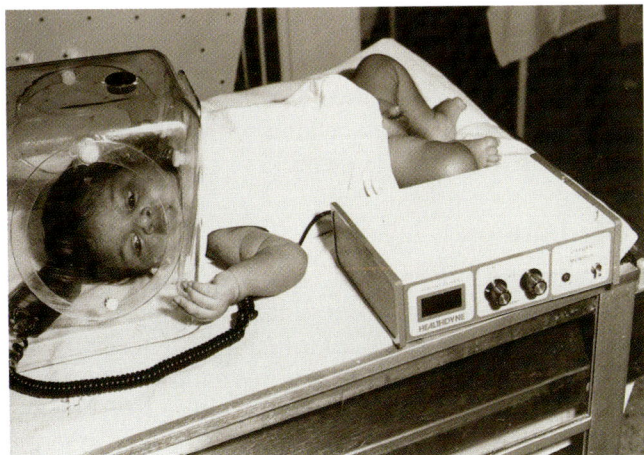

Figure 26.3 Oxygen head box. It is useful to achieve high ambient oxygen concentration around the face and minimize the wastage of oxygen. The concentration of oxygen in the box should be periodically checked with an oxygen analyzer.

administered through a nasal catheter or twin-holed nasal prongs affixed infront of nostrils by using low oxygen flow rate (<1.0 L/min). In infants with ventilation-perfusion abnormalities, oxygen can be administered through a continuous positive airway pressure (CPAP) system to ensure effective delivery of oxygen to the alveoli even during expiration. However, uncontrolled CPAP should not be provided by using high flows of oxygen through nasal cannulas.

Non-breathing infant or 'tiring' infant due to severe respiratory distress syndrome. In babies with apneic attacks, intermittent positive pressure respiration with a bag and mask is enough unless the episodes are very frequent or prolonged. When prolonged ventilation is anticipated, nasal or oral endotracheal tube should be inserted and baby attached to a ventilator. Oxygen should be administered through heated humidifiers whenever oxygen delivery system bypasses the nose and upper airways or when high flow rates (>1.0 L/min) are used.

What Parameters should be Monitored during Oxygen Therapy?

Oxygen is one of the most commonly administered drugs in the neonatal intensive care unit. It is life-saving when used as per recommended guidelines but can cause disabling adverse effects when used without proper monitoring. The various parameters to ensure safe administration of oxygen, like ambient oxygen concentration (FiO_2), arterial oxygen saturation (SpO_2 or SaO_2), arterial oxygen tension (PaO_2), duration of oxygen therapy and fundus examination should be documented in the case records.

Both hypoxia and hyperoxia are dangerous in newborn babies. There are no known clinical signs of hyperoxemia but high concentrations of arterial oxygen tension may cause retinopathy of prematurity. Table 26.2 provides target oxygen saturation guidelines to prevent

TABLE 26.2 Recommended target oxygen saturation guidelines

Gestational age	SpO₂ (percent)	PaO₂ (mm Hg)
<32 weeks	88–92	50–70
32–36 weeks	90–95	60–80
≥37 weeks	90–98	60–90

SpO_2: Arterial oxygen saturation is assessed with a hand-transcribed or handheld pulse oximeter.

PaO_2: Arterial oxygen tension

In general, SpO_2 should be maintained between 85 and 95% to prevent hypoxia and hyperoxia. The goal of oxygen therapy is to achieve adequate delivery of oxygen to the tissues without causing any oxygen toxicity.

Miscellaneous Conditions

26

hypoxia and hyperoxia in neonates of different gestational maturity.

Ambient oxygen concentration Air–oxygen blender, which mechanically blends pressurized oxygen and air, is ideal to deliver appropriate concentrations of FiO_2. Stand alone dedicated blenders are not frequently used in our country except as integral component of ventilators and CPAP systems. When a blender is not available, a venturi device can be used. The oxygen is forced through an adjustable jet orifice of the venturi which causes entrainment of room air to provide different concentrations of oxygen shown as graded markings of FiO_2 on the venturi device. The control of ambient oxygen concentration has two pitfalls. The maintenance of ambient oxygen at a concentration of less than 40% may be insufficient to prevent brain damage or at times may lead to retinopathy of prematurity. Therefore, a critical balance between the possible damage due to hypoxia versus damage due to oxygen toxicity should be maintained. The ambient oxygen concentration should be maintained 5 to 10% higher than the cyanotic threshold of the infant. During recovery, the concentration of ambient oxygen should be reduced by 10% every hour to wean off the infant.

Oxygen analyzer is a useful device to assess the concentration of ambient oxygen in the head box. It should be periodically calibrated with room air which has FiO_2 of 21% or 0.21. When oxygen analyzer is not available, rough estimate of oxygen concentration in the oxihood can be made by closing the side holes of the box. When oxygen at 5 liters/minute is allowed to flow through the oxihood, it provides ambient oxygen concentration of 30% (FiO_2 0.3) when both the holes are kept open. When one hole in the box is closed, FiO_2 approximates 60% but when both the holes are occluded, the ambient concentration of oxygen reaches around 90%.

Arterial oxygen tension The arterial PO_2 should be maintained between 50 and 80 mm Hg although preductal arterial oxygen tension of even up to 160 mm Hg is safe for the retina. The above recommendation (PaO_2 of 50–80 mm Hg) is made keeping in mind that the opening up of right-to-left shunts during hypoxemia lowers the oxygen tension of abdominal aorta, while the preductal blood coursing through the carotids may have much higher PaO_2. It would appear that for this reason temporal, brachial and radial arteries are better sampling sites though technically more difficult. If infant is receiving more than 40% oxygen, it is desirable to monitor arterial oxygen tension every 4-hourly.

Tanscutaneous oxygen tension A non-invasive transcutaneous PO_2 electrode is available for continuous monitoring of oxygen tension. The transcutaneous PO_2 values are comparable to simultaneously monitored PaO_2 values. In a healthy newborn, $tcPO_2$ is about 10% higher than the corresponding PaO_2 due to local hyperthermia induced by the transcutaneous sensor. The transcutaneous arterial oxygen tension, however, may be unreliable in a baby with severe hypothermia and shock because local vasodilation beneath the sensor cannot be effectively achieved.

Arterial oxygen saturation Availability of pulse oximetry has simplified the assessment of oxygen status by monitoring hemoglobin oxygen saturation (SpO_2 or SaO_2). Unlike transcutaneous oxygen monitors, pulse oximeters are convenient to use because they do not require any preparation of skin or the sensor and there is no hazard of skin burns at the site of sensor. The accuracy of both $tcPO_2$ monitor and pulse oximeter is perfusion dependent, while using pulse oximeter, there should be an agreement between infant's heart rate as displayed by pulse oximeter and by auscultation of the heart. The pulse oximeter is extremely sensitive to identify hypoxia but hyperoxia may be over looked due to shift of the oxygen dissociation curve to the left in newborn babies. The sensor must be shielded from direct light (phototherapy or procedure light) by covering it effectively. The oxygen saturation of the patient should be maintained between 88 and 92% by setting alarm limits between 86 and 94%.

Hyperoxia Test

Because of easy availability of point-of-care echocardiography, the hyperoxia test is rarely used to differentiate between cyanosis due to pulmonary causes *vs* congenital heart diseases. Moreover, hyperoxia and hyperventilation are associated with serious risks of oxygen toxicity and alkalosis.

PGE_1 Infusion

Neonates with deep cyanosis, especially those with acidosis should be immediately started on PGE_1 infusion. Intravenous PGE1 infusion, in a dose of 0.05–0.4 µg/kg/min typically improves and maintains oxygen saturation. The infusion dose is guided by the degree of oxygen saturation. The availability of PGE_1 infusion has revolutionized the management of neonates with cyanotic CHD, especially TGA. PGE_1 infusion is useful in almost all neonates with cyanotic CHD except when associated with severe pulmonary venous hypertension (PVH) due to obstructed TAPVC, HLHS, mitral atresia with restrictive ASD and rarely TGA with intact ventricular septum and restrictive ASD. Clinical worsening following PGE_1 infusion provides a clue towards the existence of one of these malformations. Approximately 10–12% neonates receiving PGE_1 infusion have side effects, most serious being apnea which is dose dependent and may need mechanical ventilation.

There is no definite oxygen saturation or PaO_2 that defines adequate oxygenation in a child. The emphasis must be placed on avoiding tissue hypoxia and metabolic acidosis. Cyanosis related to CHD occurs as a result of intracardiac right-to-left shunt and there is only a slight improvement in oxygen saturation with administration of oxygen. Nonetheless, oxygen supplementation increases dissolved oxygen which is undoubtedly helpful for a child with severe hypoxia. Oxygen supplementation, by causing pulmonary vasodilatation sometimes results in clinical worsening in a patient with increased pulmonary blood flow (PBF). Oxygen supplementation, therefore, must be restricted to neonates with severe hypoxia and should not be used routinely.

Humidifier

Unheated bubble humidifier containing sterile or boiled water is suitable for delivery of low flow rates of oxygen (0.5–1.0 L/min). A bubble humidifier not only produces water vapor but also creates aerosol mist which can disperse infectious particles. Humidification of air-oxygen mixture is mandatory when nasal and oral passages are bypassed by tracheal intubation or tracheostomy. Most ventilators and CPAP systems are provided with a servo-controlled humidification chamber to deliver high gas flow rates at the desired temperature and humidity.

Duration of therapy The oxygen should be considered as a potentially toxic drug and it should not be given any minute longer than needed for the baby. When supplemental oxygen is not required, it should be gradually weaned off.

Environmental temperature The hypoxic infant must be nursed in a thermoneutral environment to conserve oxygen, because during thermal stress oxygen is required for metabolic thermogenesis.

Fundus examination The oxygen therapy cannot be reliably monitored by observation of retinal arteriolar constriction because it is difficult to evaluate it clinically. If unequivocal arteriolar constriction is seen, it suggests that retinal damage has already occurred.

Fundus examination should be routinely done by an ophthalmologist in all low birth weight babies (gestation <32 weeks and/or birth weight <1500 g) in accordance with ROP protocol.

Oxygen Toxicity

Oxygen is toxic because it produces oxygen-free radicals. The formation of oxygen radicals is mediated through hypoxanthine–xanthine oxidase system. The oxygen-free radicals are highly reactive and can cause damage to cell membranes by lipid peroxidation, inactivation of enzymes, injury to DNA and degradation of structural proteins in several organs. The body is equipped with a series of defence mechanisms to guard against damage due to oxygen-free radicals. Several vitamins (A, C and E) have antioxidative properties. Serum bilirubin is endowed with antioxidant capabilities and may prevent cellular damage due to oxygen-free radicals. The important endogenous antioxygen enzymes are superoxide dismutase (SOD), catalase and glutathione peroxidase. Glutathione peroxidase is selenium-dependent and, therefore, selenium is an important trace element to provide natural defence against free radicals. In hypoxia, the hypoxanthine concentration may rise extremely high thus initiating a cascade of chemical reactions to generate free radicals. It is believed that a number of diseases in the newborn may occur as a consequence of oxygen-free radicals, e.g. retinopathy of prematurity, bronchopulmonary dysplasia, necrotizing enterocolitis and patent ductus arteriosus.

RETINOPATHY OF PREMATURITY (ROP)

Retinopathy of prematurity, which was previously called as retrolental fibroplasia (RLF), is characterized by abnormal proliferation of small retinal blood vessels due to a variety of causes. The complication is related to high oxygen tension in the arterial blood rather than the concentration of oxygen in the inspired air. The condition is, by and large, limited to preterm babies with a birth weight of less than 1750 g or gestational age of less than 34 weeks. Out of about 25 million annual live births in India, approximately 8.5% of newborns are <2000 g in weight. This would imply that almost 2 million newborns are at risk for developing ROP. The overall incidence of ROP varies between 35 and 60% in babies weighing less than 1750 g. Almost 80% of infants weighing less than 1000 g are reported to develop ROP. At lower gestational ages, large areas of the retina are avascular and is vulnerable to develop abnormal vascular proliferation due to a variety of triggering factors. In the industrialized

Miscellaneous Conditions

26

countries, ROP is one of the leading causes of blindness in children. The incidence of disease is relatively low in developing countries due to lack of adequate ventilatory facilities, extremely high mortality of VLBW babies and lack of awareness and ophthalmologic monitoring of babies in the NICU. However, it is becoming increasingly more common in India because of increasing use of assisted ventilation and improving outcome of "at-risk" preterm infants. It is emerging as one of the leading causes of preventable childhood blindness globally.

Pathophysiology

Retinopathy of prematurity is an ischemia-induced proliferative retinopathy. The process of retinal neovascularization in ROP is complex and involves angiogenic factors, such as vascular endothelial growth factor and basement membrane components. During the acute phase of hyperoxia, there is vaso-obliteration and ischemia of some areas of anterior retina. The subsequent hypoxic or chronic phase is characterized by proliferation of vascular or glial cells, arteriovenous shunt formation and retinal damage with permanent cicatricial changes. During fetal life, vascular endothelial growth factor (VEGF) is credited to promote normal retinal angiogenesis. During the acute or first phase of ROP, the retinal synthesis of VEGF is reduced leading to vasoconstriction while during the second phase, the inadequate retinal oxygenation triggers abnormal angiogenesis as a compensatory mechanism which goes overboard leading to development of pathological changes of ROP.

Risk Factors

A large number of factors other than hyperoxia have been implicated in the pathogenesis of ROP which is limited to very LBW infants (<1500 g or gestation <32 weeks). High ambient light, vitamin E deficiency, shock, sepsis, apneic attacks, hypoxia, acidosis, anemia, blood transfusion, PDA and prolonged ventilatory support (especially when accompanied by episodes of hyperoxia and hypocapnia) have been associated with ROP. Breastfeeding is protective against development of ROP. Infants born to mothers with pregnancy-induced hypertension have a reduced risk of developing ROP due to accelerated fetal maturity of retinal vessels. Till date, a direct relationship between PaO_2 and ROP has not been established and ROP has occurred in premature infants who had never received supplemental oxygen therapy and in infants with cyanotic congenital heart disease in whom

PaO_2 levels never exceeded 50 mm Hg. On the other hand, ROP has not developed in some premature infants even after prolonged period of hyperoxia. Moreover, continuous close monitoring of transcutaneous oxygen tension has not resulted in a decrease in the incidence of ROP. It would appear that ROP is not entirely preventable in some extremely LBW babies despite close monitoring of oxygen therapy.

Screening Protocol

At lower gestational ages, large areas of retina are avascular and preterm infants are vulnerable to develop abnormal vascular proliferation due to large number of triggering factors. The clinically detectable fundal changes of ROP are seen after 4 weeks of birth. All infants with a birth weight of <1750 g or gestational age of <34 weeks should be screened by a pediatric ophthalmologist with indirect ophthalmoscopy (Figure 26.4A–C). More mature infants (1750–2000 g or 34–36 weeks) should also be screened, if they suffered from severe RDS or apneic attacks and received prolonged oxygen therapy or assisted ventilation. After the initial screening at 4 weeks or 30 days of life or postconceptional maturity of 32–34 weeks (whichever is later), the subsequent screening is done after every 2 weeks until the retina is completely vascularized up to ora serrata. Infants <1200 g or <28 weeks of gestational age should be first screened after 2–3 weeks of age because they are at an increased risk to develop early and aggressive posterior ROP (AP–ROP) (Table 26.3). At least two fundus examinations should be performed after pupillary dilatation by using binocular indirect ophthalmoscopy by an experienced ophthalmologist. When ROP is diagnosed, the frequency of examination depends upon the severity and rapidity of progression of disease. Infants are examined more frequently until their retinopathy regresses and full maturity of retinal vessels is achieved or until they reach a threshold for treatment. A register should be maintained in the NICU and date of first screening to be done must be mentioned clearly, if screening has not been done prior to discharge.

The procedure is performed by a pediatric ophthalmologist in the controlled ambience of NICU under the supervision of a neonatologist so that complications can be handled promptly. The pupils are dilated with a mixture of phenylephrine 2.5% and tropicamide or cyclopentolate 0.5% instilled 3 times at 10–15 minutes intervals about one hour before the scheduled examination. The examination should be done at least one hour after the last feed to reduce the risk of vomiting and aspiration. A non-dilating pupil is suggestive

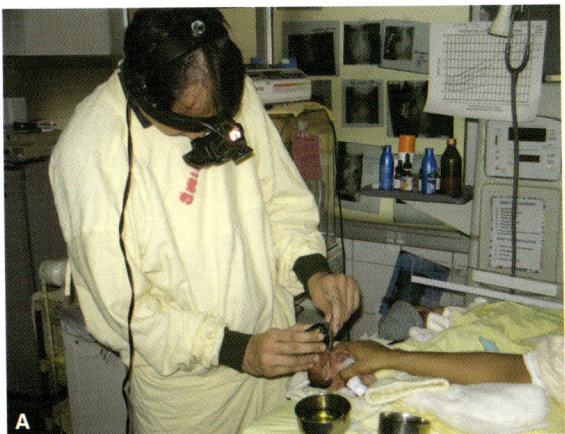
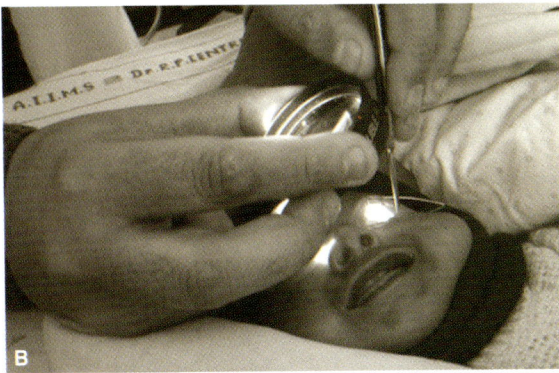
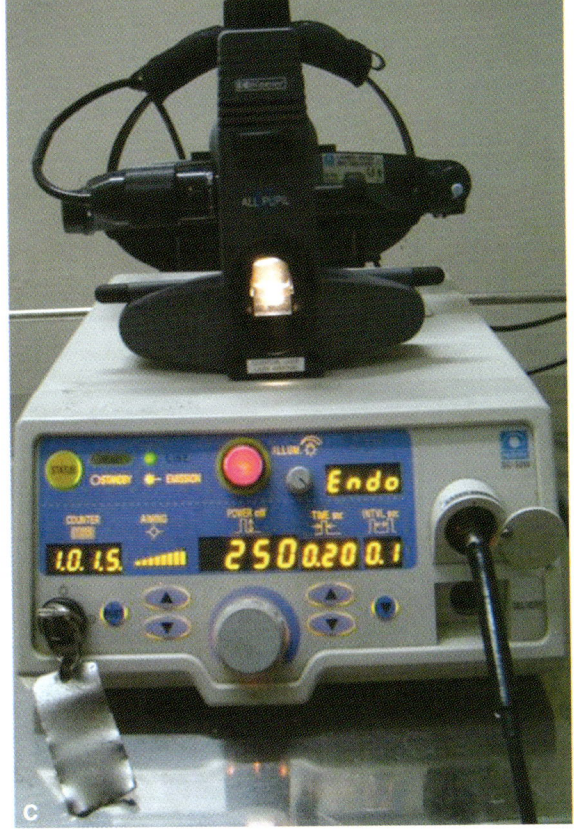

Figure 26.4 (A) and (B) Indirect ophthalmoscopy for screening of ROP, (C) Laser machine used for treatment of ROP.

TABLE 26.3 Protocol for ROP screening

Subjects

All infants with birth weight <1750 g or gestational age of <34 weeks. More mature infants (1750–2000 g or 34–36 weeks) are also screened, if they suffered from RDS or apneic attacks, hemodynamically unstable, or received prolonged oxygen therapy or assisted ventilation.

First screening

i. 4 weeks after birth or post conceptional maturity of 34 weeks (which ever is later).
ii. Infants <1200 g or <28 weeks, first screening is done between 2 and 3 weeks of age because of high risk of aggressive posterior ROP (AP-ROP).

Frequency of screening

It depends upon the extent and severity of retinal findings on the basis of ICROP guidelines

Zone of retinal findings	Stage of retinal findings	Follow-up interval
Zone 1	Immature vascularization	1–2 weeks
	Stage 1 or 2	1 week or less
	Regressing ROP	1–2 weeks
Zone 2	Immature vascularization	2–3 weeks
	Stage 1	2 weeks
	Stage 2	1–2 weeks
	Stage 3	1 week or less
	Regressing ROP	1–2 weeks
Zone 3	Stage 1 or 2	2–3 weeks
	Regressing ROP	2–3 weeks

Termination of screening

It is advised to screen the baby every 1–2 weeks until infant is 38–40 weeks of postmenstrual age and when full retinal vascularization has occurred, and/or ROP is showing regressive changes.

ICROP: International classification of retinopathy of prematurity guidelines.

of tunica vasculosa lentis which should be ruled out to avoid excessive medication for dilatation of pupils. Indirect ophthalmoscopy is performed with 20D or 30D condensing lens by using a fresh set of sterile instruments. Topical anesthetic agent should be used to reduce discomfort to the infant. Infant is swaddled in a blanket and given 1.0–2.0 mL sucrose 20% orally by a syringe to provide comfort and relieve pain. A nurse immobilizes the infant's head and a pediatric wire speculum is used to keep the eyelids apart. The nursery illumination is reduced and both the chambers of the eye and all the zones of retina are examined. Scleral depression is useful to stabilize the eye, rotate it, indent and contrast the retina. A mobile self-contained RETCAM system with a portable fundus camera can be used to provide real-time video display

Miscellaneous Conditions

26

of wide field digital images (WFDI) and capture photographs to document the retinal abnormalities.

Classification

According to the revised international classification of retinopathy of prematurity (ICROP), the severity of disease is assessed by (i) area of the retina involved, (ii) stages or severity of the disease and (iii) plus and threshold disease.

Site and Extent of Disease

The retina is divided into three equal concentric zones around the optic disc and not the macula. Zone I encloses both the optic disc and macula and its radius is twice the distance from the disc to the center of the macula. Zone II extends from the edge of Zone I to the nasal ora serrata. Zone III is the residual crescent of retina temporal to zone II and is the last to vascularize in preterm babies (Figure 26.5). The extent of involvement of retina is graded by the "clock hours" or "quadrants" by considering retina as the dial of a clock.

Stages of the Disease

Stage 1 (Demarcation line). A flat demarcation line of abnormal branching of vessels exists between the vascular and avascular zones, representing an early vascular shunt.

Stage 2 (Ridge). The vascular shunt is ridge-like, elevated above the plane of retina.

Stage 3 (Ridge with extraretinal fibrovascular proliferation). Neovascularization invades the vitreous producing scars which may cause traction on the retina or optic disc.

Stage 4 (Partial retinal detachment). There is subtotal or partial retinal detachment; stage 4A is partial detachment that spares macula; and stage 4B refers to partial detachment involving macula with risk of blindness. *Stage 5* (Total or funnel-shaped retinal detachment). There is complete retinal detachment. The detached retina assumes a funnel-like appearance with anterior and posterior ends that may be open or closed.

Pre-plus disease When "plus" changes affect up to two quadrants of posterior pole or changes are milder than definitive plus disease.

Plus disease It is characterized by vascular dilatation and tortuosity of the posterior retinal vessels involving at least two quadrants of the eye and indicates severe degree of progressive ROP. It may be associated with vascular engorgement of iris, poor pupillary dilatation (rigid pupils) and vitreous haze.

Threshold disease Involvement of five or more contiguous or 8 non-contiguous clock hours of retina (30-degree sectors) of stage 3 with plus disease in either zone 1 or 2. The risk of blindness is 50% when ROP reaches this severity and it demands therapeutic intervention.

Aggressive-posterior ROP (AP-ROP) In VLBW babies, a progressively severe form of ROP involving posterior zone, may rapidly progress to stage 5 disease within a short period. It is characterized by abnormal closed-loop vessels (instead of dichotomous branching pattern) with mild tortuosity that progresses to full blown picture in less than a week. In the past, this condition has been designated as type 2 ROP or "Rush disease".

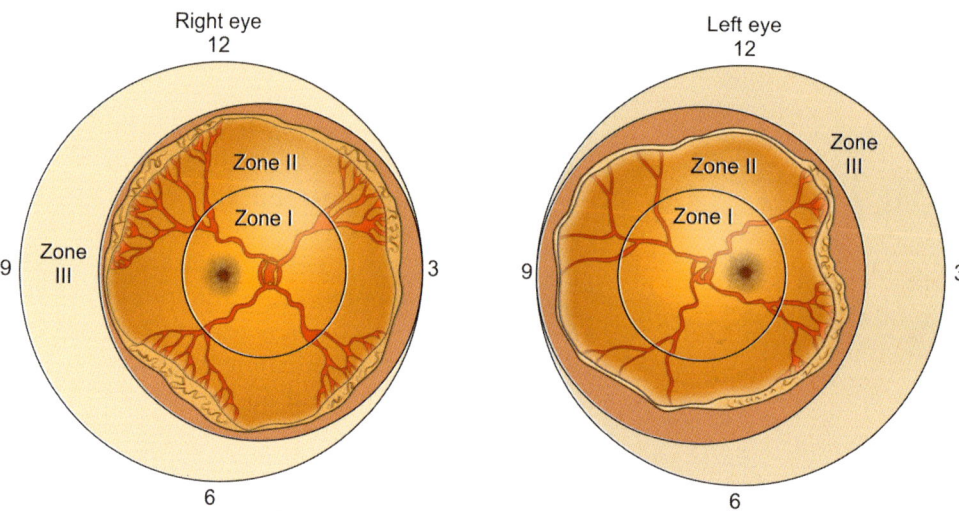

Figure 26.5 Zones of the retina for classification of extent of ROP.

Prevention

Oxygen should be considered as a potentially toxic drug in preterm babies and should be used when indicated. It should be used in the lowest ambient concentration to treat hypoxia and therapy should be withdrawn immediately when there is no valid indication to administer oxygen. Oxygen therapy should be closely monitored to maintain PaO_2 between 50 and 80 mm Hg and SaO_2 between 90 and 93%. Newborn babies should not be exposed to bright light. The characteristic oxygen dissociation curve of adult hemoglobin (shifted to the right) leads to excessive release of oxygen to the tissues including the retinal vasculature, resulting in oxidative damage. Blood transfusion should be given only when absolutely indicated. Arterial blood gases and acid–base parameters should be maintained within the narrow range of normality by vigilant monitoring and prompt therapeutic interventions. Feeding with human milk should be promoted as it reduces the risk of ROP.

The prophylactic utility of administration of high doses of vitamin E and D-penicillamine is controversial and may be associated with toxic side effects. There is recent evidence to suggest that treatment with near-infrared (NIR) light can prevent the development of ROP. The pediatrician should have the confidence and expertise to screen preterm babies for ROP. Pupils should be dilated by instilling a combination of tropicamide 0.5% and phenylepherine 2.5% eye drops on three occasions at an interval of 10–15 minutes. Fundus should be examined with a direct ophthalmoscope. The presence of dilated veins and tortuous arteries are useful markers of ROP for seeking expert opinion by an ophthalmologist. High-risk infants and infants below 1750 g or less than 34 weeks of gestation should be closely followed by an ophthalmologist as per standard protocol for early identification and management of ROP.

Treatment

Early detection of ROP is important so that avascular peripheral retina can be touched with transscleral cryopexy to prevent further spread of ROP. Cryotherapy is indicated, if stage 3 disease is identified in more than 5 contiguous clock hours or more than 8 total clock hours in zone 1 or 2 in the presence of "plus" disease. Cryopexy can be done under local anesthesia and sedation or general anesthesia. The cryoprobe is applied to the sclera and entire avascular areas of the retina are frozen to prevent further spread of disease. Laser photocoagulation therapy for ROP is preferred and has replaced cryotherapy in many centers. Both argon and infrared diode laser coagulation have been successfully used in infants with severe ROP. Laser photocoagulation is technically simpler and easier procedure with less pain and discomfort to the baby. The aim of treatment is to ablate the entire avascular retina up to ora serrata in a near confluent burn pattern reaching as close to the edge of the ridge as possible. There is reduced risk of chemosis and edema of conjunctiva and lids with better visual outcome. Scleral buckling is useful for treatment of stage 4 ROP. A combined lensectomy–vitrectomy is performed in stage 5 disease. Algorithm for management of ROP is shown in Figure 26.6. Retinal reattachment procedures have been used with limited success for treatment of stage 5 ROP. The prognosis for vision is hopeless when infant presents with leukocoria or white pupillary reflex. The quality measures for treatment of ROP are summarized in Table 26.4. Recent studies have documented that shining gentle near-infrared light (NIR) at 670 nm is a potential treatment for ROP that is less invasive, inexpensive and free of side effects.

Prognosis

Most cases of stage 1 and stage 2 of ROP are likely to regress although progression is unpredictable until vascularization is complete. These stages have been associated with higher incidence of refractive errors, amblyopia, cataract and strabismus. Stage 3 ROP

TABLE 26.4 Quality measures for treatment of retinopathy of prematurity (ROP)

Quality measure Are preterm babies routinely screened for ROP in accordance with the recommended screening protocol?

Data components
Numerator Number of neonates eligible for ROP screening in whom first eye examination by indirect ophthalmoscopy was done at 28 ±2 days of birth.
Denominator Number of neonates eligible for ROP screening as per national guidelines.

Specifications: Data to be compiled from the ROP screening proforma at the time of (i) discharge from the NICU and (ii) at 38 weeks postmenstrual age.

Analytic model: No baseline risk adjustment is needed*. Calculate proportion of neonates eligible for ROP screening in whom first eye examination by indirect ophthalmoscopy was done at 28 ±2 days of birth.

Data analysis It is presented as a proportion summarized for each quarter.

*Risk adjustment is needed if baseline risk of the index condition varies across different health care facilities.

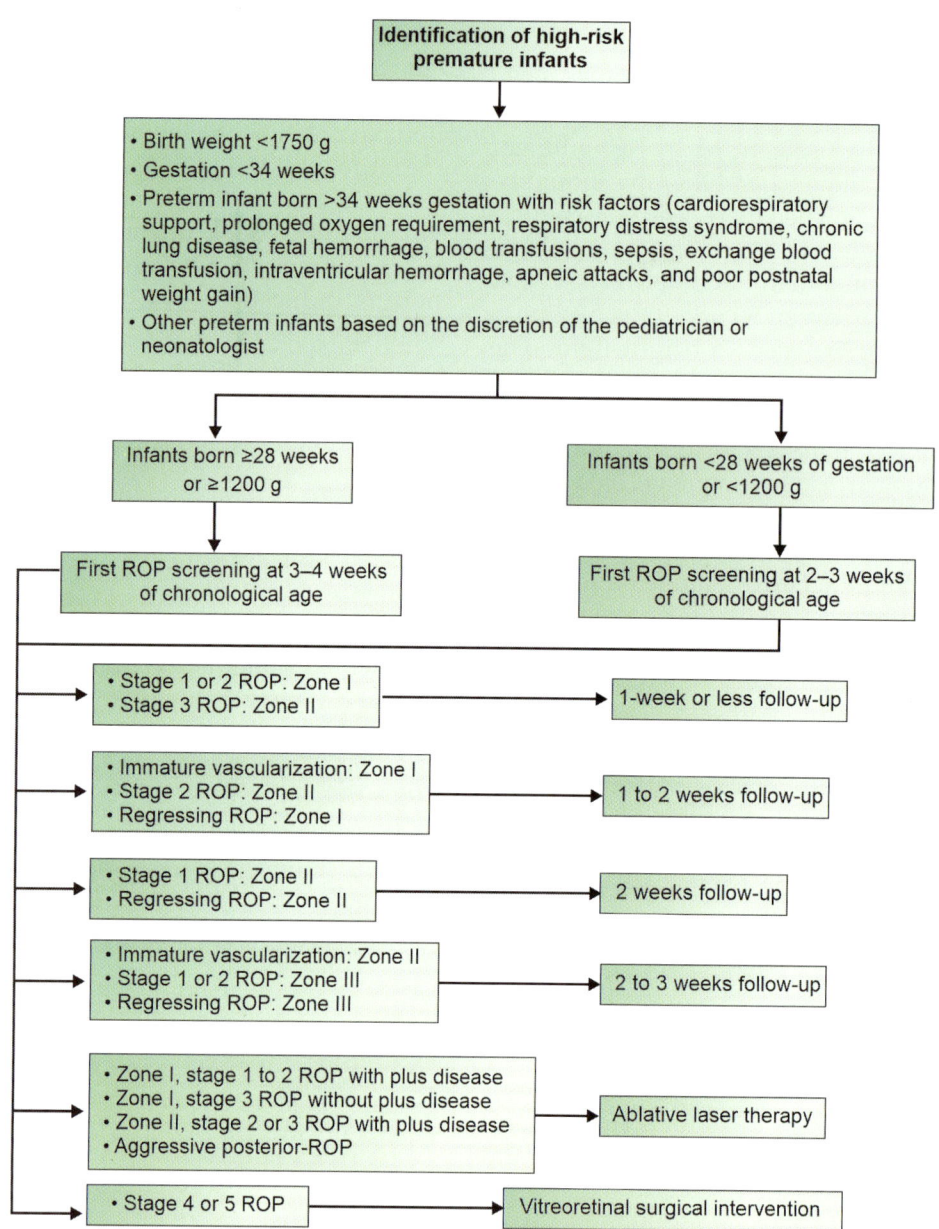

Figure 26.6 Algorithm for management of retinopathy of prematurity.

results in a high incidence of refractive errors and strabismus. Stage 4 B and stage 5 ROP have grave risk of development of acute glaucoma, retinal detachment and blindness. Visual rehabilitation should be offered to all visually challenged ROP babies.

BRONCHOPULMONARY DYSPLASIA (BPD)

It has been recognized that babies with respiratory distress syndrome who require assisted ventilation with oxygen concentration in excess of 70% for a period of at least 5 to 6 days are predisposed to develop this complication. It is controversial whether the pulmonary damage is solely because of oxygen toxicity or

as a result of barotrauma because of positive pressure ventilation. It has been claimed that negative pressure ventilators do not lead to this complication even though high concentrations of oxygen may be used for prolonged periods of time. The various predisposing and etiological factors include prematurity, mechanical ventilation, high PIPs or MAPs, barotrauma, hyperoxia, PDA, fluid over load and pulmonary edema. The affected babies pose difficulties during weaning from the respirator and their respiratory distress may continue for a couple of days or weeks and may terminate fatally. Pathological changes are characterized by patchy squamous metaplasia, peribronchiolar muscular thickening and eosinophilic exudates. For detailed discussion on bronchopulmonary dysplasia, refer to Chapter 19.

Irritability of the Central Nervous System

Cerebral vasocontriction due to hyperoxemia may cause vertigo, nausea, convulsions, coma and death.

EDEMA AND HYDROPS FETALIS

Edema is a relatively common finding in normal preterm babies but it is rather rare in term infants. It is recognized either because it is visible and palpable or evidenced by sudden gain in weight of more than 100 g per day. Edema may be localized to certain parts of the body or generalized as manifested by puffiness, edema of feet, legs and sacrum. The presence of generalized edema in association with ascites is designated as hydrops fetalis.

Physiology

The largest component of human body is water. Total body water decreases with gestational maturity. At 12 weeks of gestation, fetus is composed of 90% water which decreases to 85% at 28 weeks and 75% at term. The ratio of extracellular to intracellular water is 55 : 45 at birth which gradually reverses during neonatal period. Preterm infants have relatively larger volume of extracellular fluid as compared to term infants. Most of the excess extracellular water is distributed in the skin and subcutaneous tissues accounting for approximately 16% of the infant's body weight as opposed to 8% in an adult. In normal circumstances, balance exists between forces which tend to force and suck the water out and back into the vascular compartment. The Starling forces are so balanced that there is slight overall net flow of water from the blood into tissues which is subsequently removed by lymphatics or reabsorbed by the capillaries.

The exchange of water takes place through the whole length of capillaries and is bidirectional. Rise in capillary hydrostatic pressure either due to active increase of pressure at the arteriolar head or due to venous congestion as a result of congestive heart failure tends to force the water out of capillaries. Capillary damage due to hypoxia and hypothermia may enhance their permeability resulting in leakage of fluid into interstitial space. The colloid osmotic pressure of plasma tries to maintain adequacy of blood volume. Albumin which accounts for 80% of the oncotic pressure of the plasma proteins is the major differential force across the capillaries favoring flow of interstitial fluid into the capillaries. The osmotic pressure generated by crystalloids is tremendous (5,100 mm Hg) but because of their equidistribution throughout the extracellular space, their contribution to water exchange is minimal. It has been estimated that when colloid osmotic pressure falls below 20 cm H_2O, fluid leaks into the interstitial space resulting in generalized edema. Regulatory mechanisms also operate in the interstitial gel. Apart from oncotic pressure of proteins, macromolecules and solutes, the interstitial gel has inherent affinity for water. When water content in the interstitial space increases, gel network swells up thus restricting further uptake of water from the vascular compartment.

The lymphatics play an important role in draining water and colloids that have seeped into interstitial space. In those organs where capillaries are more permeable, such as the liver and lungs, lymphatic drainage assumes critical importance. The pumping effect of lymphatics generate negative hydrostatic pressure in the interstitial gel. The constancy of intracellular water is governed by the cellular colloid osmotic pressure and integrity of the energy dependent sodium pump of the cell membrane. Osmotically active metabolites are released into and around the cell membranes during asphyxia, acidosis, hypoglycemia and hypothermia, thus damaging the biomechanics of cell membranes.

Localized Edema

Presenting part Edema is due to obliteration of venous return and compression of the presenting part during delivery, e.g. caput succedaneum, edema of one hand in cases of hand prolapse, and edema at the site of forceps application.

Inflammatory edema Edema is invariable in association with cellulitis and abscess.

Turner's syndrome Edema is limited to dorsa of hands and feet in these 45 XO female babies. It is usually lymphatic edema and non-pitting in character.

Milroy's disease Unilateral non-pitting progressive edema of one extremity due to lymphedema as a result of congenital malformation of lymphatics is seen in this condition. The condition is inherited as autosomal dominant.

Generalized Edema

An excessive accumulation of interstitial or intracellular water generally manifests as pitting edema. In cases of generalized edema, there is increase in total body water in addition to maldistribution among the body compartments.

Edema of Prematurity

Several physiological handicaps predispose preterm infants to develop edema. Infants who suffer from intrapartum asphyxia and/or develop serious respiratory distress are more prone to develop edema. The release of catecholamines and vasoactive agents during the process of birth leads to rise in capillary hydrostatic pressure. The preterm infant is equipped with low quota of plasma albumin and hence reduced colloid osmotic pressure. Capillary permeability is increased among preterm infants due to their increased vulnerability to damage by hypoxia, hypothermia, shock and acidosis. The interstitial gel of preterm babies has greater affinity for water because of its higher albumin content. Due to poor muscle mass, reduced muscular tone and relative immobility of limbs, the lymphatic drainage is sluggish in the preterm infant. Preterm infants are also prone to develop cellular edema due to accumulation of osmotically active metabolites inside the cells due to cellular disturbances induced by asphyxia, acidosis and hypoglycemia.

Edema among preterm infants may occur on the first day or any time during intensive care or after a few weeks of life. *The incidence of early-onset edema is related to the adequacy of perinatal care of immature infants.* It commonly follows perinatal asphyxia, hypothermia, acidosis and shock at birth. Generalized edema, many weeks after birth, has been reported in association with protein and vitamin E deficiency in preterm infants. During excessive solute load, especially when sudden change from a low solute to a high solute formula is made, immature kidneys may fail to adapt resulting in fluid retention.

Hydrops Fetalis due to Rh-Isoimmunization

Prior to the advent of anti-D globulin prophylaxis, severe Rh-hemolytic disease of the newborn used to be the commonest cause of hydrops fetalis. In India, because of lack of universal anti-D globulin prophylaxis, hydrops fetalis due to erythroblastosis is still seen. Edema is contributed by severe anemia and hypoproteinemia. It has been shown that plasma oncotic pressure is reduced out of proportion to the degree of hypoproteinemia in these infants. Rarely severe anemia due to ABO-hemolytic disease or even minor blood groups incompatibility (Kell) may produce hydrops fetalis.

Non-Immune Hydrops Fetalis (NIHF)

This entity has assumed greater importance because of reduced incidence of hydrops fetalis due to Rh-isoimmunization. Maternal diabetes mellitus,

polyhydramnios, anemia and toxemia of pregnancy are recognized correlates of hydrops fetalis. Its incidence is reported to be 1 in 3,500 deliveries. When polyhydramnios is suspected during antenatal period, ultrasound examination is advisable to rule out hydrops fetalis and associated anomalies. It has been possible to diagnose fetal cardiac malformations by two-dimensional and M-mode echocardiography during pregnancy. Fetal tachyarrhythmias and heart block can be picked up during cardiotocography. Most cases of hydrops fetalis have congestive heart failure, anemia, hypoproteinemia or a combination of these factors. However, hydrops fetalis is a difficult diagnostic puzzle and even after autopsy no cause may be found in over one-third of cases. Infant is born with generalized edema and ascites. Almost one-half of affected infants are stillborn. Those born alive, pose serious resuscitation and adaptation difficulties at birth. They have shock and its consequences including disseminated intravascular coagulopathy or manifest signs of circulatory overload due to congestive heart failure. The main causes of non-immunologic hydrops fetalis are listed in Table 26.5.

Severe anemia Homozygous alpha-thalassemia is characterized by severe anemia and hepatosplenomegaly in the absence of Rh-isoimmunization. The alpha chain production is deficient while excess gamma chains combine to form Bart's hemoglobin which has very high affinity for oxygen which is not released to the tissues thus resulting in fetal hypoxia. Most infants are stillborn or die within few hours or days after birth. It is limited to populations with Oriental ethnic background and certain parts of South-East Asia where homozygous alpha-thalassemia is the commonest cause of hydrops fetalis. Hydrops fetalis occurs in association with chronic severe anemia, hypoproteinemia and cardiac decompensation.

Congenital malformations Over 40% cases of non-immunologic hydrops fetalis are associated with a variety of congenital malformations. In infants with congenital cardiac defects, hydrops fetalis can be explained on the basis of fetal congestive heart failure. In some cases of congenital malformations, hypoproteinemia or lymphatic abnormalities may explain pathogenesis of hydrops, while in majority of cases its mechanism remains unexplained.

Intrauterine infections They may cause hydrops fetalis by virtue of myocarditis, hepatitis and nephritis for which evidences should be looked for on laboratory investigations. Parvovirus B19 is implicated in the causation of 10% cases of fetal non-immunologic hydrops. The virus has special predilection for P blood

TABLE 26.5 Causes of non-immunologic hydrops fetalis on the basis of major associations

Conditions	Causes
■ **Anemia**	Homozygous alpha-thalassemia, chronic twin-to-twin or fetomaternal hemorrhage, G-6-PD deficiency and osteopetrosis.
■ **Congenital malformations**	
Cardiac	Subaortic stenosis, hypoplastic left heart syndrome, premature closure of foramen ovale or ductus arteriosus, endocardial fibroelastosis, paroxysmal atrial tachycardia and complete heart block.
Pulmonary	Chylothorax, pulmonary hypoplasia, lymphangiectasis, adenomatoid hamartoma, congenital lobar emphysema.
Renal	Finnish type congenital nephrosis, renal vein thrombosis.
Skeletal	Chondrodystrophies, asphyxiating throcic dystrophy, osteogenesis imperfecta.
Chromosomal or multiple system anomalies	E-trisomy, Down syndrome, Turner syndrome, triploidy and aneuploidy.
■ **Intrauterine infections**	Syphilis, toxoplasmosis, cytomegalovirus disease, herpes, rubella, parvovirus infection, leptospirosis and Chagas disease.
■ **Miscellaneous**	Chorioangioma of placenta, hemangioendothelioma of placenta, arteriovenous malformations of fetus or placenta, umbilical or chronic venous thrombosis, choriocarcinoma *in situ*, Gaucher's disease, glycogen storage disease, fetal neuroblastosis, congenital disorder of glycosylation, lysosomal storage disorders and CNS abnormalities like absent corpus callosum, holoprosencephaly, encephalocele.
■ **Idiopathic**	20% cases

group antigen which is widely distributed in several tissues especially erythrocytes, liver and myocardium. The congenital infection leads to severe anemia due to aplasia of erythrocytes along with hepatitis and myocarditis leading to hydrops fetalis.

Miscellaneous conditions A number of placental disorders may be associated with hydrops fetalis though their role in the etiopathogenesis of the condition is uncertain. Placenta must be examined thoroughly and preserved for histopathological examination in all cases of hydrops fetalis.

Diagnosis

Most infants with hydrops fetalis are associated with cardiac failure, severe anemia, and hypoproteinemia due to cellular damage to placenta or liver. Erythroblastosis fetalis due to rhesus isoimmunization is the commonest cause of generalized edema. Among non-immunological cases of hydrops fetalis, no cause is identified in about 30% of patients. Placenta should be examined for its size, angiomatous malformation, choriocarcinoma and transplacental infections. Investigations should be conducted to exclude rhesus isoimmunization, alpha-thalassemia, anemia due to any cause, nephrosis, hepatitis, and cardiac disorders. Specific immunological tests are necessary to confirm the diagnosis of intrauterine infections.

Management

It is essential that intrapartum asphyxia, postnatal hypoxia, acidosis, hypothermia and shock are prevented or managed promptly to prevent the development of edema of prematurity. Effective monitoring of fetus *in utero*, and satisfactory postnatal management of preterm infants has substantially reduced the incidence of skin edema in developed countries. Adequate intake of protein and vitamin E should be ensured to prevent the occurrence of late-onset edema associated with their deficiency states. Solute content of the milk formula should be restricted to prevent sodium and water retention. Overhydration can be prevented by using infusion burrettes or electronic infusion pumps. Monitoring of arterial blood pressure of sick preterm babies and rapid correction of shock with transfusion of blood, plasma or albumin is desirable for their improved outcome and reduction in the incidence of overt edema.

The presence of subcutaneous edema may be associated with tissue dysfunction especially in the lungs, brain and liver. Diuretics have been recommended for its treatment. Furosemide (1–2 mg/kg/dose) produces diuresis even in sick preterm infant but it further depletes intravascular compartment and aggravates hypotension. To safeguard against this hazard, it is recommended that a sick edematous preterm infant should be administered 1.0 g/kg salt-free albumin in conjunction with furosemide. Albumin would elevate the plasma colloid osmotic pressure and support the intravascular compartment.

The treatment of hydrops fetalis depends upon the underlying cause. Fetal tachyarrhythmia can be managed by administration of digoxin and propranolol to the mother. Exchange blood transfusion is indicated,

Miscellaneous Conditions

26

if cord blood hemoglobin is less than 10 g/dL. Central venous pressure should be monitored to avoid overloading of circulation. Resuscitation of a hydropic baby is difficult and demands high level of expertise. Endotracheal intubation should be done by a skilled operator by using a fiberoptic scope. The respiratory distress due to massive ascites and pleural or pericardial effusion would require tapping of fluid with a 20-gauge angiocatheter attached to a three-way stop cock and syringe. Paracentesis should preferably be done in the left iliac fossa to avoid damage to the enlarged liver. Low solute intake and furosemide are useful non-specific measures.

ASCITES

In most cases of ascites, there is associated generalized edema as seen in cases of hydrops fetalis. Isolated ascites may occur in the following situations.

Obstructive Uropathy

The most common cause of isolated ascites in the newborn is lower urinary tract obstruction. Bladder neck obstruction due to uretheral valve leads to back pressure with dilatation of urinary bladder and leakage of urine in the peritoneal cavity. Three masses may be palpable in the abdomen, two kidneys and urinary bladder. The urea content of the ascitic fluid would be high. It may be associated with absent abdominal musculature. The condition is best managed by bilateral nephrostomies followed by relief of obstruction.

Chylous Ascites

The congenital obstruction at the level of cisterna chyli and malformation of mesenteric lymphatics results in chylous ascites due to rupture of intestinal lymphatics. The diagnosis is suggested by the milky appearance and high cholesterol and protein content of the ascitic fluid. The cloudy appearance of ascitic fluid appears only after milk feedings have been established. The condition responds to repeated paracenteses, presumably due to establishment of collateral lymphatic pathways.

Peritonitis

Peritonitis may occur following perforation of gut, appendicitis, paracentesis and intraperitoneal transfusion. Peritoneal exudates are generally minimal and clinical picture is dominated by rigidity, guarding, paralytic ileus and evidences of septicemia. Fetal meconium peritonitis is characterized by calcification.

Biliary Ascites

It is rare and may occur in association with extra-hepatic biliary atresia and following percutaneous hepatic cholangiography.

DERMATOLOGICAL DISORDERS

Sclerema

Sclerema and scleredema are often interchangeably used terms to describe peculiar hardening of skin which is stretched and cannot be pinched but may pit on pressure, if edema is present. The condition is peculiar to newborn babies. It starts from the face and legs and spreads centrally. It is often associated with hypothermia, Gram-negative septicemia and hypernatremia. Its onset signifies grave outcome. The involvement of the thoracic skin results in respiratory difficulty and death. Histologically, the trabecular fat is broadened and fat spaces are diminished in sclerema. The cellular infiltration is absent. The use of high doses of corticosteroids and treatment of underlying condition may result in recovery in some cases. Exchange blood transfusion with fresh blood is recommended by some workers.

In subcutaneous fat necrosis due to cold injury, firm, sharply circumscribed, reddish or purple flat localized solidified areas may appear over the cheeks, buttocks, thighs and arms. The lesions may calcify and heal spontaneously with atrophy producing pronounced skin depressions.

Vesiculobullous Skin Eruptions

Vesiculobullous skin lesions in the newborn may occur due to a variety of conditions. Infant may be born with vesicles or they may appear any time during neonatal period. Vesiculobullous skin lesions may be the sole manifestation of a disease process or it may be a transient phase during the course of the disease (mastocytosis and incontinentia pigmenti). The clinical appearances of a blister may provide a clue to the possible site of lesion within the skin layers. Blisters localized to epidermal layers are thin-walled, flaccid and prone to rupture easily. Subepidermal vesicles are tense, thick-walled and sturdy. Skin biopsy is often diagnostic because location of cleavage of skin is constant and often characteristic of various conditions producing vesiculobullous eruptions. The biopsy must be taken from the most recent and intact blister. Various conditions producing vesiculobullous skin lesions in the newborn are listed in Table 26.6.

TABLE 26.6 Causes of vesiculobullous skin lesions in the newborn

- **Infections**

Bacterial	Bullous impetigo, staphylococcal scalded skin syndrome, *Pseudomonas aeruginosa, Klebsiella pneumoniae, Listeria monocytogenes*
Spriochetal	Congenital syphilis
Viral	Herpes simplex, chickenpox
Fungal	Candidiasis

- **Developmental disorders**
  Epidermolysis bullosa
  Incontinentia pigmenti
  Urticaria pigmentosa

- **Miscellaneous conditions**
  Erythema toxicum
  Transient neonatal pustular melanosis
  Burns

Bacterial Infections

Impetigo or superficial pyoderma due to Gram-positive organisms is common in tropical countries especially during summer months. The skin lesions appear after 48 hours of age in the form of thin-walled vesiculopustules surrounded by erythematous macules. They are mostly distributed over scalp, neck, axillae and groin. Hexachlorophene skin prophylaxis is effective to prevent the infection from assuming epidemic proportions. After applications of hexachlorophene, effective rinsing of skin is mandatory to prevent its systemic absorption and toxicity. Scattered or isolated lesions should be punctured and painted with triple dye. Infants with multiple or intractable lesions and those having constitutional symptoms should be treated with oral administration of erythromycin or beta-lactamase resistant penicillins.

Staphylococcal scalded skin syndrome (Ritter's disease) The characteristic skin manifestations due to staphylococci are produced by elaboration of two exotoxins, epidermolytic toxins A and B. There is sudden appearance of generalized erythema and large flaccid bullae. Large sheets of epidermis peel off spontaneously or following mild pressure (positive Nikolsky's sign), exposing moist, glistening-pink denuded area resembling boiled lobster (Figure 26.7). Facial edema, perioral crusting and generalized desquamation are characteristic. The site of blister cleavage in scalded skin syndrome is in the granular layer thus accounting for the rapid healing of denuded areas. Aspirate from intact bulla is often sterile. The condition should be differentiated from boric acid poisoning, toxic epidermal necrolysis (which is rare in the newborn) and epidermolysis bullosa. Skin should be kept moistened with sterile normal saline

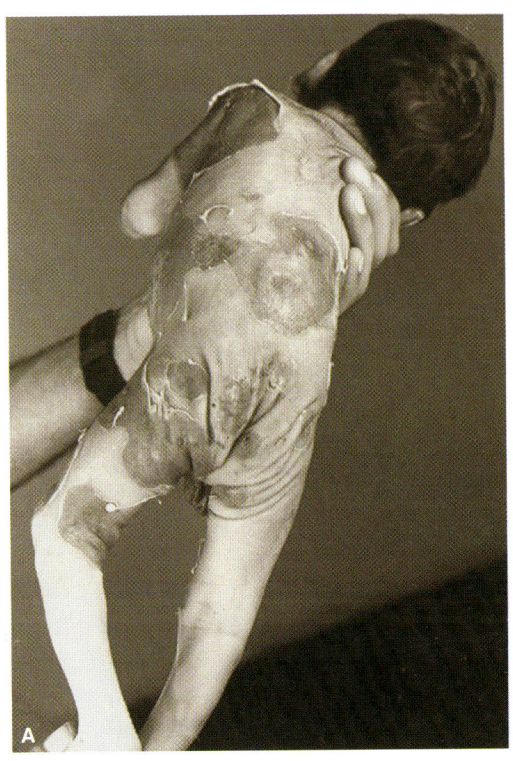

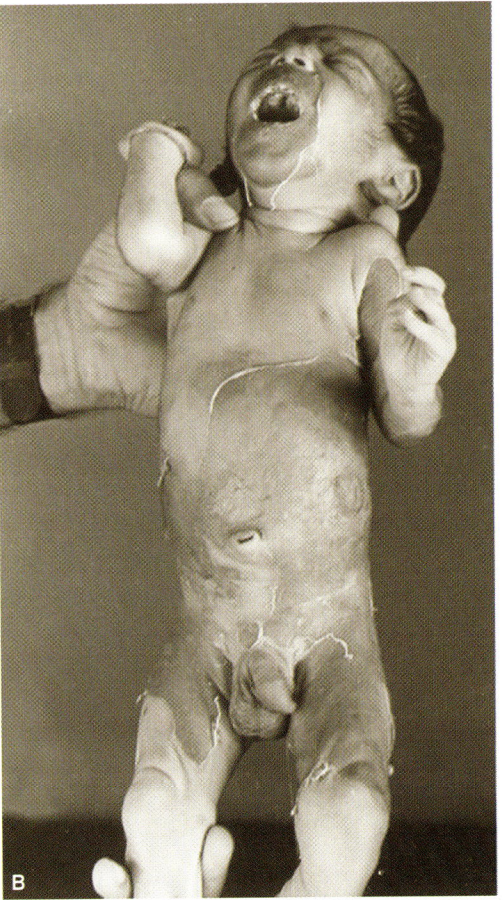

Figure 26.7A and B Typical appearances of scalded skin syndrome due to staphylococcal infection.

or 0.01% potassium permanganate compresses. Losses of fluids, electrolytes and plasma should be replaced and baby nursed in a thermoneutral range of environmental temperature. Antistaphylococcal agents in combination with an aminoglycoside should be administered parenterally.

Pseudomonas aeruginosa and Klebsiella pneumoniae may produce grayish-black vesicular, ulcerative or gangrenous skin lesions over peripheral parts of the extremity and perianal area during the course of septicemia. The appearance of skin lesions herald poor outcome.

Listeria monocytogenes infection *in utero* may manifest as fetal diarrhea, vesiculo-erythematous skin eruption and mild respiratory distress at birth. Response to ampicillin therapy is generally excellent.

Congenital syphilis The clinical features of congenital syphilis are analogous to the secondary stage of acquired syphilis and are characterized by appearance of mucocutaneous lesions. Erythematous muculopapular skin rash with vesicular or bullous lesions and desquamation is classically distributed over hands and feet but may involve whole body. Wart-like condylomatous moist lesions at the mucocutaneous junctions of mouth, anus and vulva may be rarely seen. Skin lesions are highly contagious and may recur over a period of weeks and months. Snuffles (noisy breathing), jaundice, hepatosplenomegaly and osteochondritis when associated provide diagnostic clues. Administration of procain penicillin 50,000 units/kg/day intramuscularly or aqueous crystalline penicillin G 100, 000–150, 000 units/kg/day q 12 hours IM or IV for 10 to 14 days is curative. Infant should be closely followed till treponemal serologic tests are negative.

Herpes simplex Herpes simplex type II infection may occur *in utero* through transplacental route or during the course of vaginal delivery in a mother having herpetic vesicles over external genitals. Infant may be born with vesicles or develop them subsequently. Isolated or cluster of vesicles may be distributed along a dermatome. Skin lesions may show relapses and recurrences over several months. Life-threatening systemic manifestations are seen in two-thirds of infants. Keratoconjunctivitis, meningoencephalitis with chorioretinitis, and hepatitis dominate the clinical picture of viremia. Herpetic blister is intraepidermal. Tzanck smear should be made for identification of giant cells and isolation of herpes virus. In a mother with known genital herpes infection, infant should be delivered by cesarean section preferably before the rupture of membranes. The localized HSV infection is treated by administration of acyclovir 20 mg/kg/dose IV every 8 hours for 10–14 days. Infants with disseminated or CNS infection with HSV should receive acyclovir 20 mg/kg/dose IV every 8 hours for at least 21 days.

Chickenpox Maternal chickenpox during first trimester of pregnancy is associated with risk of abortion and fetal malformations. Affected infants are characterized by intrauterine growth retardation, hypoplastic limbs or digits, cicatricial skin lesions, microcephaly, ocular abnormalities and delayed motor development. Like mumps, varicella embryopathy is rare. Infants born before 5 days of onset of rash in the mother, may present with fulminant manifestations of chickenpox during newborn period. Vesicular lesions appear like dewdrops, distributed mostly over trunk and are pleomorphic in their evolution. History of maternal infection would clinch the diagnosis. Infants born to mothers who have had varicella near the time of delivery should receive varicella zoster immune globulins (VariZIG) 125 units/kg IM or alternatively 400 mg/kg of pooled immune globulin for prophylaxis. Neonatal varicella should be treated by administration of acyclovir 20 mg/kg/dose IV every 8 hours for 7 days.

Candidiasis Intrauterine candidal infection is rare but can occur through transplacental route or by ascending infection from vagina. Skin lesions, which may be present at birth, are characterized by erythema, moist erosions and vesiculopustules with erythematous base. The entire body including palms and soles may be affected. Yellow-white nodules may be seen over the umbilical cord and placenta. The diagnosis can be confirmed by identification and isolation of *C. albicans* with KOH preparation and culture of material obtained from active lesions. Disseminated candidiasis is a life-threatening disorder and best managed by intravenous administration of amphotericin B. Isolated skin lesions respond to local application of gentian violet or nystatin. During infancy, candidal infection commonly involves diaper and intertriginous areas of skin.

DEVELOPMENTAL DISORDERS

Epidermolysis Bullosa

A heterogenous group of hereditary disorders associated with congenital blisters following mechanical trauma are categorized under this entity. The basic defect is unknown but blisters are produced by heat or mechanical trauma to skin. Blisters are distributed over those areas of skin which are vulnerable to pressure or irritation viz; bony prominences or extensor surfaces of joints. Nikolsky's sign is usually positive, i.e. skin peels off on rubbing with pressure.

Epidermolysis bullosa simplex It is a non-scarring autosomal dominant disorder. The bullae are intra-epidermal and mostly distributed over hands, feet, elbows, knees, legs and scalp (Figure 26.8). Nails may be dystrophic. It is a benign condition and as the child grows, the propensity for blister formation decreases.

Epidermolysis bullosa lethalis Though nonscarring, it produces serious morbidity and often proves lethal. Blisters are large producing moist erosive plaques with characteristic sparing of hands and feet. Dystrophic nails, growth retardation and resistant anemia are common. Blisters are subepidermal with cleavage plane between the plasma membranes of the basal cells and the basement membrane. Therapy consists in prevention or early management of infections, provision of adequate calories and iron and administration of blood transfusion.

Dystrophic epidermolysis bullosa Dystrophic epidermolysis bullosa with dominant mode of inheritance is a mild disease characterized by formation of blisters over hands, feet and sacrum. The lesions heal promptly with formation of soft wrinkled scars, and

pigmentation. The blister is subepidermal with separation beneath the basement membrane. Recessive dystrophic epidermolysis bullosa is most incapacitating and characterized by extensive blister formation, erosions and scarring. Scarring of buccal mucosa and esophageal strictures are associated with feeding difficulties and starvation. Joints are ankylosed and hands are often reduced to mittens. The subepidermal bullae are located beneath the basement membrane and anchoring fibrils are absent. Therapy is mostly supportive but corticosteroids have been used with variable success. Prognosis is poor.

Incontinentia pigmenti (Bloch-Sulzberger disease) It is a rare multisystem hereditary disorder transmitted as sex-linked dominant trait. Affected males die *in utero*. The skin manifestations are characterized by appearance of erythematous linear streaks and plaques of vesicles mostly distributed over the limbs. The linear configuration of vesicles is characteristic. Lesions heal by scarring and pigmentation manifesting as warty linear areas along Blaschko's lines after 3 months of age. The skin pigment is distributed in macular whorls, reticulated patches, flecks and linear streaks. Intraepidermal vesicle is characteristically filled with eosinophils and there is eosinophilia in the peripheral blood. Affected infants may have associated alopecia, seizures, developmental retardation, spasticity, delayed dentition and ocular defects. Prognosis is related to the type and severity of associated anomalies because skin lesions are benign and often disappear during later childhood.

Urticaria pigmentosa (mastocytosis) Aggregation of mast cells with release of histamine and heparin manifests as recurrent urticarial or bullous lesions with hyperpigmentation. Dermographism and Darier's sign are positive, i.e. stroking of skin is followed by appearance of erythema and wheal formation. Demonstration of mast cells in skin biopsy is diagnostic. Prognosis is good as spontaneous involution occurs in majority of patients by 2 years of age.

Miscellaneous Conditions

Erythema toxicum (urticaria neonatorum) It is characterized by erythematous blotches with central pale papule or vesicle giving a semblance of wheal formation. It affects about 40–55% of term infants. Infants less than 1500 g or less than 32 weeks gestation rarely manifest erythema toxicum. Skin rash appears on second day of life and involves face, neck and trunk. The condition is transient and resolves spontaneously within a few days. The exact cause is

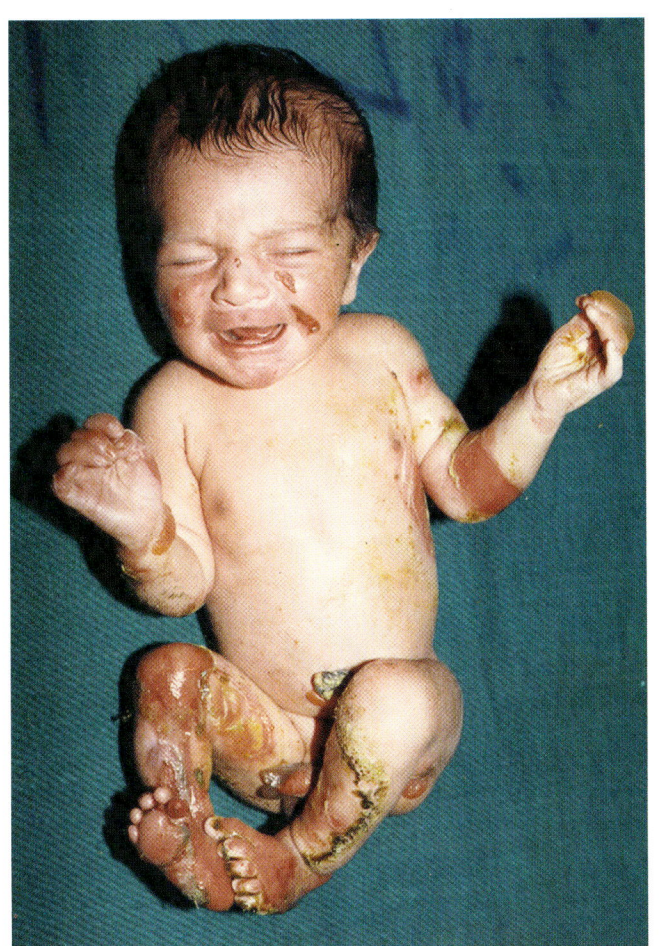

Figure 26.8 Epidermolysis bullosa simplex.

unknown but it appears to be a marker of atopy. The scrapings from skin lesions show plenty of eosinophils.

Transient neonatal pustular melanosis It is a benign, self-limited condition in which vesiculopustular eruption with pigmented macules is present at birth over the forehead, neck, back and extremities. The pustules are flaccid, superficial and fragile without any erythema. The smear from skin lesions may show neutrophils. It is a transient condition and eruption disappears within 2 to 3 days. The recovery is followed by appearance of hyperpigmented macules which disappear slowly over next 3 weeks to 3 months.

Burns Newborn babies are vulnerable to develop thermal or chemical (due to extravasation of intravenous medications and fluids) burns because of their delicate skin. Thin flaccid intraepidermal bullae appear at the site of injury. The use of hot water bottles should preferably be avoided but if ever used, the care should be taken that they do not come in contact with infant's skin.

NEONATAL ERYTHRODERMA

Erythroderma or "red baby" syndrome is defined as an inflammatory skin disorder affecting more than 90% of body surface. A large number of conditions manifest as life-threatening erythroderma in newborn babies (Table 26.7). Inflammatory erythrodermic skin disorders must be differentiated from atopic dermatitis or eczema because of different therapeutic implications.

Infections

Staphylococcal scalded skin syndrome (Ritter's disease, pemphigus neonatorum) is caused by exfoliative toxin (ETA and ETB) released by staphylococci causing focal infections, like conjunctivitis or omphalitis. These exotoxins act as "superantigens" by stimulating a large number of T cells to release lymphokines (interleukin-2, tumor necrosis factor). It is characterized by generalized erythematous rash, ruptured bullae with exudation, crusting and generalized exfoliation. Nikolsky sign is positive, i.e. skin easily peels off on rubbing. Toxic shock syndrome is caused by other exotoxins (TSST-1 and TSST-2) released by staphylococci. Toxic shock syndrome toxin is a superantigen with a size of 22 kDa produced by 5–25% of *Staphylococcus aureus* isolates. The manifestations occur early either due to intrauterine or intrapartum infection. It is characterized by fever, hypotension, shock and extensive erythematous skin rash. A similar clinical picture can be produced by

TABLE 26.7 Causes of neonatal erythroderma

Infections
Staphylococcal scalded skin syndrome
Toxic shock syndrome
Candidiasis

Immunodeficiency disorders
Omenn's syndrome
Graft-versus-host reaction
Ichthyosis
Non-bullous ichthyosiform erythroderma
Conradi-Hunermann syndrome
Bullous ichthyosiform erythroderma
Netherton's syndrome

Metabolic disorders
Disorders of biotin metabolism
Essential fatty acid deficiency

Drugs
Ceftriaxone
Vancomycin

Miscellaneous conditions
Infantile seborrheic dermatitis
Atopic dermatitis
Psoriasis
Pityriasis rubra pilaris
Generalized mastocytosis

streptococcal exotoxins. There may be evidences of concomitant maternal infection with *S. aureus*. Congenital cutaneous candidiasis occurs by ascending infection because vaginal candidiasis occurs in 20–25% of pregnant women. It is characterized by widely scattered macules, papules and pustules. The skin lesions become confluent and lead to development of exfoliative erythroderma. There is no oral thrush or bottom rash but it is usually associated with paronychia and dystrophy of nails. The course is usually benign.

Immunodeficiency Syndromes

Omenn syndrome is an autosomal recessive form of severe combined immunodeficiency (SCID). It is characterized by exfoliative erythroderma with diffuse alopecia, lymphadenopathy, hepatosplenomegaly, recurrent infections and failure to thrive. Laboratory findings include leukocytosis with eosinophilia, increased number of T lymphocytes and decreased number of B lymphocytes, hypogammaglobulinemia and raised IgE levels.

Graft-versus-host reaction is mainly seen in infants with T cell immunodeficiency but can occur in immunocompetent newborn babies due to transplacental passage of maternal lymphocytes during fetal life or following postnatal blood transfusion. It is characterized by fever, macular skin rash which may progress to erythroderma, lymphadenopathy, hepatosplenomegaly, lymphocytosis and eosinophilia.

Ichthyosiform Erythroderma

Non-bullous and bullous ichthyosiform erythroderma manifests at birth with variable degrees of erythroderma. Non-bullous variety manifests as collodion baby with "sausage-like" skin, ectropion, lip eversion and nasal obstruction. Bullous ichthyosiform erythroderma is characterized by superficial blisters with generalized erythema which can be mistaken with staphylococcal scalded skin syndrome and epidermolysis bullosa.

Netherton's syndrome is characterized by a triad of generalized erythematous exfoliative dermatitis, sparse "bamboo hair" and atopic features. There are no specific immunological abnormalities but serum IgE levels are elevated. Conradi-Hünermann syndrome may present at birth with erythroderma, skeletal abnormalities (chondrodysplasia punctata with epiphyseal stippling), cataracts and short stature. It is associated with EBP gene.

Metabolic Disorders

Holocarboxylase synthetase deficiency presents in neonatal period with erythroderma and alopecia. These infants may manifest with life-threatening ketoacidosis, dehydration and coma. Biotinidase deficiency presents after 3 months of age with lethargy, hypotonia, alopecia, seizures and skin lesions resembling acrodermatitis enteropathica. Essential fatty acid deficiency is known to present as ichthyosiform erythroderma.

Drugs

Erythroderma may occur in infants receiving ceftriaxone and vancomycin. Vancomycin when administered as a bolus may lead to generalized erythema ("The red man syndrome") due to release of histamine.

Miscellaneous Conditions

Infantile seborrheic dermatitis and atopic dermatitis are difficult to differentiate and may evolve through identical pathogenetic mechanisms. Atopic dermatitis spares nappy area and there is family history of atopy with encrusted eczema of scalp and face. There may be mild elevation of serum IgE levels. Diffuse cutaneous mastocytosis is characterized by numerous orange papules or diffuse erythema and generalized blistering of skin which mimics staphylococcal scalded skin syndrome. Darier's sign is positive, i.e. stroking of skin with a sharp object is followed by formation of wheal and flare reaction. Infiltration of mast cells at extracutaneous sites may manifest as diarrhea, vomiting, abdominal cramps, wheezing, pruritus and hypotension.

Management

Neonatal erythroderma is a medical emergency and often poses as a diagnostic and therapeutic challenge. Massive transcutaneous exudation may lead to hypernatremic dehydration, hypoalbuminemia, fever and shock. Hydration and electrolyte status should be maintained by adequate oral or parenteral fluid intake. Topical application of emollients (white soft paraffin) hydrates the skin and prevent fissuring. Diffuse blistering and exudative lesions should be treated by application of 0.01% potassium permanganate or normal saline soaks. Medicated creams containing salicylic acid or lactic acid should be avoided due to risk of transcutaneous absorption. Topical steroids should be sparingly used after confirming the diagnosis of atopic dermatitis. Intravenous antibiotic therapy with amoxycillin-clavulanic acid, cloxacillin or vancomycin is recommended for treatment of scalded skin syndrome and toxic shock syndrome. Intravenous immunoglobulins (IVIG) are recommended for management of latter condition. Congenital condidiasis is treated with topical and systemic antifungal therapy with amphotericin B and fluconazole. Oral biotin (5–10 mg/d) is useful for the treatment of holocarboxylase synthetase deficiency. Topical application of linoleic acid (sunflower seed oil) promptly clears skin lesions due to essential fatty acid deficiency. Mastocytosis is treated with oral administration of sodium cromoglycate and H_1 and H_2 antagonists. Bone marrow transplant is curative for treatment of Omenn syndrome and graft-versus-host reaction in infants with combined immunodeficiency disorder.

ICHTHYOSIS

Ichthyosis is an inherited skin disorder characterized by excessive scaling of the skin. The prevalence of disorder is around 5 to 8 per 1000 preschool children. Except in ichthyosis vulgaris, the characteristic severe scaling of skin is present at birth in the other three variants of ichthyosis.

Ichthyosis vulgaris The condition is inherited as an autosomal dominant. Scaliness of skin usually appears around one to two years of age and mostly affects buttocks and legs. Dry horny plugs around hair follicles are present. Palms and soles show an increased number of skin creases.

X-linked ichthyosis Infant is born with thick scales over the whole body except palms and soles which are spared. Corneal opacities may be seen on slit-lamp examination, both in the patient and carrier mother. Severely affected infant may present like a collodion baby.

Lamellar ichthyosis (congenital non-bullous ichthyosiform erythroderma) It is an autosomal recessive trait, characterized by broad thick scales and bright-red erythematous skin at birth. Some of the severely affected infants may appear like collodion baby as if a thick cellotape has been firmly applied over the whole skin. The skin is tightly stretched causing respiratory difficulty and eversion of eyelids (ectropian) and lips (eclabium). Thick scales and rounded small oral opening give a characteristic fish-like appearance to these babies (Figure 26.9). The skin of palms and soles is usually markedly thickened.

Epidermolytic hyperkeratosis (congenital bullous ichthyosiform erythroderma) This is an autosomal dominant disorder characterized by extensive scaling

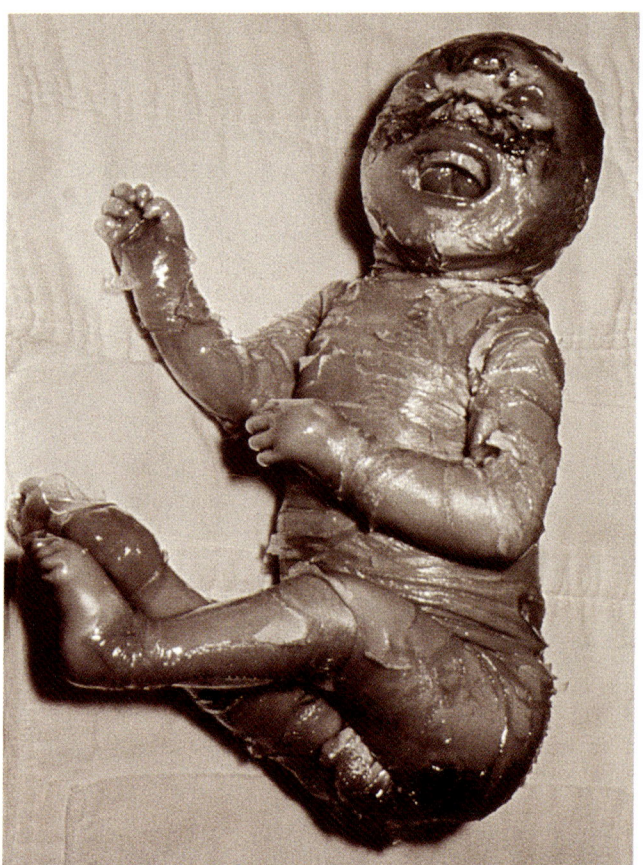

Figure 26.9 Typical appearances of a collodion baby.

of skin at birth, erythroderma and recurrent formation of skin bullae. The blisters appear due to lysis of epidermal granular layer and secondary infection with staphylococci is invariable producing pustular lesions. As the child grows, thick, warty, dirty-yellow malodorous skin lesions are seen over the palms, soles, elbows and knees.

Treatment

There is no satisfactory specific treatment. Collodion baby may be stillborn or die due to respiratory embarrassment. Skin should be protected against infection by strict asepsis. Application of liberal amounts of sterile lubricants and emollients is advised. The use of lactic acid 5% ointment applied once daily is often helpful in the more severe forms of ichthyosis. The therapeuctic utility of orally administered retinoids is still experimental.

VASCULAR NEVI

Vascular birth marks are hamartomas or benign tumor-like malformations composed of admixture of vascular components. They may be visible at birth or appear later during infancy. The vascular birth marks are classified into flat (macular) nevi and elevated (papular, nodular or tumor-like) nevi. They may spontaneously regress (involuting-type lesions) or persist as non-involuting lesions.

Flat Vascular Nevi

Involuting Type

Salmon patch (nevus simplex, stork bite) They are most common and found in almost 40% neonates and invariably disappear. They present as dull pink macules over the nape of neck, forehead and upper eyelids. They usually fade away during infancy, except nuchal erythemas which may persist much longer.

Spider nevus (nevus araneus) It is a small telangiectatic lesion consisting of a central arteriole from which superficial blood vessels radiate peripherally. The radiating vessels collapse when central punctum is pressed with a pinhead. They usually involute spontaneously.

Cutis marmorata telangiectasia congenita (congenital phlebectasia) It produces a mottled, marbled pattern of blue or dusky red erythema usually on an extremity. The skin surface overlying these lesions is depressed. There may be gradual increase in the size of lesions during early infancy followed by static or regressive phase. The condition should be distinguished from mottling of skin following exposure to cold which is a transient vasomotor phenomenon. The livedo reticularis pattern of collagen vascular disease (neonatal lupus erythematosus) is flat or macular (not depressed) and invariably bilateral in distribution.

Non-Involving Type

Portwine stain (nevus flammeus) It presents as deep red or purple-red macules over the face, neck or extremities with unilateral and segmental distribution. The color is usually light pink during infancy but tends to darken to become purple hued as age advances. Portwine stain over the extremity may be associated with enlargement of the soft tissues and hypertrophy of the underlying bone. The presence of the portwine stain over the face affecting the skin innervated by the ophthalmic branch of trigeminal nerve (level of eyelids and above) may be associated with Sturge-Weber syndrome. The syndrome is characterized by portwine stain, ipsilateral congenital glaucoma and leptomeningeal cerebral calcification due to meningeal angiomatosis by 2 years of age. Angiomatous malformation can be identified early by CT scan of brain. Glaucoma occurs in about one-half of patients with Sturge-Weber syndrome. Nevus flammeus is a recognized component of Rubinstein-Taybi syndrome (spinal arteriovenous malformation), Beckwith-Wiedemann and 13-trisomy syndromes. Portwine stain is best managed by camouflaging cosmetics. Excision, irradiation and cryosurgery are not recommended. The flash-lamp-pulsed laser therapy is the treatment modality of choice.

Raised Vascular Nevi

Involving Type

Hemangiomas (infantile hemangioma, strawberry nevus capillary hemangioma, hemangioma simplex) The lesions may not be present at birth and generally appear after 3 to 4 weeks of age. The reported incidence of infantile hemangioma is around 10% in infants below one year of age. The typical lesion is a dark-red or pinkish like a strawberry raised above the skin surface and compressible on pressure. Multiple skin hemangiomata may be associated with visceral hemangiomas in liver, lungs, gastrointestinal tract and central nervous system. It may be associated with hypertrophy of the underlying soft tissues and bones (Klippel-Trenaunay syndrome). During first 5 to 7 months, these nevi rapidly grow in size along with the somatic growth of the baby. This is followed by

involuting phase after the age of one year when central area of the lesion starts becoming pale and atrophic. The lesions may be complicated by ulceration, bleeding and infection. Cautery, irradiation, cryotherapy and CO_2 laser excision is not recommended because natural involution is followed by much better cosmetic outcome. Therapy with corticosteroids (prednisolone 1–2 mg/kg/day for 4 to 6 weeks) or topical/oral beta blocker (propranolol hydrochloride 0.5–1.0 mg/kg/day q 6–8 hr for 4–6 weeks) is indicated, if hemangioma is affecting a vital function (swallowing, breathing, vision, etc.), producing congestive heart failure or entrapping platelets and cause consumptive coagulopathy producing Kasabach-Merritt syndrome. It is associated with generalized bleeding tendency, large ecchymoses especially around hemangioma and visceral bleeding. Topical application of a cream containing corticosteroids or a beta blocker (tenolol) is associated with rapid involution of the lesion.

Non-Involving Type

Pyogenic granulomas and lymphangiomas are classified in this group but they are not truly vascular nevi. Lymphangiomas typically produce skin-colored dermal or subcutaneous diffuse, ill-defined mass containing dilated lymphatics. The lesion often hangs loosely, is compressible and transilluminant and feels like a bag of worms. They do not regress and are managed by surgical excision.

DISORDERS OF PIGMENTATION

Disorders of pigmentation of skin may be present at birth or appear subsequently. They may be present *de novo* or follow resolution of maculopapular skin lesions. They may provide useful clues to the underlying systemic disorders.

Hyperpigmentation

Flat Lesions

Mongolian spots Bluish pigmentation involving lumbosacral region, back and buttocks is seen at birth in over 80% of Asian children. At times bluish patches may be seen over shoulders, extremities and even face. They occur due to infiltration of melanocytes deep in the dermis. Their incidence is related to ethnic origin but they have no clinical significance. They gradually fade as child grows and may disappear by 2 to 3 years of age. They have no relationship to mongolism or Down syndrome.

Café au lait spots They are flat brown (coffee with milk color), round or oval skin lesions and may be present any where on the body. The spots may be present at birth or appear subsequently and persist throughout life. Large-sized café au lait spots (>5 cm) or when they are present in significant numbers (>5 spots) are suggestive of underlying neurofibromatosis. The skin biopsy of lesions shows differences in the appearances of melanosomes within the melanocytes. The presence of giant pigment granules is characteristic of neuro-fibromatosis. Apart from neurofibromatosis, tuberous sclerosis and other neuroectodermal disorders may be associated with café au lait spots.

Neurofibromatosis (von Recklinghausen's disease)

It is an autosomal recessive disorder characterized by development of multiple mixed neural and fibrous tumors in childhood. Café au lait spots are seen in over 90% of cases which may be present at birth or develop during infancy. The presence of large sized (>5 cm) or large number (>5 spots) of spots which are distributed in the axillary area has a very high association with underlying neurofibromatosis.

Junctional nevi They are brown or black nevi which are flat or slightly raised and usually present at birth. They occur at the junction of epidermis with the dermis as nests of cuboidal cells within melanocytes. The lesions are benign but may be excised for cosmetic reasons.

Albright syndrome During newborn period, the affected subject may have large, irregular, ragged, pigmented areas over the skin measuring 8 to 12 cm in size. The skin lesions are often limited to one side of the body. The syndrome is common among girls who present with polyostotic fibrous dysplasia, sexual preco-city, mental retardation and seizures during childhood.

Peutz-Jeghers syndrome The neonatal marker of this syndrome includes multiple, scattered hyperpigmented macules especially around the mouth, mucous membranes of mouth, hands and fingers. The typical manifestations of syndrome due to hamartomatous polyposis of the small bowel appear later in childhood in the form of bleeding per rectum and episode of intussusception. It is an autosomal dominant genetic disorder.

Raised Lesions

Giant hairy nevus (bathing trunk nevus) These are large, leathery rough, dark drown or black hairy nevi raised above the surface (Figure 26.10). They may involve 20–30% of body surface and may be associated with other pigmentary or CNS abnormalities. They have a tendency to progress to malignant melanoma later in life. Surgical excision though technically difficult, may be attempted for cosmetic reasons.

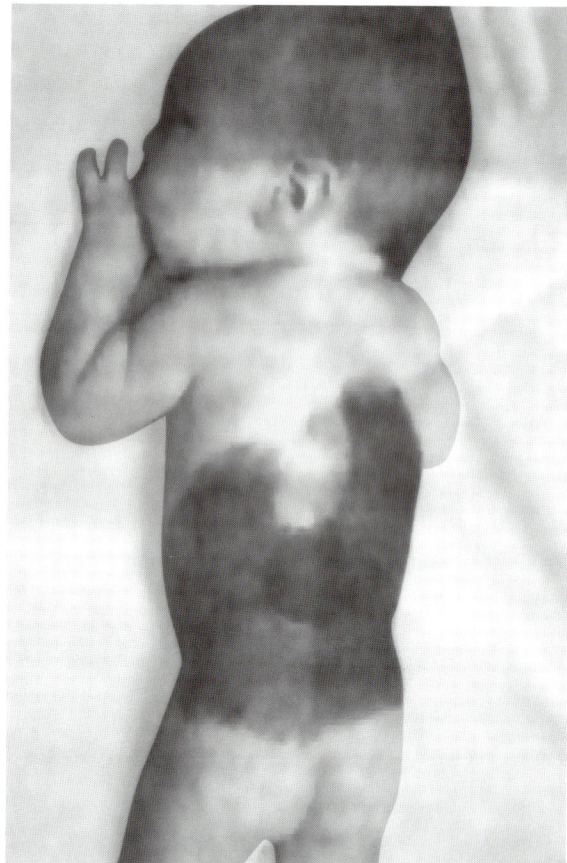

Figure 26.10 Giant pigmented hairy nevus.

Compound nevi They are large junctional nevi composed of melanocytes. They are slightly raised above the surface. Surgical excision is advised at the age of 5–6 years because of potential risk of malignant transformation later in life.

Diffuse hyperpigmentation Generalized hyper-pigmentation of skin may be seen due to racial/ethnic background, melanism, progressive familial hyper-pigmentation, generalized hereditary lentiginosis, congenital Addison's disease, Fanconi's syndrome and androgen excess due to congenital adrenal hyperplasia.

Hypopigmentation

Albinism It is an autosomal recessive disorder due to deficiency of tyrosinase enzyme. There is genera-lized and profound hypopigmentation involving skin, hair and eyes (red reflex in eyes). There is no specific treatment but skin should be protected from ultra-violet light and dark glasses worn to protect against photophobia.

Partial albinism (piebaldism) It is an autosomal recessive disorder with decreased penetrance. The skin and hair are involved in a patchy manner. There is a white "forelock" of hair. The condition may be associated with systemic disorders which should be looked for.

Waardenburg syndrome is characterized by lateral displacement of inner canthi and puncta of eyes, heterochromia of irides, deafness, white forelock and patchy pigmentation of skin. In Chediak-Higashi syndrome, partial albinism is associated with recurrent gingivitis, periodontitis, skin and respiratory infections due to neutrophil granule defects.

Vitiligo It is an autoimmune disorder characterized by patchy areas of decreased or absent pigmentation (leukoderma or "milk-like" patches) which may be present at birth but usually develop later in life. The skin lesions are seen mostly on the face, around the eyes and mouth, genitalia, hands and upper chest. The discolored patches may involve hair and mucous membranes. The condition may be aggravated by deficiencies of vitamin B_{12}, folate, copper and zinc. The condition is more commonly associated with hyperthyroidism, adrenal insufficiency, diabetes mellitus and pernicious anemia. Biopsy of the skin lesions show few or no melanocytes in the junctional layer.

Hypopigmented macules (white spots) There are white depigmented areas of skin with irregular border. They may be present at birth or appear subsequently. They are commonly associated with tuberous sclerosis.

Nevus anemicus The nevus consists of solitary or multiple, sharply delineated, pale macules that are mostly present on the trunk. The pale patches are generally present at birth but may not be detectable until early childhood. Firm stroking evokes an erythematous line and flare response in areas of pigment loss. It has been postulated that the persistent pallor may represent a sustained localized adrenergic vasoconstriction.

TWINS

Twin gestation occurs in 1 in 80 pregnancies. Over the years, the incidence of multiple births has increased due to late marriages, use of ovulation inducing drugs, intrauterine insemination and *in vitro* fertilization. The incidence of monozygous or identical twinning is constant at approximately 1 per 250 pregnancies and it results from single ovulation. Ultrasonography can detect multiple gestational sacs at 5 weeks and identify separate cardiac activity of each fetus at 6 weeks of gestation. Dizygous or non-identical twins result from double ovulation and are associated with higher gonadotropin secretion rates and administration of drugs (clomiphene) that induce ovulation. About two-thirds of all twins are dizygous and its incidence is influenced by heredity, race and maternal age. Family history of twinning among close relatives is usually present. Twin pregnancy is associated with higher incidence of pre-eclampsia, hemolysis, elevated liver enzymes and thrombocytopenia (HELLP), polyhydramnios, placenta previa and premature delivery. Multiple births are associated with higher risk of chromosomal anomalies and limb deformities, such as club feet, dislocated hips and craniosynostosis due to overcrowding of the intrauterine environment.

In normal circumstances, uterus is able to sustain the growth of two babies up to 33 weeks of gestation. Subsequently, the weight of each twin is lower than the singleton though their combined weight is more. The mean weight of monochorionic twins is lower as compared to the dichorionic twins but there may be marked discordance in the weight of monochorionic twins due to inter-twin transfusion syndrome.

Twin pregnancy must be diagnosed before labor so that adequate management is provided during delivery to improve their survival. Two pediatricians should be available to resuscitate the babies. Cord prolapse, entangling of two cords (monoamniotic twins) and rupture of vasaprevia are recognized complications of twin pregnancy. The second twin is at an increased risk of hypoxia, operative intervention, bleeding, hyaline membrane disease and intracranial hemorrhage (due to lack of molding). The second twin must be born within 15 minutes of delivery of the first baby for improved survival. The incidence of congenital anomalies in twins is twice compared to singletons. Due to crowding of uterine environment, there is greater risk of limb deformities, like club foot in multiple pregnancy. Twin-to-twin transfusion syndrome may occur in monochorionic twins due to arteriovenous anastomoses. The donor twin is pale and growth retarded while recepient twin is polycythemic and large in size. During early pregnancy, large arterial anastomoses between monochorionic twins may rarely cause vascular disruption sequence leading to low-pressure blood flow through the umbilical artery perfusing the upper part of the body. This may lead to development of a rare syndrome of acardia which is characterized by multiple congenital malformations of upper part of the body, like anencephaly, holoprosencephaly, rudimentary facial features, anomalies of upper limbs, thorax and abdominal organs.

Antenatal diagnosis of twin-to-twin transfusion syndrome (TTTS) can be made by sonographic evidences of discordance in fetal size (abdominal circumference difference of >20%), discrepancy in amniotic fluid volume of two sacs and the "stuck twin" sign (one twin is "stuck" to the uterine wall despite changes in the maternal position due to oligohydramniotic sac) and evidences of hydrops or congestive heart failure in one of the twins. The complications in the donor twin include anemia, hypovolemia, growth restriction, ischemic lesions in brain, renal insufficiency with oligohydramnios, lung hypoplasia and limb deformities. The clinical problems in recipient twin include polycythemia, polyhydramnios, fetal hyrops, thrombosis, cerebral emboli and disseminated intravascular coagulation. The outcome can be improved by serial amniocentesis to reduce polyhydramnios, microseptostomy of intertwin membrane and more recently by occlusion of vascular anastomosis by placental vascular Nd:YAG laser photocoagulation.

Zygosity of Twins

The zygosity can be determined on the basis of sex, examination of placenta, blood groups and HLA typing. Twins of different sexes are dizygous. If the placenta is monochorionic, the twins are monozygous. In dichorionic identical-sexed twins, zygosity can be established by blood grouping or HLA typing. It is important to establish the zygosity of twins which provides useful clues to the genetic basis of malformations or diseases, and is crucial for transplantation and skin grafting. About 5–10% of monochorionic twins are likely to have twin-to-twin transfusion syndrome.

Management

Perinatal morbidity is at least six to seven times among twins as compared to singletons. Delivery should be conducted by an experienced obstetrician and attended by two pediatricians to provide prompt attention to both the babies. The infants and placenta should be examined carefully for gestational maturity, growth disparity, twin-to-twin transfusion and zygosity. The disparity in the birth weight of more than 25% and in hemoglobin of more than 5 g/dL among the twins are suggestive of twin-to-twin transfusion. The perinatal mortality has been reported to be as high as 70% in twin-to-twin transfusion syndrome. The anemic twin should receive slow transfusion of packed red blood cells while polycythemic twin should be exchanged with plasma or physiological saline to reduce the complications due to hyperviscosity.

Twin babies impose considerable strain to the mother to look after their day-to-day problems, physiological and nutritional needs. Mother needs guidance, assurance and emotional support. Some mothers may be able to exclusively breastfeed both the babies though supplementary feeds are often required in most cases. The infant should be alternately fed on the breast and bottle/*paladay* so that neither of the baby is discriminated against and both obtain the nutritional and biological advantages of human milk. The follow-up studies of twins have shown that grossly smaller twin (weight at least 25% less than the bigger twin) is likely to remain significantly smaller in size and retarded in neuromotor development. If one of the monozygotic twins with vascular anastomoses die *in utero*, the surviving twin has a high risk of development of cerebral infarction, renal, hepatic and cutaneous damage due to hypotension and disseminated intravascular coagulation. The incidence of neurological sequelae is high and occurs in 25% of the surviving twin.

Conjoint Twins

Conjoint twins are rare with an overall reported incidence of 1 per 50,000–100,000 deliveries. These twins attract overwhelming public interest and pose numerous diagnostic, technical, ethical and emotional problems. The live born conjoint twins are extremely rare because majority of them terminate as abortions or stillbirths. The vast majority of live born conjoint twins die before or soon after separation. The external fusion may take place at any site. The ventrally fused conjoint twins at chest (thoracopagus) and/or abdomen are the most common accounting for 73% cases (Figure 26.11). The other conjoint twins include pyopagus (sacral) 19%, ischiopagus (pelvic outlet) 6% and craniopagus (cephalic) 2%. The conjoint twins are uniovular in origin. The female conjoint twins are 3 to 10 times more common than males. Polyhydramnios is associated in 50% cases and may require amnioreduction. Delivery should be conducted by elective cesarean section. The famous siamese twins, Chang and Eng were born of Chinese parents in Siam and lived from 1811 to 1874.

The successful surgical separation of conjoint twins depends upon the site of fusion, and extent of sharing of body organs. At times sacrifice of one baby is unavoidable which must be explained to the parents. The investigations are conducted to determine the extent of fusion of internal organs and cross-circulation between the two babies to assess the chances of their independent existence and viability. Medical management is directed to maintain asepsis, ensure adequate nursing and feeding to prepare them for surgical separation. Medications, when indicated, are administered separately to each twin. The successful

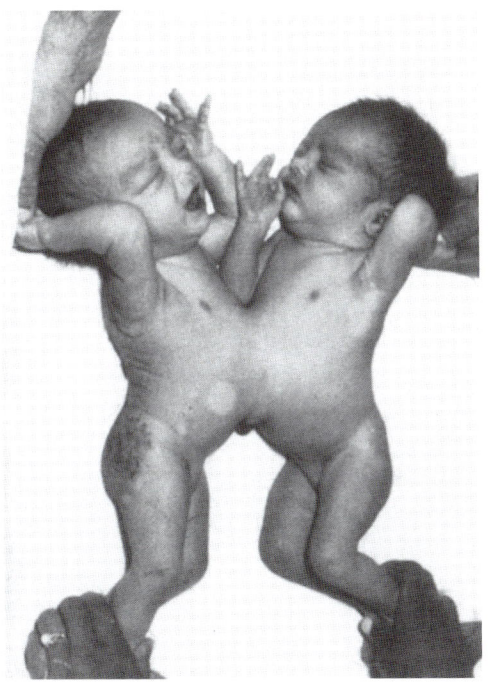

Figure 26.11 Thoracopagus siamese twins. They were successfully operated.

management demands a close interaction and cooperation between the neonatologist, pediatric surgeon, anesthetist, radiologist, radionuclear specialist and other experts depending upon the associated major problems.

IATROGENIC DISORDERS

Iatrogenic disorders refer to development of "disasters of our good intentions" as a consequence of treatment by the physician or surgeon. It includes all adverse outcomes of diagnostic and/or therapeutic interventions whether due to lack of physician's skills, inherent hazards of intervention or susceptibility of the host due to the severity of the underlying disorder. Due to rapid strides and advances in medical technology, the patients are being exposed to newer therapeutic agents and instruments, thus resulting in increased incidence of iatrogenic disorders. Because of anatomical and physiological immaturity, newborn babies are at a greater risk to suffer damage from drugs and a host of new electronic monitoring gadgets. The incidence

From inability to let well alone, too much zeal for the new and contempt for what is old, from putting knowledge before wisdom, science before art and cleverness before common-sense, from treating patients as cases, from making the cure of the disease more grievous than endurance of the same, good Lord deliver us.

Sir Robert Hutchison

of physician-induced morbidity is related to the experience of the physician and his team in the use of newer therapeutic regimes and instruments. It is desirable to assess or consider benefit-to-harm ratio of any modality of therapy introduced for management of sick newborns. The iatrogenic disorders may be preventable but at times they are unavoidable.

Fetal and Neonatal Disorders due to Maternal Medications

Fetus and newborn baby may be unavoidably exposed to the hazards of drugs administered to pregnant or lactating mothers. Due to biochemical and metabolic handicaps, fetus and newborn babies are extremely vulnerable to toxic effects of drugs which may be entirely safe for the adults.

Fetal Drug Hazards

Unavoidable transplacental fetal medication as a result of administration of drugs to pregnant women result in abortion, congenital malformations and several neonatal disorders (*see* Table 5.1 in Chapter 5). The list of chemotherapeutic agents which may be hazardous to the fetus is ever increasing. From fetal standpoint, no drug is entirely safe during pregnancy. As far as possible, all drugs should be avoided during first trimester of pregnancy which is characterized by embryogenesis or organogenesis and exposure to drugs during this phase may cause developmental defects. A drug which may be abortifacient in a large dose, may induce congenital malformation when taken in an optimal dose during critical phase of fetal development. While prescribing any medicines to the pregnant women, it is mandatory to ask oneself a few questions. Is medication indicated? Is the disease more dangerous as regards fetal safety when compared to the known hazards of the therapeutic agent? Has the drug withstood the test of time? The newer therapeutic agents are not recommended for use during pregnancy unless their teratogenic potentiality has been ruled out by studies in experimental animals. The expectant mothers should be advised to avoid self-medications and told about hazards of various addictions to their unborn child. Among married women, the diagnostic radiological studies should be restricted to the 2 weeks of post-menstruation period during which one is certain that she is not pregnant. Pelvic X-rays should not be taken during first trimester of pregnancy.

Neonatal Drug Hazards

Most chemotherapeutic agents taken by the lactating mothers are excreted in her milk though generally in small or insignificant concentrations. *Therefore, by and large, what is safely tolerated by the nursing mother, is generally safe for her suckling infant.* Drugs which should be avoided by nursing mother are listed in Chapter 5. Medications to sick newborn babies are also fraught with dangers of toxicity because they have hepatic and renal immaturity to detoxify and excrete the drugs. Hyperbilirubinemia and/or acute bilirubin encephalopathy may occur at relatively lower serum bilirubin levels during therapy with synthetic vitamin K, sulfisoxazole, salicylates, caffein, lobeline, cedalinid, novobiocin and gentamicin. Chloramphenicol when administered in a dose exceeding 75 mg/kg per day may lead to development of 'gray baby syndrome' characterized by grayish circumoral cyanosis, abdominal distension, vomiting and circulatory collapse. Tetracyclines have been shown to cause growth retardation and brownish discoloration of deciduous or primary teeth by virtue of their chelation with calcium. Streptomycin, kanamycin, neomycin and colistin may cause respiratory paralysis by blockage of muscle end-plate when applied locally over large raw surfaces or after intraperitoneal instillation. Bolus administration of intravenous sodium bicarbonate may be associated with intraventricular hemorrhage and acute left heart failure with pulmonary hemorrhage. Sodium bicarbonate 7.5% solution has an approximate osmolarity of 2000 mOsm/L. It must be diluted with equal volume of distilled water or double volume of 5% dextrose and administered at a rate of 0.1 mEq/kg/minute. Hexachlorophene skin applications, without effective rinsing, can result in diarrhea, dehydration, shock, seizures and neuromuscular disturbances. Boric acid application over large raw areas may lead to diarrhea, vomiting, generalized skin rash, hepatic necrosis and renal failure.

It is desirable that drugs in the newborn should be used when absolutely indicated and only those agents which have been well tried in the newborn period should be prescribed. Disorders due to developmental peculiarities and physiological handicaps do not require any therapy. Overdosage by accidental use of vials intended for adults, e.g. vitamin K and nalorphine, should be avoided. It is desirable to use insulin or tuberculin syringes for ease and accuracy of administration of drugs. The proprietary combinations should be avoided because of risk of inadvertent over-dosage of one of the agents. Due to prolongation of half-life of most of the drugs because of hepato-renal immaturity, dosage schedule of 8 to 12 hourly is sufficient and desirable during neonatal period.

Oxygen Toxicity

The occurrence of retinopathy of prematurity (ROP) and blindness as a result of increased oxygen concentration of arterial blood in premature babies is well known. When PaO_2 values exceed 90 mm Hg, vaso-obliteration of immature arteries may lead to ROP and its cicatricial consequences. It is estimated that about 35–65% of infants weighing less than 1500 g may develop ROP. Bronchopulmonary dysplasia or chronic lung disease due to interaction of ambient oxygen toxicity, ventilator barotrauma and left-to-right shunt through PDA can occur in low birth weight infants.

To prevent iatrogenic damage due to oxygen therapy, it is desirable that FiO_2 should be maintained between 0.4 and 0.6 and PaO_2 should be monitored and kept between 50 and 80 mm Hg. Vitamin E is a biologic antioxidant that inhibits the peroxidation of membrane lipids by free radicals, such as superoxide. There are conflicting reports regarding the prophylactic utility of vitamin E for protection against ROP and bronchopulmonary dysplasia.

Disorders due to Procedures

A large number of diagnostic and therapeutic procedures carry potential risk to the fetus and newborn. Amniocentesis may cause premature labor, amnionitis, fetomaternal hemorrhage with enhanced Rh-iso-immunization, if there is Rh-incompatibility between the mother and the fetus. Oropharyngeal and endotracheal suction of the newborn at birth should be gentle, intermittent and limited to a negative pressure of 100 mm Hg (1.0 mm Hg = 1.36 cm H_2O) otherwise mucosal bleeding, bradycardia and cardiac arrest may occur. Gastrointestinal bleeding may occur from esophagus and stomach due to indwelling catheters and vigorous suction. During resuscitation, an endotracheal tube placed too far into right bronchus, may obstruct the left main bronchus causing atelectasis of left lung. Rectal perforation, hemorrhage and peritonitis have been reported due to faulty insertion of rectal thermometer. To avoid rectal perforation, it is mandatory that thermometer should be directed slightly posteriorly and should not be inserted beyond 2 cm. Skin burns due to hot water bottle though uncommon is a potential hazard, if due caution is not exercised in its use. Intravenous infusions are fraught with dangers of local infection, extravasations and over or under infusion.

Administration of 30–40 mL of excess infusate may lead to circulatory overload and peripheral congestion. Exchange blood transfusion is associated with dangers inherent to umbilical cannulation and mismatched transfusion. There may be shock or over loading of circulation, hypothermia, apnea, cardiac arrest, electrolyte and biochemical changes. Necrotizing enterocolitis (NEC) may occur due to vasospasm and ischemia of gut. Umbilical vein catheter should be placed in the thoracic inferior vena cava, otherwise injection of hypertonic glucose or sodium bicarbonate may cause focal hepatic necrosis. Umbilical artery catheterization is associated with risk of blanching, discoloration and gangrene over the buttock or leg. Parenteral nutrition is associated with hazards of sepsis, biochemical, metabolic and electrolyte disturbances, deficiency of vitamins and trace elements, cholestatic jaundice and bleeding manifestations. The intravenous fluids and TPN solutions should be prepared under a laminar hood and strict asepsis should be maintained during insertion of catheter. Intralipid should preferably be infused through a "Y" connector and frequent biochemical monitoring should be ensured. The tubings and parenteral nutrients are a potential source of nosocomial septicemia and candidemia.

Iatrogenic anemia may occur as a result of frequent blood sampling for various investigations. It is generally not appreciated that removal of 10 mL of blood from 1500 g neonate constitutes a loss of about 8% of his blood volume (equivalent to about 400 mL of blood in an adult). It is desirable to establish ultra-microbiochemical techniques in the nursery as a safeguard against iatrogenic anemia. Apart from hazards of mismatched blood transfusion, it is associated with potential risk of transmission of life-threatening diseases, like malaria, syphilis, AIDS, CMV, and hepatitis (due to HBV and HCV). Avoidance of professional blood donors and availability of adequate screening facilities in all blood banks can reduce this complication. There is a potential risk of development of graft-versus-host reaction unless irradiated blood is used.

Hazards due to Intensive Care Equipment

Over the past two decades or so, there has been tremendous growth of biomedical engineering technology resulting in the production of a large number of sophisticated electronic gadgets. The electronic engineers have fabricated a variety of mini-transducers, microprocessors and mini-pumps which have revolutionized the intensive care of the newborn. Though non-invasive and extremely useful, some of the monitoring and therapeutic gadgets do carry

certain avoidable hazards and risks. They are a potential source of nosocomial infections which should be guarded against by vigorous aseptic routines and use of disposable materials as far as possible. Incubators and ventilators pose grave risk of nosocomial infections because of warmth and humidity. There is a risk of electrical shock and fire hazard which should be safeguarded by proper insulation and grounding. Failure of alarm system may result in hyperthermia, over-infusion and hyperoxia. In a servo-controlled incubator or open care system, if sensor is dislodged, the baby may get overheated, if it lacks an alarm system. Extensive air leaks, pneumothorax and bronchopulmonary dysplasia may occur following mechanical ventilation with continuous positive airway pressure (CPAP) or positive end expiratory pressure (PEEP). Bronchopulmonary dysplasia is a recognized complication due to exposure of air passages to high concentrations of oxygen and barotrauma. Necrotizing tracheobronchitis may occur in infants managed with high frequency jet ventilation. Burns often occur at $tcPO_2$ sensor sites which must be changed every 2 to 3 hours. There is a risk of noise hazard to the infant which is difficult to quantify or evaluate.

However, the advantages of intensive care equipment far outweigh their hazards which can be minimized by proper care and vigilance during their use. Equipment worth millions of rupees is useless and often dangerous, if there are no experienced and trained medical and nursing personnel to use them. It is desirable to consider benefit to harm ratio of every new modality of monitoring or therapeutic regimen. The avoidable hazards should be identified and safeguarded. By and large, over zealous therapeutic attempts should be curbed and tampered by one's own experience, expertise and resources. For example, it is certainly more desirable to reduce risk of nosocomial infections before contemplating to purchase ventilators and $tcPO_2$ monitors.

BIBLIOGRAPHY

American Academy of Pediatrics, American Association for Pediatric Ophthalmology and Strabismus, American Academy of Ophthalmology. Screening examination of premature infants with retinopathy of prematurity. *Pediatrics* 2006, 117(2): 572–576.

Askie LM, Henderson-Smart DJ, Ko H. Restricted versus liberal oxygen exposure for preventing morbidity and mortality in preterm or low birth weight infants. *Cochrane Database of Systematic Reviews* 2009, issue1. Art. No. CD 001077.

26

Barnes SE, Bryan EM, Harris DA, Baum JD. Edema in the newborn. In Molecular aspects of Medicine. Baum D and Gergely J (Ed.) *Pergamon Press, Oxford* 1977, 1: 222.

Cleary-Goldman J, D'Alton ME, Berkowitz RL. Prenatal diagnosis and multiple pregnancy. *Semin Perinatol* 2005, 29: 312–320.

Cordero I, Franco A, Joy SD. Monochorionic monoamniotic twins: Neonatal outcome. *J Perinatol* 2006, 26: 170–175.

Dogra MR, Katoch D, Dogra M. An update on retinopathy of prematurity (ROP). *Indian J Pediatr* 2017, 84(12):930–6.

Fagan IDG. Iatrogenic problems in neonatal intensive care. In: Fetal and Neonatal Pathology. Baron AJ (ed.) *Eastbourne Praeger,* 1982.

Finer NN. Nasal cannula use in the preterm infant: Oxygen or pressure? *Pediatrics* 2005, 116: 1216–1217.

Gilbert C, Foster A. Childhood blindness in the context of vision 2020—the right to sight. *Bull World Health Organ* 2001, 19: 227–232.

Gupta SK. Clinical approach to a neonate with cyanosis. *Indian J Pediatr* 2015, 82(11):1050–60.

Harigopal S, Satish HP, Taktak AF, *et al.* Oxygen saturation profile in healthy preterm infants. *Arch Dis Child Fetal Neonatal (Ed)* 2011, 96: F339–F342.

Harrison MR, Filly RA, Globus MS, *et al.* Fetal treatment. *N Engl J Med* 1982, 307: 1651.

Hoeger PH, Harper JI. Neonatal erythroderma: Differential diagnosis and management of a "red baby". *Arch Dis Child* 1998, 79: 186–191.

International Committee for Retinopathy of Prematurity. The international classification of retinopathy of prematurity revisited. *Arch Ophthalmol* 2005, 123 (7): 991–999.

Jacobs AH. Vascular nevi. *Pediatr Clin N Amer* 1983, 30: 465.

Jain L, Vidyasagar D. Iatrogenic disorders in modern neonatology. *Clin Perinatol* 1989, 16: 255.

Jalali S, Anand R, Kumar H, *et al.* Programme planning and screening strategy in retinopathy of prematurity. *Indian J Ophthalmol* 2003, 51(1): 89–99.

Jalali S, Hussain A, Matalia J, Anand R. Modification of screening criteria for retinopathy of prematurity in India and other middle-income group countries. *Am J Opthalmol* 2006, 14(5): 966–968.

Lees MH. Cyanosis of the newborn infant : Recognition and clinical evaluation. *J Pediatr* 1970, 77: 484.

Longhead JL. Congenital staphylococcal scalded skin syndrome. *Pediatr infect Dis J* 1992, 11: 413

Lopriose E, Vandenbussche FPHA, Tiersma ESM, *et al.* Twin-to-Twin transfusion: New perspectives. *J Pediatr* 1995, 127: 675–680.

Machin GA. Differential diagnosis of hydrops fetalis. *Am J Med Gen* 1981, 9: 341–50.

Madathil S, Anand P, Deorari AK, *et al.* Non-immune hydrops in neonates: A tertiary care center experience. *Indian Pediatr* 2020, 57:321–23.

Makhamreh MM, Cottingham N, Ferreira CR, Berger S, Al-Koutly HB. Nonimmune hydrops fetalis and congenital disorders of glycosylation: A systematic literature review. *J Inherit Metabol Dis* 2019, 43(2):480–5.

Moise KJ Jr. Dorman K, Iamvu G, *et al.* A randomized trial of amnioreduction versus septostomy in the treatment of twin-to-twin transfusion syndrome. *Am J Obstet Gynecol* 2005, 193: 701–707.

Photographic Screening for ROP Cooperative Group. The photographic screening for ROP study. *Retina* 2008, 28: S47–S54.

Quiram PA, Capone A. Current understanding and management of retinopathy of prematurity. *Current Opin Ophthalmol* 2007, 18: 228–234.

Ramamurthy RS, Reveri M, Esterly NB, *et al.* Transient neonatal pustular melanosis. *J Pediatr* 1976, 88: 831–835.

Raval DS, Barton LL, Hansen RC, Kling PJ. Congenital cutaneous candidiasis: a case report and review. *Pediatr Dermatol* 1995, 12: 355–358.

Robertson NRC, Gupta JM, Dahlenburg GW, Tizard JPM. Oxygen therapy in the newborn. *Lancet* 1968, 2: 1323.

Saugstad OD. Oxygen toxicity in the neonatal period. *Acta Paediatr Scand* 1990, 79(10): 881–92.

Shukla R, Murthy GVS, Mukpalkar S. Operational guidelines for ROP in India: A summary. *Indian J Ophthal* 2020, 68(supple 1):S108–S114.

Singh M. Iatrogenic disorders of the fetus and the newborn as a result of maternal medications. *Indian Pediatr* 1975, 12: 603.

Tin W, Gupta S. Optimum oxygen therapy in preterm babies. *Arch Dis Child Fetal Neonatal Ed* 2007, 92(2): F143–F147.

Tizard JPM. Indications for oxygen therapy in the newborn. *Pediatrics* 1964, 34: 771.

Vhing MR. Management of birth injuries. *Clin Perinatol* 2005, 32: 19–38.

Vinekar A, Dogra MR, Sangtam T, *et al.* Retinopathy of pre-maturity in Asian Indian babies weighing greater than 1250 g at birth: Ten year data from a tertiary care center in a developing county. *Indian J Opthalmol* 2007, 55(5): 331–336.

Xiao Q, Li Q, Zhang B, Yu W. Propranolol therapy of infantile hemangiomas: Efficacy, adverse effects and recurrence. *Pediatr Surg Int* 2013, 29: 575–81.

Zhao CY, Murrell DF. Blistering diseases in neonates. *Current Opin Pediatr* 2016,28(4):500–6

Assisted Ventilation and Advanced Life Support

During the last three decades or so, the technology has revolutionized the care of extremely small and critically sick newborn babies. It is essential and mandatory to establish neonatal advanced life support facilities in neonatal intensive care unit to enhance newborn survival. Availability of optimal neonatal resuscitation facilities can go a long way to ensure intact survival of babies with perinatal hypoxia and birth asphyxia. Many critically sick babies who develop life-threatening apnea or cardiovascular collapse from a variety of causes, need cardio-pulmonary resuscitation. Infants with progressive respiratory distress with impending respiratory failure or tiring respiratory muscles, can be supported and saved by assisted ventilation facilities. Mechanical ventilation and advanced life support facilities demand optimal infrastructure, essential monitoring and therapeutic equipment and specially trained pediatricians and nurses to provide state-of-the-art facilities and expertise to look after babies admitted in the NICU.

BAG AND MASK VENTILATION (BMV)

It is a very effective procedure for cardiopulmonary resuscitation of asphyxiated or apneic newborn babies. It is a life-saving procedure and all the health personnel concerned with the care of newborn babies should be skilled to provide effective bag and mask ventilation. The anesthesia bags (flow-inflating bags) are more effective to deliver higher concentrations (almost 100%) of oxygen but they are more difficult to use and require high flow rates of oxygen. Most pediatricians are conversant with self-inflating Ambu or Laerdal bags which are more convenient to use. It is possible to deliver 90% oxygen by attaching a corrugated tube or a rubber bladder as a reservoir to the self-inflating bag.

Equipment

The pediatricians should be familiar with the type of bag and mask being used in their institution. The self-inflating, as the name implies, inflates automatically without flow of oxygen or compressed air source. The salient components of self-inflating bag are shown in Figure 27.1. The capacity of bag for use in newborn babies should not exceed 750 mL (250–750 mL). Term neonates require 20–30 mL air with each ventilation (tidal volume being 5–8 mL/kg). The air inlet is the largest opening, having one-way valve, and is located at the rear end. The oxygen reservoir (either corru-gated tube or a closed rubber bladder) can be attached at the air inlet to increase the concentration of oxygen being delivered to the infant. The oxygen inlet is located near the air inlet. It is a small nipple or projection to

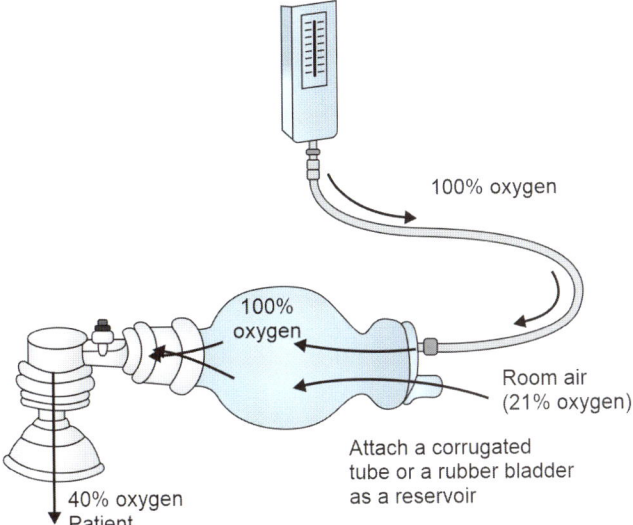

Figure 27.1 Salient components of a self-inflating bag. Attachment of oxygen reservoir at the air inlet is essential to ensure delivery of high concentration of oxygen to the baby.

which oxygen tubing can be attached. The bag can, however, be used in an emergency without attaching oxygen but it will deliver only 21% of oxygen contained in the atmosphere. The air-oxygen mixture is forced out from the patient outlet to which an appropriate sized mask or endotracheal tube is attached. The one-way valve assembly is positioned between the bag and patient outlet. It allows delivery of oxygen to the outlet when bag is squeezed but closes as soon as the bag is released so that exhaled air cannot re-enter the bag. Due to the presence of valve assembly, the self-inflating bag cannot be used for providing free-flow oxygen.

The self-inflating bags should have at least one of the two safety mechanisms. The pop-off valve (pressure-release valve) can be set to actuate when inflation pressure exceeds 30–35 cm H_2O. In some self-inflating bags (especially Laerdal variety), there is a provision to attach a pressure gauge at a point located near the patient outlet. The gauge allows the person using the bag to control the pressure of the air or oxygen being delivered to the patient. The silicone-rubber bags and masks of Laerdal make are more sturdy and can withstand autoclaving and can be readily cleaned with antiseptic solutions. The self-inflating bag and masks available in the Indian market are unsatisfactory due to poor quality of rubber and inflatability of bag, lack of oxygen inlet and absence of any safety features including pop-off valve.

Different types, shapes and sizes (Ambu OA, Rendell-Baker, Bennet, Laerdal, Ohio) of face masks are available. Soft circular masks with cushioned rim are preferable because they can form an effective seal on the face, and are less likely to leak or cause damage to infant's eyes. The moulded triangular (anatomically shaped) masks are not preferred. The correct size of the mask for each infant should be chosen so that it snugly encloses the nose and mouth of the infant. The siliconized rubber masks can be more easily cleaned and sterilized as they can withstand boiling and autoclaving. The bag and mask assembly should be checked before hand while anticipating delivery of an asphyxiated baby. The bag should be squeezed while making an airtight seal of face mask with the palm of your hand to assess functioning of valve assembly, pop-off valve and leakage or tears in the bag. After attaching the pressure gauge you can practice and train yourself to deliver desired inspiratory pressures for initial breaths (30–40 cm H_2O), subsequent breaths (15–20 cm H_2O) and for ventilation of neonates with reduced lung compliance (20–40 cm H_2O). One should be completely familiar with the types of bags and masks and other equipment being used in their unit.

Indications

Bag and mask ventilation is indicted, if an asphyxiated baby fails to establish satisfactory ventilation and cardiac status (heart rate <100/min) despite adequate suctioning and clearing of airways and tactile stimulation. Most asphyxiated neonates can be effectively resuscitated with a bag and mask ventilation alone. It is also indicated for cardiopulmonary resuscitation of critically sick neonates who are unable to maintain effective ventilation or develop prolonged apneic attacks. The infant is supported with bag and mask ventilation during brief periods while changing or suctioning the endotracheal tube in ventilated babies. Bag and mask ventilation is contraindicated in infants with diaphragmatic hernia because hernial contents will get overinflated by the procedure, resulting in further displacement of mediastinum and respiratory embarrassment. The meconium-stained babies should be bagged only after effective tracheal suctioning has been done to suck out all the meconium from the air passages. BMV is ineffective, if there is complete obstruction of upper airway. When prolonged positive pressure ventilation is required, it is best to intubate the infant and attach him to a ventilator.

Procedure

The infant should be positioned supine and neck slightly extended by placing a thin roll of towel under the shoulders. The operator should stand beyond the head end of the infant or to one side and should have unobstructed view of the chest and abdomen. After slightly lifting the jaw, apply a proper sized mask to snuggly enclose the nose and mouth of the baby. The mask is held in place by the non-dominant (left hand in a right-handed person and *vice versa*) hand with the help of thumb and index finger while ring finger holds and lifts the chin of the baby. There should be no pressure either on the eyes or trachea. The face mask must establish an airtight seal with the face. Start compressing the bag with your finger tips (after connecting it to an oxygen source and attaching oxygen reservoir) at a rate of 40/min (say one, two, squeeze to maintain this rate). Avoid squeezing the bag with the palm of whole hand due to the risk of pneumothorax. There should be noticeable rise and fall of chest with each inflation. It should be associated with good air entry on both sides of the chest, improvement in color and heart rate. If the chest does not expand adequately, reconfirm that face mask is forming an effective seal, airway is open and enough pressure is being applied on the bag which does not have any leakage or tears. Oropharyngeal airway may be inserted, if a large tongue or glossoptosis and nasal obstruction (bilateral choanal atresia) are posing difficulties. When prolonged (>5 minutes) bag and mask ventilation is contemplated, it is preferable to insert 8 Fr orogastric tube to aspirate the stomach contents in order to prevent abdominal distension.

During bag and mask ventilation of an asphyxiated baby at birth, check heart rate after every 15–20 seconds. To save time, heart rate is checked for 6 seconds only and multiplied by 10 to get heart rate/min. If despite adequate bag and mask ventilation with 100% oxygen (as evidenced by adequate bilateral expansion and deflation of chest with each bagging) the heart rate is not picking up and remains below 60/min, it is best to intubate the child (to provide bag and tube ventilation) and start external cardiac massage.

TRACHEAL INTUBATION

It is one of the most skilled and often a life-saving procedure which every pediatrician must learn; practice and achieve perfection. It is a difficult skill to maintain unless it is practiced regularly. It can be learnt on a manikin having resuscitation head or on stillborn and dead newborn babies.

Indications

- Bag and mask ventilation is ineffective to resuscitate an asphyxiated baby.
- Tracheal suctioning is required (meconium or milk aspiration).
- Ventilation of infants with diaphragmatic hernia.
- Prolonged positive-pressure ventilation (hypoxic-ischemic encephalopathy, hyaline membrane disease, pulmonary hypertension or persistent fetal circulation, prolonged apneic attacks and postoperatively).

Equipment

Pencil handle laryngoscope with straight blade (0 and 1 size) with extra set of batteries and bulb, disposable gamma-irradiated endotracheal tubes with an internal diameter of 2.5 mm, 3.0 mm, 3.5 mm and 4.0 mm, suctioning device, shoulder roll, adhesive tape, scissors, and resuscitation bag and mask should be available. The endotracheal tubes with a uniform diameter throughout the length (as opposed to tubes with tapered end) are preferred. The presence of vocal cord guide, as a black line near the tip of the tube, is useful to ensure that tip of the ET tube is at the optimal level. When vocal cord guide is placed at the level of vocal cords, the tip of the tube shall be just above the bifurcation of trachea. Table 27.1 gives guidelines for the approximate size and length of ET tubes required in babies of different sizes.

TABLE 27.1 Guidelines for endotracheal tube sizes and lengths

Birth weight (g)	Internal diameter (mm)	Tube length* to be inserted from lips (cm)	Tube length** to be inserted beyond vocal cords (cm)
< 1000	2.5	6.0	2.2
1000	3.0	7.0	2.4
1500	3.0	7.5	2.4
2000	3.5	8.0	2.6
2500	3.5	8.5	2.6
3000	4.0	9.0	2.8
> 4000	4.0	10.0	2.8

*Can be calculated by adding 6 to the weight of the baby in kg

**For nasotracheal intubation, the length of tube to be inserted is about 1–2 cm more compared to orotracheal intubation

Procedure

In most situations, orotracheal intubation is done which is easier but the tube can get dislodged readily. Nasotracheal intubation is more difficult and cumbersome but is preferred when prolonged ventilation is required. The availability and working of all the equipment required should be checked. An appropriate sized ET tube should be selected and shortened to 13 cm size so that no more then 4 to 5 cm of the tube projects beyond the infant's lips. The shortening of the tube reduces the dead space and prevents kinking. The ET tube connector should be fitted on the cut end of the tube. The suction source should be readily available to provide 100 cm H_2O negative pressure.

Orotracheal Intubation

Place the infant supine with head slightly extended by placing a roll of towel under the shoulders. Stand beyond the head end of the baby which is placed near the edge of the table. Before intubation, improve the oxygenation and condition of the baby by administration of 100% oxygen through bag and mask ventilation for 3 to 4 minutes. Turn on the laryngoscope light and hold the laryngoscope in your left hand (both for right- and left-handed individuals) with the blade pointing away from you. Stabilize the infant's head with your right hand. The laryngoscope blade is inserted and slided over the tongue. The tip of the blade is advanced beyond the base of the tongue till it rests in the vellecula (area between the base of the tongue and the epiglottis). At this point, the entire blade is lifted by pulling it forwards in the direction of the handle and not by tilting the handle backwards (Figure 27.2).

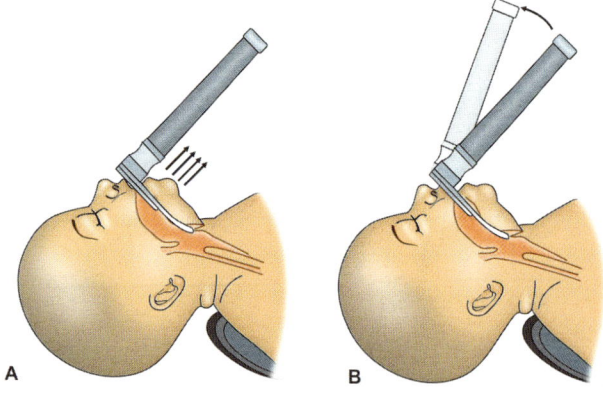

Figure 27.2 Endotracheal intubation. Note the correct procedure of lifting forward the laryngoscope blade to expose the glottic opening (A). The handle of the laryngoscope should not be tilted backwards (B).

By lifting the epiglottis by tip of the blade and by applying gentle pressure over the cricoid area (by the little and ring finger of the hand holding the laryngoscope or by an assistant), the glottic opening with all its landmarks is exposed to the view. The secretions, if any, should be sucked before the ET tube is inserted. Hold the ET tube in your right hand and introduce it into the right side of the infant's mouth. Keep the glottis in view and insert the tube until the vocal cord guide is at the level of the vocal cords. Hold the tube firmly at the lips with fingers of your right hand while keeping the baby's head stabilized. Gently remove the laryngoscope without displacing the tube. Note the centimeter mark on the tube at the level of the lips as a future guide so that it is readily identified when tube slips out.

Connect the ET tube to a bag and ventilate the infant. There should be visible rise of the chest with each ventilation with equal intensity of breath sounds on both sides of the chest (nipple level) and without any air entering the stomach or abdominal distension. Ascertain the correct position of the ET tube by taking a skiagram of chest when prolonged assisted ventilation is required. If the breath sounds are unilateral or unequal on two sides, the tube should be withdrawn by 1 cm and its placement rechecked. It is not unusual for the ET tube to enter the esophagus, when no breath sounds are heard in the chest and air is heard entering the stomach and causing abdominal distension. The procedure should be repeated again to insert the tube into the trachea. In order to minimize the dangers of hypoxia, intubation attempt should be limited to 20 seconds. The infant should be stabilized in between the attempts by ventilating with a bag and mask.

Nasotracheal Intubation

It is technically more difficult but may be required when prolonged ventilation is anticipated. Polyvinyl ET tube is inserted through one of the nostrils and visualized in the pharynx with the help of laryngoscope. The glottis and its landmarks are identified as described *vide supra*. The ET tube is grasped with McGill forceps and guided through the glottis into the trachea for the desired length. End-tidal carbon dioxide ($ETCO_2$) monitor is useful to confirm the tracheal location of the tube but it does not provide any information regarding the depth of insertion of ET. The tip of endotracheal tube should lie within 0.5–1.0 cm from upper border of arch of aorta as assessed by point-of-care ultrasonography or between T_2 and T_3 vertebral bodies as confirmed by chest radiograph taken with a portable bed side 100 mA radiograph machine.

Complications

In experienced hands, endotracheal intubation is a safe procedure. Trauma to soft structures in the mouth, hypopharynx, larynx and esophagus may occur by rough handling especially in large struggling infants. The procedure is technically easier and less likely to cause any trauma in hypoxic depressed infants. Hypoxia may be perpetuated by unsuccessful attempts at intubation. Reflex bradycardia and apnea may occur due to vagal stimulation. Overzealous attempts at ventilation especially when the tube is placed in one of the main bronchus (usually the right) may lead to pneumothorax. Strict asepsis and use of disposable ET tubes is mandatory otherwise infection may be introduced by hands and equipment. The laryngoscope blade must be sterilized before it is used for the next patient.

CHEST COMPRESSIONS (External Cardiac Massage)

Effective circulation is essential to deliver the oxygen from lungs to various tissues of the body. External cardiac massage is indicated in infants with cardiac arrest or when adequate circulation cannot be maintained in an asphyxiated newborn baby despite effective ventilation because of poor contractility of the heart and severe bradycardia (heart rate <60/min). Chest compressions must always be accompanied by ventilation with 100% oxygen.

Procedure

It is accomplished by rhythmic compressions of the sternum to compress the heart against the spine to increase intrathoracic pressure in order to ensure

effective circulation of the blood to the vital organs. The infant should be positioned on a flat firm surface and neck slightly extended. The pressure is applied to the lower sterum (below the imaginary line drawn to join the two nipples) by taking care to avoid compressing the xiphoid cartilage. The pressure can be applied either by thumbs of both hands or by two-finger technique. In the first method, the chest is encircled with both hands and thumbs are placed on the lower third of sternum side by side or one over the other in a small infant. The thumbs are used to compress the sternum while fingers provide support to the back of chest. The chest should not be squeezed by the hands but sternum should be compressed with the thumbs (Figure 27.3). Two-thumbs encircling hand technique is preferred as it generates higher peak systolic and coronary perfusion pressures than two-finger technique. Two-finger technique is preferred when access to the umbilicus is required during insertion of an umbilical catheter.

In the second technique, tips of middle and index fingers of one hand are used to compress the sternum. The finger tips are placed vertically (you cannot do it if you have long nails!) over the lower third of the sternum. The infant should be placed on a firm surface otherwise you provide support to the infant's back with your other hand. Press the sternum to a depth of 1 to 2 cm at a rate of 120/min, i.e. two compressions per second. The thumbs and tips of your fingers (depending upon the method being used) should remain in contact with the sternum all the time and they should not be lifted off during release of compression. Maintain a steady rate and depth of compressions. Check the heart rate after every 15–20 seconds and chest compressions may be stopped when heart rate exceeds 80 beats/min.

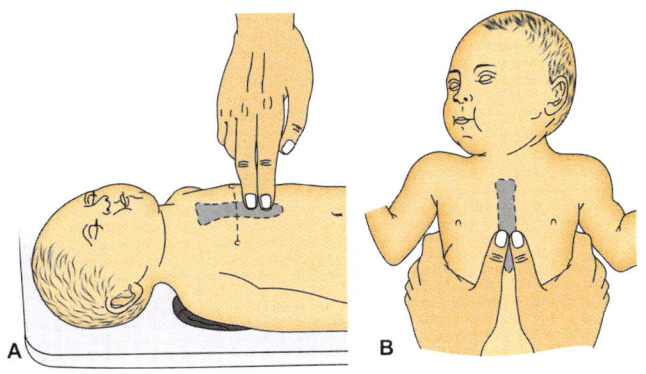

Figure 27.3A and B Technique of external cardiac massage. *See* text for details.

Complications

The ribs of a newborn baby are fragile and can be readily fractured unless due care is taken. The sharp edge of the ribs may puncture the underlying organs causing hemorrhage and pneumothorax. The compression of xiphoid process, which is spear shaped, can cause laceration of the liver.

CONTINUOUS POSITIVE AIRWAY PRESSURE (CPAP)

During normal breathing, the end expiratory pressure is approximately 3 cm H_2O which maintains the functional residual capacity (FRC) to ensure gas exchange during expiration. Infants with severe respiratory distress (HMD, pneumonia) develop "grunting" (by exhaling through partially closed glottis) during each expiration to elevate physiologic positive end expiratory pressure (PEEP) in order keep the alveoli open during expiration and improve ventilation. Continuous positive airway pressure (CPAP) or continuous distending pressure (CDP) is a modality of respiratory support in which increased pulmonary pressure is provided artificially (during both phases of breathing) in a spontaneously breathing neonate.

Physiologic Benefits

CPAP results in increased functional residual capacity (FRC) of lungs thus decreasing ventilation-perfusion (Q/V) mismatch and ensuring better alveolar gas exchange. There is improvement in minute ventilation and decreased work of breathing. It is associated with increased oxygenation, better wash out of carbon dioxide and correction of respiratory acidosis. It stabilizes the chest wall and enhances production of surfactant. It splints the upper airways and stimulates J receptors by stretching the lungs/pleura thus providing positive feed back to the respiratory center by Hering-Breuer reflex. The recycling of surfactant and functioning of pneumocytes-II is enhanced leading to early recovery from HMD. Animal experiments have shown that CPAP is associated with increased DNA and protein synthesis in the alveoli with improved compliance of premature lung. Unlike assisted ventilation, CPAP modality is safer with minimal risk of ventilator-induced lung injury (VILI) and complications due to endotracheal intubation.

Indications

In resource poor countries, CPAP is being increasingly exploited because it is cost-effective, less technology-intensive and demands lower level of skills. It can be provided with nasal prongs without undertaking endotracheal intubation. CPAP should be used early with or without exogenous surfactant in the course of RDS to reduce the need and duration of mechanical ventilation.

1. Preterm (HMD, pneumonia) and term (TTNB, MAS, pneumonia) infants with tachypnea, retractions and grunting.
2. Inability to maintain PaO_2 above 50 mm Hg despite ambient FiO_2 of 0.4.
3. Prolonged apneic attacks of prematurity. Nasal intermittent positive pressure ventilation (NIPPV) is currently considered as more effective than nasal CPAP (nCPAP or BiPAP) for management of apnea of prematurity.
4. Prophylactically in extremely preterm babies.
5. Postoperative neonates.
6. Post-extubation respiratory support during weaning.

Contraindications

In critically sick or grossly malformed babies, assisted ventilation is preferred over CPAP. It is contraindicated in following situations:

1. Poor or absent respiratory efforts.
2. Hemodynamically unstable baby.
3. Arterial pH less than 7.25 and $PaCO_2$ >60 mm Hg.
4. Congenital malformations like diaphragmatic hernia, tracheoesophageal fistula, choanal atresia and cleft palate.

CPAP Delivery Systems

Ventilator is the ideal system to provide CPAP but it is 3 times more expensive than stand alone CPAP devices. It has a blender for oxygen-air mixture, FiO_2 dial, warm humidifier, read out for various pressures, safety features and alarms. Most ventilators have a CPAP mode and they are convenient to use.

CPAP can be administered through a simple indigenously fabricated equipment by interposing water column in the expiratory circuit which blows off at the desired pressure depending upon the extent of PEEP required (Figure 27.4). It should be provided with an air-oxygen blender to vary oxygen concentration and it should never be used to deliver 100% oxygen.

CPAP system with continuous gas flow and variable or dual flow are available in Indian market. Bubble CPAP is commonly used and is a safe and effective device. The humidified air-oxygen mixture from blender flows through a heated humidifier. The distal end of the expiratory tubing is immersed in

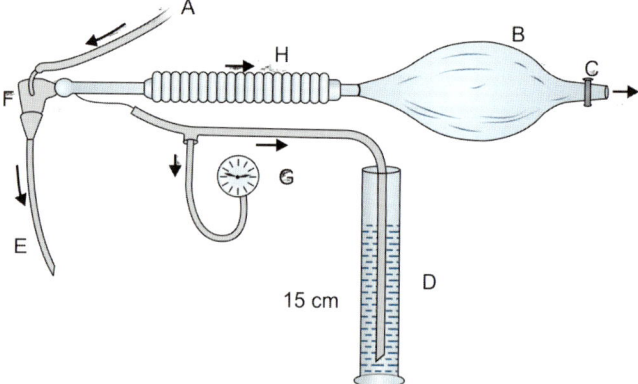

Figure 27.4 Indigenously fabricated system for applying continuous positive airway pressure (CPAP). A = gas flow, B = bag, C = screw clamp, D = underwater pop-off, E = endotracheal tube, F = modified T-piece, G = aneroid pressure gauge, H = corrugated anesthesia hose. Arrows indicate direction of gas flow.

sterile water (containing acetic acid as a bacteriostatic agent) which regulates the desired level of CPAP (Figure 27.5). Bubble CPAP has the combined effects of CPAP and pressure oscillations from the bubbles which provides protection to the lungs with reduced risk of chronic lung disease (CLD). The pressure oscillations of bubble CPAP reverberate back into the infant's airway which enhance gas exchange through the principle of facilitated diffusion. It is believed that bubble CPAP is more effective than ventilator CPAP.

Variable or dual flow CPAP devices have an integrated nasal interface and pressure generator but they are designed to use a higher gas flow. The most commonly used device is a variable flow device or infant flow driver (IFD). The pressure in the system is created at the level of the nasal device (generator) which is attached to the short twin or binasal prongs. The pressure generated in the device is controlled by adjusting the gas flow which is usually maintained above 8 L/min to achieve CPAP of about 5 cm H_2O. The expiratory limb of IFD device is kept open to the atmosphere. The baby can inspire high gas flow than that delivered through the inspiratory limb because infant can draw extra gas from the expiratory limb (variable flow). Bubble CPAP and IFD devices are equally effective in delivering CPAP and have an identical safety profile.

Patient Interfaces for Delivery of CPAP

CPAP can be provided through a face mask, nasal mask, nasopharyngeal tube or long nasopharyngeal prongs but these devices are unsatisfactory due to potential leakages and inability to maintain desired

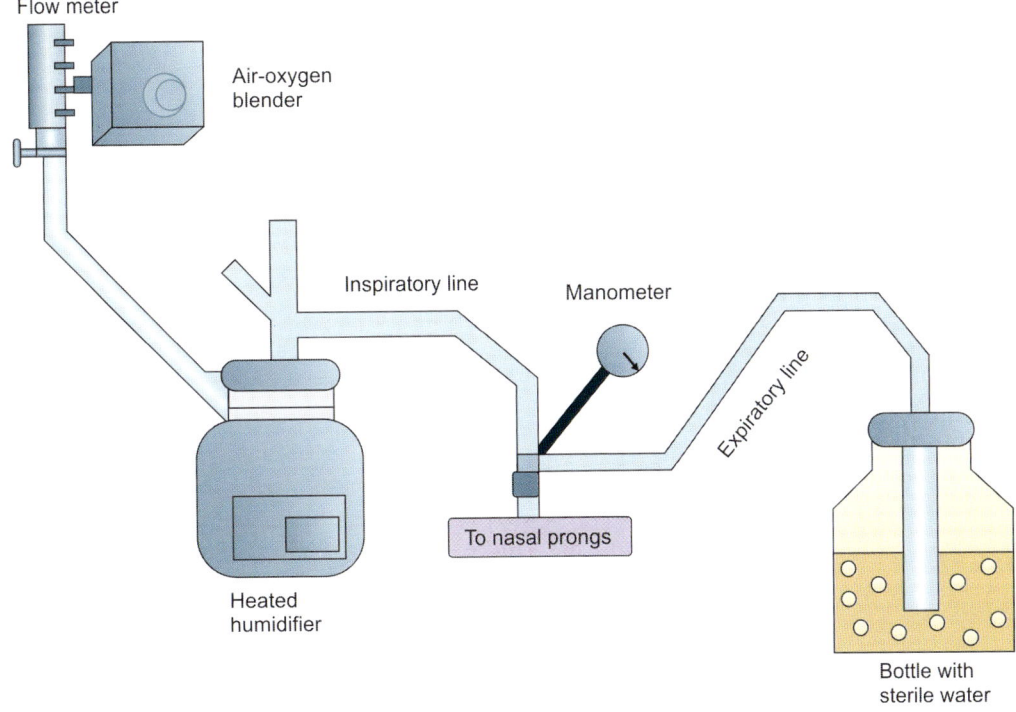

Figure 27.5 The components of bubble CPAP.

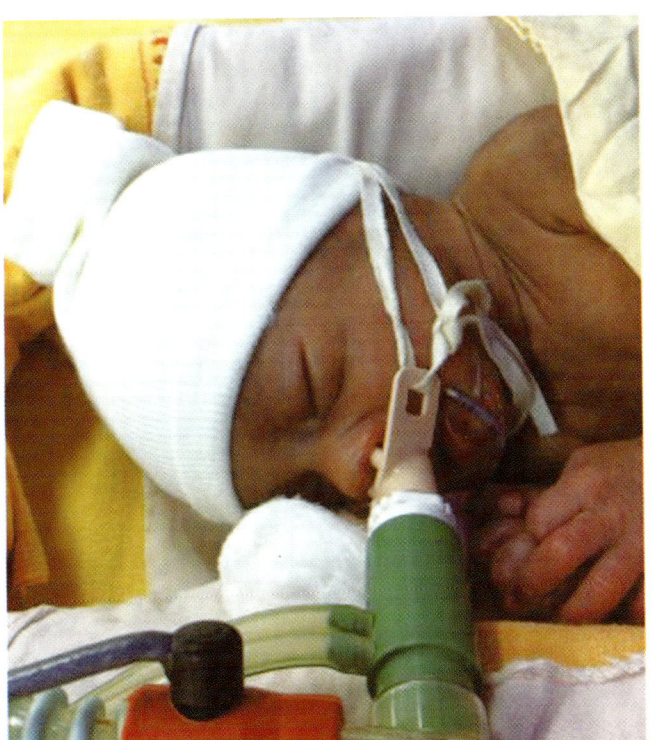

Figure 27.6 Infant with nasal CPAP lying in side position.

pressure of gases. Short binasal prongs of appropriate size (depending upon the birth weight of the baby) snugly affixed with the help of a dedicated cap are most useful and are commonly used **(Figure 27.6)**.

They are available as a dedicated attachment with a bubble CPAP and IFD devices. Ventilator-triggered CPAP is usually provided after endotracheal intubation so that baby can be readily promoted to assisted ventilation in the event of CPAP failure.

Procedure

The best fitting short binasal prongs are inserted and fixed with an appropriate sized cap provided by the manufacturer. The head of the neonate is stabilized to prevent dislodgement of nasal prongs. The circuit of CPAP machine is connected by attaching inspiratory limb with the nasal prongs and expiratory limb with the bubble chamber. Orogastric tube is inserted and its outer end is kept open and maintained above the level of stomach to constantly deflate it. The device is put on by keeping PEEP at 5 cm H_2O in case of RDS or pneumonia and at 4 cm H_2O for management of apnea of prematurity. PEEP is gradually increased by increments of 1.0 cm with the help of the knob or by increasing the depth of immersion of expiratory limb in the bubble chamber. The air-oxygen mixture is allowed to flow at a rate of 2–5 L/min and FiO_2 is kept at the minimum level to ensure negligible chest retractions and adequate expansion of lungs as evidenced by visibility of 6–8 posterior rib spaces on skiagram of chest. It is ideal to maintain PEEP between 6 and 8 cm H_2O and FiO_2 between 40 and 60%.

In general, CPAP and FiO_2 go hand in hand, e.g. 5 cm H_2O–50%, 7 cm H_2O–70% and so on. In order to ensure effective gas exchange in the lungs, initially PEEP should be gradually increased followed by increase in FiO_2. The flow of air-oxygen mixture should be kept at the minimum with visible bubbling in the bubble chamber. When surfactant deficiency is strongly suspected, nCPAP can be preceded by administration of surfactant by INSURE modality. It refers to IN (intubation) → SUR (surfactant) → E (extubation). This protocol comprises of intubation solely for administration of surfactant, followed by immediate extubation and start of nasal CPAP. When baby is stable, enteral feeds are given through orogastric tube by gravity, the outer end of the tube is kept closed for 30 minutes after delivery of feed to prevent regurgitation.

Adequacy of CPAP

CPAP is considered as adequate, if a baby is comfortable and has minimal or no chest retractions. The capillary refill time and blood pressure should be normal. The SpO_2 should be maintained between 87 and 93%, PaO_2 between 50 and 80 mm Hg, $PaCO_2$ between 40 and 60 mm Hg and pH 7.35 and 7.45.

Weaning from CPAP

When a baby is stable and has recovered from the underlying condition, the infant is gradually weaned off. The first step is to decrease FiO_2 by decrements of 5% to a level of 30%. The PEEP is gradually reduced in steps of 1.0 cm to a level of 4 cm H_2O. When a baby is on a PEEP of 4 cm H_2O and FiO_2 of less than 40%, has no or minimal chest retractions and is able to maintain arterial blood gases and pH within the normal range, he can be weaned off. Heated humidified high-flow nasal cannula (HHFNC) has a potential role as an alternative to nCPAP in post-extubation setting because of its ease of application and reduced risk of nasal trauma.

Failure of CPAP

CPAP is considered as a failure when FiO_2 of 60% and PEEP of 7–8 cm H_2O is unable to relieve chest retractions or normalize arterial blood gases. Infant should be promoted to mechanical ventilation, if despite maximal CPAP settings, the baby is unable to achieve SpO_2 >85%, PaO_2 >50 mm Hg, $PaCO_2$ <60 mm Hg and pH of >7.25.

Side Effects

CPAP is a safer modality of respiratory support compared to assisted ventilation. The risk of gastric distension can be reduced by insertion of an orogastric tube. There is some evidence that CPAP may lead to increase in pulmonary vascular resistance with risk of right-to-left shunts. There is controversial evidence for increased risk of pneumothorax or air leaks and its consequences like BPD, PVL and IVH. The procedure may compromise venous return and reduce cardiac output. Engorgement of cerebral veins may raise intracranial pressure and predispose to the development of intraventricular hemorrhage. Neonates receiving nCPAP should be monitored by sonography to detect intraventricular hemorrhage and periventricular leukomalacia and screened for retinopathy of prematurity. Prolonged nCPAP may lead to scarring nasal injury. Proper fixation of the interface, use of physical barrier between skin and interface, and good nursing care can reduce the incidence of nasal trauma. The risk of sepsis is substantially lower during CPAP compared to babies receiving mechanical ventilation.

Nasal Intermittent Positive Pressure Ventilation (NIPPV)

NIPPV is a form of non-invasive ventilatory assistance using a nasal interface to deliver IPPV to provide respiratory support. It is a non-invasive respiratory support that combines nCPAP and intermittent mandatory ventilation (IMV). Any ventilator capable of providing nCPAP and IMV modes of ventilation in neonates can be used for the NIPPV mode of respiratory support. NIPPV may be synchronized (SNIPPV) or non-synchronized (NNIPPV) with infant's breathing efforts. NIPPV may be used in the primary or secondary modes. In primary mode, NIPPV is used soon after birth with or without a short period (≤2 hours) of intubation for administration of surfactant, followed by extubation (INSURE). In secondary mode, NIPPV is used for weaning from a longer duration of conventional IPPV (>2 hours to several days of intubation) followed by SNIPPV and nCPAP.

Indications

NIPPV is not a replacement for endotracheal ventilation. It should be viewed as an enhancement or "step up strategy" over NCPAP. It can be considered for preterm infants soon after birth along with INSURE protocol. Other indications include apneic attacks and to facilitate the process of weaning after conventional ventilation. Neonates on SNIPPV should never be sedated because respiratory drive is essential for the success of NIPPV.

Contraindications

- Diaphagmatic hernia
- Tracheoesophageal fistula
- Choanal atresia
- Cleft palate
- Cardiovascular instability
- Poor or no respiratory drive
- Infant with rapidly progressive respiratory failure with increasing $PaCO_2$, decreasing pH and progressive hypoxemia.

Interface

Short binasal prongs are recommended.

Initial Settings

SNIPPV (Primary mode)	
Frequency	30–40/min
PIP	4 cm H_2O higher PIP than that required during manual ventilation
PEEP	4–6 cm H_2O
Inspiratory time (IT)	0.45 s
FiO_2	Titrate to maintain SpO_2 between 88 and 92% (alarm limits 87–93%)
Flow	10–12 L/min

SNIPPV (Secondary mode)	
Frequency	15–25 /min
PIP	2–4 cm H_2O more than 1 MV setting, adjust it to maintain effective aeration on auscultation
PEEP	5 cm H_2O
FiO_2	Tetrate to maintain SpO_2 between 88 and 92% (alarm limits 87–93%)
Flow	10–12 L/min

During weaning from conventional IPPV after intubation to SNIPPS, caffein should be given for promotion of respiratory drive.

Advantages

NIPPV whether synchronized or non-synchronized is superior to nCPAP in keeping infant off intubation. It is a safer modality with a lower risk of bronchopulmonary dysplasia.

Weaning

The neonate should be brought to the minimal settings of SNIPPV as listed below.

- Frequency <20/min
- PIP <14 cm H_2O
- PEEP ≤4 cm H_2O
- FiO_2 <0.3
- Flow 8–10 L/min
- Blood gases within normal limits

When minimal settings of NIPPV are reached, the infant is weaned to nCPAP mode as follows:

- Gradually reduce CPAP from 6 to 4 cm H_2O and then to 2 cm H_2O
- Adjust airflow to 1–2 L/min
- Titrate FiO_2 to maintain SpO_2 beween 88 and 92% (alarm limits 87–93%).

MECHANICAL VENTILATION

Modern neonatal care has been revolutionized by the availability of a large number of computerized ventilators to provide assisted ventilation. Ventilators are sophisticated electronic air pumps. The type of ventilator used is not as important as the level of training and experience of the personnel using them.

Based on their working principle, there are basically two types of ventilators. They are either pressure-limited (Baby Bird, Healthdyne, Sechrist, Bourns BP 200, Biomed) or volume-limited (Bennett, Engstrom, Bear Cub, Infant Star, Babylog, etc.). The pressure-limited ventilators generate a predetermined inspiratory or inflating pressure irrespective of the tidal volume. They are able to maintain an effective delivery of gases despite leakage around the uncuffed endotracheal tube used in neonates. The tidal volume in pressure-limited ventilator, depends upon the compliance of lungs and resistance of airways. There is thus likelihood of hypoventilation and over inflation when lungs become less or more compliant respectively. They are, however, simple in design, easy to operate and relatively cheaper. The peak inspiratory pressure (PIP), the key parameter related to bronchopulmonary dysplasia, is directly controllable.

In a volume-limited (volume-controlled or volume-targeted) ventilator, desired tidal volume can be delivered (though at times at extremely high peak inspiratory pressures when compliance is low) and there is no risk of under or over inflation. The tidal volume being small (tidal volume = 5–8 mL/kg body weight) in neonates, it may be lost in the ventilator circuit. They are more complicated in design, difficult to operate and exorbitantly priced. The inspiratory and expiratory timings are not directly controllable in a volume-limited ventilator. Their cycling is governed by the preset inspiratory and expiratory times.

Most ventilators also provide continuous flow of gases throughout the respiratory cycle and they are termed as constant-flow generators. They provide stable and consistent tidal volume and minute ventilation, independent of the lung compliance. This provides an "auto-weaning" feature, i.e. when lung compliance improves, the ventilator automatically adjusts by lowering the inspiratory pressure. By and large, there is not much to choose among different types of ventilators because success of ventilator therapy is dependent upon the experience of personnel and quality of supportive facilities. Practical experience and thorough understanding of the use of a ventilator is more important than the theoretical knowledge of various ventilators or acquisition of more expensive ventilators. Regardless of the type of ventilator, essential accessories such as humidifier, probe for recording temperature of air-oxygen mixture, air-compressor, and infusion pump must be purchased.

When to Establish Mechanical Ventilation Facilities?

The following strategies are useful and should be implemented before trying to establish ventilatory facilities. Instead of wasting resources in trying to acquire the most expensive state-of-the-art ventilators, it is more cost-effective to strengthen the infrastructure and improve the nursing coverage and the level of their expertise.

1. The neonatal mortality rate should be brought down to less than 20/1000 live births by ensuring optimal care of babies at birth, prevention of hypothermia and bacterial infections, promotion of feeding with human milk and providing optimal management to common neonatal disorders before launching assisted ventilation facilities.

2. Establish good infrastructural facilities like adequate space, centralized supply of oxygen, suction and compressed air, electronic monitoring equipment, microchemistry and ABG facilities, in-house portable X-ray and ultrasound machine, satisfactory parenteral nutrition capabilities and liberal supply of disposables.

3. Adequately trained, motivated and devoted health team comprising of neonatologists, nurses, chest physiotherapist, equipment manager, medical social worker and development psychologist is mandatory. The core medical and nursing staff must be provided with hands-on training regarding mechanical ventilation in an active and busy tertiary care center. Availability of adequate number of specially trained nurses, who are by and large permanently stationed in the NICU (occasional transfer of nurses between neonatal-ICU and pediatric-ICU may be permitted), is the most crucial requirement for optimal functioning of NICU. It must be remembered that one nurse is required round-the-clock to look after a baby receiving assisted ventilation.

4. It is desirable to first develop necessary skills and expertise to effectively and efficiently handle the conventional ventilation of newborn babies. The health team should develop confidence to handle the conventional ventilators with ease and utmost concern towards safety of their patients. The more sophisticated and complex ventilators providing PTV, SIMV, A/C, PSV modes should be purchased during the second stage of development. Only after having developed the state-of-the-art infrastructure, expertise and skills to handle the above mentioned modalities of ventilation, should a quantum leap be taken to acquire and learn high frequency ventilation, nitric oxide inhalation, liquid ventilation and ECMO.

5. It is futile to save babies without showing any concern regarding the quality of life among those who survive. It is mandatory that adequate follow-up facilities must be established to assess the physical growth, neuromotor development, cognition and integrity of special sense organs of nursery graduates. Apart from infrastructure and equipment required for follow-up program, we need a team of dedicated specialists comprising of neonatologist, pediatric surgeon, pediatric neurologist, public health nurse, medical social worker, child psychologist, development physician, ophthalmologist, audiologist, physiotherapist and occupational therapist.

Indications for Mechanical Ventilation

1. *Delivery room*
   i. Failure to establish adequate spontaneous ventilation despite positive pressure ventilation with a bag and mask.
   ii. Neonates with congenital diaphragmatic hernia.
   iii. To administer prophylactic or early rescue surfactant in extremely preterm babies.
2. Respiratory distress syndrome with hypoxemia (PaO_2 ≤50 mm Hg or SaO_2 <85% with FiO_2 >40%) but without respiratory acidosis can be managed by administration of oxygen and continuous positive airway pressure (CPAP). If despite maximal CPAP settings (PEEP 8 cm H_2O and FiO_2 0.6) infant is having chest retractions or is unable to normalize arterial blood gases (unable to maintain SpO_2 >85%, PaO_2 >50 mm Hg, $PaCO_2$ <60 mm Hg and pH of >7.25), he is promoted to assisted ventilation.

3. Respiratory failure associated with carbon dioxide retention and acute respiratory acidosis ($PaCO_2$ >60 mm Hg and pH <7.25).
4. Central apnea. Obstructive apnea responding to CPAP delivered through nasal prongs or nasal cannulae.
5. To reduce the work of breathing and fatigue of respiratory and myocardial muscles in infants with severe respiratory distress due to any cause.
6. Septic and cardiogenic shock to decrease systemic and myocardial oxygen consumption.
7. To reduce intracranial pressure through controlled hyperventilation.
8. General anesthesia requiring neuromuscular blockade.
9. To secure an airway in neonates with depressed sensorium, poor airway reflexes, intracranial hemorrhage, during recovery from general anesthesia and during transport of a sick neonate.
10. Postoperative neonate with depressed ventilatory functions.

PHYSIOLOGIC BASIS OF ASSISTED VENTILATION

The flow of gas in the air passages and alveoli is governed by the airway pressure gradient between the airway entry point and the alveoli. The airway pressure gradient is required to overcome the elastic properties of the lung parenchyma and chest wall as well as the resistance to airflow.

Compliance

Compliance refers to the elasticity or distensibility of the lungs and chest wall. It is expressed as the change in volume per unit change in pressure, as follows:

$$\text{Compliance (L/cm H}_2\text{O)} = \frac{\text{Volume (L)}}{\text{Pressure (cm H}_2\text{O)}}$$

Therefore, when compliance is normal or high, the volume expansion of lungs is greater per unit pressure. The relationship between pressure-volume (PV) loop and compliance is shown in Figure 27.7.

In neonates, the chest wall is soft and easily distensible and does not contribute to significant elastic load or compliance as compared to the lungs. Respiratory system compliance in infants with normal lungs ranges from 0.003 to 0.006 L/cm H_2O. In neonates with RDS, the lungs are stiff and the most striking abnormality of pulmonary mechanics is decreased lung compliance, which ranges from 0.0005 to 0.001 L/cm H_2O. Therefore, in infants with RDS, the airway pressure

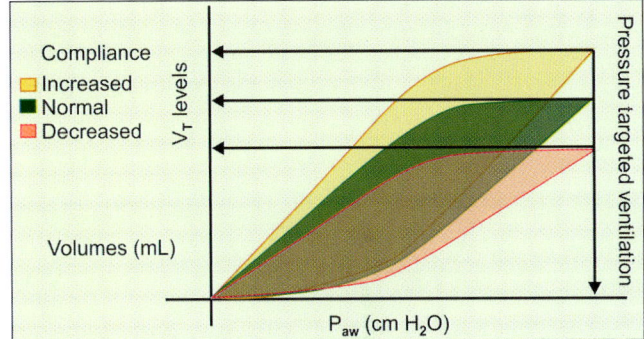

Figure 27.7 The slope of pressure-volume relationship indicates compliance. The decreased lung compliance of the infant with RDS manifests as a decreased volume change for the same change in pressure.

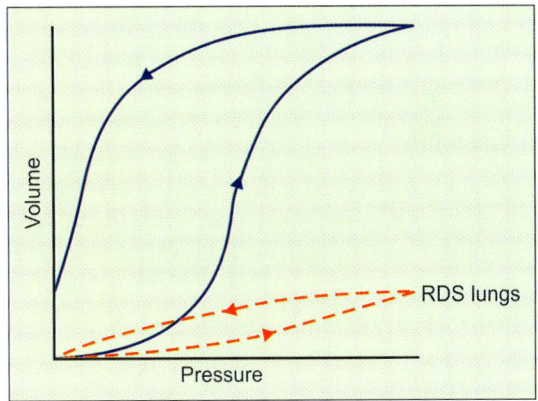

Figure 27.8 The slope of pressure-volume relationship indicates compliance. The decreased lung compliance of the infant with RDS manifests as a decreased volume change for the same change in pressure.

would have to be increased in order to maintain a normal tidal volume (Figure 27.8). In infants with meconium aspiration syndrome, compliance is minimally reduced.

Resistance

The pressure is not only required to overcome the elasticity of the respiratory system but it is also needed to overcome and surpass the resistance provided by the airways and lung tissue. The resistance to the flow of air through a long narrow tube is directly proportional to the length of the tube and inversely proportional to the 4th power of radius. Resistance is expressed as the change in airway pressure per unit change in the airflow, as follows:

$$\text{Resistance (cm H}_2\text{O/L/sec)} = \frac{\text{Pressure (cm H}_2\text{O)}}{\text{Flow (L/sec)}}$$

The total pulmonary resistance (airways + lung tissue) for normal newborn infants ranges between

TABLE 27.2 Compliance (CL), resistance (R) and time constant (KT) in normal and abnormal states in the newborn

Condition	CL (L/cm H$_2$O)	R (cm H$_2$O/L/sec)	KT (sec)
Normal	0.005	20	0.10
HMD	0.001	20	0.02
MAS	0.003	100	0.30

HMD: hyaline membrane disease
MAS: meconium aspiration syndrome

20 and 40 cm H$_2$O/L/sec. The total pulmonary resistance in intubated infants ranges between 50 and 150 cm H$_2$O/L/sec because endotracheal tube contributes to additional resistance. The pulmonary resistance is not significantly altered in infants with RDS, but it is grossly elevated in infants with meconium aspiration syndrome (Table 27.2).

Time Constant

Time constant refers to the time taken for a step change in the airway pressure (e.g. square pressure wave form during pressure-limited ventilation) to equilibrate throughout the lungs. It will depend upon the compliance of lungs and resistance of airways. Once pressure is equilibrated throughout the lungs, there will be no further airflow and thus no further volume changes. The time constant of the respiratory system refers to the time taken for the alveolar pressure to reach 63% of the change in airway pressure. Almost five time constants are required to achieve 99% equilibration (Figure 27.9). It is defined as the product of resistance and compliance, as follows:

Time constant (sec) = Resistance (cm H$_2$O/L/sec)
× compliance (L/cm H$_2$O)

The longer the duration is allowed for equilibration, higher is the percentage of equilibration that will take

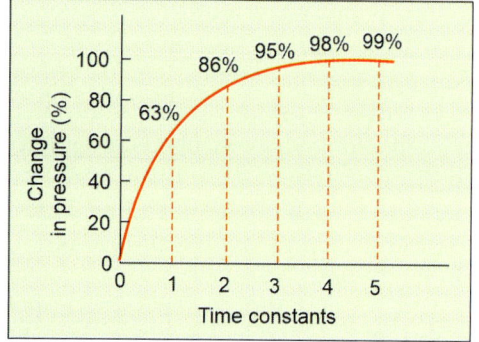

Figure 27.9 Percentage change in pressure in relation to the time allowed for equilibration. After five time constants, 99% equilibration in pressure occurs.

place. However, the time taken for the lungs to inflate and deflate will depend upon their mechanical characteristics, especially resistance and compliance. For example, in a healthy infant with a resistance of 30 cm H$_2$O/L/sec and compliance of 0.004 L/cm H$_2$O, one time constant would be 0.12 second. For complete equilibration pressure (five time constants or 5 × 0.12 sec), an inspiratory or expiratory phase of 0.6 second will be necessary. In contrast, since infants with RDS typically have a decreased lung compliance, their time constant and corresponding time for pressure equilibration will be shorter. The lungs with decreased compliance (or decreased resistance) will complete inflation and deflation in a shorter time than normal lungs. Therefore, infants with RDS would require short inspiratory and expiratory times for assisted ventilation during the period of peak severity of their disease. During recovery, when compliance improves, higher inspiratory and expiratory times would be more appropriate.

Gas Exchange

The aim of assisted ventilation is to accomplish effective gas exchange at the alveoli.

Carbon Dioxide (CO$_2$) Elimination

Carbon dioxide readily diffuses from blood into alveoli and its elimination largely depends upon the total amount of air that passes in and out of the alveoli. Since some of the tidal volume is distributed to the parts of the lungs, such as airways, that are not involved in gas exchange (dead space), alveolar ventilation is calculated as follows:

Alveolar ventilation = (Tidal volume – Dead space)
× Breathing rate/min

Since dead space stays relatively constant, CO$_2$ elimination and reduction of PaCO$_2$ is mostly achieved by increase in tidal volume or increase in frequency of breathing. In a volume-controlled ventilator, the delivered volume is preset although some of this volume may be lost in the delivered system and airleaks around the uncuffed endotracheal tube. In a pressure-limited ventilator, tidal volume depends on the lung compliance and pressure gradient (pressure difference between airway opening pressure and alveolar pressure) or peak inspiratory pressure (PIP) minus positive end-expiratory pressure (PEEP). Reducing PEEP or increasing expiratory time (T$_e$) may improve CO$_2$ elimination but is likely to reduce MAP and oxygenation.

Oxygen (O_2) Uptake

Increasing the fractional concentration of inspired oxygen (FiO_2) improves oxygenation but it fails to affect V/Q matching and may cause direct toxicity to lungs. The oxygenation by and large depends on fraction of inspired oxygen (FiO_2) and mean airway pressure (MAP or Paw). MAP is the measure of airway pressure to which the lungs are exposed during the respiratory cycle. It is calculated by dividing the area under the airway pressure curve by the duration of the cycle, or from the following equation:

$$MAP = K (PIP - PEEP) [T_i/(T_i + T_e)] + PEEP$$

$$MAP = \frac{(T_i \times PIP) + (T_e \times PEEP)}{T_i + T_e}$$

where K is a constant that depends on the rate of rise of the airway pressure curve, T_i is inspiratory time and T_e is the expiratory time (Figure 27.10).

The mean airway pressure can be agumented by increasing any of the following parameters:

i. Inspiratory flow rate (it will increase K by ensuring "square wave")
ii. Peak inspiratory pressure (PIP is "critical opening" pressure that improves V/Q)
iii. Ratio of inspiratory time to expiratory time (I:E ratio)
iv. Positive end-expiratory pressure or PEEP (prevents collapse of alveoli by maintaining FRC)
v. Rate (lowers Pi but increases the risk of inadvertent PEEP)

MAP as low as 5 cm H_2O may be sufficient in infants with normal lungs, whereas 20 cm H_2O or more may be necessary in infants with severe RDS. MAP is usually maintained between 8 and 12 cm H_2O. In general, increase in MAP is associated with improved oxygenation with certain reservations. For an identical increase in MAP, increase in PIP and PEEP are more effective in enhancing oxygenation compared to change in I:E ratio. Changes in PEEP beyond a certain level (greater than 7–8 cm H_2O) do not further enhance oxygenation. Marked elevation in MAP is counter productive because it causes over distension of alveoli, leading to right-to-left shunting of blood in the lungs. Markedly elevated MAP is transmitted to the intra-thoracic structures leading to decrease in cardiac output and thus despite adequate oxygenation, oxygen delivery (arterial oxygen content × cardiac output) to the tissues may decrease. It is an important correlate of barotrauma.

TYPES AND MODES OF MECHANICAL VENTILATORS

Time-Cycled Pressure-Limited Versus Volume-Cycled Ventilators

Pressure-limited ventilators are designed to deliver a volume of gas until a preset limiting pressure is reached. The remainder of the gas volume in the unit is then discharged into the atmosphere. Therefore, the volume of the gas delivered will vary from breath-to-breath but pressure reached would remain constant in case of pressure-limited ventilators. In contrast, the volume-controlled ventilators deliver a preset volume of gas with each breath regardless of the pressure required which may vary from breath-to-breath. They are thus preferred in situations where consistency of tidal volume delivery is critical. Since the introduction of ventilation facilities, neonatologists and respiratory therapists have debated on the relative merits of volume vs pressure-controlled ventilation. However, no studies have demonstrated any distinct benefits for either modality in all forms of neonatal respiratory disease. Each type of ventilator can provide satisfactory ventilator support if the basic physiological principles are understood well. The salient differences between pressure controlled and volume controlled ventilators are shown in Table 27.3.

When a volume-controlled ventilator is used for ventilation of an infant with atelectasis or obstructed airways, much of the volume is likely to be preferentially delivered to the more compliant healthier areas resulting in over distension and risk of air leak syndrome. There is likely to be loss of some volume around the uncuffed ET tube and in

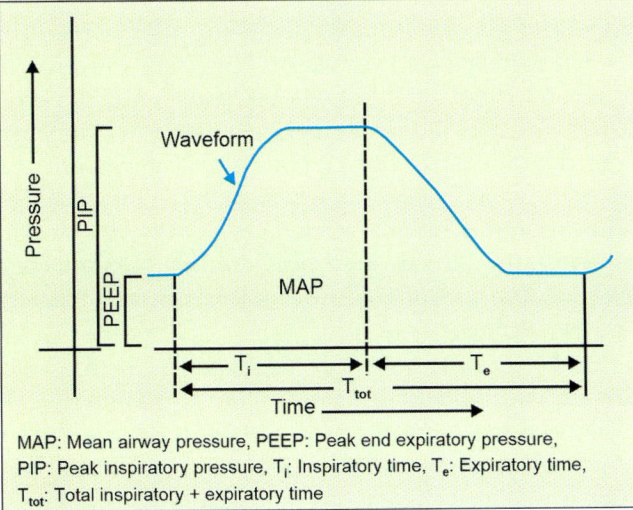

MAP: Mean airway pressure, PEEP: Peak end expiratory pressure, PIP: Peak inspiratory pressure, T_i: Inspiratory time, T_e: Expiratory time, T_{tot}: Total inspiratory + expiratory time

Figure 27.10 Ventilator controls in relation to the respiratory cycle.

Assisted Ventilation and Advanced Life Support

27

TABLE 27.3 Salient differences between pressure controlled and volume controlled ventilators

Parameter	Pressure controlled	Volume controlled
Different variables		
Tidal volume	Variable depending upon lung mechanics	Constant
PIP	Constant	Variable depending upon lung mechanics
Peak alveolar pressure	Constant	Variable
Flow pattern	Decelerating	Preset
Peak flow	Variable	Constant
Common variables		
Inspiratory time (T_i)	Preset	Preset
Minimum rate	Preset	Preset
Modes	IMV, SMV, A/C	IMV, SMV, A/C
Advantages	Lower risk of barotrauma because PIP remains constant throughout the cycle.	Lower risk of volutrauma because of constant tidal volume.
	It is more effective for ventilating stiff and atelectatic lungs because of decelerating flow pattern and front ended breaths.	It is useful in high volume or heterogeneous lung states because of back-ended loaded breaths. Auto-weaning of pressures as compliance improves
Disadvantages	Tidal volume delivery is variable. Risk of volutrauma, if PIP is not decreased when compliance improves.	Fixed inspiration flow may lead to increased work of breathing, if there is a need for high flow. Risk of barotrauma in infants with low compliance, if PIP is not monitored.

A/C: Assist/control
IMV: Intermittent mandatory ventilation
SIMV: Synchronized intermittent mandatory ventilation
PIP: Peak inspiratory pressure

the ventilator circuit tubing so that preset tidal volume may not be actually delivered to the lungs. Newer ventilator monitors are now able to measure the volume loss by comparing the inspiratory flow and expiratory return through the ET tube adapter. In infants with bronchopulmonary dysplasia, where atelectasis is changing on a day-to-day basis, the controlled tidal volume delivery is useful to prevent episodes of oxygen desaturation which are commonly seen in these infants. The variations in the peak inspiratory pressures from breath-to-breath in case of volume-controlled ventilators has been a source of concern in the past. It has now been realized that during volume-controlled ventilation the peak inspiratory pressure may automatically "wean" off as the lung compliance improves either spontaneously or in response to surfactant therapy.

In pressure-controlled ventilation, the gas volume delivered depends upon the compliance of lungs and chest wall. When the lungs are stiff due to markedly reduced lung compliance (as in case of RDS), the preset pressure is reached more rapidly and a significant portion of tidal volume is released to the atmosphere. Ventilatory failure may set in unless volume loss is compensated by increasing the peak inspiratory pressure. The common belief that pressure-limited ventilators cause less barotrauma than volume-cycled ventilators is probably an oversimplification and not based on facts. If ventilator-induced lung injury occurs due to "volutrauma", it may be argued that control of tidal volume delivery may actually protect the lungs against trauma because of rapidly changing pulmonary compliance.

In view of the relative benefits and hazards of either type of above referred ventilators, it is recommended that the choice of ventilator should be based on the experience, training and skills of the NICU team members and the credibility and after sales service capabilities of the supplier. Recently, several sophisticated ventilators have been introduced that can be operated both as a volume-controlled or pressure-controlled time-cycled ventilators offering considerable flexibility of choice to the operator to serve the specific needs of a patient. Even those babies who are started on time-cycled pressure-limited mode of ventilation, the desired tidal volume (4–6 mL/kg) and minute volume can be delivered to maintain "target" ABGs.

Most of the last generation ventilators were designed to provide intermittent mandatory ventilation (IMV). In IMV, a mechanical breath is delivered at a preset interval irrespective of the spontaneous efforts of the baby thus causing asynchrony, i.e. the baby "bucking" or "fighting" with the ventilator. Asynchrony has been shown to cause air trapping and pneumothorax, thus increasing pulmonary morbidity and delaying the recovery. Preterm babies breathing asynchronously with the ventilator have been shown to have increased risk of IVH due to greater variability and irregularity in the cerebral blood flow. A number of state-of-the-art new generation ventilators have been introduced to synchronize the spontaneous breaths of the baby with the mechanical breaths delivered by the ventilator to create perfect harmony between the baby and the machine.

NEWER MODALITIES OF ASSISTED VENTILATION

The rationale to use newer forms of assisted ventilation is to optimise synchronization between the ventilator and patient (reduce work of breathing), facilitate or reduce the duration of ventilation, and avoid undesirable pulmonary, cardiovascular and systemic side effects. The advances in microprocessor based technology has lead to the production of more complex, sophisticated, user friendly and versatile ventilators with enhanced efficacy and safety. They are equipped with pulmonary graphics and can give warning for misadventures like tube leakage and accumulation of secretions.

Patient-Triggered Ventilation (PTV)

Instead of conventional intermittent mandatory ventilation (IMV) wherein spontaneous breathing of the infant is superimposed on the ventilator cycles, a number of advanced ventilators are now available where ventilator breaths and patient's spontaneous breaths are synchronized without any bucking. Synchronized ventilatory modes are characterized by delivery of mechanical breaths in response to a signal derived from the patient's spontaneous inspiratory effort (patient triggered) and are available in both pressure-limited and volume cycled ventilators. The patient-triggered ventilation is a form of "partial ventilation" where the patient has to partly contribute to the work of breathing.

Synchronized Intermittent Mandatory Ventilation (SIMV)

In this mode of ventilation, the mechanical breaths are delivered at a fixed rate but are synchronized to the onset of the patient's own breath. This prevents the infant from "fighting" the ventilator, a sequence that happens when the infant is exhaling while the ventilator delivers a breath. However, if the inspiratory times are not identical, the patient may terminate

his own effort and begin exhalation while the ventilator is still in the inspiratory phase, resulting in partial asynchrony. The flexibility of SIMV in providing a wide range of ventilatory rates makes this modality useful both as a primary means of ventilatory support and as a modality to assist weaning. However, a low set SIMV rate is undesirable when the patient's ventilatory demands are high. Similarly reducing the SIMV to a very slow rate (<30 bpm) may adversely affect the process of weaning by imposing significant work of breathing in an intubated baby. The disadvantage of slow rate SIMV can be compensated by additional means of breath support such as pressure support ventilation.

Assist-Control Ventilation (A/C)

The ventilator delivers a positive pressure breath in response to the patient's inspiratory effort (assist), provided it exceeds the safety rate set by the operator (back up control). The back up control rate ensures a minimum mandatory minute ventilation in case patient stops making spontaneous breathing efforts. It is probably the best mode to use in a premature infant during the acute phase of illness because it requires least amount of effort on the part of the patient and produces improved oxygenation at the same mean airway pressure. PTV reduces the duration of time from weaning to extubation. The infants on PTV or A/C have reduced duration of exposure to oxygen at a lower ventilatory pressure with reduced risk of BPD and IVH. The available neonatal PTV systems with their characteristics are depicted in Table 27.4. All PTV systems provide both SIMV and A/C except the Sechirst SAVI module which provides A/C alone. The initial PTV settings are maintained as follows:

- PIP — 15–20 cm H_2O
- PEEP — 3–5 cm H_2O
- FiO_2 — 0.4 to 1.0
- Ti — 0.4 sec (0.2 to 0.5 sec)
- I:E ratio — 1:2
- Back up breathing rate — 30–40/min

The main limitations of PTV system are major swings in ventilation of apneic infants, delay in triggering mechanism and autocycling.

Pressure-Support Ventilation (PSV)

Pressure-support ventilation is defined as patient-controlled ventilation which is generally flow-cycled. This is designed to assist patient's spontaneous

TABLE 27.4 Characteristics of available PTV systems

PTV	Sensor	Response time	Modes	Features
Babylog 8000 plus	HWA flow sensor	95 ±24 ms	IPPV, IMV, SIMV, PSV and A/C, HFV (optional)	■ Ventilator adjusts the pressure to achieve the "guaranteed" volume ■ HWA sensor built into the Y- piece ■ Fully integrated, easy to use ■ Graphic display of pressure or flow waveform. Displays tidal and minute ventilation data, air leak size.
Bear Cub NVM-1 TV Monitor and Bear CEM	HWA flow sensor	65 ± 6 ms	SIMV and A/C	■ NVM-1 displays tidal and minute ventilation data, airway leak size ■ NVM-1 alarm limits can be set ■ CO_2 retention often evident, requiring an increase in PIP or ventilator rate
Bird-VIP Gold and partner TV monitor	VOP flow sensor	30–70 ms	SIMV and A/C and PSV	■ It provides volume-assured pressure support (VAPS) ■ Partner displays tidal and minute ventilation data, air leak size. Graphic display is optional ■ Can terminate positive pressure when inspiration ends. ■ Low rate of autocycling
Infant Star and Star synch	Graseby capsule detects abdominal movements	52 ±13 ms	SIMV and A/C	■ Displays spontaneous T_i and RR ■ Audible signal during inspiration aids correct capsule placement ■ No sensitivity setting is required
Sechrist IV HP CR monitor and SAVI module	Chest leads impedance	40–80 ms	A/C	■ CR gram aids correct lead placement and sensitivity setting ■ Terminates positive pressure on active expiration
SLE HV2000	VOP flow sensor	40–100 ms	SIMV and A/C	■ Combined HFOV with graphic display
SLE 5000	VOP flow sensor	40–100 ms	CPAP, CMV, PTV, SIMV, PSV, HFOV	■ Touch screen display ■ HFOV and targeted tidal volume delivery
Stephan Sophie (Figure 27.11)	VOP flow sensor	10 ms	CPAP, SIMV, PSV, A/C. HFOV with pressure/ volume control	■ Ventilator equipped with volume guarantee ventilation ■ Graphic display on in-built display monitor ■ Proportional assist ventilation (PAV) is a unique feature in this model ■ In-built humidification system

HWA: Hot wire anemometer, VOP: Variable-orifice pneumato tachometer, ms: Milliseconds. IPPV: Intermittent positive pressure ventilation, IMV: Intermittent mandatory ventilation, SIMV: Synchronized intermittent mandatory ventilation, PSV: Pressure support ventilation, A/C: Assist control, HFV: High frequency ventilation, PTV: Patient-triggered ventilation, HFOV: High frequency oscillatory ventilation.

breathing with an inspiratory pressure "boost". And once the breath is triggered by the patient's inspiratory effort, a preset system pressure is rapidly achieved and maintained throughout inspiration by the adjustment of the inspiratory flow by the machine. The inspiration ends when the inspiratory flow falls below a preset level. PSV is better customized to support and synchronize with patient's effort because

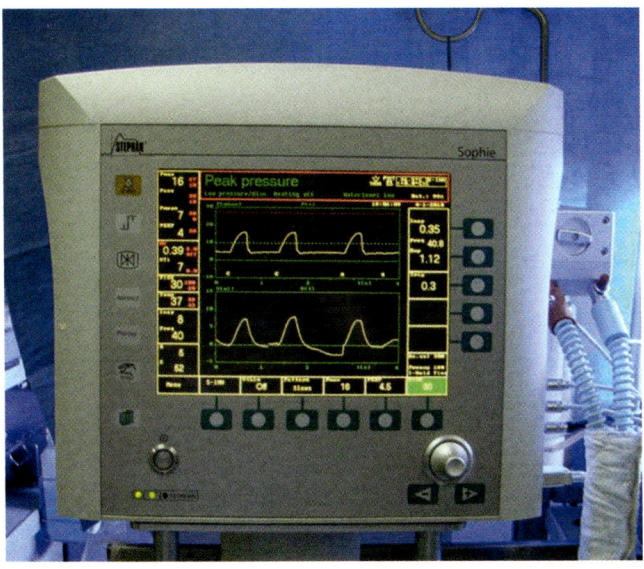

Figure 27.11 Stephan Sophie ventilator with pulmonary graphics.

the patient has the control of both the inspiratory flow rate and inspiratory time. PSV reduces the work of breathing created by the resistive forces of endotracheal tube and ventilator's circuit. It is mostly used as a weaning mode, but can be used as a primary modality in patients with ventilatory failure in the presence of respiratory drive. In most cases PSV is used in conjunction with volume-cycled SIMV during the process of weaning. PSV is also used with advantage in infants who are chronically ventilator-dependent and in those with evidences of bronchopulmonary dysplasia.

High Frequency Ventilation (HFV)

High frequency ventilation refers to that mode of assisted ventilation which employs small tidal volume (often less than dead space) and much higher frequencies than those used by conventional methods. The main advantage of HFV is that it maintains adequate minute ventilation using relatively low mean airway pressure. The risk of barotrauma to the lungs is minimized. HFV produces vibratory energy, which facilitates gas exchange and helps to mobilize and dislodge pulmonary secretions. However, it is not possible to monitor pulmonary mechanics and tidal volume with HFV. Table 27.5 summarizes the salient features of high frequency ventilators.

Indications to use HFV

1. Failure of conventional ventilation despite use of surfactant in infants with RDS
2. RDS with persistent pulmonary hypertension (PPHN)
3. Pulmonary air leaks

TABLE 27.5 Comparison of various techniques of high frequency ventilation

Features	HFPPV	HFJV	HFOV
■ Waveform	Variable	Triangular	Sine wave
■ Frequency/min	60–150	150–600	300–3000
■ Tidal volume	>Dead space	>Dead space	<Dead space
■ I:E ratio	Variable	Variable	Constant
■ Expiration	Passive	Passive	Active
■ Gas entrainment	None	Possible	None

HFPPV: High frequency positive pressure ventilation
HFJV: High frequency jet ventilation
HFOV: High frequency oscillatory ventilation

4. Pulmonary hypoplasia
5. When extremely high MAPs (>12–14 cm H_2O) are required for adequate oxygenation with continuous mandatory ventilation.

High Frequency Positive Pressure Ventilation (HFPPV)

The conventional ventilation with low compliance tubings and connectors are used for this mode of high frequency ventilation. Adequate tidal volume is delivered despite short inspiratory times and high frequencies of 60–150/minute. In HFPPV, PEEP is set to zero to avoid inadvertent PEEP.

Indications for a trial of HFPPV HFPPV mode is used for ventilation if following criteria are met in an infant who is receiving conventional ventilation:

1. PaO_2 is very labile or <50 mm Hg on FiO_2 of 1.0
2. $PaCO_2$ >70 mm Hg
3. PIP >30 cm H_2O (to achieve visible chest excursions)
4. Significantly lobored breathing efforts despite IMV rate of 60/min

The following ventilatory settings are usually adequate for HFPPV:

■ Rate	100/min (150/min in <1000 g)
■ T_i	0.3 sec
■ Flow rate	10 L/min
■ PIP	Decreased by 5 cm H_2O from conventional setting
■ MAP	1–2 cm higher than conventional ventilator
■ PEEP	0

High Frequency Jet Ventilation (HFJV) (Bunnel Life Pulse)

HFJV delivers gases from a high-pressure source through a small-base cannula. It uses a special trilumen endotracheal tube (Hi-lo jet) and pinch valve to deliver pulses of gas into the trachea. Tracheal pressures are monitored and regulated by a servocontrol mechanism through a small-cannula lumen in the endotracheal tube. The end-expiratory pressure is provided and adjusted by a conventional ventilator connected in tandem at the endotracheal tube. The conventional ventilation provides the intermittent breaths that interrupt the jet pulses. The HFJV is initiated at the following settings:

■ Frequency	
Term infants	420/min (7Hz)
Preterm infant	360/min (6Hz)
■ T_i	20 ms (range 20–34 ms)
■ I:E ratio	1:6 at 20 ms at 7Hz
■ PIP	8–50 cm H_2O
■ PEEP	2–4 cm below the MAP on either CMV or HFOV after the conversion
■ MAP	MAP on jet should be equal to the MAP on either CMV or HFOV prior to conversion. After conversion, if jet MAP is >2 cm H_2O above the CMV/HFOV MAP before conversion, than decrease PEEP 1 cm H_2O at a time until the MAP on the jet is equal to the MAP before conversion or stop at a MAP 1 cm H_2O higher, if there is a need to improve oxygenation.

ms: milliseconds

The PIP on conventional ventilator should be kept 10 cm higher than HFJV PIP. The breathing rates of conventional ventilator should be reduced to 2–10/min. Oxygenation during HFJV depends upon MAP while carbon dioxide elimination primarily depends upon tidal volume (difference between PIP and PEEP).

High Frequency Oscillatory Ventilation (HFOV) (Sensor-Medics 3100 A f, SLE 5000, Stephan Sophie, Draeger Shreeyash, Vision Alpha, Bunnel LifePulse jet ventilation)

HFOV delivers extremely small volumes (even less than dead space) of oxygen-air mixture at very high frequencies (up to 3000/min) with the help of a piston pump or acoustic speaker. The oscillations are unique because expiration is actively generated by the machine. HFOV is initiated with following settings

■ Frequency	
Term infants	600/min (10 Hz)
Preterm infant	900/min (15 Hz)
■ T_i	Set at 33% (22 ms at 15 Hz, 41 ms at 8 Hz, 55 ms at 6 Hz)

■ I:E ratio	1:2 for 3–15 Hz at 33% IT
■ PIP	Start with a value 2–4 higher than PIP on the conventional ventilator and adjust to achieve adequate "wiggling" of the chest
■ MAP	2–4 cm above the MAP on conventional mechanical ventilator

ms: milliseconds

The oxygenation depends upon MAP which is augmented by recruitment of sigh breaths. MAP is reduced once FiO_2 requirement is <0.7. Carbon dioxide elimination is achieved by increasing amplitude, reducing frequency to 600/min (10 Hz) and increasing inspiratory time to 50% (I:E ratio of 1:1)

Protocol for Weaning

The steps of weaning from HFJV or HFOV are summarized below:

■ Start weaning when oxygenation and $PaCO_2$ levels are satisfactory with FiO_2 of ≤0.5, unless the lung fields are over inflated.

■ Decrease both PIP and PEEP by 1 cm H_2O every 4–8 hours. When FiO_2 is ≤0.30–0.35, decrease PIP and PEEP by 1–2 cm H_2O every 2–4 hours to avoid over inflation (e.g. PIP 16 cm H_2O and PEEP 10 cm H_2O are decreased to 15 cm H_2O and 9 cm H_2O, respectively).

■ When MAP and PEEP range between 4 and 8 cm H_2O at FiO_2 ≤0.4, infant is shifted to IMV mode at low breathing rates (15–20 bpm) followed by extubation and promotion to NIPPV or nCPAP mode to safeguard against risk of apneic attacks.

Advantages of HFV

■ Enhanced carbon dioxide elimination in infants with RDS

■ Early resolution of pulmonary air leaks

■ Reduced need for ECMO in infants with PPHN

■ Reduced risk of bronchopulmonary dysplasia

■ There are no adverse effects on the cardiovascular system and cardiac output is well maintained.

Disadvantages and Complications of HFV

The results of clinical trials till date have not shown conclusively that HFV is more effective (or safer) as compared to conventional ventilation for first-line management of premature infants with RDS. The common side effects of HFV are listed below:

■ Inadvertent PEEP (especially with HFJV)

■ Intracranial hemorrhage

- Necrotizing tracheobronchitis
- Hypotension?

VENTILATOR VARIABLES

The currently available mechanical ventilators are provided with a large number of variables or controls with audiovisual alarms for prompt attention in case of malfunctioning (Table 27.6). Most ventilators have a CPAP (continuous positive airway pressure) mode for providing continuous distending airway pressure to a baby who is breathing spontaneously. The ventilator generates a constant positive pressure throughout the respiratory cycle without producing any ventilatory breath. The ventilator is more often used to provide intermittent positive pressure ventilation (IPPV) or intermittent mandatory ventilation (IMV). The IMV mode is used during weaning (or for a baby who is having active breathing efforts) so that the child can breathe "around" the ventilator at the same FiO_2 and PEEP without any bucking or fighting the ventilator. The key settings that regulates the pressure-limited ventilators include inspired oxygen concentration (FiO_2), peak inspiratory pressure (PIP), respiratory rate, positive end expiratory pressure (PEEP), inspiratory to expiratory ratio (I:E) and flow rate. Mean airway pressure (MAP) is the net outcome of all the parameters except FiO_2 and respiratory rate. The mean airway pressure is the true measure of average

TABLE 27.6 Characteristics and specifications of settings of an ideal ventilator

Ventilator variables	Range of specifications
FiO_2	0.21–1.0
PIP	0–80 cm H_2O*
PEEP	0–20 cm H_2O
RR	0–120 bpm
T_i	0–3 seconds
T_e	0–60 seconds

Alarms
FiO_2
PIP, PEEP, MAP fall
Loss of gas supply or leakage in the system
Humidity level
Inspired gas temperature
Power loss

Mechanical characteristics
Low compliance of ventilator circuit
Low compliance of humidifier circuit
Waveform control

*1.0 cm H_2O = 0.735 mm Hg

pressure actually being perceived by the airways (depending upon the compliance of the lungs) and is altered by changes in a number of ventilator parameters (PIP, PEEP, inspiratory time, duration of cycle, etc.). It should be maintained between 8 and 12 cm H_2O.

Inspired Oxygen Concentration (FiO_2)

In normal circumstances, environmental or ambient oxygen concentration of 21% (FiO_2 of 0.21) is adequate and comfortable, if there is no cardiopulmonary compromise. In respiratory (and cardiac) disorders, higher concentrations of ambient oxygen are required to sustain life. FiO_2 refers to fraction of oxygen in the inspired air-oxygen mixture (i.e. FiO_2 of 0.7 refers to 70% oxygen). Ambient oxygen concentration is regulated by blenders that mix oxygen and compressed air into precise concentrations as required by the infant. Unlike older models, many newer ventilators have built-in blenders. These are generally accurate but periodic checks are necesary to confirm the accuracy of the oxygen concentration being delivered. Several portable oxygen analyzers or in-line sensing devices can be used to check the oxygen concentration being delivered to the patient. FiO_2 should be kept at the minimum level to maintain SpO_2 of 90–95% in term and near term infants and 85–93% in preterm and PaO_2 between 50 and 80 mm Hg. When FiO_2 requirement is >60%, it is desirable to increase MAP. If FiO_2 requirement is <30–40%, one should try to decrease the MAP. In children with cyanotic congenital heart disease, SpO_2 between 70 and 75% is acceptable, if tissue oxygenation is good. The initial FiO_2 should be set at 0.5. Higher ambient oxygen concentration can lead to hyperoxia which is known to cause retinopathy of prematurity.

Tidal Volume

This is the primary parameter to be set in volume controlled ventilation. The initial set tidal volume (V_T) is 4–6 mL/kg in preterm infants and 6–8 mL/kg in term infants. Inappropriately low (<3 mL/kg) V_T leads to atelectasis, hypoxemia and hypercarbia, while excessive V_T (>8 mL/kg) can cause volutrauma. High volume lung injury occurs when V_T is above the upper inflection point of the pressure volume curve and low volume lung injury results from ventilation beginning below the inflection point (Figure 27.12). When the expired tidal volume measured by the ventilator is less than the set V_T, it indicates presence of an air leak through endotracheal tube, ventilator circuit or bronchopleural fistula.

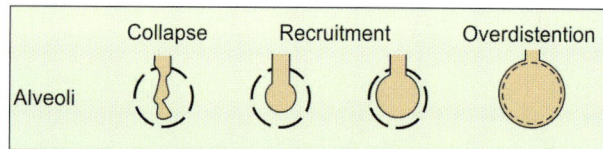

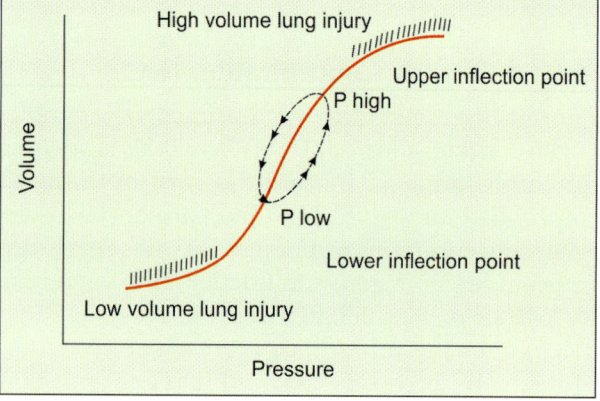

Figure 27.12 Pressure volume curve. Appropriate selection of tidal volume and pressures (PIP and PEEP) is essential to avoid lung injury.

Peak Inspiratory Pressure (PIP)

A normal breath necessitates intrapleural pressure to drop from –1 to –7 cm H_2O, i.e. a pressure change of 6 cm H_2O. A pressure of 6 cm H_2O is required to drive the gases through the ventilator circuitry. Thus a neonate with normal lungs requires a PIP of about 12 cm H_2O for ventilation. However, most neonates requiring ventilation are likely to have poor compliance of varying severity due to the underlying disease (HMD, pneumonia). Depending upon the severity of underlying lung disease, higher PIP is required for ventilation. In most cases, it is appropriate to start ventilation with a PIP of 18–20 cm H_2O and modify it subsequently depending upon the severity of lung disease. It is advisable to hand-ventilate the baby using anesthesia-type bag connected to an endotracheal tube and to estimate the PIP on a manometer. The inflating pressure that results in adequate chest expansion should be taken as the initial setting for PIP. It is the primary variable that determines tidal volume in a pressure-limited time-cycled ventilator. The minute ventilation (tidal volume × respiratory rate) is increased by increasing the tidal volume resulting in wash out of carbon dioxide. Mean airway pressure is increased by increasing the PIP leading to better oxygenation. Low PIPs may not be able to provide adequate tidal volume leading to hypoxia and hypercapnia while high PIPs are associated with the risk of pulmonary barotrauma in the form of air leaks and bronchopulmonary dysplasia. The increase in intrathoracic pressure may decrease venous return to the heart.

Positive End Expiratory Pressure (PEEP)

Adequate PEEP prevents alveolar collapse, maintains lung volume at the end expiration and improves ventilation–perfusion relationships. PEEP is the most effective parameter that increases MAP. Both extremely high and low PEEPs are associated with retention of carbon dioxide. It is important to remember that though both PIP and PEEP increase MAP and improve oxygenation, but PEEP has opposite effect on carbon dioxide. The normal physiologic PEEP is approximately 3 cm H_2O. The initial PEEP is usually kept at 4–5 cm H_2O and it should not exceed 8 cm H_2O in most situations. The PEEP range of 4–8 cm H_2O is safe and effective. Excessive elevation of PEEP may decrease lung compliance manifesting as decreased tidal volume on a pressure-limited time-cycled ventilator or an increased PIP on a volume ventilator. High PEEP may cause overdistension, gas trapping, barotrauma, hypercarbia, air leaks, impede venous return to the heart and increase pulmonary vascular resistance and intracranial tension.

Respiratory Rate (RR)

It is the main determinant of minute ventilation (Minute ventilation = Tidal volume × RR). Higher respiratory rate is useful for carbon dioxide wash out and to increase minute ventilation. By increasing respiratory rate, lower PIP can be used to reduce the risk of barotrauma. The ventilator rate is based on the decision whether the ventilator is taking over the work of breathing completely or partially. Since in most situations, at the start of mechanical ventilation, the disease process is still evolving, it is logical to take over the respiration completely. To achieve this, the ventilator rate is kept within the normal range or higher than the normal spontaneous respiratory frequency of the neonate.

The spontaneous respiratory rate of healthy neonates is usually between 40 and 50/min, the rate being higher for smaller or preterm babies. Higher respiratory rates are set in infants with restrictive lung disease (RDS, ARDS) where the time constant is less allowing for quick filling and emptying of lung units. Lower breathing rates are set in infants with high airway resistance like chronic lung disease, meconium aspiration syndrome and asthma where it is necessary to allow adequate time for expiration and some degree of permissive hypercapnia is acceptable. Hyperventilation is used in the treatment of PPHN in an effort to produce alkalosis thus reducing right-to-left shunting with marked improvement in PaO_2 without increasing MAP.

Inspiratory-Expiratory Ratio (I:E Ratio)

It primarily affects MAP and oxygenation. The physiological I:E ratio of 1:1.5 or 1:2 is used in most clinical situations and is desirable. Reversed I:E ratio (3:1 or 2:1) increases MAP and improves oxygenation so that FiO_2 and PEEP can be reduced accordingly to safer levels. Inverse breathing ratios improve V/Q matching and decrease shunting but can lead to air trapping and reduction in venous return. It is contraindicated in infants with increased pulmonary vascular resistance. Prolonged expiratory I:E ratios (1:2, 1:3) are indicated in ventilation of infants with meconium aspiration syndrome and during weaning. Infants with MAS are ventilated with high flow rates and reduced PIP and inspiratory time (to reduce air trapping) which may compromise their tidal volume and oxygenation.

Flow Rate

In neonates, flow rate of oxygen-air mixture of 4–8 L/minute is usually sufficient to ensure adequate CO_2 washout and maintain high PIP, shorter T_i and increased RR (and hence high MAP). Flow rate above 10 L/min is seldom required and increases the risk of barotrauma and pulmonary air leaks. High flow rate without adequate expiratory time may result in gas trapping due to inadvertent PEEP. The volume-targeted modes of ventilation offer a choice for various flow wave patterns. It is possible to choose a square (usually preferred), accelerating, decelerating or a sine waveform for a given VT and I:E ratio.

The Goals of Mechanical Ventilation

The efficacy and safety of assisted ventilation during neonatal period is well established. It is being liberally used these days even during relatively early stages of the disease process and in some centers even routinely in infants weighing less than 1000 g. This is largely done to reduce the work of breathing and enhance intact survival.

The goal of management of infants with respiratory disorders is to maintain PaO_2 between 50 and 80 mm Hg, $PaCO_2$ 35 and 45 mm Hg and pH 7.35 and 7.45. Infants with severe RDS as evidenced by marked tachypnea (>80/min), severe chest retractions, cyanosis in FiO_2 of 0.6 and prolonged apneic attacks will generally need assisted ventilation. The laboratory criteria for IPPV include PaO_2 <50 mm Hg despite CPAP with FiO_2 1.0, $PaCO_2$ >50 mm Hg and pH <7.20. In extremely premature neonates or a baby with severe HMD, assisted ventilation may be instituted before the appearance of severe abnormalities in blood gases and acid–base parameters. The outcome of respiratory therapy is better if ventilation is initiated at the right time before the advent of respiratory failure.

ESTABLISHMENT OF ASSISTED VENTILATION

A ventilator along with its circuit, accessories, and resuscitation equipment should be available, in working order and duly sterilized, all the time so that there is no delay in initiating assisted ventilation whenever it is required. The infant should be placed on an open care system under the servo-control mode to provide thermoneutral environment. After adequate suctioning of airways, the baby should be stabilized with a bag and mask ventilation with 100% oxygen. The infant should be attached to a multichannel vital sign monitor and pulse oximeter (Figure 27.13). Endotracheal intubation should be done as described on p 563. Nasal intubation allows greater stability of the endotracheal tube but it is more difficult and time consuming. Orotracheal intubation is satisfactory especially in emergency situations. Moreover, there is less risk of postintubation atelectasis following orotracheal intubation as compared to nasotracheal intubation because newborn babies are obligatory nose breathers. The tube should lie just above carina and its position checked by auscultation of chest. Skiagram of chest, with head in the neutral position, should show that lower end of the tube is 1 cm below C_7 or just below the medial ends of clavicles (Figure 27.14). Bag to endotracheal tube ventilation should be done, preferably with an anesthesia bag having a provision for attachment of a pressure manometer to assess lung compliance. The ventilatory pressures required for

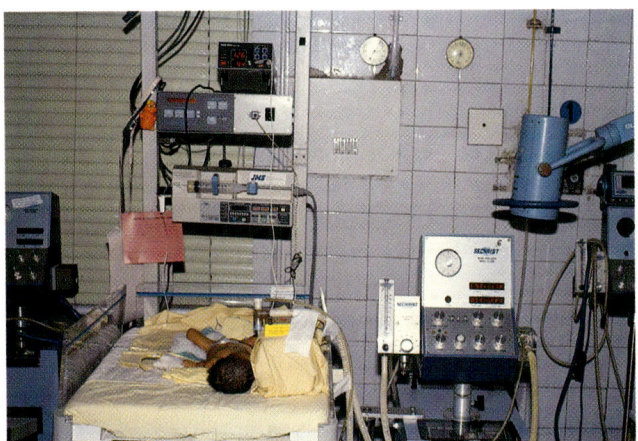

Figure 27.13 The baby on assisted ventilation. Note the use of extensive monitoring equipment.

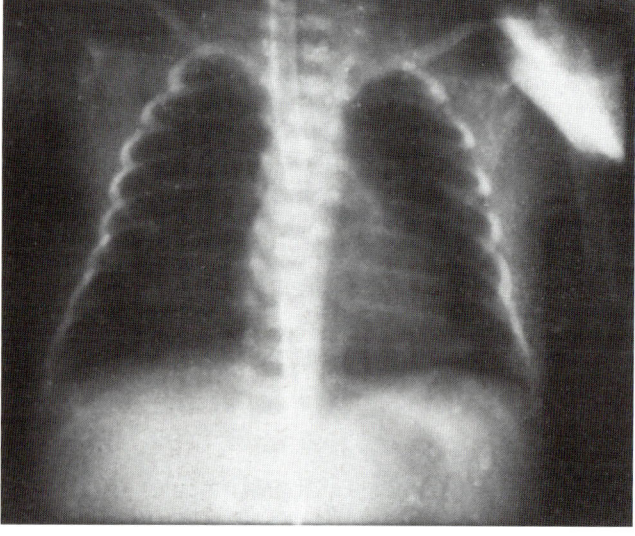

Figure 27.14 Skiagram of chest showing that endotracheal tube is too low and should be pulled out.

adequate movements of the chest wall shall provide useful guidelines for the initial setting of PIP on the ventilator. The ultimate settings of the ventilator depends upon the age of the patient, nature of the disease and status of arterial blood gases. The air-oxygen mixture should be warmed to 37°C and humidified to 70–100%.

Initial Ventilator Settings

The ventilator settings shown in Table 27.7 are usually adequate to start assisted ventilation during the first hours of life. In a patient with meconium aspiration syndrome, prolonged I: E ratio of 1:2 or 1:3 and lower PIP are used to facilitate expiration and prevent air trapping. The infant is observed for movements of chest wall, retractions, cyanosis and breath sounds. If ventilation is inadequate, increase PIP by 1.0 cm H_2O every few breaths until air entry appears adequate (maximum PIP is usually 30 cm H_2O). If oxygenation is inadequate as evidenced by cyanosis or poor saturation on pulse oximeter, increase FiO_2 by 0.05 (5%) and PEEP by 1.0 cm H_2O (maximum PEEP

8–10 cm H_2O) until cyanosis is abolished or oxygen saturation is maintained between 90 and 95%. After initial stabilization, draw arterial blood sample for gasometry. Umbilical artery should be catheterized in extremely premature or severely sick babies who are likely to need prolonged ventilation.

How to Adjust Ventilator Settings

During acute stage of the disease, ventilator settings are always in a dynamic state and require frequent alterations. Judicious clinical monitoring along with pulse oximetry and periodic blood gas analyses are crucial for the success of ventilatory therapy. The parameters indicating the adequacy of ventilation are listed in Table 27.8.

Depending upon the clinical condition of the patient and status of blood gases, appropriate changes should be made in the ventilator settings (Table 27.9). The changes in the ventilator settings must be made in short steps. PIP and PEEP should be altered only by 1.0 cm H_2O at a time, rate 2 breaths/ min, FiO_2 in steps of 0.05 (5%) and T_i in instalments of 0.05 seconds. Blood gas estimation should preferably be done after 20–30 minutes of each change in setting.

Adjuncts to Mechanical Ventilation
Sedation

Pain, discomfort and agitation should be reduced by conducting the procedures gently, providing soothing touch, reducing nursery light and noise and

TABLE 27.8 Clinical and laboratory indices of adequate ventilation
Clinical parameters
Pink color
Adequate chest expansion on both sides
Absence of retractions
Adequate air entry
Prompt refilling of capillaries (within 2 sec)
Normal blood pressure
Adequate urine output (>1.0 mL/kg/hr)
Pulse oximetry
Oxygen saturation between 90 and 95% in term babies and 85–93% in preterm babies
Blood gases
PaO_2 50–80 mm Hg
$PaCO_2$ 40–50 mm Hg (in a chronic disease permissive hypercapnia up to 60 mm Hg)
pH   7.35–7.45

TABLE 27.7 Suggested initial ventilator settings		
Settings	*Infants with normal lungs*	*Infants with RDS*
▪ FiO_2	0.5	0.5
▪ Rate	30–40 per minute	40–50 per minute
▪ PIP	12–18 cm H_2O	18–20 cm H_2O
▪ PEEP	2–3 cm H_2O	4–5 cm H_2O
▪ T_i	0.3–0.4 sec	0.4–0.5 sec
▪ Flow rate	4–6 L/min	6–8 L/min

TABLE 27.9 Blood gas abnormalities and changes in the ventilator settings to correct them

Blood gas abnormality	Corrective measure					Comments
	FiO_2	Rate	PIP	PEEP	T_i	
■ Hypercapnia ($PaCO_2$ >50 mm Hg)	—	↑	↑	—	—	Increase flow rate, T_e, reduce dead space and make sure there is no auto PEEP phenomena
■ Hypocapnia ($PaCO_2$ <35 mm Hg)	—	↓	↓	—	—	Reduce flow rate and increase dead space
■ Hyperoxia (PaO_2 >100 mm Hg)	↓	—	↓	↓	↓	Reduce FiO_2
■ Hypoxia (PaO_2 <50 mm Hg)	↑	—	↑	↑	↑	If chest excursions are adequate, it is better to increase FiO_2
■ Total ventilatory failure ($PaCO_2$ too high and PaO_2 too low)	Depends upon the underlying cause					Check that chest is moving equally on both sides with each ventilation and nasotracheal tube is not blocked. Check for air leaks and ventilator malfunction. Correct acidosis and gradually increase the settings.

promoting synchronized IMV ventilation. Morphine (0.05–0.1 mg/kg) or fentanyl (1–3 µg/kg) can be used but may cause neurologic depression. In more mature babies, lorazepam (0.05–0.1 mg/kg/dose q 4–6 hr) or midazolam (0.05–0.1 mg/kg/dose q 2–4 hr) can be used for a prolonged period.

Muscle Relaxants

Muscle relaxants may be used in large infants who "fight" with the ventilator and when high FiO_2 (>0.75) or PIP (>30 cm H_2O) are required for effective ventilation. They are routinely used during ventilation of babies with tetanus neonatorum. Pancuronium bromide (0.05–0.1 mg/kg/dose) is given intravenously every 1–4 hours as needed. Prolonged muscle relaxation may lead to fluid retention and may cause deterioration in lung compliance.

VENTILATOR SETTINGS IN COMMON DISEASE STATES

Respiratory Distress Syndrome (RDS)

Most of the preceding discussion on assisted ventilation has been focussed on the management of newborn babies with RDS or hyaline membrane disease, which is the commonest indication for neonatal ventilation. The recommended ventilation protocol in infants with hyaline membrane disease is shown in the Box. The following ventilation-related pulmonary complications need special management to prevent further damage to the lungs.

Initial ventilator settings for RDS

- Early institution of therapeutic nasal CPAP
- Early rescue surfactant administration
- Rapid breathing rate — 60/min
- Moderate PEEP — 4–5 cm H_2O
- Low PIP — 10–20 cm H_2O
- Short T_i — 0.25–0.4 sec
- Low tidal volume — 3–6 mL/kg
- Early extubation to nasal CPAP

Pulmonary Interstitial Emphysema (PIE)

The main principles for ventilation of infants with air leaks or PIE are to reduce MAP (by reducing either PIP, T_i or PEEP) and increase expiratory time to minimize over distension of lungs to reduce further air leaks. The FiO_2 is kept high (even up to 1.0) to maintain satisfactory oxygenation and the $PaCO_2$ is controlled by increasing the rate rather than PIP. The following ventilator settings are recommended:

Ventilatory settings in PIE

PIP	12–15 cm H_2O
PEEP	0–2 cm H_2O
Rate	50–60/min
I:E ratio	1:2 to 1:3

If pneumothorax occurs, it should be drained and ventilation continued with the same settings as before. Occasionally a high PIP is required to compensate for further loss of compliance but it should be used with due caution. If facilities are available, high frequency ventilation is the treatment of choice for management of infants with PIE. As in conventional ventilation, the ventilatory goal in air leak syndromes is to decrease MAP and rely on FiO_2 to improve oxygenation. High frequency jet ventilation (HFJV) or high frequency flow interrupter (HFFI) are ideal by maintaining PEEP at a lower level (4–6 cm H_2O) and by giving few or no sigh breaths.

Bronchopulmonary Dysplasia (BPD)

Although BPD is believed to have a multifactorial etiology but barotrauma appears to be the root cause. The ventilation therapy is continued to maintain adequate arterial oxygenation with the lowest possible MAP. The FiO_2 is usually maintained around 0.5 while PIP and rate are modified to prevent gross retention of carbon dioxide. However, in chronic lung disease it is acceptable to have $PaCO_2$ level up to 60 mm Hg provided the pH is normal. In the management of infants with BPD, efforts should be maintained to reduce PIP, PEEP and T_i while maintaining PaO_2 between 50 and 80 mm Hg, $PaCO_2$ up to 60 mm Hg and pH above 7.25. Weaning should be attempted extremely slowly by decreasing rate by 1–2 breaths per minute and PIP by 1.0 cm decrements everyday. Refer to Chapter 19 for supportive management of infants with BPD.

Birth Asphyxia

In birth asphyxia, apnea is usually due to cerebral edema and lack of respiratory drive while lungs are usually normal, if infant is term and amniotic fluid is clear. The following initial ventilator settings are recommended:

Ventilatory settings in birth asphyxia	
PIP	12–15 cm H_2O
PEEP	4–6 cm H_2O
Rate	20–40/min
I:E ratio	1:1.5
Tidal volume (VT)	5–8 mL/kg

Sodium bicarbonate administration is recommended, if severe metabolic acidosis persist despite adequate ventilation. Correction of acidosis may dramatically improve oxygenation by reducing right-to-left shunting of blood. High breathing rates are commonly used to improve oxygenation and ensure carbon dioxide wash out in order to reduce intracranial pressure and cerebral edema. Inotropic support to the heart is useful to improve cardiac output and systemic circulation. Most infants with terminal apnea due to birth asphyxia need short-term ventilation. When ventilation support is required for more than 12 hours, neuromotor disability due to brain damage is invariable.

Meconium Aspiration Syndrome (MAS)

The condition is by and large limited to term babies and is characterized by respiratory distress with air trapping (obstructive emphysema) due to ball valve effect of meconium. The resistance to airflow is markedly increased while compliance is normal or minimally decreased. These infants are vulnerable to develop PPHN with perpetuation of hypoxia due to right-to-left shunting of blood through foramen ovale or PDA. The incidence of air leaks, either spontaneous or following ventilation, is very high.

Infants who are stable and without any evidences of respiratory failure, do well with low to moderate CPAP through nasal prongs or nasopharyngeal catheter. CPAP stabilizes collapsed terminal airways and improves atelectasis. Surprisingly, CPAP does not increase the risk of air leaks in infants with MAS. When assisted ventilation is indicated, following ventilator settings are recommended:

Ventilatory settings in MAS	
PIP	15–20 cm H_2O
PEEP	0–3 cm H_2O
Rate	40–60/min
I:E ratio	1:2 to 1:3 (T_i 0.2 to 0.3 sec)

Since infants with MAS are vigorous, large babies with strong respiratory efforts and high risk of pulmonary air leaks, it is desirable to paralyze them before initiating assisted ventilation. In order to prevent further air trapping, minimal PEEP and short inspiratory times should be used. Carbon dioxide elevation is common in severe cases of MAS and is managed by increasing the rate and reducing I:E ratio. The FiO_2 is usually maintained at 1.0 and PIP is raised, only if there is persistent hypoxemia or hypercarbia. Refractory hypoxia secondary to PPHN is treated with hyperventilation and use of pulmonary vasodilators. Infants with PPHN should preferably be paralyzed with pancuronium bromide to prevent "fighting" with ventilator and for its therapeutic utility to relax the pulmonary vascular bed. For further details regarding management of PPHN, refer to Chapter 20.

Pneumonia

Due to rarity of GBS-pneumonia in India, ventilaory therapy is required in an occasional case of severe late-onset pneumonia which develops acute respiratory failure. Unlike HMD, the compliance of lungs is almost normal in neonates with pneumonia. The initial ventilator settings in an infant with pneumonia are as follows:

Ventilatory settings in pneumonia

PIP	20–25 cm H_2O (depending upon the weight of infant)
PEEP	3–5 cm H_2O
Rate	40–50/min
I: E ratio	1:2 (T_i 0.3–0.4 sec)
VT	6–8 mL/kg

The subsequent changes in the ventilatory settings are made on the basis of clinical signs and ABG findings. Because of excessive inflammatory exudates, frequent suctioning of endotracheal tube and chest physiotherapy are advised.

Recurrent Apnea

Recurrent apnea of prematurity or prolonged apnea in term babies (birth asphyxia, cerebral edema, intractable seizures, postoperative stabilization, etc.) demands assisted ventilation in an infant with normal lungs. MAP is readily transmitted to the intrathoracic veins because lung compliance is normal. The cardiac output may be reduced due to decreased venous return to the heart. Hyperventilation is easily achieved in normal lungs and should be avoided because of potential risk of reducing cerebral blood flow. The following ventilator settings are recommended to initiate mechanical ventilation:

Ventilatory settings in recurrent apnea

PIP	10–15 cm H_2O
PEEP	3–4 cm H_2O
Rate	30–40 /min
I:E ratio	1:1 (T_i 0.5 sec)

The breathing rate and I:E ratio can be progressively reduced as the infant regains his own spontaneous respiratory efforts.

Interstitial Pulmonary Edema

Pulmonary edema, hydrops fetalis, and massive pulmonary hemorrhage have identical pulmonary characteristics demanding similar approach in their management with assisted ventilation. The initial ventilatory settings are recommended as follows:

Ventilatory settings in pulmonary edema

PIP	30–40 cm H_2O
PEEP	4–6 cm H_2O
Rate	30–40/min
I:E ratio	1:1 (T_i 0.5 sec)

High peak inspiratory pressures should be used despite the potential risk of causing pneumothorax and obstruction to venous return to the heart. The associated pleural effusion and ascites should be drained to improve movements of the chest and expansion of lungs. Intravenous administration of furosemide is useful for rapid clearance of interstitial pulmonary edema. The PIP should be reduced as soon as lung edema clears and chest radiographic appearances show improvement.

Hypoplastic Lungs

Hypoplastic lungs with ineffective ventilation are associated in infants with diaphragmatic hernia, renal agenesis and oligohydramnios. The progressive attempts to inflate the lungs is associated with grave risk of development of pneumothorax. The PIP should be kept below 20 cm H_2O to prevent damage to the alveoli of contralateral lung. The following initial ventilator settings are recommended:

Ventilatory settings in hypoplastic lungs

FiO_2	0.5 to 1.0
PIP	up to 20 cm H_2O
PEEP	3 to 5 cm H_2O
MAP	<12 cm H_2O
T_i	0.35 sec
Rate	50–60/min

High frequency oscillatory ventilation and assist control mode of ventilation are ideal for these infants. In intractable cases, ECMO and nitric acid inhalation therapy are associated with improved survival.

Postoperative Ventilatory Support

Many infants require respiratory support following major surgery for life-threatening congenital malformations. The ventilatory assistance may be required due to respiratory depression following general anesthesia, use of muscle relaxants or narcotic analgesics. Infants undergoing thoracotomy for tracheoesophageal fistula or surgical correction of diaphragmatic hernia invariably require postoperative ventilatory support. Assisted ventilation support is also required for all infants undergoing open heart surgery. It is desirable

27

to administer narcotic analgesics postoperatively for relief of pain and infant should be partially paralyzed with pancuronium bromide to prevent struggling and bucking during ventilation. CPAP alone with 3 to 5 cm H_2O may be enough in a breathing infant with hypoventilation to expand localized areas of atelectasis. When positive pressure ventilation is required, the following initial ventilator settings are recommended:

Settings in postoperative ventilatory support	
PIP	15–20 cm H_2O
PEEP	4–6 cm H_2O
Rate	20–30/min
I:E ratio	1:1.5

Chest Physiotherapy

Infant's position should be changed from one side to the other every 2 hourly. If baby is enterally fed, physiotherapy should be done just prior to feeding. Oral cavity and posterior pharynx should be sucked before and after doing chest physiotherapy. Percussion is carried out with a vibrator, Bennet's face mask or two fingers or cupped hand. The chest is shielded with a cotton sheet to reduce the impact of pressure to the chest wall (Figure 27.15). Chest physiotherapy is recommeded every 6 to 8 hourly. More frequent physiotherapy is carried out, if there are excessive secretions or massive collapse or consolidation of the lung. The duration of physiotherapy depends upon the tolerance of the baby and should not exceed 10–15 minutes. Postural drainage, percussion and vibration over the chest are applied by a trained chest physiotherapist to loosen the tracheobronchial secretions. The procedure is done with due care and gentleness and should be abandoned immediately, if baby gets stressed and becomes unstable. Chest physiotherapy is contraindicated in the presence of pulmonary air leaks, critically sick and unstable babies, ELBW babies and infants with IVH.

Tracheobronchial Suctioning

The endotracheal tube by-passes the glottis, eliminates physiological PEEP and interferes with humidification, effective coughing and elimination of bronchial secretions. Chest physiotherapy should precede suctioning. The tracheobronchial toilet should be done every 2–4 hours with a proper sterile technique, using surgical gloves and disposable sterile packs containing suction catheters and a bowl (Figure 27.16). The size of suction catheter depends upon the size of the endotracheal tube. The catheter should not completely block the endotracheal tube to safeguard against massive atelectasis. Before the procedure, the infant should be ventilated with a bag using 100% oxygen. The suction is carried out in three positions of the head namely straight, right rotation and left rotation. The suction catheter should be introduced gently and suction (80 cm H_2O) is applied only while withdrawing the catheter. The suctioning should be limited to periods of 10 seconds followed by hyperventilation with oxygen. The suctioning of thick secretions may be facilitated by instillation of 1–2 mL of normal saline or acetylcysteine, if secretions are thick and viscid. The baby is hand ventilated for 60 seconds after instillation of saline or acetylcysteine before suctioning is done. The tracheal secretions should be periodically sent for culture and antibiotic sensitivity pattern. During the procedure, the infant should be closely watched and should be attached to a pulse oximeter and cardiac monitor.

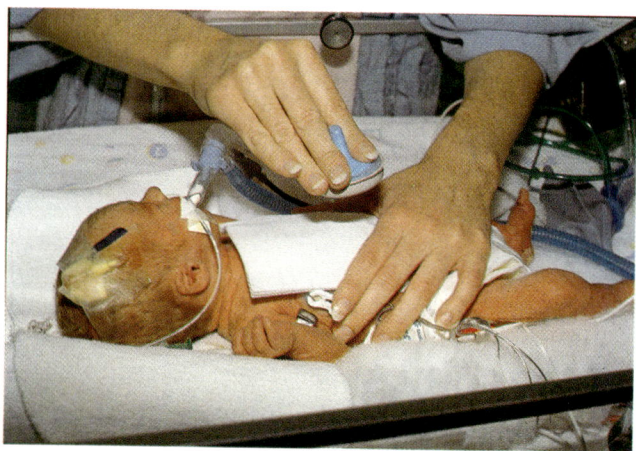

Figure 27.15 Chest physiotherapy. See text for details.

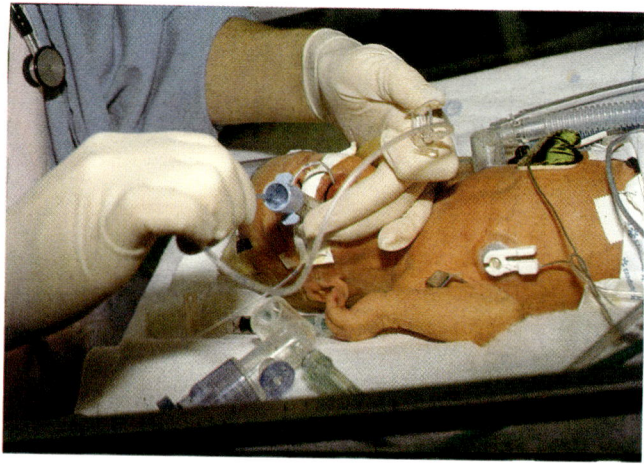

Figure 27.16 Suction of endotracheal tube with strict aseptic precautions.

VENTILATOR EMERGENCIES

The common causes of sudden deterioration in the condition of a ventilated child can be remembered by the acronym DOPE.

D Displacement of the tube
O Obstruction of the tube
P Pneumothorax
E Equipment failure

Common problems that can be encountered during the course of mechanical ventilation are listed below.

1. **Acute respiratory distress** This manifests as tachypnea, increased work of breathing, chest retractions, use of accessory muscles of respiration, tachycardia and hypotension. Possible causes include equipment failure, endotracheal tube issues and disease-related causes. If patient shows improvement after being removed from the ventilator and on hand bagging, an equipment failure is likely. If there is no improvement after being bagged, check tube position. Displacement of the tube above the vocal cords or into the right main stem bronchus or obstruction of the tube by secretions are the common tube problems. Bronchospasm, pneumonia, pulmonary edema and air leaks like pneumothorax can lead to dyspnea and patient discomfort. Clinical examination and skiagram of chest can help in making a diagnosis. Appropriate interventions include use of bronchodilators, treatment of the underlying condition that may have caused pulmonary edema like control of cardiac failure, fluid restriction, diuretics and needle aspiration or chest tube drainage in cases of symptomatic pneumothorax.

   Another cause of increased work of breathing is dynamic hyperinflation (DH) or auto-PEEP. If the ventilator delivers a breath before the patient has exhaled fully, this leads to air trapping and the lung cannot empty to the functional residual capacity (FRC). In normal circumstances, the end expiratory pressure equals atmospheric pressure. In the presence of dynamic hyperinflation, the alveolar pressure remains positive relative to atmospheric pressure. The DH may occur as a consequence of short expiratory time, higher respiratory rate or higher tidal volume. When DH exists, the work of breathing is high because the patient has to generate pressure equal to the level of auto-PEEP plus the negative inspiratory flow to trigger the ventilator. Strategies for decreasing DH include facilitating expiration by increasing the expiratory time, decreasing the rate of breathing and accepting a higher $PaCO_2$ (permissive hypercapnia). Finally, adding external PEEP (equal to 75–85% of the auto-PEEP) can decrease work of breathing and reduce distress of the patient. Another important cause for a patient fighting the ventilator is inadequate pain relief or inadequate sedation. However, before using sedatives or muscle relaxants one should rule out potentially remediable and life threatening aforementioned causes.

2. **Hypoxemia and hypercarbia** The approach is similar to a patient presenting with acute respiratory distress.

3. **Hypotension** Common causes of hypotension include hypovolemia, myocardial dysfunction, and impairment of venous return due to higher mean airway pressure and sepsis or systemic inflammatory response syndrome. Medications like sedatives and muscle relaxants can also produce hypotension by decreasing the vascular tone. Treatment should be aimed at correcting the underlying cause. In cases where higher MAP is needed for adequate oxygenation, adequate volume replacement and use of inotropes should be considered.

4. **Pulmonary hemorrhage** The main causes include pulmonary edema, trauma to trachea due to repeated suctioning, necrotizing pneumonia, tracheobronchitis, pulmonary embolism, bleeding disorders and pulmonary artery catheters. Treatment is based on the underlying cause. Conditions that lead to a decrease in lung compliance like pulmonary edema or pneumonia need a higher PEEP to maintain oxygenation.

5. **Pneumothorax** Risk factors for the development of pneumothorax in mechanically ventilated patients include use of high MAP, prolonged T_i, patient ventilator asynchrony and the presence of an underlying lung condition like MAS, PIE and pulmonary hypoplasia. Occurrence of pneumothorax in mechanically ventilated patients is manifest by an acute onset of respiratory distress, cyanosis, episodes of apnea or bradycardia, decreased air entry in the affected side, mediastinal shift and hypotension. Transillumination may reveal increased transmission of light on the affected side. However, identification of pneumothorax may be difficult in ventilated patients. During volume-controlled ventilation, the peak airway pressure progressively increases producing a high pressure alarm. In pressure-controlled ventilation, the delivered tidal volumes decrease progressively since peak airway

27

pressure remains constant. Attention to the peak airway pressures and delivered VTs and appropriate setting up of alarms are essential for early detection of complications. Iatrogenic pneumothorax due to positive pressure mechanical ventilation may lead to the development of a bronchopleural fistula or tension pneumothorax (Figure 27.17). These patients require urgent needle aspiration or chest tube insertion.

Needling of the chest is performed using a butterfly needle or intravenous cannula in the second intercostal space in the midclavicular line. The anterior to midaxillary line between the 4th or 5th intercostal space (Buelau position) is safe for performing thoracostomy in preterm and term infants. Appropriate sized chest tube is 10 Fr in small infants, and 12 Fr for bigger infants. Although single and two bottle drainage units are available, the commercially available three compartments water-seal pleural drain unit (PDU) offers more advantages. In this arrangement, one compartment acts as a fluid collection bottle, the second as a water seal that prevents aspiration of air back into the pleural space and the third as a pressure-regulating chamber, all incorporated into one disposable plastic unit.

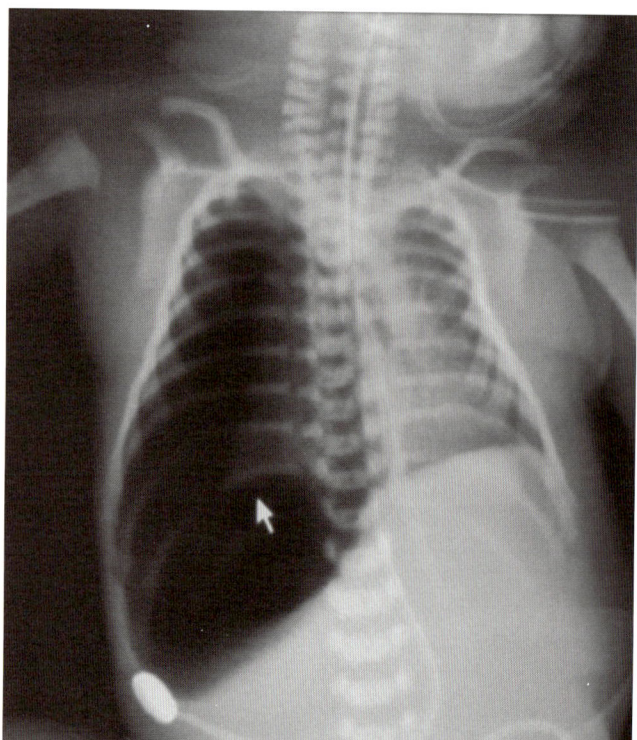

Figure 27.17 Tension pneumothorax on the right side in an infant on assisted ventilation.

Patients requiring chest tube drainage while on a mechanical ventilator need close monitoring. There should be constant bubbling in the pressure regulating chamber, otherwise the amount of suction applied to the system is unknown. Air does not bubble from the water seal chamber unless there is a persistent airleak (pneumothorax, bronchopleural fistula). Leaks in the chest tube system can also produce bubbling in the chamber in the absence of air leaks.

Patients on positive pressure ventilation are at an increased risk of tension pneumothorax, if the tube is clamped or obstructed. Hence clamping the chest tube should be done only under close monitoring prior to chest tube removal. If clamping does not result in worsening of pneumothorax, the chest tube can be safely removed.

WEANING FROM THE VENTILATOR

Weaning is a difficult and delicate procedure and should be undertaken with due caution. The clinical condition of the infant, status of blood gases and natural history of the disease dictates the possible age and time when weaning can be initiated. For example, in hyaline membrane disease, there is no question of weaning after 1–2 days and it is attempted after 3rd or 4th day especially at a time when maximum diuresis is observed which heralds the onset of recovery. It is important to reduce the settings of ventilator at this stage otherwise air leaks would occur due to improvement in the compliance of lungs. The weaning should not be unduly delayed because if the infant is not taken off the ventilator by 5th–8th day, he is more likely to develop bronchopulmonary dysplasia. On the other hand, babies with uncomplicated meconium aspiration or pneumonia can be weaned off much earlier. The baby should be stable for at least 24 hours before weaning is attempted. There is an accepted sequence and certain principles are followed while bringing down the settings of the ventilator. The first setting to be reduced is PIP by 1.0 cm H_2O decrements till it is brought down to 25 cm H_2O. High PIP is the predisposing factor for development of bronchopulmonary dysplasia. At this stage, PIP and FiO_2 (decreased by 0.05 or 5%) are reduced alternately till a relatively safe levels of 20 cm H_2O PIP and 0.6 FiO_2 are reached.

At this stage, the weaning process moves through 3 simultaneous channels (Figure 27.18). The FiO_2 and PEEP should be decreased hand in hand (i.e. at 0.6 FiO_2 the PEEP should be 6 cm H_2O and at 0.3 FiO_2

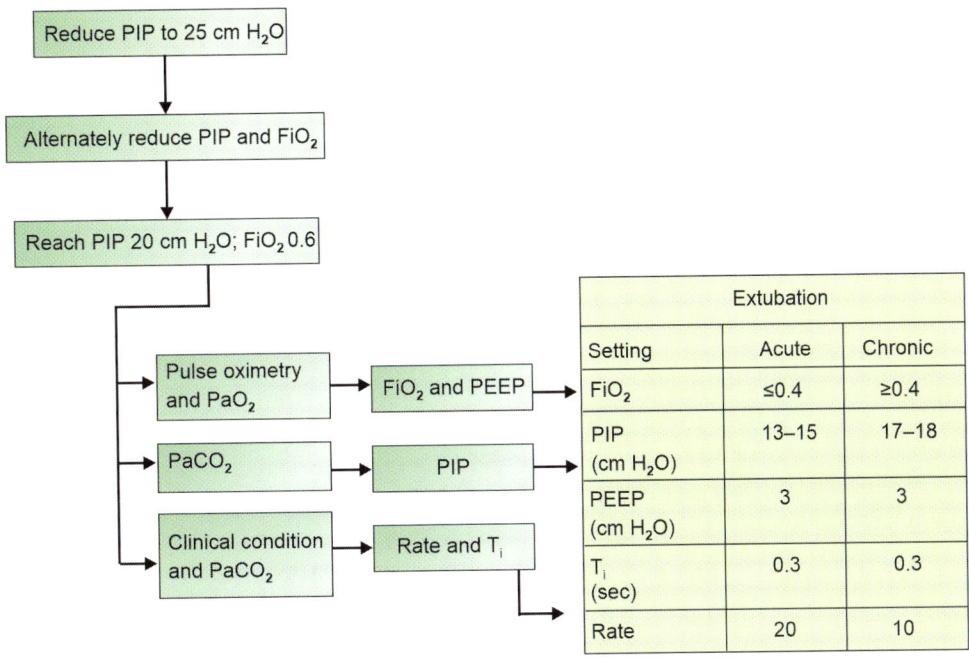

Principles

1. Ensure adequate tidal volume (V_T) of at least 4 mL/kg to overcome work of breathing.
2. Ensure normal minute ventilation, i.e. 4 mL/kg × 60 = 240 – 360 mL.
3. Avoid fatigue by supporting the spontaneous breaths.
4. Ensure slow weaning to provide adequate rest and sleep.
5. Correct underlying factors that impede the weaning process, i.e. anemia, poor nutrition, excessive sedation, airway secretions, pneumonia, bronchopulmonary dysplasia and electrolyte disturbances.

Figure 27.18 Summary of guidelines for weaning from positive pressure ventilation.

PEEP should be 3 cm H_2O and so on) depending upon the oxygenation status. PIP should be reduced by decrements of 1.0 cm H_2O every 15–20 minutes by titrating it with paCO_2 values. The ventilatory rate is now reduced in short decrements of 5 breaths/minute till it is brought down to 20 breaths/minute. The decrease in breathing rate is achieved mostly by prolonging expiratory time and providing intermittent mandatory ventilation. When ventilator settings have been brought down to FiO_2 0.4, PIP 10–15 cm H_2O (17–18 cm H_2O in BPD), PEEP 3 cm H_2O, Ti 0.3 seconds and breathing rate of 20/minute the infant can be attached to CPAP mode before extubation.

It is recommended to start intravenous aminophylline 24 hours before the expected time of extubation. Aminophylline is believed to increase efficiency of respiratory muscles especially the diaphragm and enhances minute ventilation by increasing responsiveness of respiratory center to carbon dioxide. At times, when weaning is becoming exceedingly difficult and early changes of bronchopulmonary dysplasia have set in, extubation can be primed with corticosteroid therapy. After extubation, infant should be placed in

an oxygen hood with FiO_2 of 0.4–0.5 and blood gases monitored. Skiagram of chest should be taken to exclude postextubation atelectasis.

INHALED NITRIC OXIDE (iNO)

Nitric oxide (NO) is a naturally occurring gas produced by endothelial cells. The endogenous NO or iNO delivered through the ventilator circuit, diffuses into smooth muscle cells, increases intracellular cyclic guanosine monophosphate (cGMP), relaxes the vascular smooth muscles leading to pulmonary vasodilatation. In the circulation, NO is bound with hemoglobin and biologically inactivated and therefore iNO causes little or no systemic vasodilatation or hypotension. It is a useful modality in critically sick term and near term infants with persistent pulmonary hypertension (PPHN) and respiratory failure (oxygenation index of >25). iNO is administered by conventional or preferably high-frequency ventilation in a dose of 20 parts per million (ppm). Higher doses of iNO have the potential to increase toxicity without conferring any additional benefits. iNO is most effective when administered after adequate alveolar

Assisted Ventilation and Advanced Life Support

27

recruitment by concomitant use of HFOV and/or surfactant treatment. Three FDA approved delivery devices for iNO include iNOvent (Datex-Ohmeda), iNOmax DS (Ikaria) and AeroNOx 2.0 (International Biomedical). iNO therapy can be administred to babies on conventional ventilator, high frequency ventilator and as well as babies on nCPAP. iNo ventilation is an expensive modality and is available only in select centers in India and its use is limited because of scarce availability of medical grade NO and difficulties in its calibration. Moreover, its use is restricted to a small group of term or near term infants with life-threatening PPHN (usually following MAS) and respiratory failure.

The common side effects include development of methemoglobinemia and rebound hypoxia when iNO is tapered too rapidly. Methemoglobin levels should be monitored daily during iNO ventilation and therapy should be tapered gradually until adequate oxygenation can be maintained at an iNO dose of 1 ppm. All infants with PPHN do not respond to iNO and some may deteriorate rapidly and they can be salvaged by ECMO.

Weaning from iNO

Weaning should be started when infant is stable and adequately oxygenated for 4–6 hours. FiO_2 should be less than 0.6 and/or the oxygenation index should be <10. At this stage, decrease the dose of iNO by 50% every 4–6 hours intervals. When a dose of 5 ppm is reached, further decrease in dosing should be done continuously @ 1 ppm every 4 hours. iNO is disconti-nued when infant is stable and well-oxygenated with iNO dose of 1 ppm at FiO_2 of <0.6.

EXTRACORPOREAL MEMBRANE OXYGENATION (ECMO)

ECMO is a newer modality of treatment to provide temporary life support to the neonates with life-threatening cardiorespiratory failure when standard treatment with inhaled nitric oxide (iNO) ventilation is unable to maintain adequate oxygenation. Advances in biotechnology has made the technology of cardio-pulmonary bypass fairly safe even in preterm babies undergoing open heart surgery. In this highly cost-intensive technology, the infant's blood is passed through a membrane oxygenator for extracorporeal exchange of oxygen and carbon dioxide. The availa-bility of high frequency jet ventilation and iNO-ventilation facilities have reduced the need for ECMO.

Indications

ECMO is most commonly used in neonates with persistent pulmonary hypertension (PPHN) with severe hypoxemia due to right-to-left shunting of blood through foramen ovale or ductus arteriosus. The common conditions which are associated with PPHN include meconium aspiration syndrome, congenital diaphragmatic hernia and hypoplasia of lungs. Though relatively uncommon, PPHN may be associated with severe birth asphyxia, RDS, cardiac malformations, sepsis and fulminant pneumonia. Idiopathic or primary pulmonary hypertension of the newborn is a rare entity.

ECMO should be considered only if iNO- ventilation (including newer modalities of high frequency oscillatory ventilation) are unable to sustain life. The recognized criteria for instituting ECMO are listed below:

1. Alveolar to arterial oxygen (AO_2-aO_2) gradient or AA-aDO_2 (Alveolar–arterial oxygen tension difference) of more than 600 mm Hg for 6–12 hours.

2. Arterial pO_2 to alveolar pO_2 ratio (apO_2/ApO_2) of less than 0.2.

3. Ventilation index $\dfrac{(RR \times PIP \times PaCO_2)}{1000}$ of more than 90 for 4 hours.

4. Oxygenation index $\dfrac{(MAP \times FiO_2\%)}{\text{Post-ductal } PaO_2}$ of more than 40 on conventional ventilation on two conse-cutive blood gases obtained one hour apart.

Procedure

The procedure requires sophisticated instrumentation for cardiac bypass and membrane oxygenator of an appropriate size for the infant. The blood flow is main-tained through the ECMO circuit with a non-pulsatile pump. The blood is drawn by inserting a catheter in the right internal jugular vein or right atrium. It is passed through the membrane for oxygenation and removal of carbon dioxide. The oxygenated blood is returned to the infant via right common carotid artery (venoarterial) or the femoral vein (veno-venous). The infant is kept heparinized and ventilated at resting ventilator setting like PIP of 25 cm H_2O, PEEP 5 cm H_2O, rate 10 breaths/min, inspiratory time 1.0 second and FiO_2 of 0.4. The procedure allows "lung rest" and lungs are protected from further injury due to baro-trauma and oxygen. The improved oxygenation and mild alkalosis are associated with decrease in the

Care of the Newborn

27

pulmonary artery pressure. The reduction in the intra-thoracic pressure is followed by increased venous return to the heart. Infants who are at high risk for bleeding are administered e-aminocaproic acid. All ECMO candidates are administered broad-spectrum antibiotics, furosemide and inotropes. Pain and discomfort must be relieved by administration of appropriate narcotic analgesics and sedatives. It is highly cost-intensive therapy demanding a close cooperation and coordination between the neonatologist and pediatric surgeon, nurses, perfusionist and respiratory therapist.

Contraindications

The procedure should not be undertaken in infants with irreversible lung injury, severe hypoplasia, mechanical ventilation for more than 10 days, grade 3 or 4 intraventricular hemorrhage, progressive chronic lung disease, severe coagulopathy, lethal congenital malformations, multiorgan failure, VLBW infants less than 34 weeks gestation and babies with multiple congenital malformations.

Complications and Outcome

The procedure may be complicated by bleeding, hypovolemia, dyselectrolytemia, sepsis, DIC, thromboembolic phenomenon, air emboli and IVH. The survivors have increased risk of reactive airway disease, neuromotor retardation, deafness, attention deficit and hyperactivity disorder.

SUPPORTIVE CARE DURING VENTILATION

The supportive management of critically sick pre-term infants on assisted ventilation demands availability of sophisticated technology and high quality of skills of the personnel working in the NICU. Assisted ventilation, by and large, is required for very low birth weight babies having respiratory failure due to hyaline membrane disease, pneumonia and recurrent apneic attacks. The principles of supportive and nutritional management of ventilated babies, therefore, by and large, are similar to those required for management of pre-term and very low birth weight babies with additional supervision and support for ensuring adequate and safe oxygenation by effective ventilation. The immediate and late outcome of babies on ventilation largely depends upon adequate and effective ventilation management and supportive care with due emphasis on ensuring thermoneutral environment, fluids, electrolytes and metabolic homeostasis, adequate tissue perfusion, prevention of

nosocomial infections and other complications of prolonged assisted ventilation.

Facilities Required for Assisted Ventilation

The neonatal unit must have the expertise and equipment to function as a good level II special care neonatal unit before ventilatory facilities are introduced. It is indeed lopsided and undesirable to buy ventilators without first developing suitable infrastructure to provide thermoneutral environment, ensure asepsis, satisfactory nutritional management of very low birth weight babies and availability of technology to monitor and administer oxygen to babies having respiratory problems. The neonatal mortality rate should be brought down to <20 per 1000 live births by effective use of level II newborn care facilities before it is envisaged to introduce assisted ventilation facilities. The unit must have centralized supply of oxygen, suction and compressed air along with round-the-clock facilities for monitoring blood gases, acid base parameters, taking portable skiagrams and having point-of-care ultrasonography and echocardiography facilities. There should be availability of servo-controlled open care systems, multichannel vital sign monitors including pulse oximeter and microchemistry laboratory facilities to estimate serum electrolytes, blood glucose and bilirubin on ultramicro-samples of blood. Most infants on prolonged ventilation would also require partial parenteral nutrition and some experience should be gained in this technology before embarking upon ventilation facilities (Figure 27.19).

Thermal Homeostasis

The infant should be nursed in a thermoneutral environment by using servo-controlled infant open care system to reduce energy and oxygen cost of

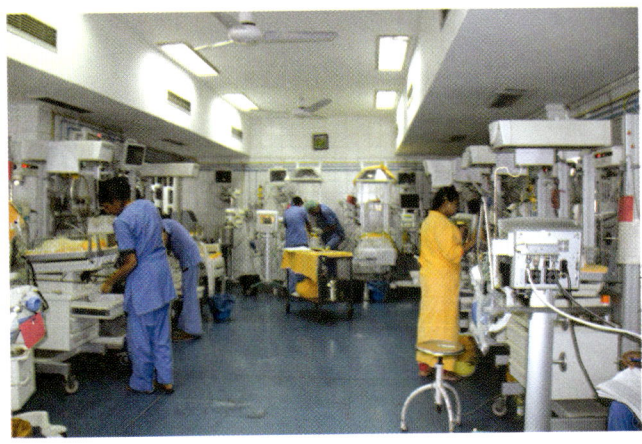

Figure 27.19 Neonatal intensive care unit equipped with state-of-the-art supportive facilities for providing assisted ventilation.

metabolic thermogenesis. The administration of cold infusates should be avoided and all the articles (including X-ray plates) with whom the baby comes in contact should be prewarmed to reduce heat loss due to conduction. The heat loss during various procedures like endotracheal intubation, blood sampling and umbilical vessel catheterisation should be prevented by using overhead radiant warmer. In extremely low birth weight babies heat and insensible water loss from skin can be reduced by draping the baby in a polythene sheet.

Fluids, Electrolytes and Nutritional Support

The maintenance requirements of fluids should be restricted in babies on assisted ventilation because insensible water losses are reduced as humidified air oxygen mixture is given and there is increased incidence of inappropriate secretion of antidiuretic hormone. Excessive fluid administration is associated with increased risk of development of patent ductus arteriosus, necrotising enterocolitis and bronchopulmonary dysplasia. During initial 48 hours, babies with a birth weight of less than 1250 g should be started on 5% dextrose infusion. The concentration of the dextrose solution may be changed depending upon the blood glucose levels because administration of 10% dextrose in extremely low birth weight babies may be associated with hyperglycemia and glycosuria. Infants with birth weight of >1250 g or gestation of >30 weeks should be administered 10% dextrose to prevent hypoglycemia.

After 48 hours, sodium (sodium chloride or sodium bicarbonate), potassium and calcium should be added to the infusate. Potassium supplements should be restricted because infants with severe RDS may develop hyperkalemia due to tissue catabolism and NSAID therapy for PDA. Acidosis should be corrected by slow administration of sodium bicarbonate. When acidosis cannot be explained on the basis of ineffective ventilation (hypoxia or hypercarbia), excessive PEEP or excessive work of breathing (infant having marked chest retractions), it is a good policy to administer 10 mL/kg of physiological saline or plasma over 20 to 30 minutes to improve tissue perfusion. Inotropic agents are indicated to correct cardiogenic shock due to persistent hypoxia and acidosis.

The energy requirements of babies on ventilation are higher to meet the increased demands due to excessive work of breathing and increased tissue catabolism. Infants with bronchopulmonary dysplasia need exceedingly high energy inputs to sustain satisfactory somatic and mental growth because energy is being diverted for hypertrophy of respiratory muscles and excessive proliferation of pulmonary tissue. Most infants on assisted ventilation should receive combined enteral feeding of expressed breastmilk through a nasogastric tube and partial parenteral nutrition. However, enteral feedings should be avoided in babies who are hemodynamically unstable or having abdominal distension or receiving CPAP through nasal prongs. When it is anticipated that assisted ventilation can be withdrawn within two to three days, enteral feedings may be withheld till infant is extubated. The enteral feeding should be started with 1–2 mL of EBM per feed and maintenance requirements should be gradually built up along with partial parenteral nutritional support. It is desirable to restrict administration of intralipids in infants having severe RDS or those with significant jaundice.

During enteral feeding, monitor abdominal girth and ensure that the volume of prefeed gastric aspirate does not exceed 50% of the volume of previous feed administered to the baby. The gastric aspirate should not be discarded but should be returned to prevent electrolyte losses in small babies. By and large, enteral feedings are well tolerated by infants receiving assisted ventilation and feeding with EBM actually reduces the risk of necrotizing enterocolitis because it provides substrate to the gut for production of enzymes, promotes peristaltic activity and reduces gastric stasis, enhances maturation of the gut and IgA in the breast milk affords local immune protection. In view of the fact that institution of TPN has several logistic and administrative problems in developing countries, it is desirable to promote enteral feeding in babies receiving assisted ventilation in order to ensure their satisfactory somatic and mental growth. The volume and caloric density of the feeds should be gradually increased to provide at least 120 kcal/kg per day to the babies on ventilation.

The maintenance requirements of intravenous fluids is monitored by accurate weighing (electronic weighing scale with a sensitivity ±1.0 g) of the baby twice a day, recording intake and urine output (ensure 2 to 4 mL/kg/hr) and maintaining normal urinary specific gravity (1005–1015), urine osmolality (150–300 mOsm/L) and plasma osmolality (280–300 mOsm/L). Urine output can be assessed with the help of a condom of test tube in a male child and urine collection bag or by placing a preweighed cotton pack under the bottom of a female infant.

Prevention of Infections

Infants receiving assisted ventilation are at an increased risk of developing nosocomial bacterial and fungal infections. Maintenance of strict asepsis and hand washing rituals are essential to reduce the risk of infection. There should not be any compromise on the use of disposable items including ventilator circuits which should not be reused. The sterility of IV sites should be ensured by effective preparation of skin and avoiding stock solutions for rinsing the intracaths. The use of bacterial filters, though expensive, are mandatory for administration of aminoacid and dextrose solutions. The solution for TPN must be prepared under a laminar flow to avoid contamination especially with *Candida albicans*. The suctioning of the oral cavity and endotracheal tubes should be done under strict aseptic conditions by wearing gloves and by using disposable sterile packs containing suction catheters and a bowl. Despite stringent efforts to protect the babies against development of nosocomial infections, it is unfortunate that some babies do develop septicemia which should be identified as early as possible by frequent monitoring of cot-side screening tests and blood cultures for septicemia. The endotracheal secretions should be sent for culture every 48 hours. In babies receiving TPN or prolonged ventilation for more than one week, there is an increased risk of development of candidemia which should be monitored by frequent examinations of urine to look for hyphae.

Monitoring and Prevention of Common Complications

Specialized monitoring charts should be prepared to enable the nurses to record various parameters such as ventilatory settings, blood gases and vital signs. The adequacy of tissue perfusion should be assessed by evaluating blood pressure, capillary refill time, difference between core and peripheral temperature and metabolic acidosis. Accurate record of fluid intake, urine output, hydration status and weight is mandatory. Frequent monitoring of blood glucose, sodium, potassium and calcium is required in all babies but especially those receiving TPN. Prolongation of QoTC (more than 0.2 sec) with the help of EKG is suggestive of hypocalcemia. Skiagrams of the chest are required every 6–12 hourly to identify any evidences of air leaks, superadded pneumonia and bronchopulmonary dysplasia.

During recovery from hyaline membrane disease, sudden decrease in pulmonary vascular resistance may be followed by development of left-to-right shunt at ductus arteriosus. The presence of bounding peripheral pulses especially dorsalis pedis, appearance of a continuous cardiac murmur and development of

congestive heart failure as evidenced by increasing hepatomegaly or sudden gain in weight are suggestive of PDA. It should be managed by restriction of fluids, administration of furosemide and if required indomethacin or ibuprofen. The occurrence of intraventricular hemorrhage is heralded by subtle seizures, sudden fall in hematocrit or rise in bilirubin, change in muscle tone and at times bulging of anterior fontanel. The availability of a portable ultrasound is useful to identify this catastrophic complication. Most infants tolerate enteral feeds without any complications but it is desirable to keep a watch on abdominal girth, gastric residuals and occult blood in the stools as early markers of necrotizing enterocolitis. The occurrence of sepsis or candidemia, which is the commonest complication in Indian set up is associated with greyish discoloration of a baby or sudden pallor due to reduced tissue perfusion, reduced activity, instability of body temperature, abdominal distension, evidences of superficial infections at IV sites, jaundice and shock. It must be identified early so that effective antibiotic therapy is administered to improve the survival of these babies. Candidemia manifests with clinical features which are akin to NEC, but without any occult blood in the stools or pneumatosis intestinalis on X-ray of the abdomen.

A large number of complications are known to occur due to the procedure of mechanical ventilation. Endotracheal intubation may be associated with trauma to soft tissues, atelectasis of left lung (due to intubation of right bronchus), perforation of trachea or esophagus, avulsion of vocal cords, subglottic stenosis (following prolonged intubation) and superinfection may occur. Acute barotrauma due to high PIP and PEEP may result in pulmonary air leaks in the form of interstitial emphysema, pneumothorax, pneumomediastinum, pneumoperitoneum and subcutaneous emphysema. Bronchopulmonary dysplasia is believed to be due to an outcome of chronic barotrauma following prolonged ventilation. High ambient oxygen concentration and hyperoxia is also associated with bronchopulmonary dysplasia and retinopathy of prematurity. Hemodynamic effects especially due to high PEEP may lead to reduced venous return and cardiac output, and increase in the cerebral pressure.

In order to reduce the risk of complications, it is, therefore, desirable that an attempt should be made to use the lowest settings of FiO_2, PIP and PEEP which are compatible with satisfactory blood gas values. The barotrauma-related complications have been reduced by introduction of high frequency jet or oscillatory ventilators. Bronchopulmonary dysplasia is suspected when there is difficulty to wean the baby from ventilator, prolonged oxygen dependence with respiratory difficulty and characteristic changes in the lungs on X-rays. The administration of corticosteroids at times facilitates weaning of the baby from ventilator and is useful during early stage of BPD. Aminophylline and caffeine are also known to increase the efficiency of respiratory muscles and may be used before extubation to facilitate weaning. The infant must be closely followed up by an ophthalmologist to make an early diagnosis of retinopathy of prematurity so that laser photocoagulation is instituted well in time as and when required. The utility of administration of high doses of vitamin E to prevent ROP and BPD is controversial.

Family Support

The parents must be constantly kept informed regarding the condition of their infant. The mother should be encouraged to establish bonding with her baby and allowed to touch and take care of the baby under supervision of the nurse. She should be encouraged to provide visual (eye-to-eye contact) and auditory stimuli (playing audio-cassette with taped music or voices of father and other siblings) to the baby. The anxiety and worry of the family should be cushioned but nevertheless they should be informed about the possible chances of recovery and future pulmonary and mental outcome in a pragmatic way. The family must be prepared both mentally and in terms of physical requirements at home before the infant is discharged from the hospital. The need for frequent contacts with the pediatrician and regular follow-up in the high-risk neonates clinic should be emphasised to the parents at the time of discharge. Home visiting by the public health nurse is mandatory for families who do not comply with the appointment schedule for follow-up.

BIBLIOGRAPHY

Amiel-Tison C. A method for neurological evaluation in first year of life. Current problems in pediatrics VII No. 1 *Year Book Medical Publishers, Chicago* 1976, pp 1–50.

Bernstein G, Mannino FL, Heldt GP, *et al.* Prospective randomized multicenter trial comparing synchronized and conventional intermittent mandatory ventilation (SIMV vs IMV) in neonates. *Pediatr Res* 1994, 216 A: 1281

Bhakoo ON. Assisted ventilation in neonates: The Indian perspective. *Indian Pediatr* 1995, 32: 1261–1264.

Bhandari V. Noninvasive respiratory support in the preterm infant. *Clin Perinatol* 2012, 39:497–511.

Buckmaster AG, Arnolda G, Foster JP, *et al.* Continuous positive airway pressure therapy for infants with respiratory distress in non tertiary care centers: a randomized controlled trial. *Pediatrics* 2007, 120: 509–518.

Carlo W. Assisted ventilation. In: Care of the High Risk Neonate. Klaus MH, Fanaroff AA (Eds.), *W B Saunders, Philadelphia,* 5th edition, 2001.

Chawla D. Continuous positive airway pressure in neonates. *Indian J Pediatr* 2015, 82(2): 107–8.

Cheema IU, Ahluwalia JS. Feasibility of tidal volume-guided ventilation in newborn infants: a randomized, crossover trial using the volume guarantee modality. *Pediatrics* 2001, 107(6) : 1323–1328.

Clark RH. High frequency ventilation. *J Pediatr* 1995, 124: 661–670.

Deorari AK, Paul VK, Singh M. Neonatal ventilation: Teething problems. *Indian Pediatr* 1994, 31: 2

De Paoli AG, Davi PG, Faber B, *et al.* Devices and pressure sources for administration of nCPAP in preterm neonates. *Cochrane Database Syst Rev* 2008, CD002977

Donn SM, Sinha SK. Invasive and non-invasive mechanical ventilation. *Respiratory Care* 2003, 48(4): 426–441.

Donn SM, Sinha SK. Newer techniques of mechanical ventilation: an overview. *Semin Neonatol* 2002, 7(5): 401–408.

Donn SM; Sinha SK. Newer modes of mechanical ventilation for the neonate. *Curr Opin Pediatr* 2001, 13(2): 99–103.

Donn SM. Neonatal ventilators. How do they differ? *J Perinatol* 2009, 29 (suppl 2): S73–S78.

Doyle LW, Ehrenkramz RA, Halliday HL. Dexamethasone treatment after the first week of life for bronchopulmonary dysplasia in preterm infants: A systemic review. *Neonatology* 2010, 98: 289–296.

Eifinger F, Lenze M, Brisken K, Welzing L, Roth B, Koebke J. The anterior to mid axillary line between 4th or 5th intercostal space (Buelau position) is safe for the use of thoracostomy tubes in preterm and term infants. *Pediatr Anesthesia* 19(6): 612–17.

Finer NN, Boyd J. Chest physiotherapy in the neonate : a controlled study. *Pediatrics* 1998, 61(2): 282–285.

Finer NN, Carlo WA, Walsh MC, Rich W, *et al.* Early CPAP versus surfactant in extremely preterm infants. SUPPORT Study Group of the Eumice Kennedy Shriver NICHD Neonatal Research Network. *N Engl J Med* 2010, 362: 1970–1979.

Fox WW, Spitzer AR, Shutak JG. Positive pressure ventilation: Pressure and time-cycled ventilators. In: Assisted Ventilation in Neonates. EOR Reynolds, Ed. *W B Saunders Co, Philadelphia* 1987, p 146–170.

Grazioli S, Karam O, Rimensberger PC. New generation neonatal high frequency ventilators: Effect of oscillatory frequency and working principles on performance. *Respiratory Care* 2015, 60(3): 363–70.

Gupta N, Saini SS, Murki S, Kumar P, Deorari AK. Continuous positive airway pressure in preterm neonates: An update of current evidence and implications for developing countries. *Indian Pediatr* 2015, 52: 319–26.

Haynes D, Baumann MH. Management of pneumothorax. *Semin Resp Crit Care Med* 2010, 31(6): 769–780.

Ichinose F, Roberts JD, Zapol WM. Inhaled nitric oxide: A selective pulmonary vasodilation. Current uses and therapeutic potential. *Circulation* 2004, 109: 3106–3111.

Keszler M. Guidelines for rational and cost-effective use of iNO therapy in term and preterm infants. *J Clin Neonatol* 2012, 1:59–63.

Keszler M, Durand J. Neonatal high-frequency ventilation: past, present and future. *Clin Perinatol* 2001, 28(3): 579–607.

Maheshwari R, Kumar H, Paul VK, Singh M, *et al.* Incidence and risk factors of retinopathy of prematurity in a tertiary care newborn unit in New Delhi. *Nat Med J India* 1996, 9: 211–214.

McNally H, Bennett CC, Elbourne D, *et al.* UK Collaborative ECMO Trial Group. United Kingdom collaborative randomized trial of neonatal extracorporeal membrane oxygenation: Follow-up to age 7 years. *Pediatrics* 2006, 117(5): e 845–e 854.

Morley CJ, Davis PG, Doyle LW, *et al.* COIN Trial Investigators. Nasal CPAP intubation at birth for very preterm infants. *N Engl J Med* 2008, 358: 700–708.

Morley CJ, Lau R, De Paoli AG, Davis PG. Nasal continuous positive airway pressure: Does bubbling improve gas exchange? *Arch Dis Child Fetal Neonatal Ed* 2005, 90: F343–F344.

Nelin LD, Potenziano JL. Inhaled nitric oxide for neonates with persistent pulmonary hypertension of the newborn in the CINRGI study: time to treatment response. *BMC Pediatr* 2019, 19:17 (https://doi.org/10.1186/s12887-018-1368-4).

Singh M, Deorari AK, Paul VK, *et al.* Three-year experience with neonatal ventilation from a tertiary care hospital in Delhi. *Indian Pediatr* 1992, 29: 1507–12.

Sinha SK, Donn SM, Gavey J, McCarty M. Randomized trial of volume-controlled versus time-cycled, pressure-limited ventilation in preterm infants with respiratory distress syndrome. *Arch Dis Child* 1997, 77(3): F202–F205.

Sinha SK, Donn SM. Weaning newborns from mechanical ventilation. *Semin Neonatol* 2002, 7(5): 421–428.

Sokol GM, Ehrenkranz RA. Inhaled nitric oxide therapy in neonatal hypoxic respiratory failure: in sights beyond primary outcomes. *Semin Perinatol* 2003, 27: 311–319.

Subramaniam P, Henderson-Smart DJ, Davis P. Prophylactic nasal continuous positive airways pressure for preventing morbidity and mortality in very preterm infants. *Cochrane Database Syst Rev* 2005: CD001234.

Assisted Ventilation and Advanced Life Support

27

Follow-up Program for High-Risk Newborns

There have been tremendous advances both in the understanding and the availability of technology for effective and rational management of high-risk newborn babies. The focus has also shifted from mere survival to intact survival and the quality of life among the survivors. The earlier passive nurse-dominated "hands off" approach in the care of premature babies has been replaced by more "aggressive" interventional strategies to enhance newborn survival. Technology-oriented approach, though beneficial in many situations, has lead to the emergence of a large number of potentially avoidable iatrogenic disorders. Over the years, the birth weight-specific survivals of newborn babies have considerably improved in the developed countries but there has been no reduction in the load of neuromotor disability and sensorineural handicaps to the society. Technology is being harnessed to save tiny babies with grossly immature organs whom nature never wanted to survive ("unnatural survivors"). The concern is often expressed, is modern specialized obstetrical and neonatal care converting deaths into disabilities? Although, the percentage of babies with neuromotor disability is lower in different birth weight groups but the load of neuromotor disability to the society is unaltered because of higher number of newborn survivors.

The neonatal intensive care is highly cost and labor intensive. It is futile and unwise to have a concern on mere survival of the babies. *It is important to remember that the aim and goal of newborn care is not only to reduce neonatal mortality but more importantly to ensure their intact survival.* It is mandatory that every neonatal unit must establish adequate facilities and a program to follow-up the nursery graduates to assess their health related quality of life and contributions to the society. Infants with neuromotor disability should be provided with early stimulation and rehabilitation services.

Apart from developing an excellent infrastructural layout and availability of adequate tools for asessment, there is a need to have a dedicated team of specialists comprising of neonatologist, pediatric neurologist, developmental physician, child psychologist, dietician, audiologist, ophthalmologist, speech therapist, physiotherapist, kinesiologist, occupational therapist, medical social worker and public health nurse.

INDICATIONS FOR FOLLOW-UP

For all practical purposes, all the nursey graduates should preferably be followed up. The following infants are at a moderate to high-risk to develop neuromotor disability and must be followed up in accordance with a set protocol.

- All infants with a birth weight of <1500 g or gestation of <32 weeks and grossly small-for-dates (<3rd centile) or large-for-dates (>97th centile) babies.
- Birth asphyxia with 5-minute Apgar score of 3 or less and/or hypoxic–ischemic encephalopathy (HIE) grade 2 and more.
- Babies on assisted ventilation.
- Babies with metabolic disorders.
- Neonatal seizures due to any cause.
- Hyperbilirubinemia requiring exchange blood transfusion.
- Neonatal sepsis with or without meningitis.
- Infants with major congenital malformations.
- Infants with major morbidities, like retinopathy of prematurity (ROP), chronic lung disease, necrotizing enterocolitis (NEC), intraventricular hemorrhage and periventricular leukomalacia.
- Infants of HIV-positive mother.
- Infants with abnormal neurological behavior during their NICU stay and at discharge.

Counseling and Documentation at Discharge

Discharge should be planned well in advance so that family can be adequately counseled. Mother should be given all the information and skills to look after the baby at home. Public health nurse should assess the home conditions before baby is discharged and medical social worker should coordinate to ensure timely follow-up and referral to various specialists. The need and importance of regular follow-up should be explained to the family. The following components of care of the baby after discharge should be explained.

- Temperature control. Proper clothing, cap, socks, mittens, kangaroo-mother care should be provided to ensure that trunk is warm to touch and hands and feet are reasonably warm and pink.
- Optimal feeding with human milk and need for nutritional supplements should be explained. Avoidance of bottle feeding should be promoted. Home-based complementary or weaning foods should be started at 6 months of corrected age.
- Prevention of infections. Handwashing, keeping the baby and mother in a room having adequate ventilation and exposure to sunlight.
- Avoidance of visitors and advising them not to touch or kiss the baby.
- Schedule of follow-up visits with their timing and place of reporting.
- Consultation schedule with specialists for screening of ROP, hearing, neuromotor development, early stimulation, physiotherapy, occupational therapy, speech therapy and special educators.
- Immunization schedule.
- Danger signs, whom to contact and where to report when baby is sick.

The following parameters should be recorded in the discharge summary to serve as useful guidelines to the follow-up team for the "intensity and periodicity of follow-up."

- Gestation at birth and discharge (postconceptional or corrected age).
- Anthropometric measurements, i.e. weight, length and head circumference at birth and discharge.
- Complete medical diagnosis, procedures undergone, medications and transfusions received.
- Details regarding assisted ventilation and oxygen therapy.
- Results of various screening tests, like ROP screen, hearing screen (OAE and BERA), sonography of brain and metabolic screening.
- Details regarding feeding, nutritional supplements and hematological parameters.
- Immunization status and protocol.
- Family characteristics and dynamics.

THE FOLLOW-UP SCHEDULE

The process of screening should begin during their stay in the NICU. Anthropometric measurements should be taken every week and recorded on the intra-uterine-postnatal growth charts. Cranial ultrasound examination should be routinely conducted on day 3, 7 and 21 to identify intraventricular–periventricular hemorrhage, ventriculomegaly, periventricular leukomalacia and hydrocephalus. In infants with abnormal USG or neurological findings, CT scan, MRI and aEEG is advised at the age of 3 months. The screening for ROP should be conducted as per the protocol outlined in Chapter 26. After discharge, physical growth, anthropometry and screening for systemic disorders should be conducted when infant reports for various immunizations. Detailed neurological examination and neuromotor development is undertaken at the corrected ages of 4 months, 8 months, 12 months and then every 6 months till 5 years of age. Medical social worker should establish a rapport with the family to ensure timely follow-up visits and help them to seek referral and appointment with various experts and specialists. Some neonatal centers follow their high-risk newborn population throughout childhood and adolescence to study their social integration and contribution towards society. During first 2 years of follow-up, the corrected age or postconceptional age should be used for comparison with norms. Therefore, their chronological age should be calculated from the expected date of delivery rather than the actual date of birth. A separate follow-up file should be maintained for each baby and it should be color-coded, blue for boys and pink for girls.

PHYSICAL GROWTH

Anthropometric evaluation should be conducted at monthly intervals during first 6 months followed by every 3 months subsequently. Most preterm babies remain below the expected weight (and occasionally for length and head circumference) during the first 2 years of life. Almost 20% of very LBW babies remain below 3rd percentile for weight at the age of 3 years. Infants with underlying systemic disorders, like bronchopulmonary dysplasia, necrotizing enterocolitis and severe CNS abnormalities are more likely to have physical stunting. Failure of normal growth of head circumference is a simple and reliable parameter of to assess the integrity of brain and neuromotor development. Babies whose head circumference is below 2 standard deviations from the mean, or when head centile is less than the length centile of the baby, they are at an increased risk of development of neurological abnormalities. Abnormalities of head shape, especially scaphocephaly or dolichocephaly, are common. The indices of physical growth, i.e. weight, length and head circumference should be charted on a combined intrauterine-postnatal growth chart (Wright's charts) up to 40 weeks of postmenstrual age and gender specific WHO growth charts subsequently to serve as ready reckoner to identify any deviations. There is gradual reduction in the velocity of growth of various anthropometric parameters as the child grows (Table 28.1).

NEUROMOTOR DEVELOPMENT AND COGNITION

Neurological Examination and Screening for Development

The pediatricians should be able to identify neurological abnormalities and early markers of neuromotor disability by clinical examination.

Assessment of muscle tone Evaluation of muscle tone is useful for early diagnosis of cerebral palsy. During fetal life, acquisition of muscle tone and motor functions evolve from lower extremities and spread upwards in the direction of head. Healthy term babies are hypertonic by adult standards. The process of muscle relaxation occurs cephalocaudally after birth. Thus the upper limbs begin to relax and acquire skills before the lower limbs. The head control appears first, followed by ability to sit, stand and finally walk by 12–18 months.

Amiel-Tison's method for assessment of muscle tone is useful for early diagnosis of cerebral diplegia. Table 28.2 gives the range of normal angles at various joints during the first year of life. Reduction of these angles occurs due to hypertonia and is suggestive of cerebral palsy. Indian babies are physiologically more hypotonic possibly due to higher incidence of intrauterine growth retardation and unsatisfactory postnatal nutrition.

There are some babies who develop transitory hypertonia during 3–6 months of age but they normalize by the age of 9 months–1 year. These infants may manifest with subtle neurological abnormalities and learning difficulties later in life.

Development screening A number of monographs are available for detailed assessment of neuromotor development. Table 28.3 gives the upper age limits of some cardinal milestones which are useful to diagnose abnormal developmental delay. A development observation card (DOC) can be given to the parents for early identification of neurodevelopment retardation.

Early markers of cerebral palsy Neurological examination and developmental assessment by the pediatrician can readily identify the following early clinical markers of cerebral palsy. In experienced hands, these parameters have a high degree of specificity and sensitivity as a screening tool.

- Episodes of inconsolable crying, chewing movements, and excessive sensitivity to light or sound.
- Persistent asymmetric neck tonic posture beyond 4 weeks.
- Clenched fists (cortical thumbs) beyond 8 weeks.
- Abnormalities in tone. Hypertonia in lower limbs and hypotonia in neck/upper limbs.

TABLE 28.1 Growth velocity of anthropometric parameters

Age	Weight gain (g/day)	Length gain (cm/month)	Head circumference gain (cm/month)
0–3 months	30	3.0	2.0
3–6 months	20	2.0	1.0
6–9 months	15	1.5	0.5
9–12 months	12	1.2	0.5
1–3 years	8	0.8	0.25

For every 10 g weight gain/day, there is 1.0 cm gain in length/month.

TABLE 28.2 Normal range of angles during infancy*

Age (months)	Adductor angle of thighs	Popliteal angle	Dorsiflexion angle of foot	Scarf sign
0–3	40°–80°	80°–100°	60°–70°	Elbow does not cross the midline
4–6	70°–110°	90°–120°	60°–70°	Elbow crosses midline
7–9	110°–140°	110°–160°	60°–70°	Elbow goes beyond anterior axillary line
10–12	140°–160°	150°–170°	60°–70°	–

*Adapted from Singh M, Pediatric Clinical Methods, CBS Publishers and Distributors Pvt. Ltd., New Delhi, sixth edition, 2020.

TABLE 28.3 Cardinal or target developmental milestones				
Upper age limit* (months)	Motor	Fine motor	Language	Social
2	–	–	–	Social smile
4	Head control	Holds objects	Cooing, turns towards sound	Recognition of mother
8	Sits without support	Transfers objects from one hand to the other	Nonsense vocalization	Laughs
12	Stands without support	Pincer grasp	Babbles syllables	Plays interactive games
18	Walks independently	Can self-feed with a spoon, makes a tower of 3–4 cubes	Jargon speech, 10–15 words vocabulary	Indicates the need for potty, and wet diaper

*Corrected or postconceptional age is used up to 2 years in preterm babies.

- Paucity or absence of fidgety, purposeless limb movements during 6–12 weeks of life.
- Persistence of automatic reflexes beyond 4–5 months.
- Slow head growth.

Formal Scales to Assess Development and Intelligence

A number of culture-specific tools have been developed to assess neuromotor development and cognition. The development is assessed in 4 domains, i.e. gross motor, fine motor, language and social. Bayley Scale of Infant Development (BSID) and Denver Development Screening Test (DDST) are widely used and have been simplified for use in our country as Baroda Development Screening Test or Developmental Assessment Scale for Indian Infants (DASII) (22 motor items and 31 mental items) and Trivandrum Development Screening Chart. DASII is the most reliable formal test for developmental assessment and should be performed on first birthday and repeated yearly till the age of 5 years. The Stanford Binet Intelligence Scale and McCarthy Scale of Children's Abilities can be used in children above 3 years of age to assess their intelligence. The Vineland Social Maturity Scale is used to assess social competence, self-help skills and adaptive behavior from infancy to adulthood. These tests require the services of a trained psychologist, soundproof room and availability of formal kits. The results of formal tests can be used to calculate developmental and intelligence quotients (developmental or intelligence age/chronologic or corrected age × 100). Detailed psychological evaluation can be done to assess the behavior, personality and learning capabilities of the child. Aptitude testing can help in providing occupational guidance keeping in mind the existence of all the neuromotor and sensory disabilities.

The intact survival of NICU graduates depends upon the quality of neonatal care provided and

TABLE 28.4 Spectrum of neurological problems in VLBW and high-risk newborn babies
Severe neurological problems
- Cerebral palsy
- Seizures (around 1%)
- Hydrocephalus or microcephaly (1–2%)
- Visual handicaps
- Deafness
- Mental retardation (IQ <70)
Subtle, minor and common neurological problems
- Transient changes in muscle tone
- Strabismus
- Fine motor coordination difficulties and clumsiness
- Attention deficit hyperactivity disorder (ADHD)
- Learning and language disabilities
- Behavior problems

vigilance and skills of health team providing the services. The incidence of CP among VLBW babies is usually reported to vary between 5 and 15%. Almost 30–50% of extremely LBW babies may require special educational resources. Table 28.4 gives the spectrum of neurological problems in VLBW and sick newborn babies. The incidence and severity of neurological handicaps are inversely related to the birth weight and gestational age of the babies.

VISION

The frequent use of assisted ventilation and improved survival of premature infants is associated with increased risk of retinopathy of prematurity (ROP) which may progress to blindness. The overall incidence of ROP varies between 25 and 55% in VLBW babies. The majority of cases resolve spontaneously but those with threshold disease can be effectively managed with cryotherapy or laser coagulation therapy. The details of protocol for monitoring and mangement of ROP are given in Chapter 26.

Follow-up Program for High-Risk Newborns

28

Ophthalmologist should evaluate the baby for vision, squint, cataract and optic atrophy at 9 months corrected age. Congenital blindness should be differentiated from global mental retardation. The blinking response to bright light, turning the head towards diffuse light or following a red moving ball or a ring are suggestive of intact vision. Pupils may be dilated and fixed in infants with optic atrophy or retinal detachment while in cortical blindness pupillary responses are preserved. Roving nystagmoid eye movements, persistent squint beyond 6 months of age, absence of opticokinetic nystagmus (tested with a rotating striped drum), lack of blink response to bright light or to sudden movement of examiner's finger towards infant's eyes are suggestive of congenital blindness. The absence of visual evoked responses provide confirmatory evidence. A blind infant is usually extra-sensitive to sound and gets easily frightened by sudden noise. Whenever indicated, the child should be provided with glasses, patching of normal eye (to stimulate the "lazy" or amblyopic eye) and corrective surgery without delay.

HEARING

According to National Sample Survey Office (NSSO), the overall population-based incidence of deafness is 6.3%. About 1.5 to 15.0% of LBW infants requring neonatal intensive care are likely to develop some degree of sensorineural hearing loss.

Risk Factors

The spectrum of risk factors for deafness is so wide that almost every infant with a prolonged stay in the NICU should be screened for hearing. When risk-based approach is followed for hearing assessment, almost 40% of hearing impaired children may be missed. *It is, therefore, recommended to follow the policy of universal screening for hearing.* The salient high-risk conditions associated with deafness are listed below.

- Family history of hearing loss in childhood. Almost 50% of hearing impairment in children is due to genetic or developmental causes.
- Birth weight <1500 g or gestation <32 weeks.
- CNS damage. Hypoxic–ischemic encephalopathy, intracranial hemorrhage, neonatal seizures, pyogenic meningitis, encephalitis, and sepsis.
- Otologic damage. Hyperbilirubinemia requiring exchange blood transfusion, assisted ventilation, ototoxic drugs (aminoglycoside, furosemide), TORCH infections (especially CMV, rubella), fetal alcohol syndrome and hyperventilation (PPHN, diaphragmatic hernia).
- Congenital malformations. Abnormalities of ear development and craniofacial anomalies.

Screening Tests

Clinical evaluation

The clinical examination for hearing in the newborn is not reliable. The baby is watched for several responses after giving a sound stimulus of a bell or 60 dB vocal sound. The sound stimulus should not be visible to the infant and it should not produce a whiff of air. The infant may give a startle response, blinking of eyes, sudden change in the activity with greater alertness, increase in breathing or heart rate, etc. The positive response indicates that hearing is intact and there is no generalized neurological disturbance while a negative response is of little significance because many variables may affect it. Many normal infants would turn towards the source of sound by the corrected age of 4 months.

The screening for hearing is based on two stages of electrophysiologic modalities. The spontaneous or sound-induced otoacoustic emissions (OAE) detect sound produced by movements of outer haircells of the cochlea while automated auditory brainstem response (ABR) measures neural response to a large number of repeated sound signals of the same pitch and intensity. Both OAE and ABR techniques are inexpensive, portable, reproducible and automated.

Transient evoked otoacoustic emissions (TEOAEs)

This test records acoustic "Feedback" or echoes from cochlea through the ossicles to the tympanic membrane and ear canal following a click stimulus. It evaluates the functioning of peripheral auditory system. The test is unreliable due to false-positive results and lack of gestation-related norms. However, it is highly cost-effective screening test and can be performed before baby is discharged from the NICU.

Auditory brainstem responses (ABRs)

The NICU graduates can be assessed by automated ABR (AABR) after 34 weeks of postconceptional maturity. The auditory threshold, the minimum intensity of sound click that produces a recognizable wave V, should be identified and compared with postconceptional age-adjusted norms. The AABR method produces a simple pass or fail result to a fixed 35–dB HL click without any need for interpretation and the test can be conducted even in the presence of background noise of NICU. In manual ABR, the intensity of stimuli is varied to determine the lowest level of sound that elicits a clear and repeatable response. The manual ABR testing allows the audiologist to determine the severity as well as nature of the hearing loss (sensorineural, conductive or neural) using both air and conduction stimuli. The hearing loss is classified into mild, moderate, severe and profound, based on lack of response to 30–40 dB, 41–60 dB, 61–80 dB and >80 dB, respectively.

Screening Protocol

All infants with abnormal AABR or EOAE at discharge from NICU should be reassessd at the corrected age of 3 months by ABR testing, auditory response cradle or Crib-o-Gram and tympanometry with a high frequency (1000 Hz) probe tone. Infants with history of neonatal seizures, perinatal viral infections and evidences of neurodevelopemental delay should be retested at 6 months of age irrespective of initial ABR results. Behavioral audiometry is best done at the age of one year. *The hearing aids should be provided by 6 months of age to improve congitive development and speech outcome.* Ideally a soundproof screening room with all the necessary tools should be available next to the NICU.

SYSTEMIC DISORDERS

Depending upon the diseases and complications encountered during their NICU stay, a number of systemic disorders may be encountered during follow-up (Table 28.5). The ongoing health problems and intercurrent illnesses should be identified and appropriately managed. Whenever indicated, the child should be admitted to the hospital on a priority basis. Bronchopulmonary dysplasia (BPD) or chronic lung disease (CLD) may lead to development of "irritable airways" and reactive airway disease with recurrent respiratory infections. Gastroesophageal reflux may lead to feeding difficulties and recurrent aspirations. Thickening of feeds, use of prokinetic agents and fundoplication may be required in some babies. NEC may lead to sequelae of bowel strictures with nutritional problems.

EARLY INTERVENTION PROGRAM

Stimulation in the NICU

Neonates in the NICU should not be treated as "objects" but provided with developmentally supportive care. Babies should be protected against bright light, loud sounds and painful procedures. They should not be unnecessarily disturbed and allowed to have peaceful and quiet periods as long as feasible without compromising their care. The bonding with mother should be promoted through kangaroo-mother care. Preterm babies can be provided non-nutritive sucking on the empty breasts of the mother. Gentle touch, massage and passive movements of joints are useful to improve

TABLE 28.5 Common non-neurologic systemic disorders in high-risk and VLBW babies

Pulmonary
- Bronchopulmonary dysplasia
- Reactive airway disease
- Recurrent respiratory infections
- Palatal grooves, enamel hypoplasia, and blocked nose
- Damage to vocal cords with speech disorder

Cardiovascular
- Systemic hypertension
- Cor pulmonale
- Pulmonary hypertension

Renal
- Nephrocalcinosis
- Renal dysfunction

Gastrointestinal
- Gastroesophageal reflux
- Feeding difficulties
- Short gut
- Nutritional disorders
- Umbilical and inguinal hernias

Reticuloendothelial
- Nutritional anemia
- Immunodeficiency state

Miscellaneous conditions
- Rickets
- Amputation of digits due to thromboembolic complications
- Scars due to procedures, like heel punctures, chest drainage, intubation, etc.

muscle tone and prevent muscle spasm. Soothing music, taped voice or heart beats of mother can be played near the baby. Rocking and oscillating water bed has been used to stimulate kinesthetic and vestibular senses.

Stimulation at Home

Early recongnition of neuromotor handicaps should be followed by a home-based stimulation program. There is evidence to suggest that early stimulation is associated with improved functioning of synapses and even regeneration of neurons because of plasticity of the brain. Gentle inputs of visual, auditory and tactile stimuli promote the maturation and development of specific areas of brain. Soothing music, soft voice, gentle touch and massage, rhythmic movements, eye-to-eye contact, caressing, cuddling and skin-to-skin contact provide useful sensory inputs to augment the process of neuromotor development. Most infants with CP are helped by passive stretching exercises and increasing the range of movements of limbs. *Massage*

TABLE 28.6 Guidelines for providing early stimulation to the infant by parents

0–2 months

Maintain eye-to-eye contact, talk and sing to the baby while doing daily chores, like body massage, bathing, dressing, feeding, nappy change, etc. Show bright lights or objects from the side, provide different sounds, like rattle, bell, and squeezing a sequeaky rubber toy. Place the baby on different surfaces and in different positions and rock the baby gently while supporting the head.

2–4 months

Lift baby by holding at the shoulders, hang bright objects about 30 cm above the crib in an arc or semicircle, talk to the child and maintain an eye contact, show bright objects to encourage the child to reach out and grasp, cuddle and caress the child after placing him on different surfaces and in various positions.

4–6 months

Place the baby flat on the mattress and encourage him to roll over, make him sit in the lap, place hands under the child's feet to encourage him to press and make pedaling movements, show a toy to reach out, sound a bell from the side to make him turn towards the sound.

6–8 months

Make the child to sit with support and place him in various positions, call him by name, encourage him to roll over by showing colorful toys from the side, give him pieces of paper to crumple and tear.

8–10 months

Encourage the child to stand with support, clap hands, look at a picture book and turn pages, drop objects into a box, place cubes one over the other.

10–12 months

Name the body parts while bathing, do simple tasks, like clapping, saying bye-bye, encourage him to pull to stand, make him stand with support, show him a mirror, let him play with other kids, show animals and birds in the park.

12–15 months

Give picture books and encourage him to turn the pages, ask him to put one cube over the other, hide a toy under a pillow and let him discover, encourage him to scribble on paper, assist him to hold small objects (strictly under observation), put objects in a box and retrieve them, motivate him to walk with support by holding on to a three-wheeled cart.

Note: The type of activities to be encouraged may be modified on the basis of developmental age of the child.

28 Care of the Newborn

is contraindicated as it may further increase the muscle tone. Parents should be instructed about ideal or functional positioning of their baby to make most effective

use of limited motor skills. At times, more intensive physiotherapy, occupational therapy, special shoes, braces or surgical intervention is required.

Mother is the best therapist for the child and she should be given the necessary guidance, skills and encouragement to stimulate the child at home. The stimulation is provided through various special senses, like touch (tactile, physical activities, kinesthetic stimulation), auditory and visual stimuli (Table 28.6). The stimulation should be done as a matter of routine in the form of a play activity and not as a ritual. The interactive play activities that both the parents and the child enjoy, is the best way to stimulate sensory system and brain of the baby.

In addition, the infant should be provided specialized stimulation services including physiotherapy and occupational therapy by specially trained personnel with the help of dedicated protocols, like Bobath neurodevelopmental stimulation program. The aim of therapy is to reduce the pathologic muscle tone and facilitate the development of integrated righting and equilibrium functions of the brain. Massage is generally contraindicated because in most cases of cerebral palsy muscle tone is increased. Early intervention is likely to prevent atrophy of muscles and reduce fixity or contractures of joints and promote functional capabilities of the child.

BIBLIOGRAPHY

Ahya KP, Suryawanshi P. Neonatal periventricular leukomalacia: Current perspectives. *Res and Reports Neonatol* 2018, 8:1–8.

American Academy of Pediatrics. Update of newborn screening and therapy for congenital hypothyroidism. *Pediatrics* 2006, 117 (6): 2290–2303.

Andrews B, Peyton C. Taking care of the nursery graduates: A team approach. *Pediatr Annals* 2018, 47(4): e140–e141.

Augustine AM, Jana AK, Kuruvilla KA, *et al.* Neonatal hearing screening: Experience from a tertiary care hospital in southern India. *Indian Pediatr* 2014, 51:179–83.

Bear LM. Early identification of infants at risk of development of disabilities. *Pediatr Clin N Am* 2004, 51:685–701.

Clarke P, Iqbal M, Mitchell SA. A comparison of transient-evoked otoacoustic emissions and automated auditory brainstem responses for predischarge neonatal hearing screening. *Int J Audiol* 2003, 42: 443–447.

Committee on Children with Disabilities. American Academy of Pediatrics. Developmental surveillance and screening of infants and young children. *Pediatrics* 2001, 108 (1): 192–195.

Costello D, Friedman H, Minich N, *et al.* Improved neurodevelopmental outcomes for extremely low birth weight infants in 2000–2002. *Pediatrics* 2007, 119: 37–45.

Downs MP, Yoshinag-Itano C. The efficacy of early identification and intervention for children with hearing impairment. *Pediatr Clin North Am* 1999, 46(1): 79–87.

Garcia-Alix A, Sanz-de Pipaon M, *et al*. Ability of neonatal head circumference to predict long term neurodevelopmental outcome. *Rev Neurol* 2004, 39 (6): 548–554.

Giuliani F, Ismail LC, Kennedy SH. Monitoring postnatal growth of preterm infants: present and future. *Am J Clin Nutr* 2016, 103(2): 635–47.

Hall JW, Smith SD, Popelka GR. Newborn hearing screening with combined otoacoustic emissions and auditory brain stem responses. *J Am Acad Audiol* 2004, 15(6): 414–425.

Johnson S, Marlow N. Developmental screen or developmental testing? *Early Hum Develop* 2006, 82(3): 173–183.

Lee E-J, Lee S-Y. The effects of early-stage neurodevelopmental treatment on the growth of premature infants in neonatal intensive care unit. *J Exerc Rehabil* 2018 14(3): 523–29.

Lim G, Fortaleza K. Overcoming challenges in newborn hearing screening. *J Perinatol* 2000; 20:S138–S142.

Nagapoornima P, Romesh, A, *et al*. Universal hearing screening. *Indian J Pediatr* 2007, 74(6): 545–549.

Nielsen KK, Kapur A, Bybjerg C. From screening to postpartum follow-up: The determinants and barriers for gestational diabetes mellitus (GDM) services, a systematic review. *BMC Pregnancy Child Birth* 2014, 14:41.

Olusanya BO, Wirz SL, Luxon LM. Community-based infant hearing screening for early detection of permanent hearing loss in Lagos, Nigeria: A cross-sectional study. *Bull World Health Org* 2008, 86: 956–963.

Qui X, Lodha A, Shah PS, *et al*. Neonatal outcomes of small-for-gestational age preterm infants in Canada. Canadian Neonatal Network. *Am J Perinatol* 2012, 29(2): 87–94.

Rai N, Thakur N. Universal screening of newborns to detect hearing impairment: is it necessary? *Int J Pediatr Otorhinolaryngol* 2013, 77:1036–41.

Sigiura T, Kouwaki M, Togawa Y, Koyama N. Neurodevelopmental outcomes at 18 months corrected age of infants born at 22 weeks of gestation. *Neonatology* 2011, 100 (3): 228–232.

Spittle AJ, Orton J, Doyle LW, Boyd R. Early developmental intervention programs; posthospital discharge to prevent motor and cognitive impairments in preterm infants. *Cochrane Database Systematic Rev.* 2007, Issue 2 Art. No. CD005495 DOI 10.1002/14651858.

US Joint Committee on Infant Hearing. Year 2007 position statement: Principles and guidelines for early hearing detection and intervention program. *Pediatrics* 2007, 120 (4):898–921.

Vohr B, Wright LL, Hack M, *et al*. Follow-up care of high-risk infants. *Pediatrics* 2004, 114 (Suppl): 1377–1397.

Procedures

The procedure may be conducted for diagnostic purposes or used as a life-saving therapeutic measure. It is important that a formal consent for the procedure should be taken from the parent/legal guardian after explaining the nature of the procedure, its likely benefits and potential side effects or hazards. The operator must have adequate skills and experience before undertaking the procedure. Strict asepsis should be observed during all procedures. Except when performing percutaneous vessel punctures and collecting capillary blood samples, strict aseptic precautions must be undertaken by wearing a mask, sterile gown and gloves.

MATERNAL AND FETAL PROCEDURES

Rapid advances in the field of perinatal medicine has led to introduction of several procedures for antenatal diagnosis and fetal therapy. These procedures are highly skill-oriented and must be performed by an experienced obstetrician. The availability of a real-time high precision ultrasound with a sector-scanner is essential to guide these procedures. In all diagnostic procedures, the benefit–risk ratio must be carefully weighed and both mother and fetus should not be exposed to unnecessary hazards.

AMNIOCENTESIS

Transabdominal amniocentesis is a relatively simple and safe procedure to collect a sample of amniotic fluid.

Indications

1. Prenatal genetic diagnosis by estimation of alpha-fetoproteins, chromosomal, biochemical and molecular studies.
2. To assess the severity of Rh hemolytic disease.

3. To assess the maturity of the baby by estimation of creatinine content, orange staining cells, lecithin to sphingomyelin ratio and phosphatidyl glycerol.

Procedure

The procedure should preferably be avoided before 14 weeks of gestation due to high incidence of failure rate and greater chances of damage to the fetus. The procedure is best performed around 15–16 weeks of gestation. The placenta and fetal parts must be localized by ultrasonography to minimize the risk of damage to the placenta or fetus. The mother should be asked to void urine. The procedure must be performed by a skilled operator. Strict asepsis should be ensured during the procedure. Spinal needle with a stylet is quite suitable. The puncture site should be determined by palpating the fetal parts. The concavity or hollowness between the fetal head and limbs on the ventral aspect of the fetus constitutes an ideal site, if placenta does not come in the way (Figure 29.1). The needle point should be directed away from the head. If uterus contracts while needle is being advanced, it is advisable to withdraw the needle 1–2 cm and wait until contractions subside. In case fresh blood is aspirated, it is better to abandon the procedure instead of manipulating the needle. A discolored fluid may indicate fetal death. About 20 mL of clear amniotic fluid should be withdrawn and collected in a sterile bottle.

Complications

In general, the procedure is quite safe, particularly when due care is exercised to avoid infection and injury to the placenta. The recognized complications are listed below:

1. Placental bleeding and fetal death in 0.5–1.0% cases.

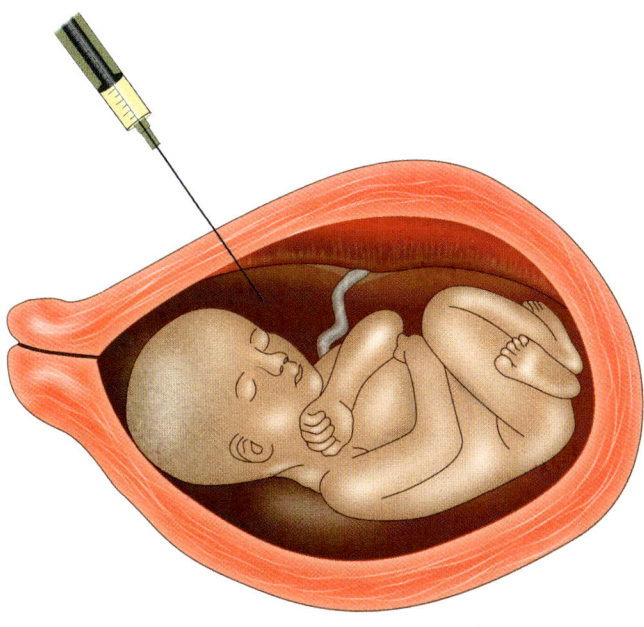

Figure 29.1 Amniocentesis. Note the site for puncture on the ventral side of fetus away from the fetal parts.

2. Fetomaternal hemorrhage with increased risk of Rh-isoimmunization. The risk can be minimized by prophylactic administration of 250 IU anti-D immunoglobulins within 72 hours of the procedure in Rh-negative women.
3. Premature onset of labor.
4. Amnionitis.
5. Rarely injury to the fetal parts may occur.
6. Postural deformities of limbs due to excessive removal of amniotic fluid.

CHORIONIC VILLUS SAMPLING

Prenatal diagnosis by obtaining fetal tissue for chromosomal, biochemical and DNA studies is being increasingly sought. In the past, fetal cells were obtained by transabdominal amniocentesis performed around 15–16 weeks of gestation. More recently, chorionic villus sampling (CVS) is gaining popularity especially for the study of those disorders which can be diagnosed by DNA probes and restriction enzyme studies. Moreover, chromosomal and biochemical analysis can be carried out directly on chorionic villus samples without the need for culture.

Indications

The indications for CVS are similar to those for amniocentesis. It is useful to screen the pregnancies of elderly mothers especially those with a previous history of birth of a child with a chromosomal or genetic disorder. The procedure is especially suitable for the

Procedure

It is a simple and relatively safe procedure which can be performed on an outpatient basis. No operative preparation is required but mother is asked to report with a full bladder so that gravid uterus is lifted up into the abdominal cavity. The procedure is ideally performed between the narrow range of 10–12 weeks of gestation because risk of complications is much higher beyond these gestations. A careful ultrasonographic study, using 5 MHz sector scanner is done to confirm that crown-rump length of the fetus corresponds to 10–12 weeks maturity. Twin pregnancy is excluded and placental site is localized. Additional contraindications include vaginitis, vaginal bleeding severe ante- or retroflexion of uterus and rhesus iso-immunization.

The procedure must be performed by an experienced obstetrician who has mastered the skill by practicing the procedure on women undergoing medical termination of pregnancy. The cervix is prepared with povidone-iodine. A polyethylene catheter (length 21–28 cm, diameter 1.0–2.0 mm) fitted with a malleable wire obturator is inserted through the cervix under continuous sonographic guidance. The catheter tip is advanced till it lies within the chorion frondosum (Figure 29.2). While the guidewire is gently removed, the catheter is advanced by 0.5 cm to ensure that it stays within the chorion. A 20 mL syringe filled with 5 mL of tissue culture medium is attached to the

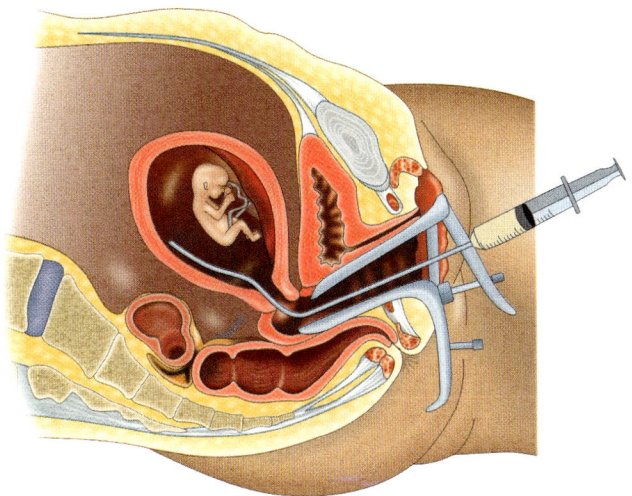

Figure 29.2 Schematic representation of chorionic villus sampling procedure. See text for details.

Procedures

29

catheter. Gentle negative suction is applied and catheter is slowly withdrawn from the placental site till catheter tip lies just above the internal os. The suction should not be applied while the catheter is traversing through the cervical canal to avoid the risk of contamination with mucus or blood. The unsensitized Rh-negative woman is administered 250 IU of anti-D immunoglobulin intramuscularly. The patient is sent home shortly after the procedure and no antibiotics are prescribed. The aspiration of 15–50 mg of trophoblastic tissue is considered as adequate. If the aspirate is unsatisfactory or procedure is unsuccessful, up to three attempts may be made by taking care that each time a fresh sterile catheter is used.

The procedure can also be performed during second trimester of pregnancy through transabdominal route under the guidance of ultrasonography. Many centers prefer to undertake transabdominal CVS due to reduced risk of infection, bleeding and abortion.

Complications

The procedure is relatively safe in experienced hands especially when it is restricted during 10–12 weeks of gestation. The overall risk of abortion is around 1.0%. The other complications include chorioamnionitis, sepsis and perforation of amniotic sac.

CORDOCENTESIS

The potentially dangerous technique of fetal blood sampling (FBS) by placentocentesis and fetoscopy has been replaced by cordocentesis or percutaneous umbilical blood sampling (PUBS). Though technically difficult, it provides an uncontaminated sample of fetal blood with acceptable risk of complications. The FBS can be obtained on several occasions after 17 weeks of gestation till delivery.

Indications

Fetal blood sample is required for prenatal diagnosis by undertaking rapid karyotyping and DNA studies in a fetus showing an abnormality on ultrasound examination. The procedure is used to establish normal reference values of hematologic indices, coagulation profile, biochemical, immunologic, endocrinologic and acid–base parameters at different gestations, and to institute fetal therapy. It is possible to measure simultaneously the maternal and fetal levels of substances to study their transplacental passage. The inborn errors of metabolism, chromosomal diseases and intrauterine infections can be diagnosed by FBS.

Procedure

The fetal blood sample is collected from umbilical vein under ultrasound guidance. No maternal sedation or preparation is required except a full bladder. High resolution real-time ultrasonography is essential to identify the point of umbilical cord insertion into the placenta. The transducer is then kept strictly immobile. Under strict aseptic conditions, the local anesthetic is injected into the abdominal wall at the anticipated puncture site. A 20-gauge spinal needle, 9 cm long, is attached to a 2 mL disposable syringe containing citrated or heparinized saline. Under continuous ultrasound guidance, the needle is introduced into the plane of ultrasound sector near the transducer. The needle tip emits clearly visible echo that is followed on the screen towards the insertion of the cord. The cord is punctured at about 1 cm from the placental insertion (Figure 29.3). Depending upon the placental position, access to the cord is gained either through the amniotic cavity or directly without penetrating the amniotic sac. As soon as first few drops of blood are obtained, the syringe is replaced with a dry empty one. According to the stage of gestation, 2 to 4 mL of blood is gently aspirated and transferred to appropriate bottles containing media or anticoagulant. The needle is gently withdrawn, puncture site in the cord is watched for any bleeding and fetus monitored for bradycardia. Repeat ultrasound examination is

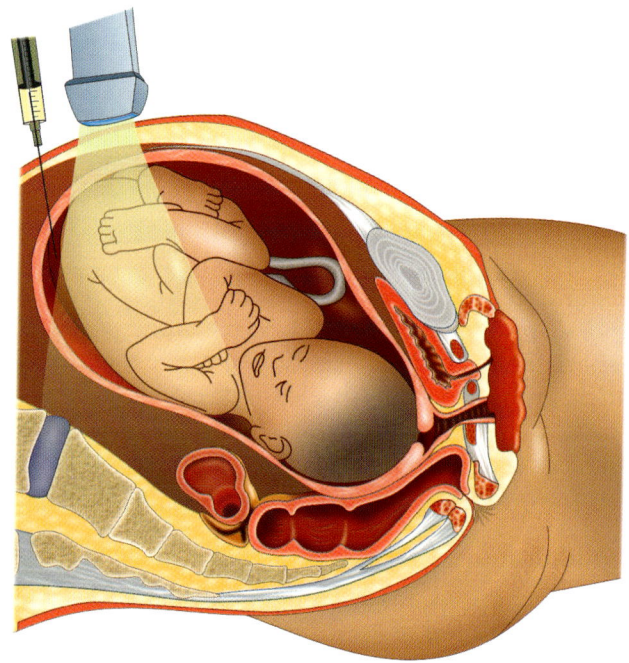

Figure 29.3 Diagrammatic representation of cordocentesis under ultrasonographic guidance.

performed after one hour to monitor the wellbeing of fetus (Manning score) and to look for any hematoma at the puncture site. The blood sample obtained should be examined for any contamination with maternal blood by Kleihauer-Betke test. The success and safety of the procedure depends upon the experience, patience and skill of the obstetrician and sonographic quality of the ultrasound machine.

Complications

The procedure may be complicated by introduction of infection, bleeding at the site of puncture, fetal bradycardia, preterm delivery in 5% and risk of fetal death in 1–2% cases.

FETAL SKIN AND MUSCLE BIOPSY

Fetal skin and mucle biopsy can be undertaken with the help of a fetoscope or under ultrasound guidance for antenatal diagnosis of those conditions which cannot be diagnosed on DNA studies. The procedure is safe and usually performed during second trimester of pregnancy. No visible scar is identified after birth due to tremendous healing capabilities of fetal skin.

Indications

The procedure is undertaken for antenatal diagnosis of lethal and dystrophic epidermolysis bullosa, ichthyosiform erythroderma, oculocutaneous albinism, Sjögren-Larsson syndrome, and ectodermal dysplasias. Some of these conditions and most of muscular dystrophies can now be diagnosed reliably and safely by DNA studies and invasive procedure of fetal biopsy is rarely undertaken.

INTRAUTERINE TRANSFUSION

The incidence and severity of erythroblastosis fetalis has declined over the years following prophylactic administration of anti-D immunoglobulins to Rh-negative women before they get sensitized. Nevertheless, several referral centers are still managing a number of pregnancies complicated by severe Rh-isoimmunization. Intrauterine transfusion is life-saving to correct severe anemia and prevent hydrops fetalis. The severity of rhesus hemolytic disease of the fetus is assessed by identification of "critical" titer of indirect Coomb's test and amniotic fluid optical density difference (ODD) at 450 mu in the Liley's zone 3 at 20 to 22 weeks of gestation or later. The titers of indirect Coombs' test and amniotic fluid optical density on spectrophotometer are evaluated after every 2 weeks to assess the need for intervention. If fetus is heterozygous Rh-positive, fetal blood type (and degree of anemia) can be determined by percutaneous cordocentesis. The intrauterine blood transfusion can be performed either by infusing blood into the peritoneal cavity of the fetus or into vascular compartment through umbilical vein. It should be remembered that intrauterine transfusion is a simple transfusion of packed red blood cells to correct the anemia and it is usually not an exchange blood transfusion.

Intraperitoneal Transfusion

It is fairly safe and simple procedure which can be performed on an out patient basis. Fresh O Rh-negative blood (preferably negative for other important antigens, like Kell, Duffy and Kidd) is packed by the standard procedure to obtain approximate hematocrit of 85 mL/dL. The blood is irradiated to destroy the white blood cells in order to eliminate the risks of chimerism and graft-versus-host disease. The procedure is guided under continuous ultrasonography with a real-time sector scanner. The procedure becomes technically simple, if fetus is lying supine presenting its anterior abdominal wall. The fetal peritoneal cavity is punctured at 90° angle with a 20-gauge spinal needle while avoiding trauma to the fetal kidneys, liver and spleen. The needle is attached with a three-way stopcock to a 10 mL syringe and packed red blood cells in a closed system. The blood is manually infused into the peritoneal cavity of the fetus in 10 mL aliquots. The volume of blood to be infused is determined by the equation: Volume = (gestation in weeks – 20) × 10. Fetal heart rate is monitored during the procedure and transfusion is withheld, if bradycardia develops. The second intrauterine transfusion is performed after one week and subsequent transfusions may be required after 1 to 4 weeks intervals depending upon the severity of the hemolytic process.

Intravascular Transfusion

In most centers, intraperitoneal transfusion procedure has been replaced by intravascular transfusion through cordocentesis. After strict aseptic precautions, a 20-gauge spinal needle is inserted into the umbilical vein near the cord insertion site under ultrasonographic guidance as described under the procedure for fetal blood sampling *vide supra*. The volume of blood to be infused is calculated according to the method of Rodeck:

$$\text{Volume} = \frac{\text{Desired HCT} - \text{Actual HCT}}{\text{HCT of donor's packed red blood cells} \times \text{Fetal blood volume}}$$

Procedures

29

The desired final hematocrit is generally taken between 40 and 45% and the hematocrit of the packed red blood cells is usually between 85 and 90%. During the manual infusion, through the closed system (as in the case of intraperitoneal transfusion), the ultrasonography monitors the flow of transfused blood though the umbilical vein and keeps a watch on the fetal heart rate. At the end of the procedure, a blood sample is obtained to check the hematocrit. At times, an overactive fetus who repeatedly obscures the cord insertion site, may have to be paralyzed by administration of 0.5 mg pancuronium directly to the fetus either intravenously or intramuscularly.

Complications

Cramping and pain during insertion of spinal needle through abdominal wall, premature labor and amniotic fluid leakage are usual complications. Fetal sepsis, and fetal bleeding due to puncture of a fetal vessel or a viscera are rare complications. There is a 2 to 5% risk of fetal death during or after the procedure. It must be remembered that the procedure is generally required for a baby which is already critically ill and has a poor chance of survival without intrauterine intervention.

FETAL SCALP BLOOD SAMPLING

Fetal wellbeing and evidences of fetal hypoxia can be monitored by observing fetal activity, variability of fetal heart rate in response to fetal movements and uterine contractions, ultrasonographic neurobehavior of the fetus and volume of the amniotic fluid. Estimation of fetal scalp pH provides a more reliable biochemical evidence of fetal hypoxia. It can be used to complement the information obtained by monitoring fetal heart rate on cardiotocometry so that delivery can be timed more appropriately and unnecessary cesarean sections can be avoided.

Indications

  i. Persistent fetal tachycardia (>160/min) or bradycardia (<120/min)
 ii. Late decelerations
iii. Decreased beat to beat variability
 iv. Persistent variable deceleration
  v. Fetal arrhythmia or sinusoidal pattern.

Contraindications

  i. HIV-positive mother
 ii. Placenta previa
iii. Umbilical cord prolapse
 iv. Brow and face presentation

  v. Chorioamnionitis
 vi. Hydrocephalus or other malformations of fetal skull
vii. Fetal hemophilia.

Procedure

The procedure can be accomplished, only if the cervix is at least 2.5 cm dilated. Patient is placed in a wide lithotomy position. Under strict aseptic precautions, the vulvar area is cleaned with providone-iodine solution. Pelvic examination is done to assess the degree of cervical dilatation and station of the presenting part. The membranes are ruptured artificially, if they are still intact. Amnioscope with an obturator of the largest convenient size, depending upon the dilatation of the cervix, is introduced along the palm and index or the middle finger of the right hand. The obturator is removed and an assistant focuses the light source into the amnioscope. After correctly angling the amnioscope, its rim is snugly applied over the scalp of the fetus. The scalp is dried with a cotton swab and sprayed with ethyl chloride to cause hyperemia. A small portion of scalp is exposed by parting the hair. A small amount of silicone gel or liquid paraffin is applied over the scalp to facilitate formation of blood drop and reduce the chances of exposure of blood to the air. The scalp is punctured to a depth of 2 mm at two points with a disposable lancet having a guard. Care should be taken to avoid making the incision over the fontanel or suture line. The blood sample is collected in a heparinized capillary tube and its ends are sealed with plasticine. Hemostasis is ensured by pressure with a cotton swab. Simultaneous capillary blood sample is obtained from the mother and both the samples are immediately analyzed for pH and acid–base parameters. Fetal blood pH value of 7.25 or more is considered as normal and it is usually 0.1 lower than the simultaneous maternal value. Fetal scalp pH of less than 7.20 suggests compromised fetus necessitating close observation and repeat sampling. Fetal scalp pH of less than 7.0 is indicative of severe asphyxia and baby should be delivered immediately.

Complications

It is an invasive procedure though the risk of complications is small. Bleeding and hematoma at the site of puncture and risk of infection are the major complications.

NEONATAL PROCEDURES

The modern neonatal care has become highly technology oriented and a large number of procedures are performed for monitoring, diagnosis and therapeutic interventions in critically sick preterm babies. The family must be informed about the procedure and formal consent should be taken. During the procedure, baby's temperature must be maintained by using a radiant heat source and if required oxygen should be administered through the head box. Excessive handling, manipulation and intervention adversely affect the oxygenation and perfusion (due to reflex bradycardia) in newborn babies. The well-recognized and time-honored principles of gentleness and minimal handling in the care of preterm babies must be practiced without denying them the essential diagnostic and therapeutic facilities of modern advances in the field of perinatal medicine. The operator must follow universal precautions, including use of gloves, gown and protective barriers to prevent exposure to blood and body fluids that may be contaminated with infectious agents.

Informed Consent

It is essential that consent is obtained from the parent/legal guardian before undertaking the procedure

- Explain the nature of the procedure in a simple language that the parents or caregiver can understand.
- Explain the information likely to be obtained from the procedure and its benefits to the patient.
- Explain the nature of sedation to be used and its likely side effects.
- The potential complications of the procedure should be explained.
- After giving the aforementioned explanations, get the consent form signed in the presences of a witness.

ANALGESIA AND SEDATION

It has been believed from times immemorial that newborn babies, especially those born preterm, do not feel pain because of lack of myelination of central nervous system, poor development of pain receptors and immaturity of the cortex. But there is now enough neuroanatomic evidence to suggest that pain pathways are well developed as early as 24–25 weeks of gestation as evidenced by the presence of nociceptive nerve endings in the skin, arborization of dendritic processes in the neocortex and synaptogenesis of thalamocortical fibers. The functional maturity of the pathways is demonstrated by fetal and neonatal EEG patterns and integrity of somatosensory evoked potentials. The pharmacological maturity of pain pathways is evidenced by the presence of various neurotransmitters and pain-related neuromodulator substances, like substance P, somatostatin, calcitonin

gene-related peptide (CGRP) and vasoactive peptides. There is no doubt that newborn babies do feel pain as evidenced by a variety of facial, behavioral, autonomic, biochemical and hormonal responses. Infact, newborn babies, not only feel pain but they also harbor the unpleasant memories of pain later in life.

Newborn babies including preterm infants do feel pain though they may not violently oppose or loudly cry during the procedure. They exhibit a variety of physical (cry, cringing posture, sweating, facial frowning and grimaces, limb withdrawal, etc.) and physiological responses, like tachycardia, sweating, elevation of blood pressure and intracranial pressure, hypoxia, hypercarbia and increase in pulmonary artery pressure with right-to-left shunting of blood. They exhibit stress-related biochemical and hormonal responses, like release of epinephrine, norepinephrine, glucagon, aldosterone, and corticosterone and suppression of insulin. There is hyperglycemia and elevation of serum lactate and pyruvate levels. Pain may cause instability of vital signs, compromise body defences and immune mechanisms and enhance metabolic stress thus adversely affecting recuperative and healing capabilities. It must be realized that even when there is lack of any physical evidences of pain (because infant is preterm or tiny), the baby is likely to experience all the adverse physiological, biochemical and immunological consequences of pain.

Minor Procedures

Heel lancing, venipunctures, establishing intravenous line, suprapubic bladder tap and lumbar puncture are commonly performed minor procedures in newborn babies. The operator should be gentle, caring and compassionate while performing these procedures. Giving sucrose or glucose 0.5–2.0 mL of 20% solution or a breastfeed two minutes before or during the procedure affords pain relief, by distraction and possibly by pharmacological effect of sucrose. Non-nutritive sucking and use of a pacifier during the procedure provides comfort. Other useful non-pharmacological modalities for relief of pain include comforting touch, stroking the baby, cuddling, caressing, swaddling and skin-to-skin contact. Several pleasant olfactory (mother's milk, vanila, lemon) and auditory (instrumental music, tick-tack sound of maternal heart) stimuli are credited to reduce the perception and adverse consequences of pain and discomfort. The non-pharmacological modalities of pain relief work not merely by distraction but also by virtue of soothing effect of sucrose and by release of endogenous feel-good neuropeptides and endorphins.

It is desirable to use mechanical lancets for heel-stick which are likely to produce less pain. Barbiturates, chloral hydrate, triclofos sodium and promethazine can be safely used for sedation of neonates undergoing imaging studies. EMLAP (Eutectic mixture of local anesthetic lignocaine 2.5% and prilocaine 2.5%) cream is now available in India and can be used for setting up IV line or before arterial punctures. Cream is applied over the intended site of puncture at least one hour before the procedure. It should be used with caution in preterm babies due to risk of development of methemoglobinemia.

Major Procedures

Endotracheal Intubation

Except emergency intubation for neonatal resuscitation, any neonate who needs elective intubation, should receive morphine 0.05–0.2 mg/kg IV before the procedure. Endotracheal administration of surfactant must be achieved under cover of a narcotic infusion. Fentanyl (2–5 µg/kg/dose IV) is a good alternative to morphine. It is more potent than morphine and readily penetrates blood–brain barrier due to high degree of lipid solubility. It is preferable to use fentanyl while intubating babies with PPHN because it prevents pain-induced elevation of pulmonary arterial pressure. Opioids should be avoided in hemodynamically unstable or hypotensive neonates due to increased risk of IVH and PVL. Till further pharmacokinetic information is available, use of midazolam should be restricted to babies weighing more than 1500 g or having a gestational maturity of 32 weeks or more.

Assisted Ventilation

Give a bolus dose of morphine (0.05–0.2 mg/kg IV) followed by steady infusion at a rate of 10–15 µg/kg/hr in preterm babies and 20–30 µg/kg/hr in term babies. Some neonatal units prefer to use fentanyl (2–5 µg/kg) because it does not cause hypotension and is preferred in infants with PPHN because of its stabilizing effect on the pulmonary arterial pressure. It can be followed by constant infusion of 0.2–0.5 µg/kg/hour. However, according to AAP guidelines on pain management, routine use of continuous infusion of morphine or fentanyl in preterm neonates with prolonged assisted ventilation, is not recommended because of short-term adverse effects and lack of long-term safety data. Endotracheal suctioning causes considerable discomfort to the baby and must be undertaken when infant is receiving constant infusion of morphine or fentanyl.

During the process of weaning, the infusion rate of morphine or fentanyl should be slowly decreased at a rate of 25–50% everyday or as tolerated by the neonate. Narcotic analgesic drugs are by and large safe especially in ventilated babies. Apart from respiratory depression, other disadvantages of narcotics include nausea, decreased gastric and intestinal motility with abdominal distension.

Thoracostomy

The tube should be inserted after local infiltration of analgesic agent, even if the baby is being ventilated and receiving morphine infusion.

Miscellaneous Conditions

Paracetamol (10–15 mg/kg/dose every 4–6 hr oral) is a useful and safe analgesic for newborn babies having painful conditions, like fracture of bones, traumatic delivery, arthritis, and osteomyelitis. Laser coagulation and cryotherapy is done under opioid cover. During circumcision, oral 20% sucrose and paracetamol is given before the procedure which can be performed under ring or dorsal penile block with 0.5 mL/kg of 0.5% lidocaine. Topical or injectable local anesthetics have a potential risk of causing seizures and abnormalities in brainstem auditory responses. Following surgical procedures, pain and discomfort should be relieved by administration of opioids and paracetamol which have synergistic effect. Chloral hydrate and triclofos sodium (10–20 mg/kg/dose) are useful sedatives to relieve distress and agitation in newborn babies. Their prolonged use should be avoided because of potential risk of hepatotoxicity.

COLLECTION OF URINE

Examination of urine, though indicated many a times, is often ignored because of difficulties in collection of a clean sample. Catheterization of bladder should be avoided because of risk of introducing infection. Whenever there is delay in plating the urine for culture, it should be kept in a refrigerator at 4°C, otherwise multiplication of bacteria at room temperature may invalidate the concept of significant colony count (10^4 organisms/mL) by giving falsely high number of bacterial counts.

Mid-stream clean catch This requires patience and luck though it is a reliable method and is devoid of any hazards to the baby. The buttocks and perineum should be washed with soap and water and dried with sterile cotton. The baby should be held with thighs abducted. Gentle pressure over the suprapubic area may help. After first few drops, urine should be collected in a sterile container.

Urine collecting bag The bag should be attached after thorough cleaning of the perineum with soap and water. The bag should be removed as soon as the urine is passed. The urine should be transferred to a sterile container by snipping one of the lower corners of the bag. It is often difficult to collect the urine in a female infant with the help of a collection bag. If the baby passes stools before the urine has been collected, he should be cleaned again and a new bag affixed. A condom or test tube may be used as a urine collecting device in male infants.

Bladder puncture This procedure should be attempted, if equivocal results have been obtained by above methods and for those ill infants in whom urine examination and culture are a matter of urgency. The puncture should be tried about one to two hours after a feed and when bladder area is dull on percussion. The procedure is contraindicated, if there is superficial infection at the intended site of puncture or baby has bleeding diathesis.

The infant should be placed in a supine posture with legs held in the frog position. The suprapubic area should be thoroughly cleaned with povidone-iodine and spirit. With a 21-gauge needle attached to a 10 mL syringe, pierce the anterior abdominal wall in the midline about 1.0–2.0 cm above the symphysis pubis (Figure 29.4). The needle should be thrust vertically backwards in one rapid movement towards infant's coccyx. The bladder is generally reached at a depth of 1.5–2.0 cm when urine can be aspirated. Tilt the syringe towards abdominal wall, if necessary, and aspirate while you withdraw the needle. Bladder puncture can also be done under ultrasound guidance.

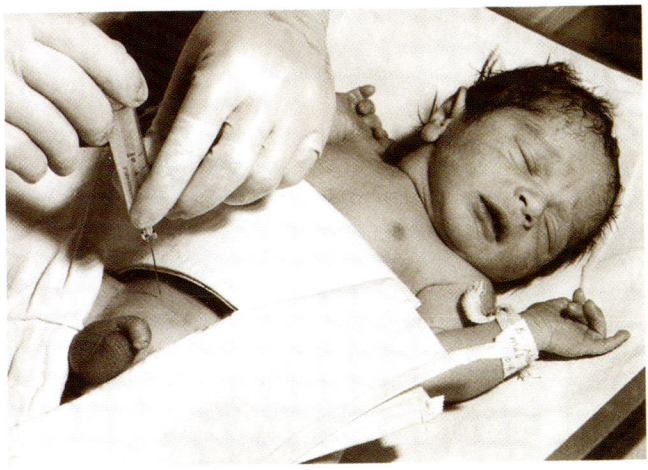

Figure 29.4 Suprapubic bladder aspiration.

Transient hematuria may occur and should be watched for.

Interpretation of Urine Results

Up to 10 white cells per cu mm in uncentrifuged specimen of urine is normal in both sexes. The cells may disappear in the alkaline urine. Bacterial counts of 10^4/mL or more are significant and suggestive of urinary tract infection, if two consecutive cultures are positive. In female babies, falsely high cell count and false positive culture may be obtained when urine is collected with a collecting bag. Any colony count is significant when urine is collected by suprapubic puncture. The findings of normal urine does not rule out urinary tract infection unless urine has been examined repeatedly because bacteriuria may be intermittent.

COLLECTION OF BLOOD SAMPLES

The site and amount of blood collected each time must be recorded. It should be remembered that 10 mL of blood from a 2 kg baby represents about 6% of his blood volume. Frequent blood sampling from a sick newborn baby is an important cause of anemia. It is important to keep an accurate record of blood withdrawn for investigations.

Cord Blood

It should be routinely collected in babies born to O group or Rh-negative mothers, antepartum hemorrhage, intrauterine infection, maternal diabetes mellitus, severe birth asphyxia, collection of stem cells, and for metabolic screening, and if there is a history of previous neonatal death(s). The umbilical vein is easier to sample due to its large diameter. However, umbilical artery blood gas analysis gives more accurate information about the fetal metabolic condition and correlates better with outcome of the neonate.

Techniques

1. Ideally while the placenta is still *in utero*, the needle should be inserted into the umbilical vein or artery and blood withdrawn.
2. While the placenta is still *in utero*, releasing the cord clamp results in free flow of blood. This blood may be unsuitable because it gets diluted and contaminated with Wharton's jelly and may give a false negative direct Coombs' test. The cord should never be milked for collection of blood sample.
3. After delivery of placenta, the blood can be obtained by puncturing one of the fetal veins overlying the

placenta. At times enough blood cannot be collected by this procedure.

4. After applying two ligatures 10 to 20 cm apart, blood can be collected from the isolated segment of umbilical artery for blood gases and acid–base parameters.

Capillary Blood

Capillary blood is suitable for determination of pH and other biochemical estimations. It is unsuitable for blood culture, PO_2 and PCO_2 determinations. The procedure is contraindicated, if infant is in shock, having local edema or infection and in cases of severe polycythemia. The heel should be warmed with a cotton wool pledget soaked in sterile water at 40°C taking care that burning of skin is avoided. With the left hand, the foot should be dorsiflexed and grasped along with the leg in such a way so that the engorged heel pulp stands out. After cleaning the skin with povidone-iodine and alcohol, it is stabbed with a lancet. After pushing lancet to a depth of about 2 mm, it should be rotated before being pulled out. Mechanical or "spring-release" lancets are preferred because they cause less pain. The first drop should be wiped away with a sterile cotton. Apply sterile liquid paraffin or silicone gel at the puncture site so that a good-sized drop of blood is formed. The subsequent-drops should be allowed to fall freely straight into a container without scraping the skin with the edge of the container. The blood should flow freely with minimal or no squeezing. The blood drops can also be sucked into capillary tubes. The alternate squeezing and releasing of calf facilitates milking out of blood. After collection, the wound should be covered with a piece of adhesive plaster or benzoin seal. Avoid inflicting punctures at the apex of heel, because painful scars may cause difficulty in walking later in life (Figure 29.5). The common complications of the procedure include cellulitis, osteomyelitis of calcaneum, abscess formation and development of painful scars.

Venous Blood

Venous blood from peripheral veins is suitable for most investigations except for estimation of PO_2 and PCO_2. Blood for culture should not be taken through umbilical catheter because of risk of contamination and false positive culture results. It is preferable to use superficial veins located at anetcubital fossa, scalp, dorsum of hands and feet though it is often difficult to obtain sufficient amount of blood by this procedure. Wash hands and wear sterile gloves. Clean the skin overlying the selected vein with alcohol-povidone

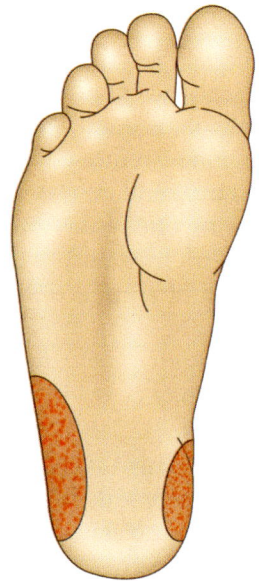

Figure 29.5 Appropriate and safe sites for obtaining capillary blood sample from the heel.

(30 sec) – alcohol. Tie a tourniquet or ask an assistant to occlude the vein proximal to the vein puncture site. Insert a 23–25 gauge needle, with bevel facing up, through the stretched skin at an angle of 20°. For collection of blood culture sample, if venipuncture attempt fails, use a new sterile needle each time. If two attempts for venipuncture are abortive, seek the help of another colleague. A relatively large needle should be used and gentle suction should be applied to obtain smooth flow. Instead of suction with a syringe, the blood may be allowed to drip out of the needle hub and collected for biochemical investigations. The hub may be broken to reduce the dead space to obtain better yield of sample. The tourniquet should be removed before removing the needle to prevent formation of hematoma. Apply local pressure with dry cotton for 3 minutes to produce hemostasis. Femoral venipuncture is not recommended due to risk of bleeding, hematoma, septic arthritis and osteomyelitis.

External jugular venipuncture The relatively short and obese neck of the newborn baby makes this procedure rather difficult. The external jugular vein courses in a line from the angle of the mandible to the middle of the clavicle. The infant is restrained in a supine position and his head and neck are suspended beyond the edge of the table. The head is rotated to one side and supported by an assistant while shoulders are maintained firmly on the table. The infant is stimulated to cry which causes engorgement of the vessel. As soon as the external jugular vein is spotted, the skin is pierced immediately over the vessel and needle is advanced into the lumen while maintaining gentle suction in the syringe. After the procedure, gentle but sufficient pressure should be applied over the puncture site and baby should be held in an upright position for two to three minutes.

Arterial Blood

Arterial blood is suitable for all investigations but is desirable for monitoring blood gases, ammonia, lactate and pyruvate levels. When repeated arterial blood samples are required, it is best to cannulate the umbilical artery for ease and convenience.

Radial artery puncture Modified Allen's test should be done to assess the adequacy of collateral circulation before radial artery is punctured or cannulation. Cold light is used to locate ulnar and radial arteries. Elevate the arm and simultaneously occlude the radial and ulnar arteries at the wrist; and rub the palm to cause blaching. Release the pressure on the ulnar artery, while keeping the radial artery compressed. If palm becomes pink within 10 seconds; it is suggestive of adequate collateral circulation. If the normal color in the palm does not return even after 15 seconds, it is suggestive of poor collateral circulation and it is best to avoid radial artery puncture in this arm. In order to improve the reliability of Allen test, laser Doppler flowmetry or pulse oximetry can be used to assess the adequacy of collateral circulation.

The radial artery is difficult to palpate in a newborn baby. It lies in the center of the lateral third of the flexor aspect of the wrist, just lateral to the tendon of the flexor carpi radialis. The artery can be located with the help of cold light or Doppler ultrasound. The dead space of the syringe should be filled with physiological saline. With bevel facing upwards, needle is inserted from peripheral side just proximal to the proximal skin crease at an angle of 25°–45°. The smallest possible needle (23–26 G) should be used to minimize trauma to the vessel. The needle is withdrawn while maintaining gentle suction till blood flows into the syringe. If the artery is missed, needle can be pushed again in either direction without withdrawing it from the skin. After collection of sample, the site must be kept pressed for at least 5 minutes to stop bleeding.

Temporal artery puncture The temporal artery is situated vertically in front of tragus of the ear and can be located by palpation or by seeing the pulsations after removing the hair from the temporal region. The artery can be punctured against the flow of blood by directing the needle from above downwards. The common complications of the procedure include distal ischemia due to arteriospasm, hematoma, thrombosis, infection and nerve damage.

Brachial artery puncture The brachial artery can be sited by palpation but because of greater depth of artery, the success rate is poor. Moreover, there is minimal collateral circulation and high risk of median nerve damage. The blood can also be obtained from dorsalis pedis and posterior tibial arteries.

INTRAVENOUS INFUSION

The infusion can be set up in a peripheral vein by percutaneous venipuncture with a small-vein or scalp-vein infusion set. It is, however, preferable to use a percutaneous venous catheter (medicath or angiocath) because of reduced risk of dislodgment and leakage. For long-term intravenous alimentation with hyper-osmolar solutions, it is advisable to use a central vein catheter to reduce the risk of thrombosis.

Small-vein set Any peripheral vein can be used for infusion but the scalp veins are easy to puncture due to relative immobility and ease of splintage. The set is attached to a syringe containing saline and flushed. Grasp the rubber finger grip (butterfly) of the needle and pierce the skin gently. The course of needle is directed just under, and almost parallel to the skin. Coming over the vein, pierce it while applying gentle negative pressure by the syringe. The bevel of needle should face upwards and it should be inserted along the direction of flow of blood. The blood would appear in the tube immediately upon entry of the vein. Sometimes with 24 to 26 gauge needle and when the patient is in shock, the blood may not show in the tubing. Slowly flush the needle with saline and look for swelling proximal to the needle tip. Secure the needle and tubing to the site with adhesive tape as shown in Figure 29.6 and adjust the flow rate. Check flow rate regularly to prevent under or overinfusion. Measured volume infusion sets (burette set) and infusion pumps are ideal to regulate the rate of infusion in newborn babies.

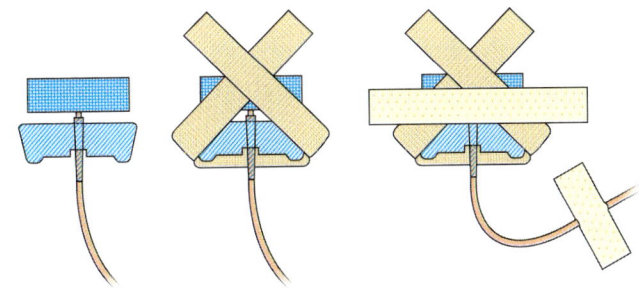

Figure 29.6 Method to securely affix the scalp vein set.

Catheter needle The catheter with 24 gauge needle (neoflon) is grasped between the thumb and forefinger with its attached syringe resting against the palm of the operator's hand. The vein may be approached from above, at a venous junction or from the side. The skin adjacent to the vein is briskly punctured with the needle-catheter held approximately 10–15° to the skin or axis of the arm. Once beneath the dermis, the angle is narrowed so that the catheter is nearly flush with the axis of the vein. When blood is seen in the needle hub, the catheter and needle are advanced along the course of the vein for additional 2 to 3 mm. If a syringe is attached to the catheter, it is aspirated to observe the free return of blood. The plastic catheter is then advanced gently into the vein while the needle is held stationary. Slight pressure may be applied at the tip of the catheter to prevent backflow of blood while advancing the desired length of the catheter. The tourniquet is released, the needle is completely removed from the catheter and an intravenous solution is attached. Sterile dressing is placed at the puncture site and the entry point of catheter. The catheter is secured by adhesive tape. The limb may be splinted with a padded wooden spatula. When scalp vein needle or catheter is removed, the site should be compressed for at least two minutes and a sterile dressing applied.

Complications

Fluid overload may occur, if measured volume burette or infusion pump is not used. Prolonged restraint is usually necessary unless the veins on the dorsum of hand are used. This interferes with the activity of the child. Local swelling and thrombophlebitis can occur. Extravasation of fluid or blood must be identified early to prevent local complications. When extravasation of a hyperosmolar or irritant solution (calcium gluconate) occurs, administer 150 µg/mL hyaluronidase in normal saline, 0.2 mL SC at 5 sites around the leading edge of the infiltrate to minimize tissue injury. In case of extravasation of vasoconstrictive agents (dopamine, dobutamine), phentolamine 1 mg/mL solution in normal saline is injected subcutaneously in aliquots of 0.2 mL at 5 separate sites around the edge of infiltration. A separate 25- or 27-gauge needle should be used for each injection. In neonates, intravenous lines constitute an important portal and source for nosocomial infections. There is some evidence to suggest that prolonged placement of polyvinylchloride based devices leach a plasticizer Di (2 ethylhexyl)-phthalate (DEHP), which may be toxic when used on long-term basis. The devices made of alternative material which is DEHP-free should be used whenever feasible.

INTRAOSSEOUS INFUSION

The use of intraosseous (IO) access during resuscitation is widely accepted and promoted in pediatric intensive care. Recently, the procedure is being recommended for use in the neonates. According to American Heart Association, if one is unable to get venous access within three attempts or 90 seconds, IO access should be established without undue delay. IO cannulation provides access to non-collapsible marrow venous plexus, which serves as a rapid, safe and reliable route for administration of crystalloids, colloids, blood products, life-saving drugs including antibiotics. The only absolute contraindication includes fracture of the tibia or long bones, which are the potential sites for insertion of the IO cannula.

Procedure

Arrow EZ-IO® battery-powered or hand-driven needles (G 15, 25, 45 mm) with a stylet are available. The conventional hypodermic needle or Jamshidi-type bone marrow aspiration needle can also be used. The infant lies supine with hip externally rotated. The common site of cannulation is anteromedial surface of the tibia 2 cm below and 1–2 cm medial to the tibial tuberosity. The site is prepared with strict asepsis by application of alcohol-povidone-alcohol. Support the leg on a firm surface. Insert the IO needle perpendicularly through the skin using gentle but firm twisting movements. The needle is directed slightly caudally towards feet to avoid injury to the joint or epiphysis. The needle is gradually advanced through the bony cortex till decrease in resistance or feeling of "give-in" is felt when bone marrow cavity is reached. The needle should stand firmly without any support in case of correct insertion. The stylet is removed and attempt is made to flush the needle. The marrow can be sent for determination of glucose level, chemistries, blood type and crossmatching, but not for a complete blood count. The needle is stabilized and 10 mL of normal saline is injected slowly. When test injection is successful and there are no signs of extravasation, the syringe is disconnected and infusion set is attached after removing any air in the connection tubing. The needle and tubing are firmly secured and leg is immobilized with a padded splint.

Complications

It is a relatively safe procedure. The extravasation of the fluids suggest misplacement of the needle with a need for reinsertion through an alternative site. Cellulitis, osteomyelitis and epiphyseal injury are rare complications in experienced hands.

PERCUTANEOUS CENTRAL VENOUS CATHETERIZATION

Central venous line is established for a long-term access for administration of intravenous fluids or parenteral nutrition. The procedure is technically difficult and should be conducted by an experienced operator with strict aseptic precautions. The cannulation can be accomplished through a peripheral or a central vein.

Subclavian vein catheterization The infant is sedated and placed supine with a towel roll between the scapulae. The head is turned away from the side of needle insertion and shoulders dropped posteriorly. The skin is prepared with spirit-betadine-spirit and infiltrated with 1% xylocaine. The introducer needle of 3 Fr silastic or silicone catheter is inserted through the skin, at a point beneath the clavicle joining outer one-third with the inner two-thirds of clavicle. The needle is kept almost parallel to the chest wall and directed towards the sternal notch. When blood flow is established, the guidewire is passed and catheter is advanced to lie at the junction of the superior vena cava with right atrium. The position of the catheter tip should be confirmed radiographically. The insertion site is covered with transparent surgical dressing. The procedure is blind and associated with risk of development of pneumothorax, hemothorax and inadvertent puncture of subclavian artery.

External jugular vein catheterization Silicon or silastic 2 Fr catheter with introducer needle is used. The site is prepared with spirit-betadine-spirit. The vein is identified with cold light and needle with catheter is inserted along the flow of blood. The catheter is advanced after removing the needle so that its tip is positioned at the junction of superior vena cava with right atrium. The position of the catheter tip is confirmed radiographically. The procedure is safe and common complications include infection, thrombosis and thrombophlebitis.

Peripherally Inserted Central Catheter

Peripherally inserted central catheters (PICC) are used for infusion of irritant or vesicant medications, hypertonic solution and prolonged administration of parenteral nutrients. It can also be used for monitoring the central venous pressure (CVP). After strict aseptic precautions, 28G polyurethane or silicone (premicath, neocath) is inserted either through upper limb (basilic or brachial vein) or lower limb (saphenous or femoral vein). The length of the catheter to be inserted is determined by measuring the distance between the site of catheter insertion to mid-sternum (upper limb entry) or xiphisternum (lower limb entry). Clean the site of entry with spirit-povidone-iodine-spirit and drape it with a sterile towel. The catheter is inserted through a breakaway needle rather than over a guidewire and catheter is advanced by holding it with forceps. The desired length of the catheter is advanced to ensure that its tip rests in superior vena cava (T4–T5) in case of insertion through the upper limb or inferior vena cava (T8–T10) when catheter is inserted through the lower limb. If the catheter tip has entered the right atrium, it should be withdrawn. Catheter can be advanced under the guidance of cot-side ultrasonography and position of the catheter tip confirmed with the help of a skiagram. The site of entry should be dressed with a sterile, transparent, semipermeable dressing (Tegaderm) by applying gentle pressure for few hours. Polyurethane catheter can be left *in situ* for 3–4 weeks while silicone catheter can be left in place for a longer duration. The insertion site should be inspected twice a day for early identification of phlebitis and dressing changed after every 3–4 days. In order to ensure the patency of catheter, the fluids should be heparinized (0.5–1.0 units heparin/mL). The catheter can be flushed with a 5 mL syringe containing heparinized saline. TPN filters must be used for prevention of infection because TPN solution provides good ground for proliferation of bacteria. PICC should neither be used for sampling nor for administration of blood and blood products.

Complications

PICCs are relatively safer compared to directly inserted central venous catheters. They are associated with following complications:

   i. Bacterial sepsis and candidemia.
  ii. Thrombophlebitis, thrombosis and embolism.
 iii. Perforation of vein and extravasation.
 iv. Catheter malposition in the right atrium with cardiac arrhythmias.

The catheter should be removed as early as possible when its use is no longer required. Other indications for catheter removal include septicemia, septic emboli, endocarditis and fungemia. Use strict aseptic precautions and pull out the catheter gradually. The exit site should be kept pressed to stop bleeding and a sterile dressing is applied. The catheter tip should be sent to the laboratory for microbiological studies.

The availability of umbilical vessels during first week of life provides a rather convenient site for blood sampling and setting up of infusion particularly for performing exchange blood transfusion. Catheterization is contraindicated, if stump is infected or abdominal surgery is contemplated. Transparent polyvinyl infant feeding tubes with rounded end and a hole at the tip are used. The catheter size Fr 4 and 5 is suitable for artery and Fr 7 or 8 for the vein. The catheter is attached to a 10 mL syringe containing heparinized saline. A loose purse-string ligature is placed around the base of the cord. The umbilical vein is usually located at about 12 o'clock position and it often gapes. The two arteries stand out laterally as small whitish protrusions with obliterated lumens.

Umbilical Vein Catheterization

Indications

It is cannulated for exchange blood transfusion, rapid replacement of blood or fluids and rarely for setting up infusion when other sites fail. The central venous pressure may be monitored but its reliability is doubtful unless catheter tip is kept at least 1.0 cm above the diaphragm. The infusion through umbilical veins should not be allowed to drip for more than 24 hours.

Technique

Restrain the infant by using a padded crucifix splint for fixing all four limbs. The infant should be placed under a radiant warmer in the servo mode to maintain skin temperature around 36.5°C. Site is prepared aseptically using alcohol-povidone-alcohol. Drape the abdomen using sterile towels. Cut the umbilical stump with the scalpel blade about 2.0 cm from the skin (Figure 29.7). The umbilical stump is held with a toothed forceps and opening of the vein is identified. Clot or debris is removed with forceps and its opening dilated with the closed point of a small artery forceps. The catheter (5 Fr for <3.5 kg and 8 Fr for >3.5 kg) is marked with a thread for the appropriate distance to be inserted (20% of crown heel length). The catheter filled with normal saline is gently pushed into the vein. If it sticks at a distance of 1–2 cm, gentle suction should be applied to suck out any additional clot followed by injection of heparinized saline. The umbilical stump is pulled downwards and catheter is gently pushed forwards with occasional rotatory movements till a free flow of blood is obtained. If catheter is intended to be left *in situ*, X-ray chest, posteroanterior and

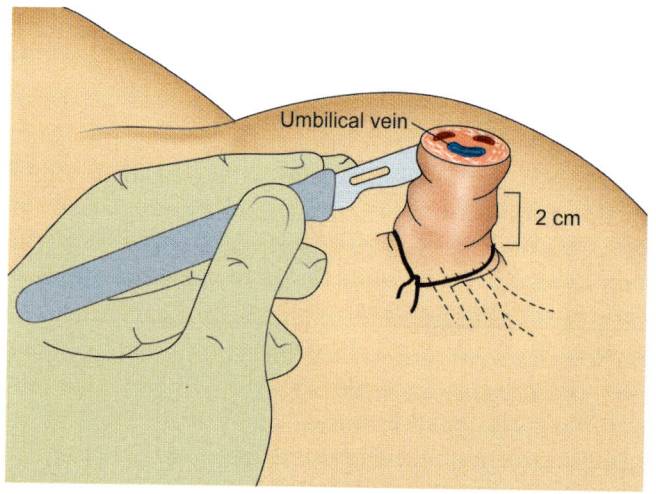

Figure 29.7 Cutting the umbilical stump about 2 cm from skin for placement of umbilical venous catheter.

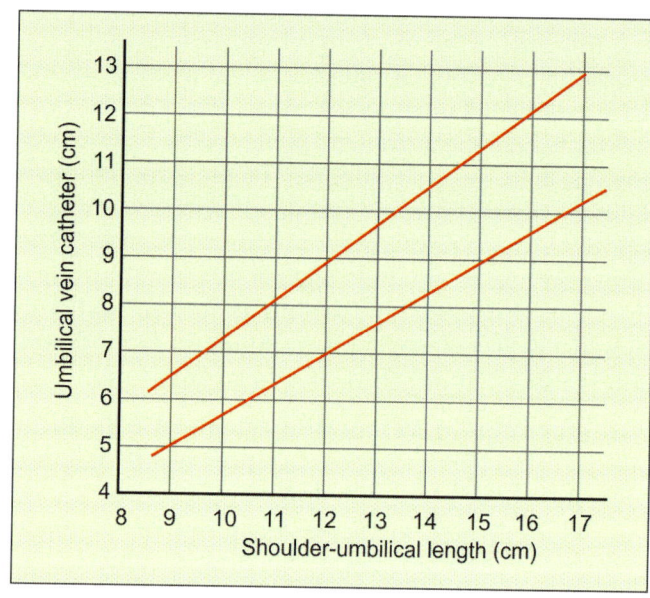

Figure 29.8 Desired umbilical venous catheter length based on the shoulder-umbilical length.

lateral views should be taken. For administration of IV fluids, the catheter tip should be passed beyond the ductus venosus to lie in the thoracic segment (T9–T10) of the inferior vena cava at the level of diaphragm. The desired length of the catheter to be inserted can be calculated by measuring the shoulder-umbilical distance (Figure 29.8). The desired UVC length in cm can be calculated by the formula: (1.5 × birth weight in kg) + 5.5 cm. Other formulae used for calculation of UVC length insertion in cm include JSS formula (6.5 + weight in kg) and revised Shukla method (3 × birth weight in kg + 9) ÷ 2. For resuscitation and exchange blood transfusion, catheter tip is kept just underneath the skin from where a good flow of blood is obtained. The venous catheter should never be left open to air for fear of air embolism. The catheter should be secured in place with a purse-string suture. The free end of the catheter should be strapped to the abdominal wall well away from the perineum to avoid contamination.

Umbilical Artery Catheterization

Indications

Indwelling arterial catheter is ideal for frequent blood gas analyses and for invasive monitoring of blood pressure.

Technique

The cord and surrounding skin up to 5 cm is prepared with alcohol-povidone-alcohol. The umbilical stump is cut clean with a scalpel under strict aseptic conditions. Squeezing the cord between thumb and index finger for 2 minutes may cause dilatation of the umbilical arteries due to hypoxia. The stump should be grasped with a toothed forceps and opening of one of the umbilical arteries should be dilated with a metallic probe. Select an appropriate sized catheter (3.5 Fr <1250 g and 5 Fr for >1250 g), fill it with heparinized saline and attach a syringe and stopcock. Insert the catheter gently towards caudal direction. Keep the umbilical artery stretched and dilated with curved iris forceps while inserting the catheter (Figure 29.9). After inserting about 2 cm of catheter, the umbilical stump should be elevated superiorly and catheter pushed caudally till the desired length is cannulated. The desired UAV length in cm can be calculated by the formula: (4 × birth weight in kg) + 7 cm. Refer to Table 29.1 and Figure 29.10 for desired length of catheter to be inserted. The tip of the catheter may be positioned at a high or low site. In the former, the catheter tip lies at the lower thoracic aorta above the diaphragm between ductus arteriosus and origin of celiac axis (between T8 and T10 vertebrae). In the lower location of umbilical artery catheter, the tip is positioned in the abdominal aorta between inferior mesenteric artery and aortic bifurcation (L3 and L4 vertebrae). The position of the catheter should be confirmed by taking an X-ray of the abdomen (Figure 29.11). The lower location of catheter is associated with greater risk of blanching, cyanosis and gangrene of buttocks and legs. During and following the procedure, the feet should be examined for any evidences of discoloration and blanching. When blanching occurs, warming the opposite leg may resolve the vasospasm. If blanching and discoloration persists, the catheter should be

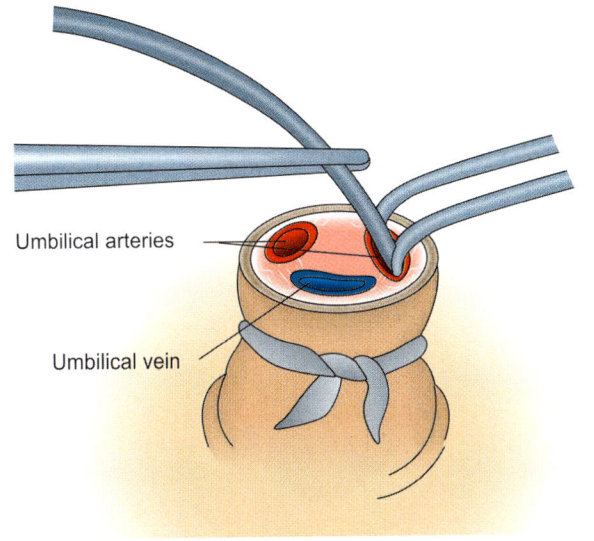

Figure 29.9 Dilatation of umbilical artery and insertion of catheter.

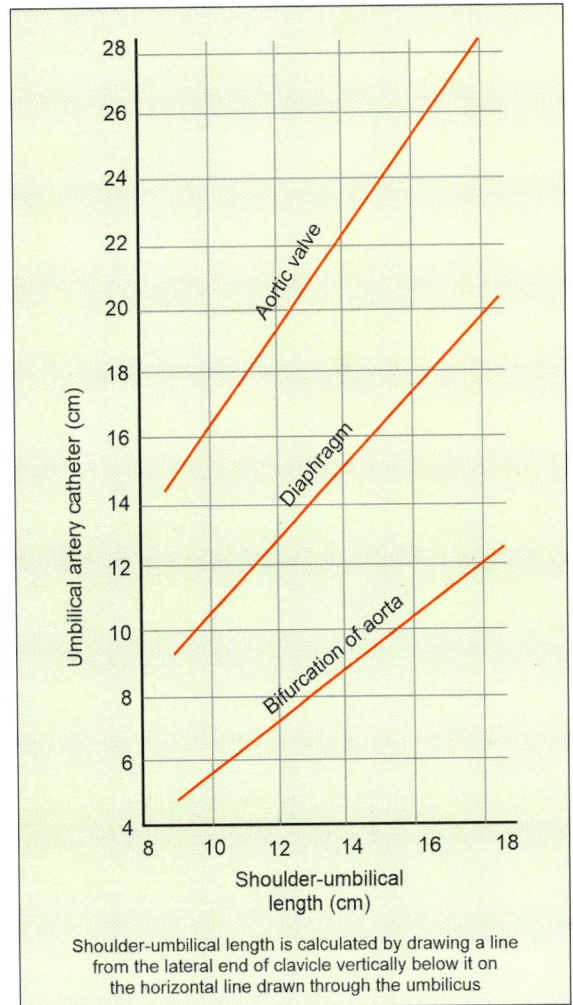

Shoulder-umbilical length is calculated by drawing a line from the lateral end of clavicle vertically below it on the horizontal line drawn through the umbilicus

Figure 29.10 Desired umbilical arterial catheter length based on the shoulder-umbilical length.

Procedures

29

TABLE 29.1 Optimal length of catheter to be passed for umbilical vessel catheterization

Crown heel length (cm)	Venous catheter to reach IVC** (cm)	Arterial catheter to reach bifurcation of aorta*** (cm)
34	5.5	5.0
36	6.0	5.5
38	6.5	6.0
40	7.0	6.5
42	7.25	7.0
44	8.0	7.5
46	8.25	8.0
48	8.5	8.5
50	9.0	9.0
52	9.5	9.5
Shoulder-umbilical length*		
10	5.5	5.5
11	6.0	6.0
12	6.75	6.75
13	7.5	7.5
4	8.25	8.50
15	8.75	9.25
16	9.5	10.0

*Shoulder-umbilical length is calculated from lateral end of clavicle to a point vertically beneath it on the horizontal line drawn through the umbilicus.

**Resistance is usually met at ductus venosus. The catheter should be passed 1–2 cm beyond the point of resistance.

***Resistance is often met at the junction of umbilical artery with internal iliac artery.

(*Adapted from* Dunn PM; Localization of the umbilical catheter by post-mortem measurements. *Arch Dis Child* 1966; 41(215): 69–75).

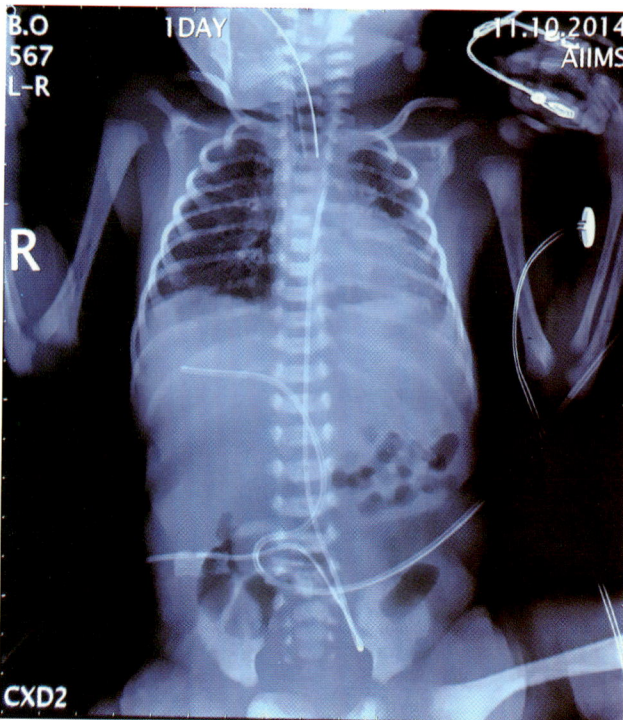

Figure 29.11 Incorrectly placed umbilical venous and arterial catheters.

Complications

Thrombosis, embolization, perforation of the vessel, air embolism, misplacement of catheter into the portal venous system, bleeding, infection, necrotizing enterocolitis and rarely extrahepatic portal hypertension in childhood may occur. In view of a large number of potential complications, umbilical artery catheters should be employed only when absolutely necessary and their tips should be positioned below the origin of the renal vessels to minimize renal artery down-stream embolization.

Removal of Catheters

Catheter should be removed as early as possible depending upon the needs of the baby. When a baby develops clinical evidences of NEC, catheter/s must be removed immediately. With due aseptic precautions, purse-string suture is applied at the base of the cord. The venous catheter can be pulled out easily and bleeding controlled by local pressure and pulling the purse-strings. After withdrawing umbilical arterial catheter to within 1–2 cm of the opening of the artery, one should wait for about one to two minutes to allow the umbilical artery to contract. After finally removing the catheter, bleeding should be stopped by local pressure at the umbilicus and abdominal wall below and to the side of the umbilicus, and tightening of artery

removed. The purse-string ligature at the base should be tightened and catheter stitched in place. The catheter is filled with heparinized saline and stoppered with a rubber cap. The patency of the arterial line is best maintained by infusing heparinized normal saline at a rate of 1.0 mL/hr with an infusion pump. The umbilical area should be sprayed with an antibiotic powder and free end of the catheter should be strapped to the abdominal wall well away from the perineum. For sampling, about 2 mL of blood and heparinized saline contained in the umbilical catheter is withdrawn, the sample should be collected in another heparinized syringe and the blood previously removed should be returned to the baby. The catheter must be adequately cleared of the infusate before withdrawing the blood sample.

forceps. The catheter tip must be sent for culture in all cases. In case a baby with indwelling catheters dies, the catheters should remain *in situ* and pathologist should be requested to ascertain the location of catheter tips and determine the possible role of umbilical catheterization regarding the death of the baby.

Peripheral Arterial Cannulation

Cannulation of peripheral arteries is generally avoided but may be required, if umbilical artery is inaccessible or has been used for a long time. Radial, posterior tibial or dorsalis pedis arteries can be cannulated. Right radial artery puncture or cannulation is done for collection of preductal blood sample for diagnosis of persistent fetal circulation. Before cannulation of radial artery, patency of ulnar artery should be assessed by the modified Allen test (refer to page 613).

The site overlying the artery to be cannulated is prepared with alcohol-povidone-alcohol. The artery is located with a cold light. The intravenous cannula (22–24 gauge) is inserted against the blood flow through the skin at an angle less than 30° to the horizontal and slowly advanced into the artery (Figure 29.12). Stylet is removed as soon as the artery is entered and catheter is advanced. Heparinized saline is infused at a rate of 1.0 mL per hour to maintain the patency of catheter (Figure 29.13). The distal part of the limb beyond cannulation should be closely watched for any change in color or temperature due to ischemia. Never administer any medications through the peripheral arterial line. For collection of blood sample, apply suction to remove saline and 1.0 mL of blood with a syringe. Collect blood sample in a heparinized syringe for ABG. Return the saline

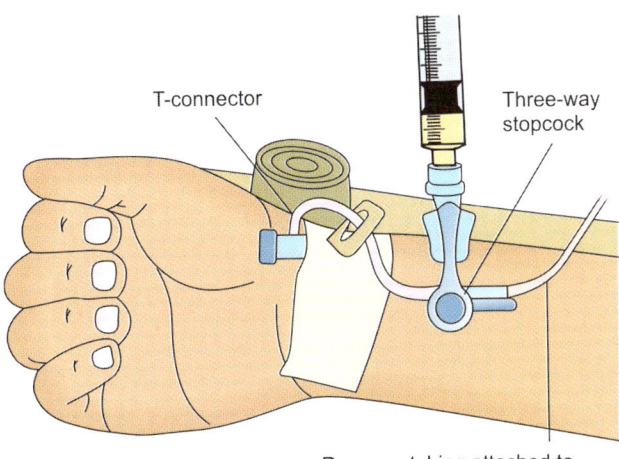

Figure 29.13 Radial artery indwelling catheter set up for continuous monitoring of arterial blood pressure and frequent blood sampling.

and dead space blood back to the baby. Maintain an accurate record of blood samples taken for various investigations. The intravenous tubing and flushing solution should be changed every 24 hours.

EXCHANGE BLOOD TRANSFUSION

Relatively small blood volume of the newborn baby makes the procedure of exchange transfusion feasible for a variety of conditions.

Indications

1. At birth. Cord hemoglobin of less than 10 g/dL or bilirubin of more than 5 mg/dL with history of severe Rh-isoimmunization in previous babies.
2. Rh-isoimmunized babies with unconjugated serum bilirubin level of more than 10 mg/dL within 24 hours or 15 mg/dL within 48 hours or rate of rise of bilirubin by >0.5 mg/dL/hour are well-known indications for exchange blood transfusion.
3. Indirect serum bilirubin level of 20 mg/100 mL or more; (or salicylate saturation index of more than 7 or HBABA binding capacity of less than 50%, or bilirubin protein ratio of more than 3.5) during first 5 days of life in term babies. Preterm infants should be exchanged at a relatively lower serum bilirubin level (when bilrubin level exceeds 1.0 mg/100 g body weight) particularly when it is associated with perinatal distress factors, viz. asphyxia, acidosis, hypothermia, hypoglycemia and respiratory distress. Refer to Chapter 18 for indications of exchange blood transfusion in preterm babies.

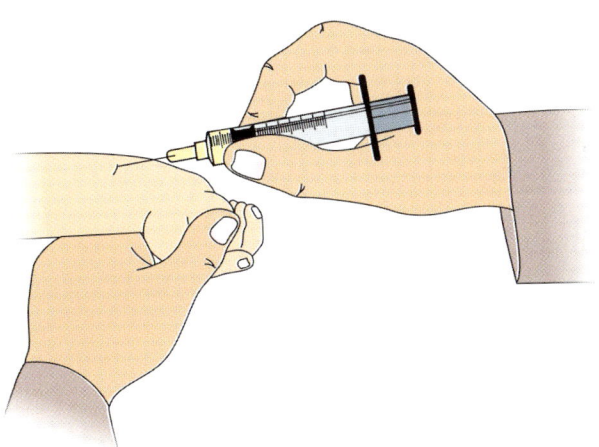

Figure 29.12 Direct puncturing of radial artery for collection of sample of arterial blood for gases.

4. Partial exchange transfusion for chronic anemia due to any cause.
5. Exchange transfusion with fresh heparinized blood for disseminated intravascular coagulation.
6. Life-threatening metabolic disorders, such as hyperglycinemias.
7. Poisoning due to accidental injection of local anesthetic into fetal scalp during paracervical block, transplacental passage of chlorpropamide and magnesium sulfate to the fetus.
8. Acute renal and hepatic failure.
9. Septicemia with sclerema.
10. Exchange transfusion with normal saline for symptomatic polycythemia.

Choice of Blood

In emergency situations, O Rh-negative blood can be used without crossmatching. When blood is arranged in anticipation of the birth of severely Rh-sensitized infant, O Rh-negative blood crossmatched against maternal serum, should be arranged. For subsequent exchange transfusions, irrespective of ABO group of the infant, group O blood crossmatched against infant's serum should be used. It is important that an Rh-negative infant or an infant with hemolytic disease of the newborn due to Rh-isoimmunization must be given Rh-negative blood.

In less severely affected cases, blood is arranged after the birth of the infant. The ABO groups of the mother and her baby should be identified. If infant's red blood cells are compatible with the mother's serum (mother and baby have identical ABO groups, or mother is AB, or infant is O group), the blood of the same ABO type as the baby, crossmatched against mother's serum, can be used for first exchange transfusion. In case infant's red cells are incompatible with the mother's serum, ABO type-specific blood crossmatched against infant's serum should be used. In hemolytic disease of the newborn due to ABO incompatibility, O Rh-specific cells with a low titer of anti-A and anti-B antibodies should be crossmatched with mother or O Rh-specific RBCs can be suspended in AB plasma.

Fresh citrate phosphate dextrose (CPD) blood (not more than 3 days old) or heparinized blood can be used for the procedure. Acid-citrate-dextrose (ACD) blood has a tendency to produce hypocalcemia, hyperkalemia and metabolic acidosis while heparinized blood carries the risk of hypoglycemia and rise in free fatty acids leading to displacement of bilirubin from albumin binding sites. CPD blood is relatively safe and free from side effects. An effective exchange is achieved by performing the procedure with double

the blood volume of the baby, i.e. about 180 mL/kg. The stored CPD-blood must be prewarmed by immersing the bottle in a water bath at 37°C. Administration of albumin, half to one hour before the exchange, is associated with more effective removal of bilirubin. Instead of albumin-primed exchange transfusion, some workers prefer addition of albumin into the donor or exchange blood itself.

Collection of Specimens

Exchange transfusion provides an opportunity for large quantities of blood being available for various investigations.

Donor blood. Hemoglobin, hematocrit, potassium and pH.

Baby's blood at the beginning. Hemoglobin, hematocrit, bilirubin, glucose, calcium, potassium, pH and various investigations for the cause of jaundice.

Post-exchange. Hemoglobin, hematocrit, bilirubin, glucose, calcium, potassium and pH.

The total affluent should also be collected for bilirubin estimation in order to calculate the total bilirubin removed.

Bacteriological specimens. Umbilical swab for culture at the beginning of the procedure and blood for culture at the end. At the time of removal of the catheter, its tip should be sent for culture.

Procedure

It should be performed in the NICU with due aseptic precautions. The baby must be kept adequately warm during the procedure with the help of a servo-controlled over head radiant heat source. The stomach contents should be aspirated. The baby is fastened on a well-padded curcifix splint. Telethermometer and electrocardiography oscilloscope or stethoscope should be attached to monitor baby's temperature and cardiac status. An exchange transfusion chart should be prepared incorporating the following information: IN/OUT volume, heart rate, respiratory rate, oxygen saturation, color of the baby and umbilical blood, temperature, venous pressure, drugs administered and any problems encountered.

After full aseptic precautions, umbilical vein should be cannulated. Some neonatologists prefer to use the umbilical artery for the procedure. The catheter is attached to two three-way taps so that their leads are connected to the umbilical catheter, syringe, donor blood and a sterile container for waste. The blood is withdrawn with gentle suction and donor's blood is injected slowly in aliquots of 10 to 20 mL depending upon the size of the baby. The blood should be prewarmed by immersing the bottle in a water bath at 37°C. It should never be heated under a hot water tap. During the procedure, the bottle of donor blood should be gently agitated from time-to-time to keep the cells and plasma mixed. The jammed syringes and blocked three-way connectors should be rinsed with heparinized saline (10 units of heparin/mL). Nurse or an assistant must maintain an accurate record of the IN/OUT and condition of the baby. Whenever any untoward signs appear, such as restlessness, grunting, distressed respirations, heart rate above 160 or below 100 per minute, fall in oxygen saturation and deterioration in the color of the baby or umbilical blood, the procedure must be withheld till baby improves.

After every 100 mL exchange, the venous pressure should be checked though its interpretation may be difficult because it is influenced by the location of the catheter tip. During exchange transfusion in an hydropic infant, the venous pressure should be monitored more frequently. The plasma proteins and intravascular oncotic pressure progressively rises in these infants as the exchange progresses. This leads to expansion of blood volume which may result in cardiac decompensation. Therefore, repeated deficits may have to be established in order to prevent vascular overload. When ACD or CPD blood is being transfused, 1 mL calcium gluconate 10% should be injected slowly after every 50 mL of exchange. The catheter should be rinsed with heparinized saline before and after the injection of calcium gluconate to avoid clotting of blood. During the injection, heart rate must be watched closely for any bradycardia. If calcium gluconate injection is poorly tolerated, it should be abandoned and baby started on oral calcium gluconate after the procedure. After completion of the procedure, the catheter should be filled with heparinized normal saline and umbilical stump sprayed with an antibiotic powder. The prophylactic use of antibiotics is not recommended though they are often given in centers where asepsis is at suspect.

Exchange Blood Transfusion through other Routes

In the presence of umbilical sepsis, umbilical route should not be used for exchange blood transfusion. When umbilical cord has fallen or umbilical vessel cannot be cannulated, cut-down should be performed by making an incision in the midline above the umbilicus. The umbilical vein lies rather deep in a trough. When umbilical vein cut-down also fails, saphenous vein below the inguinal ligment should be exposed by cut-down to cannulate femoral vein. It may be impossible to withdraw blood from this site though blood can be injected with ease. In such circumstances, radial artery should be cannulated for adequate withdrawal of blood, while blood can be injected through the cut-down established at the saphenous vein. Angiocath can be used for blind cannulation of femoral vein.

Complications

1. Complications due to catheterization of umbilical vessels are mentioned on page 618. In addition, hazards of blood transfusion in general should be kept in mind including risk of malaria, syphilis, CMV, HIV and hepatitis B and C.
2. Over-loading of circulation with cardiac failure or shock following excessive deficit.
3. Hypocalcemia, hyperkalemia, acidosis and sudden cardiac arrest or arrhythmia may occur during exchange transfusion with ACD blood. Acidosis may be followed by mild alkalosis as the citrate is metabolized.
4. Hypoglycemia and bleeding manifestations may occur following exchange transfusion with heparinized blood.
5. Oxygen toxicity may occur at a relatively lower arterial oxygen tension because adult hemoglobin (transfused blood) readily releases oxygen to the tissues by virtue of its poor affinity to bind oxygen.

PERITONEAL DIALYSIS

Peritoneal dialysis (PD) is a safe and effective procedure to manage acute renal failure in the newborn. PD is preferred over hemodialysis in the newborn because of technical difficulties in establishing vascular access in young infants. PD is also used for management of life-threatening hyperammonemia due to urea cycle defect and congenital lactic acidosis.

Indications

Unlike older children, there are no absolute criteria for undertaking PD in newborn babies.
- Oliguria or anuria of >48 hours.
- Pulmonary edema and fluid over load.
- Persistent and unresponsive hyperkalemia (>7.5 mEq/L).
- BUN >125 mg/dL or rising by 20 mg/dL everyday.
- Serum creatinine >3.0 mg/dL.
- Severe and persistent metabolic acidosis (pH <7.2).

Dialysate Solution

Neonates with acute kidney damage (AKD) are often hypoxic and cannot metabolize lactate contained in the conventional dialysis solution. It is desirable to prepare a dialysis solution where lactate is replaced by bicarbonate (Table 29.2). Since calcium may get precipitated in the solution containing bicarbonate, it should not be incorporated in such a dialysate and is administered separately intravenously. Changes are made in the composition of dialysis solution depending upon the clinical status of the infant and therapeutic requirements. Higher dextrose concentration (3% instead of 1.5%) is administered to correct fluid overload. Potassium chloride (4 mEq/L) is added to the dialysis fluid when serum potassium level falls below 4.5 mEq/L.

Procedure

Bladder should be emptied by compression or catheterization. Under thorough aseptic conditions, intravenous cannula (venflon) is introduced into the peritoneal cavity and 20–40 mL/kg of dialysis solution is injected slowly to distend the abdomen. After removing the cannula, an incision is made about 1 cm below the umbilicus after local infiltration of xylocaine. Peritoneal dialysis cannula (pediatric size) is introduced through the incision and positioned in the left or right ileac fossa. Commercially available catheters or chest drain catheter can be used in preterm babies. When prolonged peritoneal dialysis is anticipated, a Tenckhoff catheter should be used. The peritoneal dialysis fluid is warmed to body temperature and infused into the peritoneal cavity over 10 minutes. The fluid is kept in the peritoneal cavity for 30 to 45 minutes and then siphoned off over 10–15 minutes by placing the drainage bag below the level of the baby. The fluid

TABLE 29.2 Composition of dialysis solution in newborn babies

Component	Volume
One-half physiological saline (0.45%)	915 mL
Sodium chloride (2.5 mEq/mL)	12 mL
Sodium bicarbonate (1 mEq/mL)	40 mL
Magnesium sulfate (10%)	1.8 mL
Dextrose solution 50%	30 mL
Total	998.8 mL

This solution provides sodium 142 mEq/L, chloride 100 mEq/L, magnesium 1.5 mEq/L and bicarbonate 40 mEq/L. Calcium gluconate (10%) 1–2 mL/kg every 8 hours is given intravenously.

exchange is done manually or with the help of an automated peritoneal dialysis machine. Heparin 1 unit/mL is added in the dialysis fluid during the first 2 to 3 cycles. The cycles are continued till the clinical and chemical abnormalities are corrected usually by 36 to 48 hours. Careful monitoring of body weight, vital signs, urine out put and renal parameters including serum electrolytes should be repeated after every 24 hours. Microscopic examination for cell count and culture of effluent peritoneal fluid is done after completion of the procedure. The tip of the catheter should be sent for culture. Prophylactic use of antibiotics is not recommended. After removing the catheter, the entry site should be pressed with a piece of sterile gauze, sealed with Tr. benzoin and dressed.

Complications

The procedure is simple, effective and relatively safe and without any serious complications. Mortality is dependent on the underlying renal condition and associated pre-procedure complications. The common problems and complications are listed below.

1. Inadequate drainage is the commonest problem which can be resolved by ensuring that holes of the PD catheter are placed intraperitoneal. At times, catheter is reinserted to ensure free flow of effluent.

2. Intestinal perforation may occur, if abdomen is not distended before insertion of PD catheter.

3. Hyperglycemia should be monitored with dextrostix and managed by reducing concentration of dextrose or treating with insulin. Use of fructose dialysate or increasing dwelling time may correct hyperglycemia.

4. Hypokalemia is prevented by adding potassium in the dialysate, if procedure is continued beyond 24 hours.

5. Peritonitis should be ruled out by microscopic examination and culture of peritoneal effluent. It should be treated aggressively with intraperitoneal and intravenous antibiotics.

6. Depletion syndrome due to hypovolemia is managed by administration of fresh frozen plasma.

NEUROLOGICAL PROCEDURES

Lumbar Puncture

It is indicated in a neonate with convulsions and whenever pyogenic meningitis and intracranial bleeding are suspected. Serial lumbar punctures are also recommended for the management of posthemorrhagic hydrocephalus. A neonatal lumbar puncture needle (22 to 24 gauge) with stylet or scalp vein needle may be used for the procedure. The scalp vein set has the added advantage that the CSF pressure can be measured by holding the polythene tubing upright. However, some workers feel that it is not advisable to perform a lumbar puncture without stylet because implantation of a core of epidermis into the subarachnoid space may lead to the development of an epidermoid tumor in later life. The procedure is contraindicated in critically sick newborn babies with cardiorespiratory instability, lumbosacral anomalies or skin infection at the lumbar site.

It is preferable to make the baby sit up with dorsal and lumbar spines flexed as much as possible. Alternatively, baby may be made to lie on his side with spine flexed as much as possible though small and sick babies may not withstand too much flexion. Neck flexion should be avoided due to risk of compromising the airway. The spine of 4th lumbar vertebra should be identified by drawing a line joining the two iliac crests. Use thorough aseptic precautions and cleanse the local site with alcohol-povidone-alcohol. The needle should be inserted at the midpoint between L4 and L5 spines and advanced anteriorily with bevel facing headward. The subarachnoid space is reached within a depth of 1 cm but sensation of penetrating the ligamentum flavum is often absent. The stylet should be withdrawn frequently as the needle is being advanced. Slight rotation of the needle also helps to obtain the CSF. If no fluid is obtained, space between L3 and L4 spines should be tried. In a newborn baby, spinal cord comes down to L3 level, therefore, higher taps are fraught with dangers of injury to the spinal cord. Traumatic tap and unsuccessful lumbar puncture are quite common in newborn babies. If the CSF is blood-stained, following observations may help to differentiate between traumatic tap and genuinely blood-stained CSF.

1. If it was an easy clean tap without any difficulty, the red staining is likely to be due to blood in the CSF.
2. The CSF should be collected in a couple of bottles to see whether the blood staining is uniform or it gradually clears off.
3. After centrifugation, xanthochromic supernatant suggests that blood has been present in CSF for some time provided the baby is not jaundiced.
4. The presence of macrophages and crenated red blood cells on microscopic examination also suggests that CSF has been blood stained for at least few hours.

About 0.5 mL CSF is collected in an EDTA bottle for cytology and 1–2 mL in plain vial for culture and biochemistry. After withdrawing the needle, the puncture site is sealed with Tr. benzoin or micropore seal to prevent oozing. It is important that even in grossly blood-stained CSF, cell count, Gram staining and culture must be done. Simultaneous estimation of blood glucose is desirable for meaningful interpretation of cerebrospinal fluid glucose level. In normal circumstances, CSF glucose should not be less than 75% of blood glucose. CSF for cytology should be examined without any delay and preferably within 30 minutes. The normal cerebrospinal fluid findings in newborn babies are very different as compared to older children and are given in Appendix 9.

Cisternal Puncture

Puncture of cisterna magna (cerebellomedullaris cistern) should not be attempted unless examination of CSF is urgently required. It is contraindicated in babies with myelomeningocele who are likely to have Arnold-Chiari malformation. The hair from the occipital bone and back of the neck should be shaved. The baby should be held while lying on its side and neck flexed as much as possible. A little padding should be placed under the baby's neck and cheek to avoid lateral flexion of cervical spine. The point of entry is bounded above by the base of the occipital bone and below by the spine of the axis vertebra (C2) which is the highest palpable portion of the cervical spine and on either side by posterior nuchal muscles. A medium-sized lumbar puncture needle should be used and pushed horizontally forwards aiming towards a point on the forehead just above the glabella. After reaching a depth of about 1 cm, stylet should be withdrawn and needle gently rotated. If no fluid is obtained, needle should be pushed further until either the CSF is obtained or needle hits the occipital bone. When occipital bone is hit, needle should be partly withdrawn and reinserted aiming at a slightly lower point on the forehead to avoid hitting the base of the occipital bone. The usual depth to which the needle needs to be inserted is about 1.5 cm in a term baby.

Subdural Tap

This should be attempted only when subdural hematoma is strongly suspected by the presence of characteristic predisposing and associated factors. Cranial ultrasound or CT examination should be done to confirm the existence of subdural effusion or hematoma.

Procedures

29

It is desirable to use rather short and wide-bored needle as compared to lumbar puncture needle. The anterior half of the scalp should be shaved and washed thoroughly with soap and water. The baby should be held completely wrapped with his head near the edge of the table. The tap is done at two sites in the coronal suture just lateral to the lateral angles of anterior fontanel. One should wait for about half a minute or so because subdural fluid is often thick and viscid. If no fluid comes out, needle should be advanced further to a maximum depth of 1.0–1.5 cm, withdrawing the stylet frequently. The suction with a syringe should never be applied. If one side is dry, tap should be tried on the other side and even more lateral sites in the coronal suture if subdural effusion is strongly suspected. Avoid removing more than 5.0 mL of fluid or blood at a time.

Ventricular Tap

Ventricular taps may be done for the diagnosis of intraventricular hemorrhage, for administration of antibiotics for the treatment of ventriculitis in a case of bacterial meningitis and for relief of intracranial pressure in an infant with hydrocephalus pending shunt operation.

The preparation of scalp and landmarks are the same as for subdural tap. The right ventricle should be tapped as a routine by using long lumbar puncture needle. The needle should be pushed forwards and inwards directing it towards the nasion (Figure 29.14). Depending upon the size of the baby and degree of

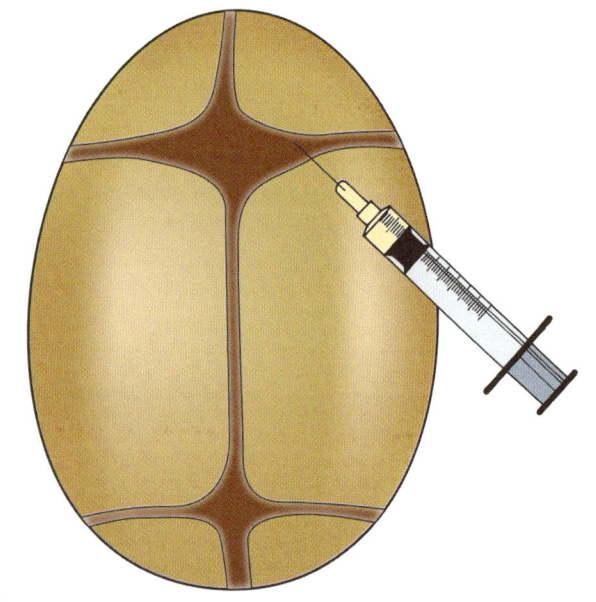

Figure 29.14 Diagrammatic representation of ventricular tap. The needle should be directed forwards and inwards towards the nasion.

ventricular dilatation, the ventricle is generally reached at a depth of 2.5 cm. As in cases of sudural tap, suction with a syringe should never be applied. After removal of needle, the baby should be made to sit up and CSF oozing stopped by local pressure.

TRANSILLUMINATION WITH COLD LIGHT

Cold light source with a fiberoptic cable is a useful equipment to have in the labor room and NICU. It provides a rapid and non-invasive method for prompt diagnosis of pneumothorax by transillumination of chest. Hydranencephaly, porencephaly and subdural hematoma can be screened by transillumination of head. Cold light is useful for illumination of the vessel wall for puncture or cannulation of a peripheral vein and artery.

Chest transillumination Darken the room by switching off all lights. Infant is positioned supine and flat. Place the tip of the scope snugly on the lateral chest wall, in the midaxillary line, at the level of the eighth rib by angling it towards the midsternal region. Repeat the procedure on the opposite side. A halo of light up to 1.0 cm around the light source is normal. In an infant with pneumothorax, the whole chest will brightly transilluminate, especially in preterm babies because of thin chest wall.

Skull transillumination In a dark room, the light source is first placed on the center of parietal bones and then over the center of the occipital bones. The size of the halo of light around the tip of light source is noted. The normal halo of light is up to 2.0 cm in the parietal region and 1.0 cm over the occipital region. In infants with hydranencephaly or porencephaly, the whole skull will be brilliantly transilluminant. The halo of light around the tip of the scope is reduced or disappears in infants with subdural hematoma.

Vessel transillumination The light source is set at low intensity and the probe is positioned against and beneath the selected vessel slightly away from the site of procedure. The sterility of the probe should be maintained by cleaning it with alcohol. The vein would be visible as a dark linear structure while artery would be pulsatile.

PLEURAL ASPIRATION

Aspiration of pleural space is life-saving in a case of tension pneumothorax and pleural effusion or empyema. Pneumothorax can be promptly suspected at cot-side by testing the transillumination of chest with fiberoptic light.

Tension pneumothorax Aspiration of pleural space is life-saving in a baby with tension pneumothorax. It is unnecessary to attempt aspiration of a small pneumothorax in the absence of any mediastinal displacement and respiratory distress. A 22- or 24-gauge intravenous catheter (angiocath) with an attached 3-way stopcock and 20 mL syringe should be inserted either at second intercostal space about 1 cm lateral to the sternal border or at the 4th intercostal space in the anterior axillary line. The air is gently aspirated with a syringe and pushed out by closing the three-way to the baby. The procedure is continued till baby improves when arrangements are made to insert an intercostal drain. When facilities are available these infants are best managed with high-frequency oscillation ventilation (HFOV).

Pleural effusion Pleural effusion and empyema are rare in the newborn baby. Chylothorax is the commonest cause of effusion in a newborn baby. The infant should be supported in a sitting position. The needle should be introduced at the point of maximum dullness or 8th intercostal space in the posterior axillary line in the back. The point of entry of the needle should be close to the upper border of the rib to avoid injury to the intercostal blood vessels. In cases of empyema, closed intercostal drainage under water seal is essential to ensure rapid expansion of the lung.

Chest drainage Strict aseptic precautions should be followed by using gown, gloves and mask. The baby is placed in a lateral position with side to be drained uppermost. Identify the site, sixth intercostal space in the midaxillary line, just above the upper border of rib. Clean the area with alcohol-povidone-alcohol. Infiltrate the puncture site with 1% xylocaine. Using the straight blade scalpel, make a small incison in the skin and intercostal muscles adjacent to upper border of the rib at the selected site. Using a trocar or an artery forceps, separate the muscle fibers along their axes. Insert the tip of cannula (8–11 Portex pneumothorax cannula) into the pleural space with the help of an artery forceps. Alternatively, 16–18 gauge angiocath can be used for drainage of pneumothorax or 10–12 Fr catheter can be inserted for constant drainage of pleural fluid. Connect the cannula with a three-way stopcock to the underwater seal. The glass tube connected with pleural drain should dip 2 cm under the surface of water. The bubbling of water suggests drainage of air and correct positioning of the cannula. The drainage bottle is provided with another short tube to serve as a vent to release extra air to prevent build up of pressure within the bottle. The drainage tube should be secured to the chest with a purse-string suture. Cover the site of tube insertion with a sterile gauze dressing and apply an adhesive tape. Attach the underwater seal system to a slow suction machine to apply a constant negative pressure of 15–20 cm H_2O to ensure effective drainage. Skiagram of chest, anteroposterior and lateral views should be taken to confirm the position of tube.

The removal of chest tube is planned when there is no further bubbling of air or any movements of water column and X-ray chest confirms total re-expansion of the lung. Prior to removal of the tube, 3-way stopcock is closed for 6 hours and baby closely observed. X-ray chest is repeated after 6 hours to check that there has been no reaccumulation of air or effusion. After removing the tube, mattress suture should be tightened and dressing applied. X-ray chest should be repeated after 2–4 hours of removing the tube.

PERICARDIOCENTESIS

Pericardiocentesis may be required to relieve cardiac tamponade due to pericardial effusion or more commonly pneumopericardium following pulmonary air leaks. Under strict asepsis, 20 to 22 gauge angiocath is introduced through subxiphoid space by directing it towards the left shoulder at an angle of 30 to 45° from skin. The needle is electrocardiographically monitored by connecting it with an alligator clamp to the chest lead. The elevation of ST-segment or appearance of ectopic beats indicate that needle has touched the epicardium. It is slightly withdrawn and air or pus is aspirated with a gentle suction through the syringe. It is best to undertake the procedure under cot-side echocardiography. The common complications include hemopericardium, arrhythmia, air embolism, infection and cardiac arrest.

ABDOMINAL PARACENTESIS

Abdominal paracentesis may be occasionally required for therapeutic purposes, if massive ascites is associated with respiratory distress or as a diagnostic procedure at times. Diagnostic abdominal tap is often indicated to exclude perforation and peritonitis in an infant with NEC. The procedure is identical to the one advocated in older children except that the tap should be done in the left iliac fossa to avoid puncturing of the liver, if it is grossly enlarged. The bladder should be drained manually or with the help of a catheter.

About 5.0 to 10 mL of fluid is removed for diagnostic purposes while 10 to 20 mL/kg should be removed for therapeutic relief. The aspirate is collected in EDTA and plain bottles for cytology, Gram staining, biochemistry and culture studies. The puncture site should be kept pressed for a few minutes and sealed with Tr. benzoin.

MEASUREMENT OF BLOOD PRESSURE

The blood pressure and tissue perfusion should be monitored in all critically sick newborn babies and during treatment with drugs known to cause hypotension (tolazoline, morphine, curare, prostaglandins) and hypertension (corticosteroids).

Indirect Measurement

The conventional technique of taking blood pressure in the newborn is often unsatisfactory due to difficulty in palpation and auscultation of peripheral arteries. The appropriate cuff width is 2.0–2.5 cm in a term neonate and its inflatable portion must be long enough to completely encircle the limb. Too wide a cuff may give falsely low readings of blood pressure while falsely high readings may be obtained with a narrow cuff. The baby must be in a quiet state. The cuff should be applied and baby either offered a feed or a pacifier to soothe him before proceeding further.

Flush method The conventional method of recording blood pressure should be tried first because, if successful, it gives a more reliable reading as compared to flush method. In flush method, the limb should be raised and squeezed or milked till hand or foot becomes pale. The cuff should be inflated to a pressure above 110 mm Hg and limb lowered and placed by the side of the baby. The pressure should be gradually and slowly released by 5 mm Hg, holding for about 5 seconds at each step. The point at which the flushing of the hand or foot is seen represents the systolic pressure which is about 5 mm Hg less than that obtained by auscultation. The diastolic pressure cannot be recorded by this technique.

Oscillometer method When the pressure in the cuff is released, the point at which oscillometer needle begins to flick regularly is the systolic pressure and the point where oscillations are maximal denotes diastolic pressure. The systolic and diastolic blood pressure values obtained by automated oscillometry correlate well with intra-arterial blood pressure recordings.

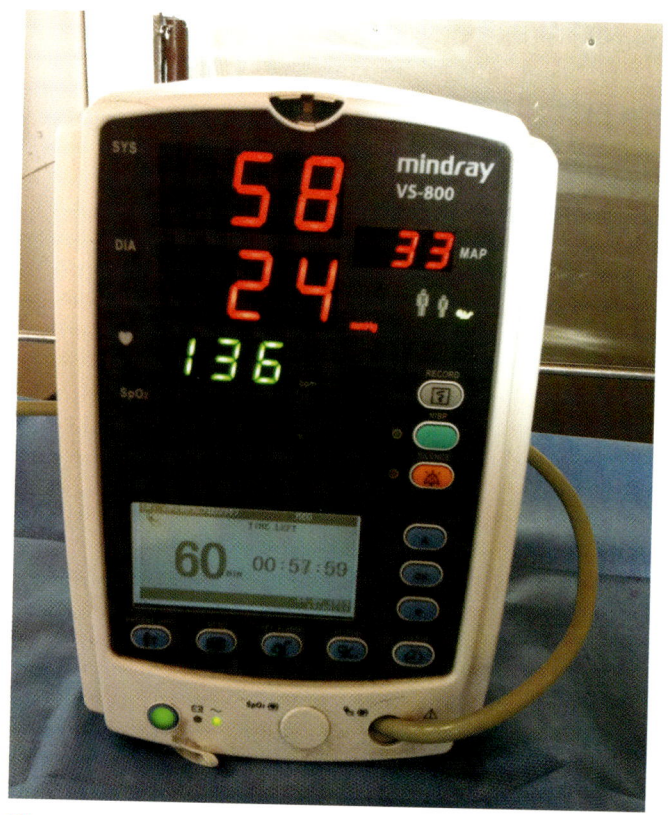

Figure 29.15 Non-invasive blood pressure and heart rate monitor.

Doppler technique Among the indirect techniques for recording blood pressure, non-invasive BP monitor is the most reliable and is comparable to the direct method. The ultrasonic waves are picked up by the transducer located in the cuff. The baby is made to lie in a supine position and an appropriate sized cuff is fitted around the arm. The instrument provides continuous display of heart rate, systolic, diastolic and mean blood pressure (Figure 29.15). There is a provision for alarm or warning signal when blood pressure falls or rises beyond certain preset limits. The blood pressure cuff should be loosened between readings and removed on and off because both radial and peroneal nerve palsies have been reported as complications of multiple blood pressure measurements. Refer to Chapter 2 for details of non-invasive blood pressure monitoring.

Direct Arterial Measurement

When an arterial catheter is in place for monitoring of blood gases, direct arterial pressure can be recorded by using a transducer. It is quite comparable to the value obtained by indirect means but arterial catheterization is never attempted for the sole purpose of monitoring blood pressure.

BIBLIOGRAPHY

American Academy of Pediatrics. Committee on Fetus and Newborn. Prevention and management procedural of pain in the neonate: An update. *Pediatrics* 2016, 137(2): e20154271.

Anand KJ. International Evidence-Based Group for Neonatal Pain: Consensus statement for the prevention and management of pain in the newborn *Arch Pediatr Adolesc Med* 2001, 155: 507–520.

Anand KJ, Aranda JV, Berde CV, *et al.* Summary proceedings from the Neonatal Pain-control Group. *Pediatrics* 2006, 117: S9–S22.

Bell JG, Weiner S. Cordocentesis. *Current Opinion Obstet Gynecol* 1993, 5: 218–224.

Bramhati B, Oldrini A, Ferraze E, Lanzani A. Chorionic villus sampling : an analysis of the obstetric experience of 1000 cases. *Prenat Diagn* 1987, 7: 157.

Carbajal R, Rousset A, Danan C, *et al.* Epidemiology and treatment of painful procedures in neonates in intensive care units. *JAMA* 2008, 300(1): 60–70.

Courtney SE, Weber KR, Breakie LA, *et al.* Capillary blood gases in the neonate. *Amer J Dis Child* 1990, 144: 168.

Daffos F. Fetal blood sampling. In: Current Therapy in Neonatal-Perinatal Medicine-2, *B.C.Decker Inc. Toronto*, 1990.

Davies PA, Robinson RJ, Scopes JW, Tizard JPM, Wigglesworth JS (Eds.). In: Medical Care of Newborn Babies. *Spastic International Medical Publications* 1972, p. 261.

De Carvalho OPS, de Luz GPM, Peterlini MAS. Placement of peripherally inserted central catheters in children guided by ultrasound: prospective randomized and controlled trial. *Pediatr Crit Care Med* 2012, 13: e 282–287.

Deorari AK, Paul VK, Scotland J, *et al.* Practical Procedures for the Newborn Nursery: A manual for physicians and nurses. *Noble Vision, New Delhi* 2001.

Deorari AK, Singh M. Emergency procedures. In: Medical Emergencies in Children. Singh M (Ed.) *Sagar Publications, New Delhi* 5th edition 2012; pp. 876–899.

Dunn PM. Localization of the umbilical catheter by postmortem measurements. *Arch Dis Child* 1966, 41: 69.

Elias S, Simpson JL. Amniocentesis. In: Essential of Prenatal Diagnosis. Simpson JL, Elias S (eds.). *Churchill Livingstone, New York* 1993, pp 27–44.

Fleming SE, Kim JH. Ultrasound-guided umbilical catheter insertion in neonates. *J Perinatol* 2011, 31:344–9.

Garges HP, Moody MA, Cotton CM, *et al.* Neonatal meningitis: What is the correlation among cerebrospinal fluid cultures, blood cultures and cerebrospinal fluid parameters? *Pediatrics* 2006, 117: 1094–1100.

Garland JS, Henrickson K, Maki DG. The 2002 Hospital Infection Control Practices Advisory Committee. Center for Disease Control and Guidelines for Prevention of Intravascular Device–related Infections. *Pediatrics* 2002, 110: 1009–1013.

Goodarzi R, Tariverdi M, Khamesan B, Zare S, Houshmandi MM. Dunn and Shukla's method for predicting length of umbilical catheters in newborns. *Asian J Med Pharma Res* 2014, 4:85–133.

Gupta JM, Robertson NRC, Wigglesworth JS. Umbilical artery catheterization in the newborn. *Arch Dis Child* 1968, 43:382.

Haggee WA, Schonberg SA, Globus MS. Chorionic villus sampling: Experience of the first 1000 cases. *Amer J Obstet Gynecol* 1986, 154: 1249.

Hall RW, Anand KJ. Pain management in newborns *Clin Perinatol* 2014, 41(4): 895–924.

Jackson L, Wapner RJ. Chorionic villus sampling. In: Essentials of Prenatal Diagnosis. Simpson JL, Elias S (eds.) *Churchill Livingstone, NewYork* 1993, pp 45–61.

Krishnegowda S, Thandaveshwar D, Mahadevaswamy M, Doreswamy SM. Comparison of JSS formula with modified Shukla's formula for insertion of umbilical venous catheter: A randomized controlled study. *Indian Pediatr* 2019, 56:199–201.

Lago P, Garetti E, Bellieni CV. Guidelines for procedural pain in the newborn. *Acta Paediatrica* 2009, 98(6): 932–39.

Lodha R, Kabra SK, Sinha A, Thukral A. In: Pediatric Procedures. CBS Publishers and Distributors Pvt. Ltd., 2014.

Scrivens A, Reynolds PR, Emergy FE, *et al.* Use of intraosseous needles in neonates: A systematic review. *Neonatology* 2019, 116:305–14.

Sheelman LP, Elias S. Percutaneous umbilical blood sampling, fetal skin sampling and fetal liver biopsy. *Semin Perinatol* 1990, 14: 456–464.

Singh M. The need for analgesia and sedation in newborn babies. *Perinatology* 2001, 3: 146–149.

Stevens B, Johnston C, Petryshen P, Taddio A. Premature infant pain profile: Development and initial validation. *Clin J Pain* 1996, 12:13.

Symansky MR, Fox HA. Umbilical vessel catheterization: Indications, management and evaluation of the technique. *J Pediatr* 1972, 80: 820.

Voigt J, Waltzman M, Lottenberg L. Intraosseous vascular access for inhospital emergency use: A systematic clinical review of the literature and analysis. *Pediatr Emergy Care* 2012, 28:185–99.

Appendices

1.1 Milligrams/Milliequivalents Conversions

$$\text{mEq/L (milliequivalents per liter)} = \frac{\text{mg per liter}}{\text{equivalent weight}}$$

$$\text{Equivalent weight} = \frac{\text{atomic weight}}{\text{valence of element}}$$

$$\text{mmoles/L (millimoles per liter)} = \frac{\text{Weight in gram}}{\text{Molecular weight}}$$

Milligrams and Milliequivalents

Radical	mEq/L	mg/dL	mg/dL	mEq/L
Sodium	1	2.30	1	0.4348
Potassium	1	3.91	1	0.2558
Calcium	1	2.00	1	0.4988
Magnesium	1	1.21	1	0.8230
Chloride	1	3.55	1	0.2817
Ammonium	1	1.80	1	0.5556
Bicarbonate	1	6.10	1	0.1639
Lactate	1	8.90	1	0.1123
Phosphorus				
Valence 1	1	3.10	1	0.3226
Valence 1.8	1	1.72	1	0.5814

Atomic Weights and Valencies

Radical	Atomic weight	Valence
Sodium	23	1
Potassium	39	1
Calcium	40	2
Magnesium	24	2
Phosphorus	31	1 and 1.8
Chloride	35.5	1

1.2 Conventional Units and SI Units

The SI system (Systems International d' Units) has now been adopted in clinical biochemistry in the United Kingdom and many other countries and has replaced the empirical or conventional units (e.g. mg/dL, mEq/L). The SI unit uses mole or its fractions per liter (or cubic decimeter) to express concentration of biochemical substances.

$$\text{Number of moles (mol)} = \frac{\text{Weight in gram}}{\text{Molecular weight}}$$

The decimal fractions of mole are millimoles (10^{-3}), micromoles (10^{-6}), nanomoles (10^{-9}) and picomoles (10^{-12}). The units of expression of concentration in SI units would be mmol/L, µmol/L, nmol/L and pmol/L. When the molecular weight of a substance being measured is unknown or uncertain, the SI units will be in g or mL/L, e.g. total serum protein of 7.0 g/dL would be expressed as 70 g/L.

Conversion of mEq/L to mmol/L

In the case of univalent ions such as Na and K, mEq/L is identical to mmol/L. For polyvalent ions, the mEq/L unit is divided by the valency to obtain mmol/L value. For example, serum calcium of 5 mEq/L is expressed as 2.5 mmol/L.

Conversion of mg/dL to mmol/L

The method for conversion is to divide mg/dL value by the molecular weight (to convert mg to mmoles) and to multiply by 10 (to convert dL to liter). For example, the molecular weight of urea is 60 and of glucose 180. The blood urea and glucose concentrations of 30 mg/dL and 90 mg/dL respectively would be expressed as 5 mmol/L in SI units for both the constituents.

The SI unit of pressure is pascal (Pa) and kilopascal (kPa); one kilopascal is equivalent to 7.5 mm Hg. The unit of energy in SI system is joules (J) and kilojoules (kJ); one kJ is equivalent to 0.238 kcal.

1.3 Conversion Factors for SI Units for Selected Constituents (*Ref. 14*)

Substance	Molecular weight	From SI units	To SI units
Bilirubin	584.7	umol/L × 0.0585 = mg/dL	mg/dL × 17.1 = umol/L
Calcium	40.08		
Plasma		mol/L × 4.008 = mg/dL	mg/dL × 0.250 = mmol/L
Urine		mmol/24 hr × 40.08 = mg/24 hr	mg/24 hr × 0.025 = mmol/L
Cholesterol	386.7	mmol/L × 38.6 = mg/dL	mg/dL × 0.0259 = mmol/L
Copper	63.54		
Plasma		umol/L × 6.35 = µg/dL	µg/dL × 0.157 = umol/L
Urine		umol/24 hr × 63.5 = µg/24 hr	µg/24 hr × 0.0157 = umol/24 hr
Creatinine	113.1		
Plasma		umol/L × 0.0113 = mg/dL	mg/dL × 88.4 = umol/L
Urine		mmol/24 hr × 0.113 = g/24 hr	g/24 hr × 8.84 = mmol/L
Glucose	180.2		
Plasma/blood		mmol/L × 18.02 = mg/dL	mg/dL × 0.0555 = mmol/L
Urine		mmol/L × 0.0180 = g/dL	g/dL × 55.5 = mmol/L
Iron and TIBC	55.85	umol/L × 5.59 = µg/dL	µg/dL × 0.179 = umol/L
Lead	207.2		
Blood		umol/L × 20.7 = µg/dL	µg/dL × 0.0483 = umol/L
Urine		umol/24 hr × 207 = µg/24 hr	µg/24 hr × 0.0483 = umol/24 hr
Magnesium	24.31		
Plasma		mmol/L × 2.43 = mg/dL	mg/dL × 0.411 = mmol/L
Urine		mmol/24 hr × 24.3 = mg/24 hr	mg/24 hr × 0.0411 = mmol/24 hr
Phosphate	30.97		
Serum		mmol/L × 3.10 = mg/dL	g/dL × 0.323 = mmol/L hr
Urine		mmol/24 hr × 0.0310 = g/24 hr	g/24 hr × 32.3 = mmol/24 hr
Salicylate	138.1	mmol/L × 13.81 = mg/dL	mg/dL × 0.0724 = mmol/L
Thyroxine	776.9	nmol/L × 0.0777 = µg/dL	µg/dL × 12.87 = nmol/L
Triiodothyronine	651.01	nmol/L × 0.651 = ng/dL	ng/dL × 1.54 = nmol/L
Triglycerides	885.4	mmol/L × 88.5 = mg/dL	mg/dL × 0.113 = mmol/L
Uric acid	168.1	mmol/L × 16.81 = mg/dL	mg/dL × 0.595 = mmol/L
Urea	60.06	mmol/L × 6.01 = mg/dL	mg/dL × 0.166 = mmol/L

APPENDIX 2. Mean Hematologic Values in Preterm and Term Newborns (*Ref. 9*)

Determination	Preterm		Term				
	28 wks	34 wks	Cord blood	Day 1	Day 3	Day 7	Day 14
Hemoglobin (g/dL)	14.5	15.0	16.8	18.4	17.8	17.0	16.8
Hematocrit (%)	45.0	47.0	53.0	58.0	55.0	54.0	52.0
Red blood cells (mm^3)	4.0	4.4	5.2	5.8	5.6	5.2	5.1
MCV (µ^3)	120.0	118.0	107.0	108.0	99.0	98.0	96.0
MCH (pg/cell)	40.0	38.0	34.0	35.0	33.0	32.5	31.5
MCHC (%)	31.0	32.0	31.7	32.5	33.0	33.0	33.0
Reticulocytes (%)	5–10	3–10	3–7	3–7	1–3	0–1	0–1
Nucleated RBCs (per 100 leukocytes)	—	—	500.0	200.0	0.5	0	0

Care of the Newborn

APPENDIX 3. Total and Differential White Blood Cell Count in Term and Preterm Newborns (*Ref. 2 and 9*)

Age	Total leukocytes		Neutrophils				Lymphocytes		Eosinophils		Basophils		Monocytes	
	Mean	Range (×10³)	Total (mean)	Seg.	Band	B/N	Total (mean)	%	Total (mean)	%	Total (mean)	%	Total (mean)	%
Term newborn														
Birth	18,100	9–30	11,000	9,400	1,600	0.14	5,500	31	400	2.2	100	0.6	1,050	5.8
12 hours	22,800	13–38	15,500	—	—	0.14	5,500	24	500	2	—	—	1,200	5.0
24 hours	18,990	9.4–34	11,500	—	—	0.14	5,800	31	500	2	—	—	1,100	6.0
7th day	12,200	5–12	5,500	4,700	730	0.14	5,000	41	500	4.1	50	0.4	1,100	9.1
14th day	11,400	5–20	4,500	3,900	6.30	0.14	5,500	48	350	3	50	0.4	1,000	8.8
Preterm newborn														
1500–2000 gm														
Day 7	13,000	6.7–14.7	8,200	7,200	1,050	0.13	4,000	29	260	2	130	1	650	5
Day 14	10,000	7.0–14.1	5,100	4,300	800	0.15	3,600	36	300	3	100	1	900	9
<1500 gm														
Day 7	16,800	61–32.8	10,240	9,000	1,700	0.11	5,000	30	330	2	168	1	1,000	6
Day 14	15,400	10.4–21.3	8,000	7,100	900	0.11	5,400	35	450	3	150	1	1,550	10

APPENDIX 4. Normal Coagulation Values in Healthy Term and Preterm Babies* (Ref. 11)

Procoagulants	Synonyms	Term	Preterm 32–36 weeks	28–31 weeks
Factor I (mg/dL)	Fibrinogen	246 ±55	244 ±55	270 ±85
Factor II[+] (%)	Prothrombin	45 ±15	35 ±12	30 ±10
Factor V (%)	Proaccelerin, labile factor	*100 ±5	*80 ±9	*76 ±7
Factor VII[+] (%)	Proconvertin, stable factor	56 ±16	40 ±15	38 ±14
Factor VIII (%)	Antihemophilic factor (AHF)	105 ±34	98 ±40	70 ±30
Factor IX[+] (%)	Plasma thromboplastin component (PTC), Christmas factor	28 ±8	NA	27 ±10
Factor X[+] (%)	Stuart Prower factor	56 ±16	40 ±15	38 ±14
Factor XI (%)	Plasma thromboplastin antecedent (PTA)	29 ±7	NA	5 ±1.8
Factor XII (%)	Hageman factor	25 ±7	30–100	NA
Factor XIII (%)	Fibrin stabilizing factor	100	100	100
Prekallikrein (PK)	Fletcher factor	33 ±6	NA	27
High molecular weight	Williams, Fitzgerald, Flaujac factor kininogen (HMWK)	56 ±12	NA	28
Platelet count (#mm³)		150–400	150–400	100–400
PT (seconds)	Prothrombin time[a]	13-20	12–21	23
APPT (seconds)	Activated partial prothrombin time	55 ±10	70	NA
FDP (µg/mL)	Fibrin degradation products	55	48	33 ±9
D-dimers (mg/L)			<0.25–1.0	0.25–0.5
Thrombin time (seconds)		10–16	11–17	16–28

*These values could differ depending on the methodology of each laboratory

[+]Vitamin K-dependent protein

[a]The international normalized ratio or INR is a calculation based on results of PT that are used to monitor patients who are being treated with the blood thinning medication.

APPENDIX 5. Normal Blood Chemistry Values in Cord Blood and Capillary Blood of Full Term Infants (Ref. 1 and 13)

Determination	Cord blood		Infant's blood 1–12 hr		12–24 hr		24–48 hr		48–72 hr	
	Mean	Range	Mean	Range	Mean	Range	Mean	Range	Mean	Range
Sodium (mEq/L)	147	126–166	143	124–156	145	132–159	148	136–160	149	139–162
Potassium (mEq/L)	7.8	5.6–12	6.4	5.3–7.3	6.3	5.3–8.9	6.0	5.2–7.3	5.9	5.0–7.7
Calcium (mg/dL)	9.3	5.2–11.2	8.4	7.3–9.2	7.8	6.9–9.4	8.0	6.1–9.9	7.9	5.9–9.7
Phosphorus (mg/dL)	5.6	3.7–8.1	6.1	3.5–8.6	5.7	2.9–8.1	5.9	3.0–8.7	5.8	2.8–7.6
Blood urea (mg/dL)	29	21–40	27	8–34	33	8–63	32	13–77	31	13–68
Total proteins (g/dL)	6.1	4.8–7.3	6.6	5.6–8.5	6.6	5.8–8.2	6.9	5.9–8.2	7.2	6.0–8.5
Blood sugar (mg/dL)	73	45–96	63	40–97	63	42–104	56	30–91	59	40–90
Lactic acid (mg/dL)	19.5	11–30	14.6	11–24	140	11–23	14.3	9–22	13.5	7–21

APPENDIX 6. Blood Chemistry Values in Premature Infants (Birth Weight 1500–1700 g) (*Ref. 13*)

Determination	1 week		3 weeks		5 weeks		7 weeks	
	Mean	*Range*	*Mean*	*Range*	*Mean*	*Range*	*Mean*	*Range*
Sodium (mEq/L)	139.6	133–146	136.3	129–142	136.8	133–148	137.2	133–142
Potassium (mEq/L)	5.6	4.6–6.7	5.8	4.5–7.1	5.5	4.5–6.6	5.7	4.6–7.1
Calcium (mg/dL)	9.2	6.1–11.6	9.6	8.1–1.0	9.4	8.6–10.5	9.5	8.6–10.8
Phosphorus (mg/dL)	7.6	5.4–10.9	7.5	6.2–8.7	7.0	5.6–7.9	6.8	4.2–8.2
Blood urea (mg/dL)	18.6	6.2–51	26.6	4.2–62.8	26.6	4.0–53	26.8	5.0–61.0
Total proteins (g/dL)	5.49	4.40–6.26	5.38	4.28–6.7	4.98	4.14–6.9	4.93	4.02–5.86
Blood sugar (mg/dL)	45	28–61	56	23–98	52	18–77	48	22–83

APPENDIX 7. Normal Blood Chemistry Values of Healthy Newborn Babies (*Ref. 1*)

Component	Age	Values	
Alanine aminotransferase (SGPT)		5–28 iu/L	
Alkaline phosphatase		20–225 iu/L	
Ammonia nitrogen			
	At birth	90–150 μg/dL	
	0–2 wks	79–129 μg/dL	
Amylase		5–65 u/L	
Aspartate aminotransferase (SGOT)		5–40 iu/L	
Bilirubin (total)		Premature (mg/dL)	Full term (mg/dL)
	Cord	2	2
	0–1 day	8	6
	3–5 days	15	12
Bilirubin (direct)		0.0–0.2 mg/dL	
C-Reactive protein		10–350 mg/mL	
Calcium		*See* Appendices 4 and 5	
Ceruloplasmin		1–30 mg/dL	
Cholesterol			
	Cord	45–100 mg/dL	
	Newborn	53–135 mg/dL	
	3 days–1 year	69–174 mg/dL	
Clotting time		*See* Appendix 3	
Complement C3		88.4 ± 11.7 mg/dL	
		99.5 ± 17.4 mg/dL	
Cortisol		1–24 μg/dL	
Creatinine			
	Cord	0.6–1.2 mg/dL	
	Newborn	0.3–1.0 mg/dL	
Creatinine phosphokinase			
	Premature	0–210 iu/L	
	Birth–3 weeks	22–267 iu/L	
	3 weeks onwards	15–134 iu/L	
Ferritin		25–200 ng/dL	

(*contd.*)

APPENDIX 7. Normal Blood Chemistry Values of Healthy Newborn Babies (*Ref. 1*) *(Contd.)*

Component	Age	Values
Fetal hemoglobin (% HbF)		
	1st day	77.0 ±7.3
	5th day	76.8 ±5.8
	3rd week	70.0 ±7.3
	6–9 weeks	52.9 ±11.0
Fibrinogen		*See* Appendix 3
Galactose		0–20 mg/dL
Glucose		*See* Appendices 4 and 5
Growth hormone		
	Cord	10–15 ng/mL
	Newborn	10–40 ng/mL
Haptoglobin		5–48 mg/dL
Hematocrit (capillary)		
	1st day	48–69%
	2nd day	48–75%
	3rd day	44–72%
	After 3rd day	28–42%
Immunoglobulins (mg/dL)		

	Age	IgG	IgA	IgM
	Newborn	631–1431	up to 8	1–21

Component	Age	Values
Osmolality		275–295 mOsmol/kg
Phospholipids (total)		75–170 mg/dL
Phosphorus		*See* Appendices 5 and 6
T4 (µg/mL)		
	Birth	6.9–16.7
	1–3 days	11–23
	1 week–1 month	9–18
Transferrin		130–275 mg/dL
Triglycerides		10–98 mg/dL
TSH (µIU/mL)		
	Birth	3–22
	24 hours	17.1 ±3
	48 hours	12.8 ±1.9
	2 weeks	<10
Uric acid		2.0–6.2 mg/dL

APPENDIX 8. Normal Blood Gas and Acid–Base Parameters in Newborn Babies (*Ref. 3, 12*)

Determination	Arterial blood	Venous blood
pH	7.35–7.45	7.30–7.40
PaO_2 (mm Hg)	90–100	45–50
$PaCO_2$ (mm Hg)	35–45	40–45
HCO_3 (mmol/L)	20–22	20–22
Base excess	–3 to –7	–3 to –7
Oxygen saturation (%)	92–95	—

APPENDIX 9. Cerebrospinal Fluid in Healthy Term and Preterm Newborns (*Ref. 8, 10 and 14*)

Determination	Premature	Term infant 0–24 hours	Day 1	Day 7
Color	Xanthochromic	Clear or xanthochromic	Clear or xanthochromic	Clear or xanthochromic
Pressure (mm CSF)	—	50–80	50–80	50–80
Red blood cells (per mm³)	—	9 (0–1070)	23 (0–620)	3 (0–48)
Polymorphs (per mm³)	—	3 (0–70)	7 (0–26)	2 (0–5)
Lymphocytes (per mm³)	—	2 (0–20)	5 (0–16)	1 (0–4)
Protein (mg/dL)	100 (50–180)	63 (32–240)	73 (40–148)	47 (27–65)
Sugar (mg/dL)	50 (30–70)	51 (32–78)	48 (38–64)	55 (48–62)
Chloride (mg/dL)	—	720 (680–760)	720 (680–760)	740 (720–760)
LDH (iu/L)	—	1.5–50.0	—	—

APPENDIX 10. Normal Biochemical Values in Urine (*Ref. 4*)

Component	Age	Values
Ammonia	1st day	0.02–0.50 mEq/kg/24 hr
	7th day	0.26–0.86 mEq/kg/24 hr
Bicarbonate		1.5–2.0 mmol/L
Calcium	1st day	0.1–0.3 mg/24 hr
	7th day	1.8–3.4 mg/24 hr
Creatinine	Premature	8.3–19.9 mg/kg/24 hr
	Term	10–20 mg/kg/24 hr
Creatinine clearance		40–65 mL/min/1.73 m²
Galactose		<60 mg/dL
Glucose	1st week	<25 mg/dL
	1st day	2–76 mg/kg/24 hr
	7th day	66–150 mg/kg/24 hr
Osmolality	At birth	79–118 mOsm/kg
	1st 24 hr	115–232 mOsm/kg
	>24 hr	150–250 mOsm/kg (Max. 600 mOsm/kg)
pH		5.1–6.8
Potassium*	1st day	0.08–0.64 mEq/kg/24 hr
	7th day	0.0–2.25 mEq/kg/24 hr
Protein		8–12 mg/24 hr
Sodium*	1st day	0.11–0.39 mEq/kg/24 hr
	7th day	0.0–4.4 mEq/kg/24 hr
Steroids	17-Hydroxycorticosteroids	0.05–0.3 mg/day
	17-ketosteroids	0.1–0.5 mg/day
	Pregnentriol	0.0–0.2 mg/day
Titrable acidity		0.3 mEq/kg/24 hr
Urea	0–2 days	39 mg/kg/24 hr
	2–4 days	52 mg/kg/24 hr
	5–7 days	73 mg/kg/24 hr

*The excretion value depends upon intake.

Appendices

APPENDIX 11. Fecal Constituents in Normal Newborns (*Ref. 4*)

Constituents	Meconium	Neonatal
Amount	70–90 g	15–25 g/d (breast milk)
		30–40 g/d (cow milk)
Bilirubin	25–102 mg/100 g	—
Iron	1.2–2.7 mg/100 g	—
Fecal fat		—
Total	0.3–1.3 g/24 hr	—
Neutral fat	0.16–0.38 g/24 hr	—
Fatty acids	0.14–0.97 g/24 hr	—
pH	5.7–6.4	4.6–5.2 (breast milk)
Potassium	1.2–5.1 mEq/100 g	0.5–1.5 mEq/24 hr
Sodium	9.0–18.2 mEq/100 g	0.5 mEq/24 hr
Water	68–82%	62–86%

APPENDIX 12. Average Systolic, Diastolic and Mean Blood Pressures (mm Hg) during First Twelve Hours of Life in Normal Newborn According to Birth Weight (*Ref. 7*)

Birth weight	Blood pressure	Age in hours											
		1	2	3	4	5	6	7	8	9	10	11	12
1001 to 2000 g	Systolic	49	49	51	52	53	52	52	52	51	51	49	50
	Diastolic	26	27	28	29	31	31	31	31	31	30	29	30
	Mean	35	36	37	39	40	40	39	39	38	37	37	38
2001 to 3000 g	Systolic	59	57	60	60	61	58	64	60	63	61	60	59
	Diastolic	32	32	32	32	33	34	37	34	38	35	35	35
	Mean	43	41	43	43	44	43	45	43	44	44	43	42
Over 3000 g	Systolic	70	67	65	65	66	66	67	67	68	70	66	66
	Diastolic	44	41	39	41	40	41	41	41	44	43	41	41
	Mean	53	51	50	50	51	50	50	51	53	54	51	50

Note: The mean arterial pressure is 30–35 mm Hg in a 1000 g infant and it increases approximately by 1.0 mm Hg for every 100 g increase in birth weight

APPENDIX 13. Normal Electrocardiographic Values in Newborn Babies (*Ref. 5*)

Parameter	Age		
	0–24 hours	*1–7 days*	*8–30 days*
Heart rate	119 (85–145)	133 (100–175)	163 (115–190)
P-R interval	0.10 (0.07–0.13)	0.09 (0.05–0.13)	0.09 (0.07–0.13)
P duration	0.051 (0.040–0.075)	0.046 (0.035–0.065)	0.048 (0.040–0.065)
QRS duration	0.065 (0.05–0.09)	0.056 (0.04–0.08)	0.057 (0.04–0.08)
P amplitude in lead II	1.5 (0.5–2.6)	1.6 (0.5–2.8)	1.6 (0.5–2.7)
QRS axis	135 (160–180)	125 (60–180)	110 (0–180)
T axis	70 (–20–180)	25 (–40–100)	35 (–20–120)
T amplitude in V4	4.3 (8.5)*	4.4 (8.5)*	5.3 (8.5)*
T amplitude in V6	2.4 (4.5)*	2.9 (4.5)*	3.5 (7.5)*
Age	30 hours	30 days	
R amplitude in V4R	8.6 (3.5–15.0)	6.3 (3.0–12.0)	
R in V1	11.9 (5.0–30.0)	11.1 (4.0–20.0)	
R in V5	9.4 (2.0–20.0)	15.0 (3.8–30.0)	
R in V6	5.4 (1.5–15.0)	10.8 (1.0–22.0)	
S in V4R	3.8 (0–12.0)	1.8 (0–9.0)	
S in V1	9.7 (0–26.0)	6.1 (0–15)	
S in V5	9.5 (5.0–22.0)	8.3 (0–30)	
S in V6	5.6 (0.2–20.0)	4.8 (0–18.0)	

*Maximum value

BIBLIOGRAPHY

1. Acharya PT, Payne WW. Blood chemistry of normal full term infants in the first 48 hours of life. *Arch Dis Child* 1965, 40: 430–5.

2. Altman PL, Dittmer DS. Blood and other body fluids. *Washington DC. Federation of American Societies for Experimental Biology*, 1961.

3. Avery ME, Norman ICS. Respiratory physiology in the newborn infant. *Anesthesiology* 1965, 26: 510.

4. Cockburn F, Drillien MC. Neonatal Medicine. *Blackwell Scientific Publications* 1974, p. 802–805.

5. Hastreiter AR, Abella JB. The electrocardiogram in the newborn period. *J Pediatr* 1971, 78: 147.

6. Hathaway WE, Bonnar J. Perinatal Coagulation. *Grune and Stratton*, New York, 1978.

7. Kiterman JA, Phibbs RH, Tooley WH. Aortic blood pressure in normal newborn infants during first 12 hours of life. *Pediatrics* 1969, 44: 959.

8. Naidoo T. The cerebrospinal fluid in the healthy newborn infant. *South Africa Med J* 1968, 42: 933.

9. Oski FA, Naiman JL. Hematologic Problems in the Newborn. *WB Saunders and Co.*, 1972, p.13.

10. Otilo E. Studies on the cerebrspinal fluid in premature infants. *Acta Paediatr Scand* 1984, 35: (suppl.) 9.

11. Pramanik AK. The bleeding neonate. In Medical Emergencies in Children. Singh M (Ed), *Sagar Publications*, New Delhi 5th edition, 2012, p 306–336.

12. Schaffer AJ. Diseases of the Newborn. *WB Saunders and Co., Phila*, 3rd edition, 1971.

13. Thomas JL and Reichelderfer T. Premature infants: Analysis of serum during the first seven weeks. *Clin Chem* 1968, 14: 272.

14. Tietz NW. In: Fundamentals of Clinical Chemistry, *WB Saunders and Co., Phila*, 3rd edition, 1987, p. 975.

15. Wolf H and Hoepffner L. The cerebrospinal fluid in the newborn and premature infant. *World Neurol* 1961, 2: 871–8.

Appendices

Index

Index

Index

Index

Index